Harald Schütz

Benzodiazepines

A Handbook

Basic Data, Analytical Methods,
Pharmacokinetics and
Comprehensive Literature

With 152 Figures

Springer-Verlag
Berlin Heidelberg New York 1982

Dr. rer. nat. Harald Schütz
Diplom-Chemiker
Institut für Rechtsmedizin der Justus Liebig-Universität
Frankfurter Straße 58, D-6300 Giessen

ISBN 3-540-11270-7 Springer-Verlag Berlin Heidelberg New York
ISBN 0-387-11270-7 Springer-Verlag New York Heidelberg Berlin

Printing and Bookbinding: Offsetdruckerei Julius Beltz KG Hemsbach
2119/3140-543210

Preface

To comment at length on the importance of the benzodiazepines seems superfluous within the scope of this preface. No other class of active substances has experienced an even approximately comparable advance in the past two decades. It is therefore not surprising that the formerly dominant barbiturates and bromocarbamides have had to give way in many fields to the benzodiazepines, which now rank first (Proudfoot and Park [1828]).
Closely linked with the great therapeutic importance of the benzodiazepines are analytical problems. Detection and the determination of blood levels can be necessary under therapeutic aspects, for instance in working out optimally effective levels in the treatment of epileptic conditions ("drug monitoring"), but also in connection with questions at issue in toxicology and traffic medicine.
A toxicological analysis can be subdivided into the following steps:

Detection (identification including screening)
Determination (e.g. blood, plasma or serum levels)
Interpretation of the analytical results.

This book is intended as a contribution to each of these chapters:
The part "Analytical Data" (pp. 1–122) gives a comprehensive collection of data, e.g. general and chromatographic data (TLC, GLC) as well as spectra (UV, IR, MS) of 19 commercial preparations, 23 important metabolites and 18 hydrolysis derivatives. Information about biotransformation and the possible formation of aminobenzophenone derivatives is also given.
The most important analytical methods are presented in an extensive review on pp. 123–204 in order to make it possible to select the optimum method on the basis of the essential data.
Another review (pp. 205–244) and several diagrams facilitate the interpretation of quantitatively determined blood, plasma or serum concentrations.
There is also a tremendous increase of the literature (see diagram on page XI). The Review of Literature and the list of References (pp. 245-426) does not only deal with "Analytical Methods and Pharmacokinetics" in the strict sense but with the literature which has appeared since the early 60's in the broadest sense, thus providing extensive reference material for numerous additional subjects of a predominantly clinical and pharmacological nature. Thus, this book is not only addressed to the analyst, pharmacokinetist or toxicologist, but to all colleagues who come into contact with the benzodiazepines, including, of course, also those clinicians and practitioners who do not make their analyses themselves but obtain their data from laboratories and who have to interpret these data in taking therapeutic measures and in consideration of connections that are often only known to them.

I wish to thank all those who have helped me in compiling this book, and I would appreciate suggestions and wishes, especially critical ones.
I am indebted to Professor G. Schewe and Professor S. Ebel for their assistance and the numerous suggestions and discussions, and to Mrs. Gisela Zimmermann for her untiring efforts in typing the sometimes difficult text.
Special thanks are also due to the different manufacturing firms (in particular Hoffmann-La Roche, Beecham, Boehringer-Ingelheim, Hoechst, Mack-Midy, Schering, Thomae, Tropon, Upjohn, Warner-Lambert and Wyeth), and to the Bund gegen Alkohol im Straßenverkehr e. V., for their support and encouragement over many years, and to the publishing house, Springer-Verlag, for their exemplary collaboration.
Last but not least I thank the many colleagues and journal editors throughout the world for giving me permission, in most cases spontaneously and accompanied by encouraging words, to use their published material for this book.

Gießen, January 1982 Harald Schütz

Contents

Preface VI

Formula Index and Melting Points 1

Biotransformation 4

Index of Treated Substances 12

Formation of Aminobenzophenones and Other Hydrolysis Products (Survey) 13

Formation of the Hydrolysis Derivatives (Formula Index) 14

Some Important Data (Molecular Weight, Molecular Formula, Mass-Spectrum Peaks) 17

TLC-Data 21
Technical Conditions 21
Data (R_f-Values and Detection) 21

GLC-Data 24
Technical Conditions 24
Data (Retention Times and Retention Index, SE-30 and OV-17) 24

Infrared- and Mass-Spectra 27

Ultraviolet-Spectra 91

Table of Absorption Maxima 91
Spectra 93

Presentation of Analytical Methods 123

Methods for the Detection and Determination of Various Benzodiazepines (Simultaneous-Methods) 123
Methods for the Detection and Determination of a Special Benzodiazepine (Mono-Methods) 144
Chlordiazepoxide 144
Diazepam (see also p. 187) 149
Oxazepam 165
Nitrazepam 168
Medazepam 175
Clorazepate 176
Lorazepam (see also p. 167) 178
Prazepam 181
Clonazepam (see also p. 155, 170, 171) 182
Flurazepam 190
Bromazepam (see also p. 199) 194

Flunitrazepam (see also p. 171) 197
Clobazam 201
Camazepam 204

Blood-, Serum- and Plasma-Levels and Other Pharmacokinetic Data from Literature 205

Chlordiazepoxide 205
Diazepam 209
Other Pharmacokinetic Data 217
Oxazepam 219
Nitrazepam 221
Medazepam 224
Clorazepate 225
Lorazepam 227
Prazepam 229
Clonazepam 230
Flurazepam 233
Bromazepam 235
Flunitrazepam 236
Clobazam 238
Camazepam 239
Ketazolam 240
Triazolam 241
Lormetazepam 242
Ranges of Maximum Concentrations After Oral Administration 243
  Chlordiazepoxide 243
  Diazepam (single dose) 243
  Oxazepam (single dose) 243
  Nitrazepam (single dose) 243
  Medazepam (single dose) 244
  Lorazepam (single dose) 244
  Bromazepam (single dose) 244
  Diazepam (multiple dose) 244
  Nordiazepam (after multiple doses of Diazepam) 244

Survey of Benzodiazepine Literature 245

Absorption 245
Benzodiazepines in Relation to Mother and Child 246
Bioavailability Studies 247
Biotransformation/Metabolism 247
Disposition 248
Effects and Interactions with Other Compounds 248
Emergency-Drug-Analysis 250
Extraction from Biological Samples (Selection) 251
Fluorescence/Fluorometry 251
Gas-Liquid-Chromatography 251
General Analytical Data 252
General Treatment 253
High-Pressure-Liquid-Chromatography 253
Hydrolysis of Benzodiazepines 253

Infrared-Spectra 253
Levels (Blood, Plasma, Serum) 254
Mass-Spectra 255
NMR-Spectra 255
Pharmacokinetics 255
Pharmacology and Clinical Investigations 257
Poisoning (Treatment, Reports, Cases) 265
Polarography 266
Protein-Binding 266
Radioactive-Labelled-Benzodiazepines 276
Radioimmunoassay and Other Immunoassays 267
Screening 268
Side-, Adverse-, Residual- and Withdrawal-Effects 268
Sleep-Effects 271
Synthesis 271
Theory of Action/The Benzodiazepine Receptor 272
Thin-Layer-Chromatography 275
Toxicity/Toxicology 276
Traffic-Medicine 276
UV- and VIS-Spectroscopy 277
Other Themes 277

References 279
Alphabetical List 1 279
Alphabetical List 2 329
Alphabetical List 3 362
Addendum 1 379
Alphabetical List 4 383
Addendum 2 427

Subject Index 429

Screening of Benzodiazepines in Urine (inside backcover)

Ring-Nomenclature for 1,4-Benzodiazepines and Benzophenones/ Ring-Nomenklatur für 1,4-Benzodiazepine und Benzophenone

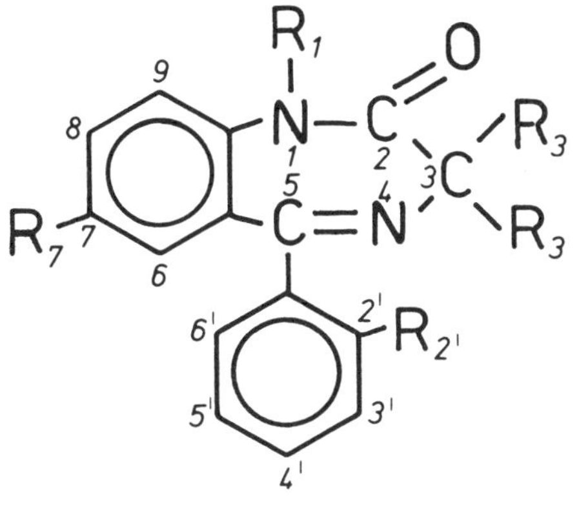

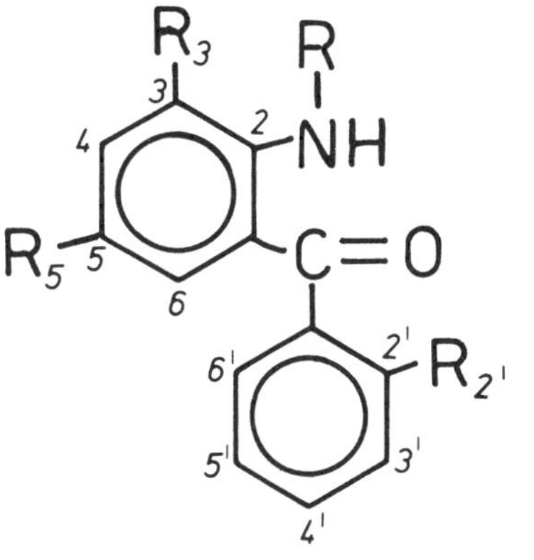

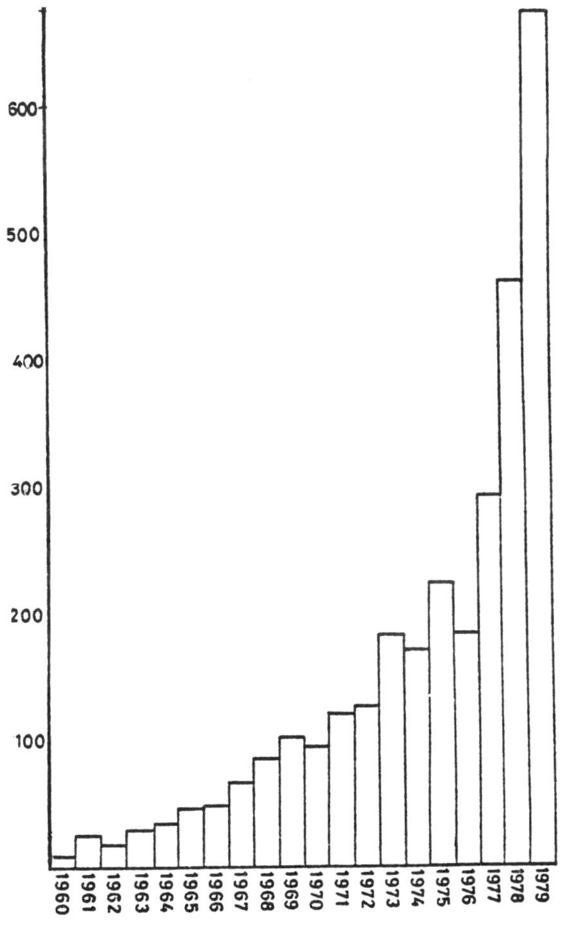

Annual Increase of the Benzodiazepine-Literature (Analytical and Pharmacokinetic Themes)
Jährlicher Anstieg der Benzodiazepin-Literatur (Analytische und pharmakokinetische Themen)

Some Abbreviations

a.c. = ac = ante cibum/vor der Mahlzeit
AUC = area under curve/Fläche unter der Kurve
b.i.d. = bd = bis in die/2 x täglich
ca. = approx./ca. (etwa)
Cl = clearance/
Cl_{tot} = total clearance/
C.V. = coefficient of variation/Variationskoeffizient
D =Diazepam
DD = N-Desmethyldiazepam (Nordiazepam)
h.s. = hs = hora somni = vor dem Einschlafen
i.m. = intramuscular/intramuskulär
i.v. = intravenous/intravenös
multiple dose/mehrfache Verabreichung
N.D. = n.d. = not detectable/nicht nachweisbar
N.M. = n.m. = not measurable/nicht meßbar
N.M. = n.m. = not measured/nicht gemessen
o.d. = omni die/täglich
OX = Oxazepam
p = significance/Signifikanz
p.o. = per os/oral
q.d. = quaque die/täglich
q.h. = quaque hora/stündlich
q.i.d. = quater in die/4 x täglich
q.x.d. = quaque x hora/alle x Stunden
S.D. = SD = standard deviation/Standardabweichung
S.E. = SE = standard error/Standardfehler
single dose/einmalige Verabreichung
$t_{1/2\,a}$ = absorption half-life/Halbwertszeit der Resorption
$t_{1/2\,\alpha}$ = distribution half-life/Halbwertszeit der Verteilung
$t_{1/2\,\beta}$ = elimination half-life/Halbwertszeit der Elimination
t.d.s. = tds = ter die summendum/3 x täglich insgesamt
t.i.d. = tid = ter in die/3 x täglich
V_d = volume of distribution/Verteilungsvolumen
1000 ug = 1 mg, 1000 ng = 1 ug, 1000 pg = 1 ng, 1 nm = 1 mu,
1lb. = 16 ounces = 453.59 g, 1 in. = 1 inch = 2.54 cm

Formula Index and Melting Points+)

Formelverzeichnis und Schmelzpunkte

No. / Nr.	Generic Names (chemical Names) / Int.Kurznamen (chem.Bezeichn.)	Formula / Formel	Melt.Point / Schmelzp.
1	Chlordiazepoxide (Librium®)	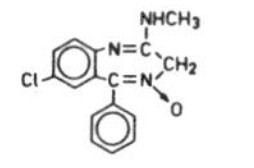	236-237°C
2	Demoxepam	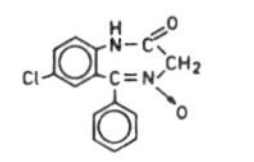	235-236°C
3	Desmethyl-Chlordiazepoxide	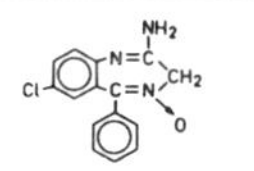	255-256°C
4	2-Amino-5-chloro-benzophenone	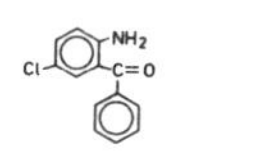	98- 99°C
5	Diazepam (Valium®)	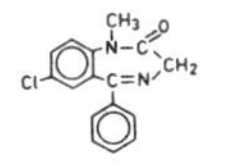	131-135°C
6	Nor-Diazepam	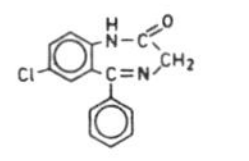	216-217°C
7	3-Hydroxy-Diazepam (Temazepam)	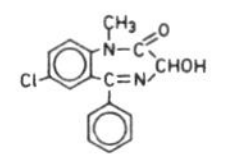	118-120°C
8	Oxazepam (Adumbran®, Praxiten®, Serax®, Serenal-D®)	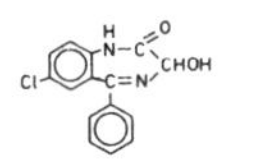	204-206°C
9	2-Methylamino-5-chloro-benzophenone	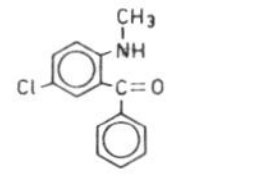	96- 97°C
10	Nitrazepam (Mogadan®, Mogadon®)	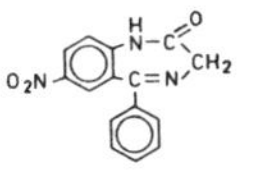	224-226°C
11	7-Amino-Nitrazepam	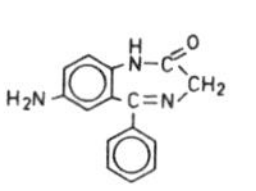	235-238°C
12	7-Acetamido-Nitrazepam	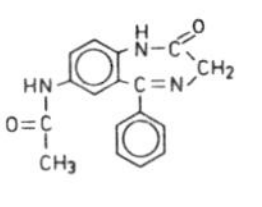	ca. 260°C
13	2-Amino-5-nitro-benzophenone	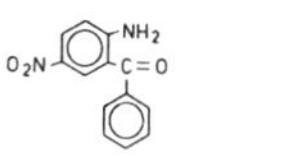	162-163°C
14	2,5-Diamino-benzophenone	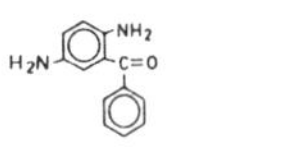	
15	Medazepam (Nobrium®)	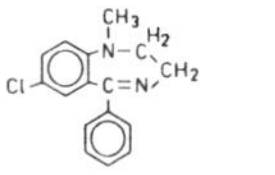	95- 97°C
16	Chlorazepate / Clorazepate (Tranxilium®, Tranxene®)	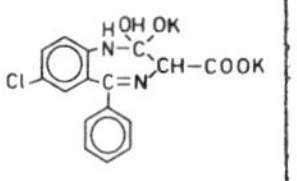	209-211°C
17	Lorazepam (Tavor®, Ativan®, Temesta®)	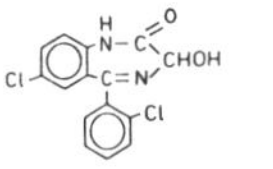	158-160°C
18	2-Amino-5,2'-dichloro-benzophenone	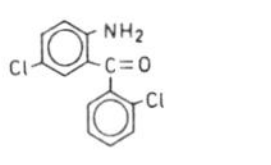	88 -89°C
19	Prazepam (Demetrin®, Verstran®)	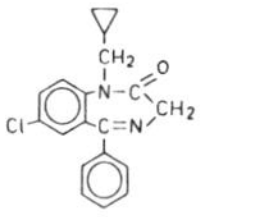	146-148°C
20	3-Hydroxy-Prazepam	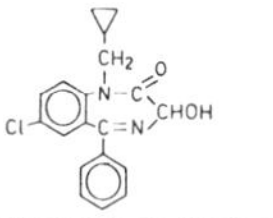	160-162°C
21	2-Cyclopropyl-methylamino-5-chloro-benzophenone	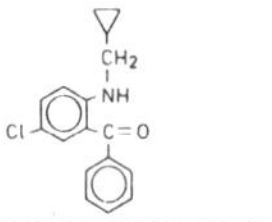	79- 81°C
22	Clonazepam (Rivotril®)	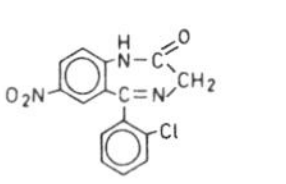	238-240°C
23	7-Amino-Clonazepam	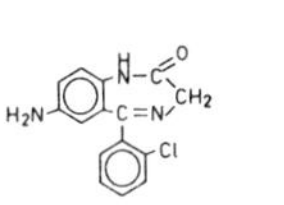	230-232°C
24	7-Acetamido-Clonazepam	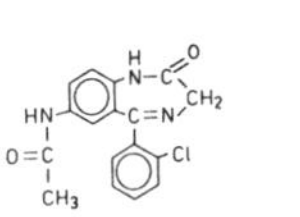	292-300°C

+) melting points from 231,233,234,236,240,241,242,244 and other sources

25	2-Amino-5-nitro-2'-chloro-benzophenone	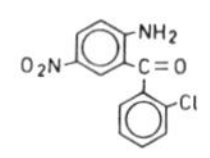	118-120°C
26	2,5-Diamino-2'-chloro-benzophenone	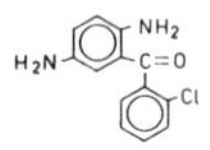	30 -40°C
27	Flurazepam (Dalmadorm[R], Dalmane[R])	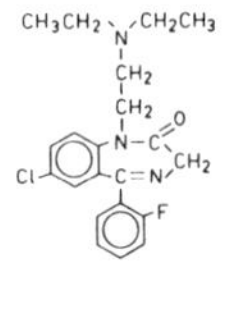	190-220° dec.
28	N-1-Desalkyl-Flurazepam	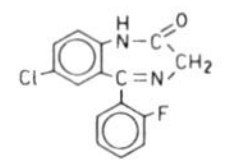	205-206°C
29	N-1-Hydroxyethyl-Flurazepam	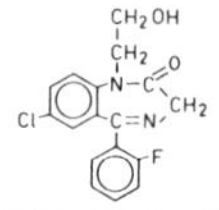	110-115°C
30	2-Diethylamino-ethylamino-5-chloro-2'-fluoro-benzophenone	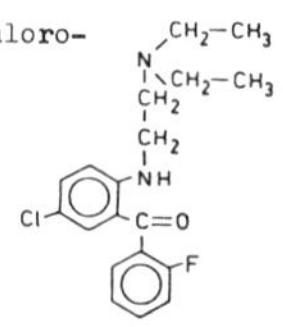	134-143°C (x HCl)
31	2-Amino-5-chloro-2'-fluoro-benzophenone	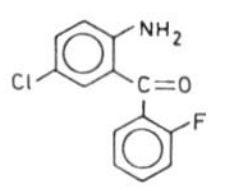	
32	2-Hydroxyethylamino-5-chloro-2'-fluoro-benzophenone	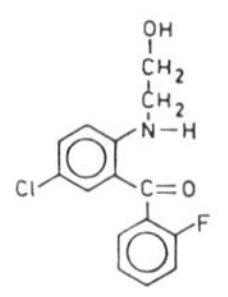	96-101°C
33	Bromazepam (Lexotanil[R], Lexotan[R])	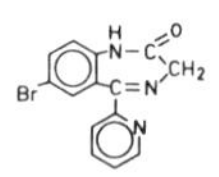	237-239°C
34	3-Hydroxy-Bromazepam	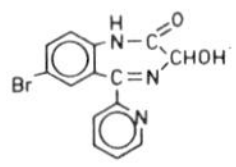	198-200°C dec.
35	2-(2-Amino-5-bromo-benzoyl)-pyridine	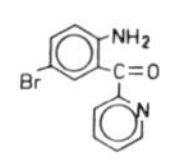	98 -99°C
36	Flunitrazepam (Rohypnol[R])	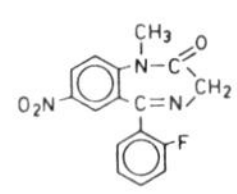	170-172°C
37	Nor-Flunitrazepam	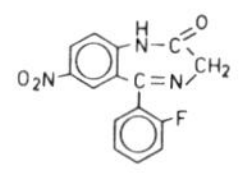	210-211°C
38	7-Amino-Flunitrazepam	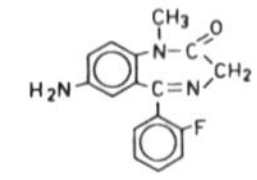	ca. 202°C dec.
39	7-Acetamido-Flunitrazepam	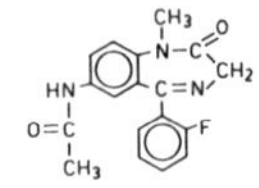	ca. 260°C dec.
40	7-Amino-Nor-Flunitrazepam	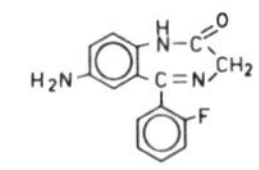	ca. 260°C dec.
41	2-Methylamino-5-nitro-2'-fluoro-benzophenone	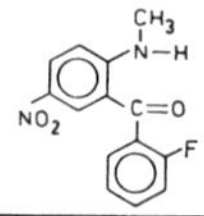	
42	2-Amino-5-nitro-2'-fluoro-benzophenone	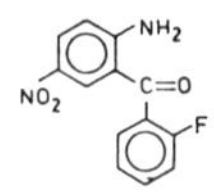	
43	2-Methylamino-5-amino-2'-fluoro-benzophenone	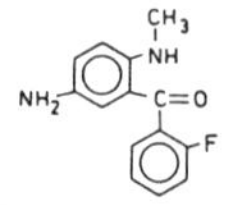	
44	2,5-Diamino-2'-fluoro-benzophenone	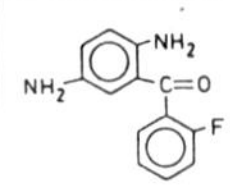	
45	2-Amino-3-hydroxy-5-chloro-benzophenone	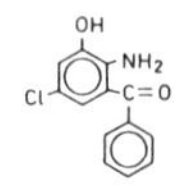	165-167°C
46	Clobazam (Frisium[R])	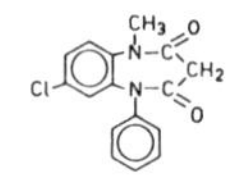	182-184°C
47	Nor-Clobazam	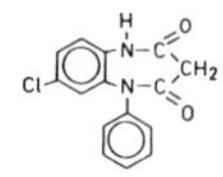	ca. 240°C dec.
48	Camazepam (Albego[R])	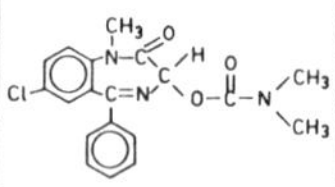	165-167°C
49	Diazepam-N-Oxide	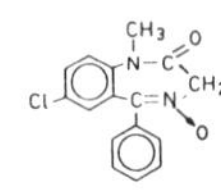	
50	3-Acetoxy-Diazepam	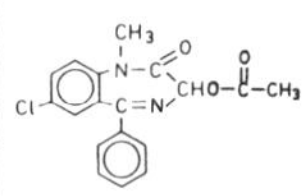	
51	Prazepam-N-Oxide	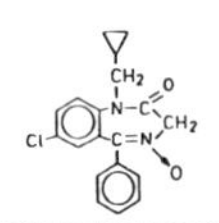	
52	3-Acetoxy-Prazepam	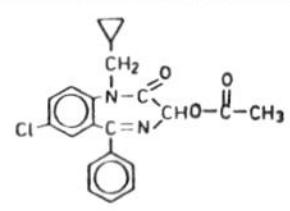	

53	Desmethyl-Medazepam	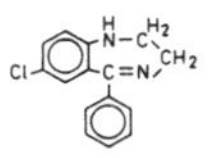	170–172°C
54	Monodesethyl-Flurazepam	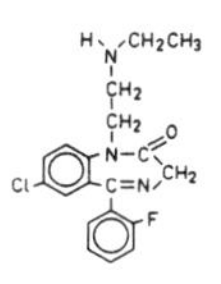	215–217°C (x 2HCl)
55	Didesethyl-Flurazepam	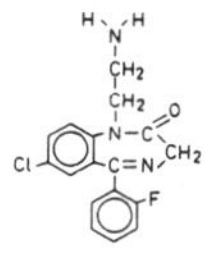	221–223°C (x 2HCl)
56	Bromazepam-N(Py)-Oxide	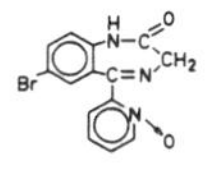	>250°C dec.
57	Ketazolam	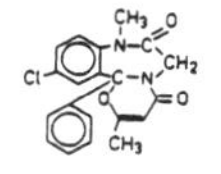	158–160°C
58	Triazolam	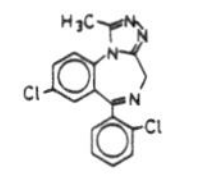	238–241°C
59	Clotiazepam	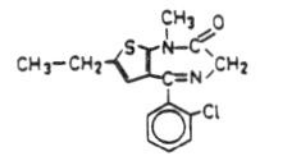	ca. 100°C
60	Lormetazepam	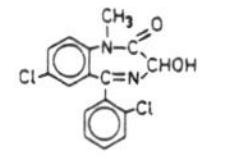	209–211°C
61	2-Methylamino-2',5-dichlor-benzophenone	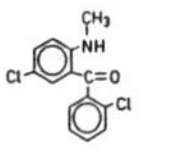	
62	Tetrazepam	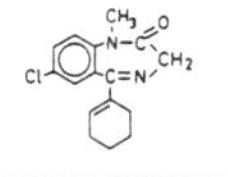	144°C
63	Nor-Tetrazepam	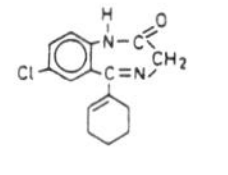	ca. 205°C

Biotransformation

Major Pathways

Symbols and Abbreviations:

e.g. 34	(number of substance, e.g. 3-Hydroxybromazepam)
B	detectable in blood, plasma or serum
(B)	see B, minor metabolite, low concentrations
U	detectable in urine
(U)	see U, minor metabolite, low concentrations
U !	suitable for screening in urine

Many compounds are excreted as conjugates, so that hydrolysis procedures (enzymatic or acid hydrolysis) are necessary prior to extraction.

Hydrolysis Conditions: (e.g.)

a) Enzymatic hydrolysis: With Arylsulfatase (EC 3.1.6.2.) / β-Glucuronidase (EC 3.2.1.31) , pH 4.6 - 4.8, 37°C , 4 - 12 hrs.

b) Acid hydrolysis (cleavage of conjugates and formation of aminobenzophenones in most cases):

A 20 - 50 ml volume of undiluted urine is transferred to a 250 ml round-bottomed flask, to which 10 ml of concentrated hydrochloric acid are added and swirled. The flask ist then placed in a water-bath maintained boiling for 30 minutes under reflux conditions. The flask is cooled to room temperature and the contents are adjusted to pH 9 - 11 by addition of ammonium hydroxyde. A 50-ml volume of diethylether or ethylacetate is added and the flask is then shaken on a reciprocating shaker for 10 minutes.

Important: Biotransformation patterns can change extremely in overdose and poisoning cases.

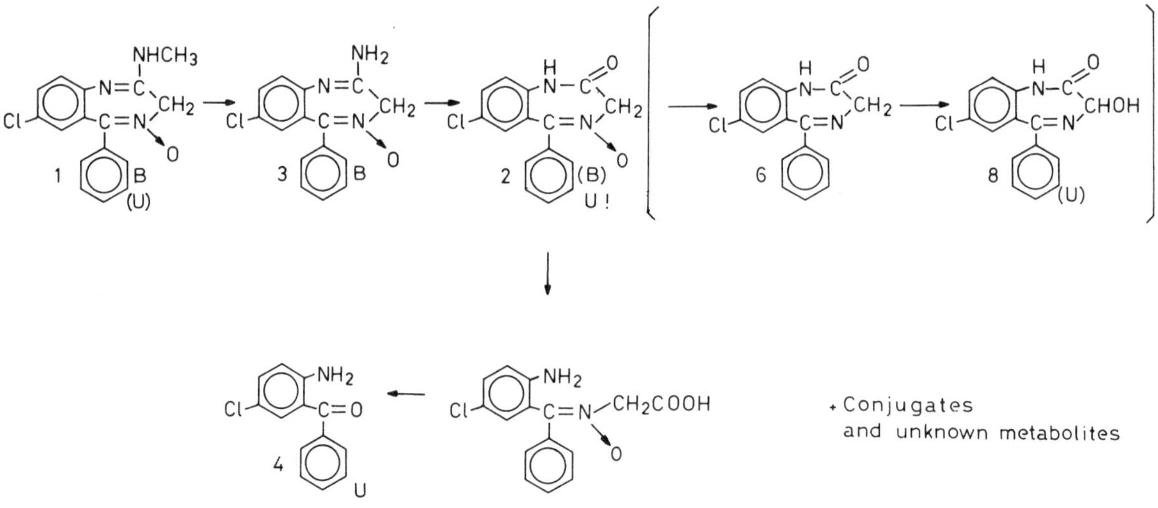

Biotransformation of Chlordiazepoxide
(Lit. 37, 598, 599, 600, 864, 999, 1002, 1003, 1004, 1006)

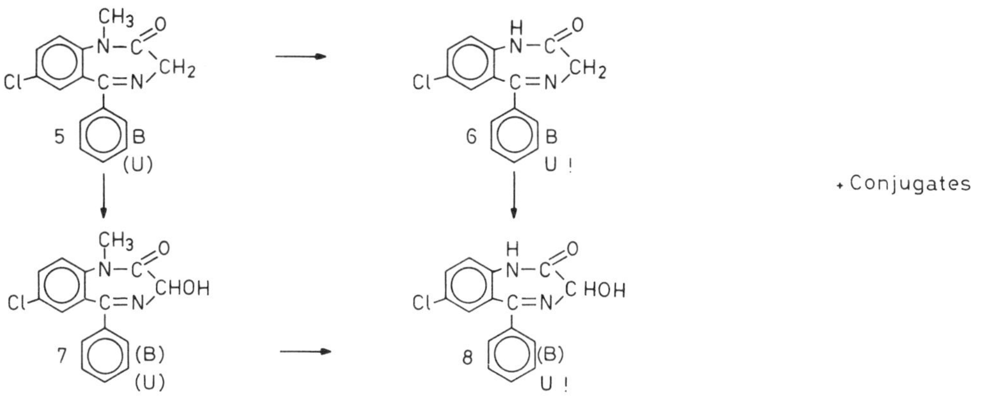

Biotransformation of Diazepam
(Lit. 238, 243, 530, 556, 923, 991, 995, 996, 1000, 1014, 1630)

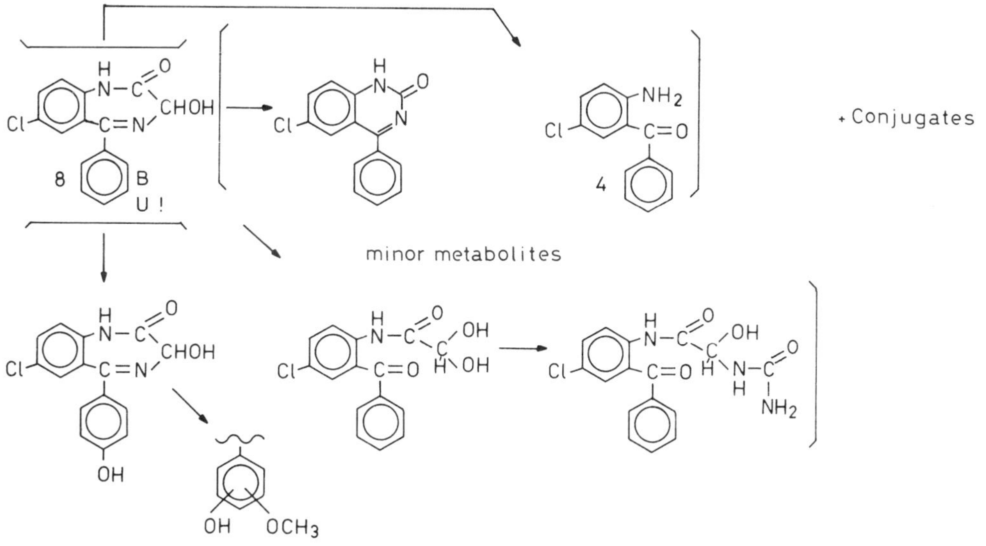

Biotransformation of Oxazepam
(Lit. 595, 1052, 1053)

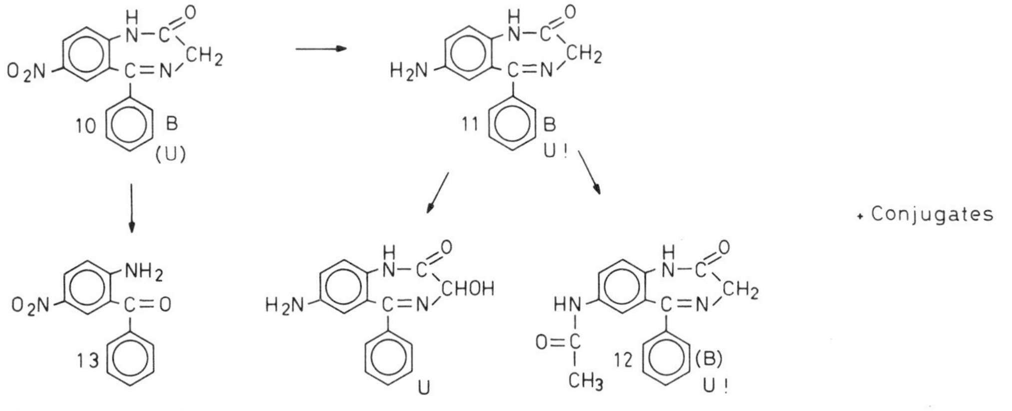

Biotransformation of Nitrazepam
(Lit. 865, 908, 909, 954, 955, 2512, 2535)

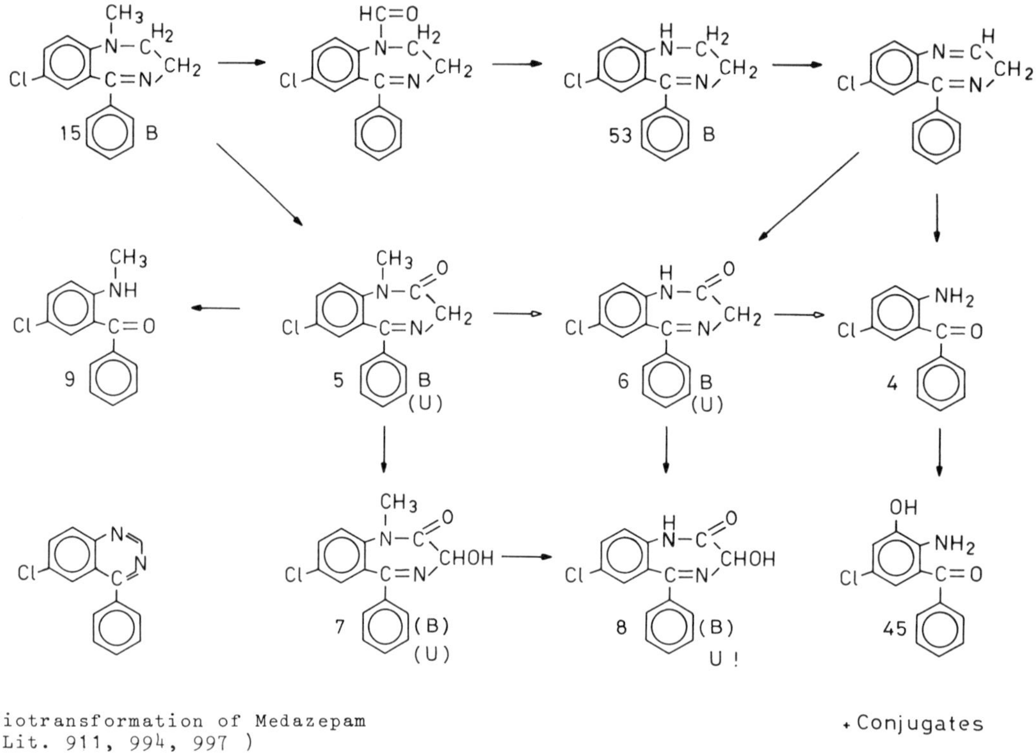

Biotransformation of Medazepam
(Lit. 911, 994, 997)

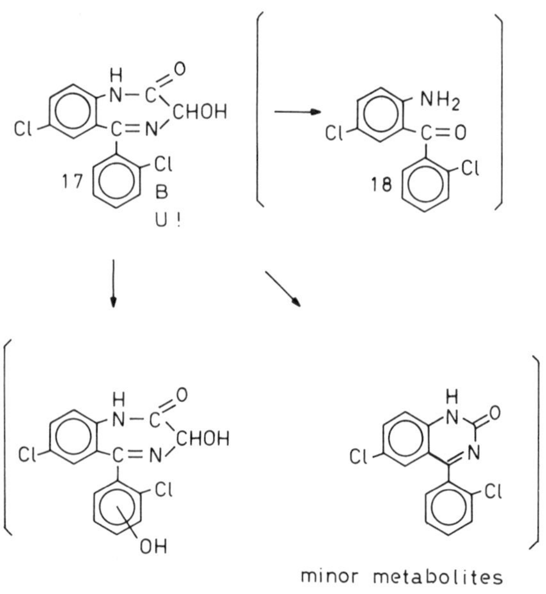

Biotransformation of Lorazepam
(Lit. 594, 961)

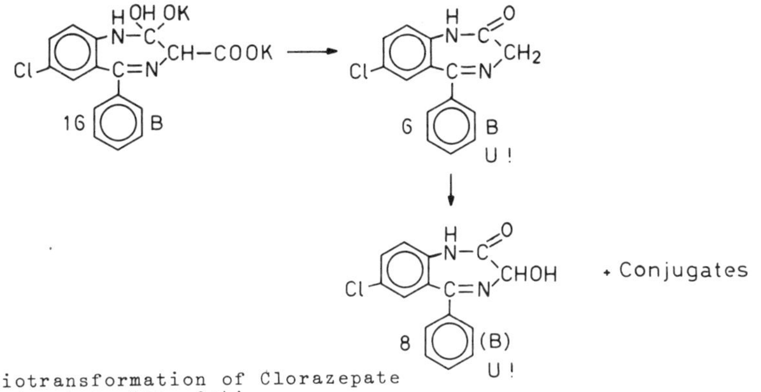

Biotransformation of Clorazepate
(Lit. 439, 893, 894)

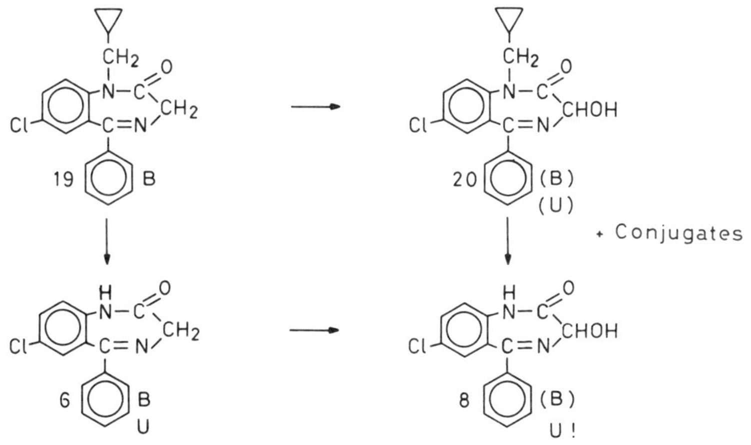

Biotransformation of Prazepam
(Lit. 253, 254, 1171, 1172, 1173)

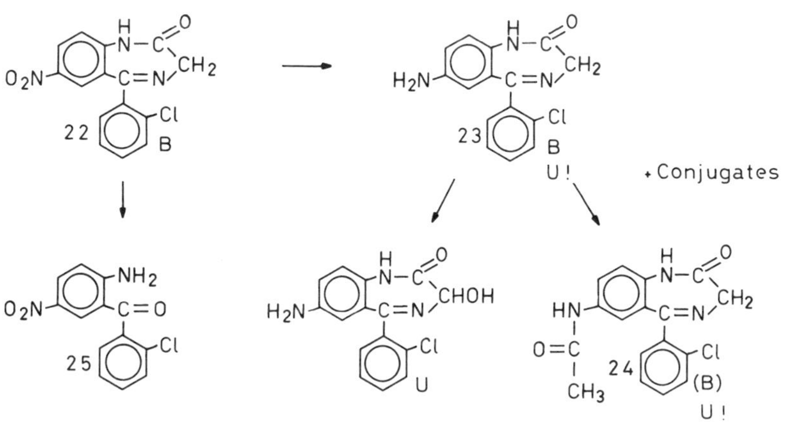

Biotransformation of Clonazepam
(Lit. 280, 298)

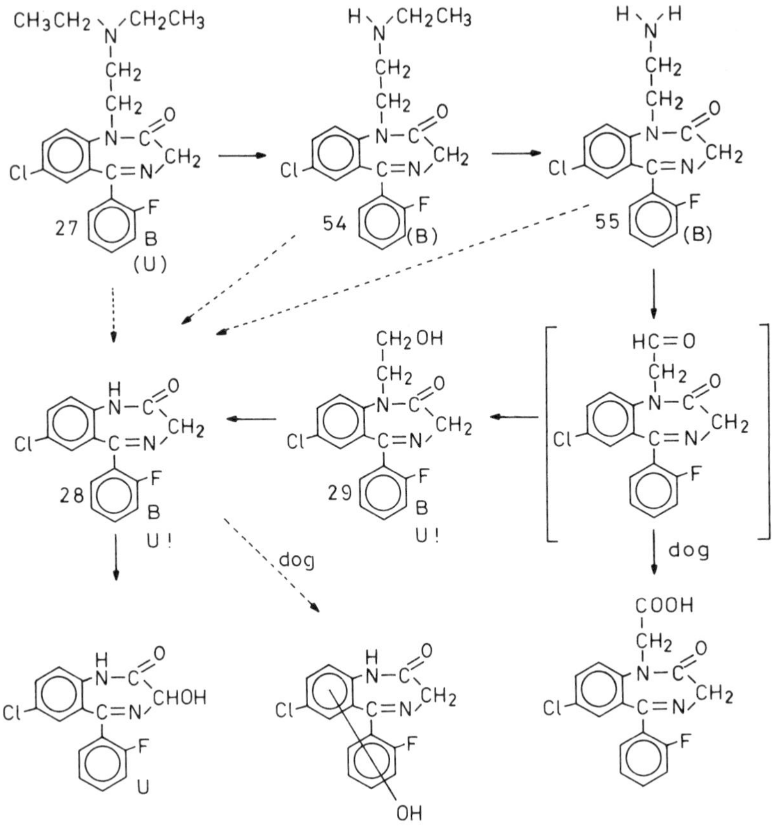

Biotransformation of Flurazepam
(Lit. 189, 244, 468, 559, 1001, 1007, 1008)

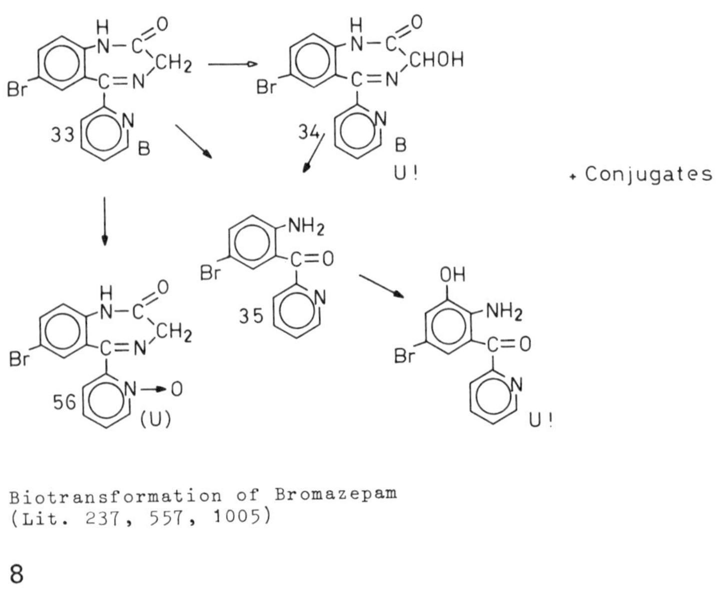

Biotransformation of Bromazepam
(Lit. 237, 557, 1005)

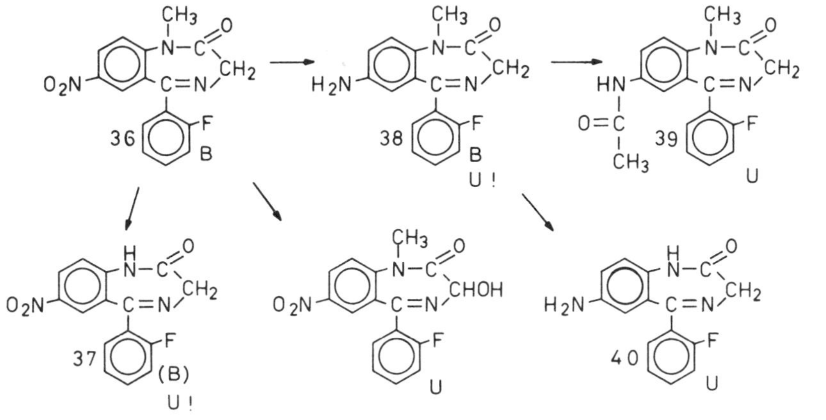

Biotransformation of Flunitrazepam
(Lit. 242, 555, 2501)

+Conjugates

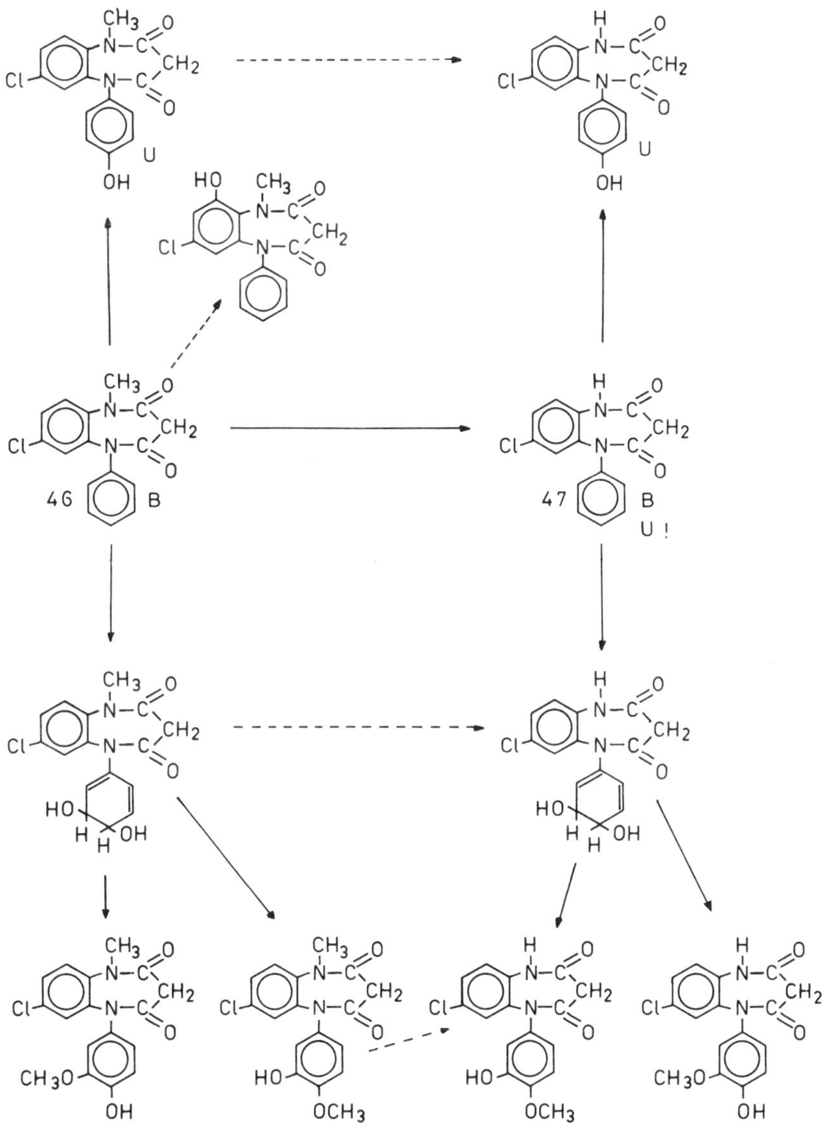

Biotransformation of Clobazam
(Lit. 2495, 2466, 2469)

+Conjugates

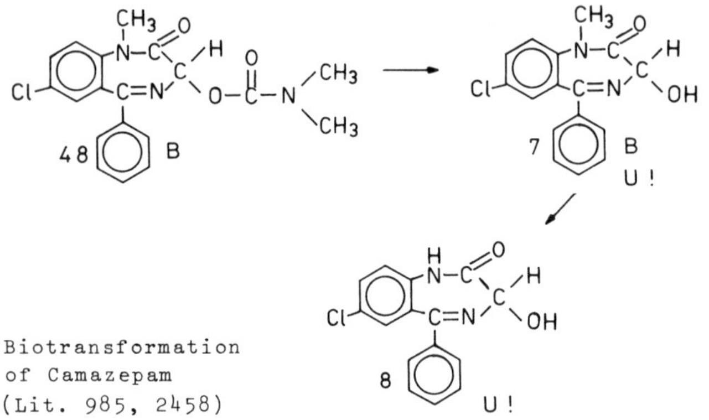

+ Conjugates

Biotransformation
of Camazepam
(Lit. 985, 2458)

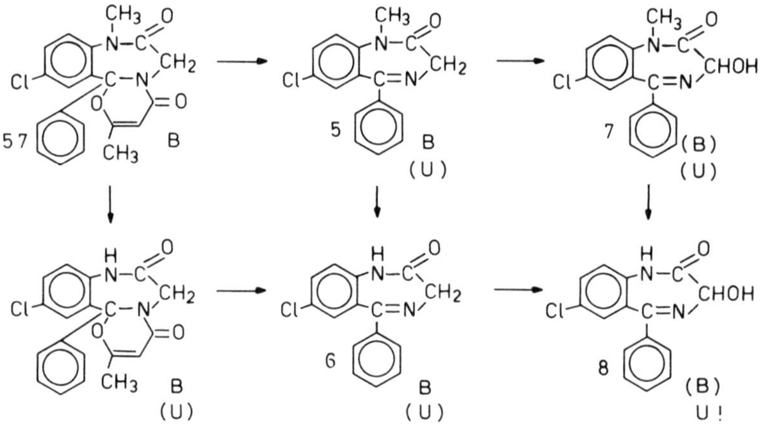

Biotransformation of Ketazolam
(Lit. 2457, 3768, 3769)

+ Conjugates

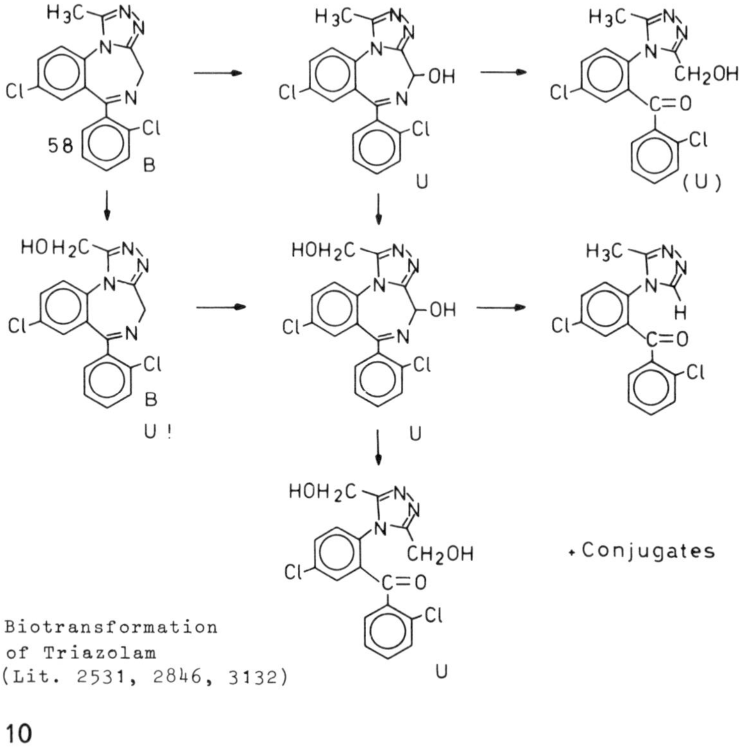

+ Conjugates

Biotransformation
of Triazolam
(Lit. 2531, 2846, 3132)

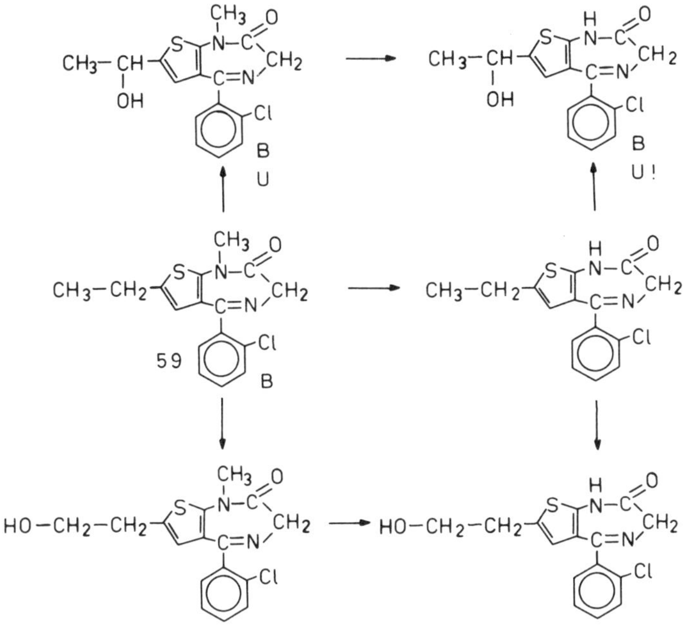

Biotransformation of Clotiazepam
(Lit. 2536, 2549)

+ Conjugates

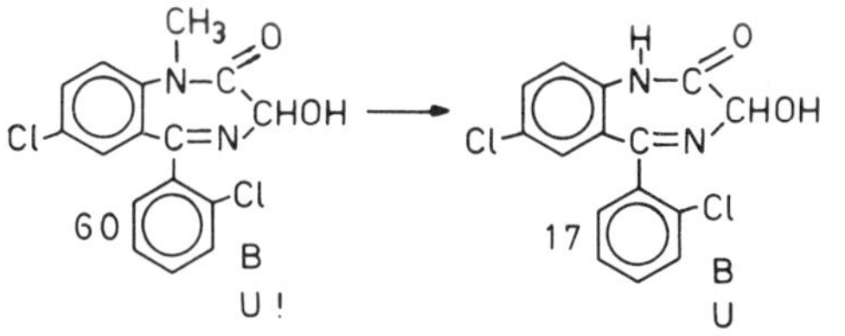

+ Conjugates

Biotransformation of Lormetazepam
(Lit. 3047, 3048)

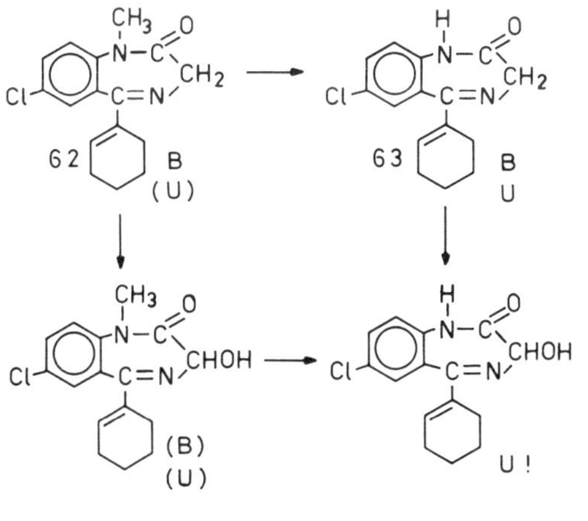

+ Conjugates

Biotransformation of Tetrazepam
(Lit. 2457, 3772)

Index of Treated Substances

Liste der bearbeiteten Substanzen

No.	Substance / Substanz
1	Chlordiazepoxide (Librium^{R})
2	Demoxepam
3	Desmethyl-Chlordiazepoxide
4	2-Amino-5-chlor-benzophenone
5	Diazepam (Valium^{R})
6	Nor-Diazepam
7	3-Hydroxy-Diazepam (Temazepam)
8	Oxazepam (Adumbran^{R}, Praxiten^{R}, Serax^{R}, Serenal-D^{R})
9	2-Methylamino-5-chlor-benzophenone
10	Nitrazepam (Mogadan^{R}, Mogadon^{R})
11	7-Amino-Nitrazepam
12	7-Acetamido-Nitrazepam
13	2-Amino-5-nitro-benzophenone
14	2,5-Diamino-benzophenone
15	Medazepam (Nobrium^{R})
16	Chlorazepate - Clorazepate (Tranxilium^{R}, Tranxene^{R})
17	Lorazepam (Tavor^{R}, Ativan^{R}, Temesta^{R})
18	2-Amino-5,2′-dichlor-benzophenone
19	Prazepam (Demetrin^{R}, Verstran^{R})
20	3-Hydroxy-Prazepam
21	2-Cyclopropyl-methylamino-5-chlor-benzophenone
22	Clonazepam (Rivotril^{R})
23	7-Amino-Clonazepam
24	7-Acetamido-Clonazepam
25	2-Amino-5-nitro-2′-chlor-benzophenone
26	2,5-Diamino-2′-chlor-benzophenone
27	Flurazepam (Dalmadorm^{R}, Dalmane^{R})
28	N-1-Desalkyl-Flurazepam
29	N-1-Hydroxyethyl-Flurazepam
30	2-Diethylamino-ethylamino-5-chlor-2′-fluor-benzophenone
31	2-Amino-5-chlor-2′-fluor-benzophenone
32	2-Hydroxyethylamino-5-chlor-2′-fluor-benzophenone
33	Bromazepam (Lexotanil^{R}, Lexotan^{R})
34	3-Hydroxy-Bromazepam
35	2-(2-Amino-5-brom-benzoyl)-pyridine
36	Flunitrazepam (Rohypnol^{R})
37	Nor-Flunitrazepam
38	7-Amino-Flunitrazepam
39	7-Acetamido-Flunitrazepam
40	7-Amino-nor-Flunitrazepam
41	2-Methylamino-5-nitro-2′-fluor-benzophenone
42	2-Amino-5-nitro-2′-fluor-benzophenone
43	2-Methylamino-5-amino-2′-fluor-benzophenone
44	2,5-Diamino-2′-fluor-benzophenone
45	2-Amino-3-hydroxy-5-chlor-benzophenone
46	Clobazam (Frisium^{R})
47	Nor-Clobazam (Clofazin)
48	Camazepam (Albego^{R})
49	Diazepam-N-Oxide
50	3-Acetoxy-Diazepam
51	Prazepam-N-Oxide
52	3-Acetoxy-Prazepam
53	Desmethyl-Medazepam
54	Monodesethyl-Flurazepam
55	Didesethyl-Flurazepam
56	Bromazepam-N(Py)-Oxide
57	Ketazolam (Contamex^{R})
58	Triazolam (Halcion^{R})
59	Clotiazepam (Trecalmo^{R})
60	Lormetazepam (Noctamid^{R})
61	2-Methylamino-2′,5-dichlor-benzophenone
62	Tetrazepam (Musaril^{R})
63	Nor-Tetrazepam

Formation of Aminobenzophenones and Other Hydrolysis Products (Survey)

Die Entstehung der Aminobenzophenone und anderer Hydrolyseprodukte

Benzodiazepine-compound Benzodiazepinverbindung		Hydrolysis-Product Hydrolyseprodukt	
No.	Subst.	No.	Subst.
1	Chlordiazepoxide	4	2-Amino-5-chlor-benzophenone
2	Demoxepam	4	2-Amino-5-chlor-benzophenone
3	Desmethyl-Chlordiazepoxide	4	2-Amino-5-chlor-benzophenone
5	Diazepam	9	2-Methylamino-5-chlor-benzophenone
6	Nor-Diazepam	4	2-Amino-5-chlor-benzophenone
7	3-Hydroxy-Diazepam	9	2-Methylamino-5-chlor-benzophenone
8	Oxazepam	4	2-Amino-5-chlor-benzophenone
10	Nitrazepam	13	2-Amino-5-nitro-benzophenone
11	7-Amino-Nitrazepam	14	2,5-Diamino-benzophenone
12	7-Acetamido-Nitrazepam	14	2,5-Diamino-benzophenone
15	Medazepam		stable / stabil
16	Chlorazepate	4	2-Amino-5-chlor-benzophenone
17	Lorazepam	18	2-Amino-5,2′-dichlor-benzophenone
19	Prazepam	21	2-Cyclopropyl-methylamino-5-chlor-benzophenone
20	3-Hydroxy-Prazepam	21	2-Cyclopropyl-methylamino-5-chlor-benzophenone
22	Clonazepam	25	2-Amino-5-nitro-2′-chlor-benzophenone
23	7-Amino-Clonazepam	26	2,5-Diamino-2′-chlor-benzophenone
24	7-Acetamido-Clonazepam	26	2,5-Diamino-2′-chlor-benzophenone
27	Flurazepam	30	2-Diethylamino-ethylamino-5-chlor-2′-fluor-benzophenone
28	N-1-Desalkyl-Flurazepam	31	2-Amino-5-chlor-2′-fluor-benzophenone
29	N-1-Hydroxyethyl-flurazepam	32	2-Hydroxyethylamino-5-chlor-2′-fluor-benzophenone
33	Bromazepam	35	2-(2-Amino-5-brom-benzoyl)-pyridine
34	3-Hydroxy-Bromazepam	35	2-(2-Amino-5-brom-benzoyl)-pyridine
36	Flunitrazepam	41	2-Methylamino-5-nitro-2′-fluor-benzophenone
37	Nor-Flunitrazepam	42	2-Amino-5-nitro-2′-fluor-benzophenone
38	7-Amino-Flunitrazepam	43	2-Methylamino-5-amino-2′-fluor-benzophenone
39	7-Acetamido-Flunitrazepam	43	2-Methylamino-5-amino-2′-fluor-benzophenone
40	7-Amino-nor-Flunitrazepam	44	2,5-Diamino-2′-fluor-benzophenone
48	Camazepam	9	2-Methylamino-5-chlor-benzophenone
57	Ketazolam	9	2-Methylamino-5-chlor-benzophenone
60	Lormetazepam	61	2-Methylamino-2′,5-dichlor-benzophenone

Formation of the Hydrolysis Derivatives

See page 4 for hydrolysis procedure.
Detection according to BRATTON and MARSHALL (139)

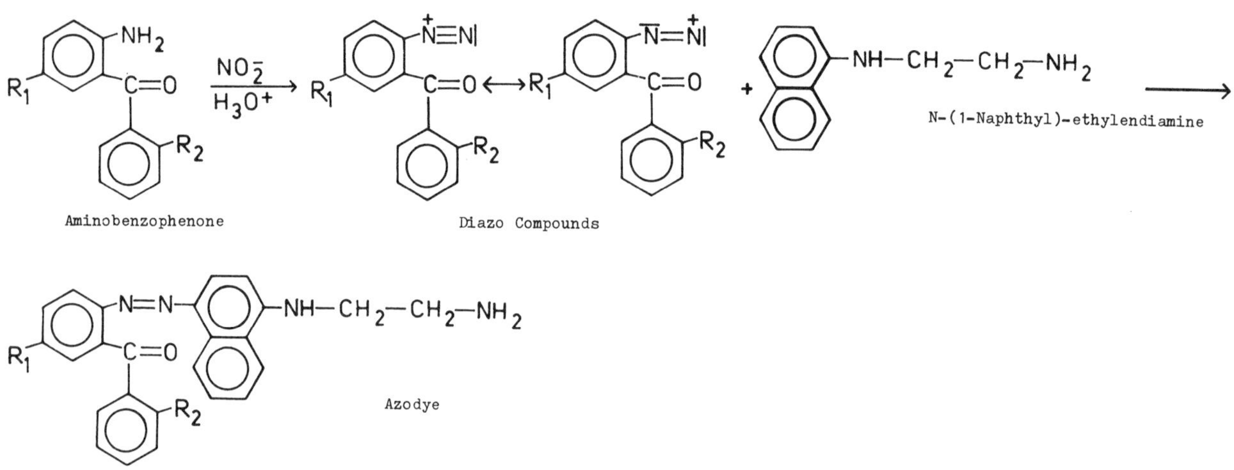

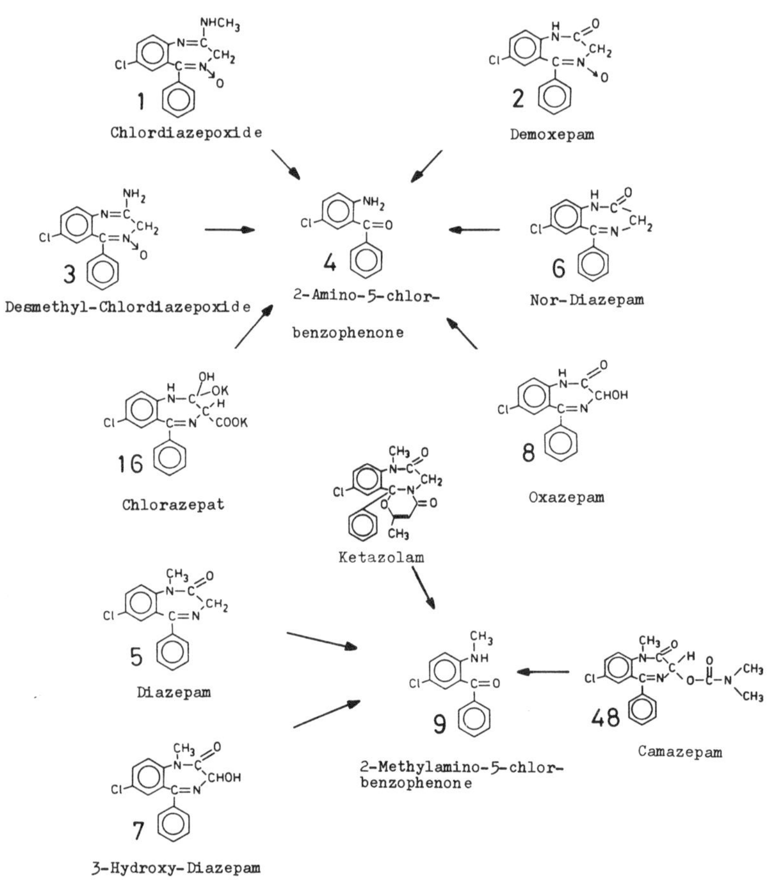

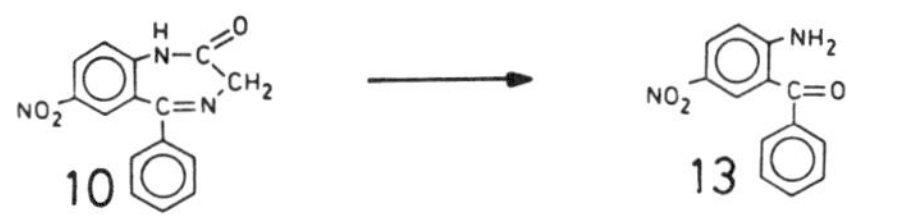

Nitrazepam — 2-Amino-5-nitro-benzophenone

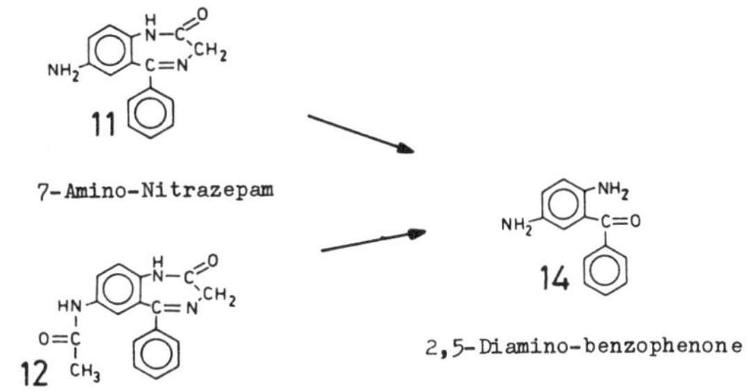

7-Amino-Nitrazepam

2,5-Diamino-benzophenone

7-Acetamido-Nitrazepam

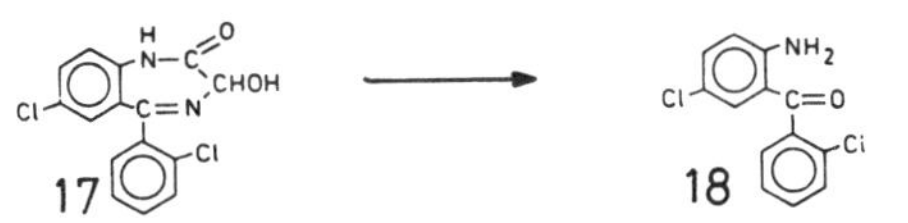

Lorazepam — 2-Amino-5,2'-dichlor-benzophenone

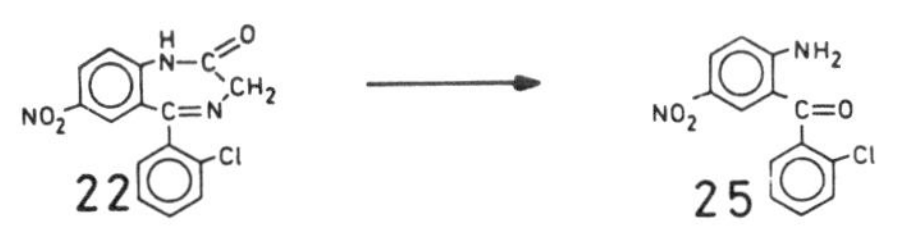

Clonazepam — 2-Amino-5-nitro-2'-chlor-benzophenone

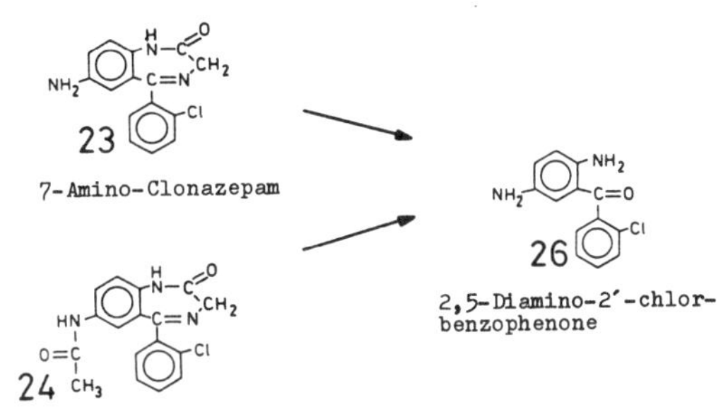

7-Amino-Clonazepam

2,5-Diamino-2'-chlor-benzophenone

7-Acetamido-Clonazepam

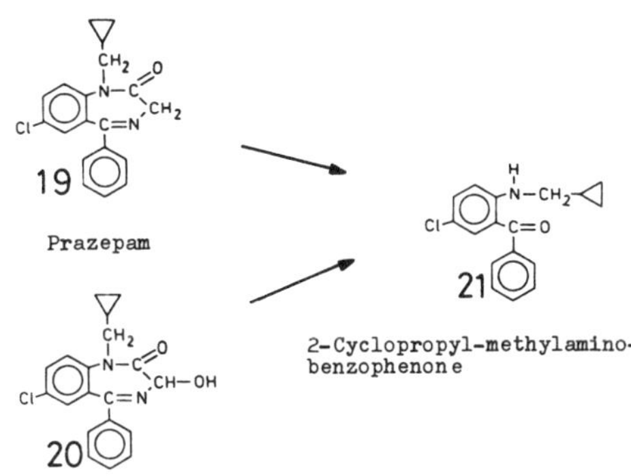

Prazepam

2-Cyclopropyl-methylamino- 5-chlor-benzophenone

3-Hydroxy-Prazepam

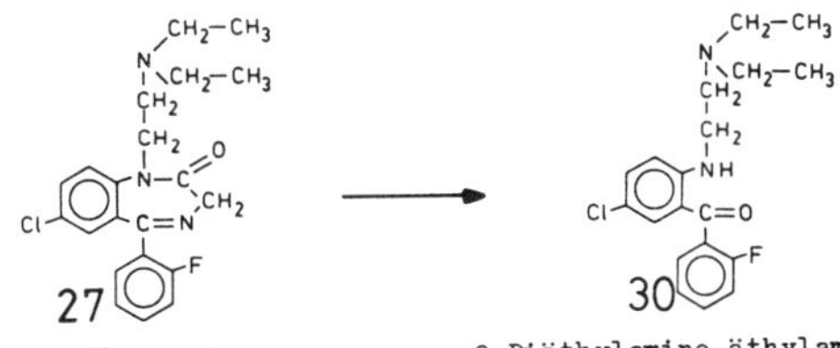

Flurazepam — 2-Diäthylamino-äthylamino-5-chlor-2'-fluor-benzophenone

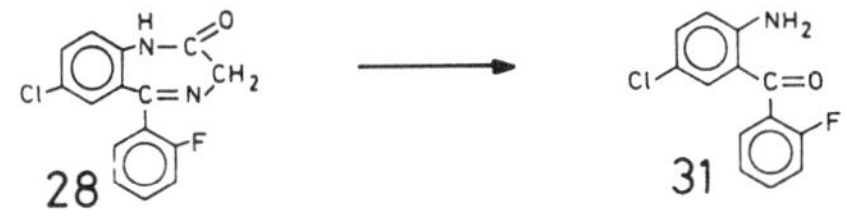

N-1-Desalkyl-Flurazepam — 2-Amino-5-chlor-2'-fluor-benzophenone

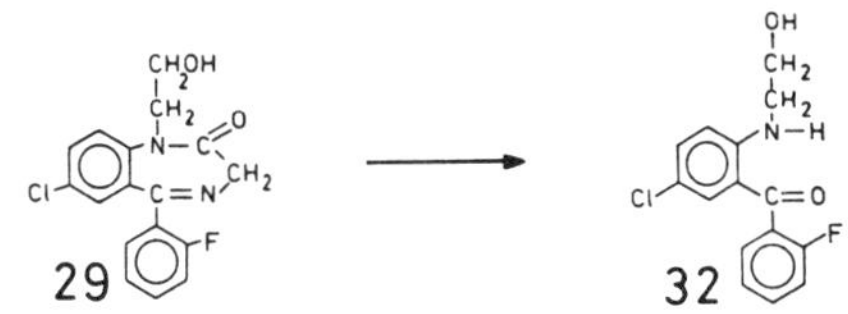

N-1-Hydroxyäthyl-Flurazepam — 2-Hydroxyäthylamino-5-chlor-2'-fluor-benzophenone

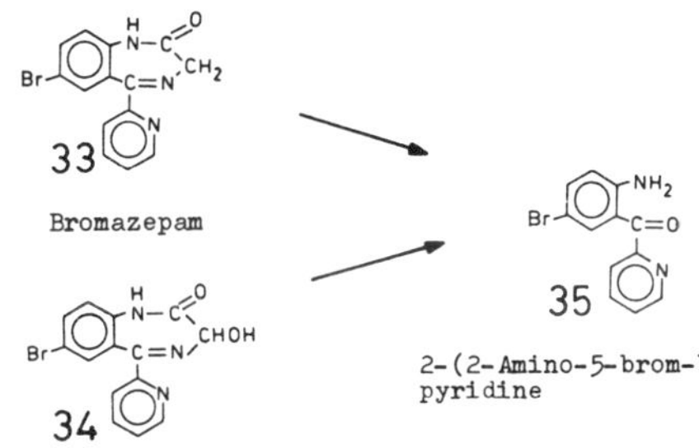

Bromazepam

2-(2-Amino-5-brom-benzoyl)-pyridine

3-Hydroxy-Bromazepam

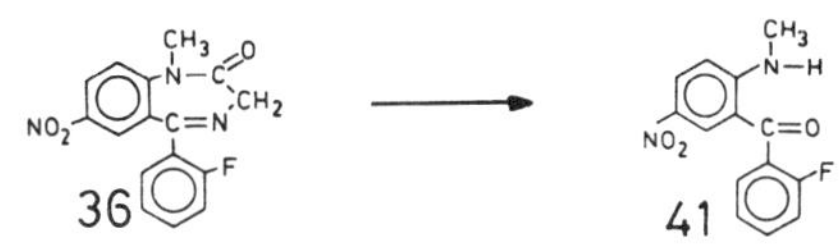

Flunitrazepam — 2-Methylamino-5-nitro-2'-fluor-benzophenone

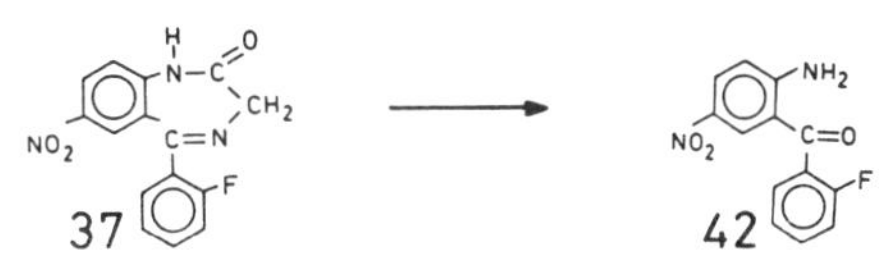

Nor-Flunitrazepam — 2-Amino-5-nitro-2'-fluor-benzophenone

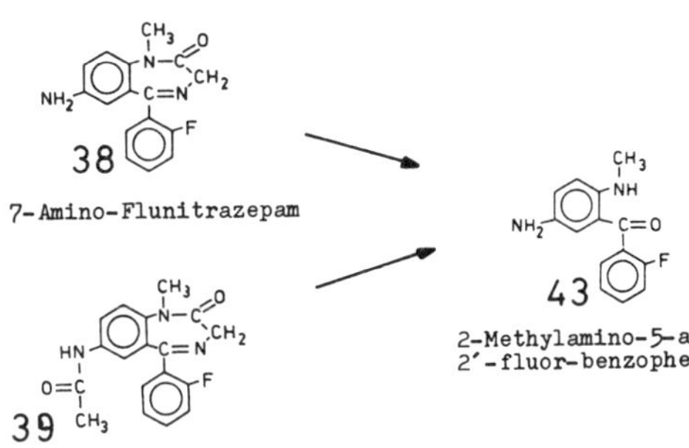

7-Amino-Flunitrazepam

2-Methylamino-5-amino-2'-fluor-benzophenone

7-Acetamido-Flunitrazepam

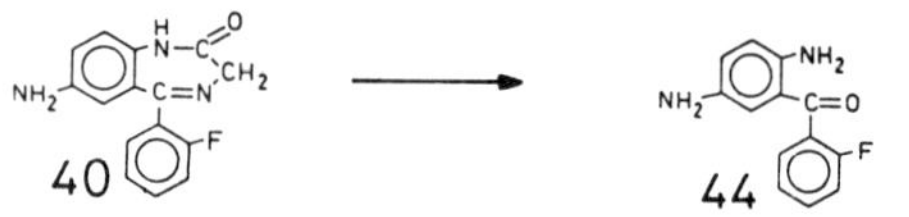

7-Amino-Nor-Flunitrazepam

2,5-Diamino-2'-fluor-benzophenone

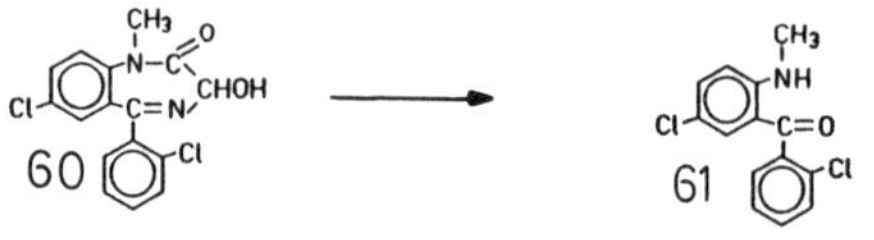

Lormetazepam

2-Methylamino-2',5-dichlor-benzophenone

Some Important Data

Einige wichtige Daten

No.	Subst.	Molec.Form. Brutto Form.	Mol.Weight Mol.Gew.	MS-Base Peak MS-Basispeak	Some other MS-Peaks Einige andere MS-Peaks
1	Chlordiazepoxide	$C_{16}H_{14}ClN_3O$	299,7	282	44,56,77,91,180,241, 247,283,284
2	Demoxepam (Nor-Diazepam-N-Oxide)	$C_{15}H_{11}ClN_2O_2$	286,7	285	77,107,152,167,180, 241,242,269,286,287
3	Desmethyl-Chlordiazepoxide	$C_{15}H_{12}ClN_3O$	285,7	285	42,43,73,77,233,268, 269,270,284,286,287
4	2-Amino-5-chlor-benzophenone	$C_{13}H_{10}ClNO$	231,7	230	44,77,105,154,195,231, 232,233
5	Diazepam	$C_{16}H_{13}ClN_2O$	284,7	256	44,57,77,78,221,255, 257,258,283,284,285
6	Nor-Diazepam	$C_{15}H_{11}ClN_2O$	270,7	242	44,45,76,77,180,207, 241,243,244,269,270,271
7	3-Hydroxy-Diazepam	$C_{16}H_{13}ClN_2O_2$	300,7	271	41,42,43,56,57,77,257, 273,300
8	Oxazepam	$C_{15}H_{11}ClN_2O_2$	286,7	257	44,51,75,77,104,205,233, 239,241,259,267,268,286
9	2-Methylamino-5-chlor- benzophenone	$C_{14}H_{12}ClNO$	245,7	245	44,51,77,105,168,193, 228,244,246,247
10	Nitrazepam	$C_{15}H_{11}N_3O_3$	281,3	280	77,103,205,234,252,253, 254,264,281
11	7-Amino-Nitrazepam	$C_{15}H_{13}N_3O$	251,3	251	43,44,84,98,103,111,195, 222,223,250,252
12	7-Acetamido-Nitrazepam	$C_{17}H_{15}N_3O_2$	293,3	293	43,44,207,212,213,263, 264,292,294
13	2-Amino-5-nitro-benzophenone	$C_{13}H_{10}N_2O_3$	242,2	241	43,44,51,55,57,77,105, 119,165,195,242
14	2,5-Diamino-benzophenone	$C_{13}H_{12}N_2O$	212,3	211	43,57,77,107,139,212
15	Medazepam-Base	$C_{16}H_{15}ClN_2$	270,7	207	43,44,57,165,206,208, 227,242,243,244,270
16	Chlorazepate Clorazepate	$C_{16}H_{13}ClN_2O_4$	332,7	242	43,57,76,77,89,103,151, 207,235,241,243,244, 269,270,271,272
17	Lorazepam	$C_{15}H_{10}Cl_2N_2O_2$	321,2	291	50,75,102,111,138,177, 239,240,273,274,275,276, 292,293,302,304,320,322
18	2-Amino-5,2'-dichlor- benzophenone	$C_{13}H_9Cl_2NO$	266,1	139	44,75,111,141,156,230
19	Prazepam	$C_{19}H_{17}ClN_2O$	324,8	269	44,55,77,91,241,242, 271,295,296,297,324
20	3-Hydroxy-Prazepam	$C_{19}H_{17}ClN_2O_2$	340,8	257	44,55,77,239,259,311, 313,340
21	2-Cyclopropyl-methylamino- 5-chlor-benzophenone	$C_{17}H_{16}ClNO$	285,8	285	44,55,77,91,105,166,180, 230,244,256,257,270,272, 286,287
22	Clonazepam	$C_{15}H_{10}ClN_3O_3$	315,7	280	43,44,51,75,76,77,89, 102,151,205,234,240, 268,287,288,289,314, 315,316,317
23	7-Amino-Clonazepam	$C_{15}H_{12}ClN_3O$	285,7	285	43,44,57,69,84,97,110, 111,220,222,250,256,257, 258,286,287
24	7-Acetamido-Clonazepam	$C_{17}H_{14}ClN_2O_2$	327,8	327	43,44,57,119,167,220, 221,250,256,257,258,264, 284,292,298,299,300,301, 326,328,329
25	2-Amino-5-nitro-2'-chlor- benzophenone	$C_{13}H_9ClN_2O_3$	276,7	241	43,44,75,111,119,139, 165,195,242,275,276,278
26	2,5-Diamino-2'-chlor- benzophenone	$C_{13}H_{11}ClN_2O$	246,7	246	43,44,55,80,107,111,210, 211,245,247,248

No.	Subst.	Molec.Form Brutto Form.	Mol.Weight Mol.Gew.	MS-Base Peak MS-Basispeak	Some other MS-Peaks Einige andere MS-Peaks
27	Flurazepam	$C_{21}H_{23}ClFN_3O$	387,9	86	42,56,58,71,86,87,99, 183,211,245,263,287, 315,387
28	N-1-Desalkyl-Flurazepam	$C_{15}H_{10}ClFN_2O$	288,7	260	44,75,85,102,112,259, 261,262,269,287,288, 289,290
29	N-1-Hydroxyethyl-Flurazepam	$C_{17}H_{14}ClFN_2O_2$	332,8	288	43,44,58,109,183,211, 245,273,287,289,290,304, 313,331,332,333
30	2-Diethylamino-ethylamino-5-chlor-2′-fluor-benzophenone	$C_{19}H_{22}ClFN_2O$	348,9	86	43,56,58,78,86,87,95, 109,123,166,348
31	2-Amino-5-chlor-2′-fluor-benzophenone	$C_{13}H_9ClFNO$	249,7	249	95,99,107,123,126,154, 230,232,248,250,251
32	2-Hydroxyethylamino-5-chlor-2′-fluor-benzophenone	$C_{15}H_{13}ClFNO_2$	293,7	262	75,95,109,123,166,168, 264,275,293,295
33	Bromazepam	$C_{14}H_{10}BrN_3O$	316,2	236	44,51,52,63,77,78,79,90, 91,103,104,179,180,207, 208,237,259,261,286,287, 288,314,315,316,317
34	3-Hydroxy-Bromazepam	$C_{14}H_{10}BrN_3O_2$	332,2	79	44,51,52,78,79,105,179, 206,302,303,304,305,314, 316,331,333
35	2-(2-Amino-5-brom-benzoyl)-pyridine	$C_{12}H_9BrN_2O$	277,1	62	43,44,45,61,62,63,88,89, 131,132,247,248,249,250, 276,278
36	Flunitrazepam	$C_{16}H_{12}FN_3O_3$	313,3	285	44,109,120,183,238,239, 248,266,286,294,312,313
37	Nor-Flunitrazepam	$C_{15}H_{10}FN_3O_3$	299,3	298	44,51,75,77,85,99,102, 109,112,170,197,223,224, 225,234,252,270,271,272, 280,299,300
38	7-Amino-Flunitrazepam	$C_{16}H_{14}FN_3O$	283,3	283	44,106,254,255,264,282, 284
39	7-Acetamido-Flunitrazepam	$C_{18}H_{16}FN_3O_2$	325,4	325	43,57,255,256,257,296, 297,306,324,326
40	7-Amino-Nor-Flunitrazepam	$C_{15}H_{12}FN_3O$	269,3	269	44,52,93,107,111,119, 120,121,213,240,241, 242,250,268,270
41	2-Methylamino-5-nitro-2′-fluor-benzophenone	$C_{14}H_{11}FN_2O_3$	274,3	274	43,44,95,123,133,179, 211,227,255,257,258, 273,275
42	2-Amino-5-nitro-2′-fluor-benzophenone	$C_{13}H_9FN_2O_3$	260,2	260	43,44,55,57,77,91,95, 119,123,195,185,213, 230,241,259,261
43	2-Methylamino-5-amino-2′-fluor-benzophenone	$C_{14}H_{13}FN_2O$	244,3	244	43,55,57,65,69,95,97, 112,121,122,123,149,225, 227,228,243,245
44	2,5-Diamino-2′-fluor-benzophenone	$C_{13}H_{11}FN_2O$	230,3	230	43,58,86,95,107,123,135, 210,211,229,231
45	2-Amino-3-hydroxy-5-chlor-benzophenone	$C_{13}H_{10}ClNO_2$	247,7	77	45,51,57,77,78,105,170, 211,230,246,247,248,249
46	Clobazam	$C_{16}H_{13}ClN_2O_2$	300,8	300	51,77,91,119,181,196, 208,214,229,231,243,255, 256,257,258,259,260,261, 283,285,301,302
47	Nor-Clobazam	$C_{15}H_{11}ClN_2O_2$	286,7	286	44,51,77,78,83,167,203, 215,216,217,218,219,220, 241,244,245,246,287,288
48	Camazepam	$C_{19}H_{18}ClN_3O_3$	371,8	271	43,44,51,55,57,58,91, 110,115,118,150,151,152, 165,177,193,221,227,255, 256,257,273,283,299,328, 343,345,371
49	Diazepam-N-Oxide	$C_{16}H_{13}ClN_2O_2$	300,7	299	43,77,105,151,152,165, 177,193,205,219,221,248, 255-258,265,271,283,284, 285,300,301,302
50	3-Acetoxy-Diazepam	$C_{18}H_{15}ClN_2O_3$	342,7	271	43,45,61,70,73,77,88, 105,165,193,221,227-230, 243,255-259,272,273,300, 302,342,343,344
51	Prazepam-N-Oxide	$C_{19}H_{17}ClN_2O_2$	340,8	55	43,44,57,69,71,77,91, 105,205,227,241,242,269, 285,295,323-326,339,340
52	3-Acetoxy-Prazepam	$C_{21}H_{19}ClN_2O_3$	382,8	257	43,44,45,55,60,77,151, 179,227,239,241,258,259, 269,296,297,311,312,313, 322,324,340,341,342,382, 383,384

No.	Subst.	Molec.Form. Brutto Form.	Mol.Weight Mol.Gew.	MS-Base Peak MS-Basispeak	Some other MS-Peaks Einige andere MS-Peaks
53	Desmethyl-Medazepam	$C_{15}H_{13}ClN_2$	256,7	193	43,51,57,63,65,75,76,77, 82,83,89,95,96,110,127, 128,142,152,163,164,165, 177,192,194,199,204,218, 219,228,229,230,238,239, 253,255,256,257,258
54	Monodesethyl-Flurazepam	$C_{19}H_{19}ClFN_3O$	359,8	246	42-44,55-59,71,75,91, 109,117,118,125,151,153, 163-165,171,183,191,192, 205,211,220,245-248,255, 257,259,273-276,289,291, 302-304,313-315,326,328, 341-343,359-361
55	Didesethyl-Flurazepam	$C_{17}H_{15}ClFN_3O$	331,8	314	42-44,51,54,63,75,109, 117,125,137-139,152,183, 191,211,223,245-248,255, 261,273,274,289,291,302-304,313-316,331
56	Bromazepam-N(Py)-Oxide	$C_{14}H_{10}BrN_3O_2$	332,2	79/80	41,42,44,50-53,62-65,75-81,83,84,88-92,99-105, 107,113-120,128-130,141-143,155-157,161,169,171, 182,183,184,195-199,209-211,225,238,239,255,262, 264,276-278,289-291,304-306,317-319,321,333-336
57	Ketazolam	$C_{20}H_{17}ClN_2O_3$	368,8	256	43,44,51,55,57,69,75,77, 84,89,91,110,117,125, 127,151,152,163,165,177, 193,199,205,221,222,228, 239,241,248,249,255-259, 268,283-286,325,327,368, 370
58	Triazolam	$C_{17}H_{12}Cl_2N_4$	343,2	342	75,77,102,105,110,111, 115,119,122,132,133,137, 138,139,153,163,177,190, 203,231,238,239,240,241, 253,266,273,279,281,286, 300,307,309,313-317,342-346
59	Clotiazepam	$C_{16}H_{15}ClN_2OS$	318,8	289	89,120,123,127,145,152, 166,198,212,213,225,228, 232,234,239,248,255,262, 268,275,277,283,289-292, 303,305,317-321
60	Lormetazepam	$C_{16}H_{12}Cl_2N_2O_2$	335,2	304	44,45,50,51,57,75,91, 102,103,111,117,118,138, 152,165,177,193,195,213, 222,227,238,254,255,261, 268,288,290,304-308,333-335
61	2-Methylamino-2′,5-dichlor-benzophenone	$C_{14}H_{11}Cl_2NO$	280,1	149	44,45,55-57,61,62,75-77, 105,111,122,125,133,139, 150,165,167,170,180,205, 209,214,215,223,227,229-231,244-246,262,264,278-283
62	Tetrazepam	$C_{16}H_{17}ClN_2O$	288,8	253	41,43,44,51,57,77,79,91, 103,154,165,167,168,180-182,195-197,225,231-233, 245-247,253-254,259-261, 273,287-291
63	Nor-Tetrazepam	$C_{15}H_{15}ClN_2O$	274,8	239	41,43,44,51,77,91,128, 140,165-168,182,183,203, 211,217,231-233,239,240, 245-247,259,261,273-277

TLC - Data

DC-Daten

Technical Notes on TLC - Conditions

TLC-plates: Precoated TLC plates, Silicagel 60 F_{254}, 20 x 20 cm, layer-thickness 0.25 mm, Merck, Darmstadt, Germany, activated for 1 hour (110°C), saturated chamber, ascenting method, length of run 10 cm, 20°C (984).

Solvent Systems:
- A: Chloroform / Acetone (90 + 10, v/v)
- B: Benzene (may be replaced by toluene)
- C: Benzene / iso-Propanol/ Ammonia Sol. 25% (85 + 15 + 1).

Detection: BRATTON-MARSHALL-Reagent (139) after diazotization.
DRAGENDORFF-Reagent according to MUNIER and MACHEBOEUF (see STAHL (1079) p. 829, reagent No. 89).
JODOPLATEAT according to SMITH (see STAHL (1079) p. 837, reagent No. 140).

The aminobenzophenones were obtained by acid hydrolysis (continuous TLC-control of the reaction). See the part Biotransformation for hydrolysis procedures.

Most of the substances were kindly supplied by HOFFMANN-LA ROCHE (Switzerland); Camazepam by BOEHRINGER INGELHEIM, Clobazam by HOECHST, Clorazepate and Tetrazepam by MACK-MIDY, Clotiazepam by TROPON, Ketazolam by BEECHAM-WÜLFING, Lorazepam by WYETH, Lormetazepam by SCHERING, Oxazepam by THOMAE, Prazepam by WARNER-LAMBERT - GÖDECKE and Triazolam by UPJOHN.

Technische Angaben zur Dünnschichtchromatographie

DC-Platten: DC-Fertigplatten, Kieselgel 60 F_{254}, 20 x 20 cm, Schichtdicke 0,25 mm, Merck, Darmstadt, BRD, aktiviert bei 110°C (1 h), Kammersättigung, aufsteigende Methode, Laufstrecke 10 cm, 20°C Kammertemperatur (984).

Fließmittelsysteme:
- A: Chloroform / Aceton (90 + 10, v/v)
- B: Benzol (ersatzweise Toluol)
- C: Benzol / Iso-Propanol / Ammoniak 25% aqu. (85 + 15 + 1, v/v/v)

Detektion: BRATTON-MARSHALL-Reagens (139) nach Diazotierung (vgl. Lit. 970 - 974).
DRAGENDORFF-Reagens nach MUNIER und MACHEBOEUF (s. STAHL (1079) S. 829, Reag.Nr. 89).
JODOPLATEAT nach SMITH (s. STAHL (1079) S. 837, Reag.Nr. 140).

Die Aminobenzophenone wurden mit Hilfe einer sauren Hydrolyse hergestellt (fortlaufende DC-Kontrolle der Reaktion). S. Kapitel Biotransformation bezüglich der Arbeitsvorschrift.

Die meisten Substanzen wurden in freundlicher und dankenswerter Weise vom Hause HOFFMANN LA ROCHE (Schweiz), Camazepam von BOEHRINGER INGELHEIM, CLOBAZAM von HOECHST AG, Clorazepat und Tetrazepam von MACK-MIDY, Clotiazepam von TROPON, Ketazolam von BEECHAM-WÜLFING, Lorazepam von WYETH, Lormetazepam von SCHERING, Oxazepam von THOMAE, Prazepam von WARNER-LAMBERT - GÖDECKE und Triazolam von UPJOHN zur Verfügung gestellt.
Eine Reihe von Metaboliten wurde mit Hilfe von Reaktionen auf der DC-Platte im Mikromaßstab gewonnen (Lit. 279, 280, 282, 283, 979 und 980).

Thin-Layer Chromatographic Data / Dünnschichtchromatographische Daten

No.	Subst.	R_f-Value in			Detection		
		A	B	C	Bratton-Marsh.	Dragend.	Jodoplat.
1	Chlordiazepoxide	0,07	0,00	0,47	neg.	orange	redviol. rotviol.
2	Demoxepam (Nor-Diazepam-N-Oxide)	0,10	0,00	0,30	neg.	orange	viol.
3	N-Desmethyl-Chlordiazepoxide	0,02	0,00	0,30	neg.	orange	viol.
4	2-Amino-5-chlor-benzophenone	0,87	0,36	0,90	viol.	orange	yellow gelb
5	Diazepam	0,52	0,00	0,74	neg.	orange	viol.
6	Nor-Diazepam	0,26	0,00	0,52	neg.	orange	viol.
7	3-Hydroxy-Diazepam	0,42	0,00	0,51	neg.	orange	viol.
8	Oxazepam	0,16	0,00	0,26	neg.	orange	viol.
9	2-Methylamino-5-chlor-benzophenone	0,93	0,67	0,95	neg.	orange	yellow gelb
10	Nitrazepam	0,24	0,00	0,48	neg.	orange	viol.

Thin-Layer Chromatographic Data / Dünnschichtchromatographische Daten (continued / Fortsetzung)

No.	Subst.	R_f-Value in A	B	C	Detection Bratton-Marsh.	Dragend.	Jodoplat.
11	7-Amino-Nitrazepam	0,08	0,00	0,30	blueviol. blauviol.	orange	viol.
12	7-Acetamido-Nitrazepam	0,04	0,00	0,18	neg.	orange	viol.
13	2-Amino-5-nitro-benzophenone	0,80	0,19	0,79	redviol. rotviol.	orange	yellow gelb
14	2,5-Diamino-benzophenone	0,35	0,00	0,61	viol.	orange	viol.
15	Medazepam-Base	0,56	0,00	0,85	neg.	orange	redbrown rotbraun
16	Chlorazepate Clorazepate	0,25	0,00	0,56	neg.	orange	viol.
17	Lorazepam	0,16	0,00	0,30	neg.	orange	viol.
18	2-Amino-5,2′-dichlor-benzophenone	0,97	0,45	0,94	viol.	orange	yellow gelb
19	Prazepam	0,63	0,00	0,79	neg.	orange	viol.
20	3-Hydroxy-Prazepam	0,56	0,00	0,61	neg.	orange	viol.
21	2-Cyclopropyl-methylamino-5-chlor-benzophenone	0,98	0,80	0,98	neg.	orange	yellow gelb
22	Clonazepam	0,27	0,00	0,48	neg.	orange	viol.
23	7-Amino-Clonazepam	0,08	0,00	0,30	viol.	orange	brownviol. braunviol.
24	7-Acetamido-Clonazepam	0,04	0,00	0,19	neg.	orange	viol.
25	2-Amino-5-nitro-2′-chlor-benzophenone	0,78	0,23	0,80	redviol. rotviol.	orange	yellow gelb
26	2,5-Diamino-2′-chlor-benzophenone	0,40	0,00	0,61	blueviol. blauviol.	grey grau	brown braun
27	Flurazepam	0,03	0,00	0,46	neg.	orange	blueviol. blauviol.
28	N-1-Desalkyl-Flurazepam	0,25	0,00	0,52	neg.	orange	viol.
29	N-1-Hydroxyethyl-Flurazepam	0,14	0,00	0,44	neg.	orange	viol.
30	2-Diethylamino-ethylamino-5-chlor-2′-fluor-benzophenone	0,08	0,00	0,74	neg.	orange	brownviol. braunviol.
31	2-Amino-5-chlor-2′-fluor-benzophenone	0,88	0,45	0,92	viol.	orange	yellow gelb
32	2-Hydroxyethylamino-5-chlor-2′-fluor-benzophenone	0,45	0,05	0,59	neg.	orange	viol.
33	Bromazepam	0,07	0,00	0,47	neg.	orange	blueviol. blauviol.
34	3-Hydroxy-Bromazepam	0,05	0,00	0,27	neg.	orange	viol.
35	2-(2-Amino-5-brom-benzoyl)-pyridine	0,66	0,04	0,73	redviol. rotviol.	orange	viol.
36	Flunitrazepam	0,51	0,00	0,64	neg.	orange	viol.
37	Nor-Flunitrazepam	0,25	0,00	0,48	neg.	orange	viol.
38	7-Amino-Flunitrazepam	0,15	0,00	0,35	redviol. rotviol.	orange	viol.
39	7-Acetamido-Flunitrazepam	0,08	0,00	0,22	neg.	orange	viol.
40	7-Amino-Nor-Flunitrazepam	0,07	0,00	0,28	redviol. rotviol.	orange	viol.
41	2-Methylamino-5-nitro-2′-fluor-benzophenone	0,90	0,41	0,93	neg.	yellow gelb	yellow gelb
42	2-Amino-5-nitro-2′-fluor-benzophenone	0,75	0,21	0,75	viol.	yellow gelb	yellow gelb
43	2-Methylamino-5-amino-2′-fluor-benzophenone	0,12	0,00	0,35	viol.	brown braun	viol.
44	2,5-Diamino-2′-fluor-benzophenone	0,07	0,00	0,12	viol.	brown braun	viol.
45	2-Amino-3-hydroxy-5-chlor-benzophenone	0,60	0,05	0,62	brownviol. braunviol.	brown braun	viol.
46	Clobazam	0,52	0,00	0,59	neg.	orange	viol.
47	Nor-Clobazam	0,22	0,00	0,45	neg.	orange	viol.
48	Camazepam	0,50	0,00	0,72	neg.	orange	viol.
49	Diazepam-N-Oxide	0,43	0,00	----	neg.	orange	viol.
50	3-Acetoxy-Diazepam	----	0,00	----	neg.	orange	viol.

Thin-Layer Chromatographic Data / Dünnschichtchromatographische Daten (continued / Fortsetzung)

No.	Subst.	R_f-Value in			Detection		
		A	B	C	Bratton-Marsh.	Dragend.	Jodopl.
51	Prazepam-N-Oxide	0,53	0,00	----	neg.	orange	viol.
52	3-Acetoxy-Prazepam	----	0,00	----	neg.	orange	viol.
53	Desmethyl-Medazepam	0,10	0,00	0,75	neg.	orange	viol.
54	Monodesethyl-Flurazepam	0,00	0,00	0,42	neg.	orange	viol.
55	Didesethyl-Flurazepam	0,00	0,00	0,22	neg.	orange	viol.
56	Bromazepam-N(Py)-Oxide	0,00	0,00	0,17	neg.	orange	viol.
57	Ketazolam	0,45	0,00	0,86	neg.	orange	viol.
58	Triazolam	----	0,00	0,86	neg.	orange	viol.
59	Clotiazepam	0,50	0,00	0,90	neg.	orange	viol.
60	Lormetazepam	0,40	0,00	0,65	neg.	orange	viol.
61	2-Methylamino-2',5-dichlor-benzophenone	0,99	0,70	0,98	neg.	orange	viol.
62	Tetrazepam	0,55	0,00	0,92	neg.	orange	viol.
63	Nor-Tetrazepam	0,25	0,00	0,80	neg.	orange	viol.

GLC - Data

GC-Daten

Technical Notes on GLC - Conditions

The gas chromatograph was a Varian Aerograph Series 2100 with a flame-ionization detector; integration was carried out with a Spectra Physics Minigrator and a Varian Aerograph Model 480 respectively.
Column: 1.5 m x 2 mm I.D. glass column packed with 3 % OV-17 or 3 % SE-30 on Chromosorb G AW DMCS (80 - 100 mesh).
Carrier gas: Nitrogen at a flow-rate of ca. 15 ml min^{-1}.

Retention indices were calculated according to the literature (Kovâts: Helv.Chim.Acta <u>41</u>, 1915 (1958) and Kaiser: Chromatographia <u>3</u>, 134 (1970) and Chromatographia <u>7</u>, 251 (1974) resp.).

When the gas chromatographic data are discussed, it must be considered that rearrangements and thermolysis are possible, especially with 3-hydroxy-benzodiazepines (334, 929).

Technische Angaben zum Kapitel Gaschromatographie

Zur Bestimmung der Daten wurde ein Gaschromatograph Varian Aerograph Series 2100 mit FID und elektronischer Integration benutzt (Spectra Physics Minigrator bzw. Varian Aerograph Modell 480).

Säule: 1,5 m x 2 mm I.D., Glas, bepackt mit 3 % OV-17 bzw. 3 % SE-30 auf Chromosorb G AW DMCS (80 - 100 mesh).
Trägergas: Stickstoff (ca. 15 ml min^{-1}).

Die Berechnung der Retentionsindizes erfolgte nach der Methode von Kovâts bzw. Kaiser (Lit.s.o.).

Bei der Interpretation der gaschromatographischen Daten ist zu berücksichtigen, daß Umlagerungen und Thermolyseeffekte auftreten können, insbesondere bei 3-Hydroxybenzodiazepinen (334, 929).

See ARDREY and MOFFAT for a critical compilation of retention indices (3774).

GLC - Data / GLC - Daten

No.	Subst.	220°C Ret.Time(s) SE-30	220°C Ret.Time(s) OV-17	220°C Ret.Index SE-30	220°C Ret.Index OV-17	250°C Ret.Time(s) SE-30	250°C Ret.Time(s) OV-17	250°C Ret.Index SE-30	250°C Ret.Index OV-17	280°C Ret.Time(s) SE-30	280°C Ret.Time(s) OV-17	280°C Ret.Index SE-30	280°C Ret.Index OV-17
1	Chlordiazepoxide					134 + 266	435 + 671	2570 + 2845	3068 + 3223	65 + 114	180 + 520	2657 + 2910	3160 + 3595
2	Demoxepam (Nor-Diazepam-N-Oxid)					135	420	2574	3058		169		3142
3	N-Desmethyl-Chlordiazepoxide					279	1234	2885	3484	114	474	2930	3590
4	2-Amino-5-chlor-benzophenone	86	233	2046	2457	55	99	2080	2516	21	47	2125	2584
5	Diazepam					102	297	2487	2948	48	127	2510	3020
6	Nor-Diazepam					120	403	2554	3060	57	162	2585	3124
7	3-Hydroxy-Diazepam					152	472	2628	3125	70	194	2675	3200
8	Oxazepam					73	198	2380	2829	40	93	2424	2888
9	2-Methylamino-5-chlor-benzophenone	95	236	2105	2490	47	91	2155	2536	20	43	2104	2570
10	Nitrazepam									96	335	2832	3455
11	7-Amino-Nitrazepam					215		2785		104	369	2870	3475
12	7-Acetamido-Nitrazepam									210	823	3205	3815
13	2-Amino-5-nitro-benzophenone	220	803	2380	2875	98	297	2433	2942	47	141	2476	2990
14	2,5-Diamino-benzophenone	127	367	2170	2604	50	156	2225	2740	30	77	2300	2800

		220°C				250°C				280°C			
No.	Subst.	Ret.Time(s) SE-30	Ret.Time(s) OV-17	Ret.Index SE-30	Ret.Index OV-17	Ret.Time(s) SE-30	Ret.Time(s) OV-17	Ret.Index SE-30	Ret.Index OV-17	Ret.Time(s) SE-30	Ret.Time(s) OV-17	Ret.Index SE-30	Ret.Index OV-17
15	Medazepam-Base	145	398	2243	2660	66	146	2286	2710	34	71	2360	2775
16	Chlorazepate						377		3070	65	163	2655	3126
17	Lorazepam					86	255	2442	2925	48	115	2514	2979
18	2-Amino-5,2'-dichlor-benzophenone	122	345	2195	2600	57	135	2240	2670	50	72	2480	2680
19	Prazepam									81	230	2717	3178
20	3-Hydroxy-Prazepam									110	358	2860	3375
21	2-Cyclopropyl-methylamino-5-chlor-benzophenone	215	539	2370	2752	85	185	2398	2807	43	86	2450	2855
22	Clonazepam									140	435	2964	3518
23	7-Amino-Clonazepam									115	470	2905	3560
24	7-Acetamido-Clonazepam									246	1200	3270	3970
25	2-Amino-5-nitro-2'-chlor-benzophenone					109	414	2538	3106	55	208	2552	3143
26	2,5-Diamino-2'-chlor-benzophenone x HCl	218	765	2334	2816	77	265	2355	2891				
27	Flurazepam x HCl									91	219	2800	3275
28	N-1-Desalkyl-Flurazepam					110	359	2500	3020	47	134	2510	3062
29	N-1-Hydroxyethyl-Flurazepam					189	638	2715	3235	74	210	2730	3255
30	2-Diethylamino-ethylamino-5-chlor-2'-fluor-benzophenone					126	278	2555	2930	51	97	2560	2940
31	2-Amino-5-chlor-2'-fluor-benzophenone	86	230	2047	2435	38	78	2090	2488				
32	2-Hydroxyethylamino-5-chlor-2'-fluor-benzophenone	265		2426		99	244	2490	2907	46	105	2500	2957
33	Bromazepam					170	695	2672	3260	85	364	2700	3353
34	3-Hydroxy-Bromazepam					121	359	2540	3019	61	180	2568	3068
35	2-(2-Amino-5-brom-benzoyl)-pyridine	142	425	2277	2734	59	175	2259	2786				
36	Flunitrazepam					162	484	2646	3168	66	181	2678	3195
37	Nor-Flunitrazepam					203	737	2735	3322	77	264	2745	3350
38	7-Amino-Flunitrazepam					198	654	2726	3278	72	236	2719	3305
39	7-Acetamido-Flunitrazepam									178	713	3113	3751
40	7-Amino-Nor-Flunitrazepam									94	425	2825	3550
41	2-Methylamino-5-nitro-2'-fluor-benzophenone	232	792	2383	2862	104	276	2436	2908	48	133	2470	2940
42	2-Amino-5-nitro-2'-fluor-benzophenone	206	769	2344	2827	87	282	2381	2886				
43	2-Methylamino-5-amino-2'-fluor-benzophenone					187	714	2703	3270	70	230	2700	3297
44	2,5-Diamino-2'-fluor-benzophenone	117	394	2152	2652	61	157	2226	2713		83		2743
45	2-Amino-3-hydroxy-5-chlor-benzophenone	217		2360		87	230	2400	2840	38	112	2382	2868
46	Clobazam					153	482	2662	3172	75	232	2646	3170

No.	Subst.	220°C Ret.Time(s) SE-30	220°C Ret.Time(s) OV-17	220°C Ret.Index SE-30	220°C Ret.Index OV-17	250°C Ret.Time(s) SE-30	250°C Ret.Time(s) OV-17	250°C Ret.Index SE-30	250°C Ret.Index OV-17	280°C Ret.Time(s) SE-30	280°C Ret.Time(s) OV-17	280°C Ret.Index SE-30	280°C Ret.Index OV-17
47	Nor-Clobazam					225	704	2814	3315	84	316	2697	3297
48	Camazepam									161	500	2965	3645
53	Desmethyl-Medazepam							2370	2855			2395	2935
54	Monodesethyl-Flurazepam							2970	3580			3030	3665
55	Didesethyl-Flurazepam							2660	2930			2505	3045
56	Bromazepam-N(Py)-Oxide							2650	3295			2735	3375
57	Ketazolam							2470	2970			2510	3030
58	Triazolam										OV-101	3110	3740
59	Clotiazepam										OV-101	2580	3080
60	Lormetazepam											3030	3690
61	2-Methylamino-2',5-dichlor-benzophenone											2185	2650
62	Tetrazepam							2460	2930			2505	3045
63	Nor-Tetrazepam							2520	3040			2570	3125

Infrared- and Mass-Spectra

Infrarot- und Massen-Spektren

Mass-Spectra: VARIAN MAT 101
electron impact energy 70 eV

Infrared-Spectra:
PERKIN ELMER 337
Grating Infrared Spectrophotometer
KBr - technique

Ultraviolett-Spectra:
LEITZ Unicam SP. 800
calibration with Holmium

Important: The UV-measurements were carried out with different concentrations in order to obtain a better differentiation.

Interpretation of Mass- and Infrared-Spectra

Mass-Spectra $(M^+ - x)$-peaks

x = 16.000	O (from N-Oxides)
16.024	NH_2 (from prim. Amines)
17.008	OH (e.g. from N-Oxides)
18.016	H_2O (N-Oxides or Hydroxy-compounds)
19.000	F (e.g. flurazepam or flunitrazepam)
27.027	HCN (e.g. from aromat. Amines)
28.011	CO (typical fragment of Benzodiazepines)
28.035	CH_2N (many Benzodiazepines)
29.019	HCO
29.062	C_2H_5
30.008	NO (rare)
31.035	CH_2=OH (Alcohols)
35.457	Cl
45.062	CH_3-CH=OH (Alcohols)
46.008	NO_2 (rare)
79.916	Br (e.g. bromazepam and metabolites)

Combination Fragments

45.019	-(CO + OH)
46.027	-(CO + H_2O)
47.011	-(CO + F)
53.473	-(Cl + H_2O)
58.019	-(CO + NO)
63.468	-(CO + Cl)
80.478	-(CO + OH + Cl)
81.484	-(CO + H_2O + Cl)
107.920	-(CO + Br)
125.936	-(CO +H_2O + Br)

Infrared-Spectra

-OH	st	3650-3200 cm^{-1}	$-CH_3$	δ	ca. 1460 cm^{-1}
-COOH	st	3550-2500 cm^{-1}	$-CH_2$	δ	ca. 1460 cm^{-1}
-NH	st	3500-3200 cm^{-1}	-CF	st	1400-1000 cm^{-1}
ar-CH	st	3080-3030 cm^{-1}	$-NO_2$	st sy	1390-1260 cm^{-1}
≡CH	st	3000-2840 cm^{-1}	-C-O	st	1330-1050 cm^{-1}
$-N^+H$	st	3000-2000 cm^{-1}	-C-O(H)	st	1260- 970 cm^{-1}
-C=O	st	1800-1650 cm^{-1}	ar-CH	δ oop	900- 650 cm^{-1}
$-NO_2$	st as	1660-1490 cm^{-1}	-CCl	st	< 830 cm^{-1}
-NH	δ	1650-1550 cm^{-1}	$-CH_2-$	γ	770- 720 cm^{-1}
ar-C-C	st	1600 cm^{-1} 1500 cm^{-1} 1450 cm^{-1}	-CBr	st	< 700 cm^{-1}

Recommended Values for Single-Ion Monitoring Procedures:

m/e =	Benzophenone derivative
139	2-Amino-5,2'-dichlorobenzophenone (hydrolysis product of lorazepam)
211	2,5-Diaminobenzophenone (hydrolysis product of 7-aminonitrazepam and 7-acetamidonitrazepam)
230	2-Amino-5-chlorobenzophenone (hydrolysis product of chlordiazepoxide, desmethylchlordiazepoxide, demoxepam, oxazepam, desmethyldiazepam and clorazepate)
230	2-Amino-5,2'-dichlorobenzophenone (hydrolysis product of lorazepam)
230	2,5-Diamino-2'-fluorbenzophenone (hydrolysis product of 7-amino-norflunitrazepam)
241	2-Amino-5-nitrobenzophenone (hydrolysis product of nitrazepam)
241	2-Amino-5-nitro-2'-chlorobenzophenone (hydrolysis product of clonazepam)
244	2-Methylamino-5-chlorobenzophenone (hydrolysis product of diazepam, 3-hydroxydiazepam = temazepam, camazepam and ketazolam)
244	2-Methylamino-5-amino-2'-fluorbenzophenone (hydrolysis product of 7-aminoflunitrazepam and 7-acetamidoflunitrazepam)
244	2-Methylamino-2',5-dichlorbenzophenone (hydrolysis product of lormetazepam)
245	2-Methylamino-5-chlorobenzophenone (hydrolysis product of diazepam, 3-hydroxydiazepam = temazepam, camazepam and ketazolam)
246	2,5-Diamino-2'-chlorobenzophenone (hydrolysis product of 7-aminoclonazepam and 7-acetamidoclonazepam)
249	2-Amino-5-chloro-2'-fluorbenzophenone (hydrolysis product of N-1-desalkylflurazepam)
249	2-(2-Amino-5-brombenzoyl)-pyridine (hydrolysis product of bromazepam and 3-hydroxybromazepam)
260	2-Amino-5-nitro-2'-fluorobenzophenone (hydrolysis product of norflunitrazepam)
262	2-Hydroxyethylamino-5-chloro-2'-fluorbenzophenone (hydrolysis product of N-1-hydroxyethylflurazepam)
274	2-Methylamino-5-nitro-2'-fluorbenzophenone (hydrolysis product of flunitrazepam)
285	2-Cyclopropylmethylamino-5-chlorobenzophenone (hydrolysis product of prazepam and 3-hydroxyprazepam)

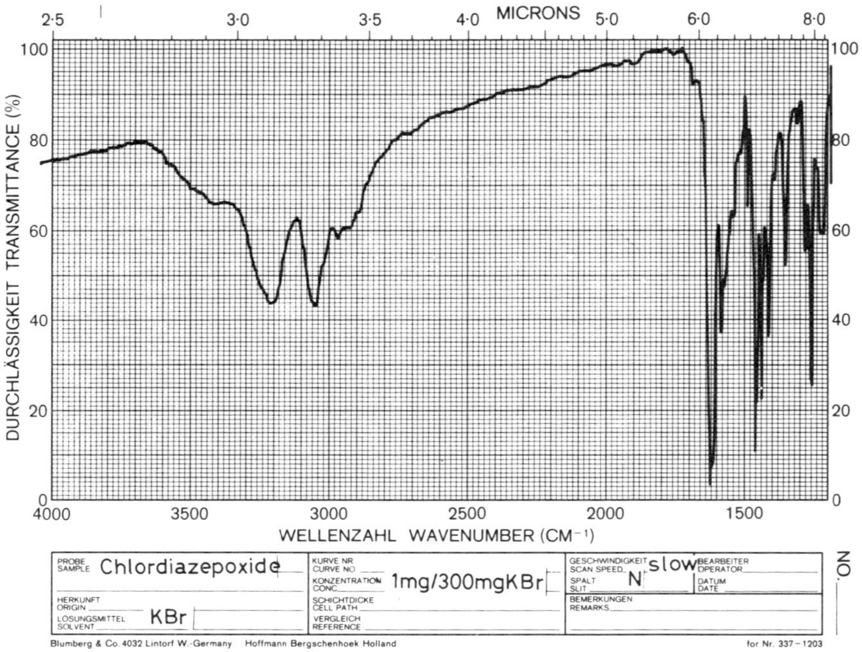

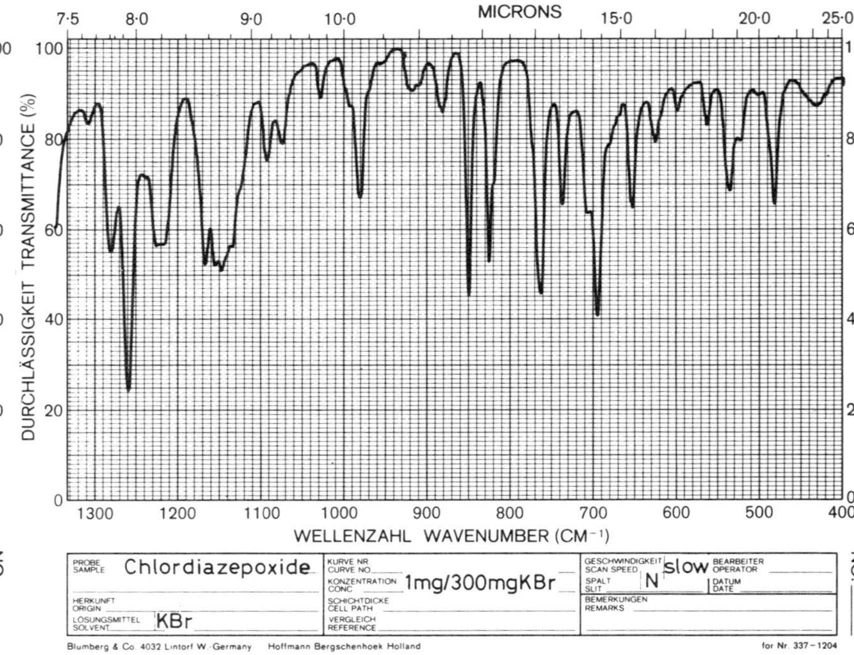

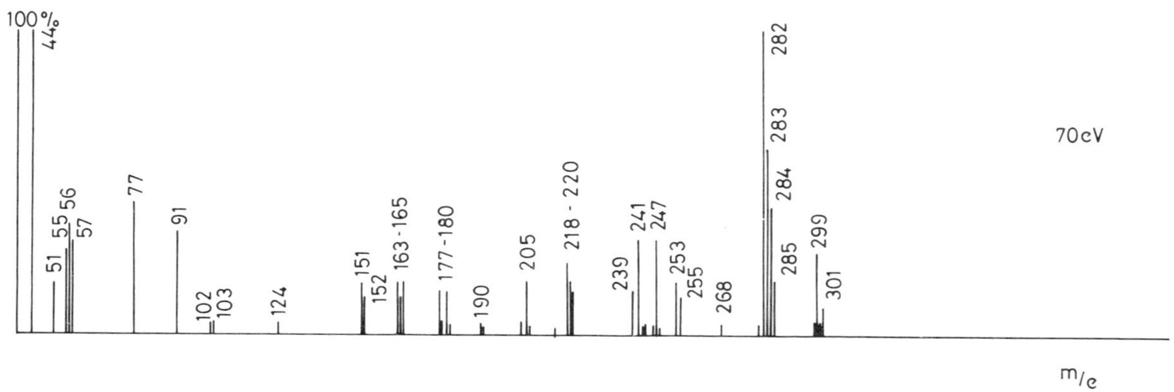

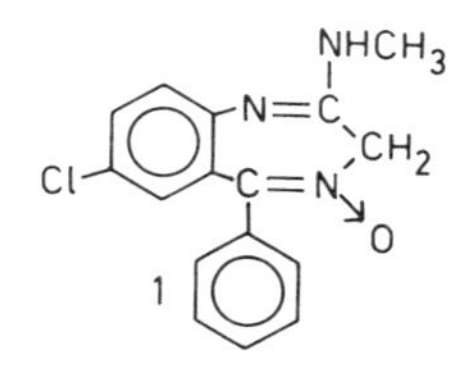

Chlordiazepoxide

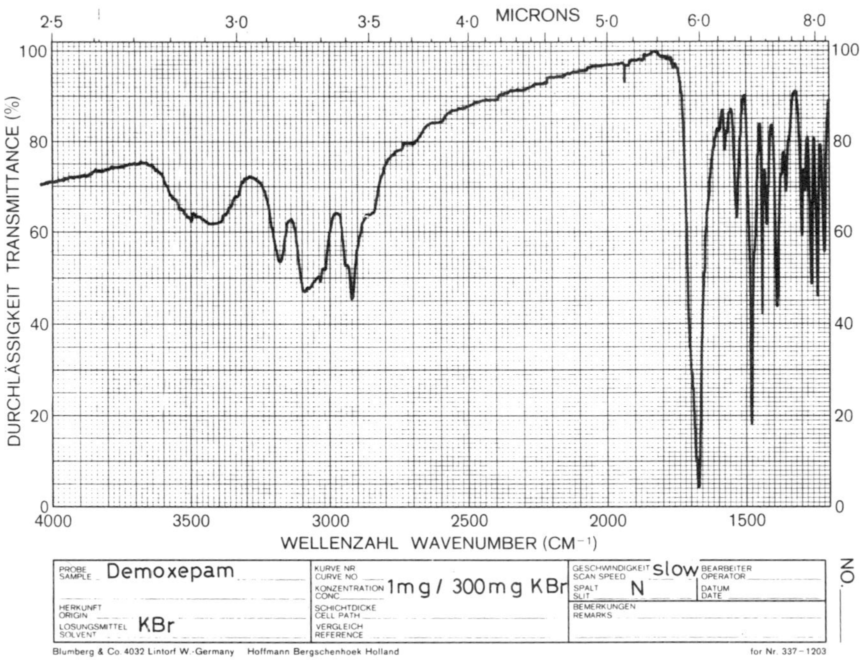
MICRONS
DURCHLÄSSIGKEIT TRANSMITTANCE (%)
WELLENZAHL WAVENUMBER (CM⁻¹)
PROBE SAMPLE Demoxepam
HERKUNFT ORIGIN
LÖSUNGSMITTEL SOLVENT KBr
KURVE NR CURVE NO
KONZENTRATION CONC 1mg / 300mg KBr
SCHICHTDICKE CELL PATH
VERGLEICH REFERENCE
GESCHWINDIGKEIT SCAN SPEED slow
SPALT SLIT N
BEARBEITER OPERATOR
DATUM DATE
BEMERKUNGEN REMARKS
NO.
Blumberg & Co. 4032 Lintorf W.-Germany Hoffmann Bergschenhoek Holland
for Nr. 337-1203

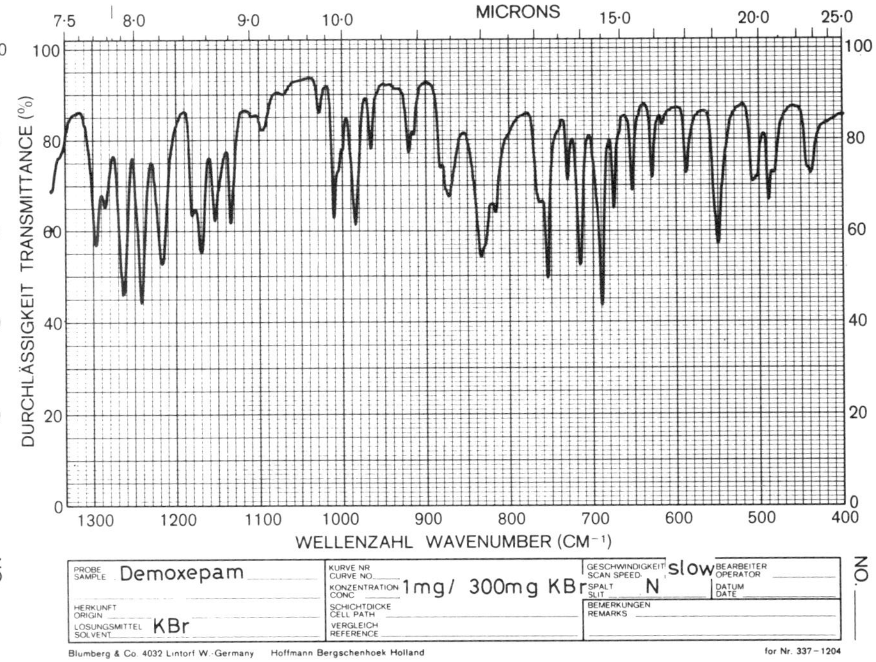
MICRONS
DURCHLÄSSIGKEIT TRANSMITTANCE (%)
WELLENZAHL WAVENUMBER (CM⁻¹)
PROBE SAMPLE Demoxepam
HERKUNFT ORIGIN
LÖSUNGSMITTEL SOLVENT KBr
KURVE NR CURVE NO
KONZENTRATION CONC 1mg/ 300mg KBr
SCHICHTDICKE CELL PATH
VERGLEICH REFERENCE
GESCHWINDIGKEIT SCAN SPEED slow
SPALT SLIT N
BEARBEITER OPERATOR
DATUM DATE
BEMERKUNGEN REMARKS
NO.
Blumberg & Co. 4032 Lintorf W.-Germany Hoffmann Bergschenhoek Holland
for Nr. 337-1204

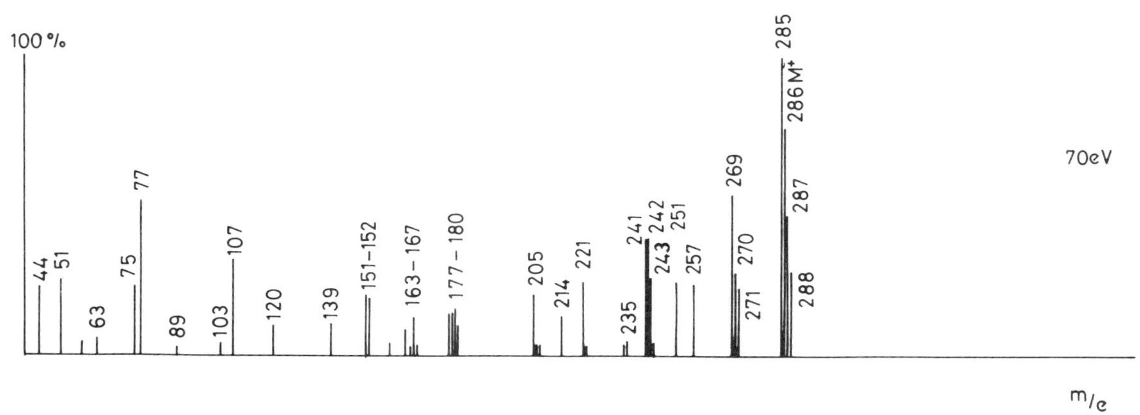
100 %
44
51
63
75
77
89
103
107
120
139
151-152
163-167
177-180
205
214
221
235
241
242
243
251
257
269
270
271
285
286 M⁺
287
288
70eV
m/e

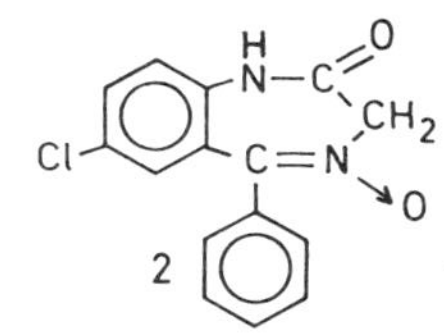

2

Demoxepam

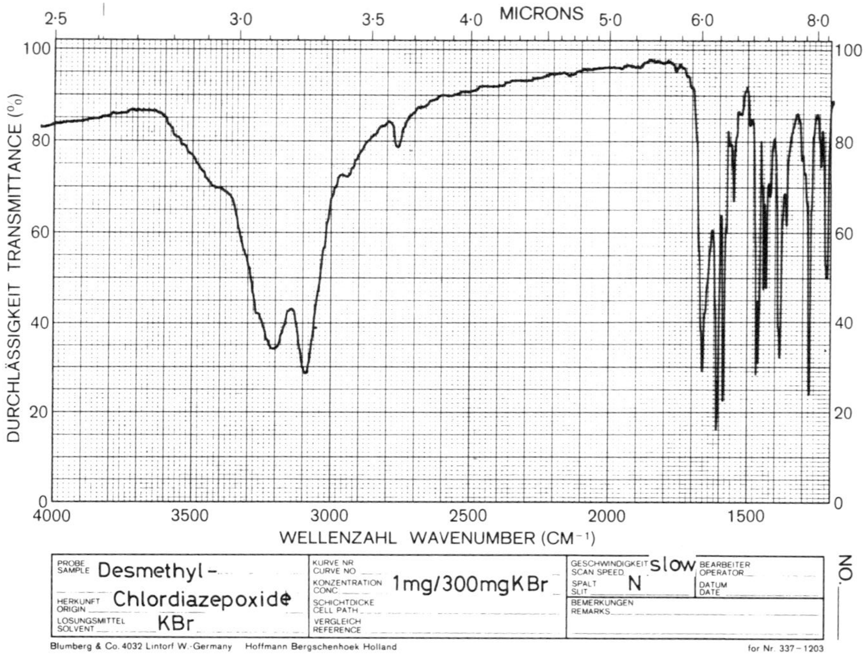

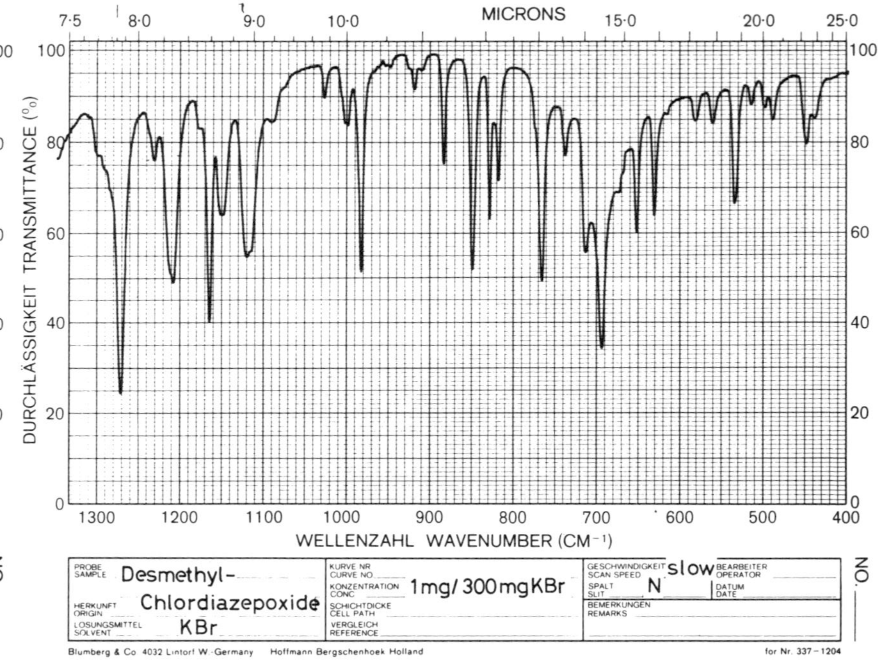

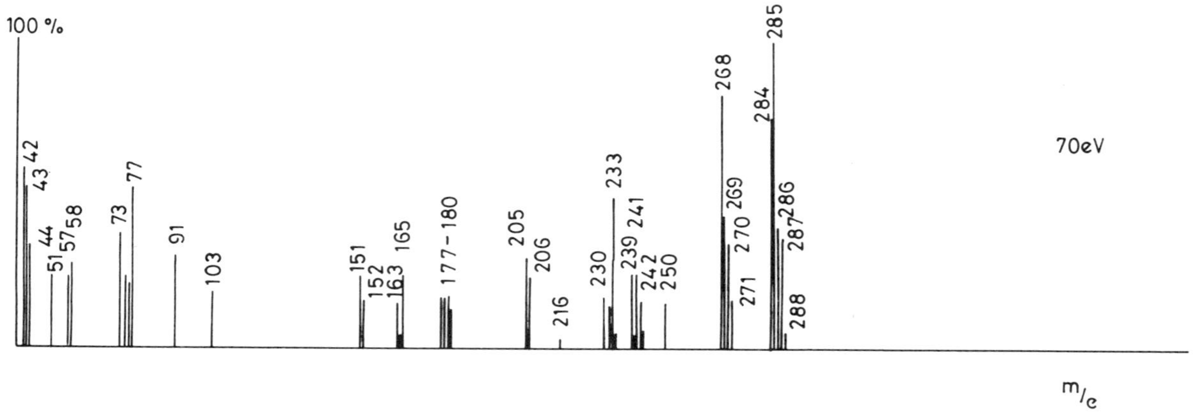

70eV

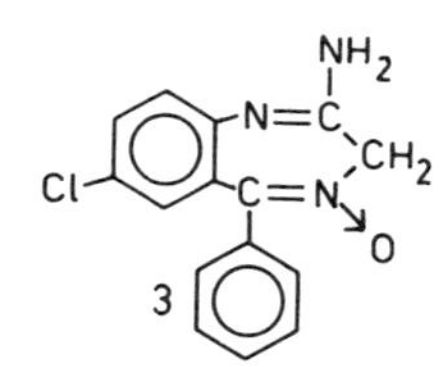

Desmethyl-Chlordiazepoxide

Base

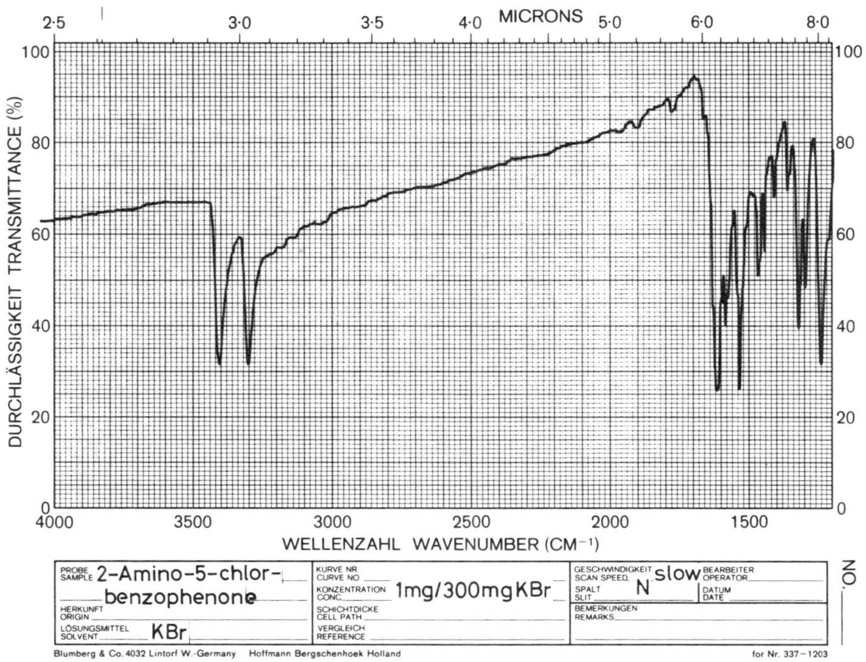

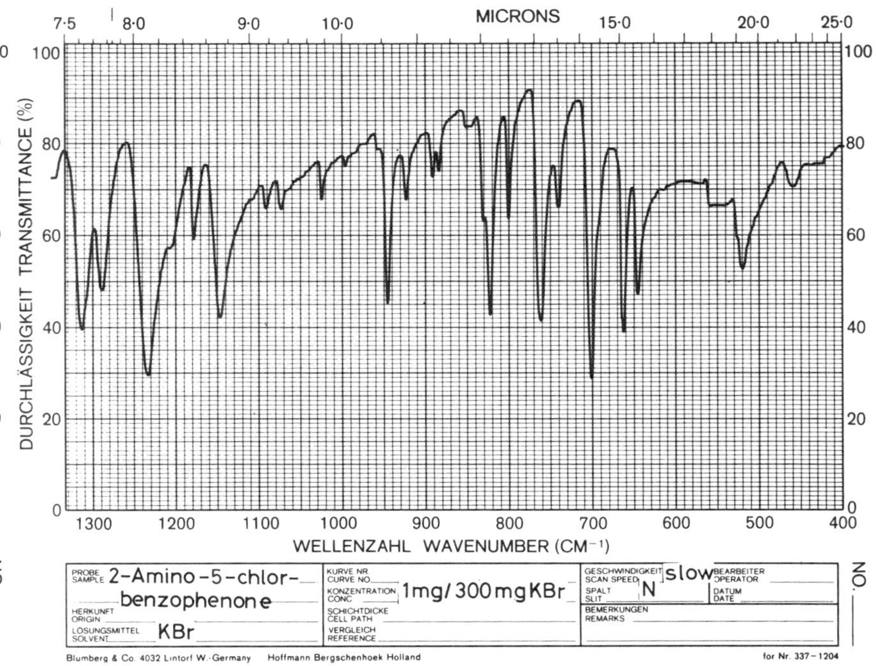

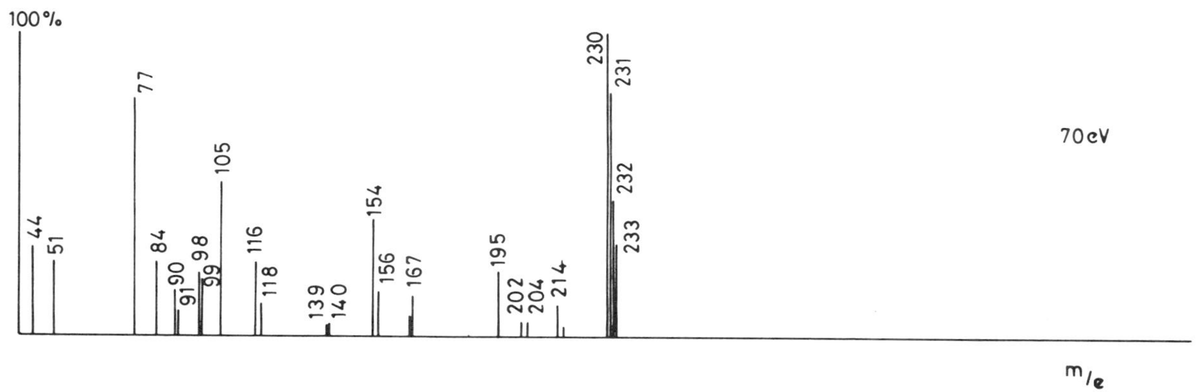

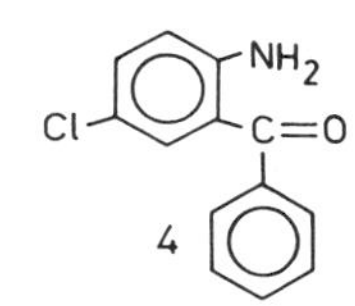

2-Amino-5-chlor-benzophenone

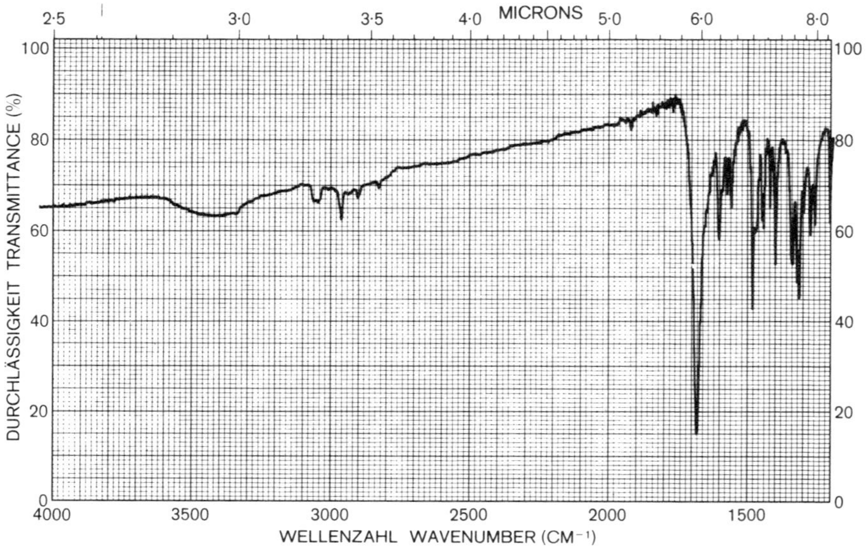

PROBE SAMPLE Diazepam | KURVE NR CURVE NO | GESCHWINDIGKEIT SCAN SPEED slow | BEARBEITER OPERATOR | NO.
HERKUNFT ORIGIN | KONZENTRATION CONC. 1mg/300mgKBr | SPALT SLIT N | DATUM DATE
LÖSUNGSMITTEL SOLVENT KBr | SCHICHTDICKE CELL PATH | VERGLEICH REFERENCE | BEMERKUNGEN REMARKS

Blumberg & Co. 4032 Lintorf W.-Germany Hoffmann Bergschenhoek Holland for Nr. 337-1203

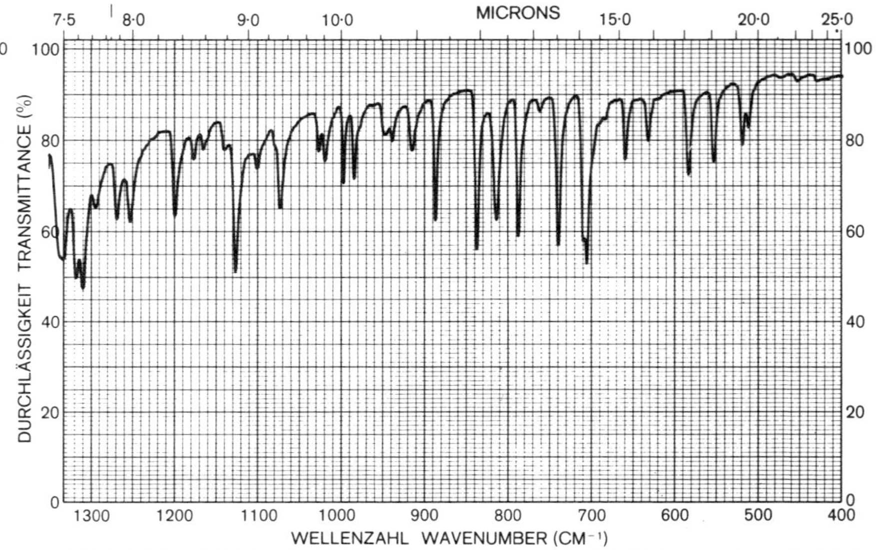

PROBE SAMPLE Diazepam | KURVE NR CURVE NO | GESCHWINDIGKEIT SCAN SPEED slow | BEARBEITER OPERATOR | NO.
HERKUNFT ORIGIN | KONZENTRATION CONC. 1mg / 300mg KBr | SPALT SLIT N | DATUM DATE
LÖSUNGSMITTEL SOLVENT KBr | SCHICHTDICKE CELL PATH | VERGLEICH REFERENCE | BEMERKUNGEN REMARKS

Blumberg & Co. 4032 Lintorf W.-Germany Hoffmann Bergschenhoek Holland for Nr. 337-1204

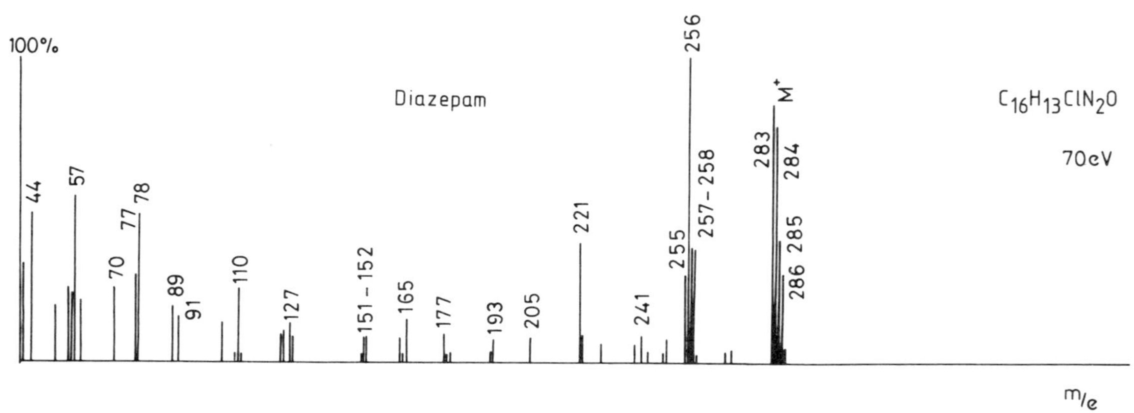

$C_{16}H_{13}ClN_2O$

70eV

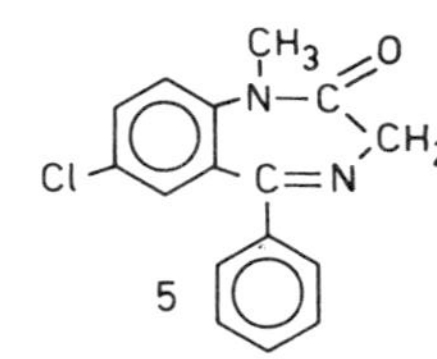

5

Diazepam

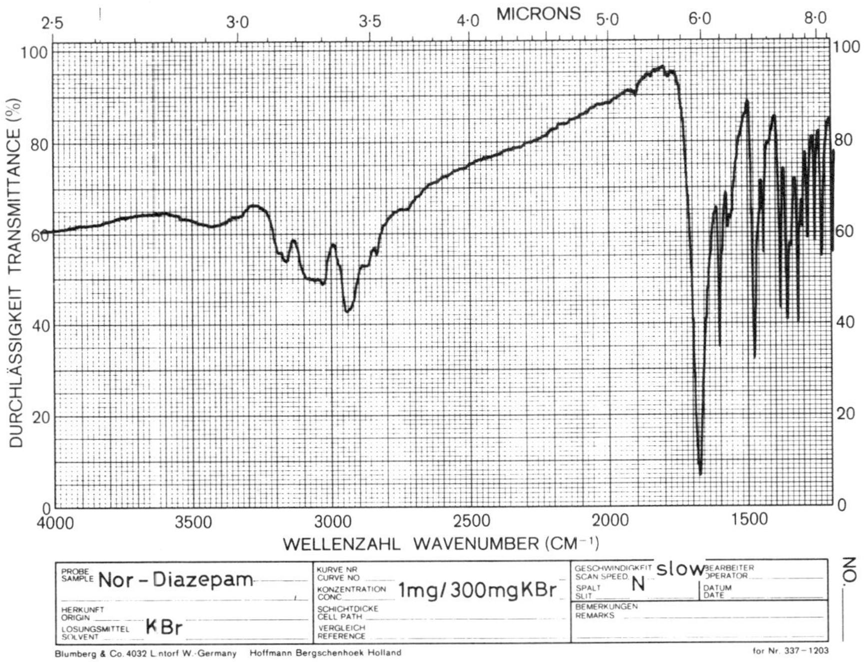

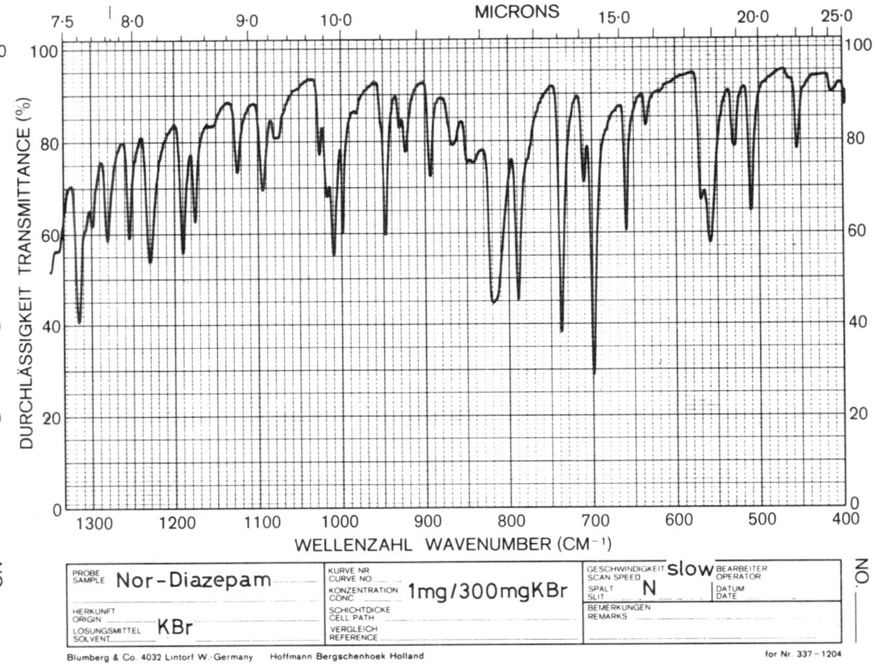

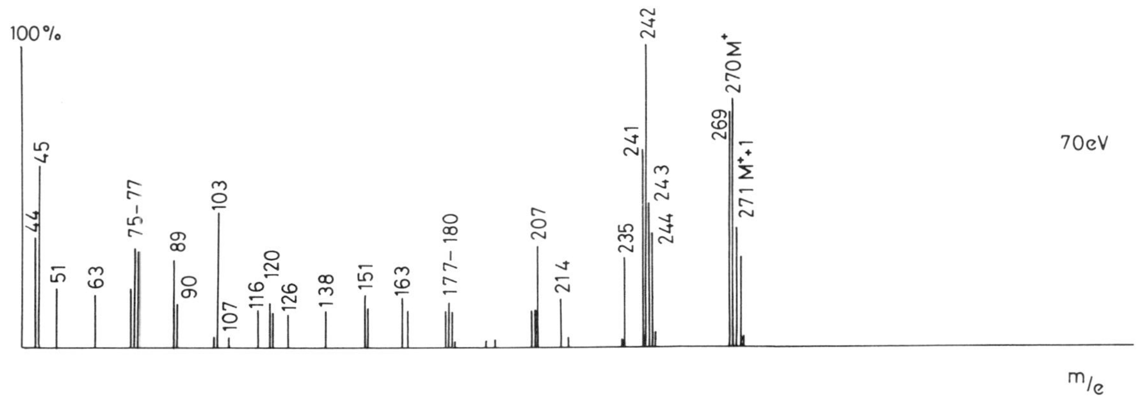

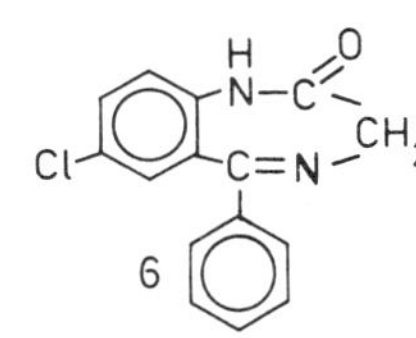

Nor-Diazepam

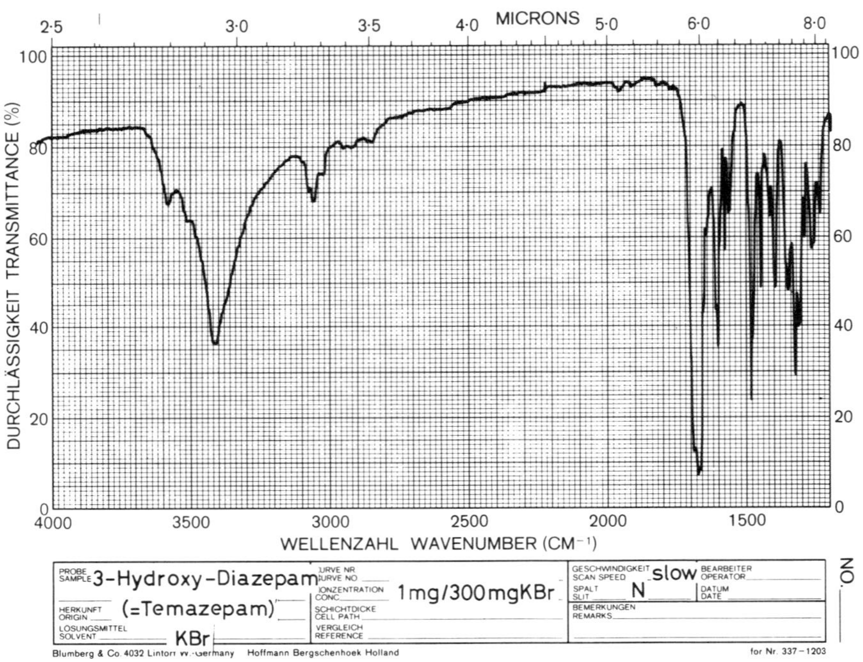

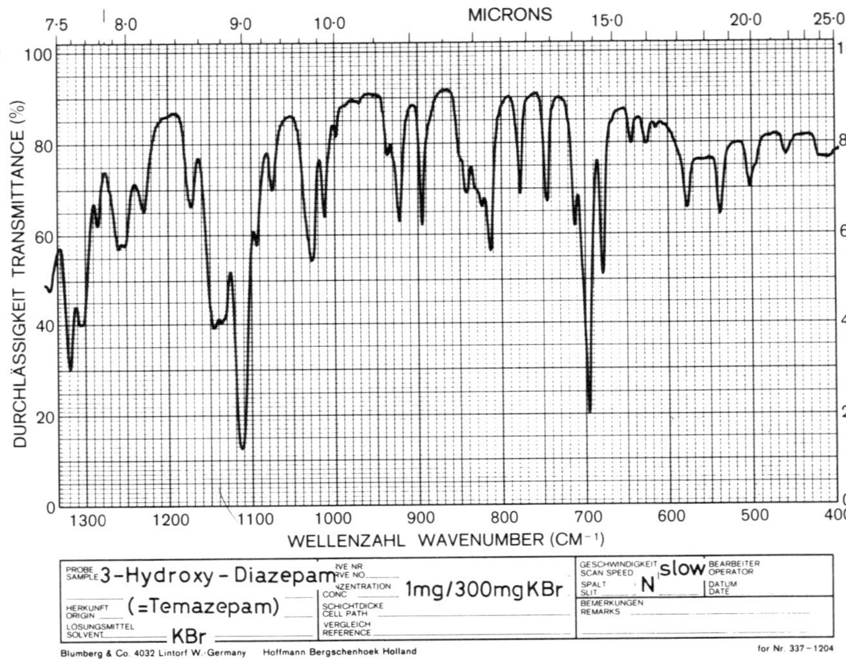

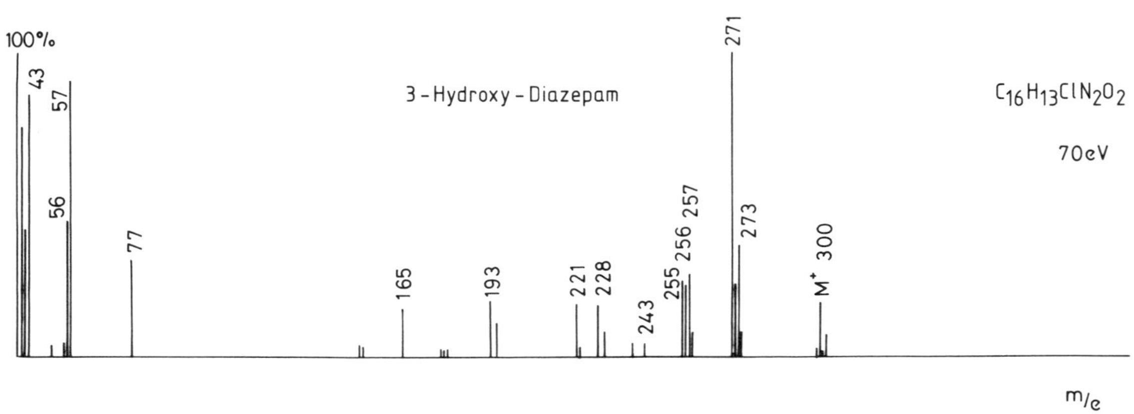

3-Hydroxy-Diazepam

$C_{16}H_{13}ClN_2O_2$

70eV

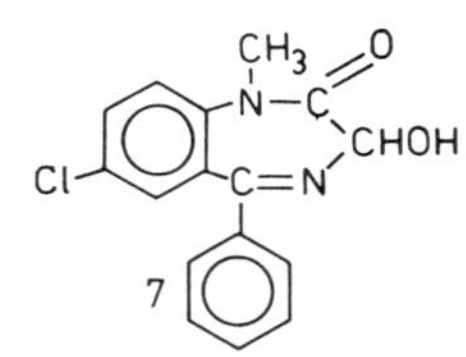

3-Hydroxy-Diazepam

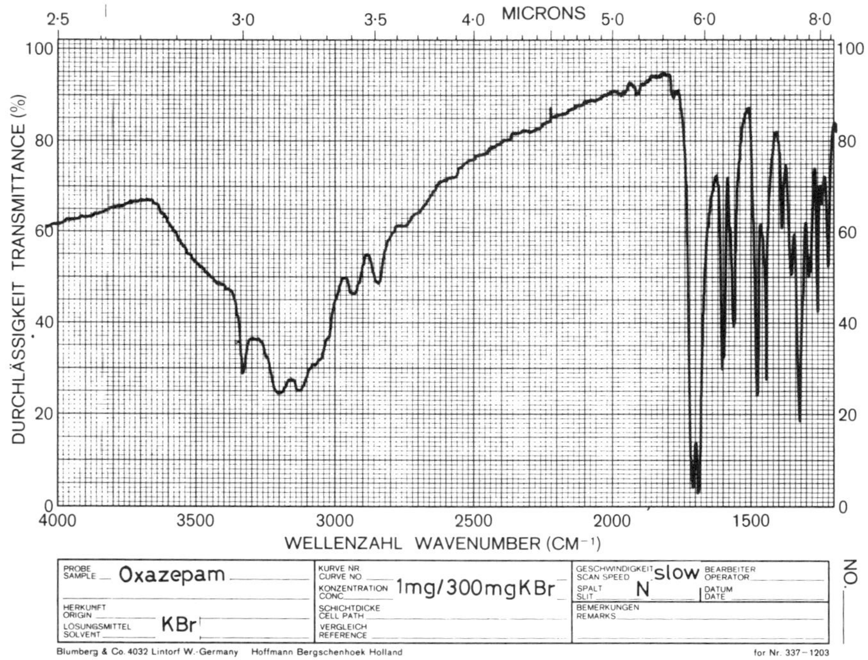
MICRONS
DURCHLÄSSIGKEIT TRANSMITTANCE (%)
WELLENZAHL WAVENUMBER (CM⁻¹)
PROBE SAMPLE Oxazepam
KURVE NR CURVE NO
KONZENTRATION CONC. 1mg/300mgKBr
GESCHWINDIGKEIT SCAN SPEED slow
BEARBEITER OPERATOR
SPALT SLIT N
DATUM DATE
HERKUNFT ORIGIN
LÖSUNGSMITTEL SOLVENT KBr
SCHICHTDICKE CELL PATH
VERGLEICH REFERENCE
BEMERKUNGEN REMARKS
NO.
Blumberg & Co. 4032 Lintorf W.-Germany Hoffmann Bergschenhoek Holland
for Nr. 337-1203

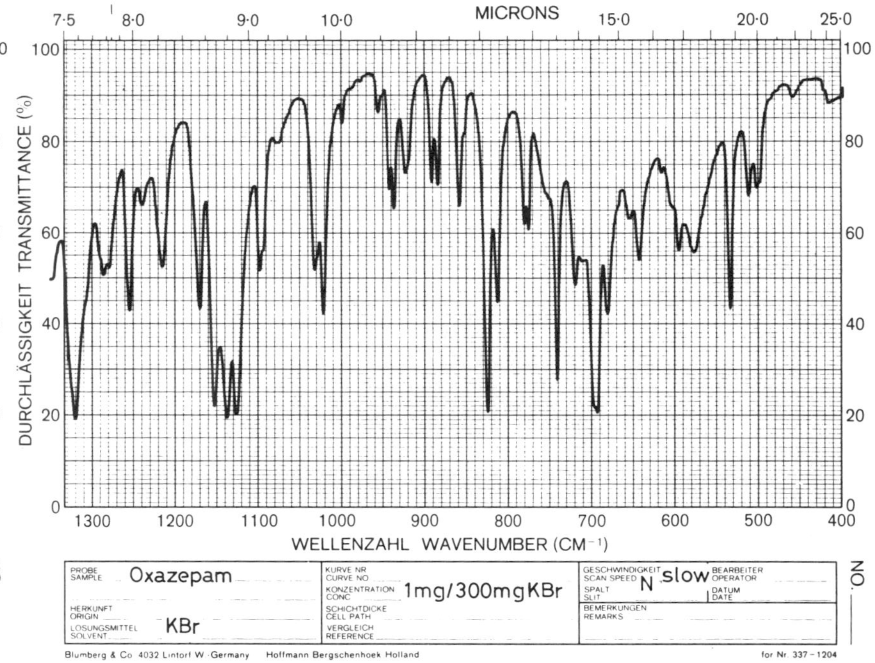
MICRONS
DURCHLÄSSIGKEIT TRANSMITTANCE (%)
WELLENZAHL WAVENUMBER (CM⁻¹)
PROBE SAMPLE Oxazepam
KURVE NR CURVE NO
KONZENTRATION CONC. 1mg/300mgKBr
GESCHWINDIGKEIT SCAN SPEED N slow
BEARBEITER OPERATOR
SPALT SLIT
DATUM DATE
HERKUNFT ORIGIN
LÖSUNGSMITTEL SOLVENT KBr
SCHICHTDICKE CELL PATH
VERGLEICH REFERENCE
BEMERKUNGEN REMARKS
NO.
Blumberg & Co. 4032 Lintorf W.-Germany Hoffmann Bergschenhoek Holland
for Nr. 337-1204

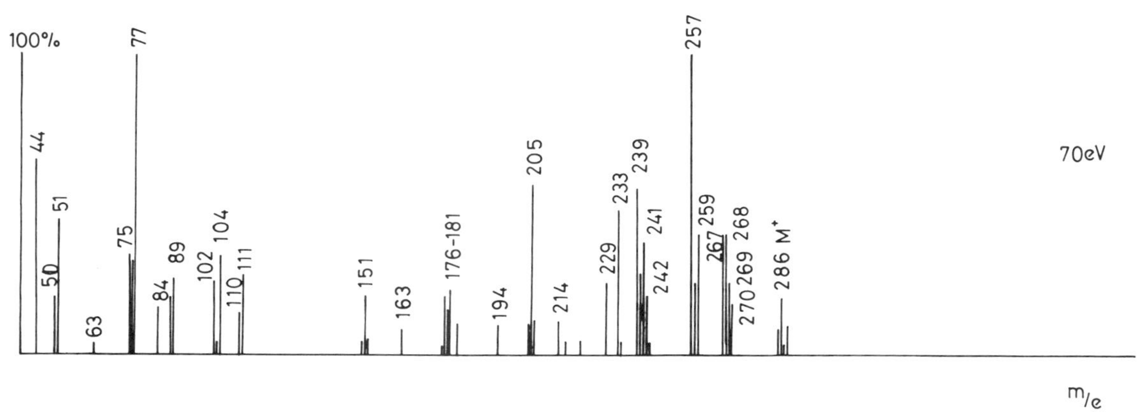
100%
44
50
51
63
75
77
84
89
102
104
110
111
151
163
176-181
194
205
214
229
233
239
241
242
257
259
267
268
269
270
286 M⁺
70eV
m/e

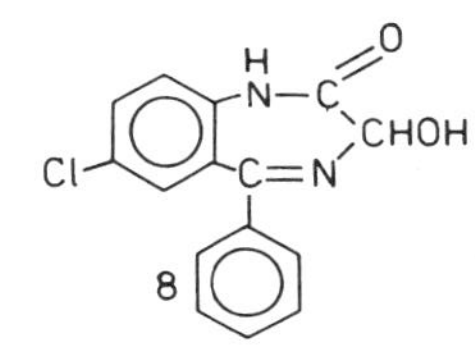
H
O
N
C
CHOH
Cl
C=N

8

Oxazepam

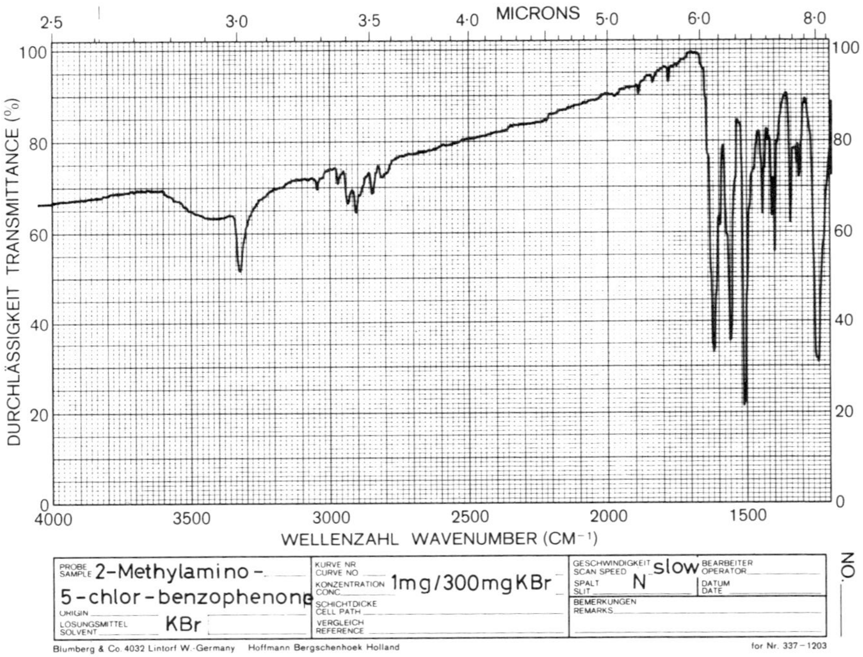

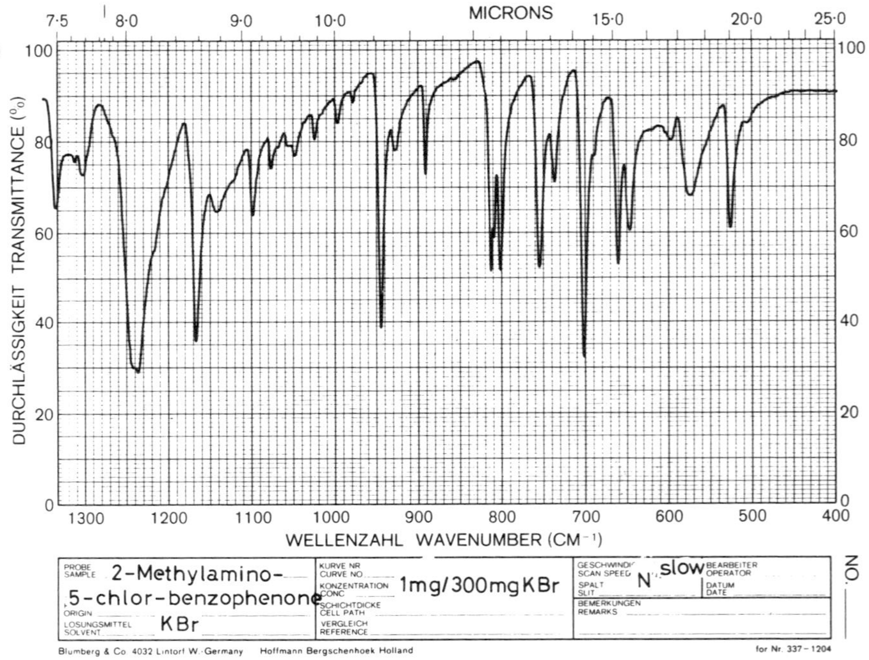

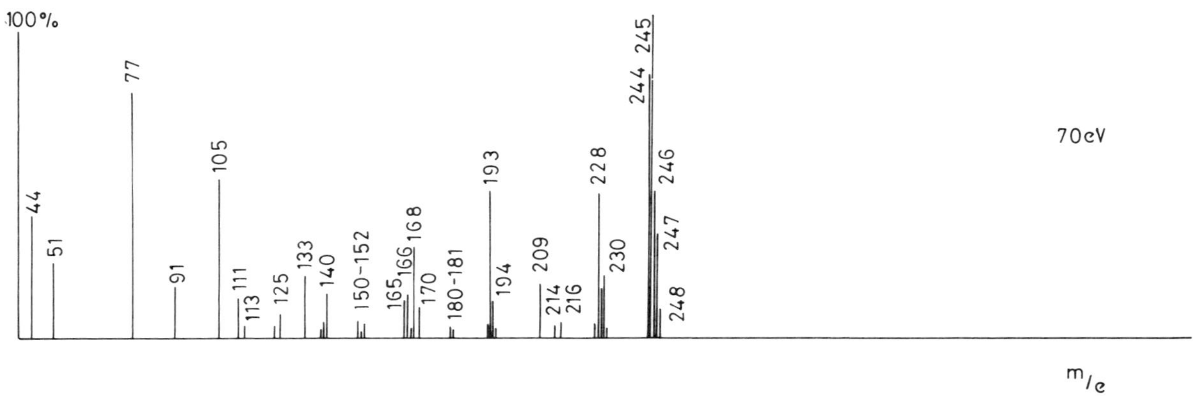

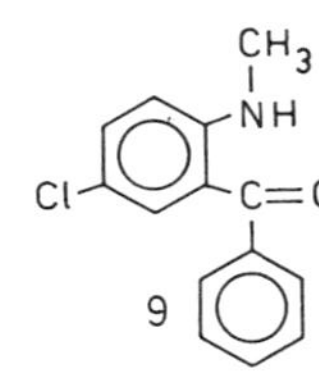

9

2-Methylamino-5-chlor-benzophenone

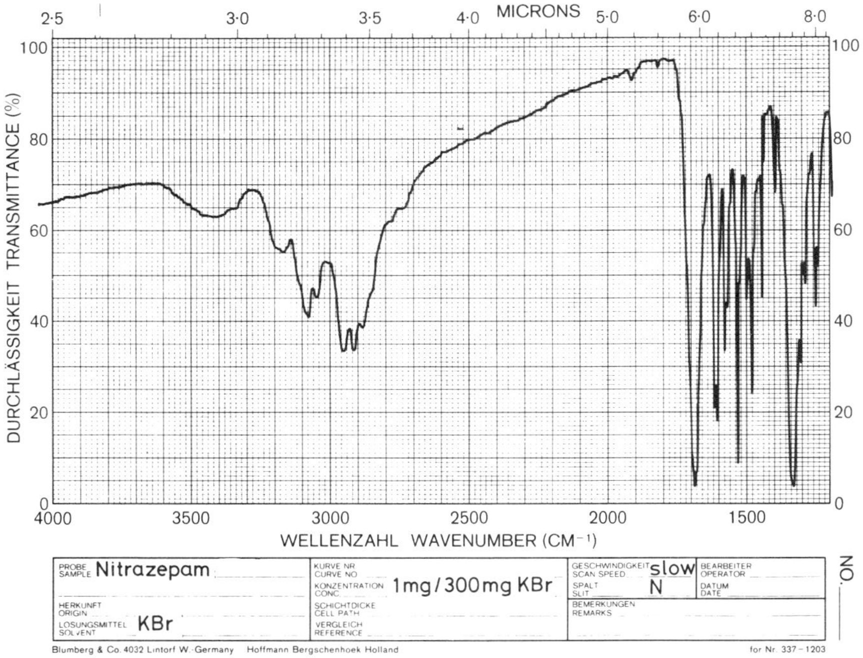

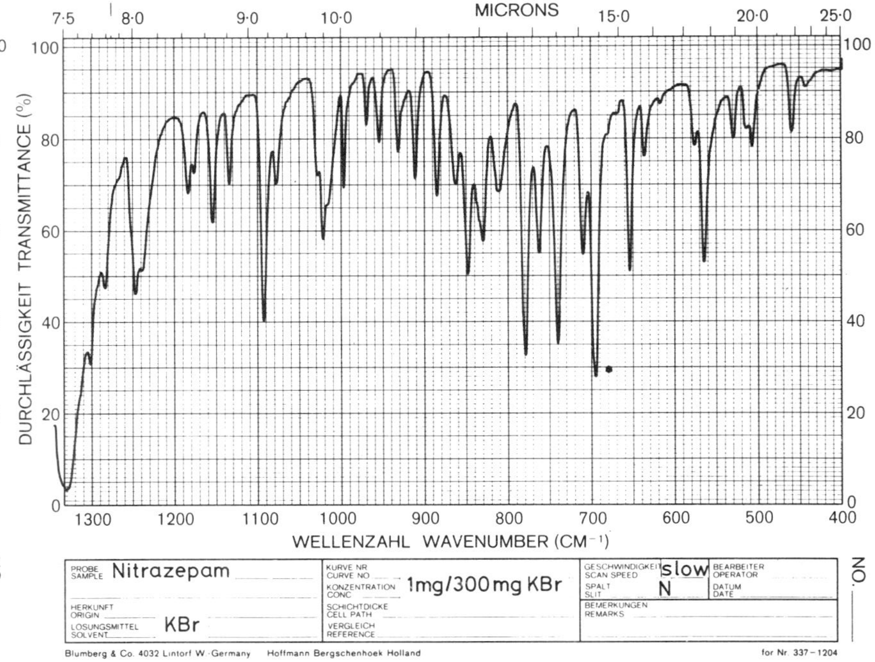

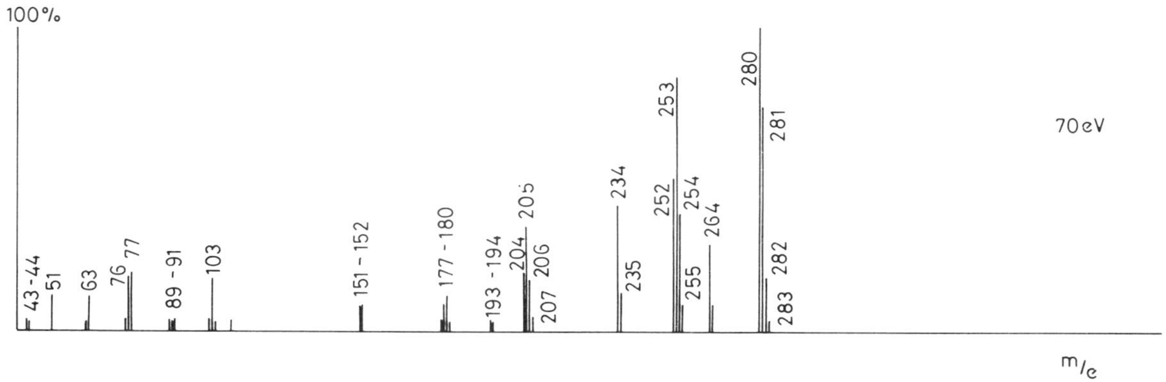

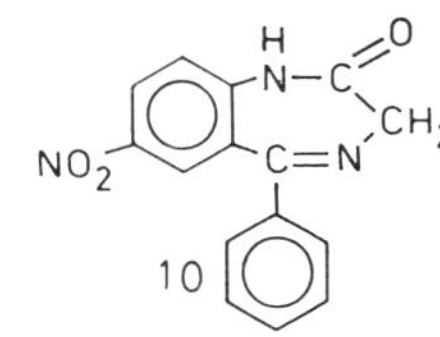

10

Nitrazepam

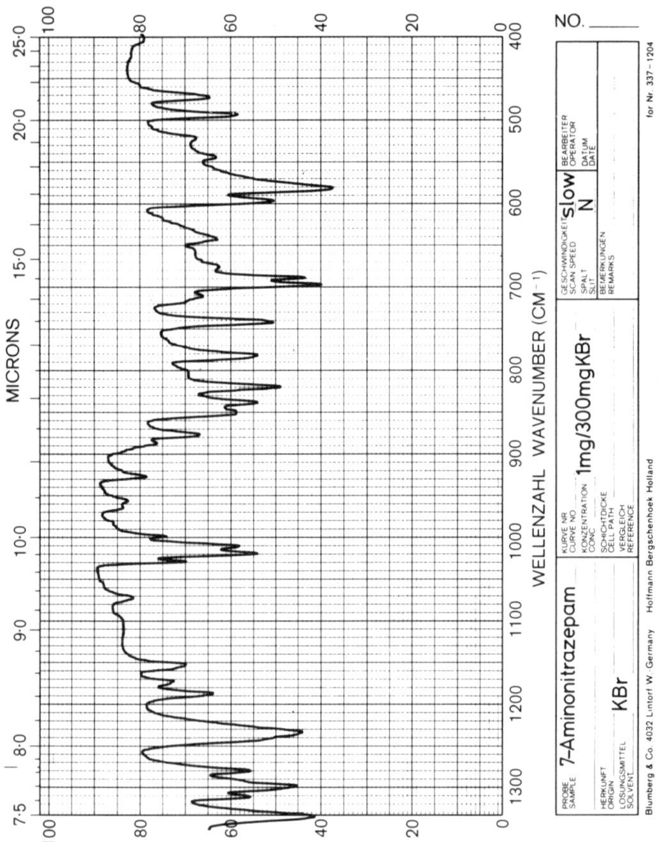

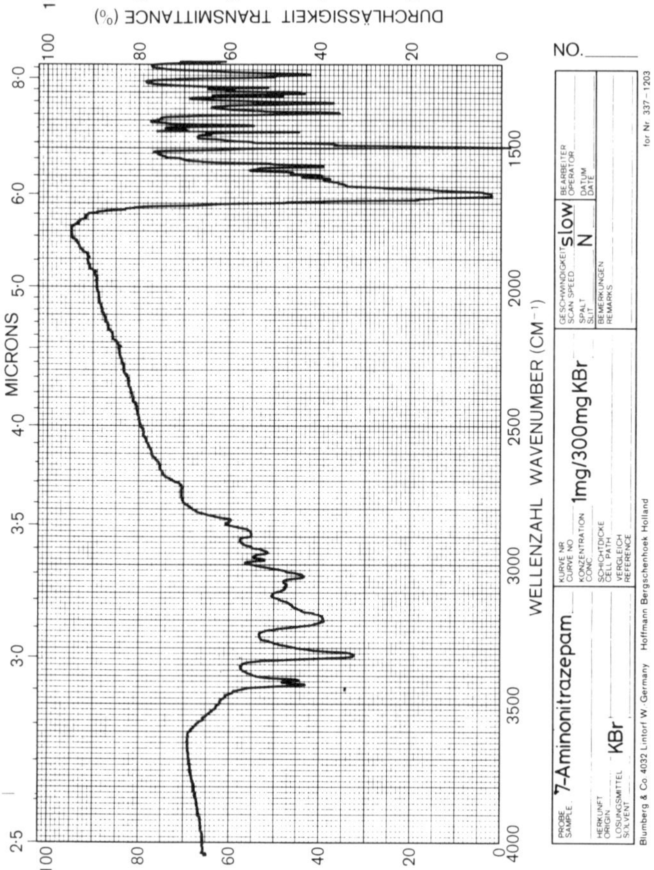

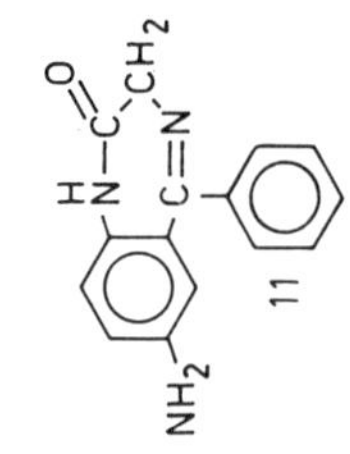

11

7-Amino-Nitrazepam

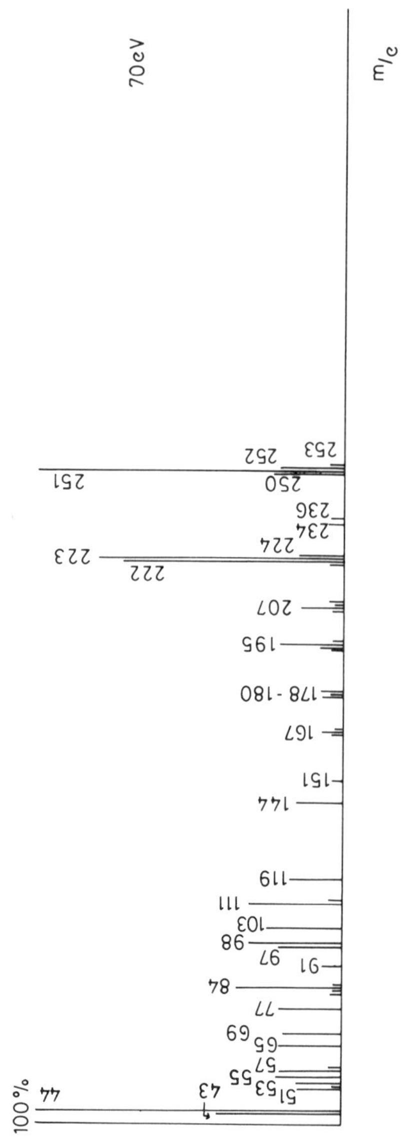

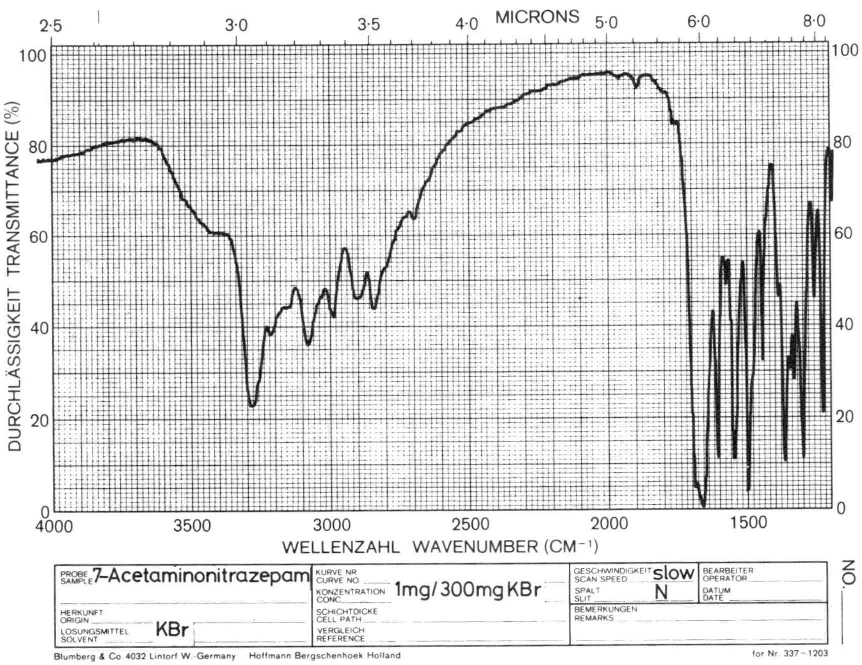

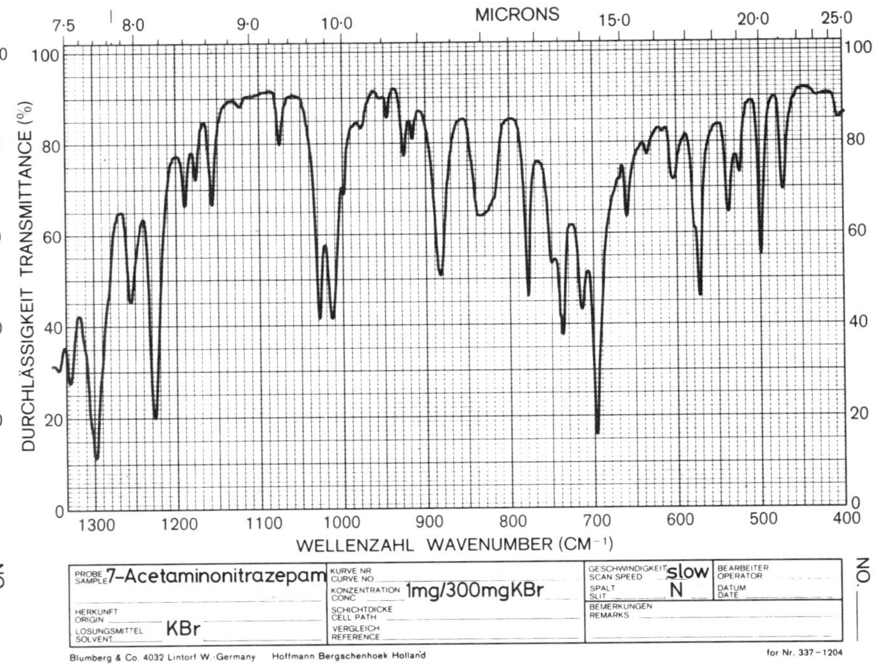

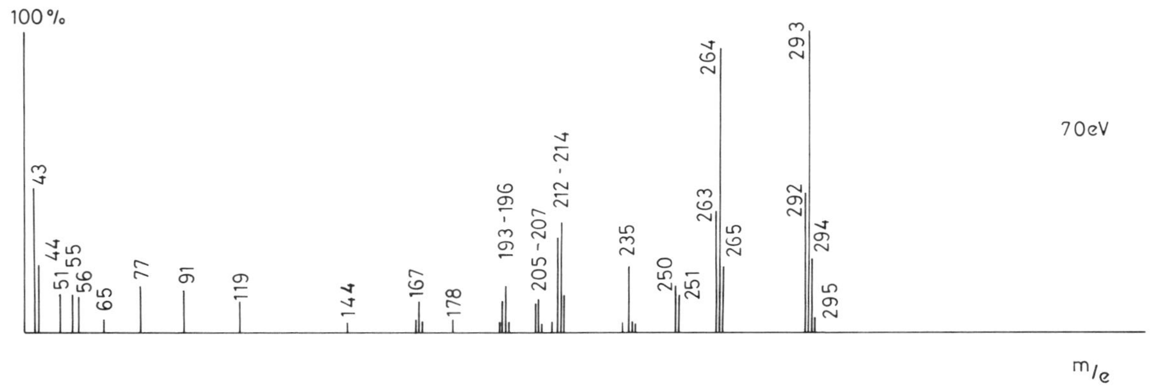

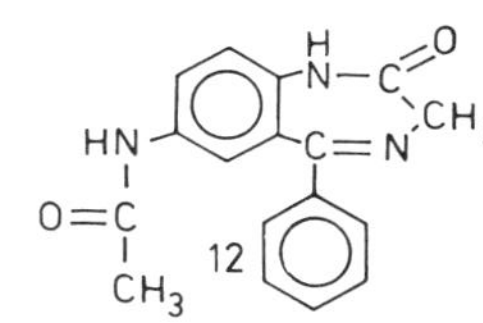

7-Acetamido-Nitrazepam

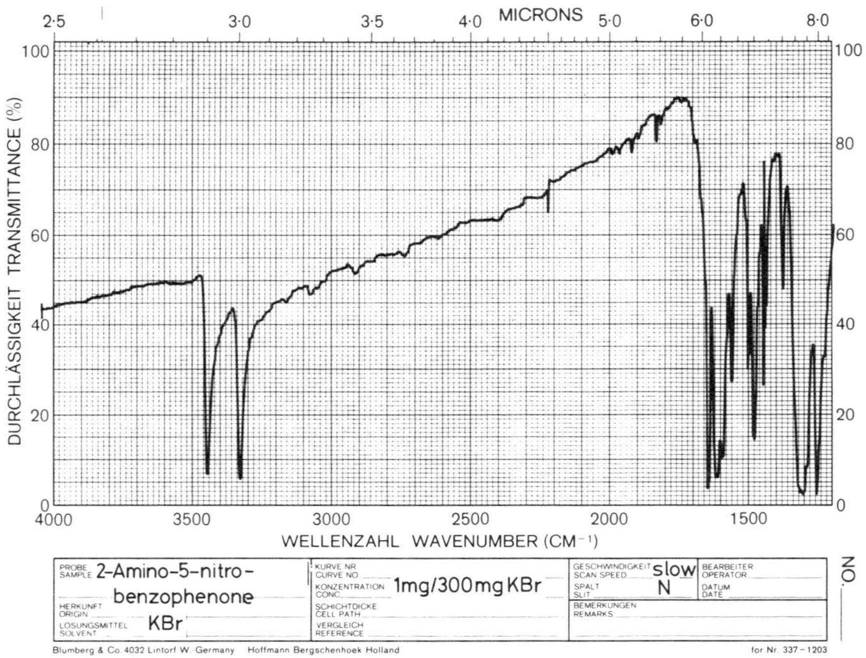

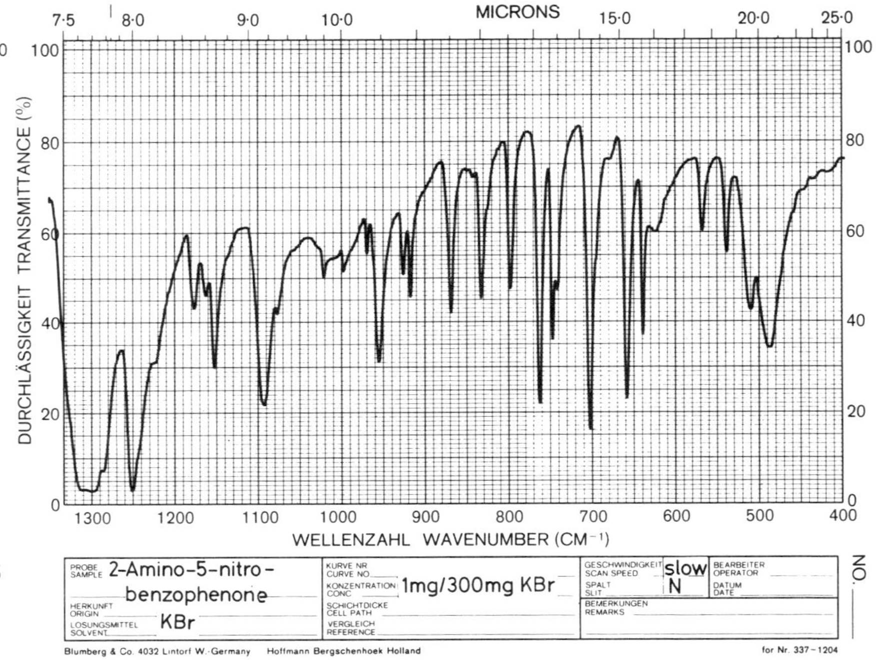

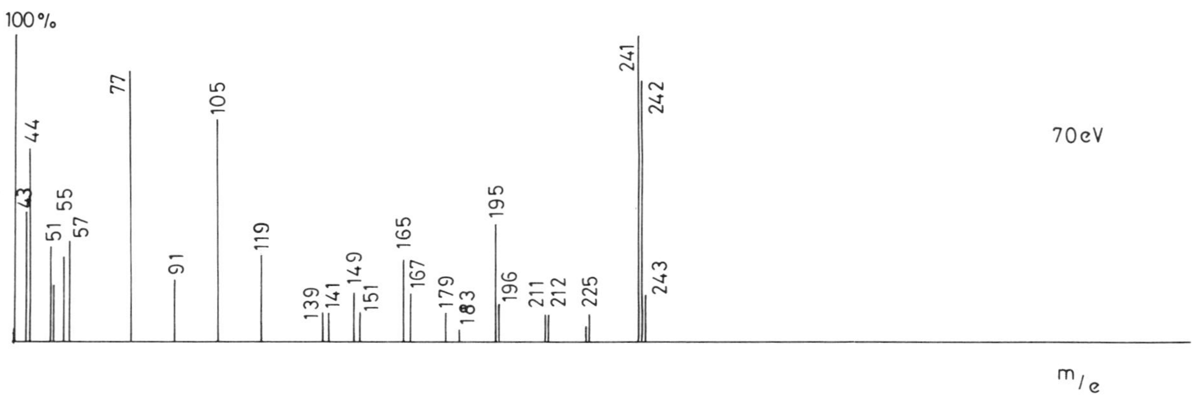

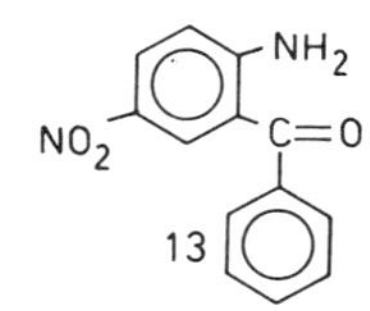

13

2-Amino-5-nitro-benzophenone

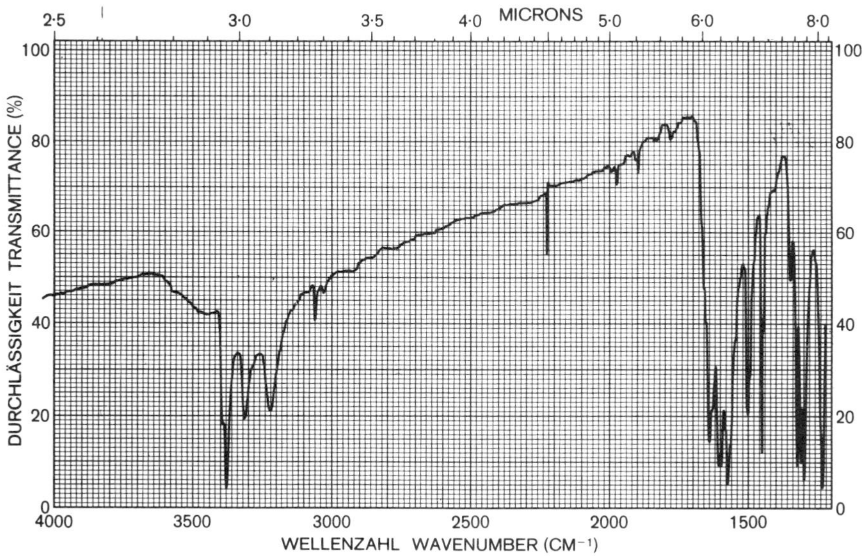

PROBE SAMPLE 2,5-Diamino-benzophenone
HERKUNFT ORIGIN
LÖSUNGSMITTEL SOLVENT KBr
KURVE NR CURVE NO
KONZENTRATION CONC 1mg/300mgKBr
SCHICHTDICKE CELL PATH
VERGLEICH REFERENCE
GESCHWINDIGKEIT SCAN SPEED slow
SPALT SLIT N
BEARBEITER OPERATOR
DATUM DATE
BEMERKUNGEN REMARKS
NO.

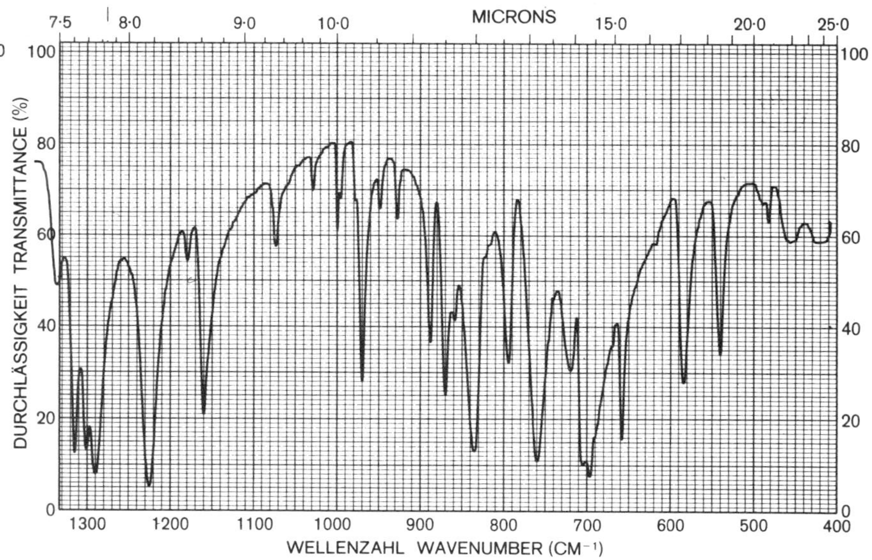

PROBE SAMPLE 2,5-Diamino-benzophenone
HERKUNFT ORIGIN
LÖSUNGSMITTEL SOLVENT KBr
KURVE NR CURVE NO
KONZENTRATION CONC 1mg/300mgKBr
SCHICHTDICKE CELL PATH
VERGLEICH REFERENCE
GESCHWINDIGKEIT SCAN SPEED slow
SPALT SLIT N
BEARBEITER OPERATOR
DATUM DATE
BEMERKUNGEN REMARKS
NO.

Blumberg & Co 4032 Lintorf W.-Germany Hoffmann Bergschenhoek Holland for Nr 337-1204

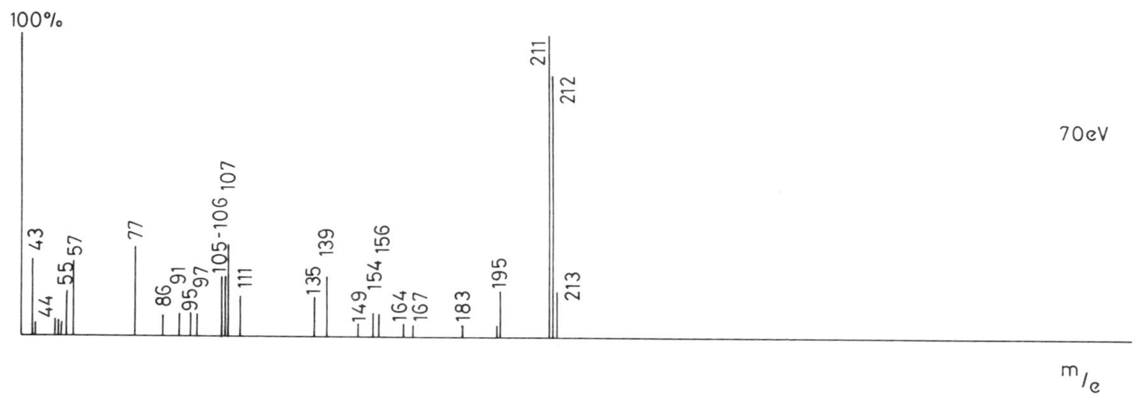

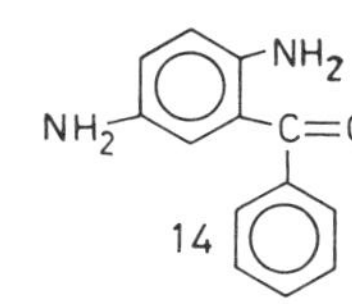

14

2,5-Diamino-benzophenone

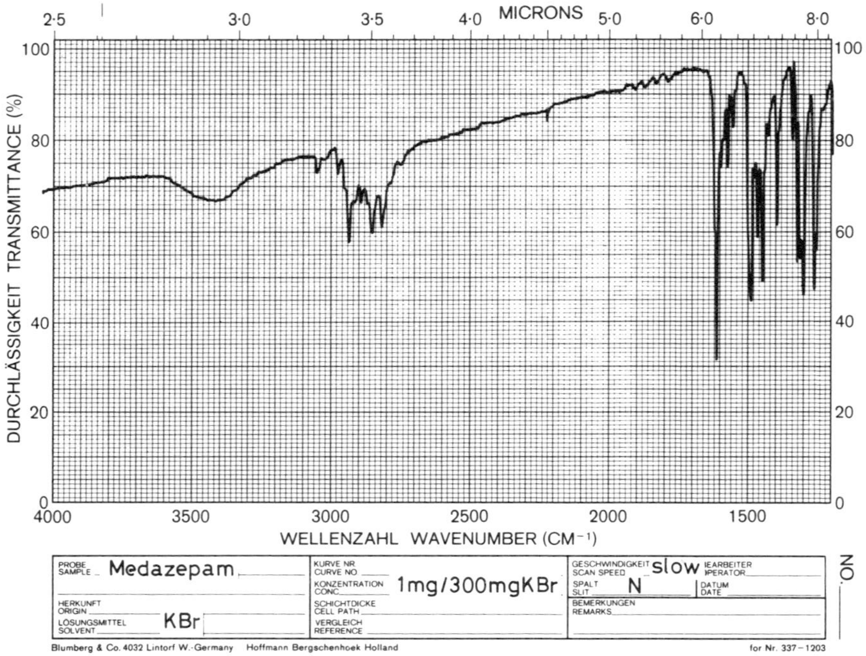

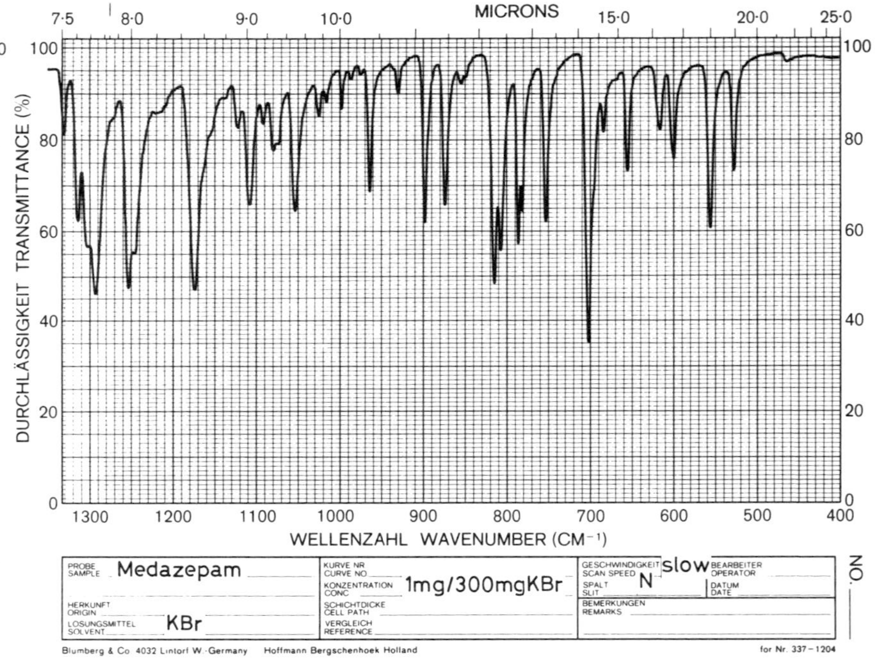

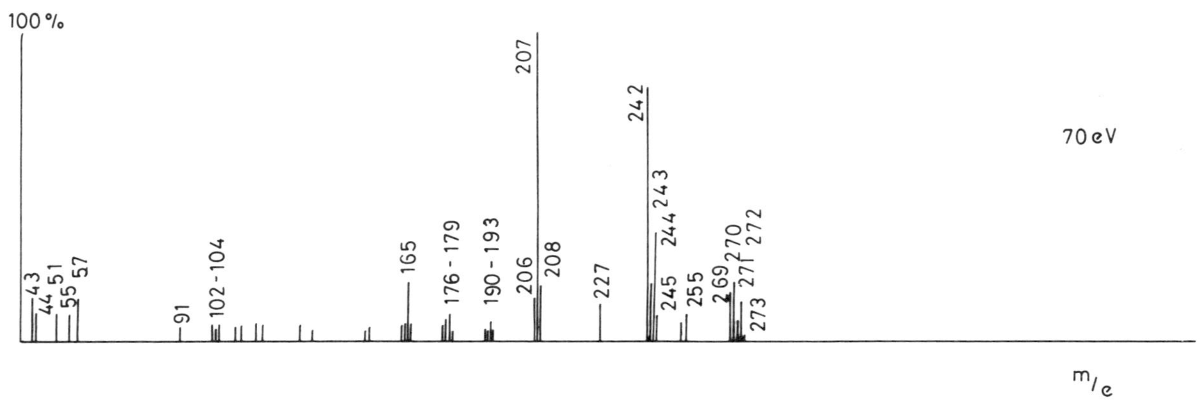

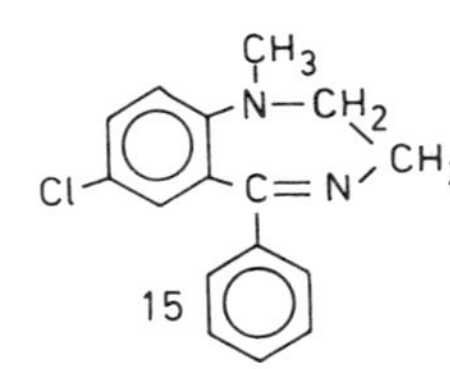

15

Medazepam-Base

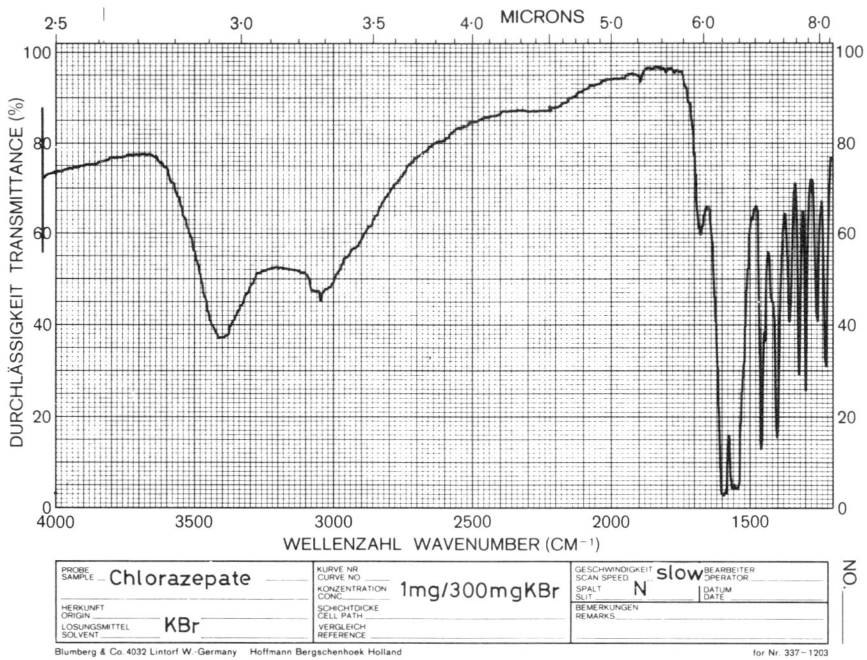

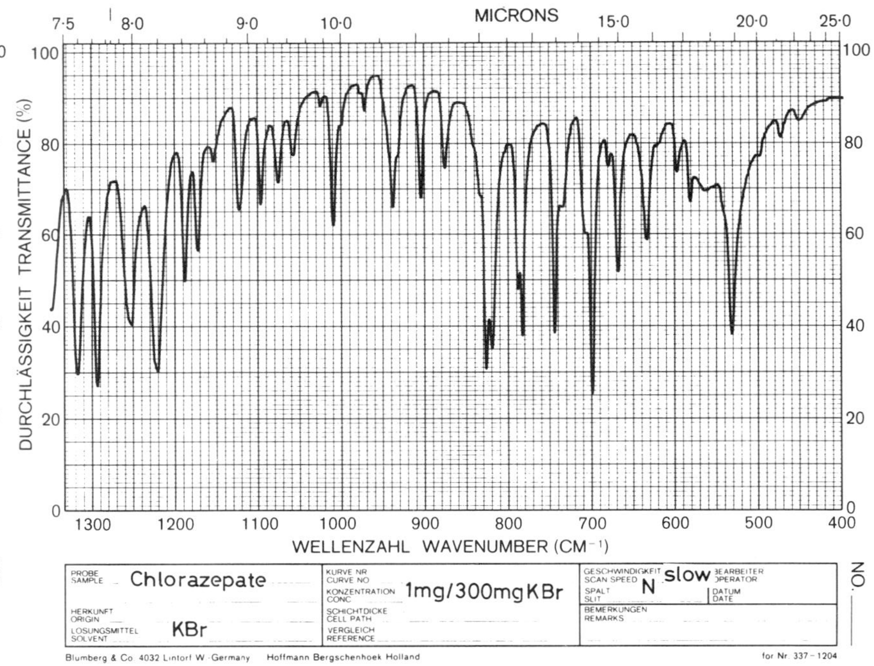

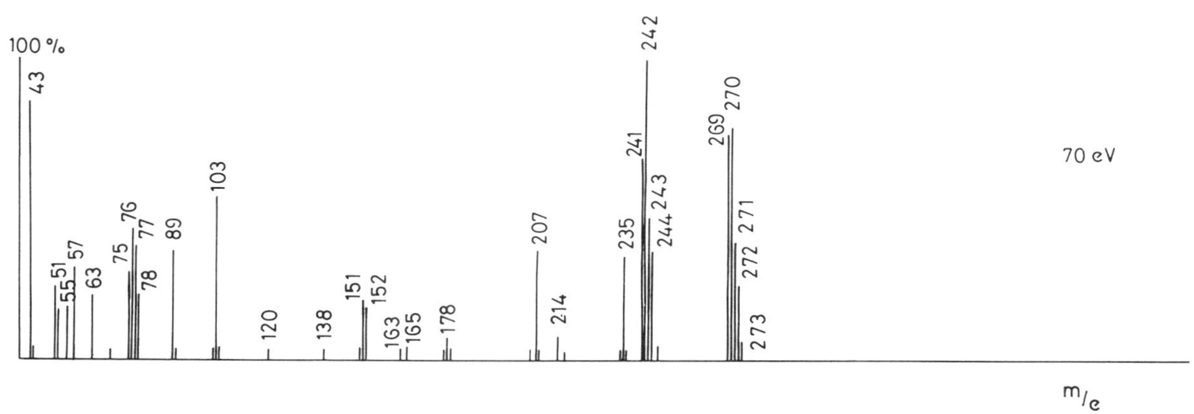

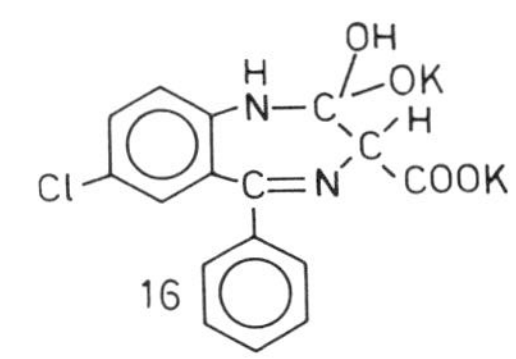

16

Chlorazepate

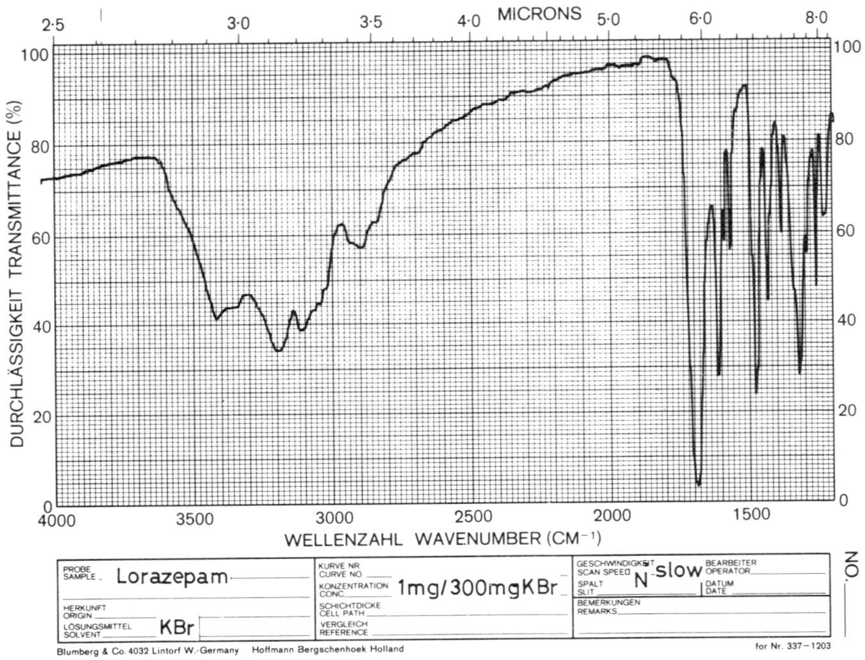
MICRONS
2·5
3·0
3·5
4·0
5·0
6·0
8·0
100
80
60
40
20
0
4000
3500
3000
2500
2000
1500
DURCHLÄSSIGKEIT TRANSMITTANCE (%)
WELLENZAHL WAVENUMBER (CM⁻¹)
PROBE SAMPLE Lorazepam
HERKUNFT ORIGIN
LÖSUNGSMITTEL SOLVENT KBr
KURVE NR CURVE NO
KONZENTRATION CONC. 1mg/300mgKBr
SCHICHTDICKE CELL PATH
VERGLEICH REFERENCE
GESCHWINDIGKEIT SCAN SPEED N-slow
SPALT SLIT
BEARBEITER OPERATOR
DATUM DATE
BEMERKUNGEN REMARKS
NO.
Blumberg & Co. 4032 Lintorf W.-Germany Hoffmann Bergschenhoek Holland
for Nr. 337-1203

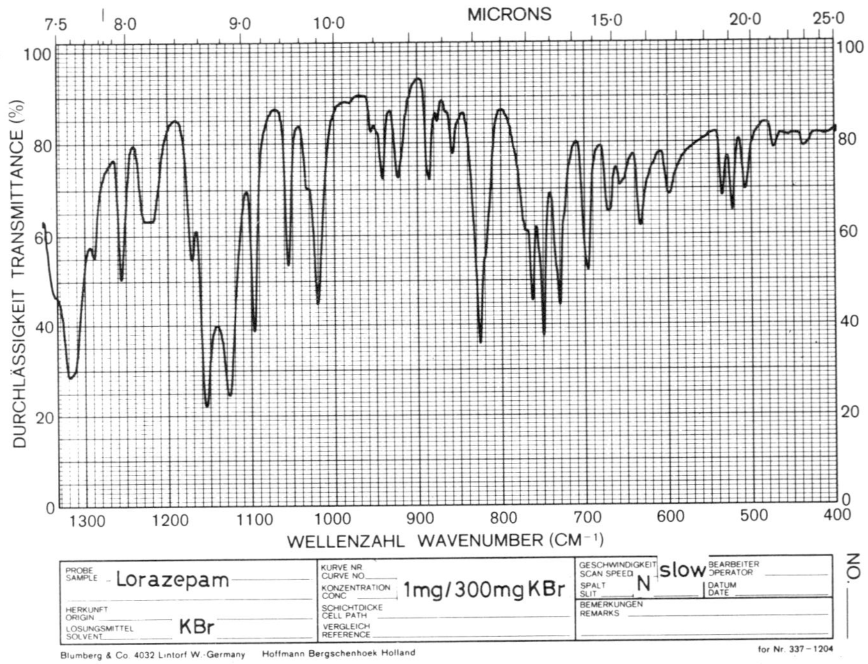
MICRONS
7·5
8·0
9·0
10·0
15·0
20·0
25·0
100
80
60
40
20
0
1300
1200
1100
1000
900
800
700
600
500
400
DURCHLÄSSIGKEIT TRANSMITTANCE (%)
WELLENZAHL WAVENUMBER (CM⁻¹)
PROBE SAMPLE Lorazepam
HERKUNFT ORIGIN
LÖSUNGSMITTEL SOLVENT KBr
KURVE NR CURVE NO
KONZENTRATION CONC. 1mg/300mg KBr
SCHICHTDICKE CELL PATH
VERGLEICH REFERENCE
GESCHWINDIGKEIT SCAN SPEED N slow
SPALT SLIT
BEARBEITER OPERATOR
DATUM DATE
BEMERKUNGEN REMARKS
NO.
Blumberg & Co. 4032 Lintorf W.-Germany Hoffmann Bergschenhoek Holland
for Nr. 337-1204

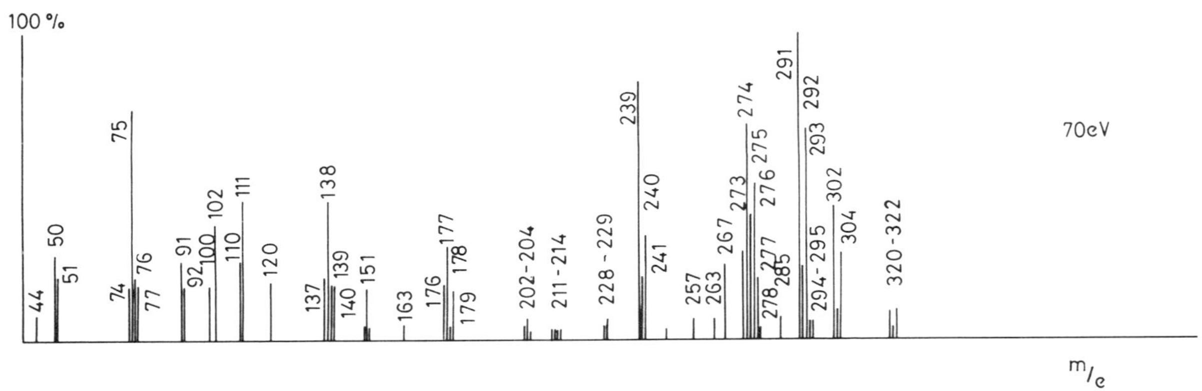
100 %
44
50
51
74
75
76
77
91
92
100
102
110
111
120
137
138
139
140
151
163
176
177
178
179
202-204
211-214
228-229
239
240
241
257
263
267
273
274
275
276
277
278
285
291
292
293
294-295
302
304
320-322
70eV
m/e

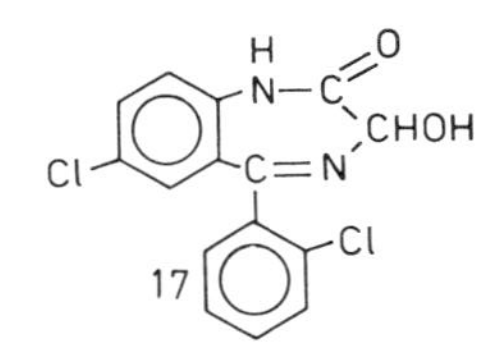
H
N
C
O
CHOH
C
N
Cl
Cl
17

Lorazepam

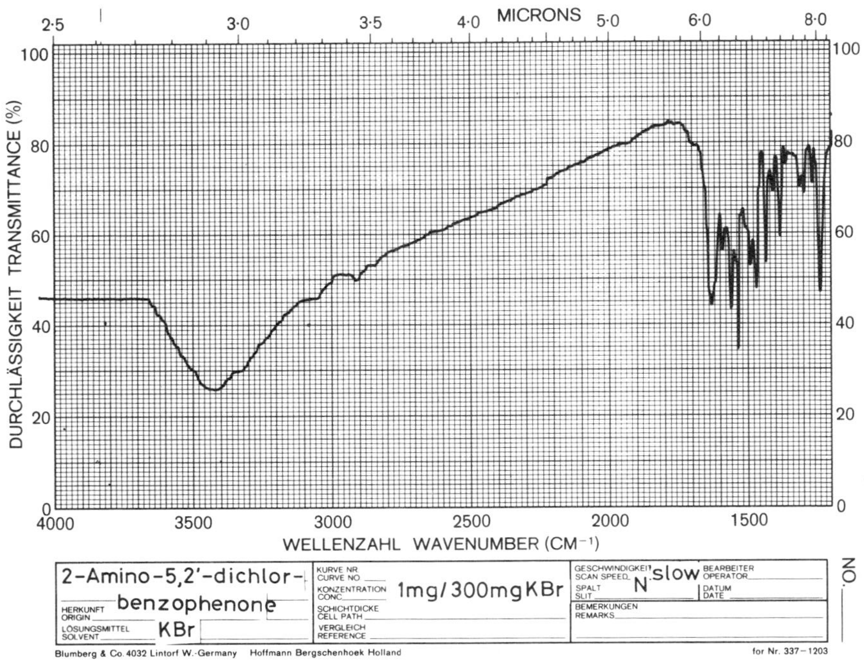

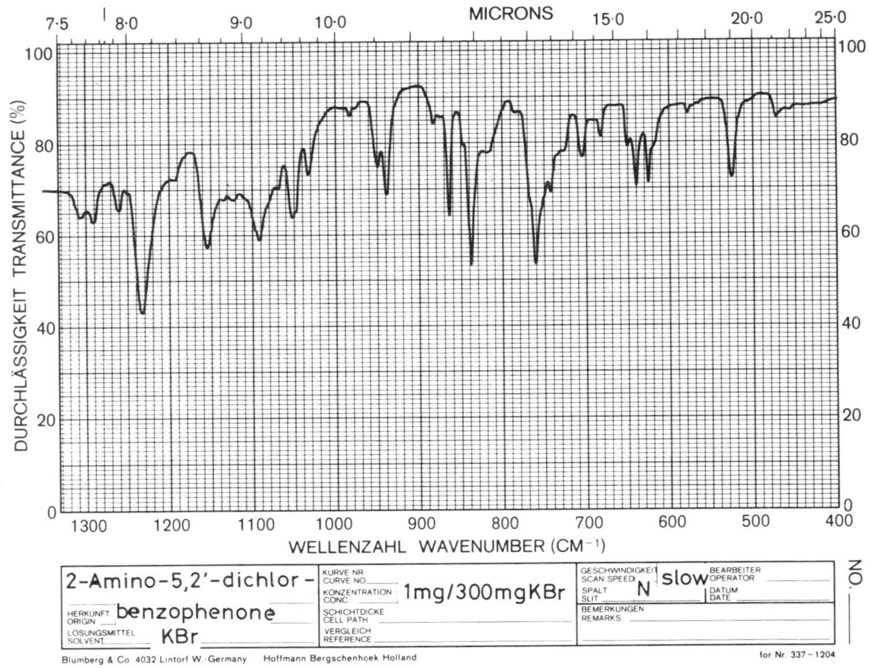

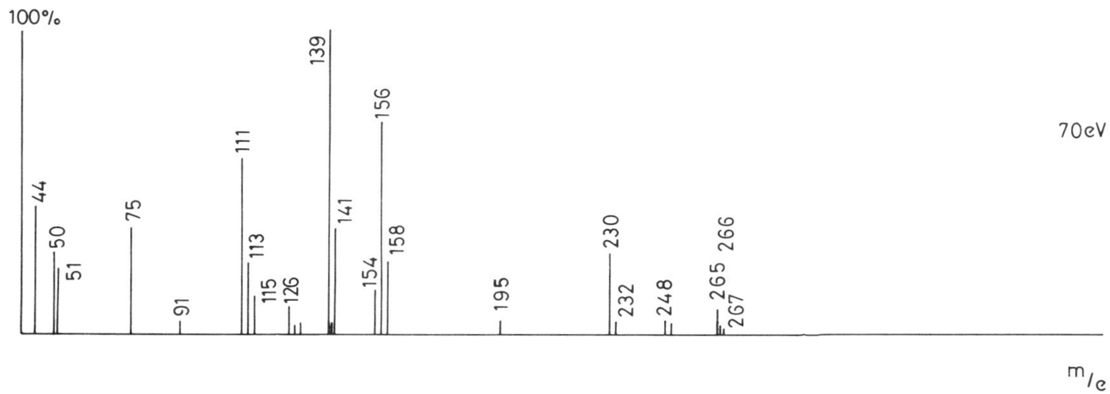

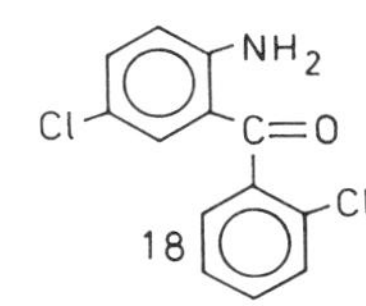

18

2-Amino-5,2'-dichlor-benzophenone

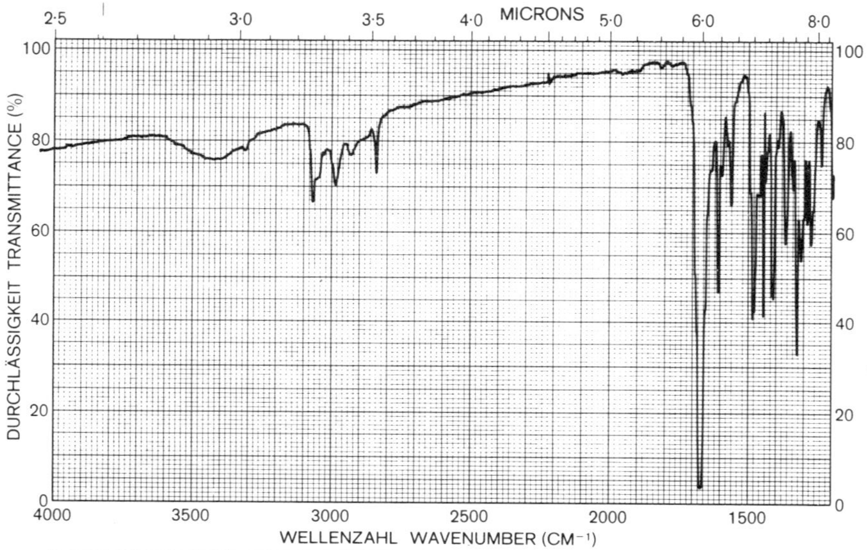

PROBE SAMPLE Prazepam
HERKUNFT ORIGIN
LÖSUNGSMITTEL SOLVENT KBr
KURVE NR CURVE NO
KONZENTRATION CONC. 1mg/300mgKBr
SCHICHTDICKE CELL PATH
VERGLEICH REFERENCE
GESCHWINDIGKEIT SCAN SPEED slow
BEARBEITER OPERATOR
SPALT SLIT N
DATUM DATE
BEMERKUNGEN REMARKS
NO.

Blumberg & Co. 4032 Lintorf W.-Germany Hoffmann Bergschenhoek Holland for Nr. 337-1203

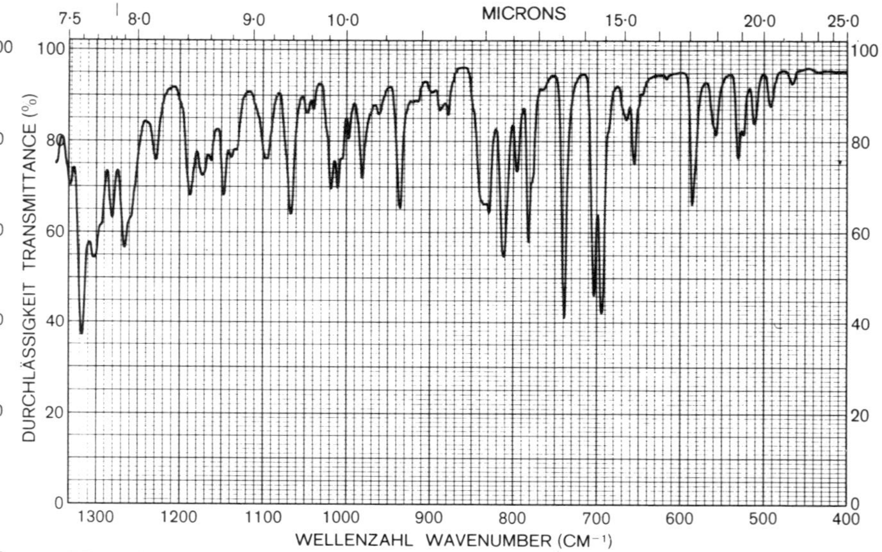

PROBE SAMPLE Prazepam
HERKUNFT ORIGIN
LÖSUNGSMITTEL SOLVENT KBr
KURVE NR CURVE NO
KONZENTRATION CONC. 1mg/300mgKBr
SCHICHTDICKE CELL PATH
VERGLEICH REFERENCE
GESCHWINDIGKEIT SCAN SPEED slow
BEARBEITER OPERATOR
SPALT SLIT N
DATUM DATE
BEMERKUNGEN REMARKS
NO.

Blumberg & Co. 4032 Lintorf W.-Germany Hoffmann Bergschenhoek Holland for Nr. 337-1204

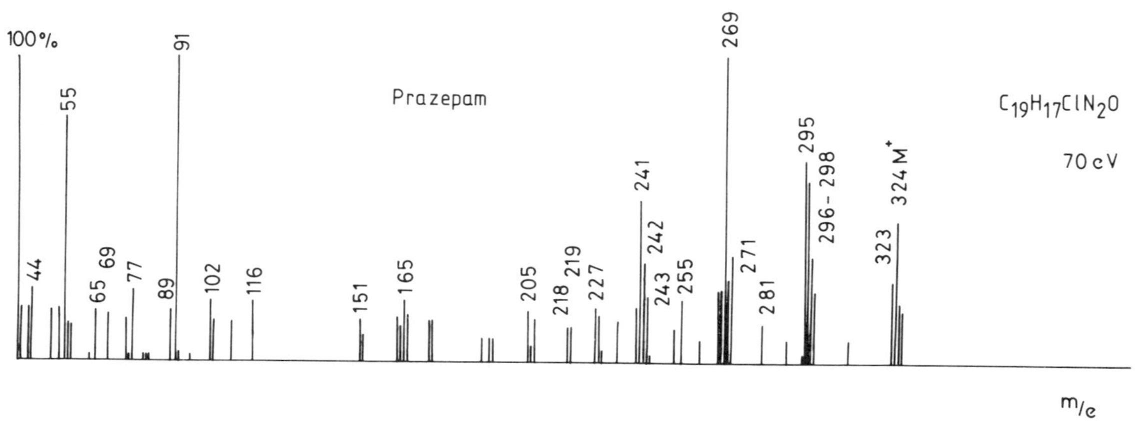

Prazepam

$C_{19}H_{17}ClN_2O$

70 eV

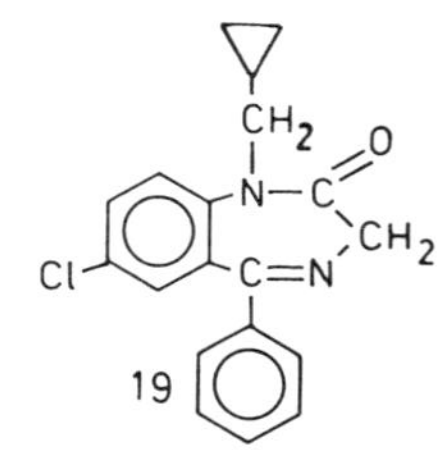

19

Prazepam

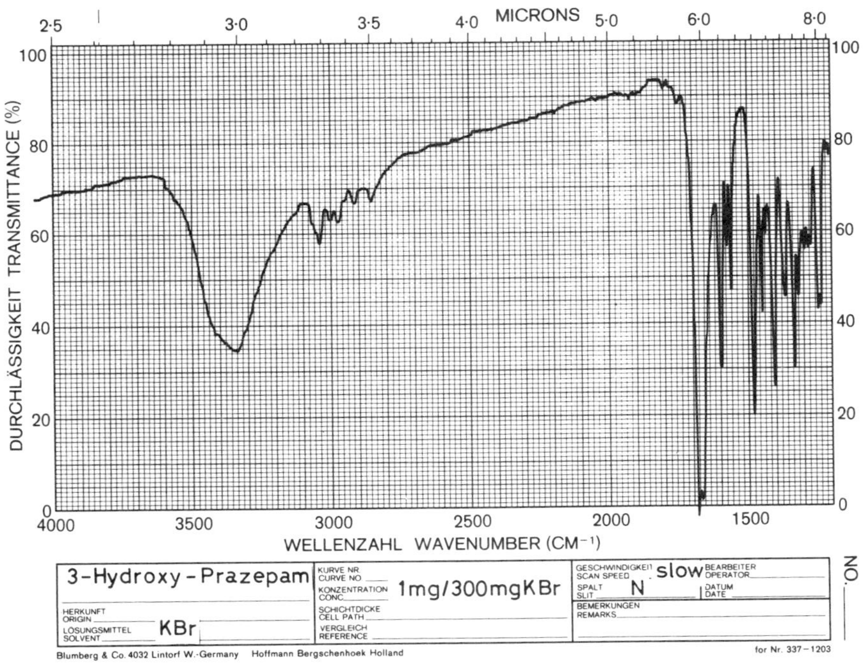

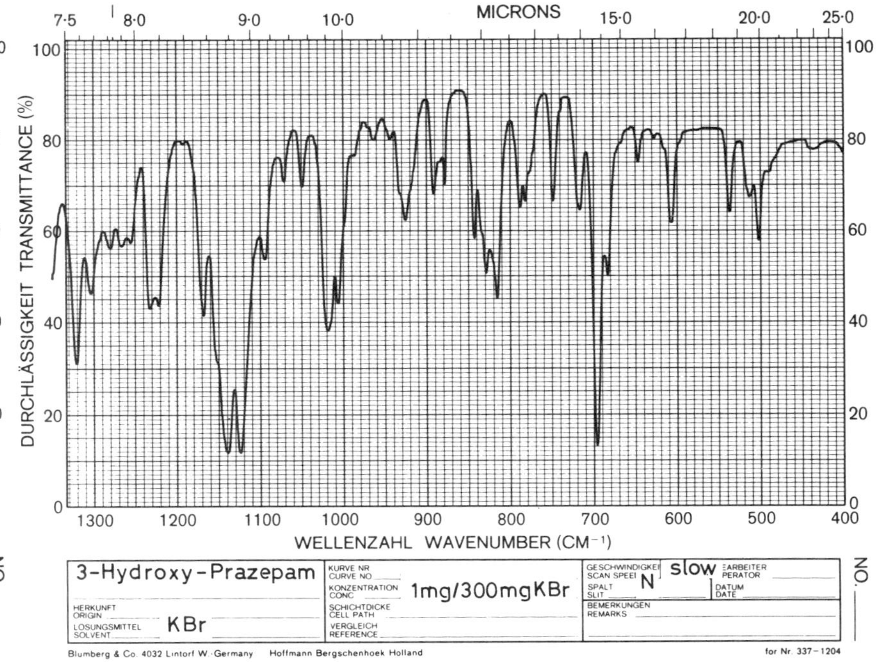

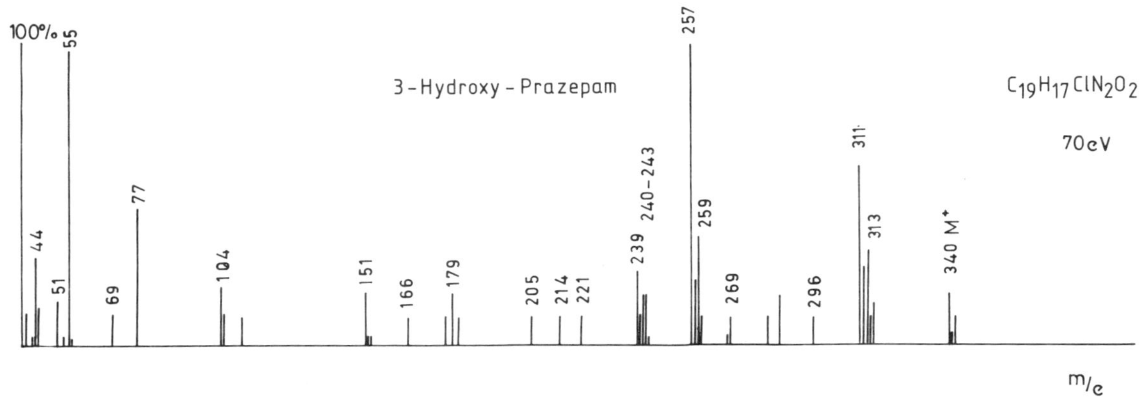

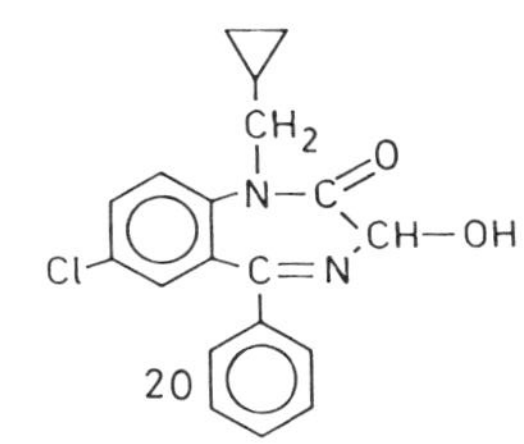

20

3-Hydroxy-Prazepam

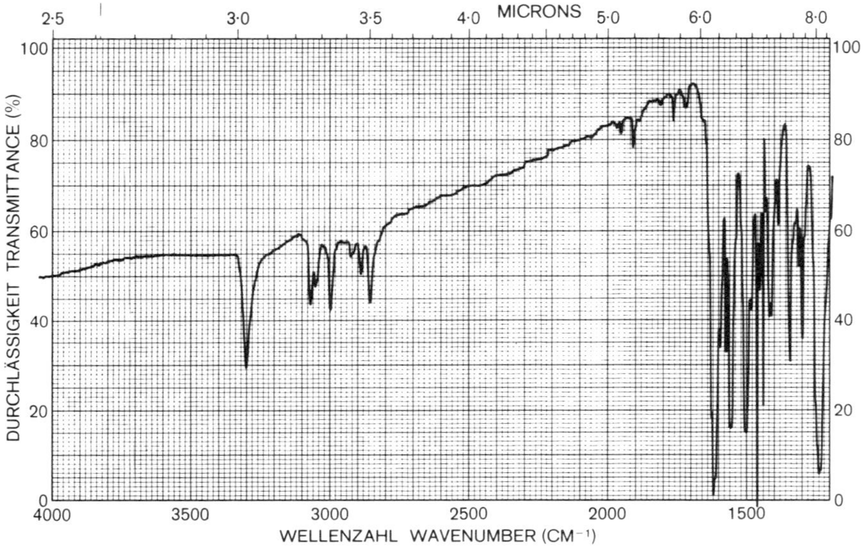

2-Cyclopropyl-methylamino-5-chlor-benzophenone

VE NR / VE NO	KONZENTRATION / CONC. 1mg/300mgKBr	GESCHWINDIGKEIT / SCAN SPEED slow
ORIGIN	SCHICHTDICKE / CELL PATH	SPALT / SLIT N
LÖSUNGSMITTEL / SOLVENT KBr	VERGLEICH / REFERENCE	BEMERKUNGEN / REMARKS
BEARBEITER / OPERATOR	DATUM / DATE	NO.

Blumberg & Co. 4032 Lintorf W.-Germany   Hoffmann Bergschenhoek Holland   for Nr. 337 – 1203

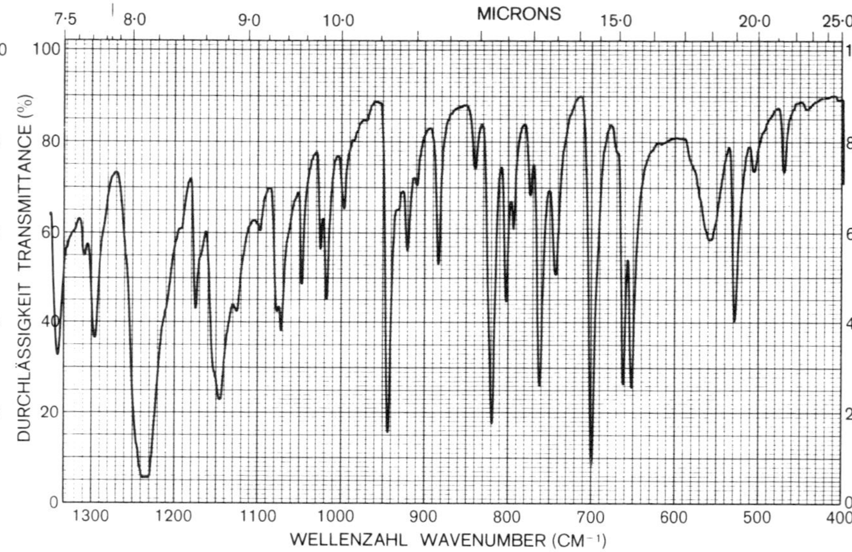

2-Cyclopropyl-methylamino-5-chlor-benzophenone

VE NR / VE NO	KONZENTRATION / CONC. 1mg/300mgKBr	GESCHWINDIGKEIT / SCAN SPEED slow
ORIGIN	SCHICHTDICKE / CELL PATH	SPALT / SLIT N
LÖSUNGSMITTEL / SOLVENT KBr	VERGLEICH / REFERENCE	BEMERKUNGEN / REMARKS
BEARBEITER / OPERATOR	DATUM / DATE	NO.

Blumberg & Co. 4032 Lintorf W.-Germany   Hoffmann Bergschenhoek Holland   for Nr. 337 – 1204

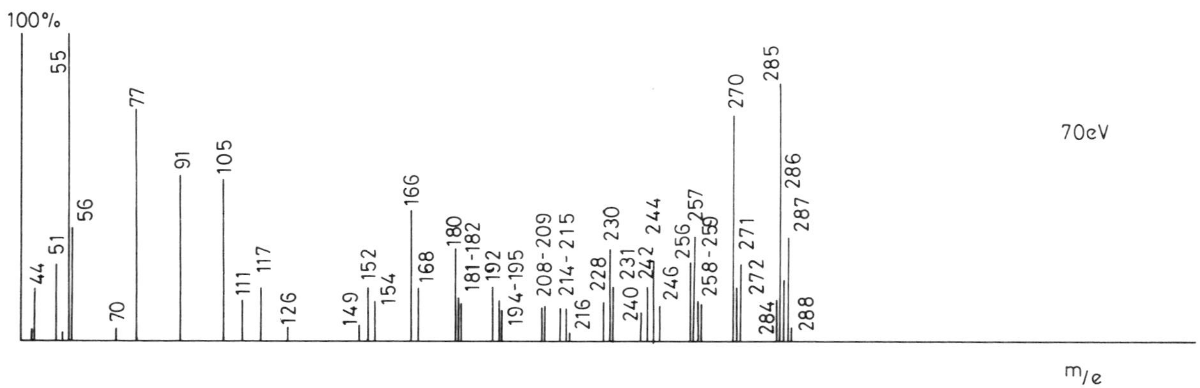

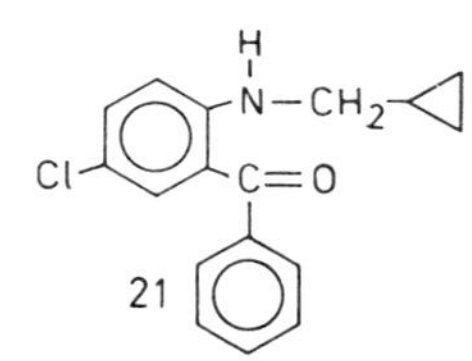

21

2-Cyclopropyl-methylamino-5-chlor-benzophenone

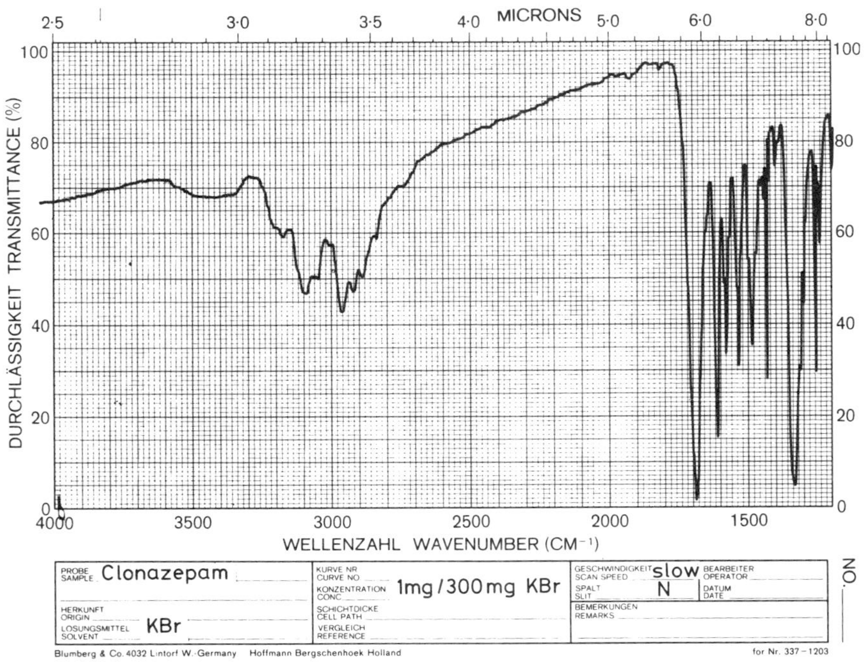
MICRONS
2·5
3·0
3·5
4·0
5·0
6·0
8·0
DURCHLÄSSIGKEIT TRANSMITTANCE (%)
100
80
60
40
20
0
4000
3500
3000
2500
2000
1500
WELLENZAHL WAVENUMBER (CM⁻¹)
NO.
PROBE SAMPLE Clonazepam
HERKUNFT ORIGIN
LÖSUNGSMITTEL SOLVENT KBr
KURVE NR CURVE NO
KONZENTRATION CONC 1mg/300mg KBr
SCHICHTDICKE CELL PATH
VERGLEICH REFERENCE
GESCHWINDIGKEIT SCAN SPEED slow
SPALT SLIT N
BEARBEITER OPERATOR
DATUM DATE
BEMERKUNGEN REMARKS
Blumberg & Co. 4032 Lintorf W.-Germany Hoffmann Bergschenhoek Holland
for Nr. 337-1203

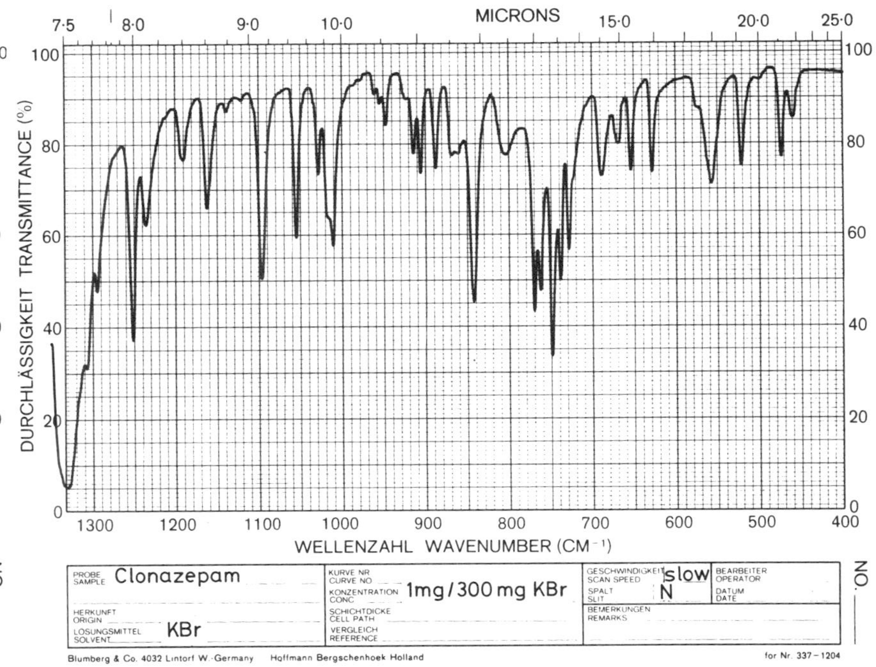
MICRONS
7·5
8·0
9·0
10·0
15·0
20·0
25·0
DURCHLÄSSIGKEIT TRANSMITTANCE (%)
100
80
60
40
20
0
1300
1200
1100
1000
900
800
700
600
500
400
WELLENZAHL WAVENUMBER (CM⁻¹)
NO.
PROBE SAMPLE Clonazepam
HERKUNFT ORIGIN
LÖSUNGSMITTEL SOLVENT KBr
KURVE NR CURVE NO
KONZENTRATION CONC 1mg/300mg KBr
SCHICHTDICKE CELL PATH
VERGLEICH REFERENCE
GESCHWINDIGKEIT SCAN SPEED slow
SPALT SLIT N
BEARBEITER OPERATOR
DATUM DATE
BEMERKUNGEN REMARKS
Blumberg & Co. 4032 Lintorf W.-Germany Hoffmann Bergschenhoek Holland
for Nr. 337-1204

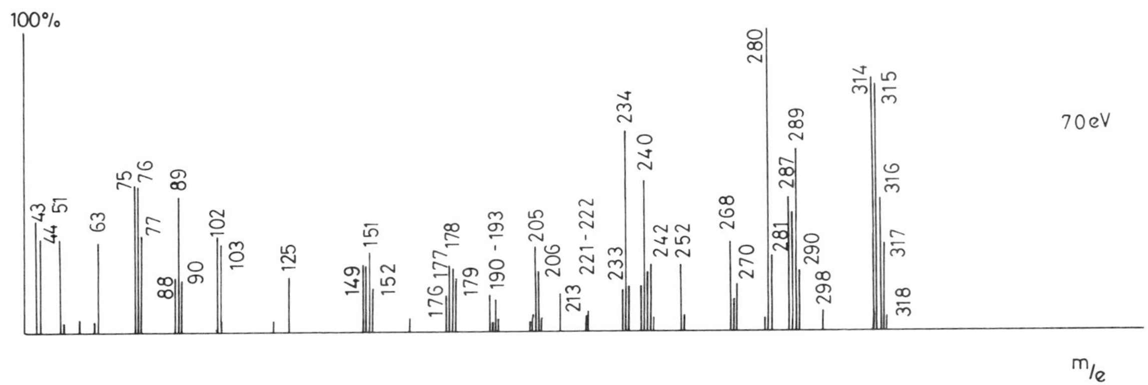
100%
43
44
51
63
75
76
77
88
89
90
102
103
125
149
151
152
176
177
178
179
190 - 193
205
206
213
221 - 222
233
234
240
242
252
268
270
280
281
287
289
290
298
314
315
316
317
318
70eV
m/e

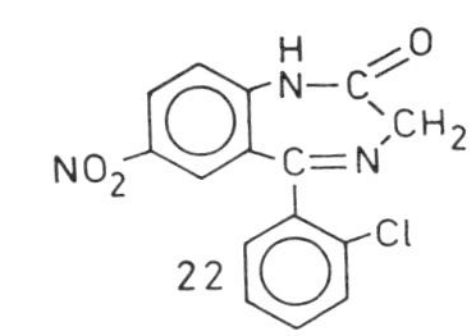
H
N
C
O
CH2
C=N
NO2
Cl
22

Clonazepam

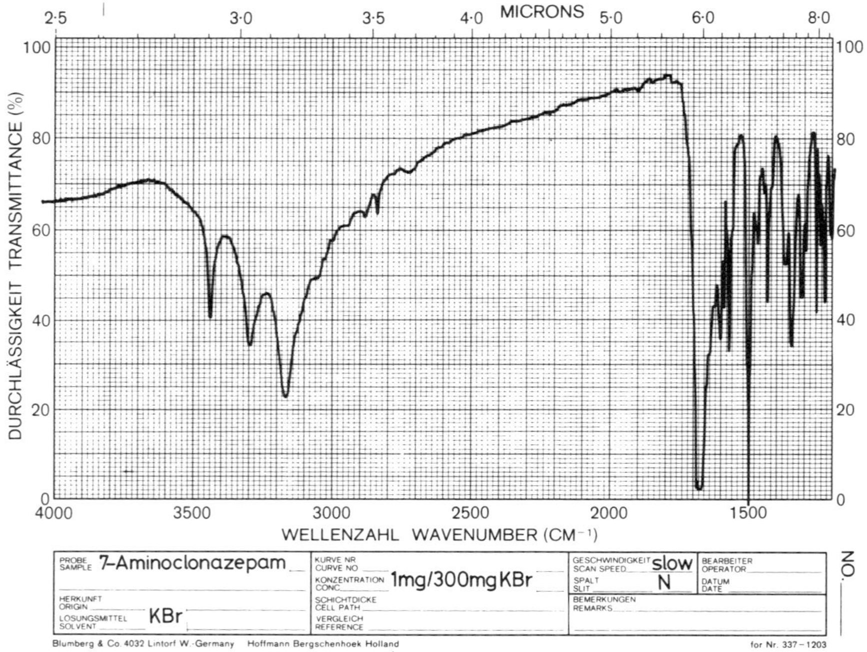

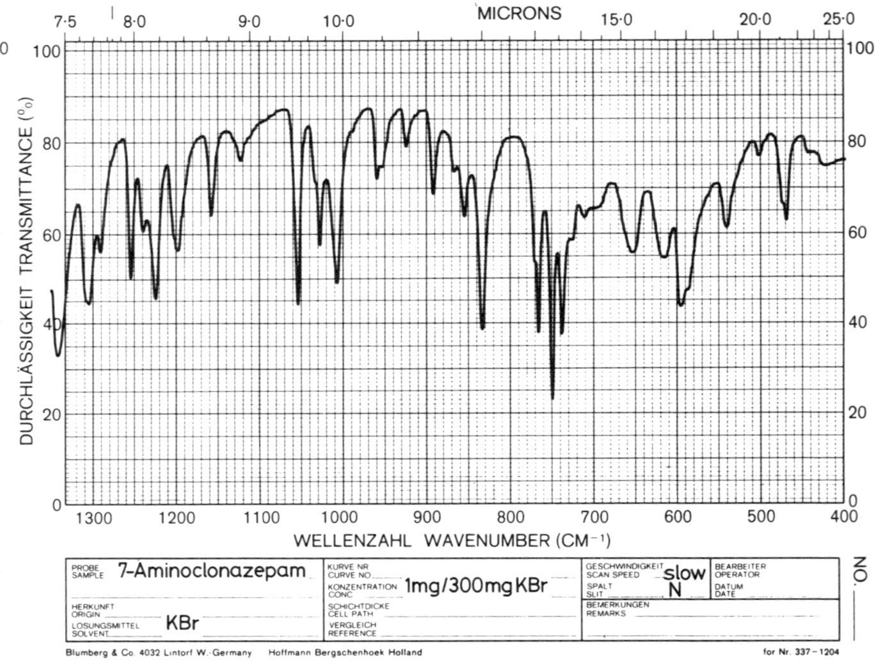

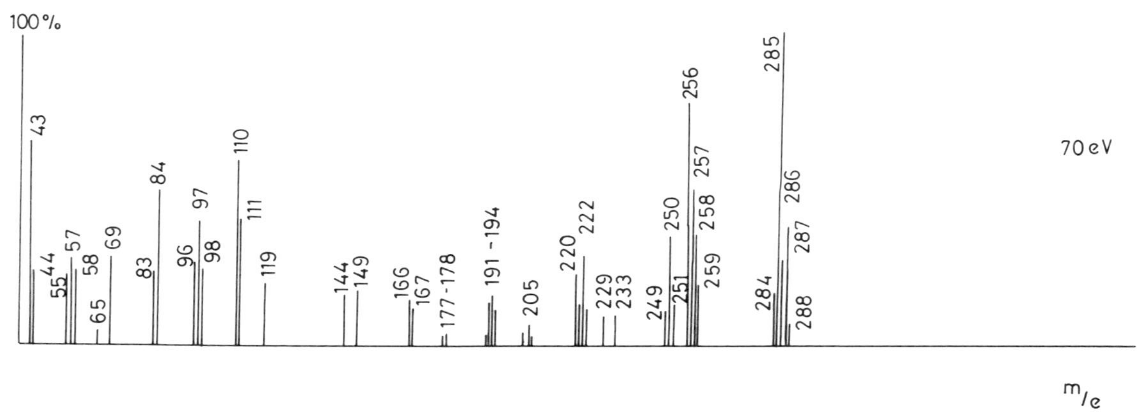

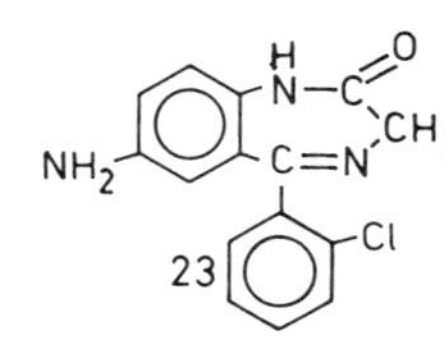

7-Amino-Clonazepam

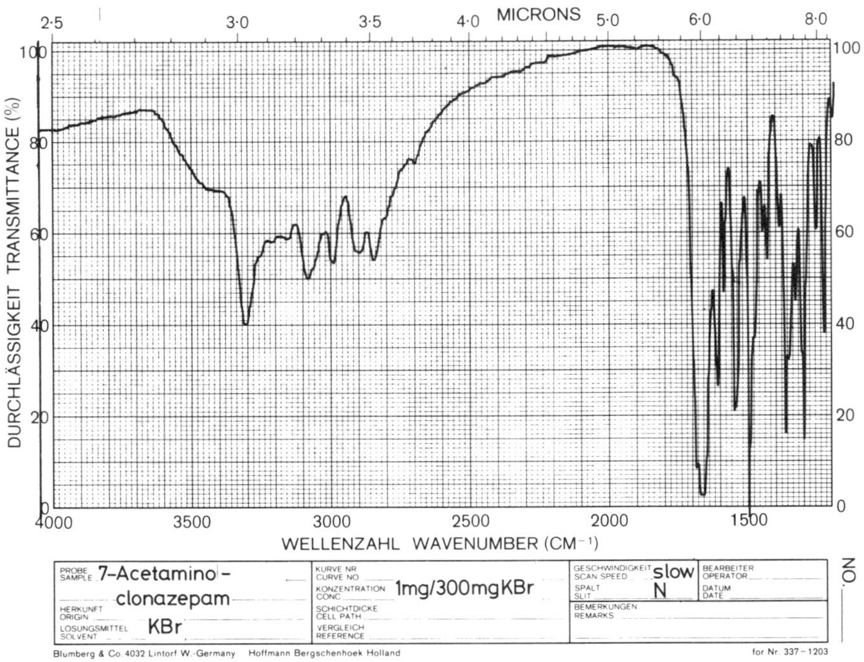

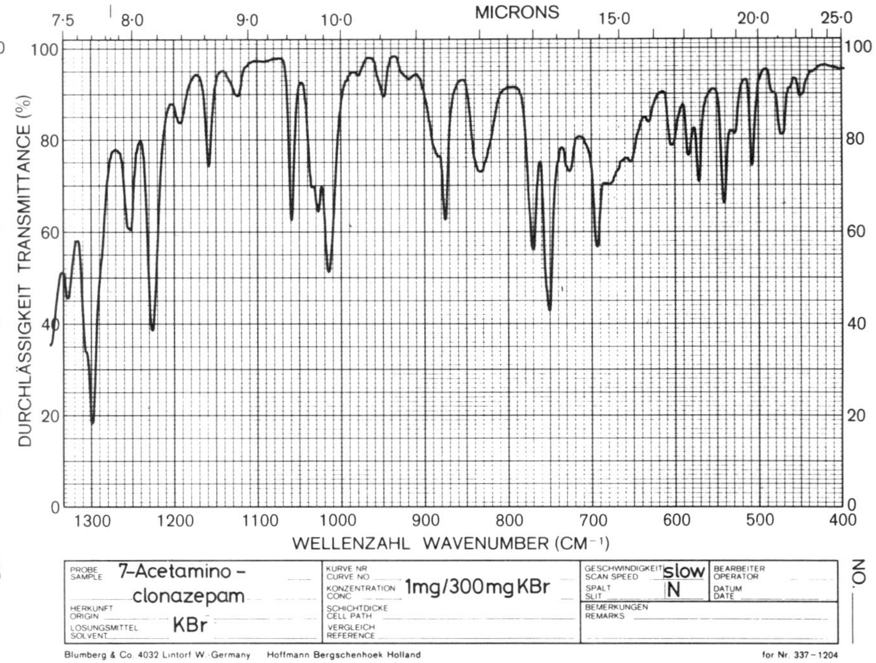

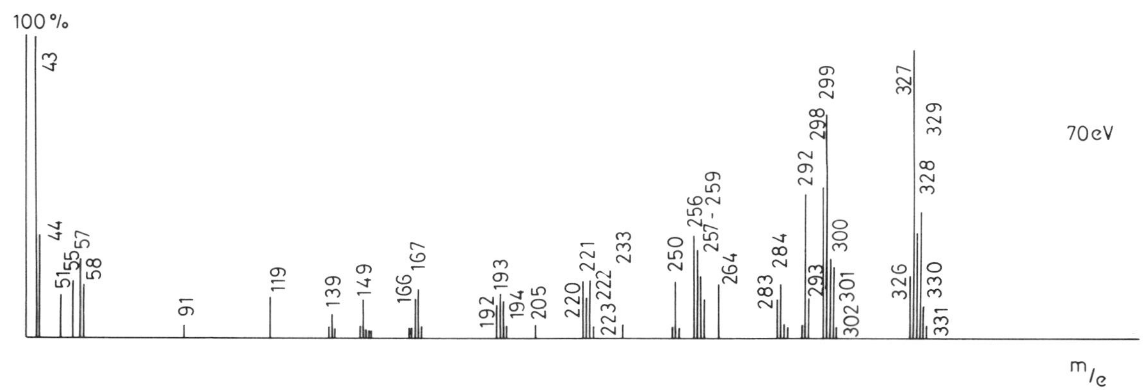

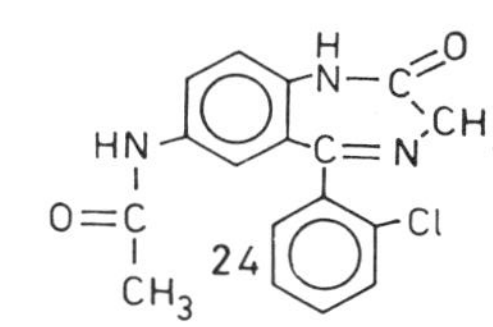

7-Acetamido-Clonazepam

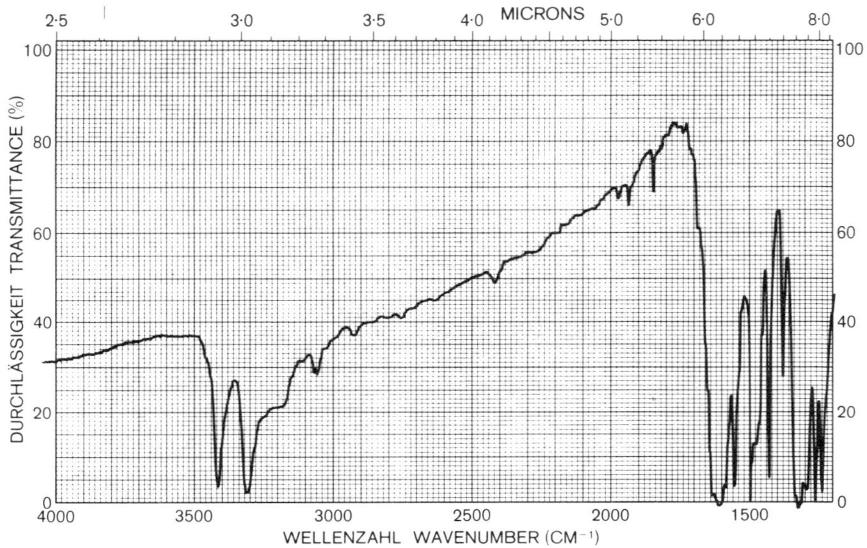

PROBE SAMPLE 2-Amino-2'-chlor-5-nitro-benzophenone
HERKUNFT ORIGIN
LOSUNGSMITTEL SOLVENT KBr
KURVE NR CURVE NO
KONZENTRATION CONC. 1mg/300mg KBr
SCHICHTDICKE CELL PATH
VERGLEICH REFERENCE
GESCHWINDIGKEIT SCAN SPEED slow
SPALT SLIT N
BEMERKUNGEN REMARKS
BEARBEITER OPERATOR
DATUM DATE
NO.

Blumberg & Co 4032 Lintorf W.-Germany Hoffmann Bergschenhoek Holland for Nr. 337-1203

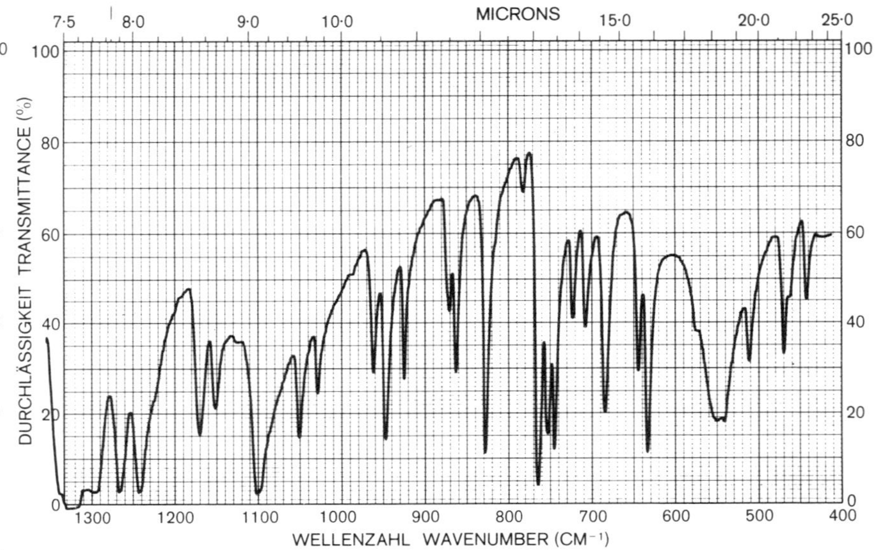

PROBE SAMPLE 2-Amino-2'-chlor-5-nitro-benzophenone
HERKUNFT ORIGIN
LOSUNGSMITTEL SOLVENT KBr
KURVE NR CURVE NO
KONZENTRATION CONC. 1mg/300mg KBr
SCHICHTDICKE CELL PATH
VERGLEICH REFERENCE
GESCHWINDIGKEIT SCAN SPEED slow
SPALT SLIT N
BEMERKUNGEN REMARKS
BEARBEITER OPERATOR
DATUM DATE
NO.

Blumberg & Co. 4032 Lintorf W.-Germany Hoffmann Bergschenhoek Holland for Nr. 337-1204

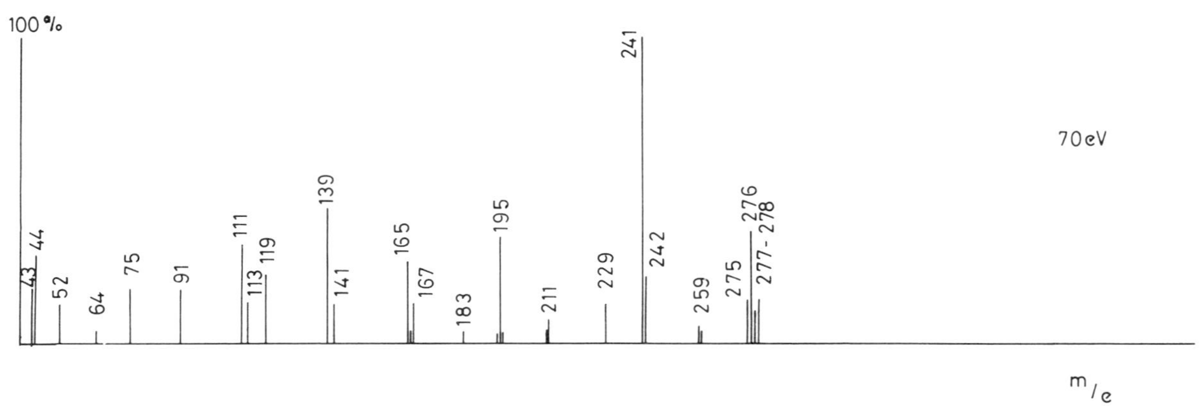

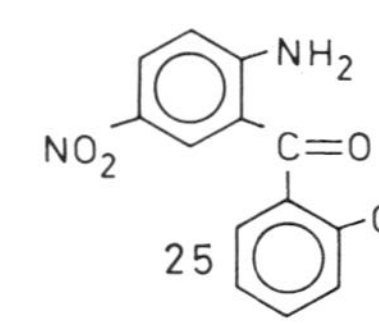

2-Amino-5-nitro-2'-chlor-benzophenone

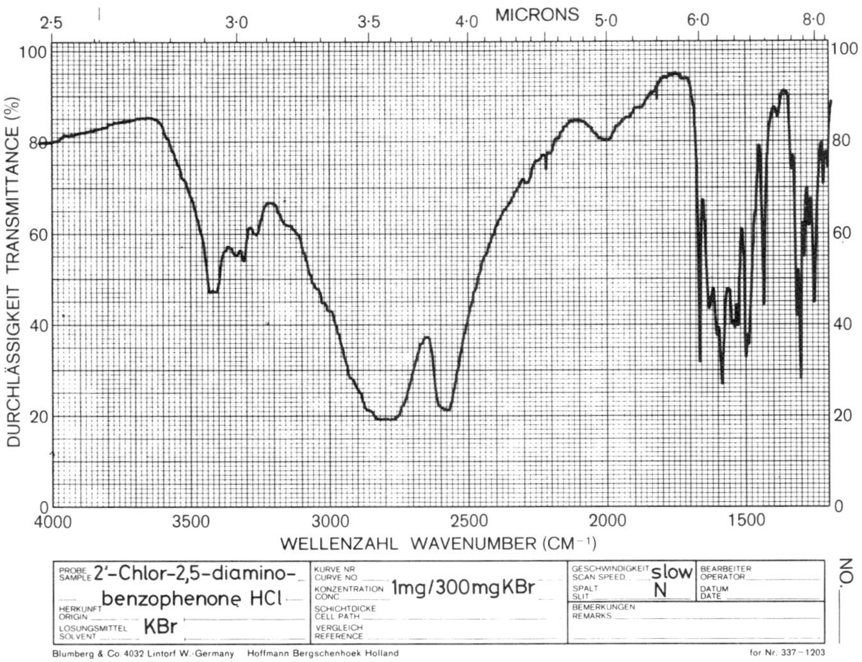

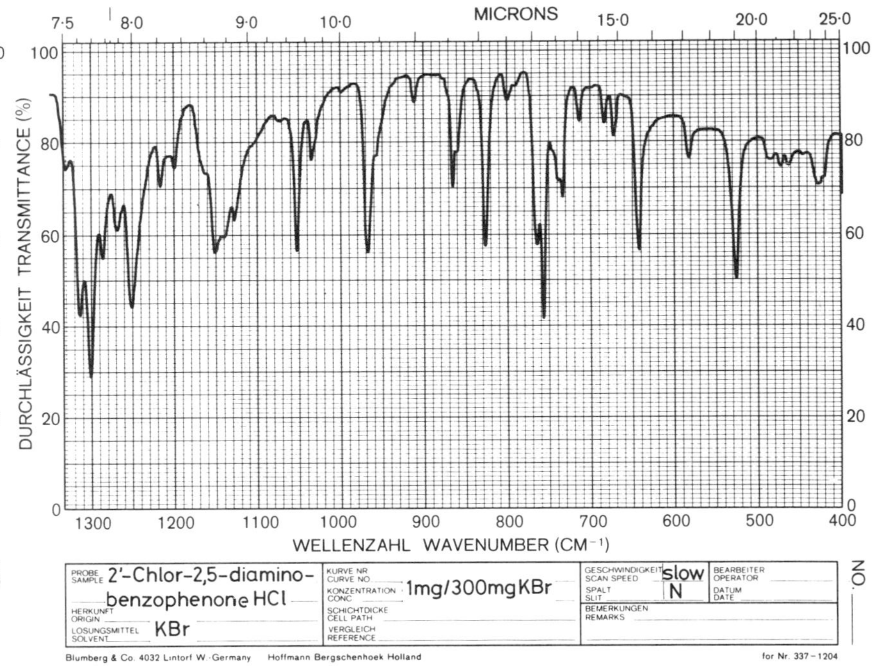

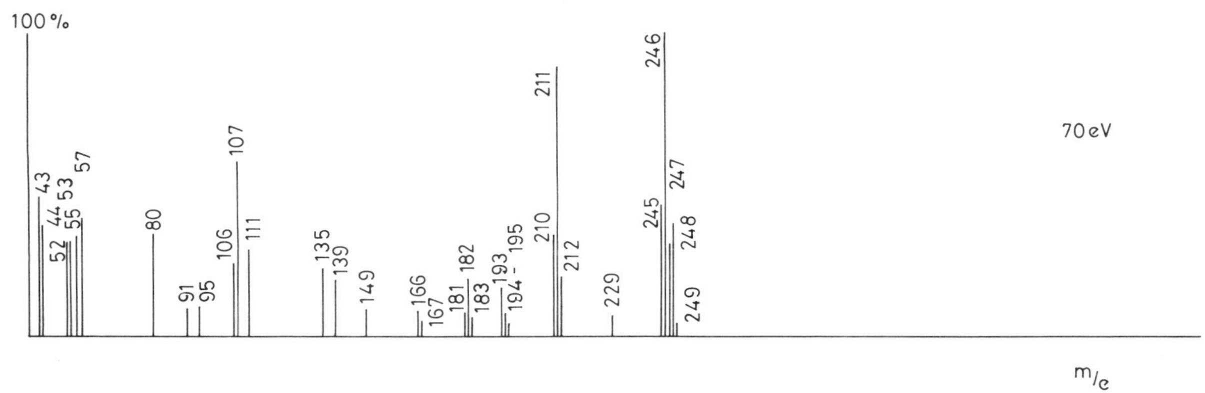

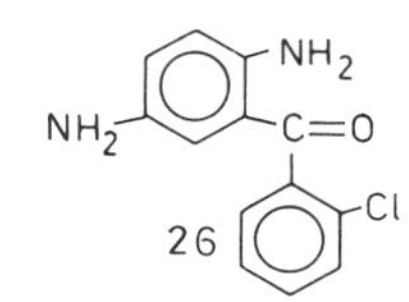

2,5-Diamino-2'-chlor-benzophenone HCl

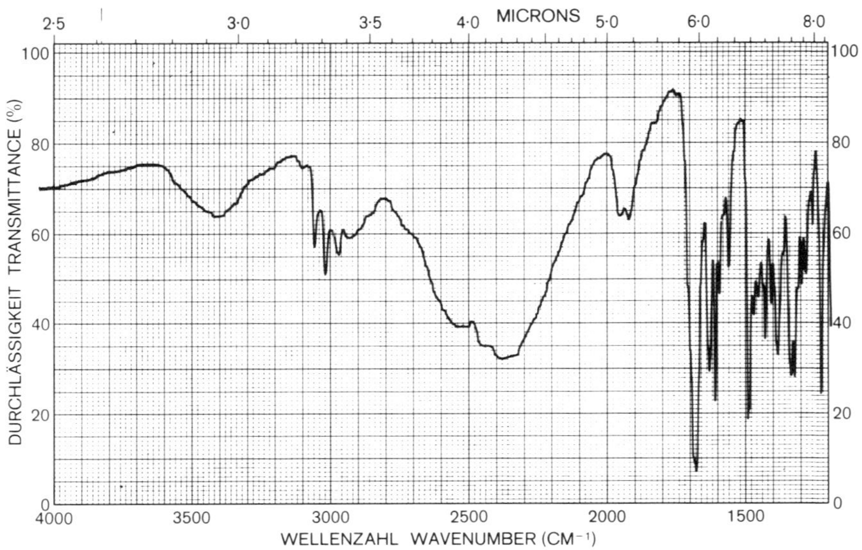

PROBE SAMPLE Flurazepam HCl	KURVE NR CURVE NO	GESCHWINDIGKEIT SCAN SPEED slow	BEARBEITER OPERATOR
HERKUNFT ORIGIN	KONZENTRATION CONC. 1mg/ 300mg KBr	SPALT SLIT N	DATUM DATE
LÖSUNGSMITTEL SOLVENT KBr	SCHICHTDICKE CELL PATH	BEMERKUNGEN REMARKS	
	VERGLEICH REFERENCE		

NO. ______

Blumberg & Co. 4032 Lintorf W.-Germany Hoffmann Bergschenhoek Holland for Nr. 337-1203

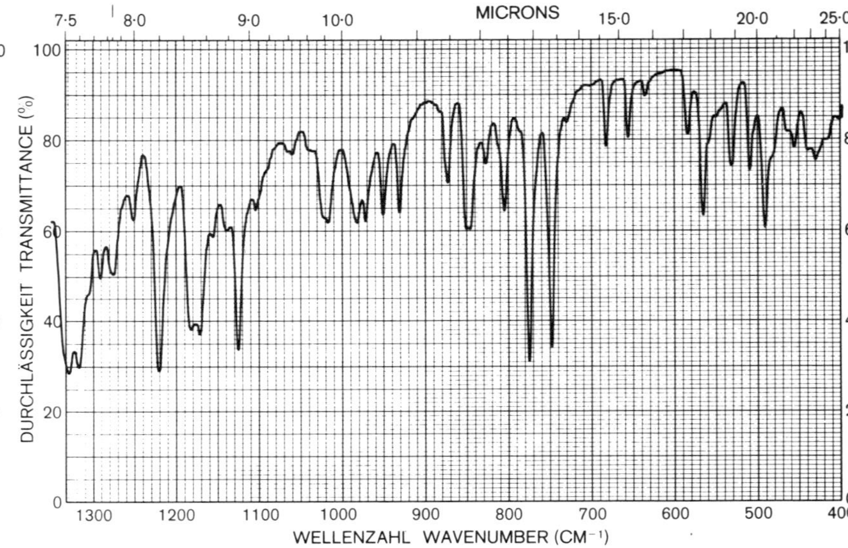

PROBE SAMPLE Flurazepam HCl	KURVE NR CURVE NO	GESCHWINDIGKEIT SCAN SPEED slow	BEARBEITER OPERATOR
HERKUNFT ORIGIN	KONZENTRATION CONC. 1mg/300mg KBr	SPALT SLIT N	DATUM DATE
LÖSUNGSMITTEL SOLVENT KBr	SCHICHTDICKE CELL PATH	BEMERKUNGEN REMARKS	
	VERGLEICH REFERENCE		

NO. ______

Blumberg & Co. 4032 Lintorf W.-Germany Hoffmann Bergschenhoek Holland for Nr. 337-1204

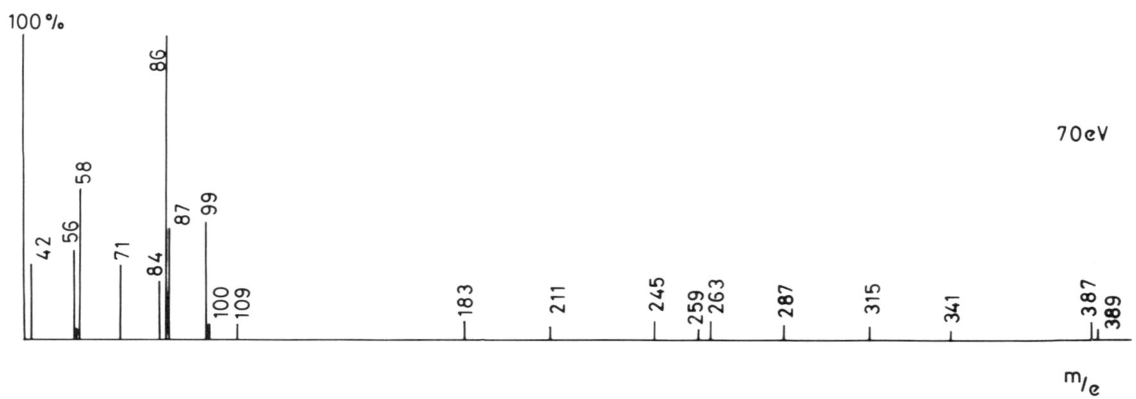

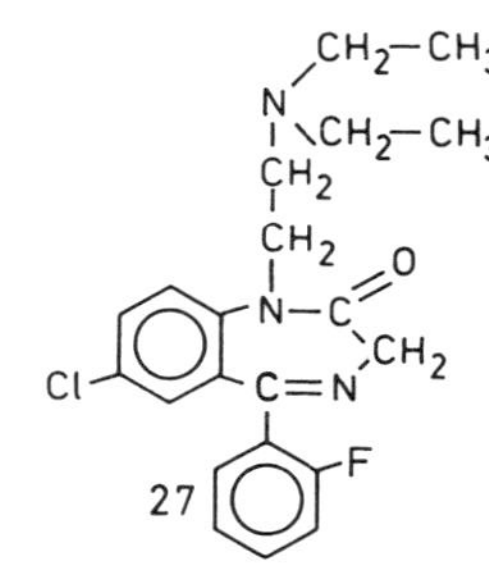

Flurazepam x HCl

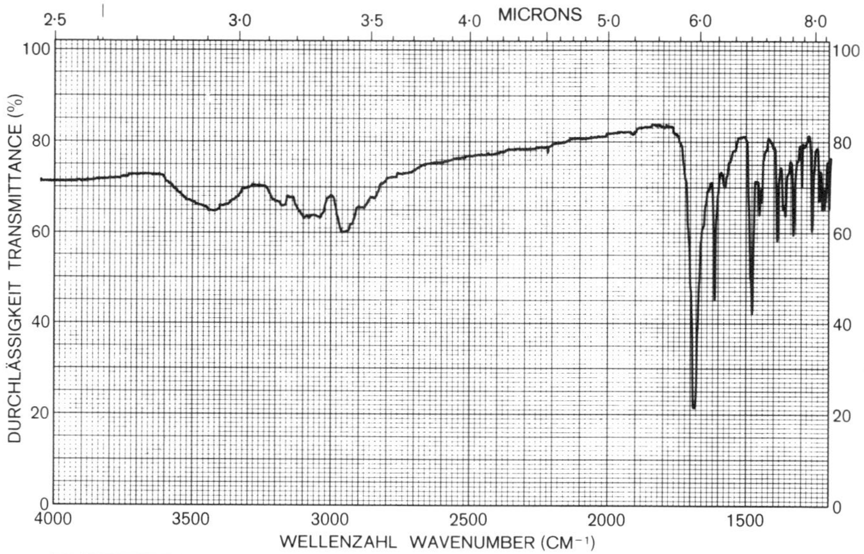

PROBE SAMPLE N-1-Desalkyl-Flurazepam | KURVE NR CURVE NO | GESCHWINDIGKEIT SCAN SPEED slow | BEARBEITER OPERATOR | NO.
HERKUNFT ORIGIN | KONZENTRATION CONC. 1mg/300mgKBr | SPALT SLIT N | DATUM DATE
LÖSUNGSMITTEL SOLVENT KBr | SCHICHTDICKE CELL PATH | VERGLEICH REFERENCE | BEMERKUNGEN REMARKS

Blumberg & Co. 4032 Lintorf W.-Germany Hoffmann Bergschenhoek Holland for Nr. 337-1203

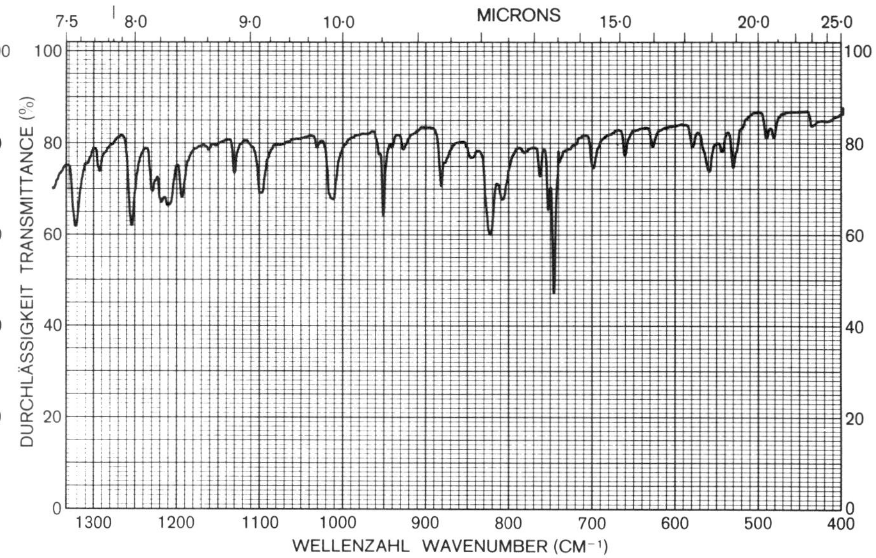

PROBE SAMPLE N-1-Desalkyl-Flurazepam | KURVE NR CURVE NO | GESCHWINDIGKEIT SCAN SPEED slow | BEARBEITER OPERATOR | NO.
HERKUNFT ORIGIN | KONZENTRATION CONC. 1mg/300mgKBr | SPALT SLIT N | DATUM DATE
LÖSUNGSMITTEL SOLVENT KBr | SCHICHTDICKE CELL PATH | VERGLEICH REFERENCE | BEMERKUNGEN REMARKS

Blumberg & Co. 4032 Lintorf W.-Germany Hoffmann Bergschenhoek Holland for Nr. 337-1204

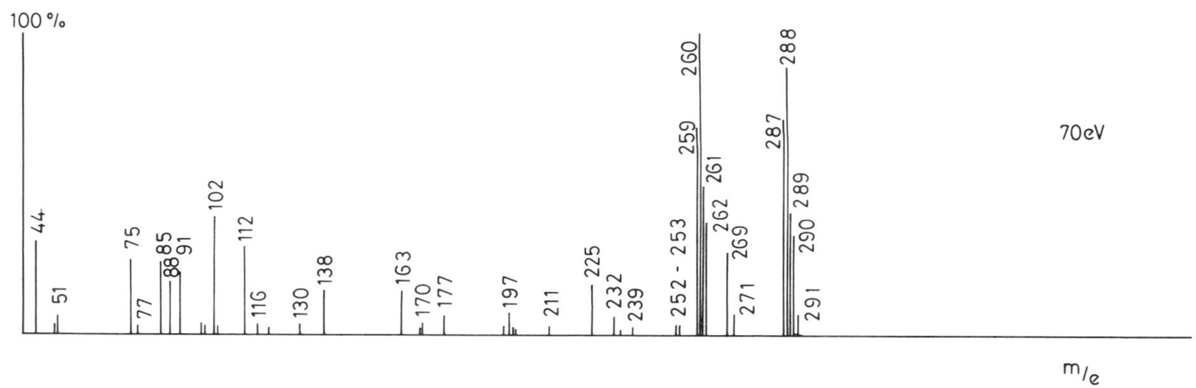

70eV

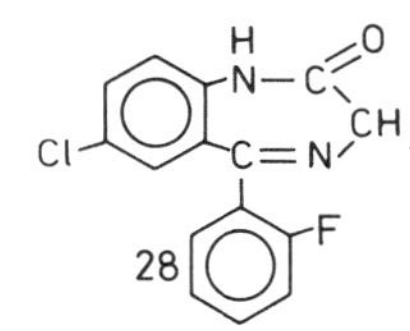

N-1-Desalkyl-Flurazepam

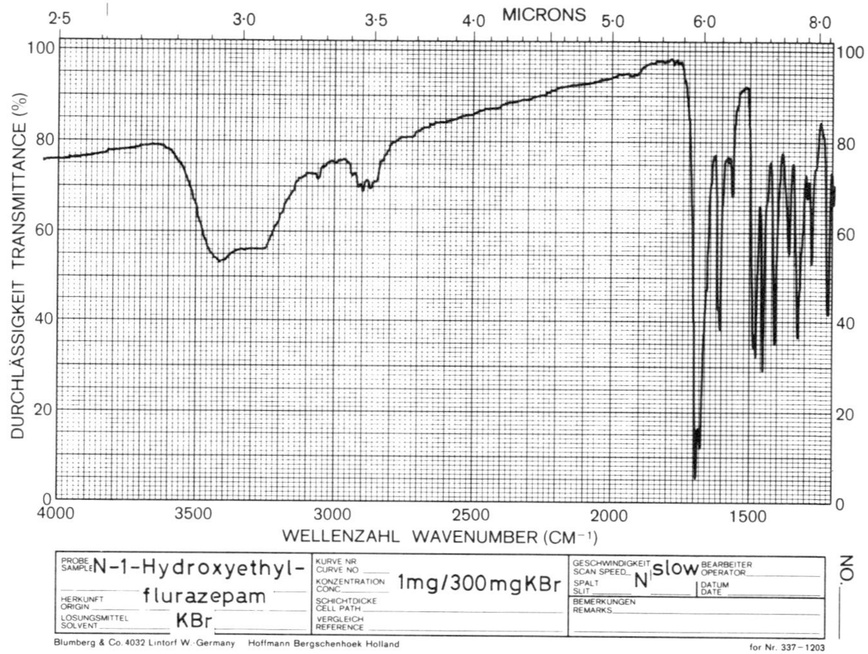

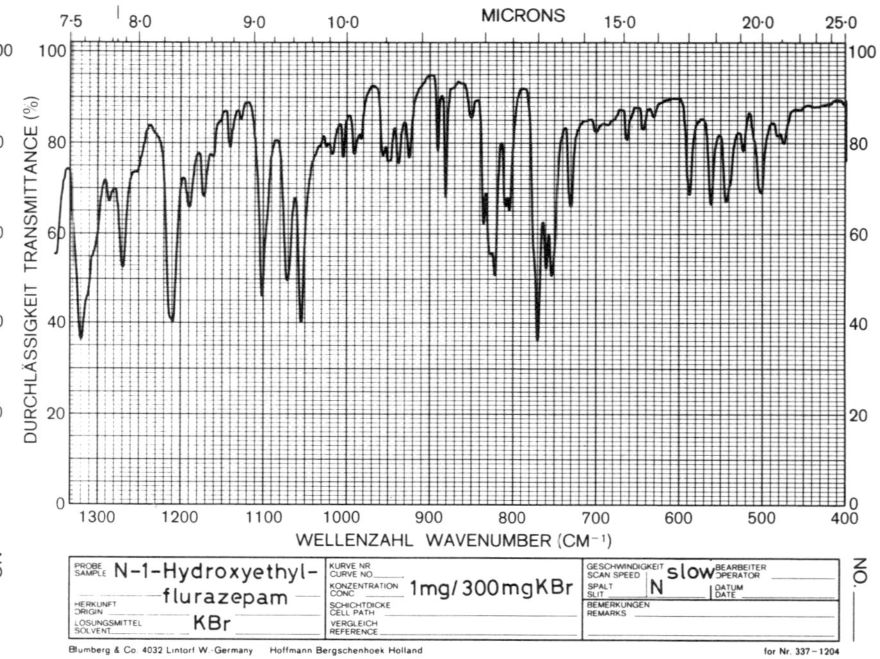

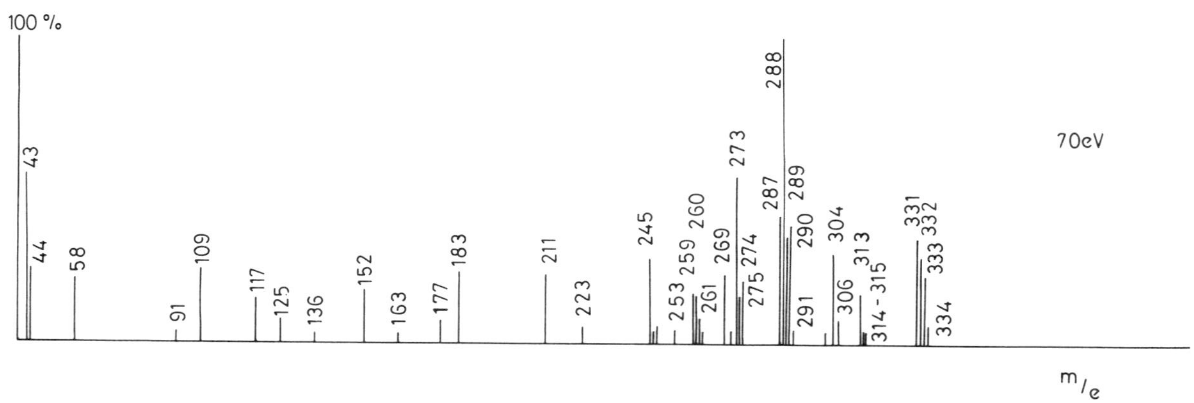

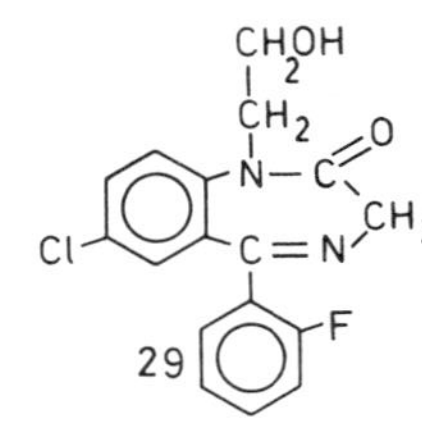

N-1-Hydroxyethyl-Flurazepam

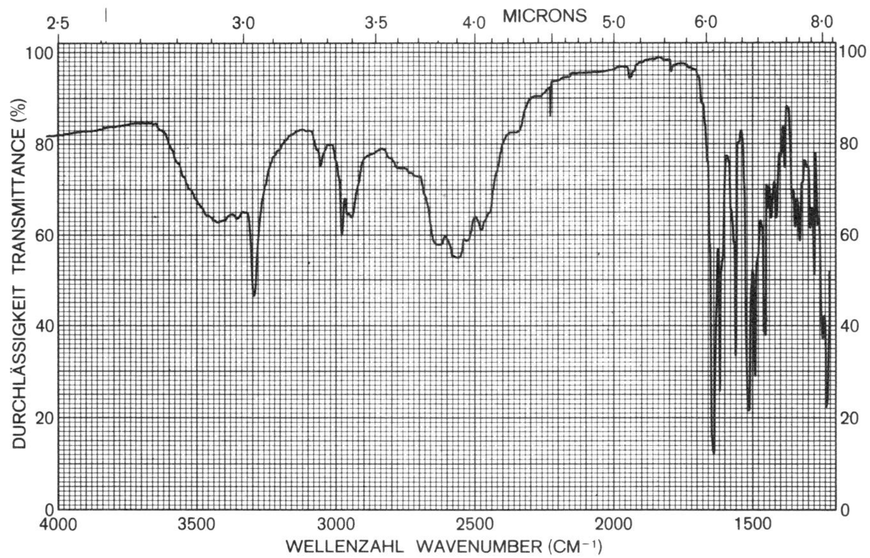

2-Diethylamino-ethylamino-5-chlor-2'-fluor-benzophenone

HERKUNFT ORIGIN
LÖSUNGSMITTEL SOLVENT KBr
KURVE NR CURVE NO
KONZENTRATION CONC. 1mg/300mgKBr
SCHICHTDICKE CELL PATH
VERGLEICH REFERENCE
GESCHWINDIGKEIT SCAN SPEED slow
SPALT SLIT N
BEARBEITER OPERATOR
DATUM DATE
BEMERKUNGEN REMARKS
NO.

for Nr. 337-1203

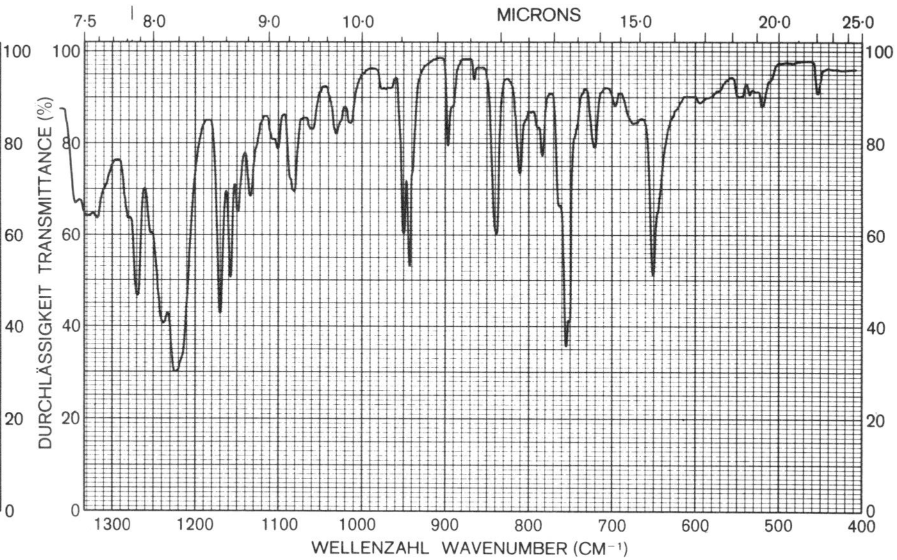

2-Diethylamino-ethylamino-5-chlor-2'-fluor-benzophenone

HERKUNFT ORIGIN
LÖSUNGSMITTEL SOLVENT KBr
KURVE NR CURVE NO
KONZENTRATION CONC. 1mg/300mgKBr
SCHICHTDICKE CELL PATH
VERGLEICH REFERENCE
GESCHWINDIGKEIT SCAN SPEED slow
SPALT SLIT N
BEARBEITER OPERATOR
DATUM DATE
BEMERKUNGEN REMARKS
NO.

Blumberg & Co. 4032 L... Germany Hoffmann Bergschenhoek Holland for Nr. 337-1204

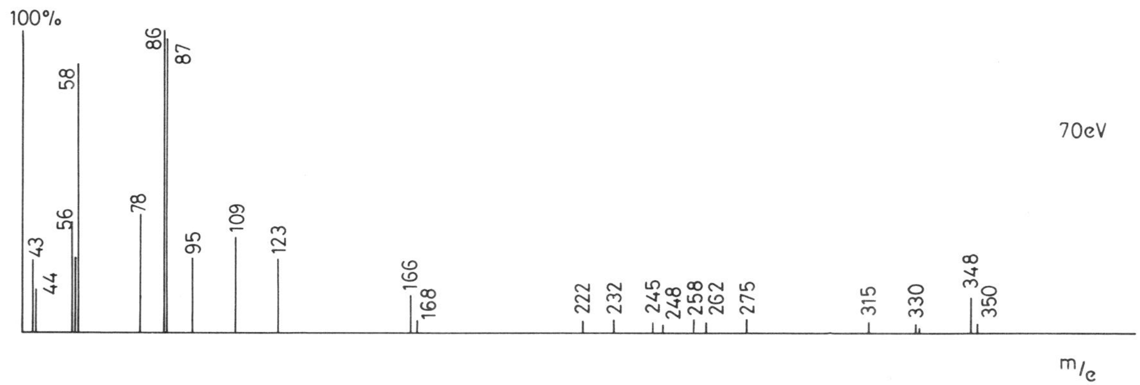

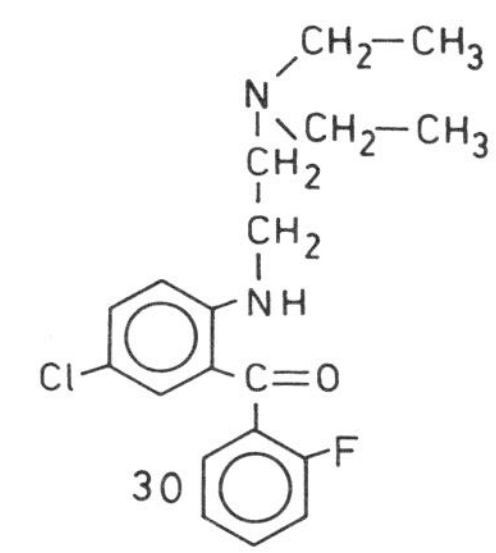

2-Diethylamino-ethylamino-
5-chlor-2'-fluor-benzophenone

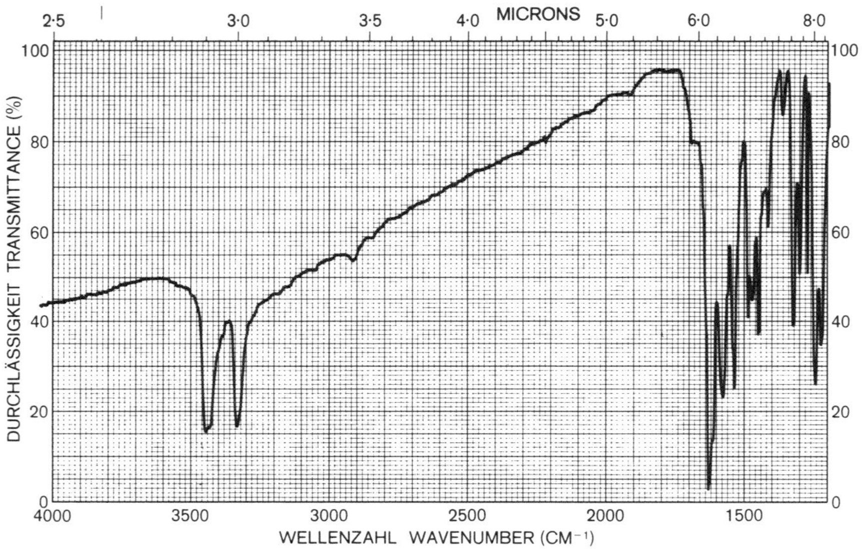

PROBE SAMPLE 2-Amino-5-chlor-2'-fluor-benzophenone
HERKUNFT ORIGIN
LÖSUNGSMITTEL SOLVENT KBr
KURVE NR CURVE NO
KONZENTRATION CONC. 1mg/300mgKBr
SCHICHTDICKE CELL PATH
VERGLEICH REFERENCE
GESCHWINDIGKEIT SCAN SPEED slow
SPALT SLIT N
BEARBEITER OPERATOR
DATUM DATE
BEMERKUNGEN REMARKS
NO.

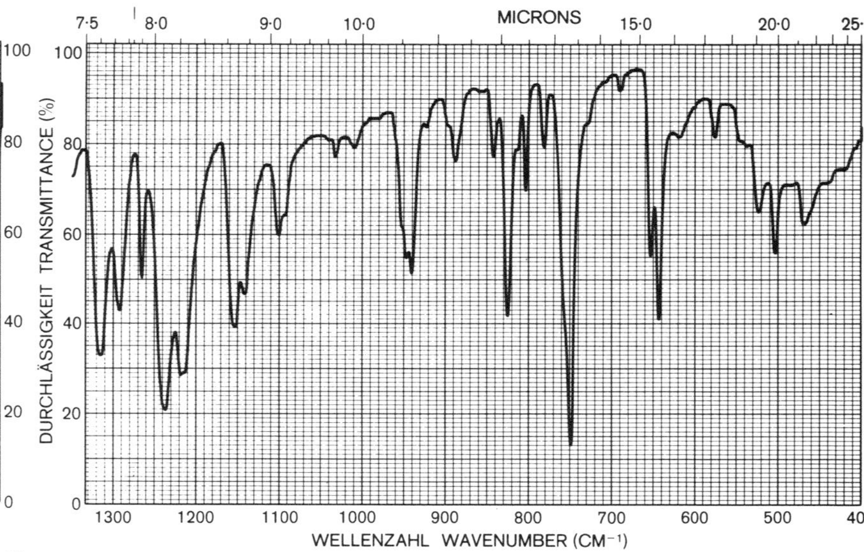

PROBE SAMPLE 2-Amino-5-chlor-2'-fluor-benzophenone
HERKUNFT ORIGIN
LÖSUNGSMITTEL SOLVENT KBr
KURVE NR CURVE NO
KONZENTRATION CONC. 1mg/300mgKBr
SCHICHTDICKE CELL PATH
VERGLEICH REFERENCE
GESCHWINDIGKEIT SCAN SPEED slow
SPALT SLIT N
BEARBEITER OPERATOR
DATUM DATE
BEMERKUNGEN REMARKS
NO.

Blumberg & Co. 4032 Lintorf Germany Hoffmann Bergschenhoek Holland for Nr. 337-1204

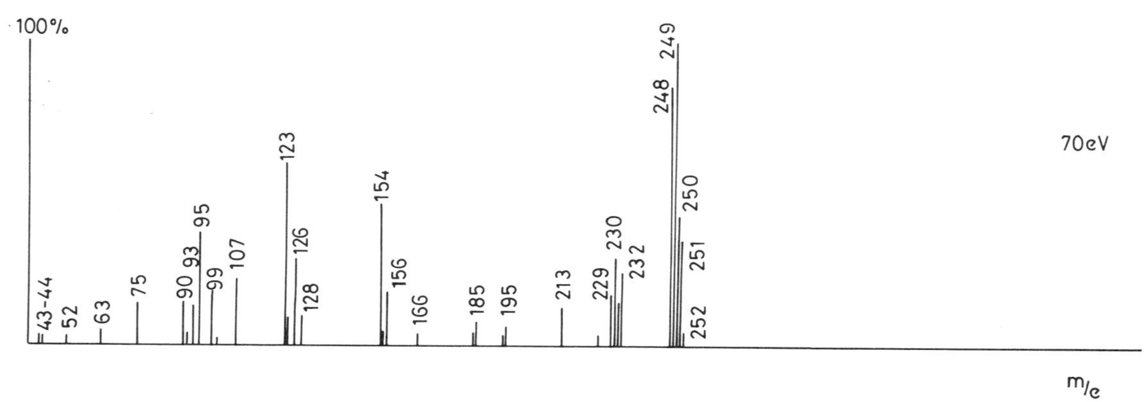

70eV

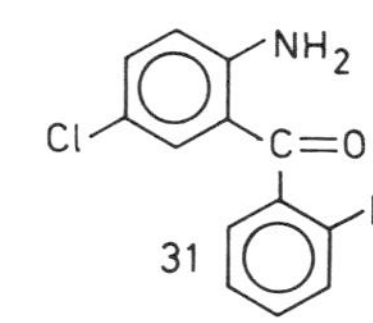

31

2-Amino-5-chlor-2'-fluor-benzophenone

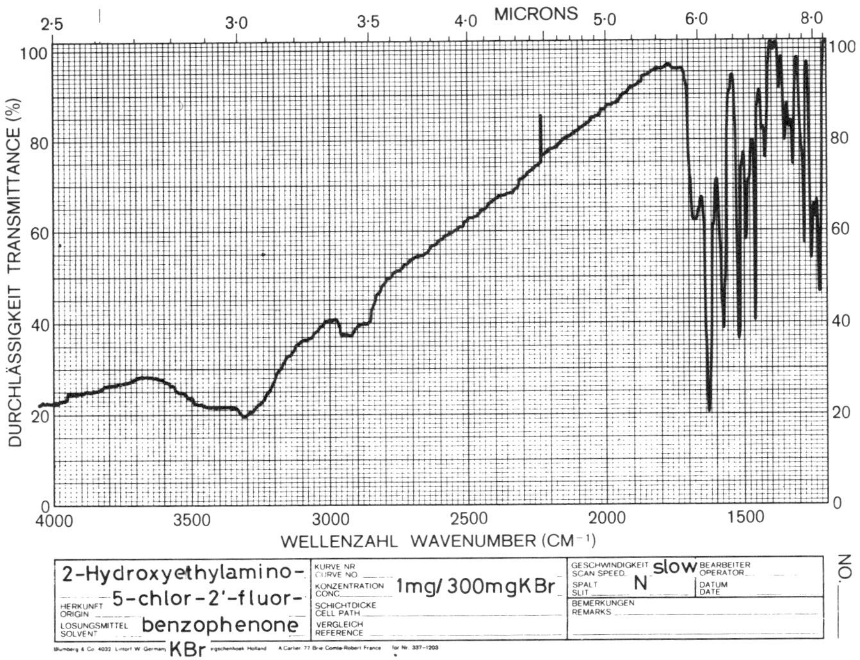

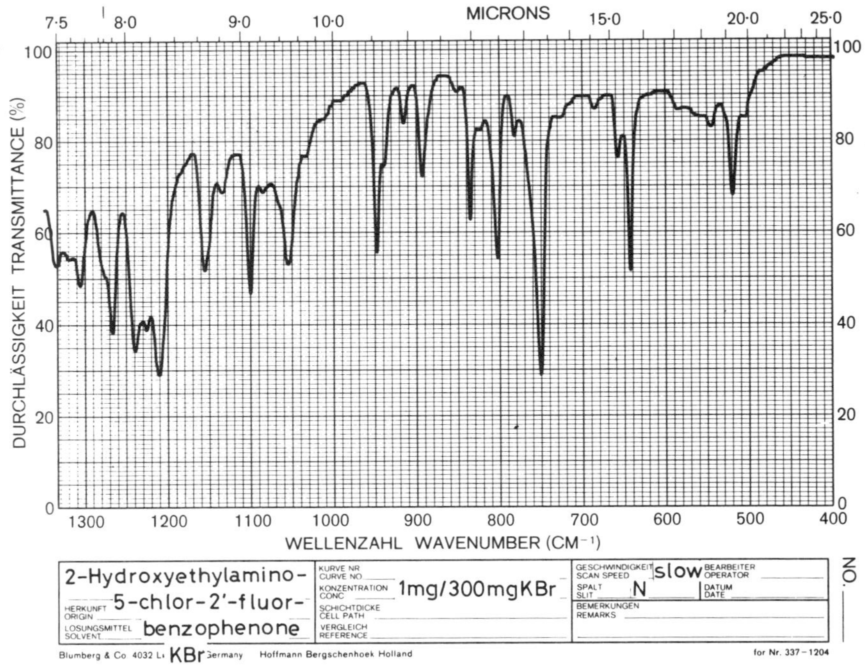

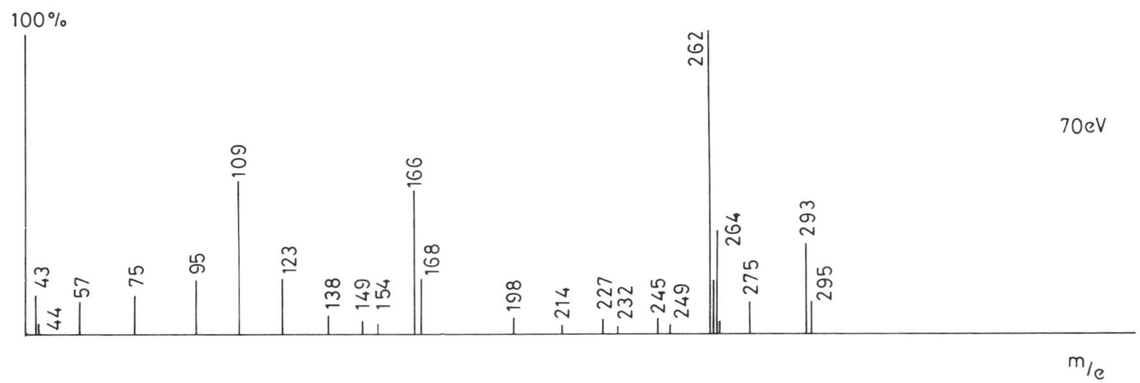

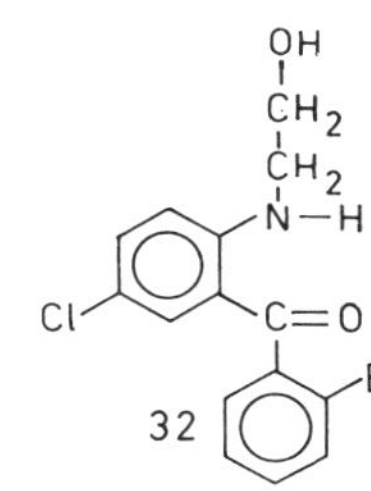

32

2-Hydroxyethylamino-5-chlor-2'-fluor-benzophenone

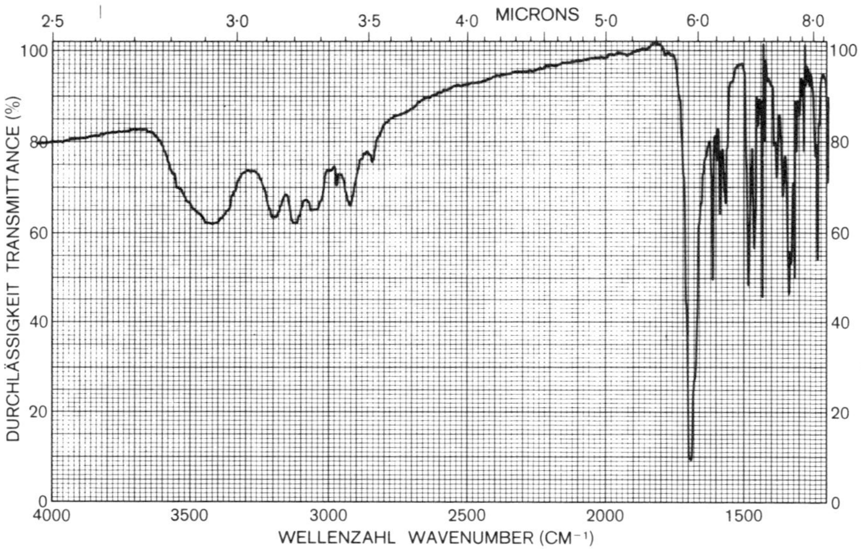

PROBE SAMPLE Bromazepam	KURVE NR CURVE NO	GESCHWINDIGKEIT SCAN SPEED slow BEARBEITER OPERATOR
	KONZENTRATION CONC 1mg/300mgKBr	SPALT SLIT N DATUM DATE
HERKUNFT ORIGIN	SCHICHTDICKE CELL PATH	BEMERKUNGEN REMARKS
LÖSUNGSMITTEL SOLVENT KBr	VERGLEICH REFERENCE	

NO.

Blumberg & Co. 4032 Lintorf W.-Germany Hoffmann Bergschenhoek Holland for Nr. 337-1203

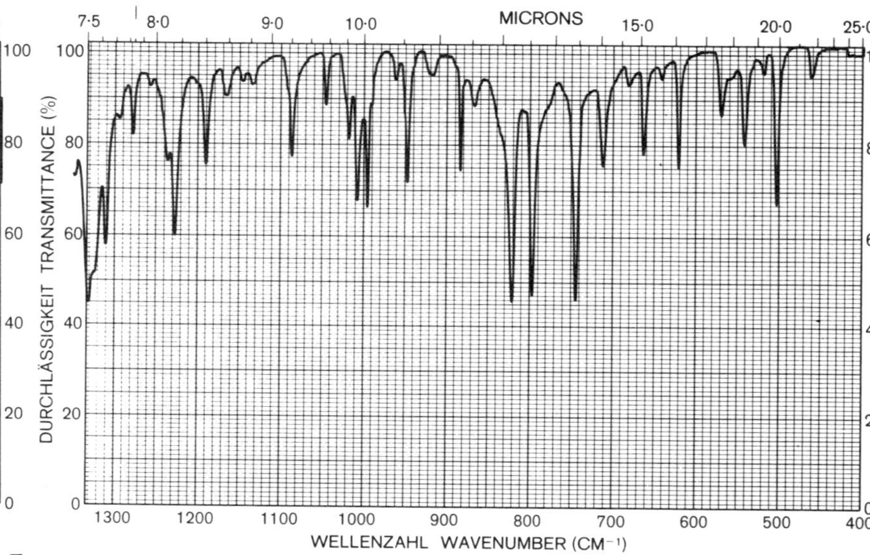

PROBE SAMPLE Bromazepam	KURVE NR CURVE NO	GESCHWINDIGKEIT SCAN SPEED slow BEARBEITER OPERATOR
	KONZENTRATION CONC 1mg/300mgKBr	SPALT SLIT N DATUM DATE
HERKUNFT ORIGIN	SCHICHTDICKE CELL PATH	BEMERKUNGEN REMARKS
LÖSUNGSMITTEL SOLVENT KBr	VERGLEICH REFERENCE	

NO.

Blumberg & Co. 4032 Lintorf W.-Germany Hoffmann Bergschenhoek Holland for Nr. 337-1204

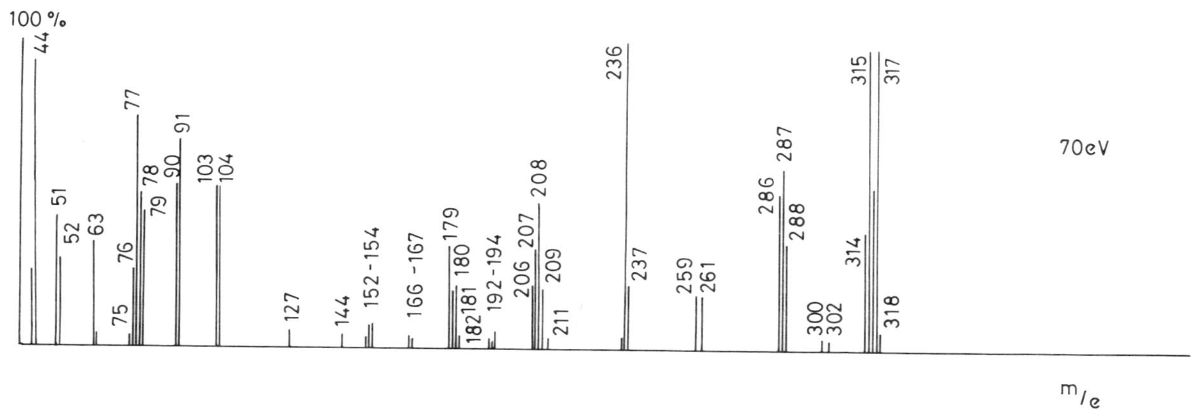

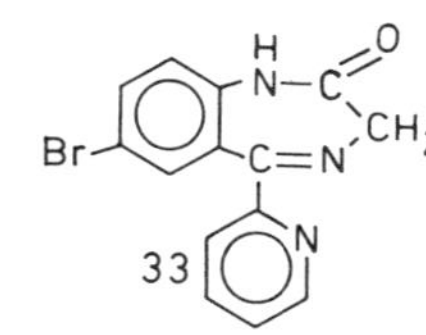

33

Bromazepam

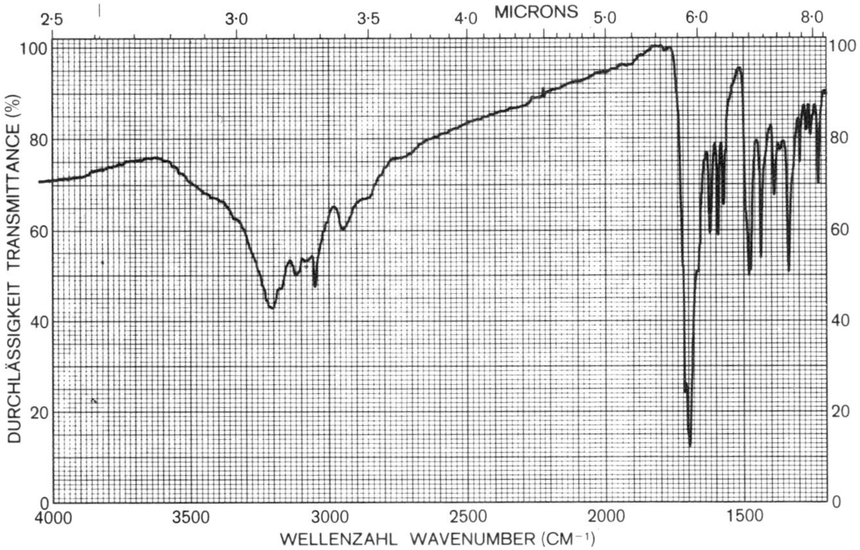

3-Hydroxy-Bromazepam | KURVE NR CURVE NO | KONZENTRATION CONC. 1mg/300mgKBr | GESCHWINDIGKEIT SCAN SPEED slow | BEARBEITER OPERATOR | SPALT SLIT N | DATUM DATE | NO.

HERKUNFT ORIGIN | LÖSUNGSMITTEL SOLVENT KBr | SCHICHTDICKE CELL PATH | VERGLEICH REFERENCE | BEMERKUNGEN REMARKS

Blumberg & Co. 4032 Lintorf W.-Germany Hoffmann Bergschenhoek Holland for Nr. 337-1203

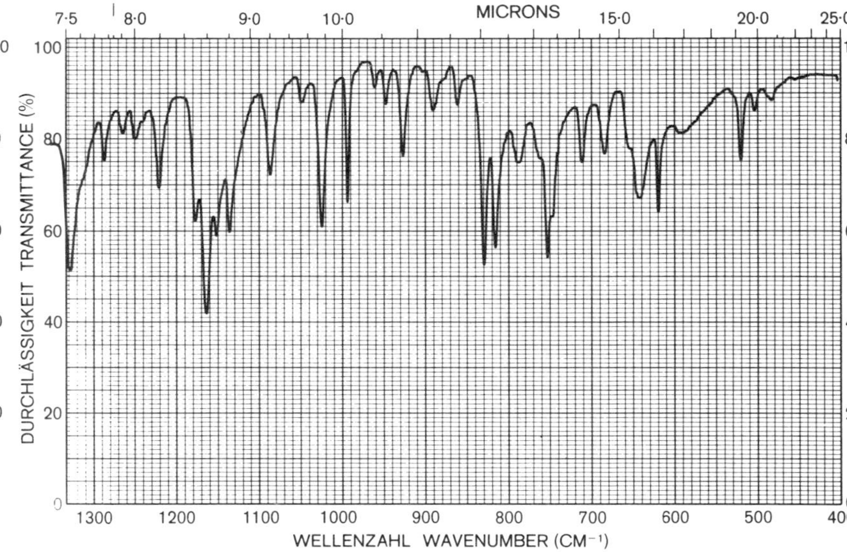

3-Hydroxy-Bromazepam | KURVE NR CURVE NO | KONZENTRATION CONC. 1mg/300mgKBr | GESCHWINDIGKEIT SCAN SPEED slow | BEARBEITER OPERATOR | SPALT SLIT N | DATUM DATE | NO.

HERKUNFT ORIGIN | LÖSUNGSMITTEL SOLVENT KBr | SCHICHTDICKE CELL PATH | VERGLEICH REFERENCE | BEMERKUNGEN REMARKS

Blumberg & Co. 4032 Lintorf W.-Germany Hoffmann Bergschenhoek Holland for Nr. 337-1204

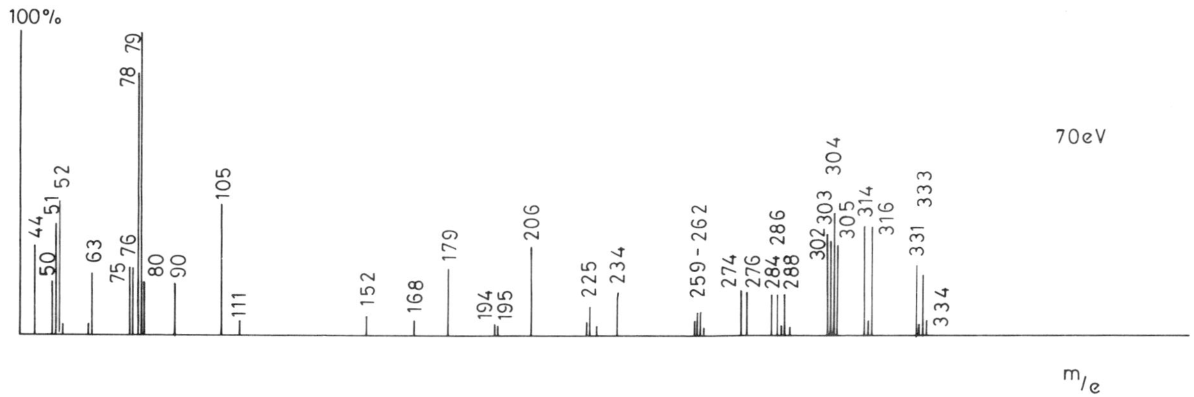

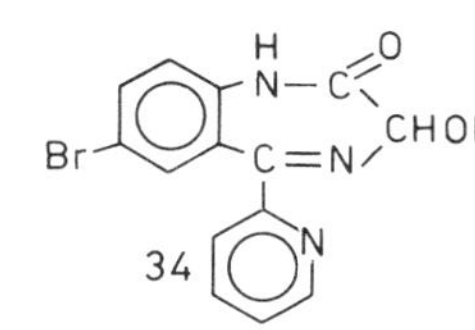

34

3-Hydroxy-Bromazepam

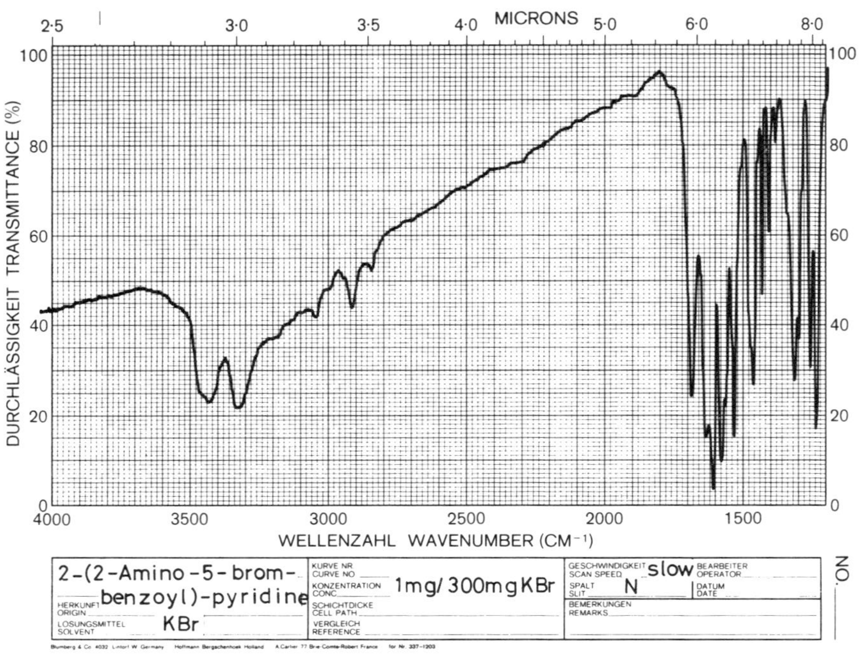

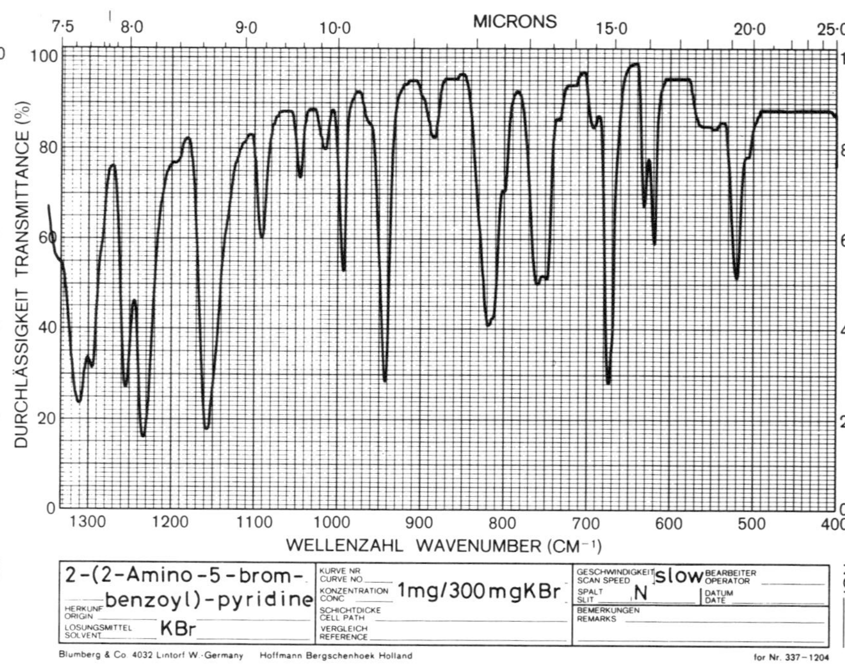

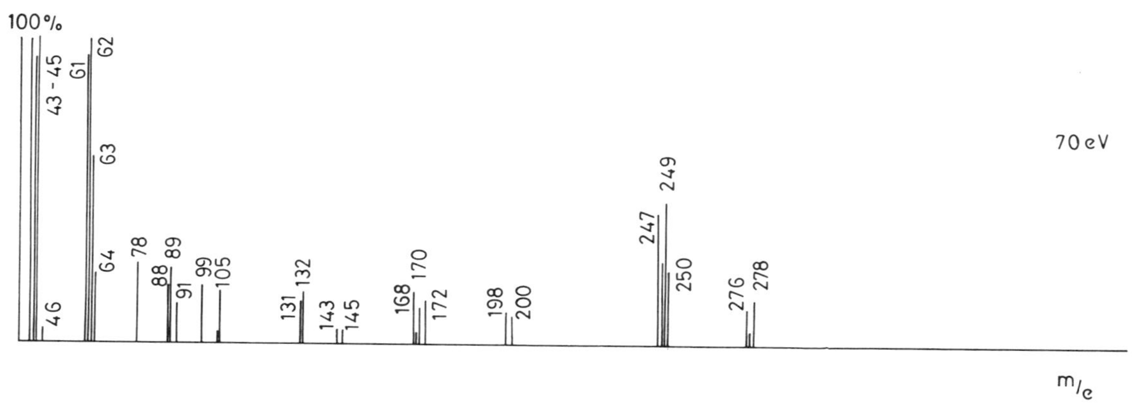

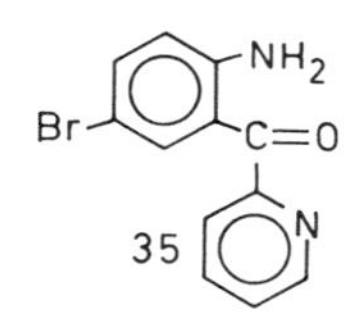

35

2-(2-Amino-5-brom-benzoyl)-pyridine

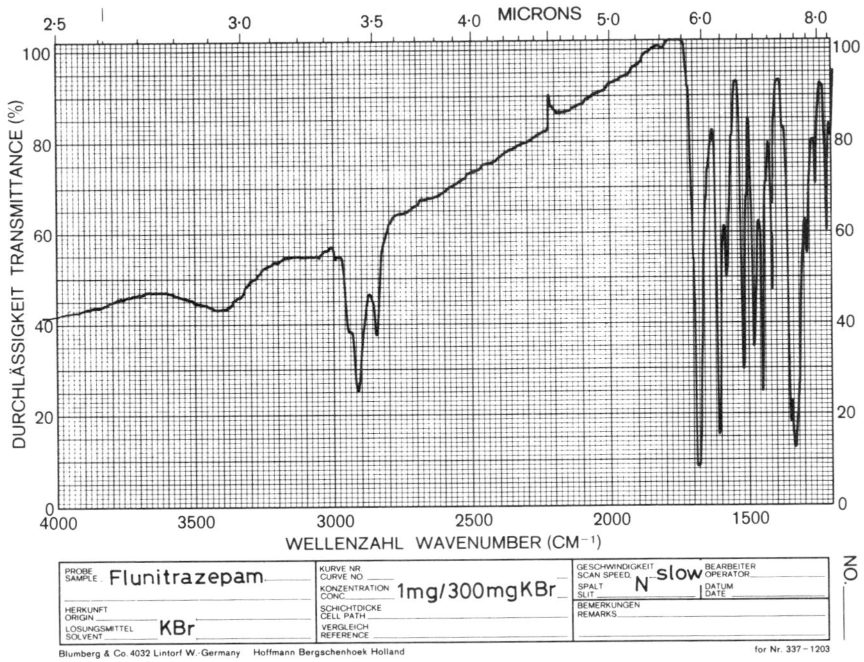

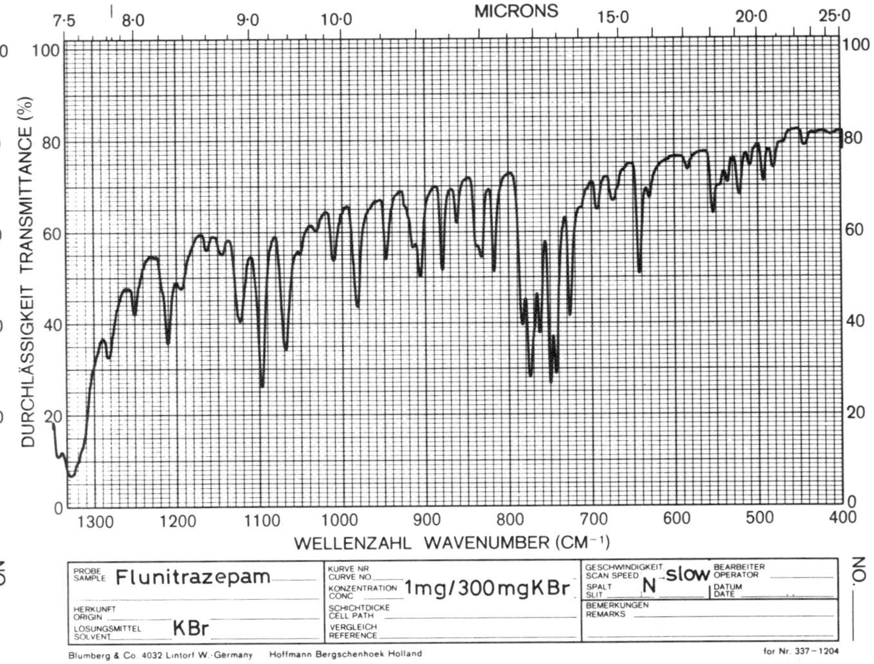

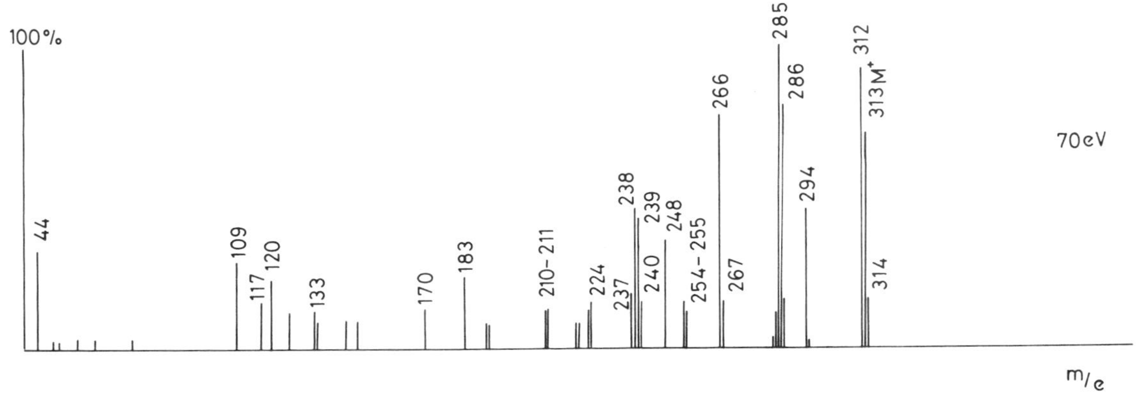

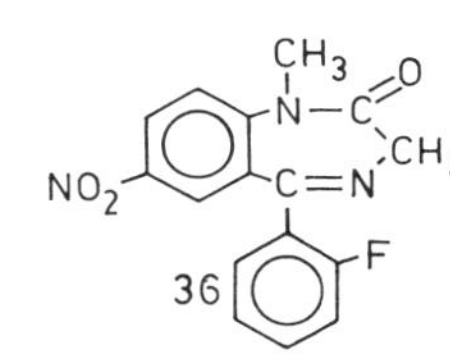

Flunitrazepam

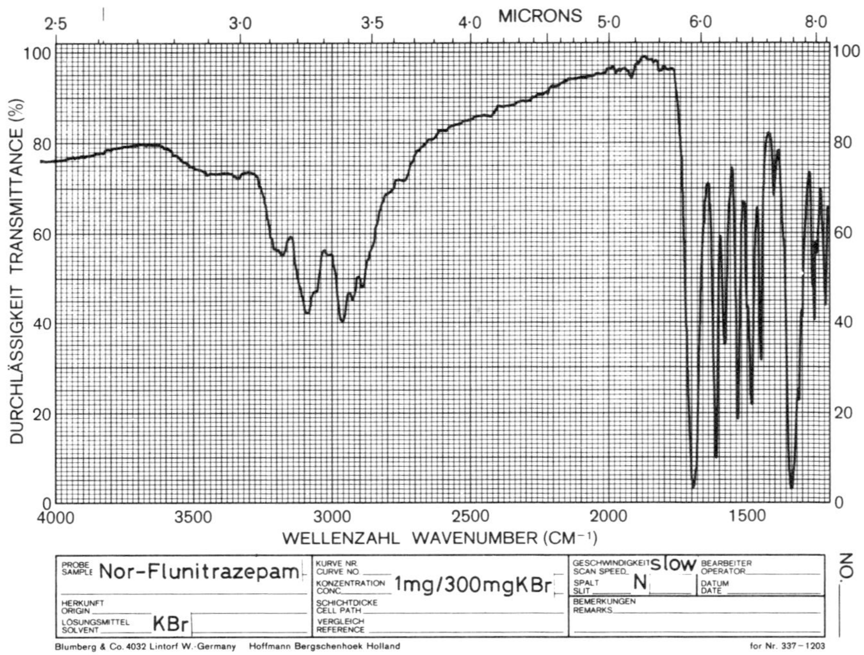

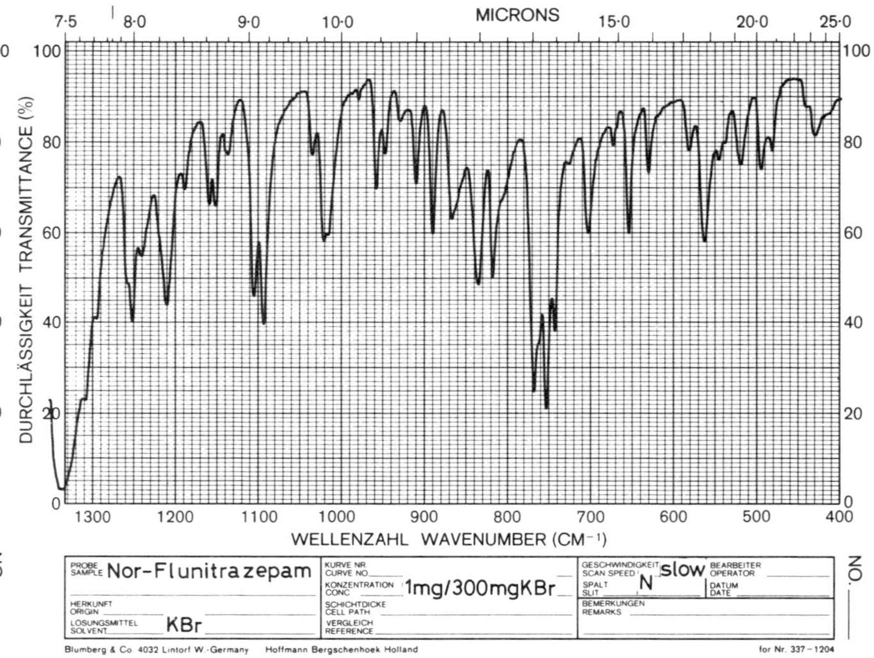

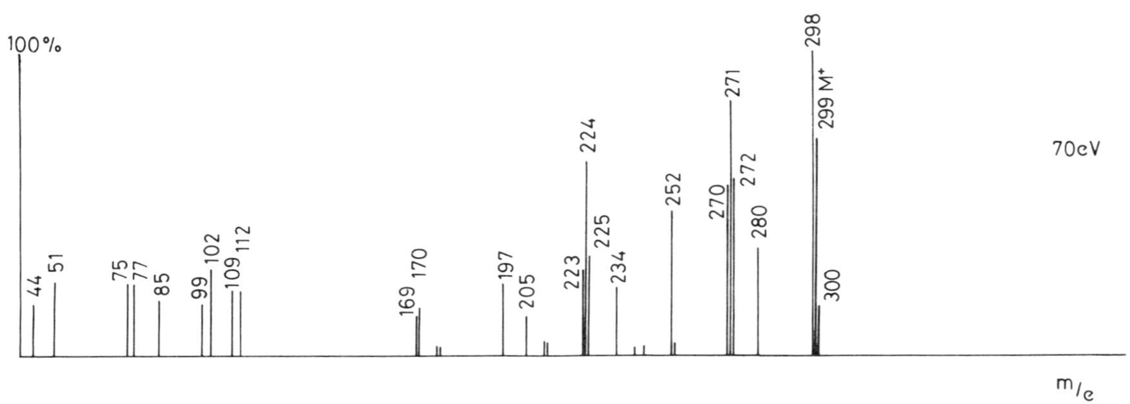

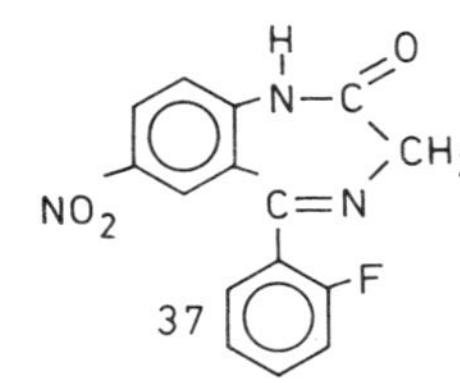

Nor-Flunitrazepam

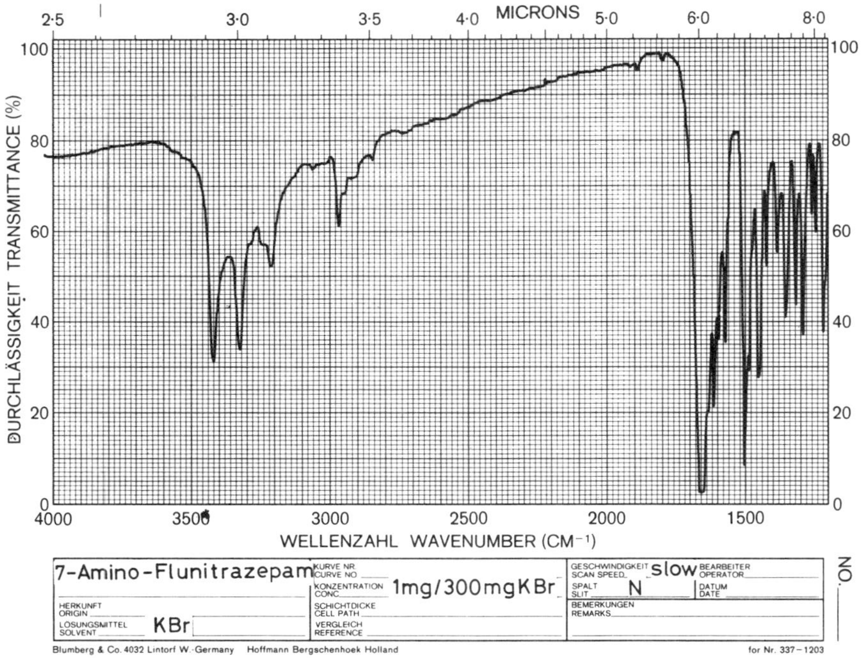

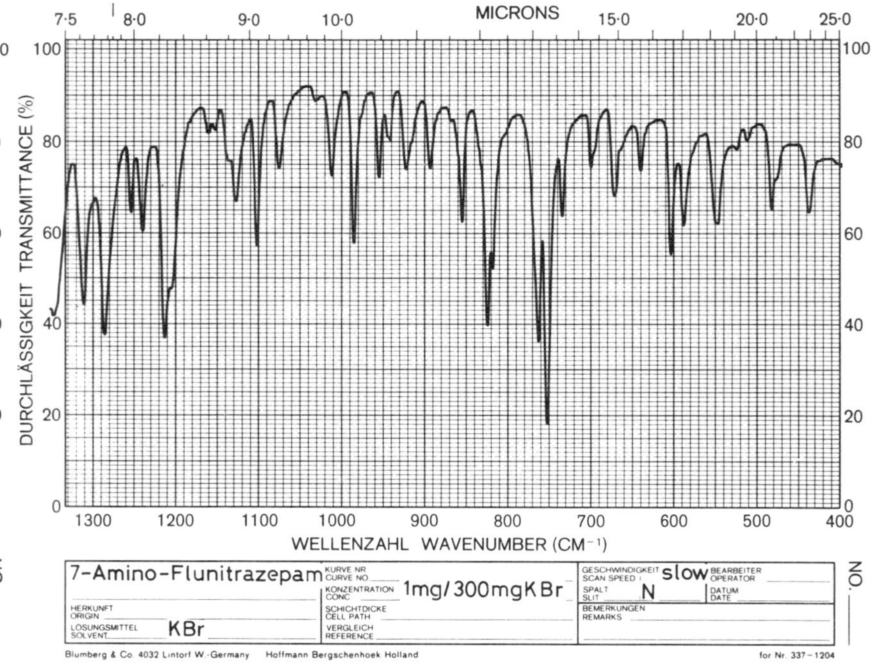

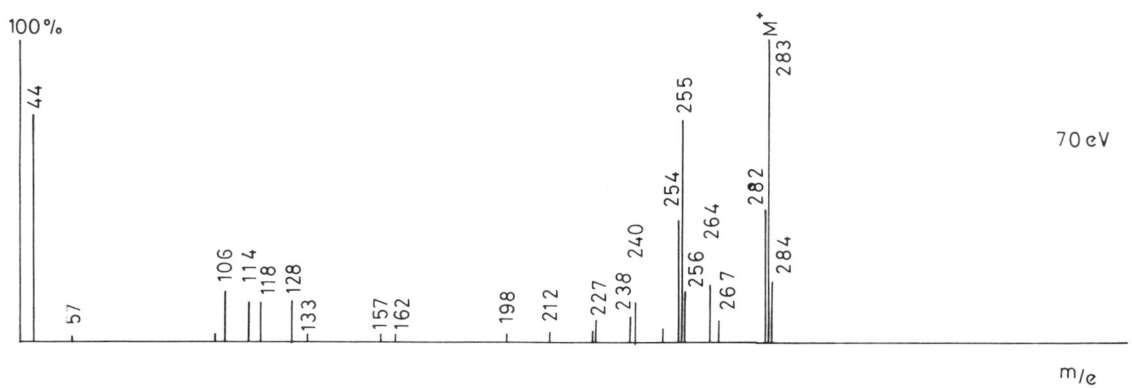

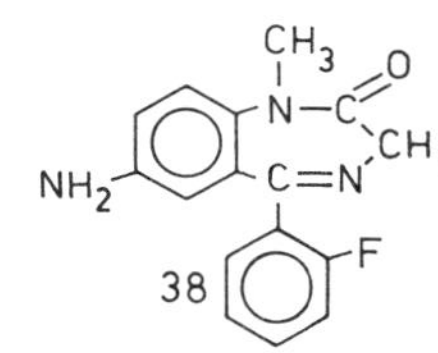

7-Amino-Flunitrazepam

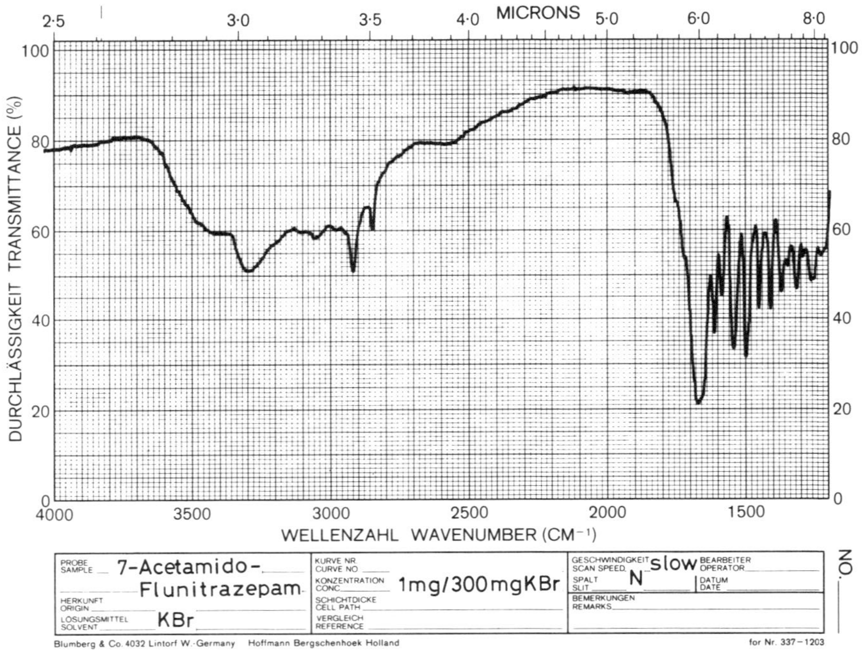

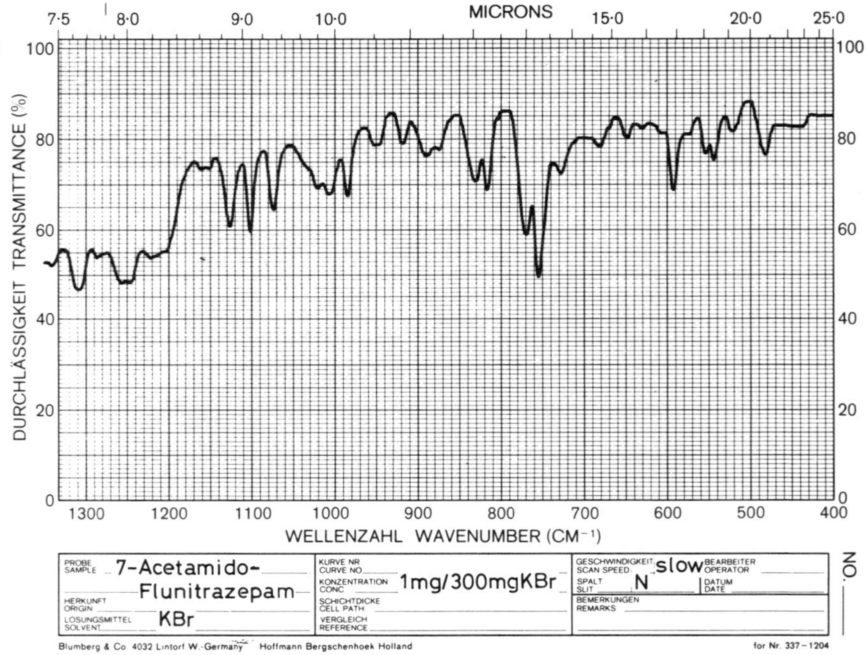

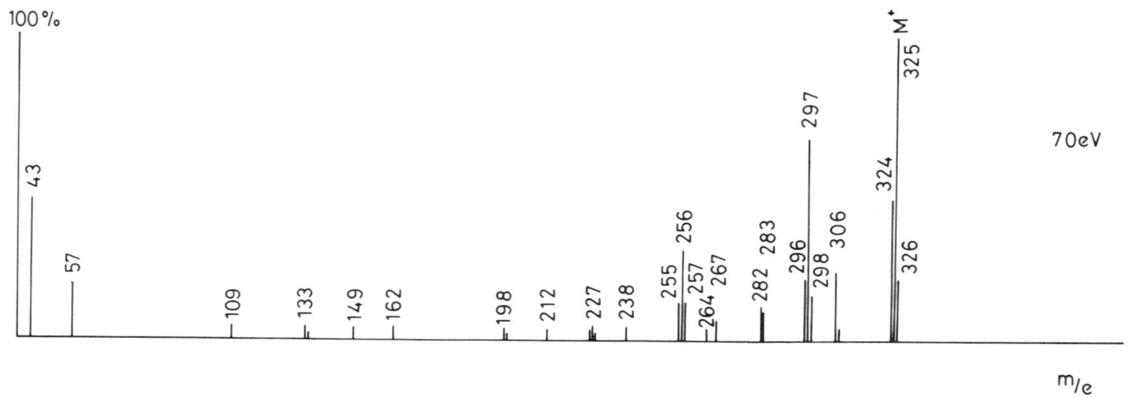

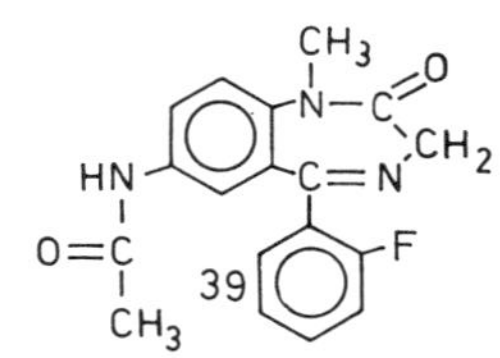

7-Acetamido-Flunitrazepam

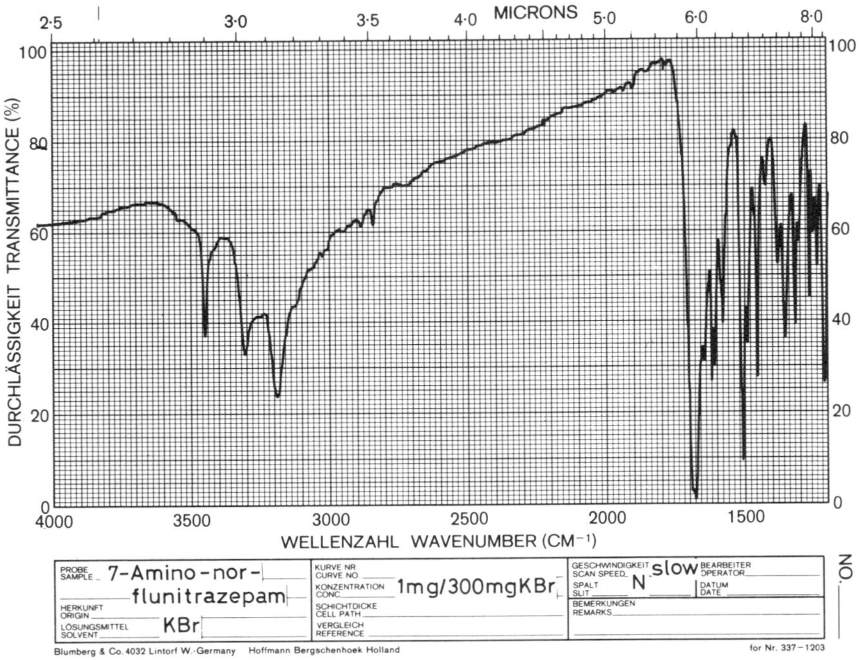

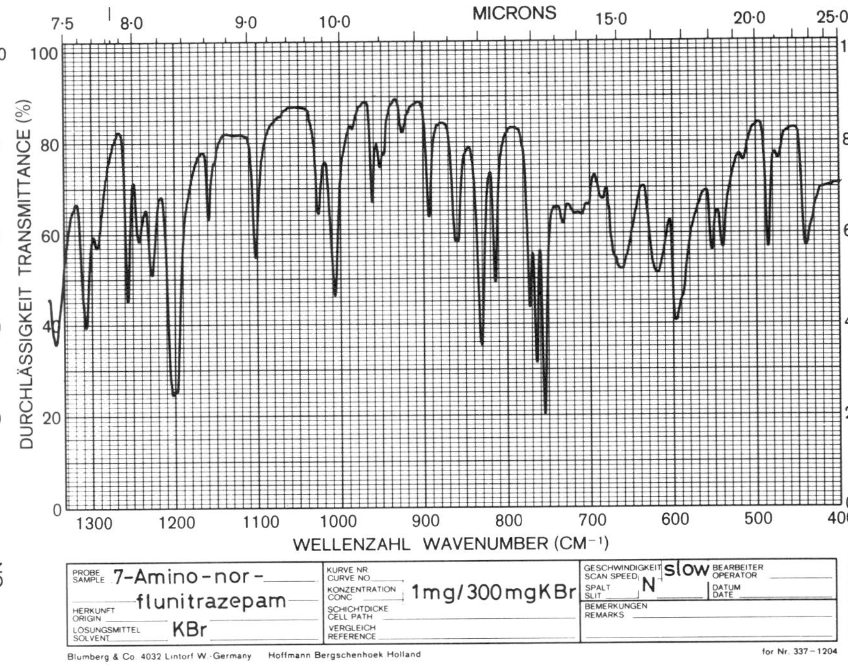

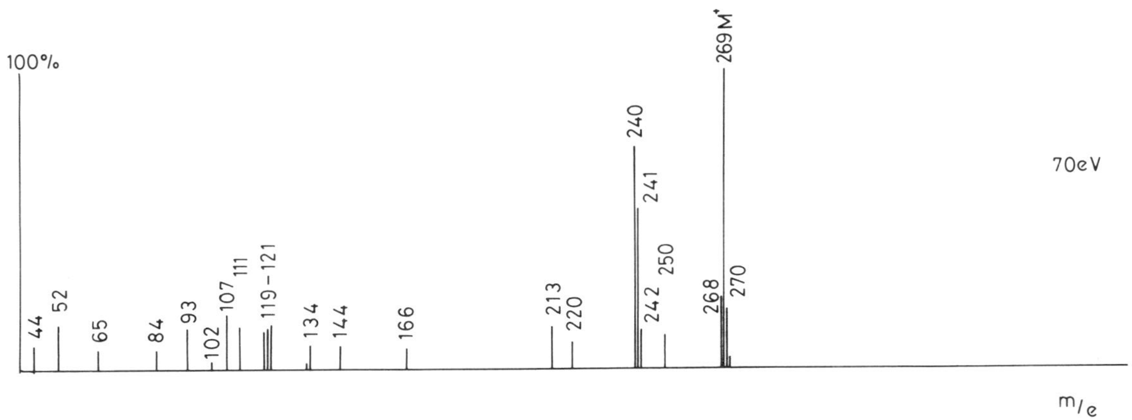

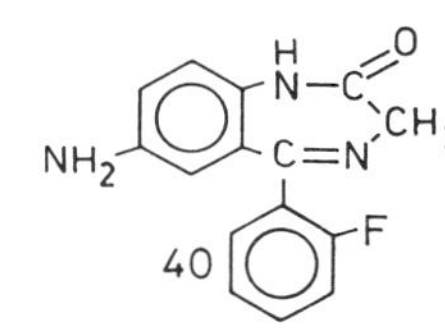

7-Amino-Nor-Flunitrazepam

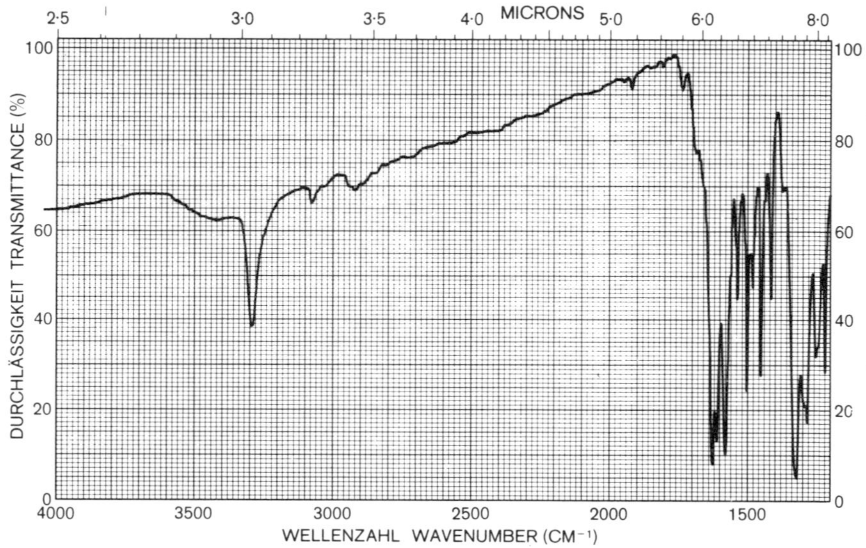

2-Methylamino-5-nitro-2'-fluor-benzophenone
KURVE NR / CURVE NO
KONZENTRATION / CONC. 1mg/300mgKBr
SCHICHTDICKE / CELL PATH
VERGLEICH / REFERENCE
LÖSUNGSMITTEL / SOLVENT KBr
GESCHWINDIGKEIT / SCAN SPEED slow
SPALT / SLIT N
BEARBEITER / OPERATOR
DATUM / DATE
BEMERKUNGEN / REMARKS
NO.

Blumberg & Co. 4032 Lintorf W.-Germany Hoffmann Bergschenhoek Holland for Nr. 337–1203

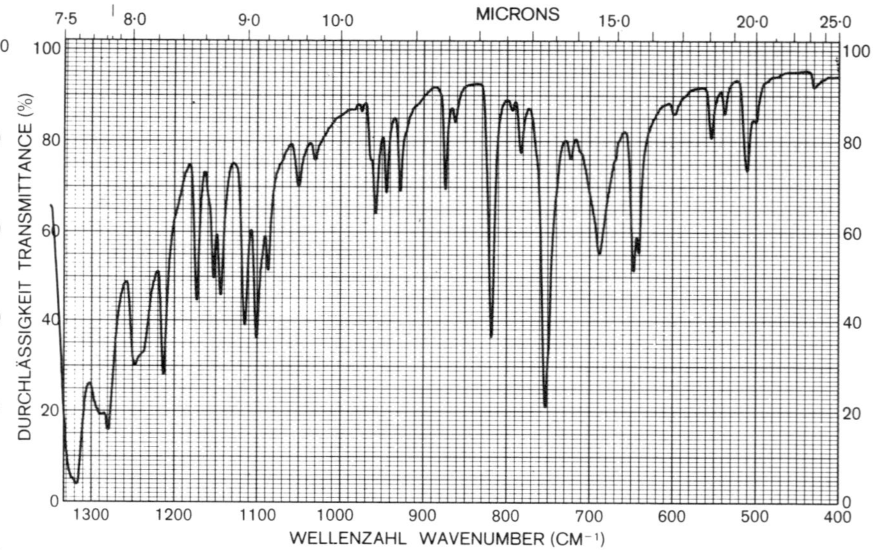

2-Methylamino-5-nitro-2'-fluor-benzophenone
KURVE NR / CURVE NO
KONZENTRATION / CONC. 1mg/300mgKBr
SCHICHTDICKE / CELL PATH
VERGLEICH / REFERENCE
LÖSUNGSMITTEL / SOLVENT KBr
GESCHWINDIGKEIT / SCAN SPEED slow
SPALT / SLIT N
BEARBEITER / OPERATOR
DATUM / DATE
BEMERKUNGEN / REMARKS
NO.

Blumberg & Co. 4032 Lintorf W.-Germany Hoffmann Bergschenhoek Holland for Nr. 337–1204

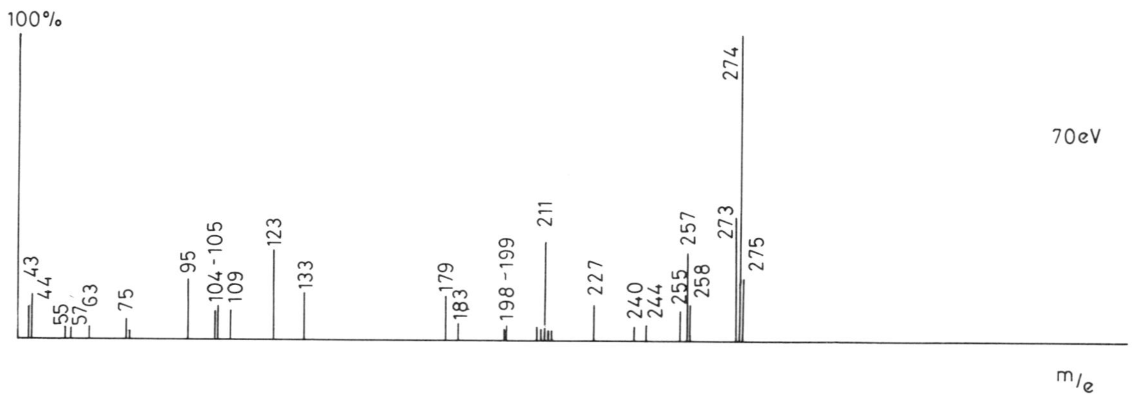

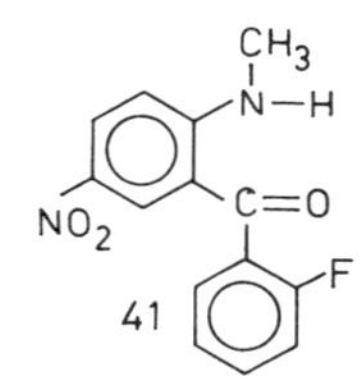

41

2-Methylamino-5-nitro-2'-fluor-benzophenone

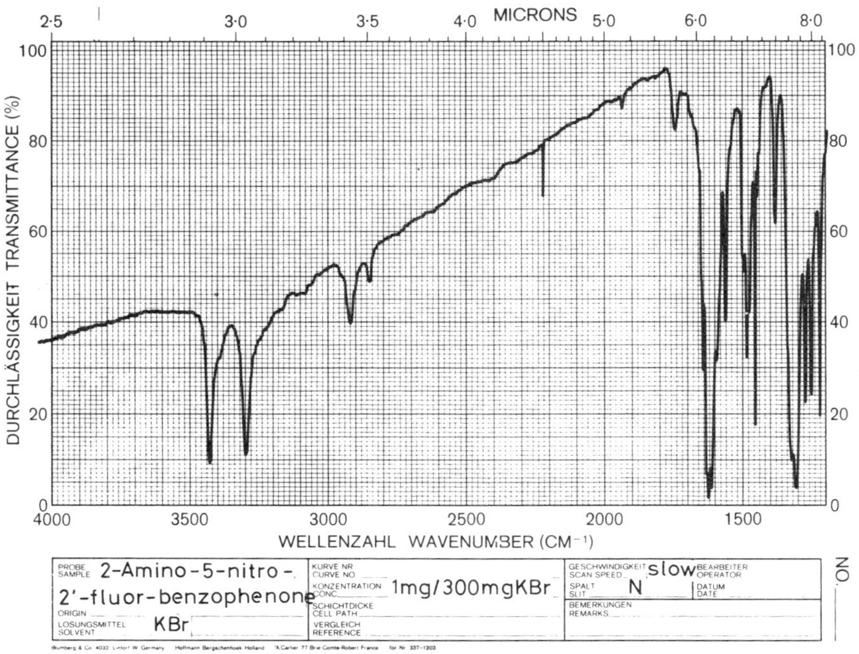

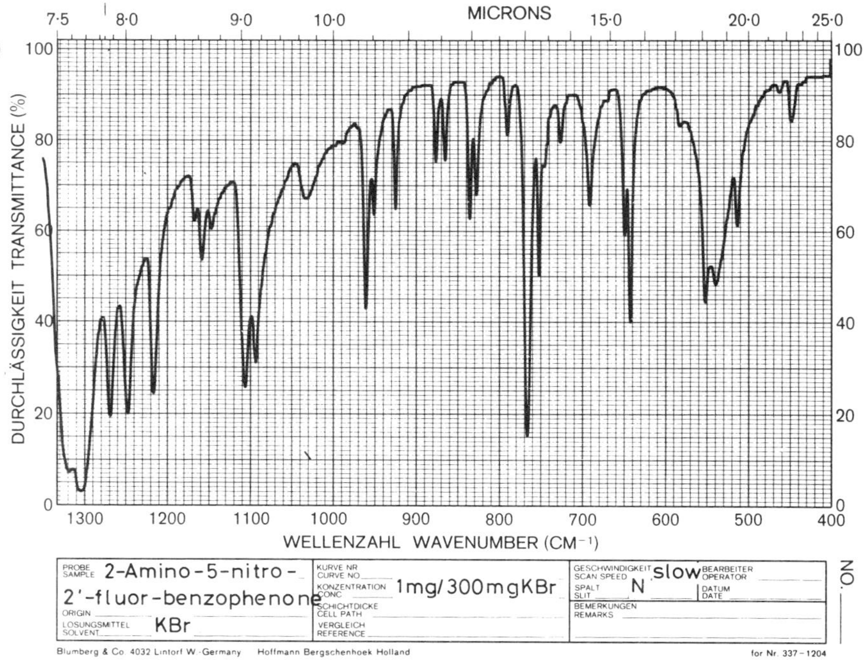

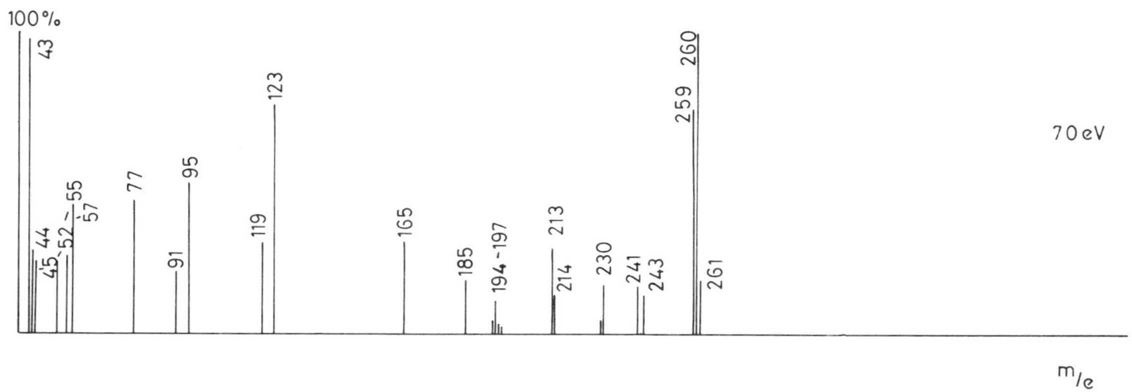

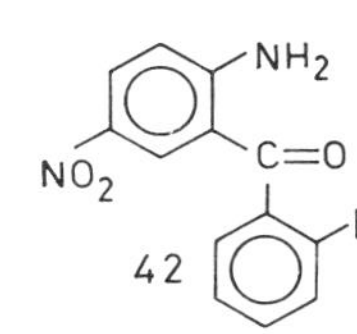

42

2-Amino-5-nitro-2'-fluor-benzophenone

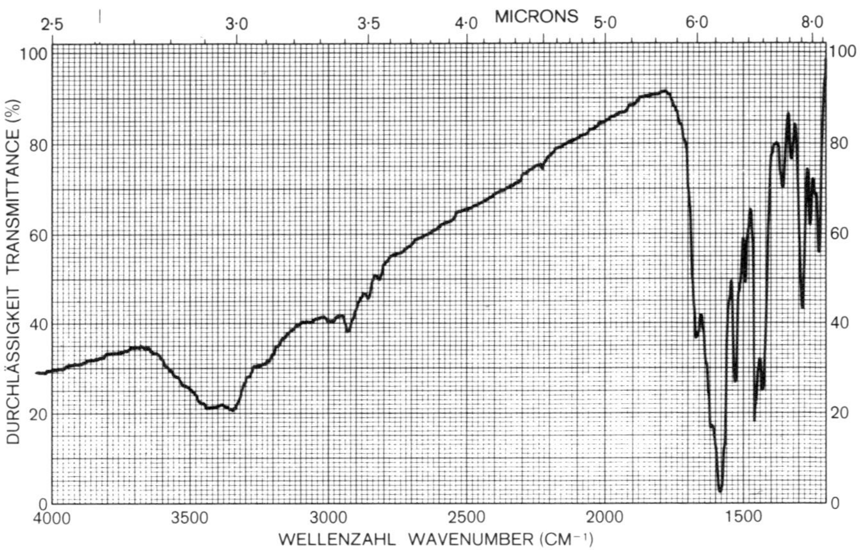

2-Methylamino-5-amino-2'-fluor-benzophenone

KURVE NR / CURVE NO	GESCHWINDIGKEIT / SCAN SPEED: slow	BEARBEITER / OPERATOR
KONZENTRATION / CONC: 1mg/300mgKBr	SPALT / SLIT: N	DATUM / DATE
SCHICHTDICKE / CELL PATH	BEMERKUNGEN / REMARKS	
LÖSUNGSMITTEL / SOLVENT: KBr	VERGLEICH / REFERENCE	

NO. \

Blumberg & Co. 4032 Lintorf W. Germany Hoffmann Bergschenhoek Holland A. Carter 77 Brie-Comte-Robert France for Nr. 337-1203

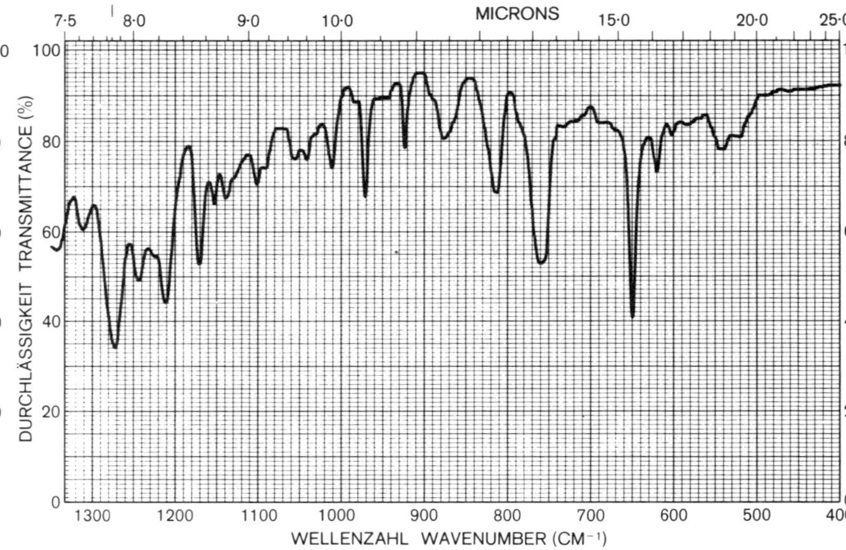

2-Methylamino-5-amino-2'-fluor-benzophenone

KURVE NR / CURVE NO	GESCHWINDIGKEIT / SCAN SPEED: slow	BEARBEITER / OPERATOR
KONZENTRATION / CONC: 1mg/300mgKBr	SPALT / SLIT: N	DATUM / DATE
SCHICHTDICKE / CELL PATH	BEMERKUNGEN / REMARKS	
LÖSUNGSMITTEL / SOLVENT: KBr	VERGLEICH / REFERENCE	

NO.

Blumberg & Co. 4032 Lintorf W.-Germany Hoffmann Bergschenhoek Holland for Nr. 337-1204

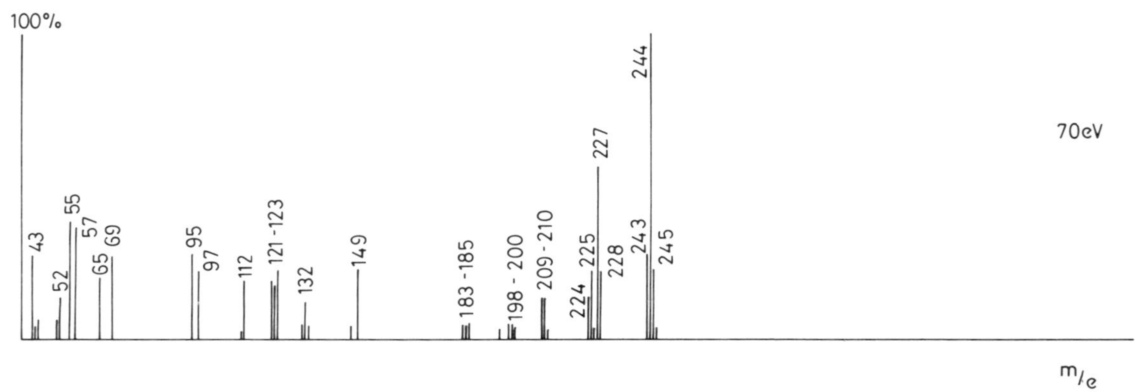

70eV

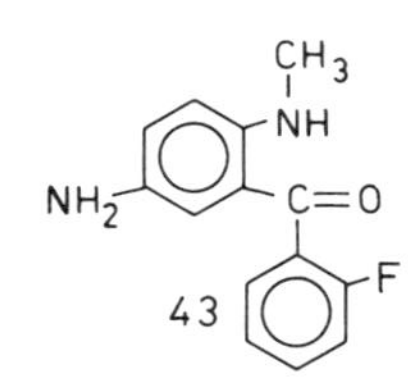

2-Methylamino-5-amino-2'-fluor-benzophenone

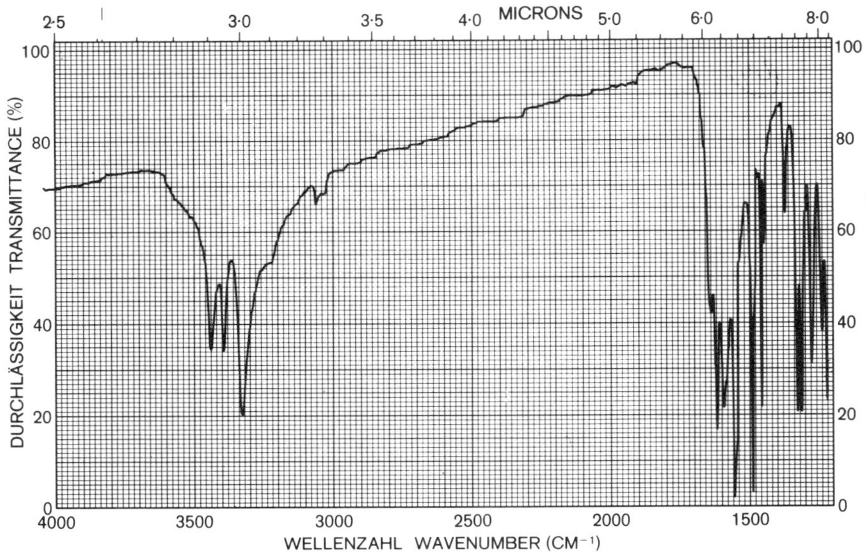

NO.

2,5-Diamino-2'-fluor-benzophenone

HERKUNFT ORIGIN

LÖSUNGSMITTEL SOLVENT KBr

KURVE NR CURVE NO

KONZENTRATION CONC 1mg/300mgKBr

SCHICHTDICKE CELL PATH

VERGLEICH REFERENCE

GESCHWINDIGKEIT SCAN SPEED slow

SPALT SLIT N

BEARBEITER OPERATOR

DATUM DATE

BEMERKUNGEN REMARKS

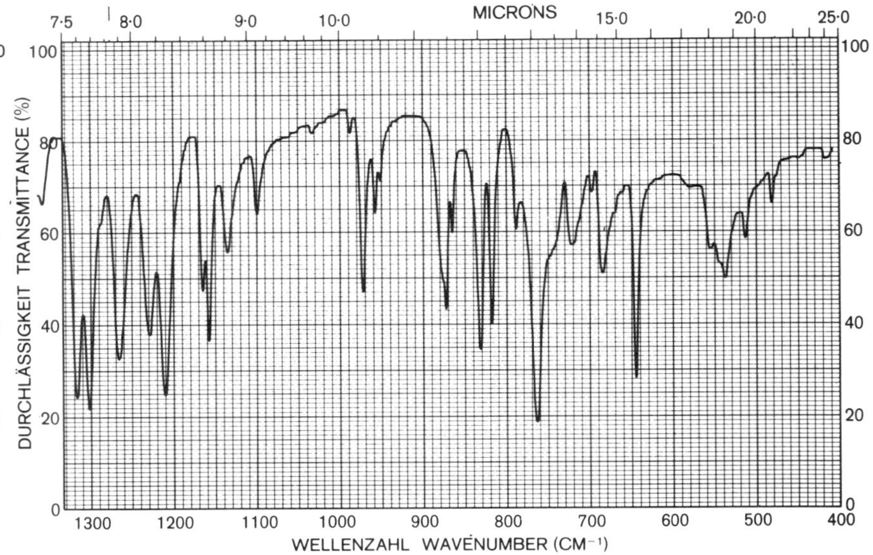

NO.

2,5-Diamino-2'-fluor-benzophenone

HERKUNFT ORIGIN

LÖSUNGSMITTEL SOLVENT KBr

KURVE NR CURVE NO

KONZENTRATION CONC 1mg/300mgKBr

SCHICHTDICKE CELL PATH

VERGLEICH REFERENCE

GESCHWINDIGKEIT SCAN SPEED slow

SPALT SLIT N

BEARBEITER OPERATOR

DATUM DATE

BEMERKUNGEN REMARKS

Blumberg & Co 4032 Lintorf W-Germany Hoffmann Bergschenhoek Holland for Nr. 337-1204

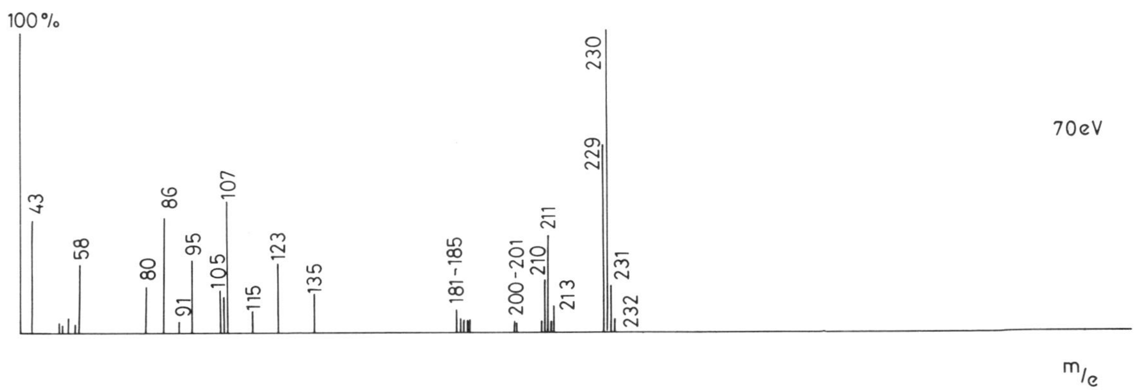

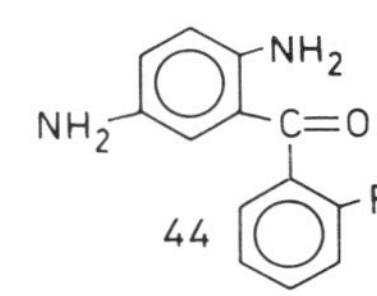

2,5-Diamino-2'-fluor-benzophenone

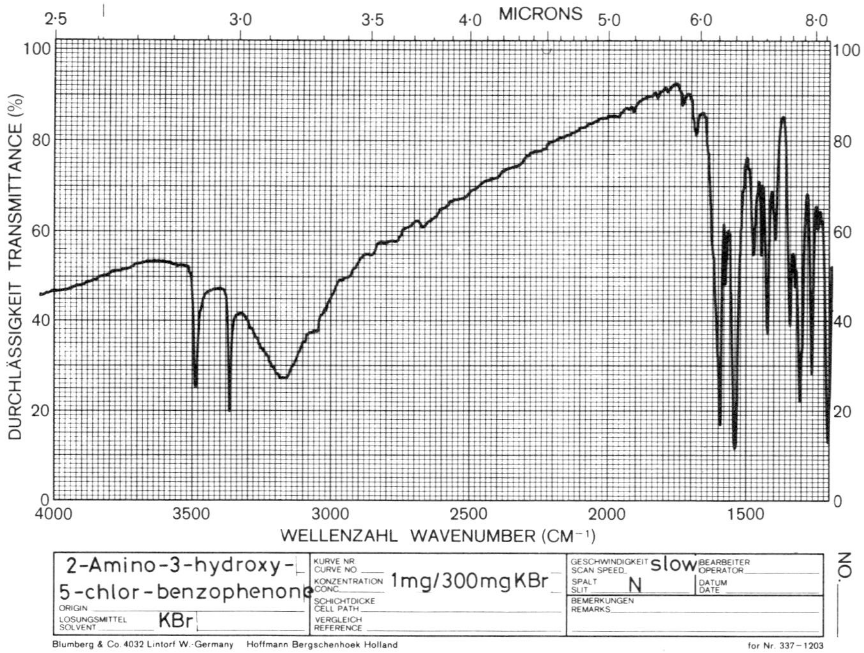

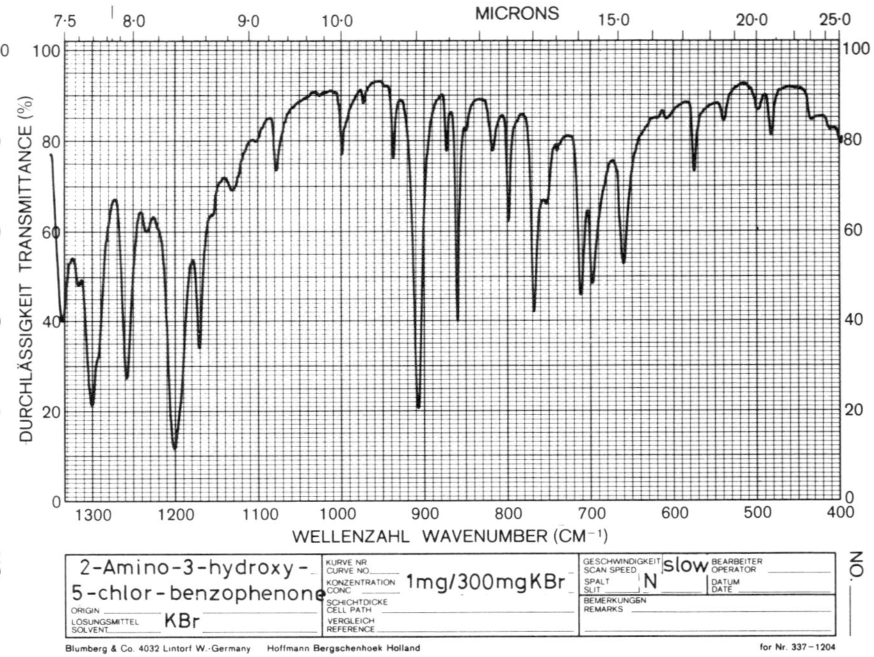

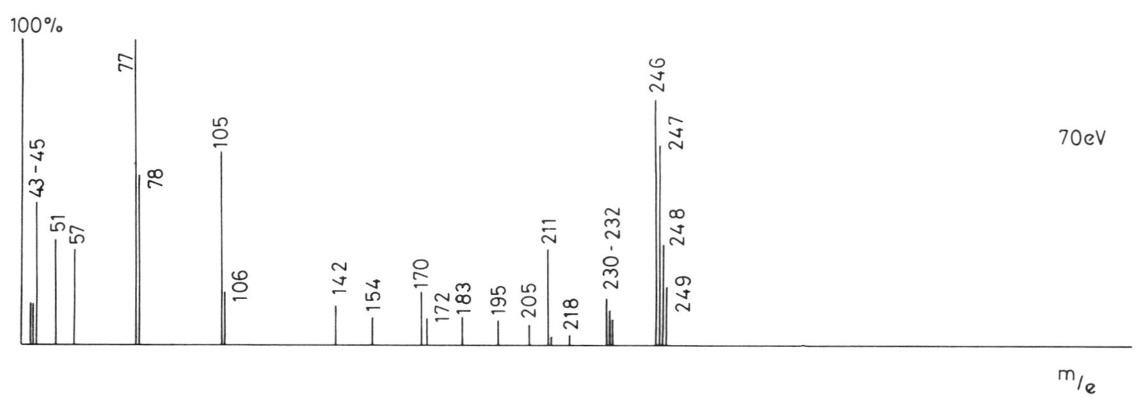

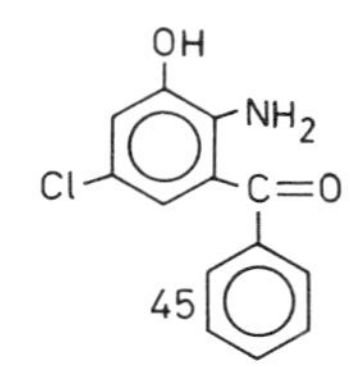

2-Amino-3-hydroxy-5-chlor-benzophenone

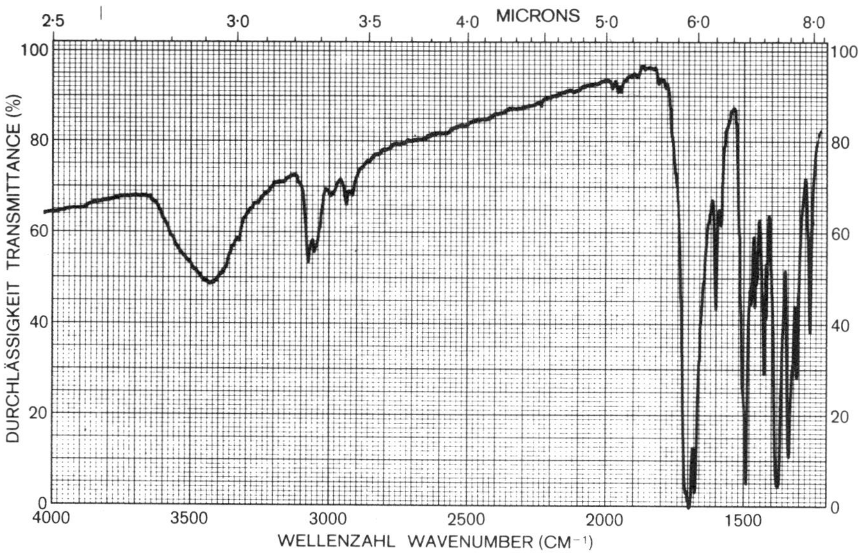

PROBE SAMPLE Clobazam
HERKUNFT ORIGIN
LÖSUNGSMITTEL SOLVENT KBr
KURVE NR CURVE NO
KONZENTRATION CONC 1mg/300mgKBr
SCHICHTDICKE CELL PATH
VERGLEICH REFERENCE
GESCHWINDIGKEIT SCAN SPEED slow
SPALT SLIT N
BEARBEITER OPERATOR
DATUM DATE
BEMERKUNGEN REMARKS
NO.

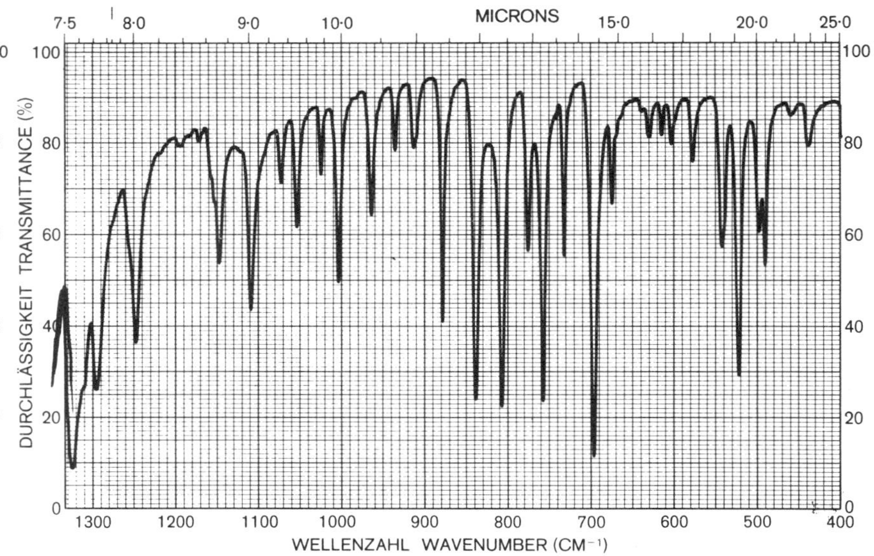

PROBE SAMPLE Clobazam
HERKUNFT ORIGIN
LÖSUNGSMITTEL SOLVENT KBr
KURVE NR CURVE NO
KONZENTRATION CONC 1mg/300mgKBr
SCHICHTDICKE CELL PATH
VERGLEICH REFERENCE
GESCHWINDIGKEIT SCAN SPEED slow
SPALT SLIT N
BEARBEITER OPERATOR
DATUM DATE
BEMERKUNGEN REMARKS
NO.

Blumberg & Co 4032 Lintorf W·Germany Hoffmann Bergschenhoek Holland for Nr. 337-1204

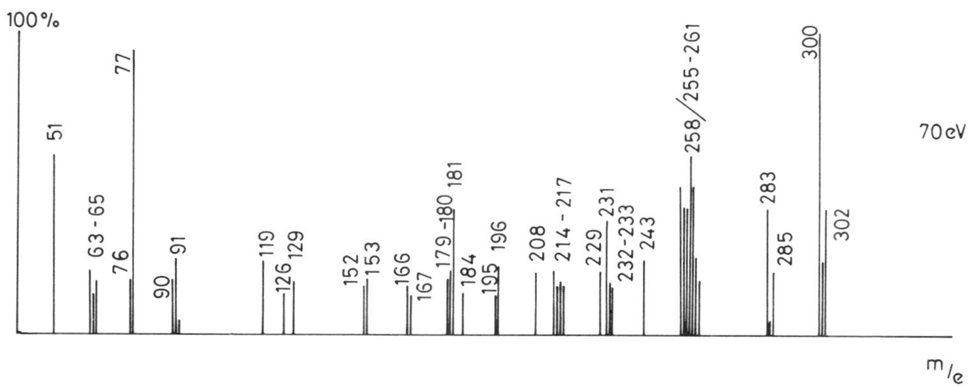

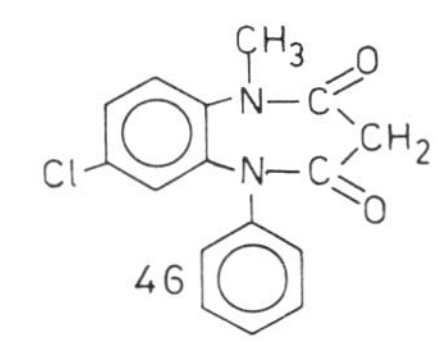

Clobazam

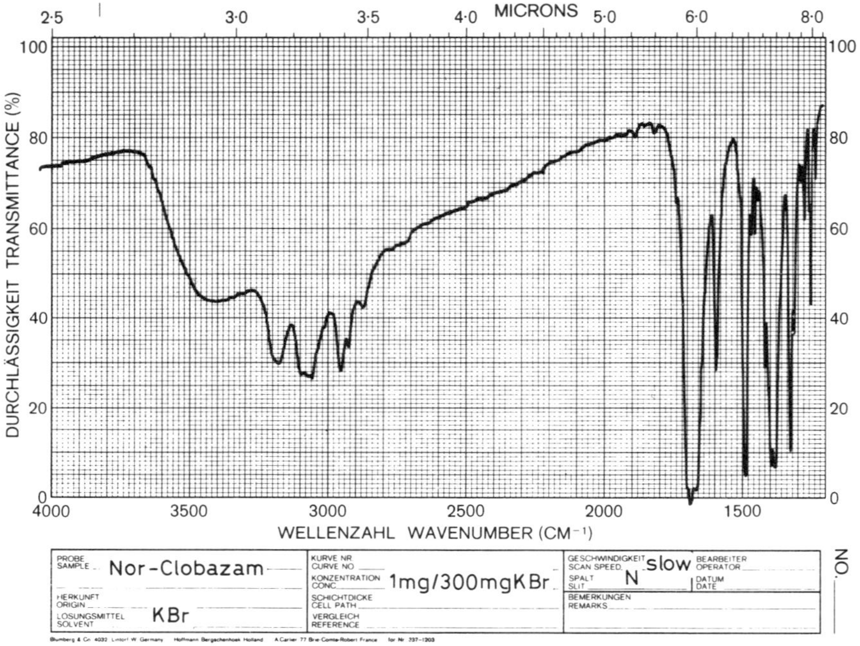

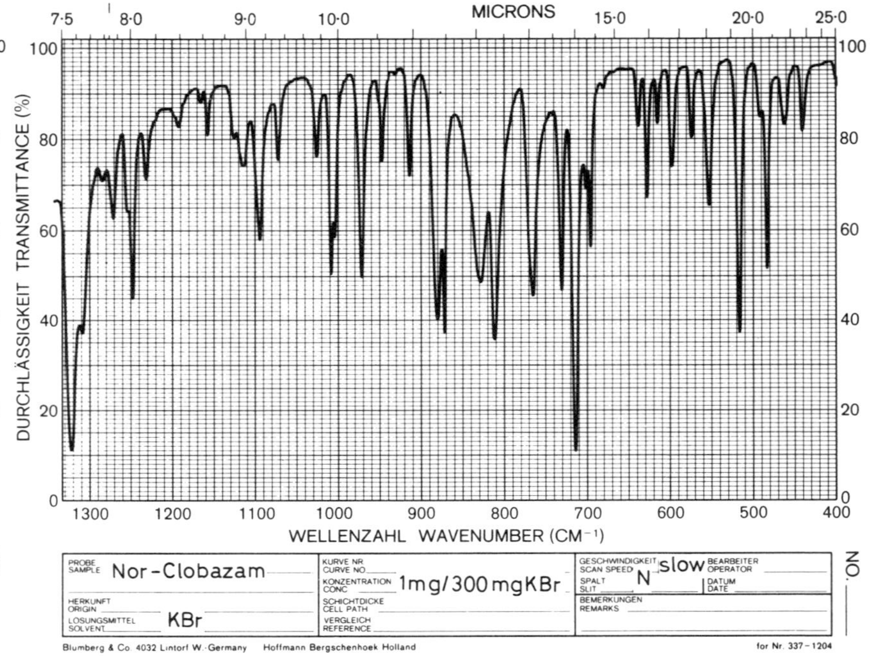

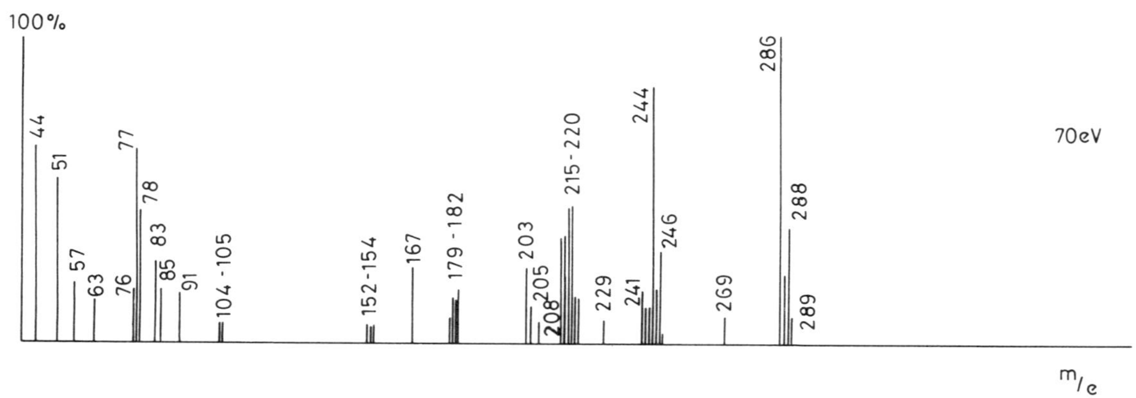

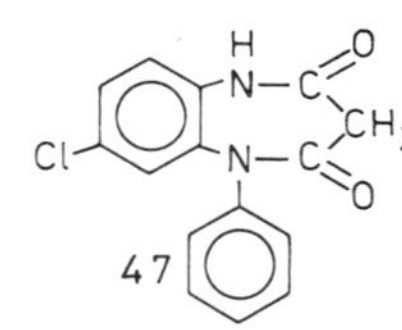

Nor-Clobazam

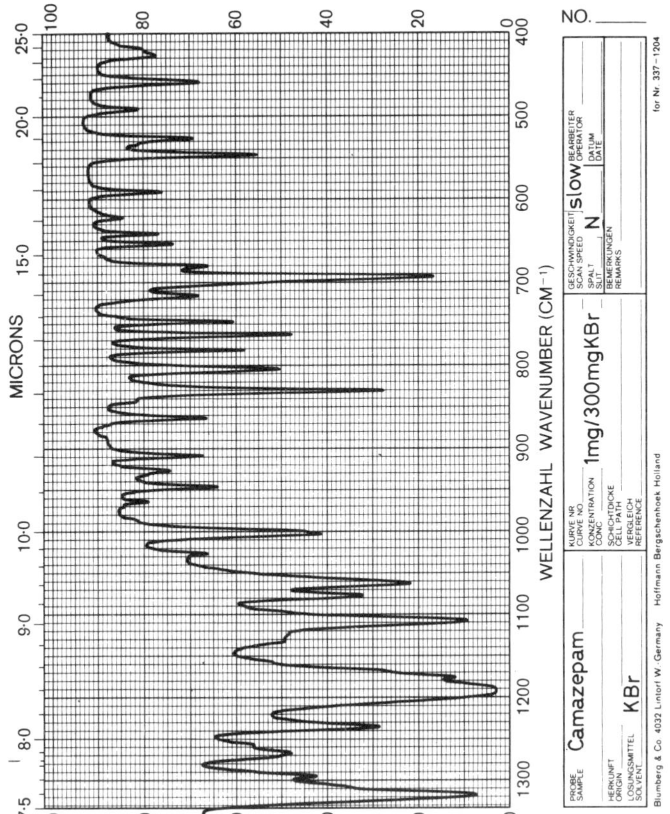

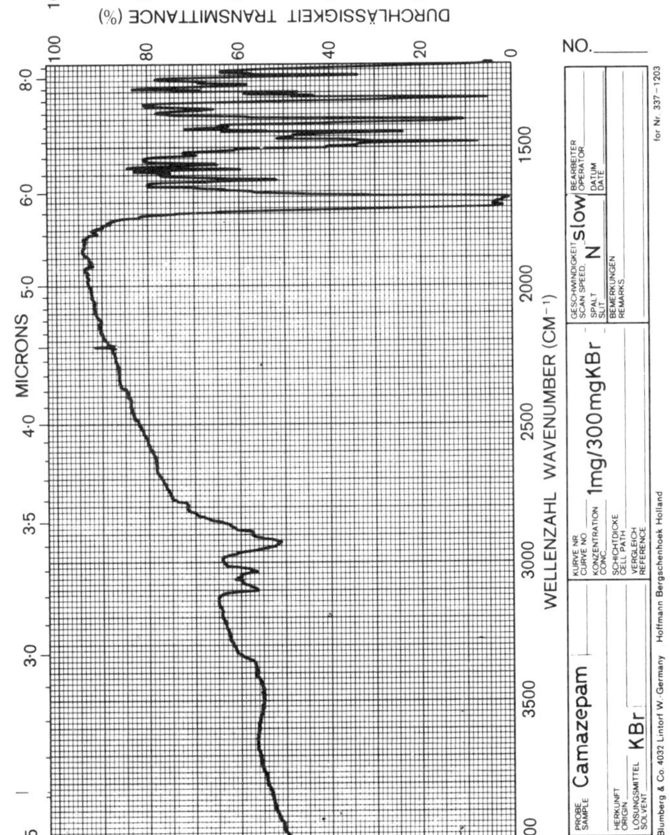

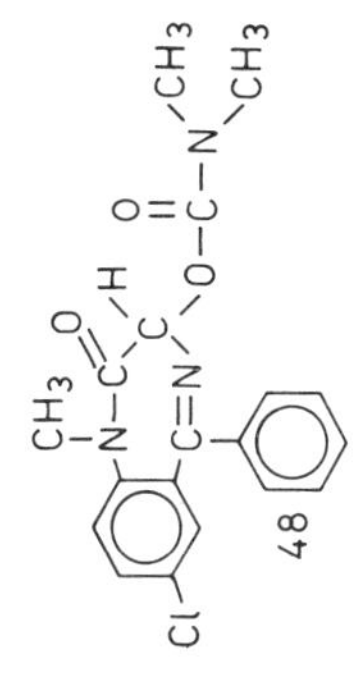

48

Camazepam

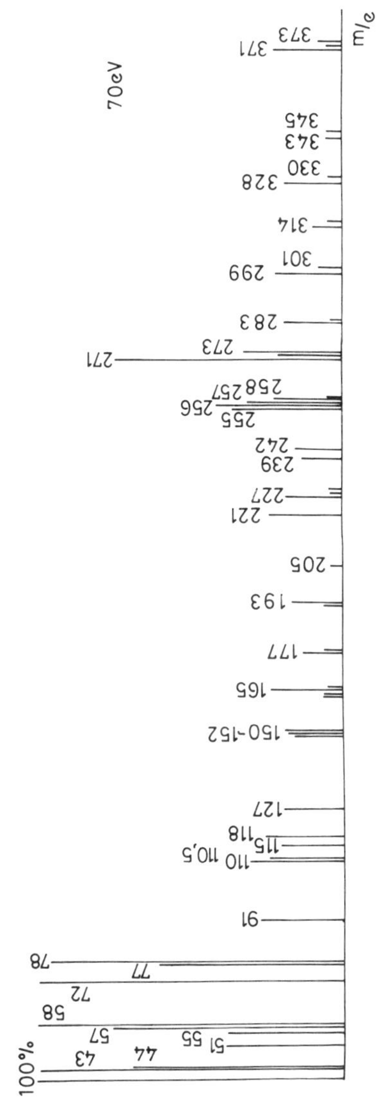

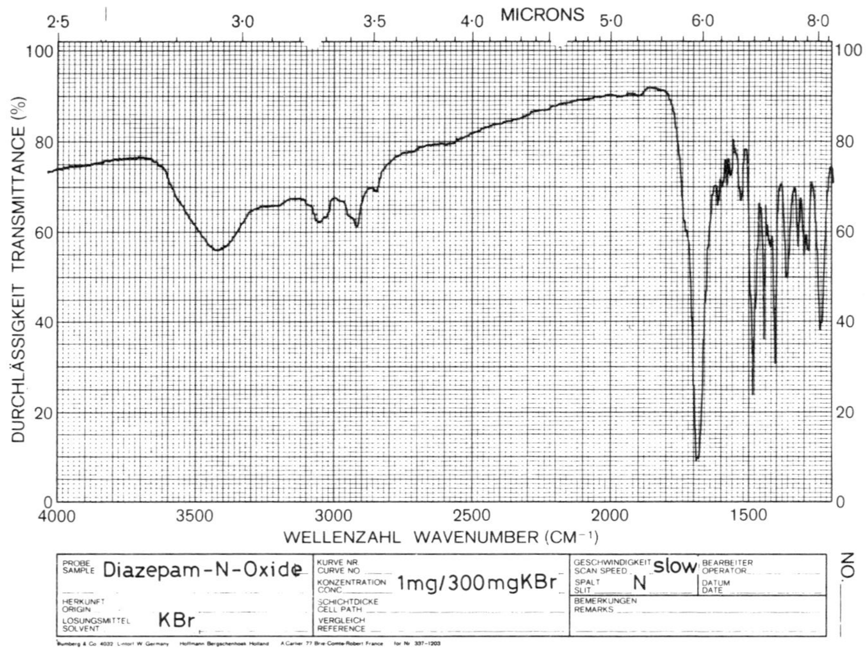

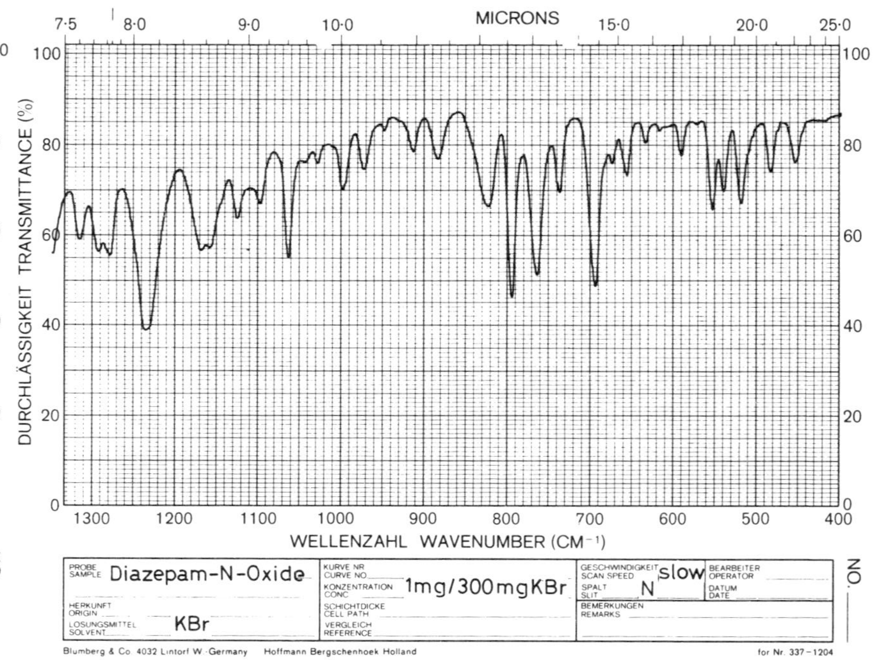

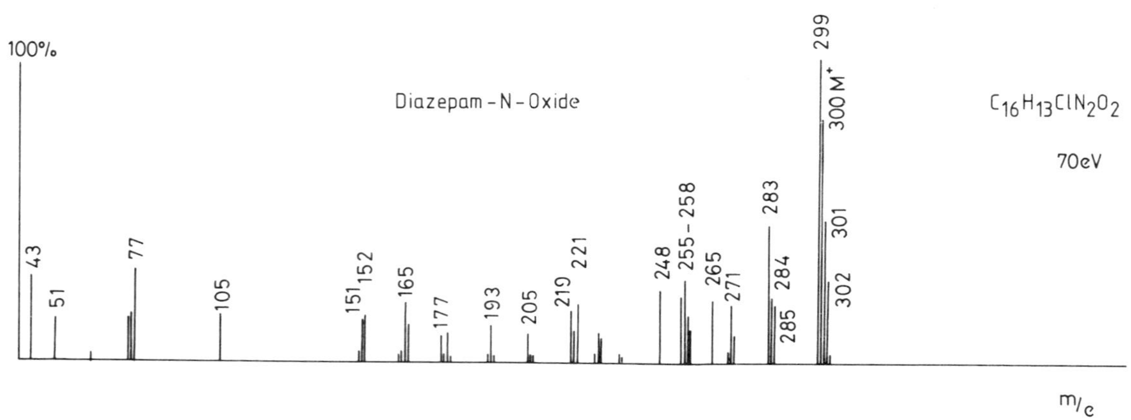

$C_{16}H_{13}ClN_2O_2$

70eV

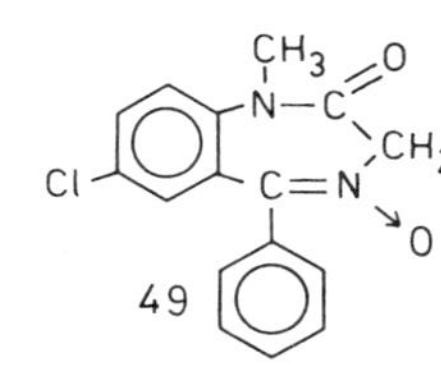

Diazepam-N-Oxide

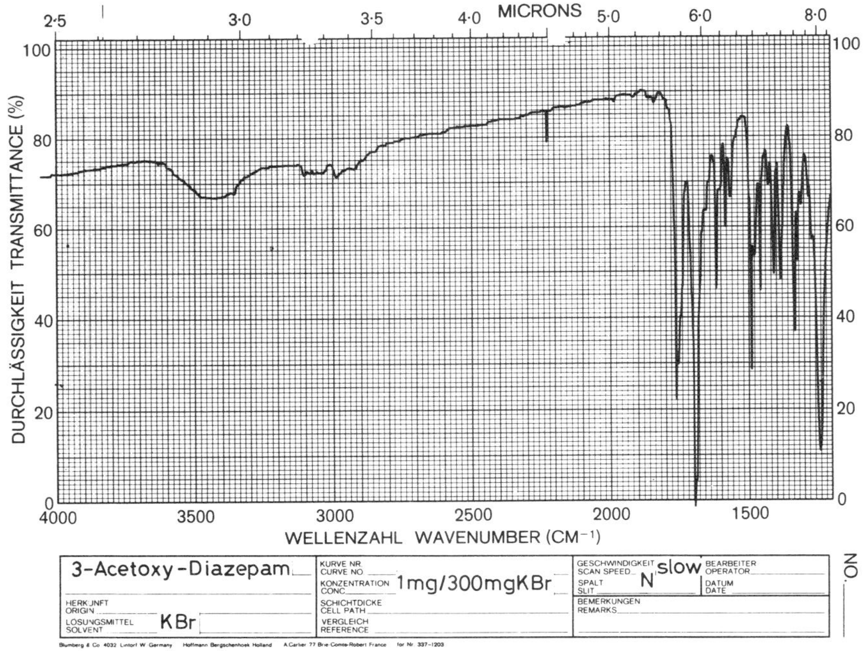

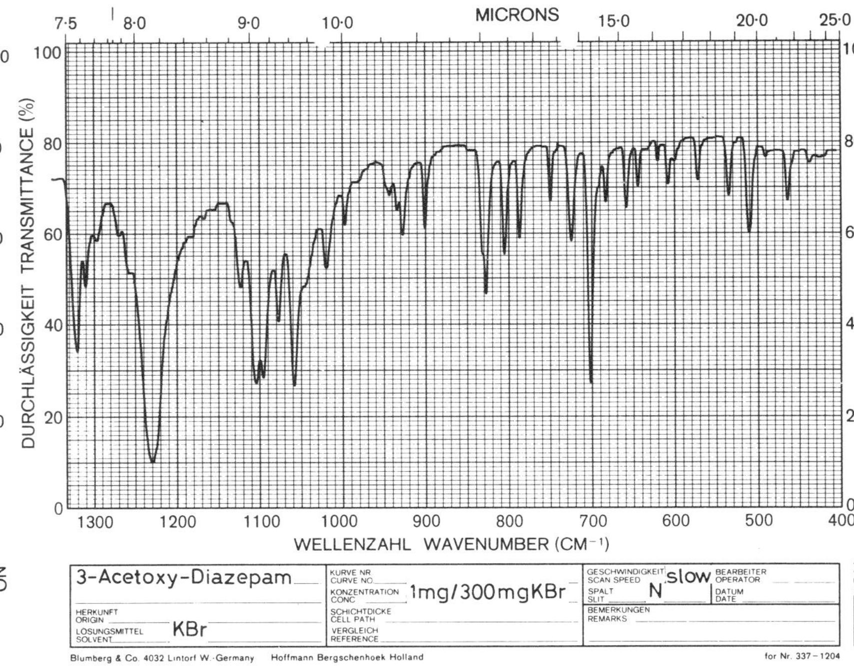

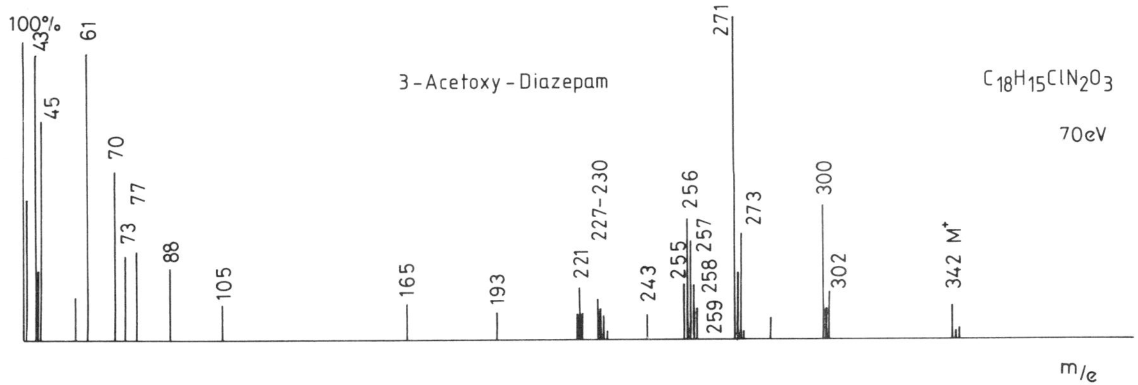

3-Acetoxy-Diazepam

$C_{18}H_{15}ClN_2O_3$

70eV

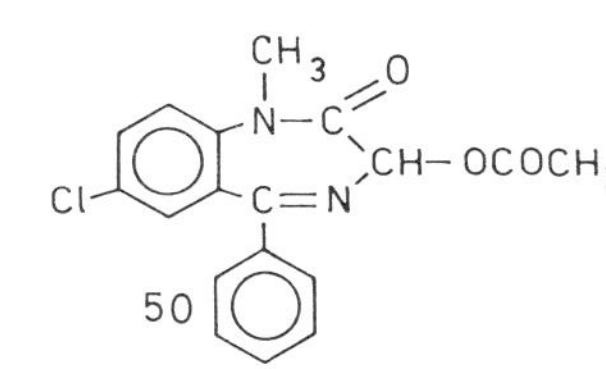

3-Acetoxy-Diazepam

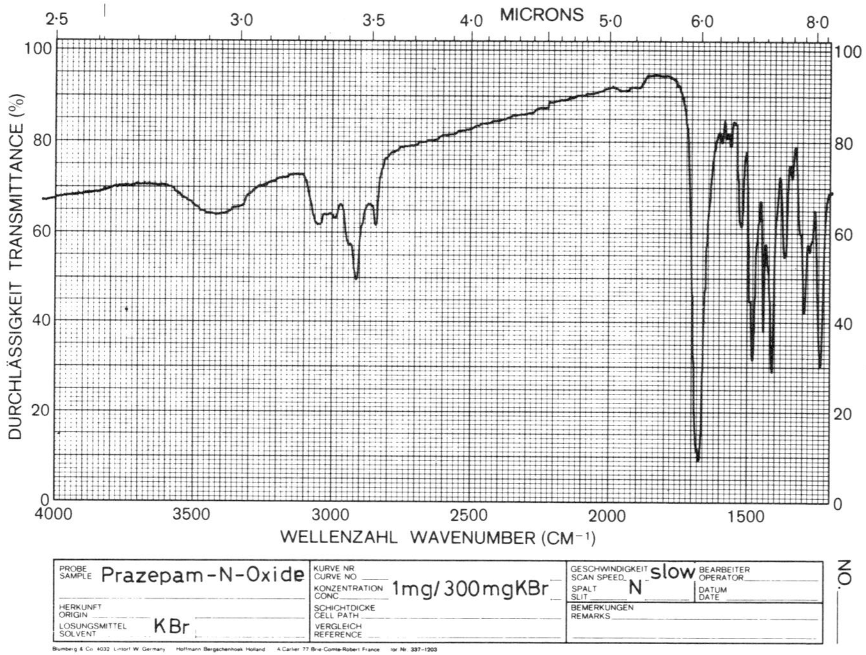

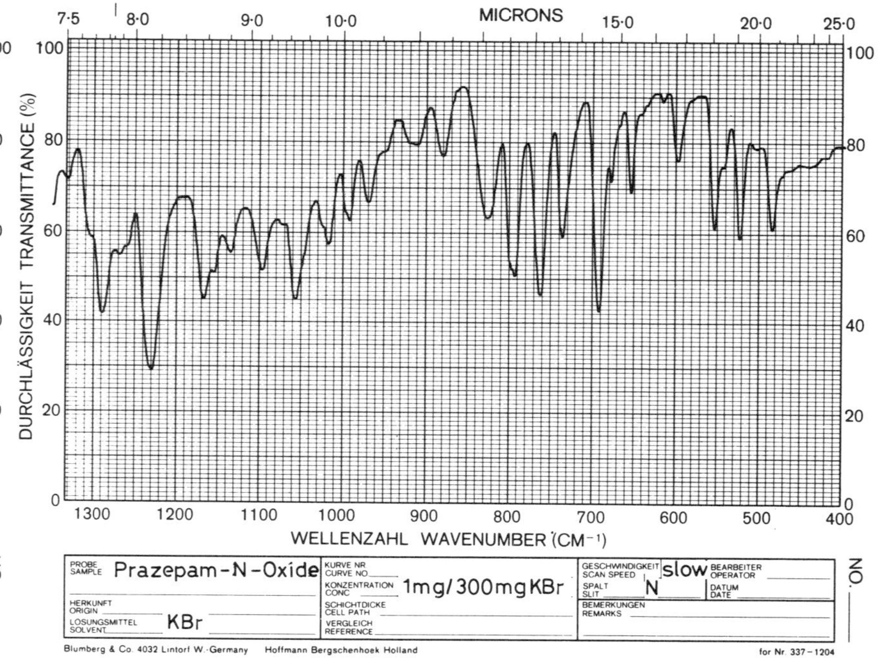

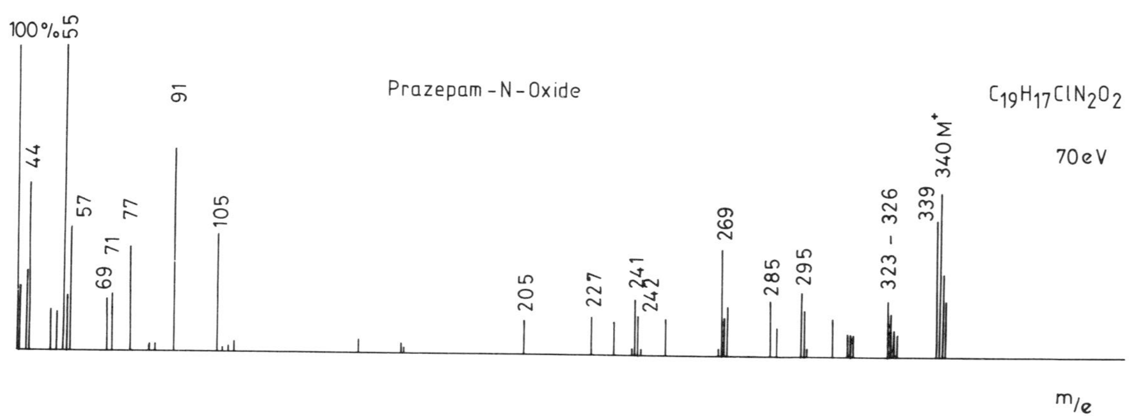

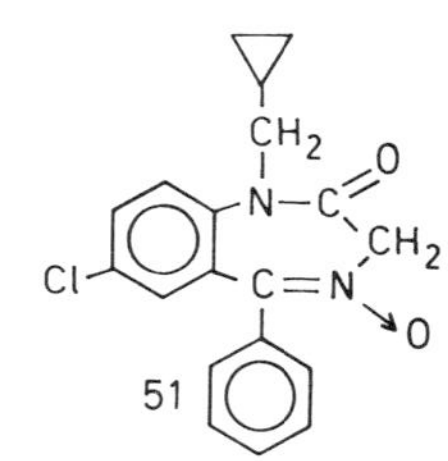

Prazepam-N-Oxide

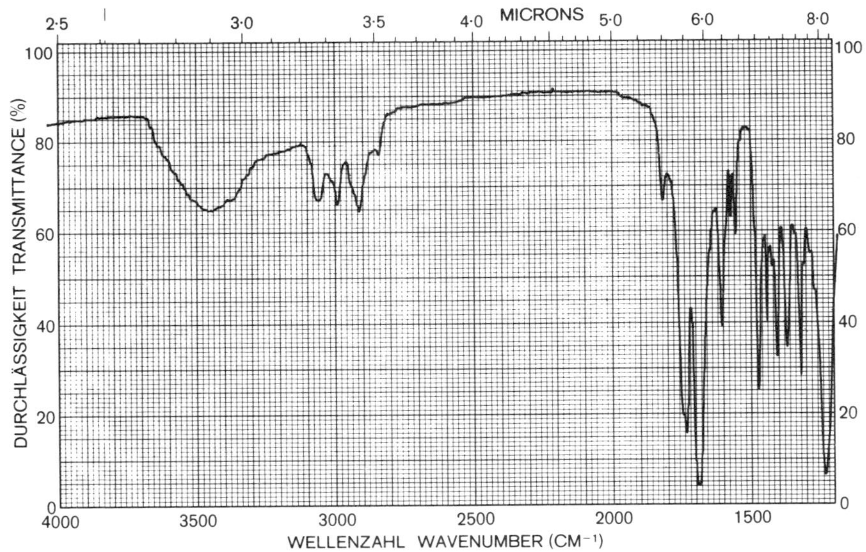

PROBE SAMPLE 3-Acetoxy-Prazepam | KURVE NR CURVE NO | KONZENTRATION CONC 1mg/300mgKBr | GESCHWINDIGKEIT SCAN SPEED slow | SPALT SLIT N | BEARBEITER OPERATOR | DATUM DATE | HERKUNFT ORIGIN | SCHICHTDICKE CELL PATH | LÖSUNGSMITTEL SOLVENT KBr | VERGLEICH REFERENCE | BEMERKUNGEN REMARKS | NO.

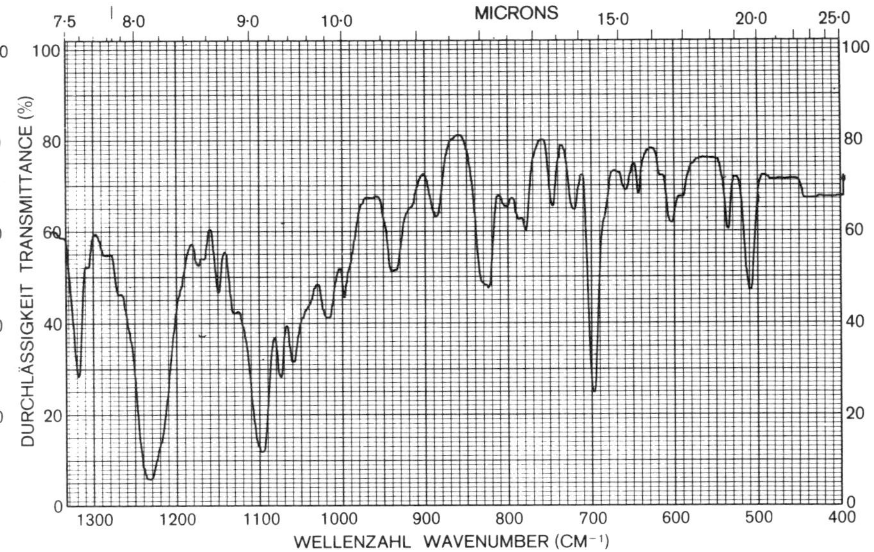

PROBE SAMPLE 3-Acetoxy-Prazepam | KURVE NR CURVE NO | KONZENTRATION CONC 1mg/300mgKBr | GESCHWINDIGKEIT SCAN SPEED slow | SPALT SLIT N | BEARBEITER OPERATOR | DATUM DATE | HERKUNFT ORIGIN | SCHICHTDICKE CELL PATH | LÖSUNGSMITTEL SOLVENT KBr | VERGLEICH REFERENCE | BEMERKUNGEN REMARKS | NO.

Blumberg & Co. 4032 Lintorf W.-Germany Hoffmann Bergschenhoek Holland for Nr. 337-1204

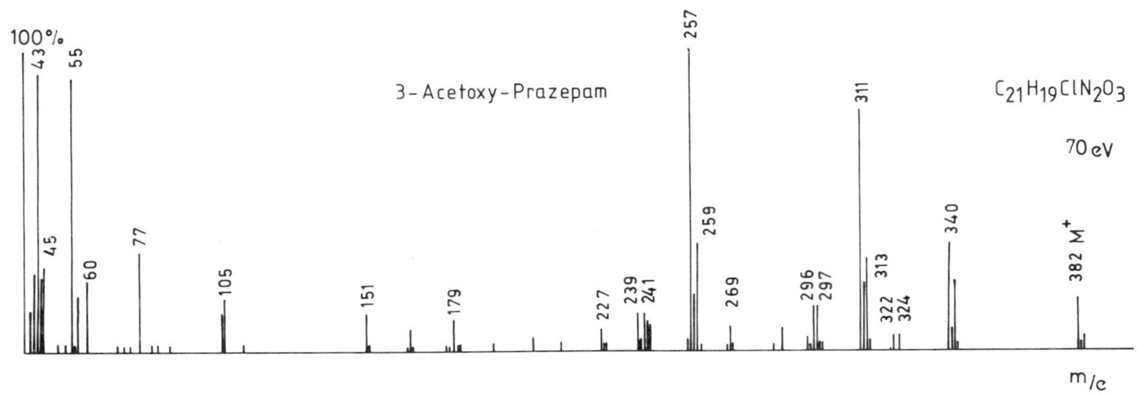

3-Acetoxy-Prazepam

$C_{21}H_{19}ClN_2O_3$

70 eV

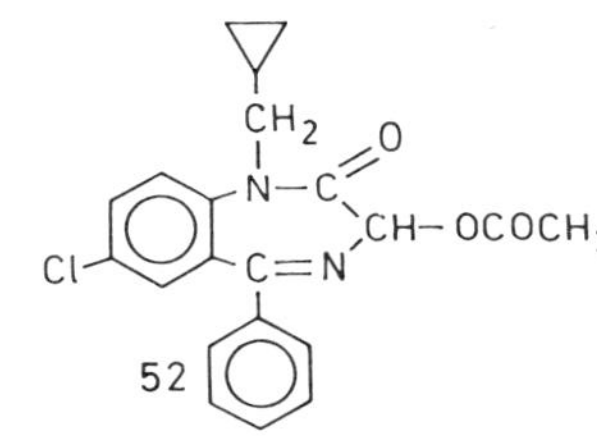

3-Acetoxy-Prazepam

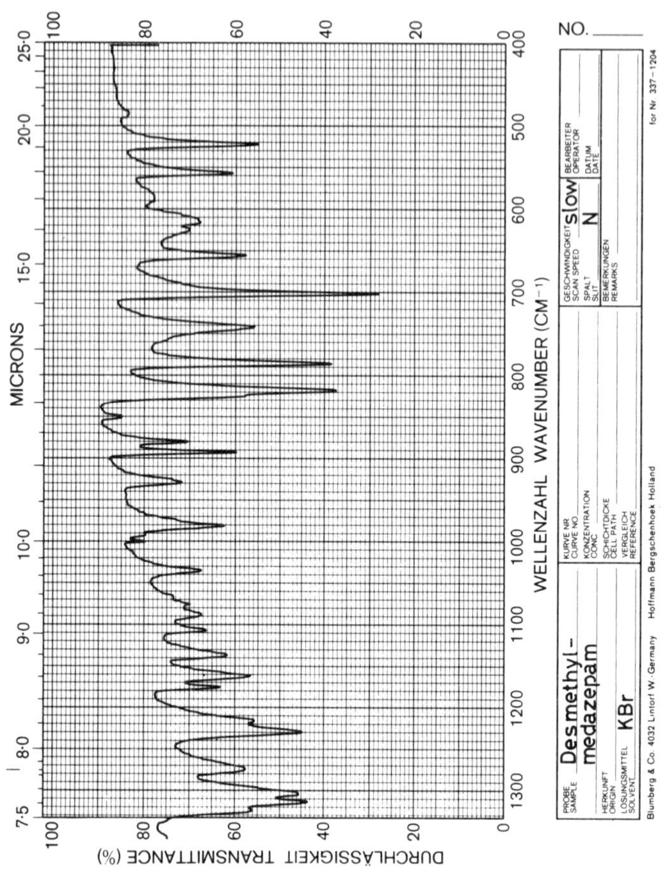

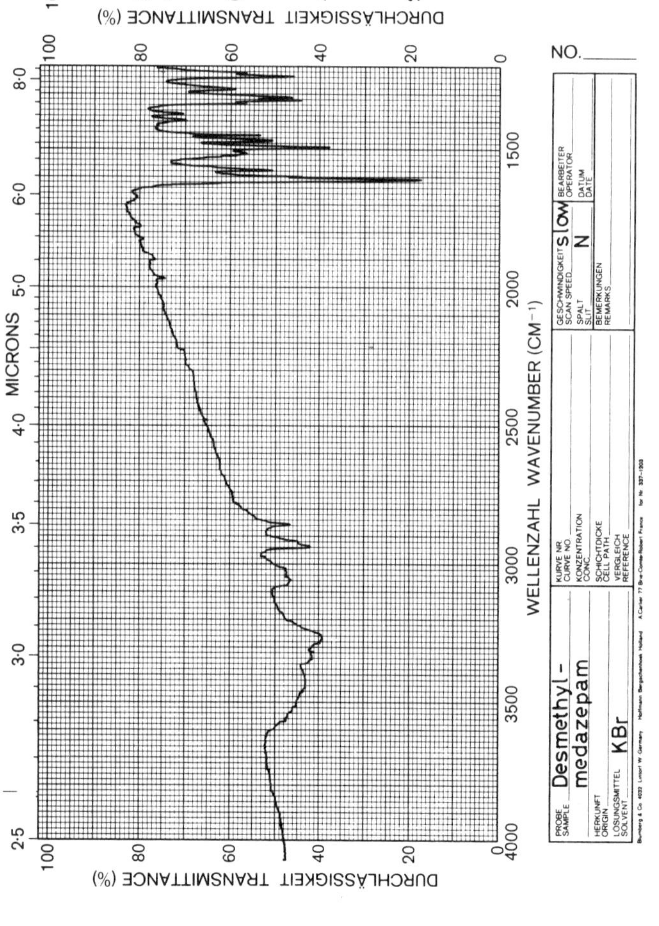

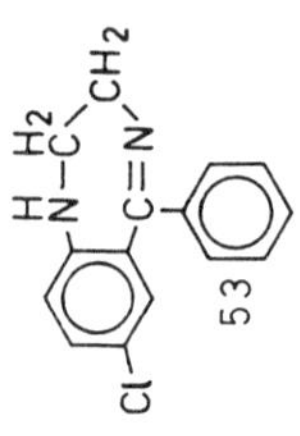

Desmethyl - Medazepam

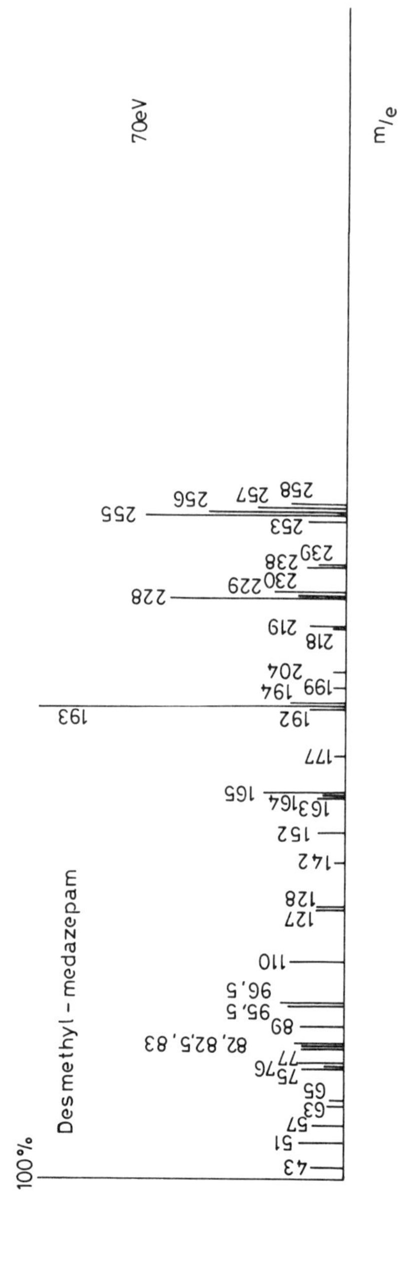

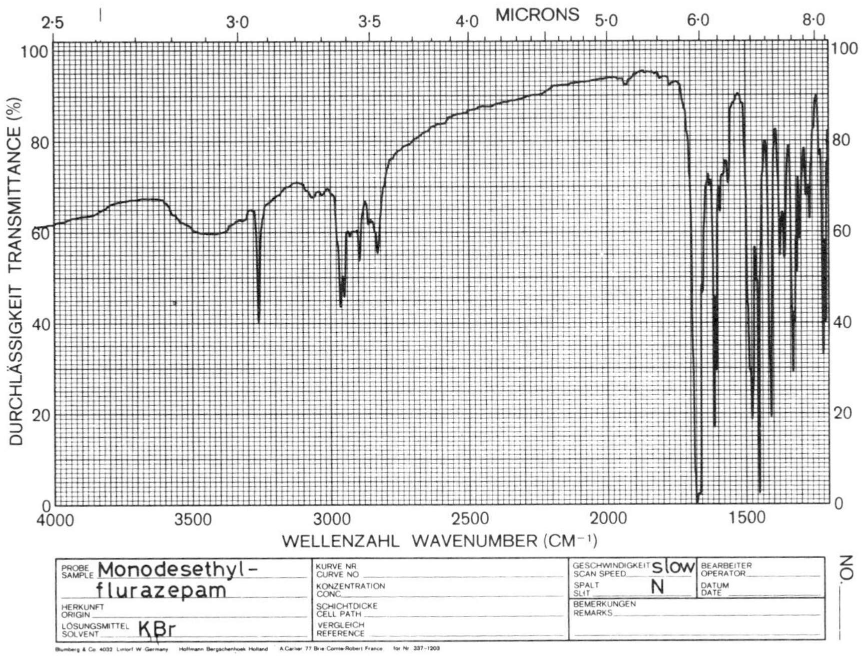

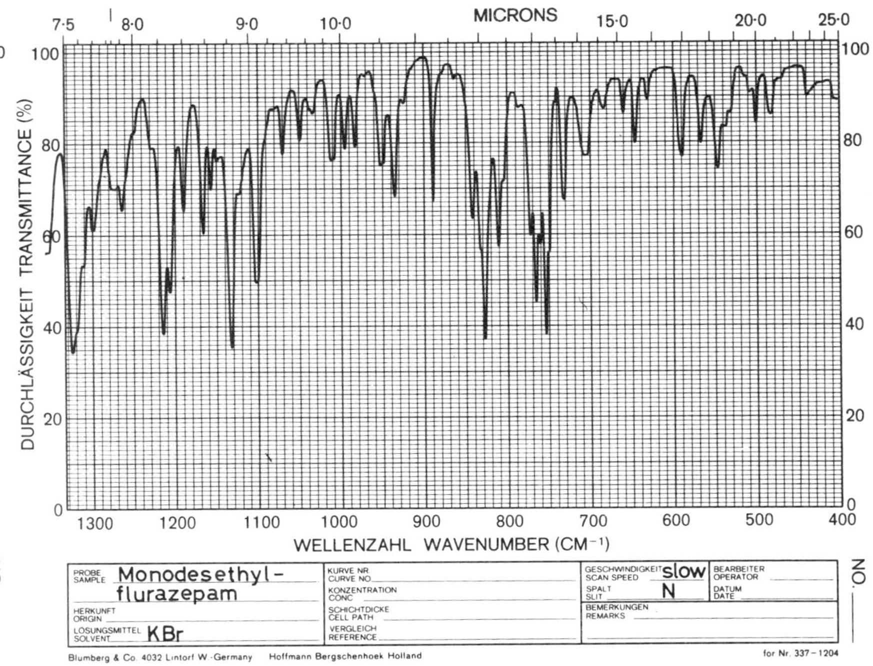

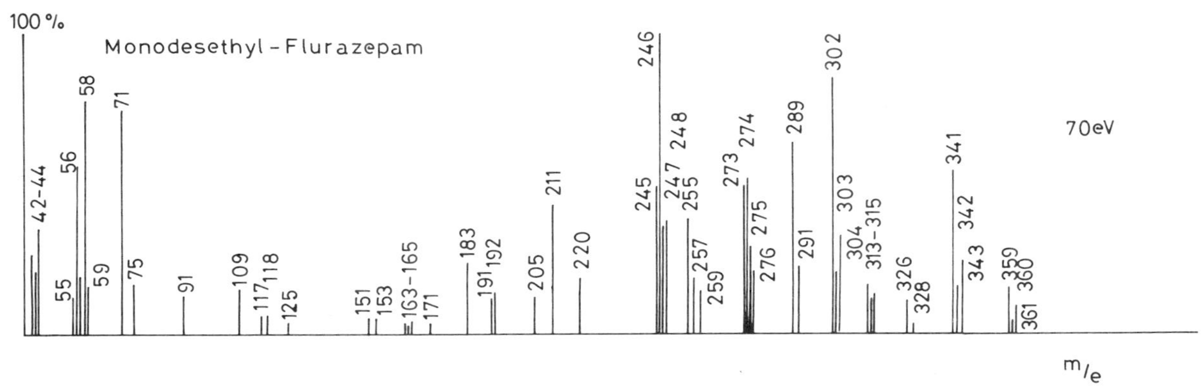

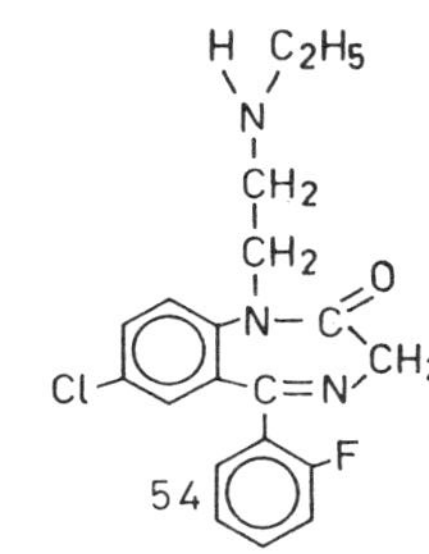

Monodesethyl-Flurazepam

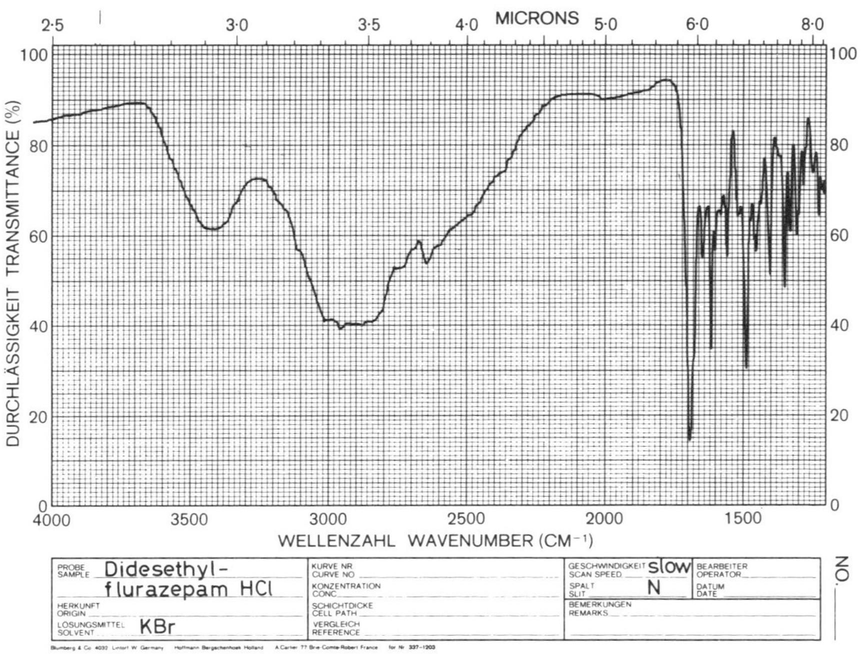

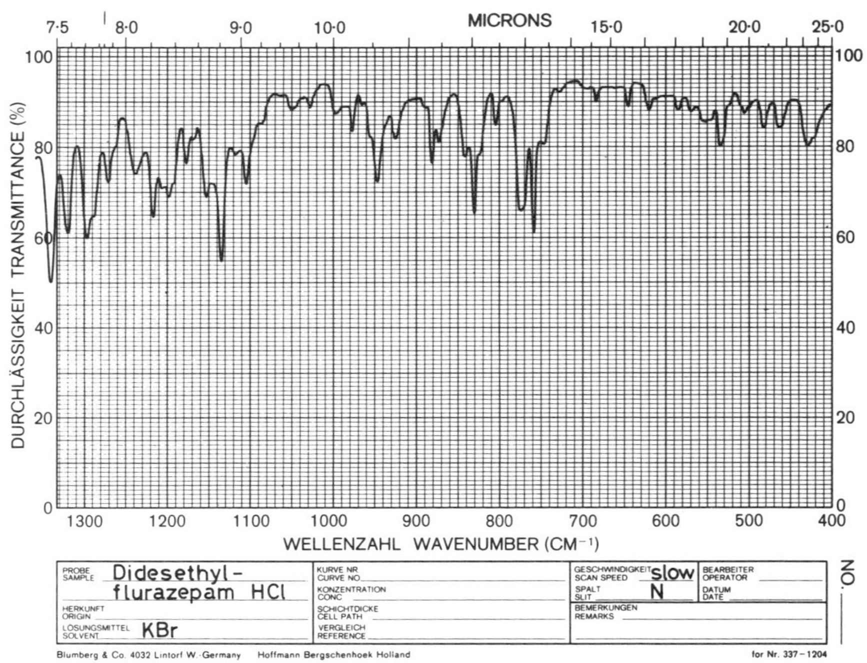

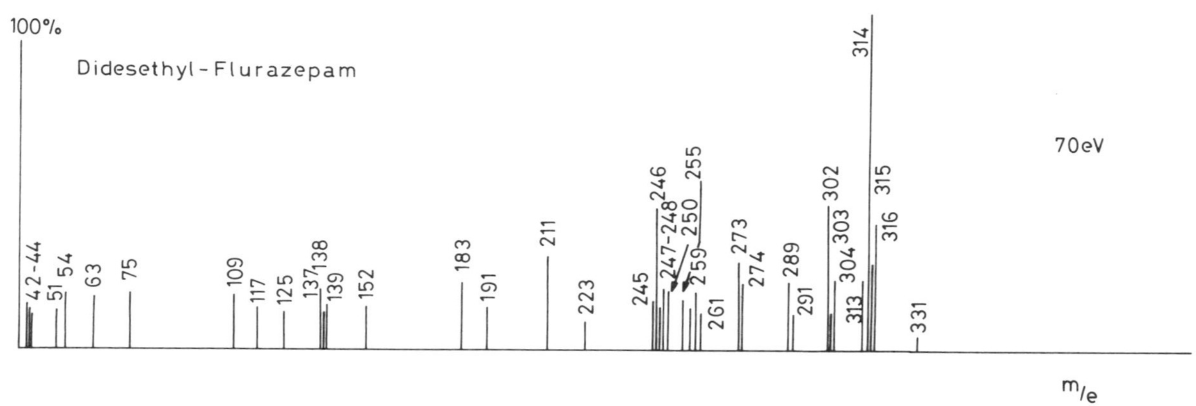

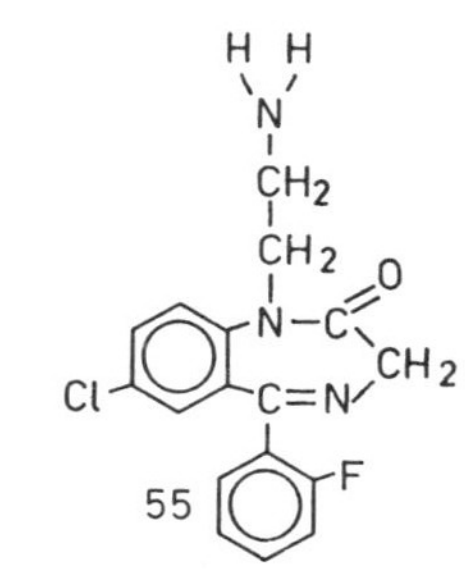

Didesethyl-Flurazepam

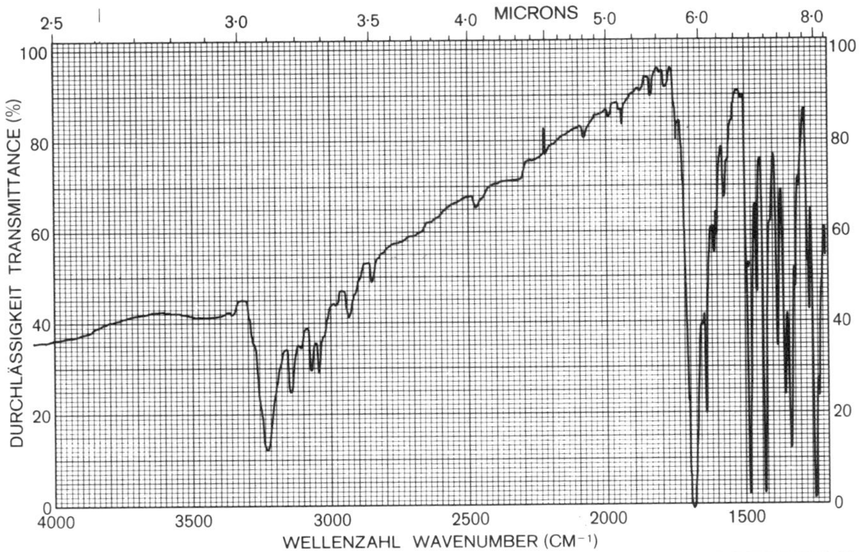

PROBE SAMPLE: Bromazepam-N(Py)-Oxide
HERKUNFT ORIGIN
LÖSUNGSMITTEL SOLVENT: KBr
KURVE NR. CURVE NO.
KONZENTRATION CONC.
SCHICHTDICKE CELL PATH
VERGLEICH REFERENCE
GESCHWINDIGKEIT SCAN SPEED: slow
SPALT SLIT: N
BEARBEITER OPERATOR
DATUM DATE
BEMERKUNGEN REMARKS
NO.

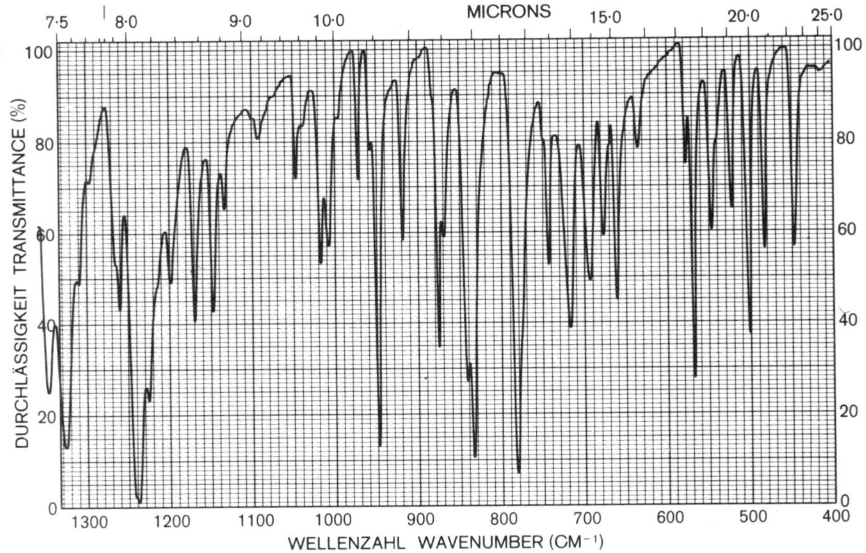

PROBE SAMPLE: Bromazepam-N(Py)-Oxid
HERKUNFT ORIGIN
LÖSUNGSMITTEL SOLVENT: KBr
KURVE NR. CURVE NO.
KONZENTRATION CONC.
SCHICHTDICKE CELL PATH
VERGLEICH REFERENCE
GESCHWINDIGKEIT SCAN SPEED: slow
SPALT SLIT: N
BEARBEITER OPERATOR
DATUM DATE
BEMERKUNGEN REMARKS
NO.

Blumberg & Co. 4032 Lintorf W.-Germany Hoffmann Bergschenhoek Holland for Nr. 337-1204

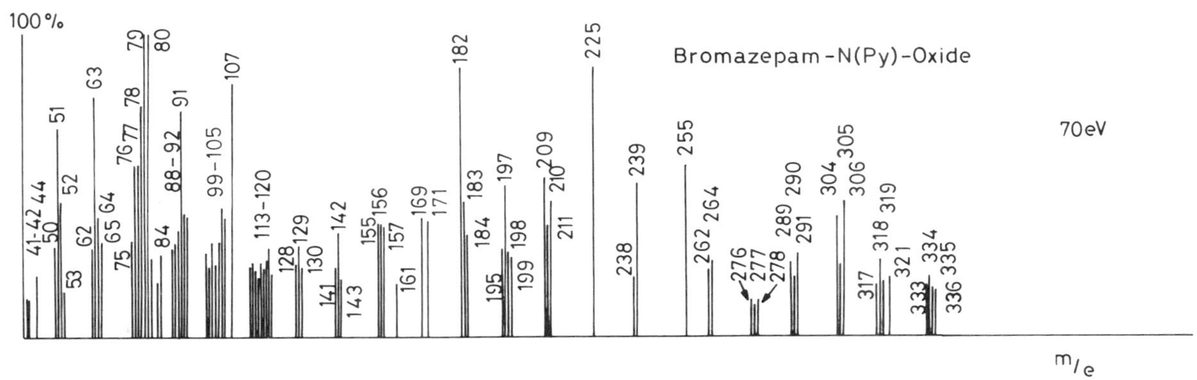

Bromazepam-N(Py)-Oxide

70eV

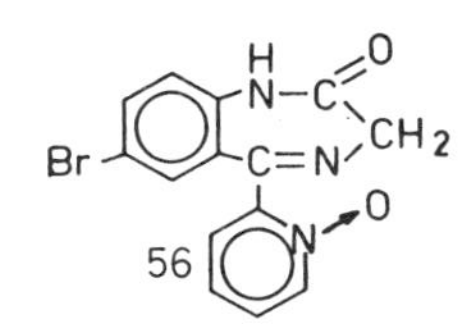

Bromazepam-N(Py)-Oxide

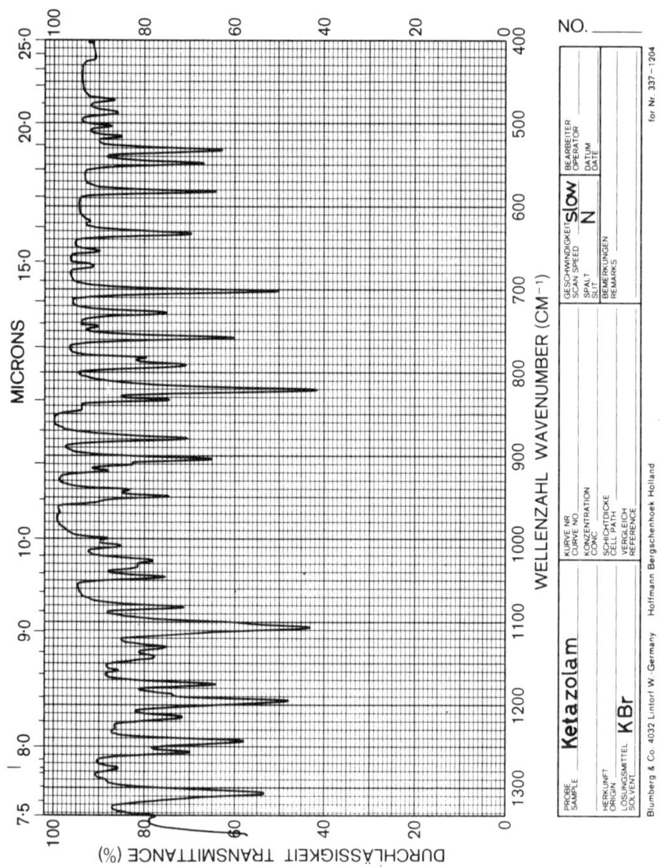

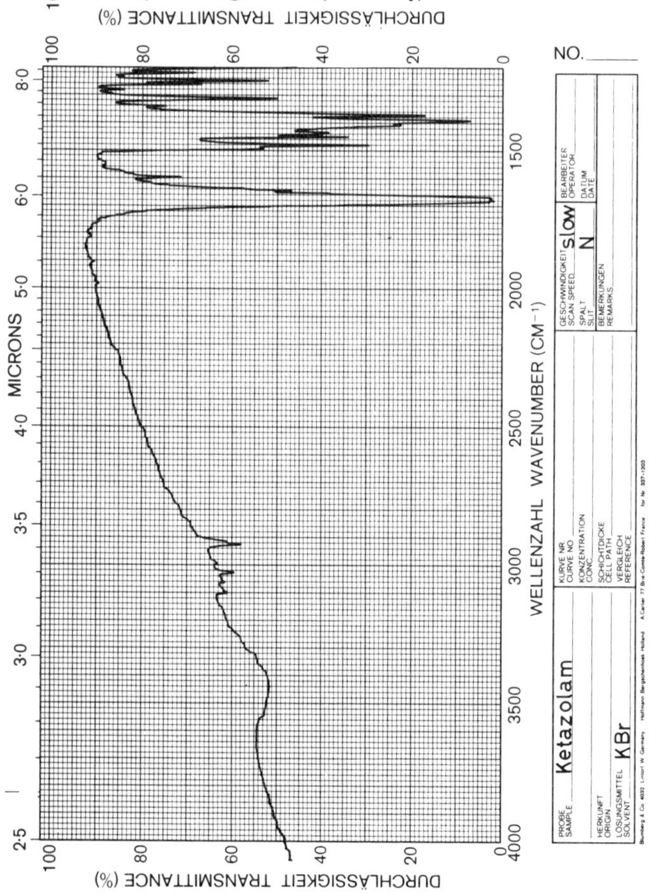

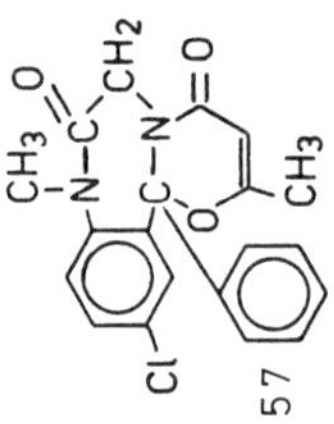

57

Ketazolam

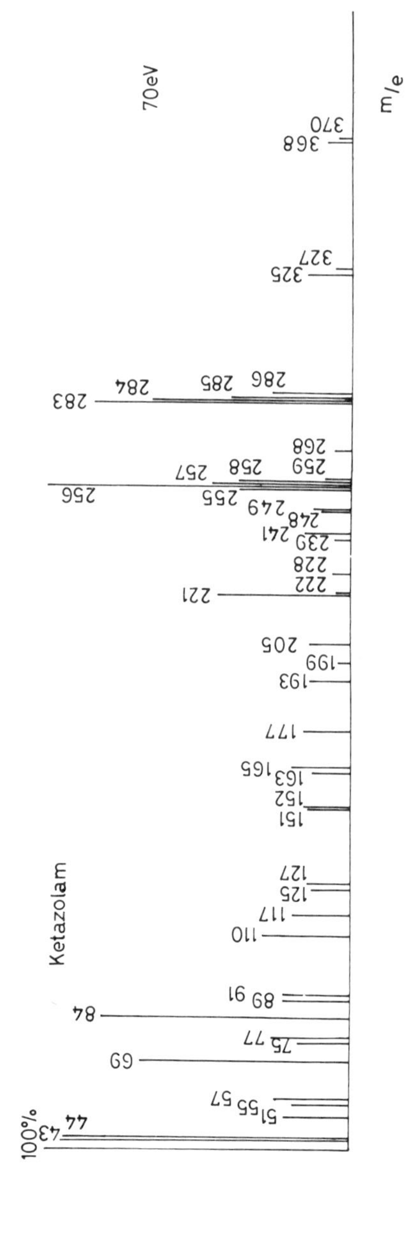

Ketazolam

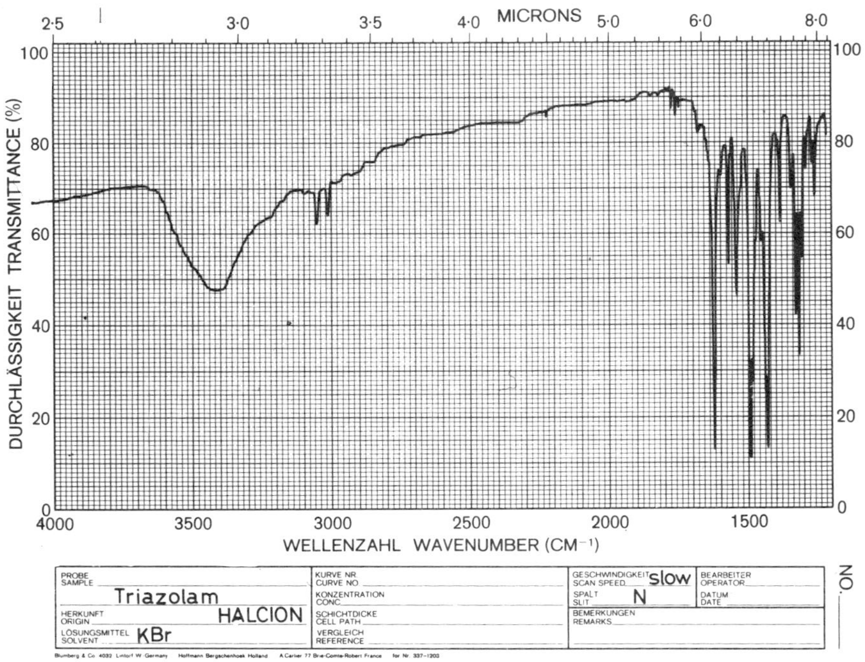
MICRONS
DURCHLÄSSIGKEIT TRANSMITTANCE (%)
WELLENZAHL WAVENUMBER (CM⁻¹)
PROBE SAMPLE Triazolam
HERKUNFT ORIGIN HALCION
LÖSUNGSMITTEL SOLVENT KBr
KURVE NR CURVE NO
KONZENTRATION CONC.
SCHICHTDICKE CELL PATH
VERGLEICH REFERENCE
GESCHWINDIGKEIT SCAN SPEED slow
SPALT SLIT N
BEARBEITER OPERATOR
DATUM DATE
BEMERKUNGEN REMARKS
NO.

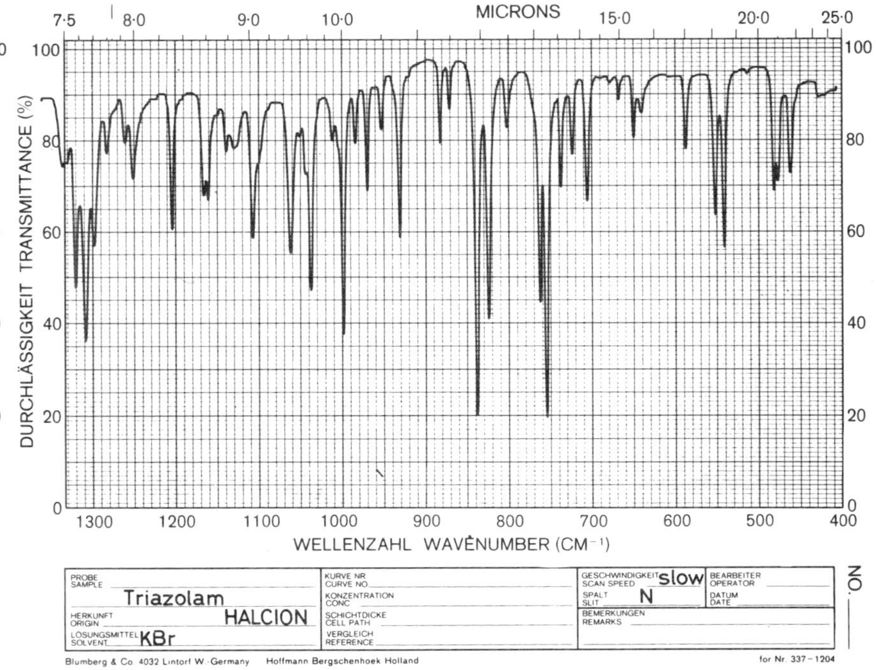
MICRONS
DURCHLÄSSIGKEIT TRANSMITTANCE (%)
WELLENZAHL WAVENUMBER (CM⁻¹)
PROBE SAMPLE Triazolam
HERKUNFT ORIGIN HALCION
LÖSUNGSMITTEL SOLVENT KBr
KURVE NR CURVE NO
KONZENTRATION CONC.
SCHICHTDICKE CELL PATH
VERGLEICH REFERENCE
GESCHWINDIGKEIT SCAN SPEED slow
SPALT SLIT N
BEARBEITER OPERATOR
DATUM DATE
BEMERKUNGEN REMARKS
NO.
Blumberg & Co. 4032 Lintorf W.-Germany
Hoffmann Bergschenhoek Holland
for Nr. 337-1204

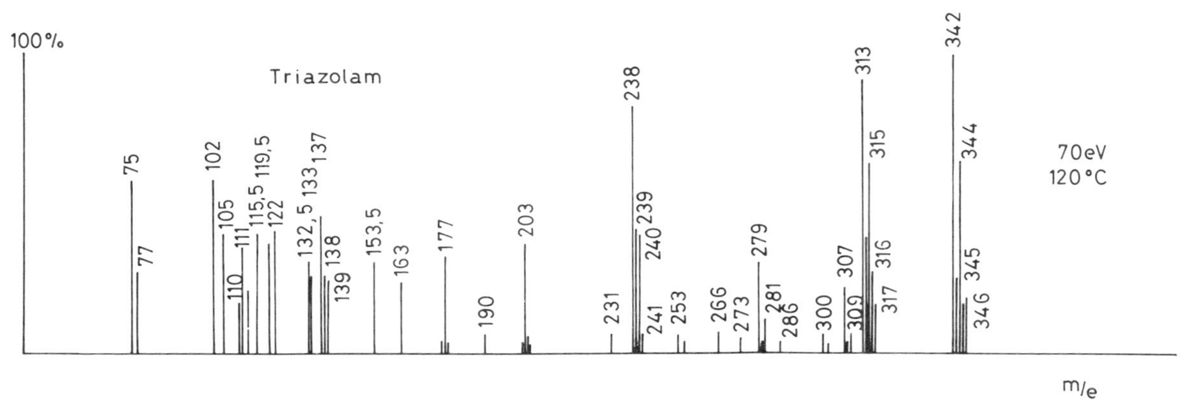
100%
Triazolam
75
77
102
105
110
111
115,5
119,5
122
132,5
133
137
138
139
153,5
163
177
190
203
231
238
239
240
241
253
266
273
279
281
286
300
307
309
313
315
316
317
342
344
345
346
70eV
120°C
m/e

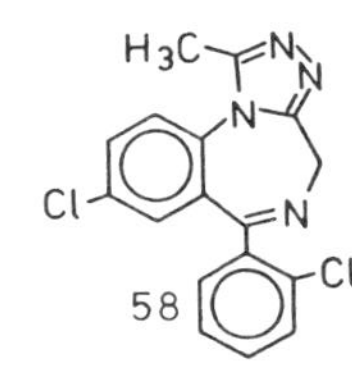
H3C
N
N
N
Cl
N
Cl
58

Triazolam

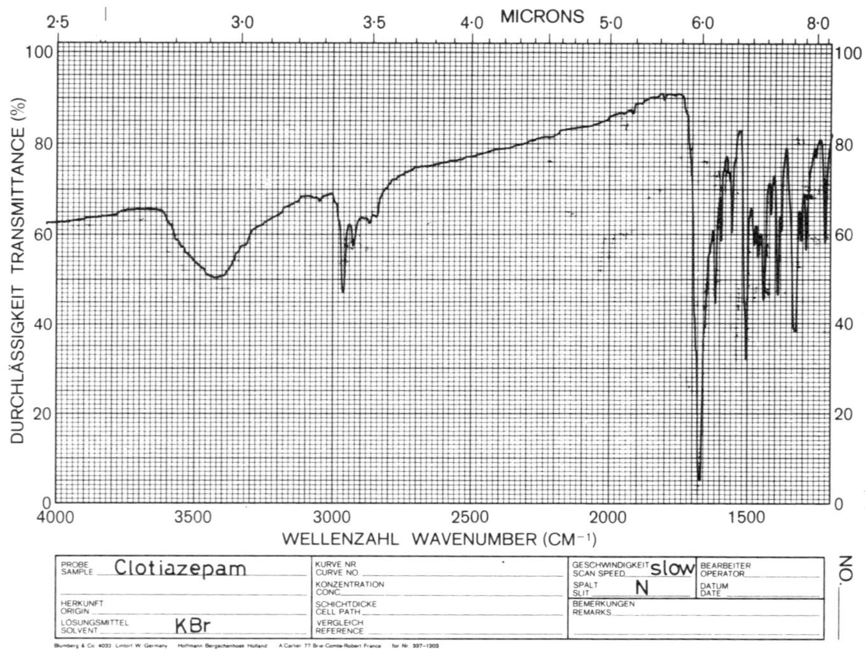

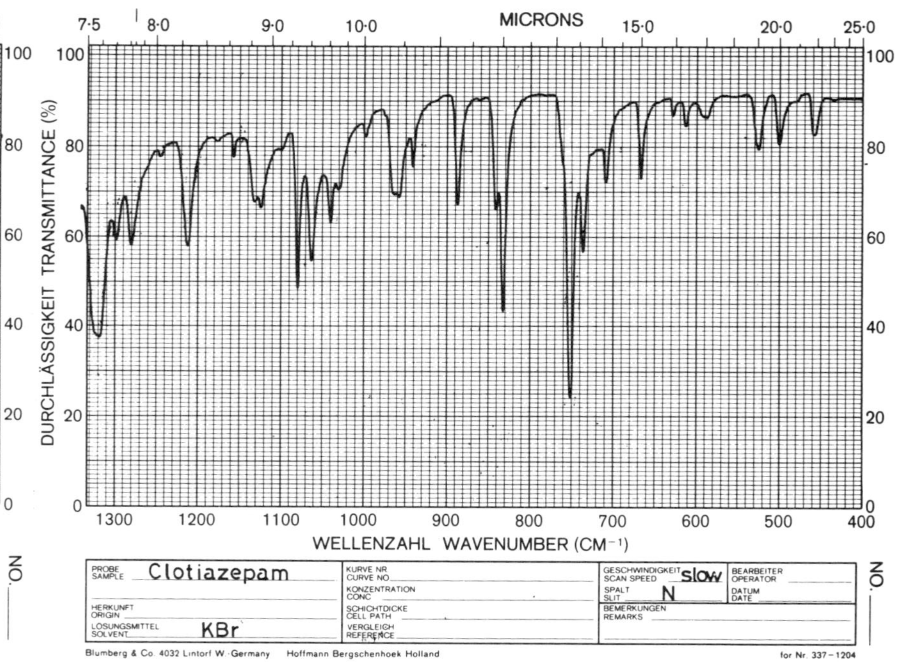

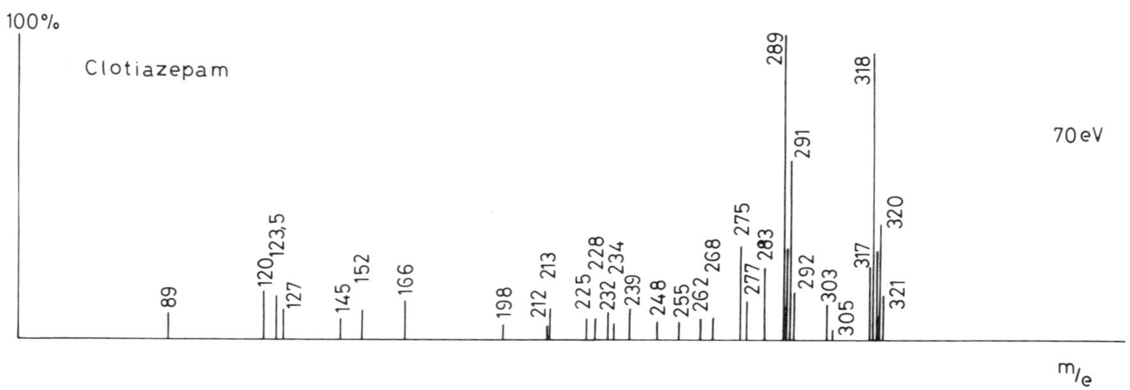

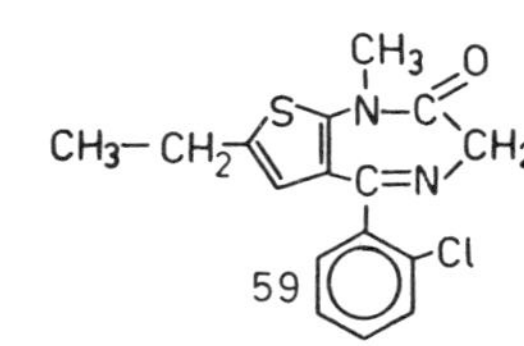

Clotiazepam

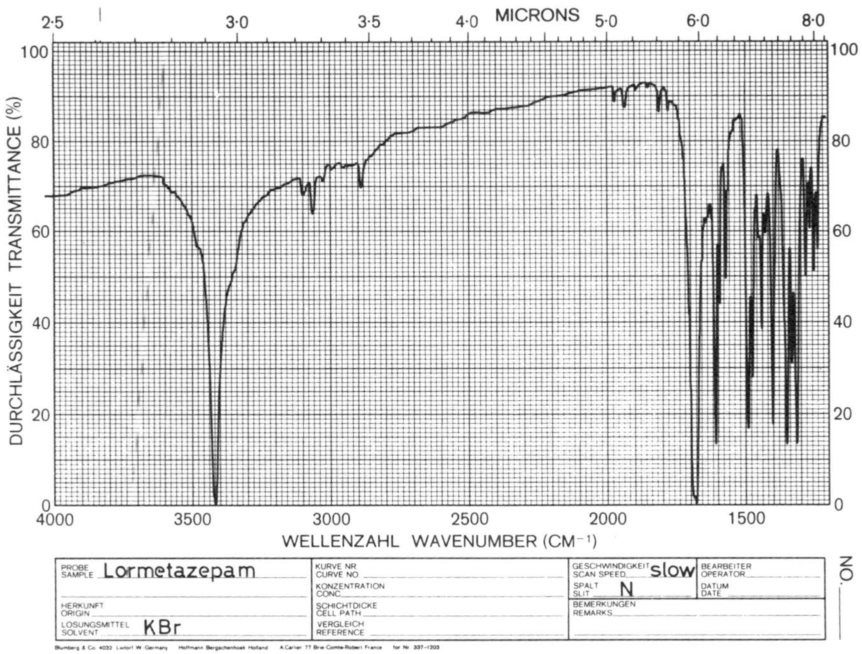

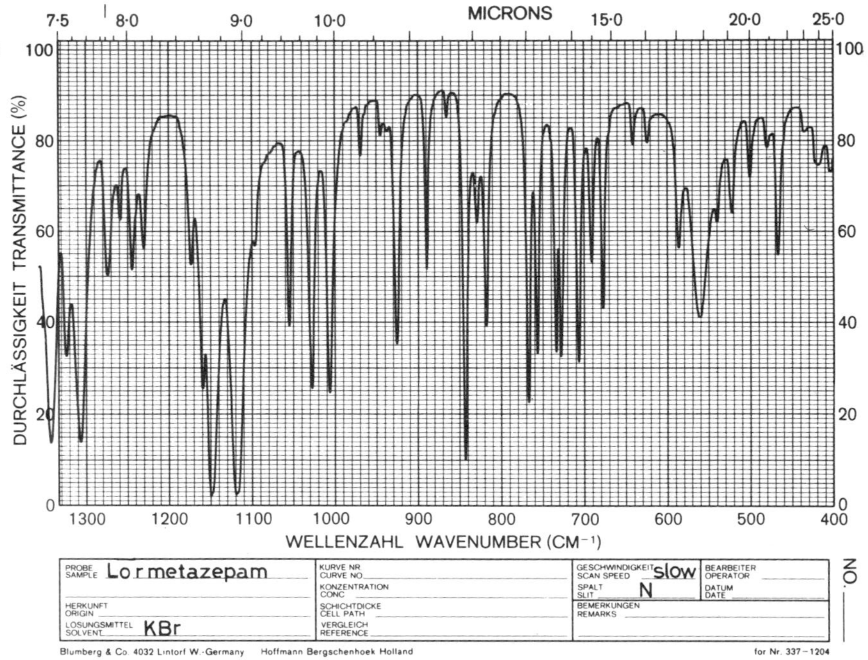

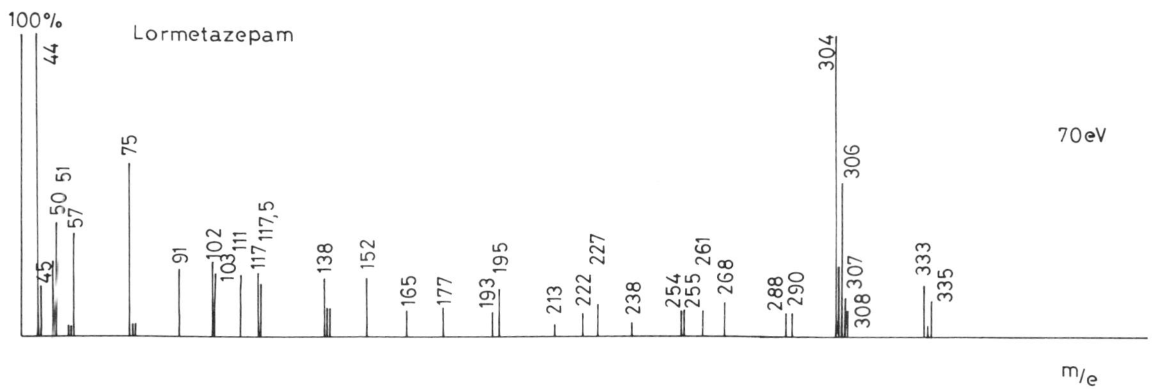

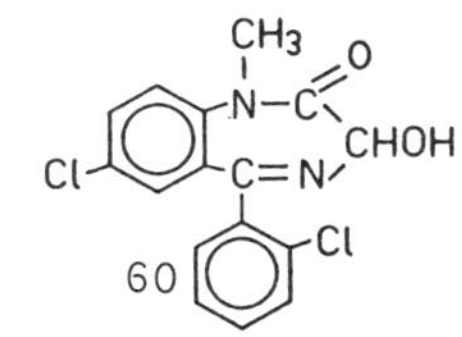

Lormetazepam

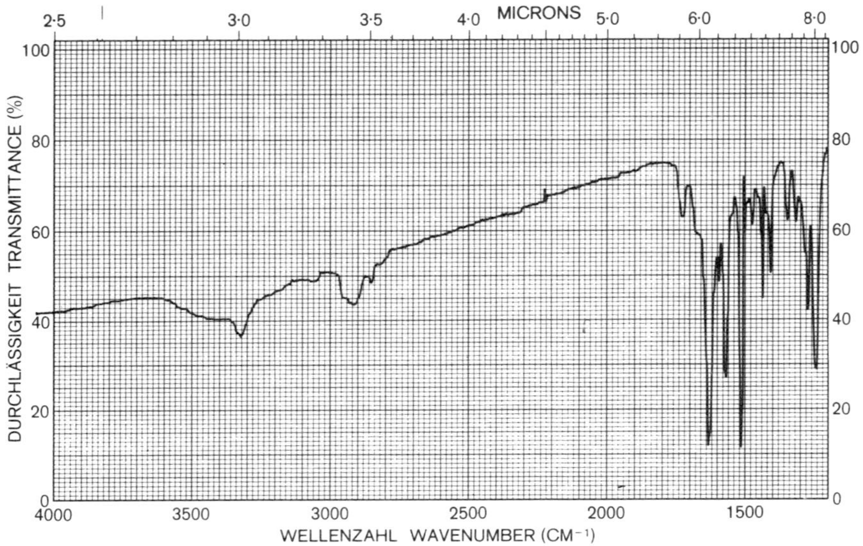

PROBE SAMPLE 2-Methylamino-2',5-dichlor-benzo-phenon	KURVE NR CURVE NO.	GESCHWINDIGKEIT SCAN SPEED slow	BEARBEITER OPERATOR
HERKUNFT ORIGIN	KONZENTRATION CONC.	SPALT SLIT N	DATUM DATE
LÖSUNGSMITTEL SOLVENT KBr	SCHICHTDICKE CELL PATH	BEMERKUNGEN REMARKS	
	VERGLEICH REFERENCE		

NO.

Blumberg & Co. 4032 Lintorf W.-Germany Hoffmann Bergschenhoek Holland A.Carlier 77 Brie-Comte-Robert France for Nr. 337-1203

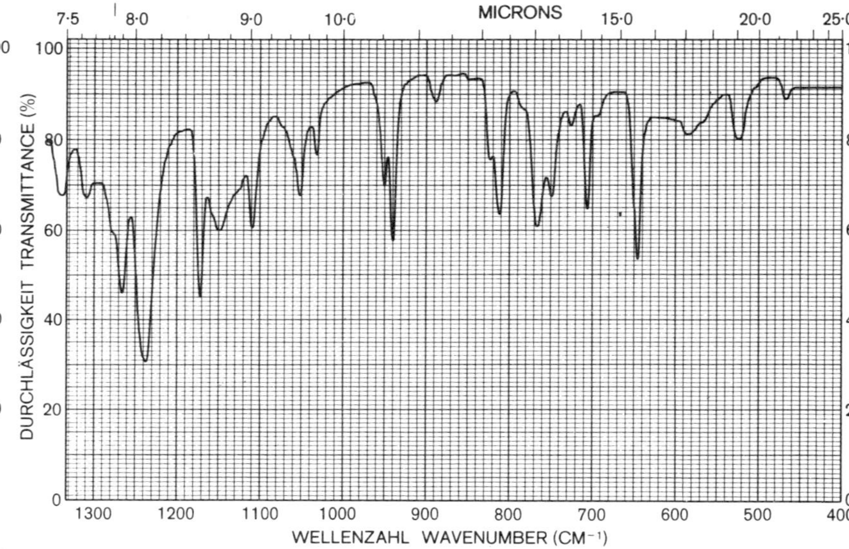

PROBE SAMPLE 2-Methylamino-2',5-dichlor-benzo-phenon	KURVE NR CURVE NO.	GESCHWINDIGKEIT SCAN SPEED slow	BEARBEITER OPERATOR
HERKUNFT ORIGIN	KONZENTRATION CONC.	SPALT SLIT N	DATUM DATE
LÖSUNGSMITTEL SOLVENT KBr	SCHICHTDICKE CELL PATH	BEMERKUNGEN REMARKS	
	VERGLEICH REFERENCE		

NO.

Blumberg & Co. 4032 Lintorf W.-Germany Hoffmann Bergschenhoek Holland for Nr. 337-1204

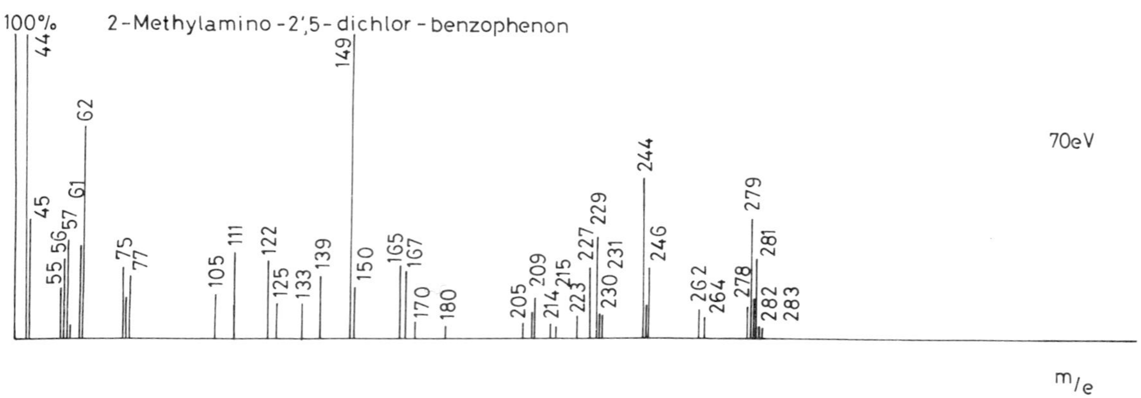

70eV

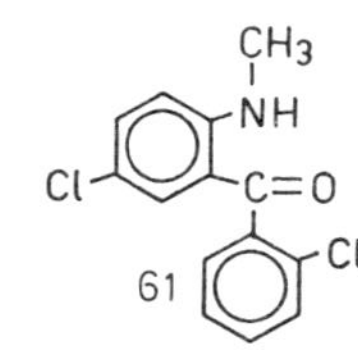

2-Methylamino-2',5-dichlor-benzophenone

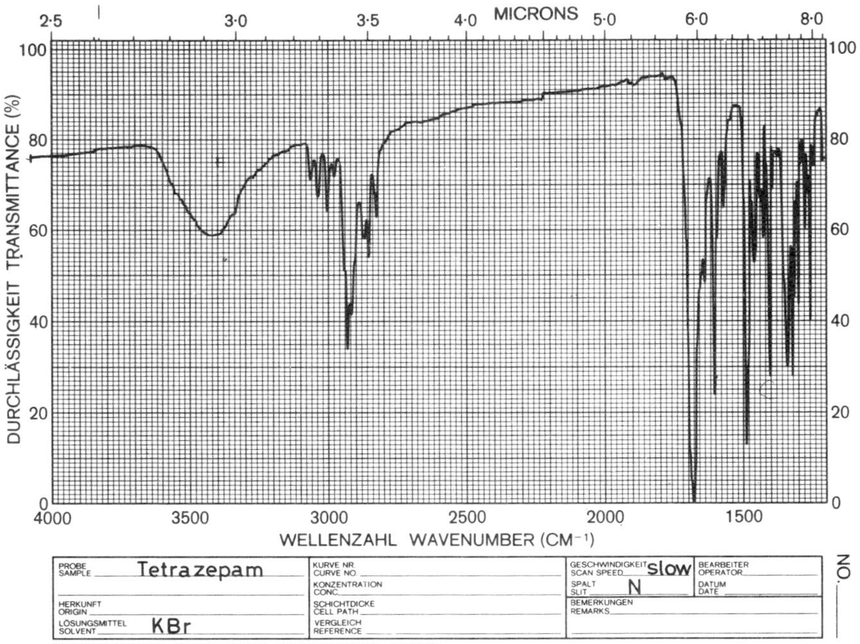
MICRONS
DURCHLÄSSIGKEIT TRANSMITTANCE (%)
WELLENZAHL WAVENUMBER (CM⁻¹)
PROBE SAMPLE Tetrazepam
LÖSUNGSMITTEL SOLVENT KBr
GESCHWINDIGKEIT SCAN SPEED slow
SPALT SLIT N
NO.

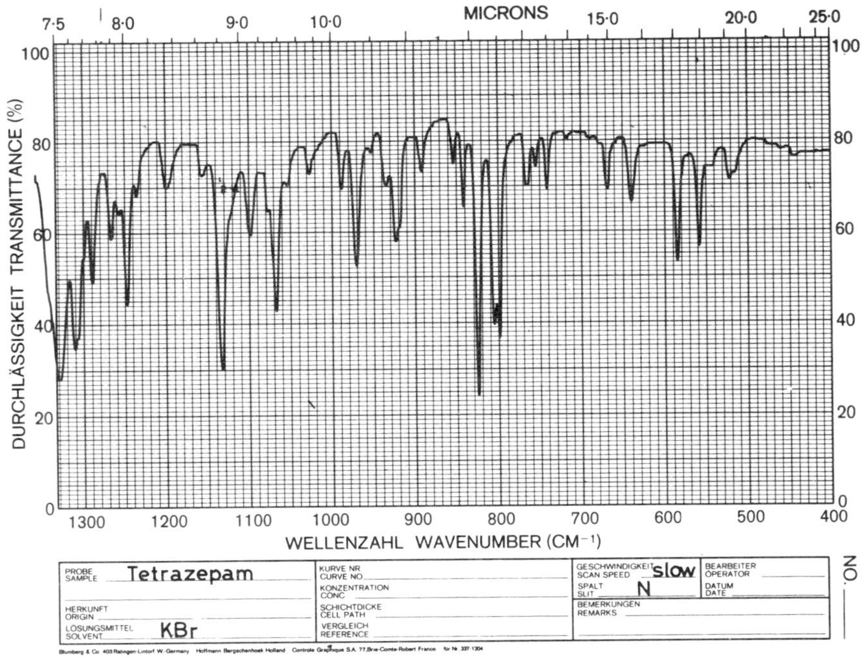
MICRONS
DURCHLÄSSIGKEIT TRANSMITTANCE (%)
WELLENZAHL WAVENUMBER (CM⁻¹)
PROBE SAMPLE Tetrazepam
LÖSUNGSMITTEL SOLVENT KBr
GESCHWINDIGKEIT SCAN SPEED slow
SPALT SLIT N
NO.

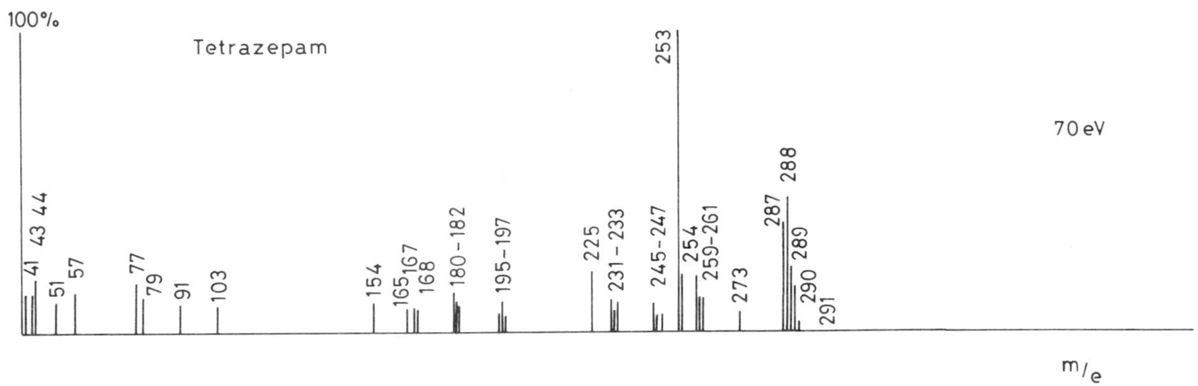
100%
Tetrazepam
70 eV
m/e
41 43 44 51 57 77 79 91 103 154 165 167 168 180-182 195-197 225 231-233 245-247 253 254 259-261 273 287 288 289 290 291

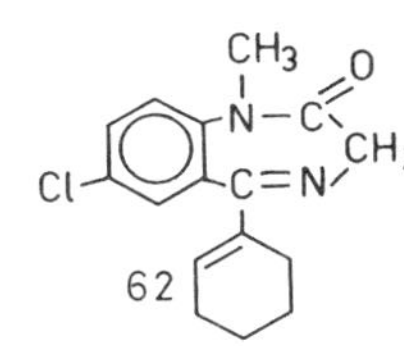
CH3
O
N
C
CH2
Cl
C=N
62

Tetrazepam

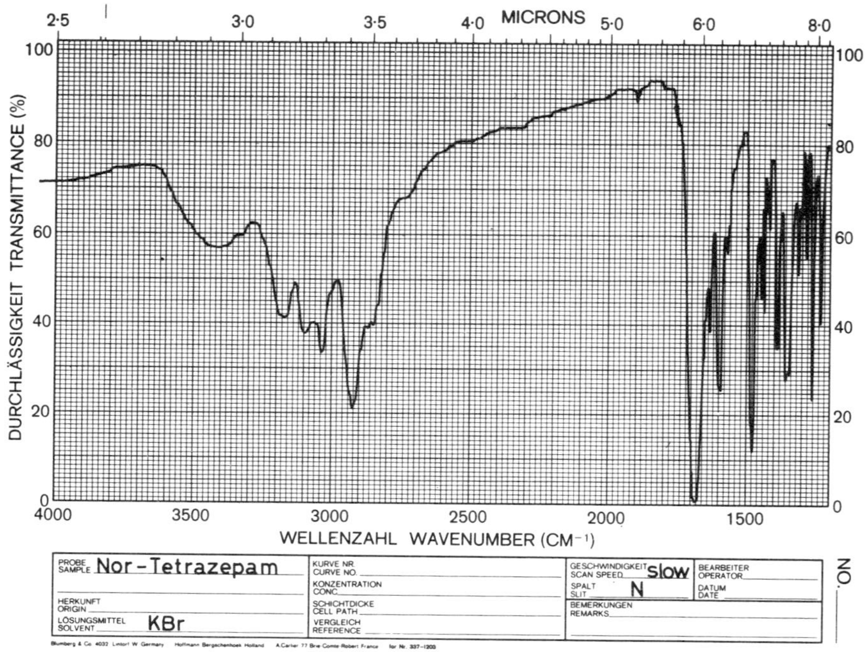

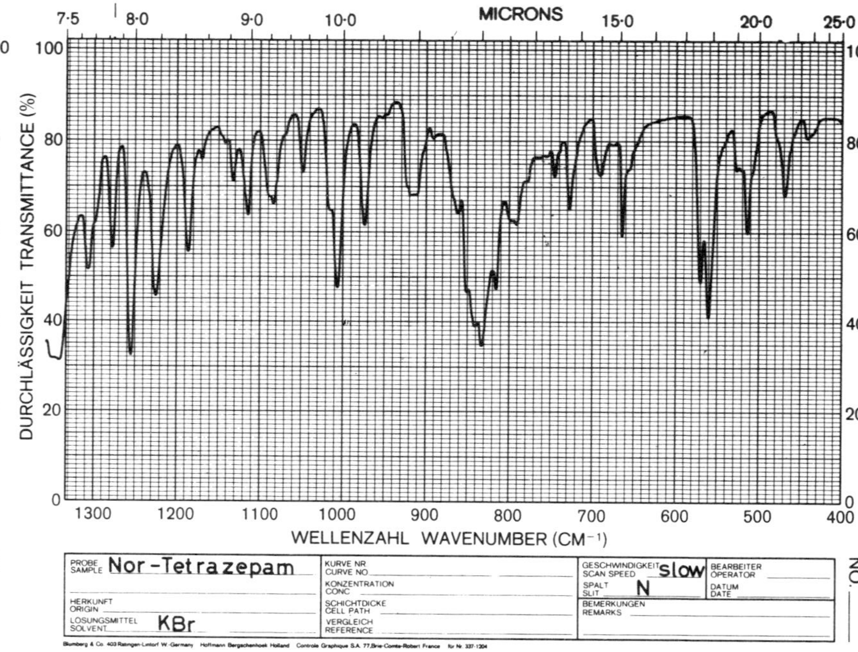

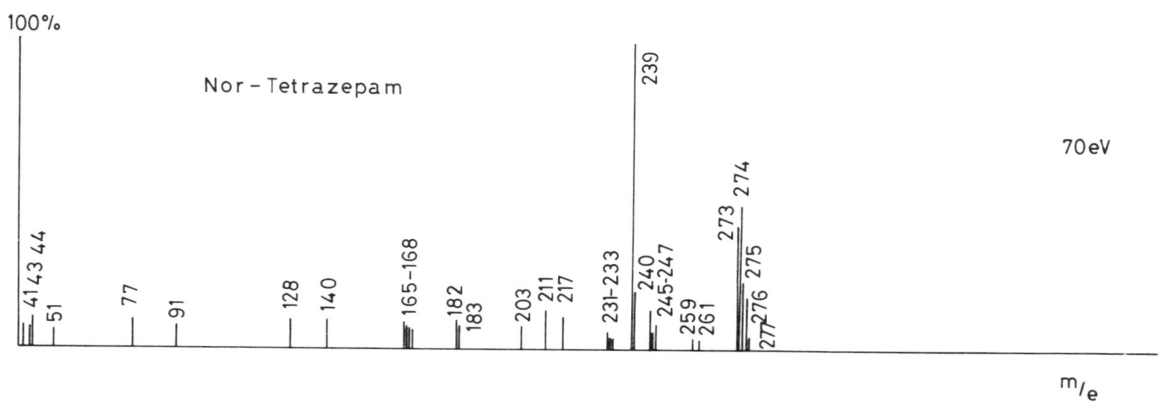

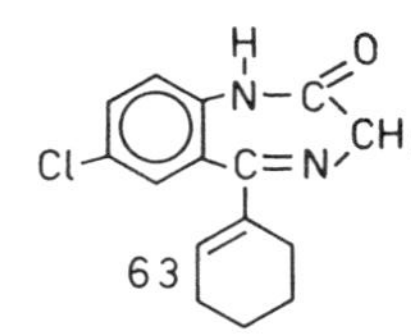

Nor-Tetrazepam

Ultraviolet-Spectra

Ultraviolett-Spektren

Absorption Maxima (UV - Spectra)
Absorptionsmaxima (UV - Spektren)

Wavelength in nanometers
Wellenlängen in Nanometer

Main Maxima underlined
Hauptmaxima unterstrichen

——————— = in Ethanol

- - - - - - - - - - - = in 0,1 N HCl

xxxxxxxxxxxxxxxxxx = in 0,1 N NaOH

Nr.	Substance / Substanz	Maxima in Ethanol abs.	/ Maxima in 0,1 N HCl	/ Maxima in 0,1 N NaOH
1	Chlordiazepoxide	245 / 267	245 / 310	261
2	Demoxepam (=Nor-Diazepam-N-Oxid)	235 / 312	235	243 / 257
3	N-Desmethyl-Chlordiazepoxide	242 / 263	246 / 310	258
4	2-Amino-5-chlor-benzophenone	237 / 392	260	----
5	Diazepam	230 / 255	241 / 285 / 360	229
6	Nor-Diazepam	228 / 325	237 / 282 / 370	340
7	3-Hydroxy-Diazepam	231 / 255 / 315	235 / 283 / 355	----
8	Oxazepam	229 / 324	234 / 281	234 / 340
9	2-Methylamino-5-chlor-benzophenone	236 / 410	270	----
10	Nitrazepam	220 / 258 / 312	280	226 / 258 / 357
11	7-Amino-Nitrazepam	242 / 350	232 / 282 / 350	238 / 350
12	7-Acetamido-Nitrazepam	247 / 330	257	237
13	2-Amino-5-nitro-benzophenone	230 / 350	355	355
14	2,5-Diamino-benzophenone	237 / 353	232 / 357	243 / 400
15	Medazepam-Base	231 / 252 / 360	254	----
16	Chlorazepat	230	238 / 286	233 / 340
17	Lorazepam	229 / 322	230	234 / 349
18	2-Amino-5,2'-dichlor-benzophenone	233 / 263 / 330 / 394	232 / 394	394
19	Prazepam	228 / 256	240 / 287 / 360	230
20	3-Hydroxy-Prazepam	229 / 255 / 315	233 / 280	----
21	2-Cyclopropyl-methylamino-5-chlor-benzophenone	237 / 410	----	----

Nr.	Substance / Substanz	Maxima in Ethanol abs./	Maxima in 0,1 N HCl /	Maxima in 0,1 N NaOH
22	Clonazepam	218 / 250 /312	270	366
23	7-Amino-Clonazepam	241 / 355	233 / 283 / 355	236 / 355
24	7-Acetamido-Clonazepam	243 / 275 / 335	257	235
25	2-Amino-5-nitro-2'-chlor-benzophenone	230 / 350	360	360
26	2,5-Diamino-2'-chlor-benzophenone x HCl	230 / 260 / 385	230 / 260 / 385	240 / 420
27	Flurazepam x HCl	228 / 315	236 / 285 / 355	230
28	N-1-Desalkyl-Flurazepam	229 / 320	238 / 282/ 360	234 / 350
29	N-1-Hydroxyethyl-Flurazepam	230	240 / 284 / 355	232 / 255
30	2-Diethylamino-ethylamino-5-chlor-2'-fluor-benzophenone	235 / 410	236 / 270 / 405	242 / 420
31	2-Amino-5-chlor-2'-fluor-benzophenone	234 / 270 / 392	----	----
32	2-Hydroxyethylamino-5-chlor-2'-fluor-benzophenone	234 / 273 / 415	237 / 415	273 / 415
33	Bromazepam	233 / 325	240 / 350	238 / 350
34	3-Hydroxy-Bromazepam	234 / 325	240 / 350	240 / 350
35	2-(2-Amino-5-brom-benzoyl)-pyridine	237 / 400	273 /420	238 / 400
36	Flunitrazepam	221 / 253 / 311	275	400
37	Nor-Flunitrazepam	221 / 250 / 303	275	225 / 365
38	7-Amino-Flunitrazepam	242 / 350	237 / 280 / 350	240 / 350
39	7-Acetamido-Flunitrazepam	246 / 325	257 / 380	241 / 325
40	7-Amino-Nor-Flunitrazepam	242 / 350	233 / 280 / 350	240 / 365
41	2-Methylamino-5-nitro-2'-fluor-benzophenone	232 / 365	250 / 382	240 / 382
42	2-Amino-5-nitro-2'-fluor-benzophenone	230 / 352	232 / 245 / 362	245 / 362
43	2-Methylamino-5-amino-2'-fluor-benzophenone	255 / 435	258 / 405	258 / 435
44	2,5-Diamino-2'-fluor-benzophenone	242 / 425	233 / 380	242 / 420
45	2-Amino-3-hydroxy-5-chlor-benzophenone	246 / 280 / 400	263	259 / 300
46	Clobazam	231 / 297	228 / 285	285
47	Nor-Clobazam	228 / 295	226	230 / 265 / 305
48	Camazepam	230 / 255 / 315	227	232
53	Desmethyl-Medazepam	230 / 375	251 / 445	
54	Monodesethyl-Flurazepam	230 / 315	237 / 282 /360	
55	Didesethyl-Flurazepam	227	236 / 281 / 355	
56	Bromazepam-N(Py)-Oxide	230		230
57	Ketazolam	242	242	242
58	Triazolam	223	223	
59	Clotiazepam	245 / 305 /395	260 / 300 / 395	239 / 340

Nr.	Substance / Substanz	Maxima in Ethanol abs.	Maxima in 0,1 N HCl	Maxima in 0,1 N NaOH
60	Lormetazepam	230 / 310	230	300
61	2-Methylamino-2',5-dichlor-benzophenone	231 / 405	232 / 405	405
62	Tetrazepam	227 / 225	240 / 283 / 345	310
63	Nor-Tetrazepam	225 / 310	237 / 282 / 350	325

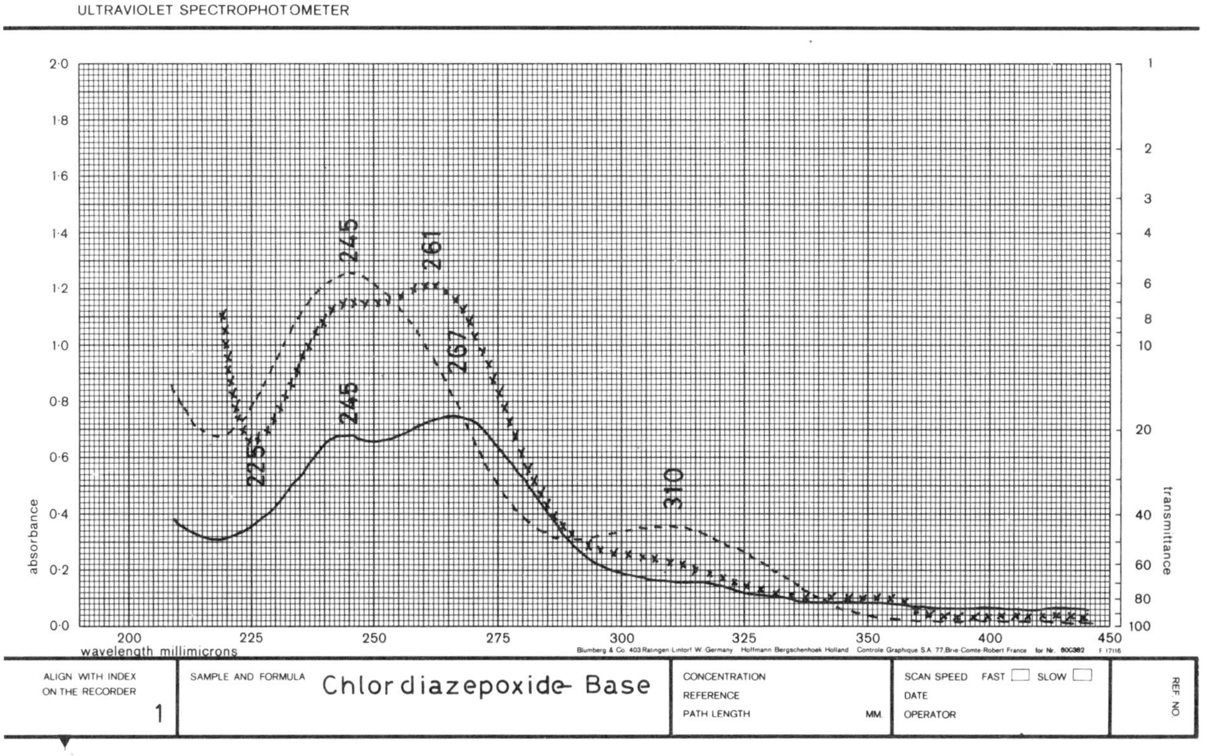

ULTRAVIOLET SPECTROPHOTOMETER

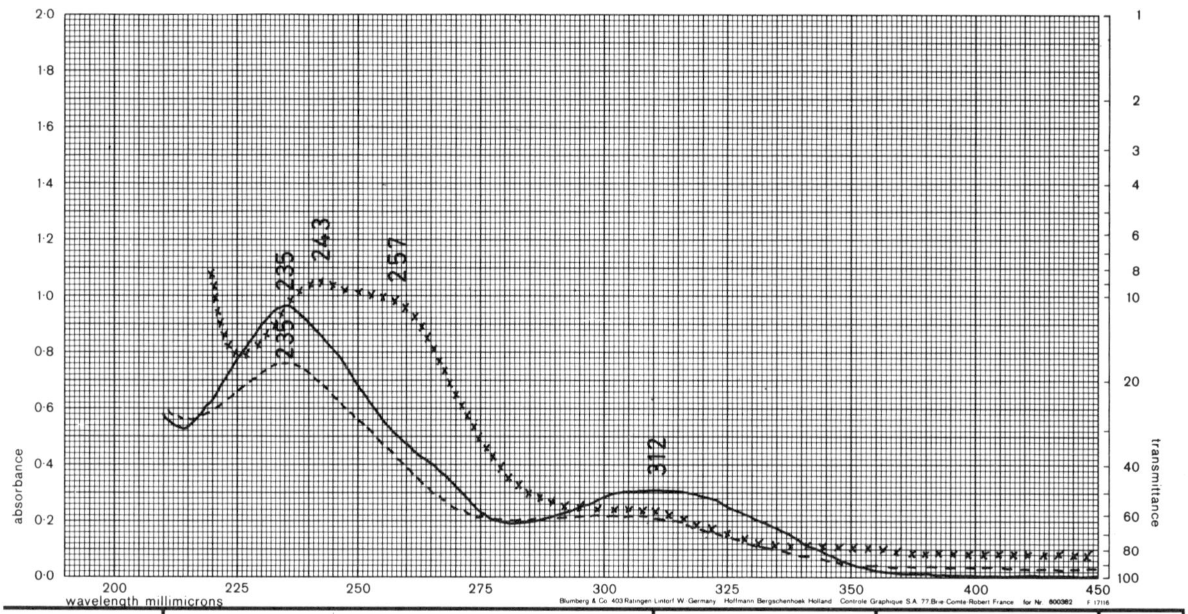

ALIGN WITH INDEX ON THE RECORDER	SAMPLE AND FORMULA	CONCENTRATION / REFERENCE / PATH LENGTH MM.	SCAN SPEED FAST ☐ SLOW ☐ / DATE / OPERATOR	REF. NO.
2	Demoxepam = Nor-Diazepam-N-Oxid			

ULTRAVIOLET SPECTROPHOTOMETER

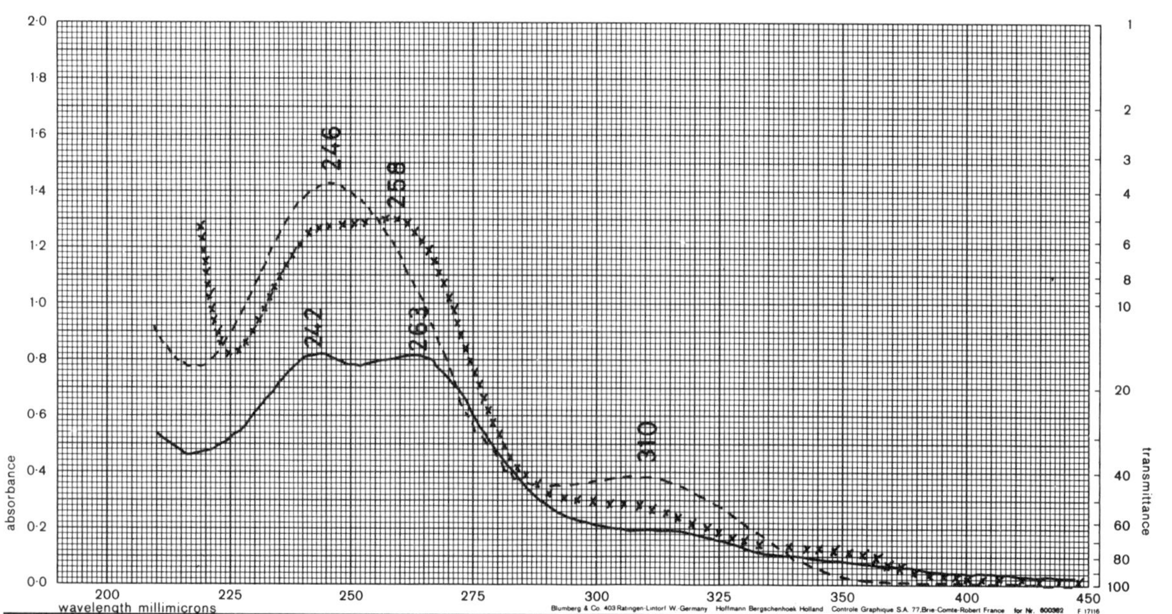

ALIGN WITH INDEX ON THE RECORDER	SAMPLE AND FORMULA	CONCENTRATION / REFERENCE / PATH LENGTH MM.	SCAN SPEED FAST ☐ SLOW ☐ / DATE / OPERATOR	REF. NO.
3	Desmethyl-Chlordiazepoxide-Base			

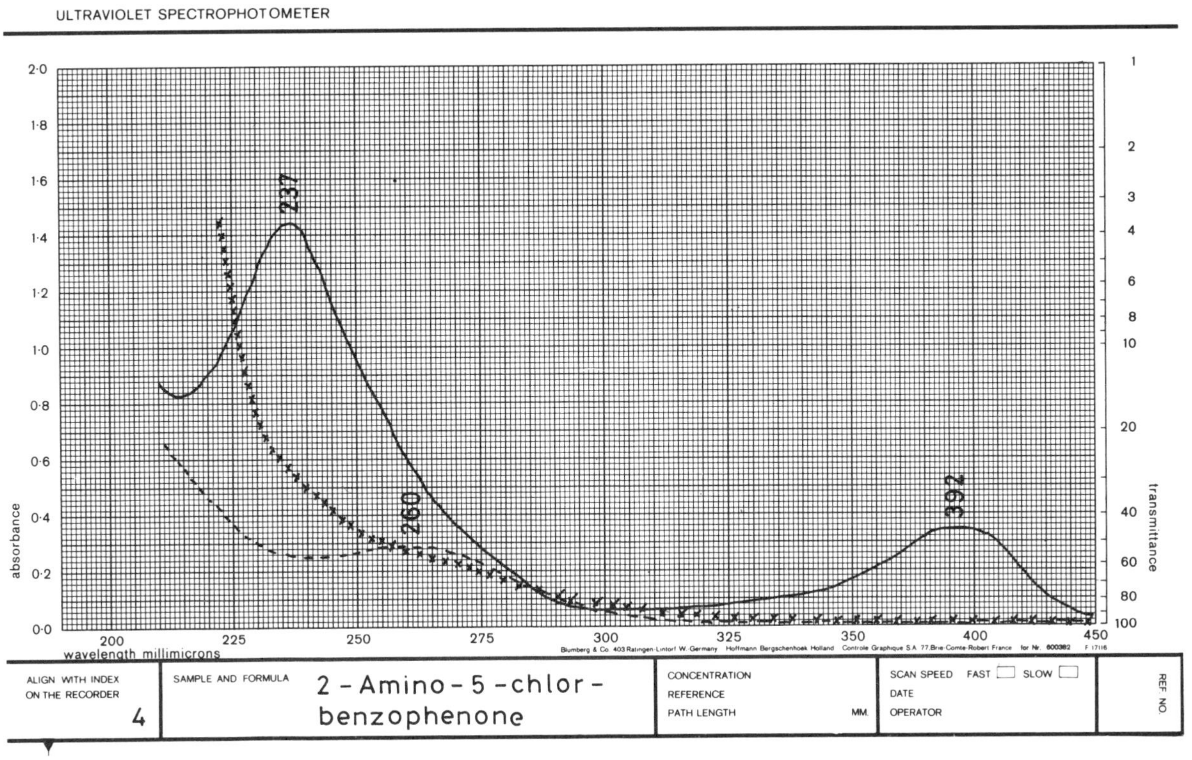
ULTRAVIOLET SPECTROPHOTOMETER
absorbance
transmittance
wavelength millimicrons
237
260
392
ALIGN WITH INDEX ON THE RECORDER
4
SAMPLE AND FORMULA
2-Amino-5-chlor-benzophenone
CONCENTRATION
REFERENCE
PATH LENGTH MM.
SCAN SPEED FAST SLOW
DATE
OPERATOR
REF NO.

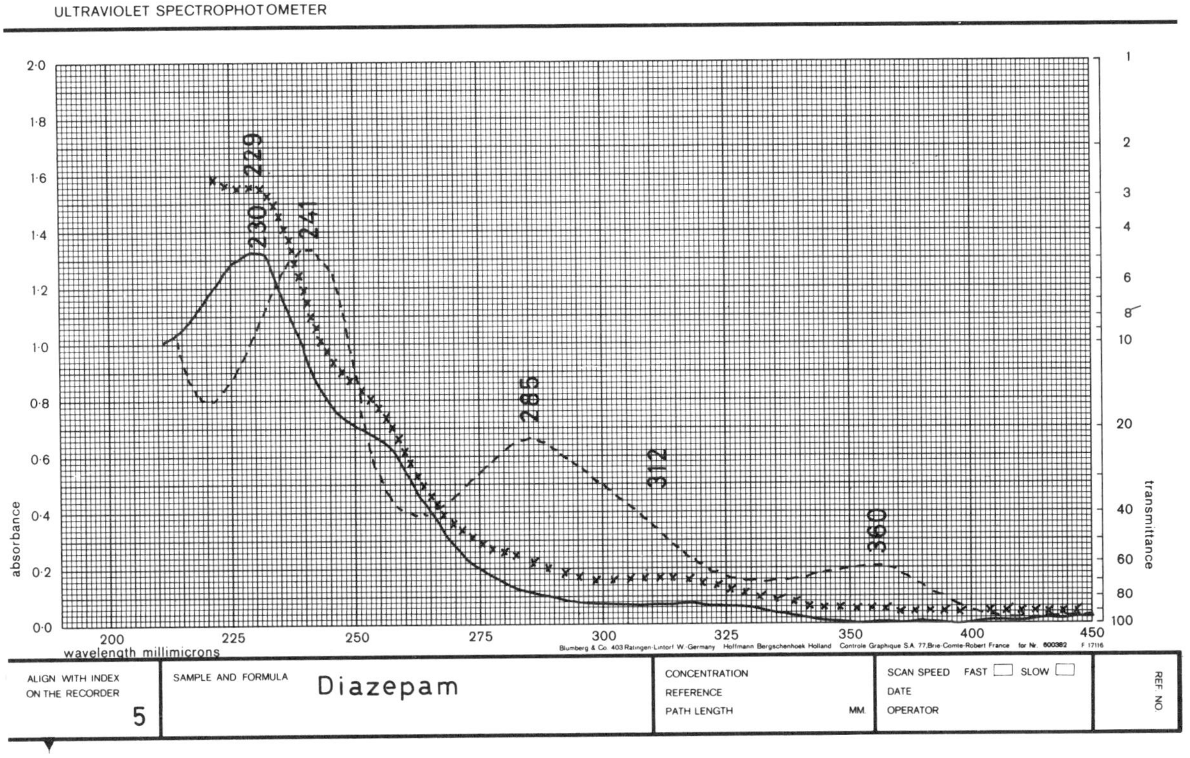
ULTRAVIOLET SPECTROPHOTOMETER
absorbance
transmittance
wavelength millimicrons
229
230
241
285
312
360
ALIGN WITH INDEX ON THE RECORDER
5
SAMPLE AND FORMULA
Diazepam
CONCENTRATION
REFERENCE
PATH LENGTH MM.
SCAN SPEED FAST SLOW
DATE
OPERATOR
REF NO.

ULTRAVIOLET SPECTROPHOTOMETER

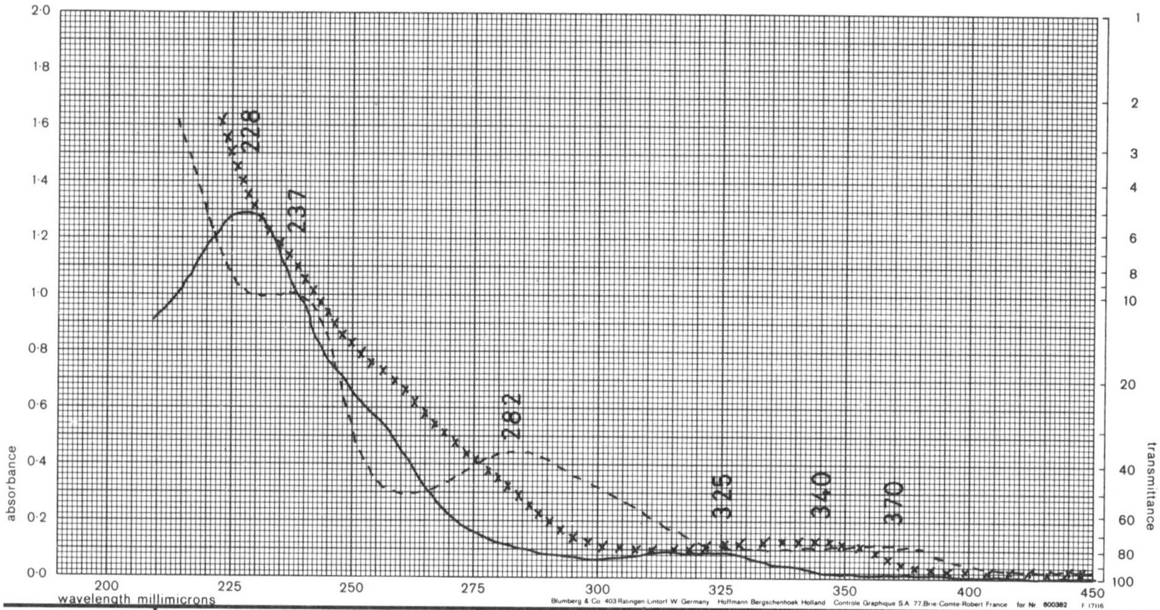

ALIGN WITH INDEX ON THE RECORDER 6

SAMPLE AND FORMULA Nor - Diazepam

CONCENTRATION
REFERENCE
PATH LENGTH MM

SCAN SPEED FAST ☐ SLOW ☐
DATE
OPERATOR

REF NO

ULTRAVIOLET SPECTROPHOTOMETER

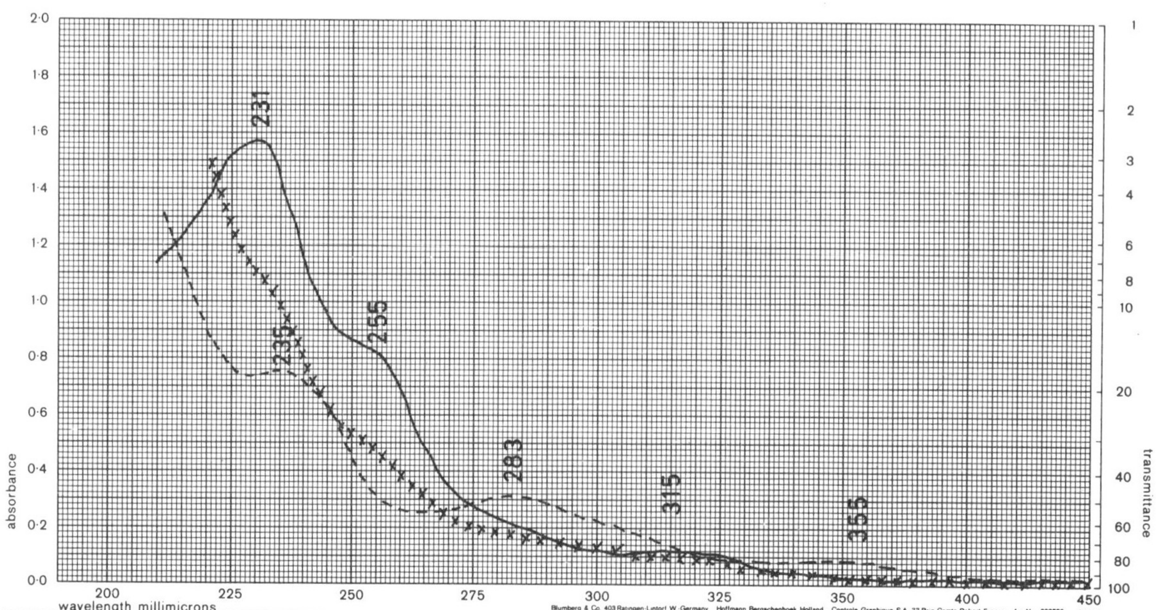

ALIGN WITH INDEX ON THE RECORDER 7

SAMPLE AND FORMULA 3-Hydroxy-Diazepam

CONCENTRATION
REFERENCE
PATH LENGTH MM

SCAN SPEED FAST ☐ SLOW ☐
DATE
OPERATOR

REF NO

ULTRAVIOLET SPECTROPHOTOMETER

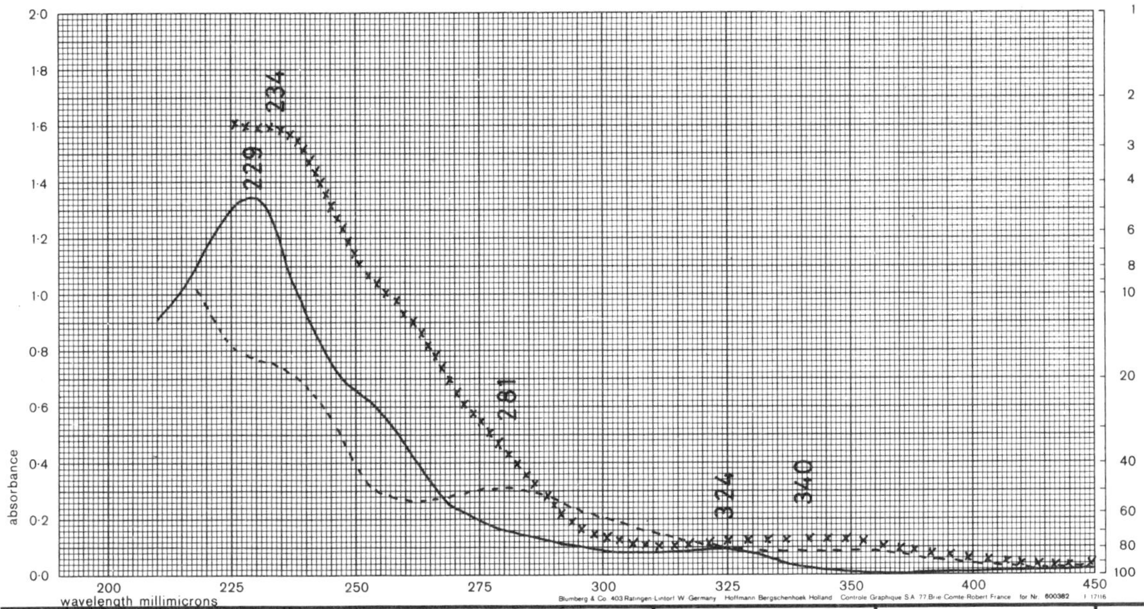

ALIGN WITH INDEX ON THE RECORDER	SAMPLE AND FORMULA	CONCENTRATION / REFERENCE / PATH LENGTH MM	SCAN SPEED FAST ☐ SLOW ☐ / DATE / OPERATOR	REF NO
8	Oxazepam			

ULTRAVIOLET SPECTROPHOTOMETER

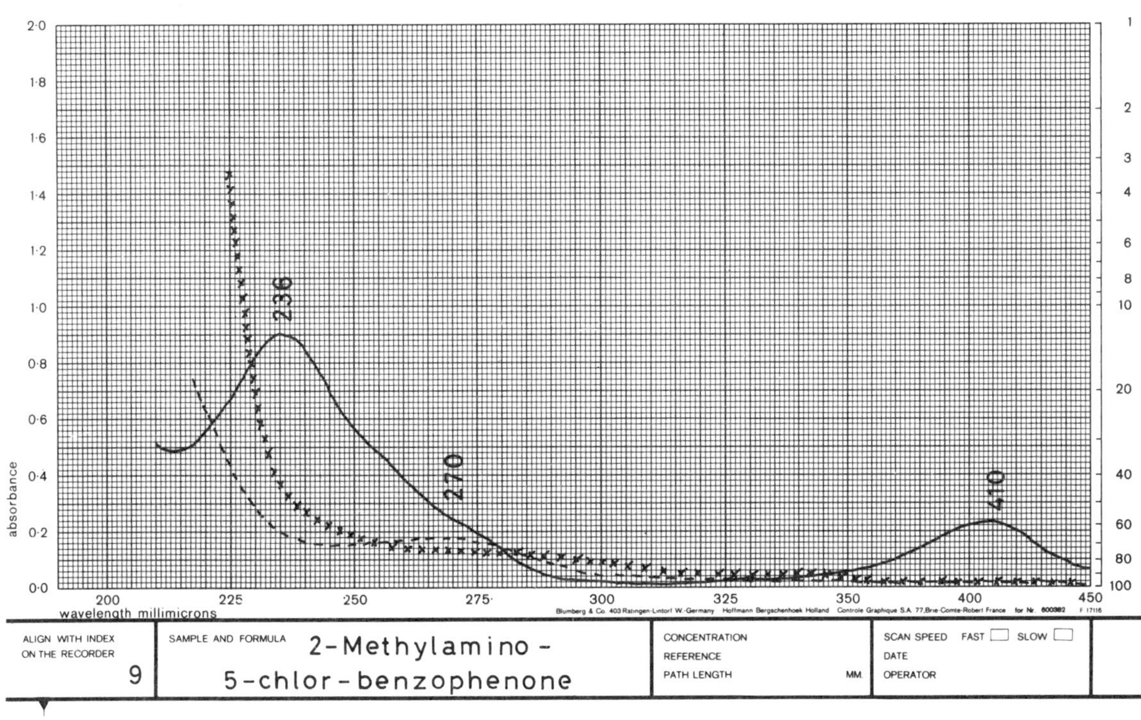

ALIGN WITH INDEX ON THE RECORDER	SAMPLE AND FORMULA	CONCENTRATION / REFERENCE / PATH LENGTH MM	SCAN SPEED FAST ☐ SLOW ☐ / DATE / OPERATOR	REF NO
9	2-Methylamino - 5-chlor-benzophenone			

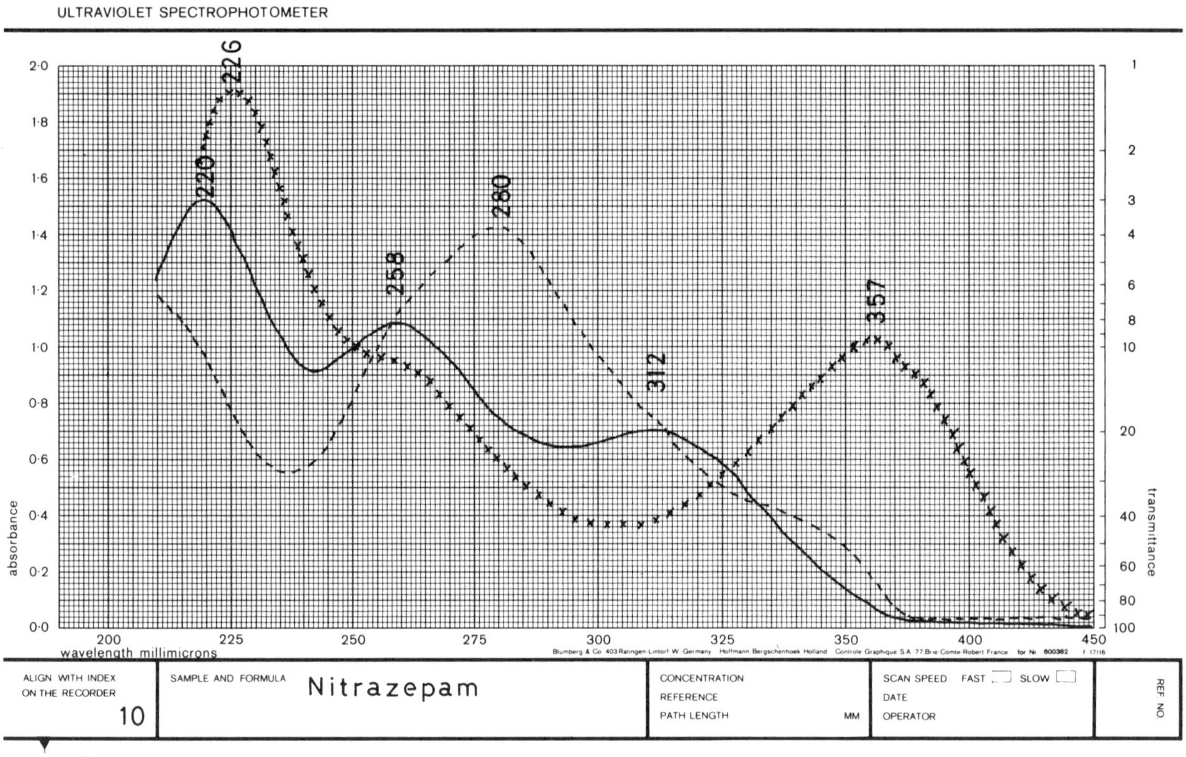
ULTRAVIOLET SPECTROPHOTOMETER
2·0
1·8
1·6
1·4
1·2
1·0
0·8
0·6
0·4
0·2
0·0
absorbance
1
2
3
4
6
8
10
20
40
60
80
100
transmittance
226
220
280
258
357
312
200
225
250
275
300
325
350
400
450
wavelength millimicrons
ALIGN WITH INDEX ON THE RECORDER
10
SAMPLE AND FORMULA
Nitrazepam
CONCENTRATION
REFERENCE
PATH LENGTH
MM
SCAN SPEED FAST SLOW
DATE
OPERATOR
REF. NO.

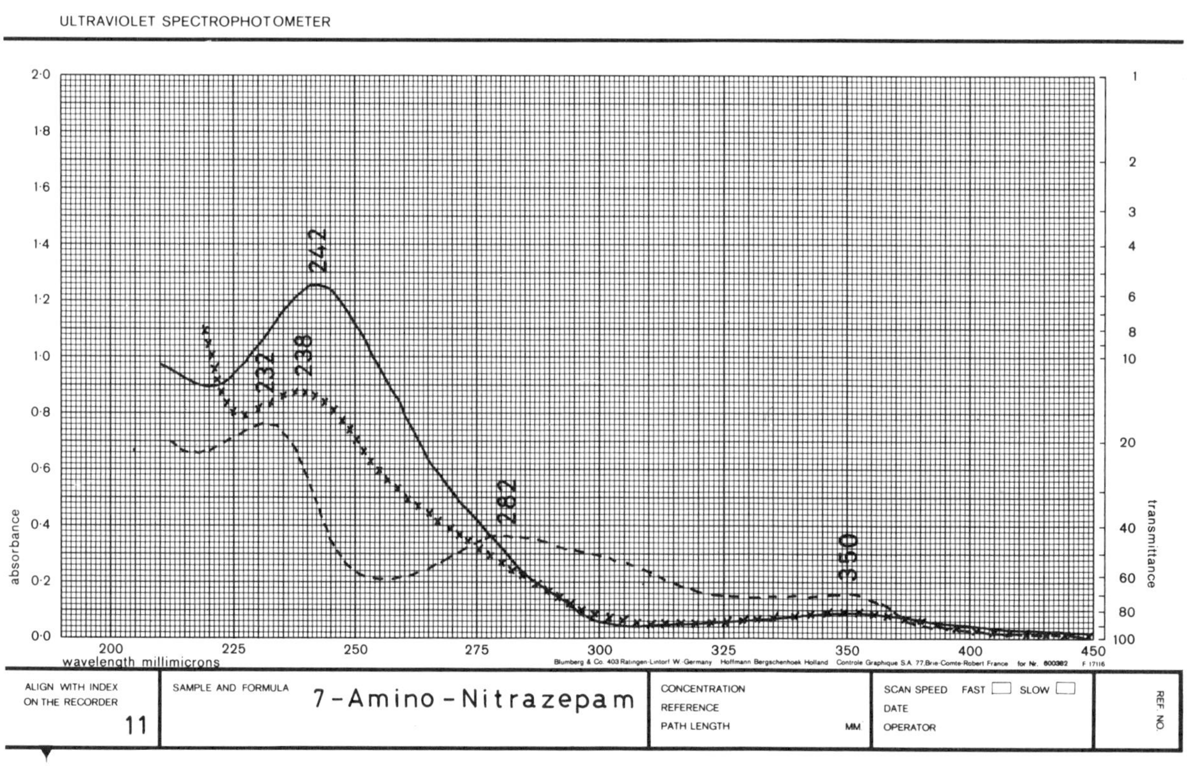
ULTRAVIOLET SPECTROPHOTOMETER
2·0
1·8
1·6
1·4
1·2
1·0
0·8
0·6
0·4
0·2
0·0
absorbance
1
2
3
4
6
8
10
20
40
60
80
100
transmittance
242
232
238
282
350
200
225
250
275
300
325
350
400
450
wavelength millimicrons
ALIGN WITH INDEX ON THE RECORDER
11
SAMPLE AND FORMULA
7-Amino-Nitrazepam
CONCENTRATION
REFERENCE
PATH LENGTH
MM
SCAN SPEED FAST SLOW
DATE
OPERATOR
REF. NO.

ULTRAVIOLET SPECTROPHOTOMETER

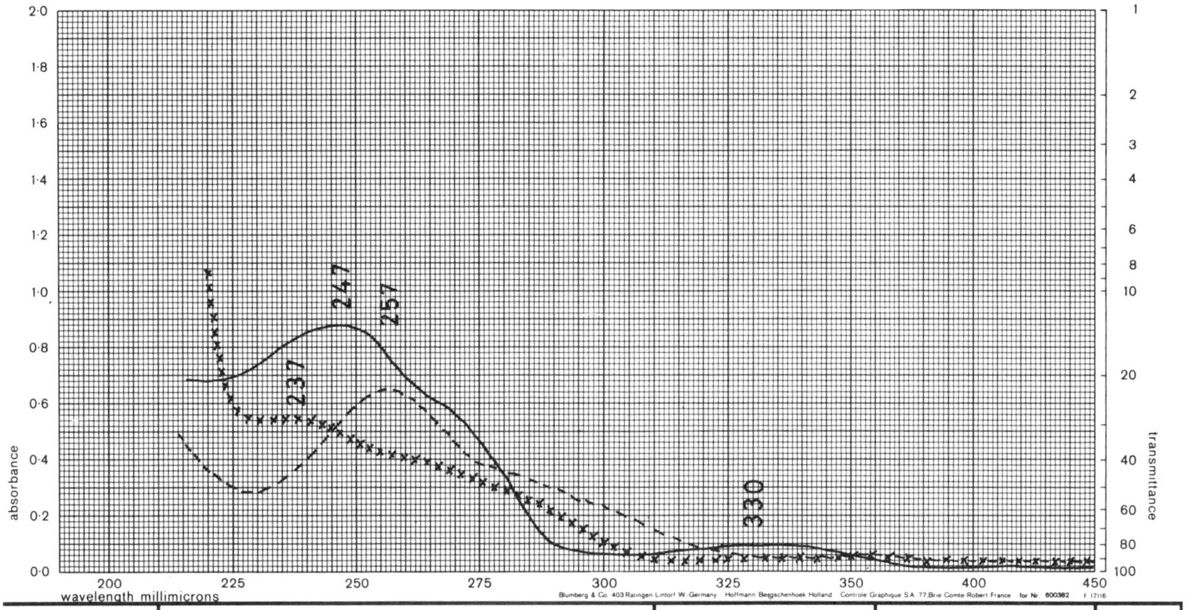

ALIGN WITH INDEX ON THE RECORDER 12

SAMPLE AND FORMULA 7-Acetamido-Nitrazepam

CONCENTRATION
REFERENCE
PATH LENGTH MM

SCAN SPEED FAST ☐ SLOW ☐
DATE
OPERATOR

REF NO.

ULTRAVIOLET SPECTROPHOTOMETER

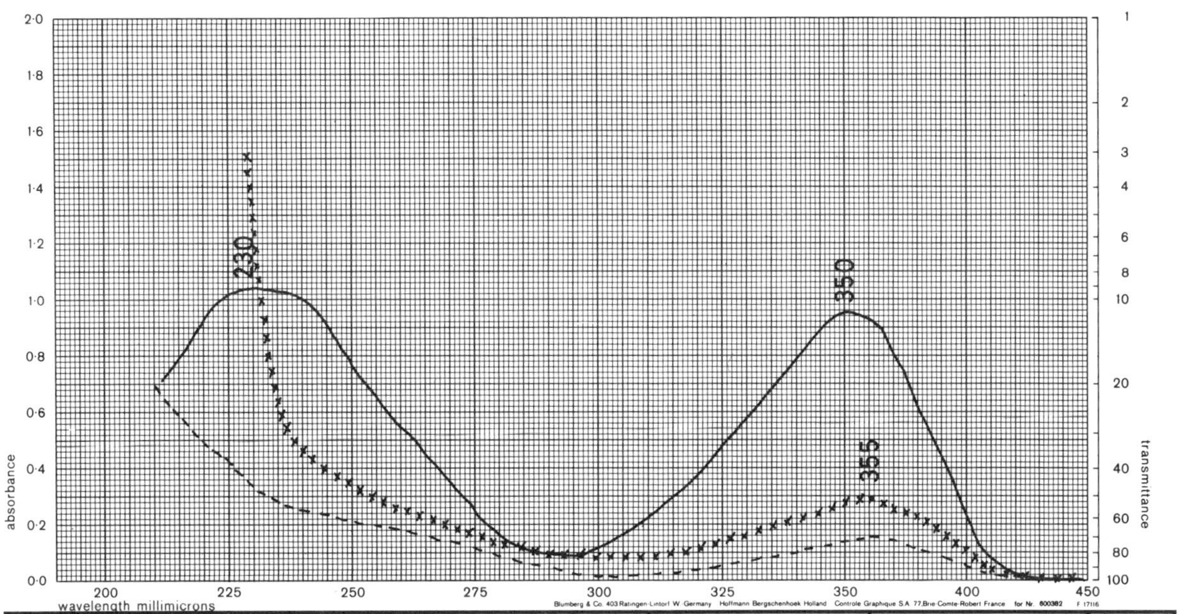

ALIGN WITH INDEX ON THE RECORDER 13

SAMPLE AND FORMULA 2-Amino-5-nitro-benzophenone

CONCENTRATION
REFERENCE
PATH LENGTH MM

SCAN SPEED FAST ☐ SLOW ☐
DATE
OPERATOR

REF NO.

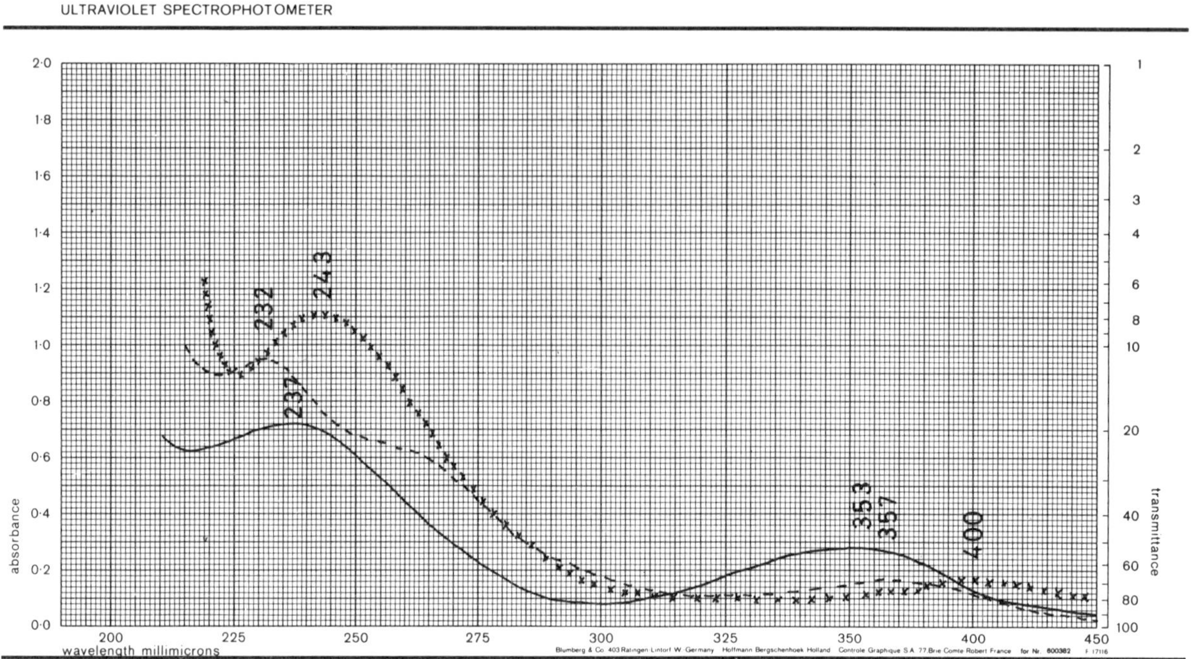

ALIGN WITH INDEX ON THE RECORDER 14

SAMPLE AND FORMULA 2,5-Diamino-benzophenone

CONCENTRATION
REFERENCE
PATH LENGTH MM

SCAN SPEED FAST ☐ SLOW ☐
DATE
OPERATOR

REF NO

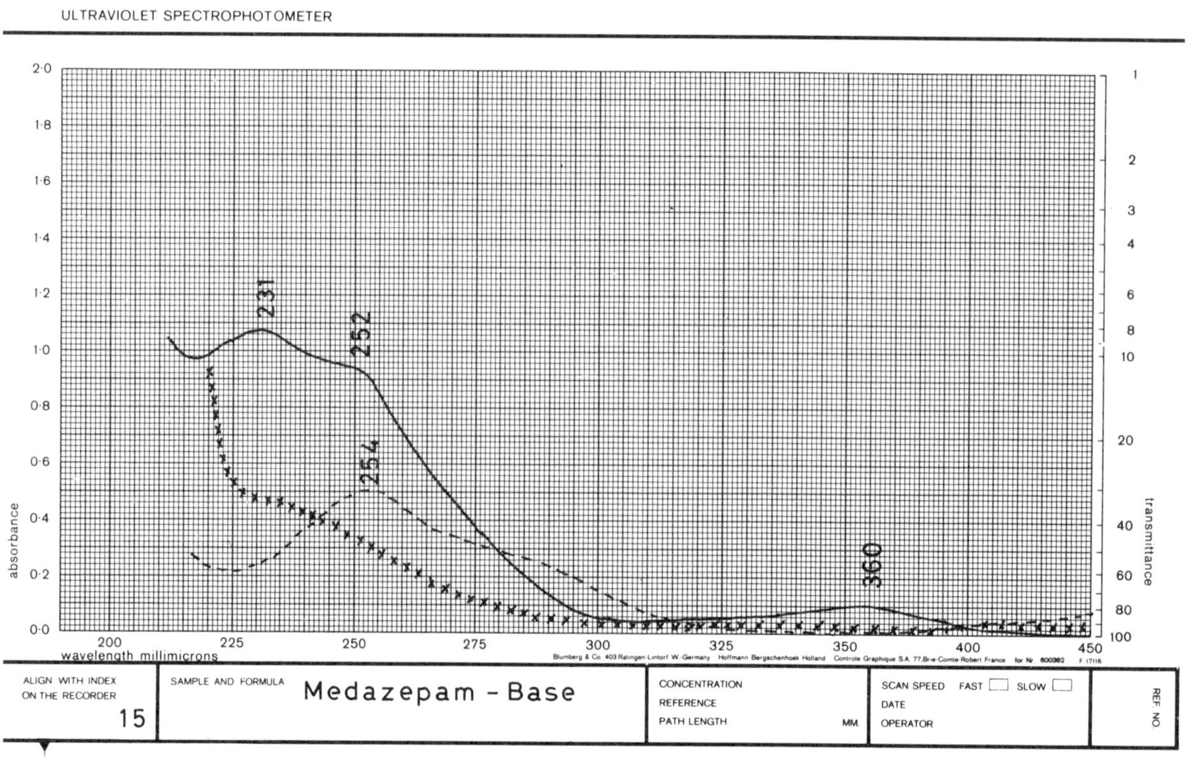

ALIGN WITH INDEX ON THE RECORDER 15

SAMPLE AND FORMULA Medazepam - Base

CONCENTRATION
REFERENCE
PATH LENGTH MM

SCAN SPEED FAST ☐ SLOW ☐
DATE
OPERATOR

REF NO

ULTRAVIOLET SPECTROPHOTOMETER

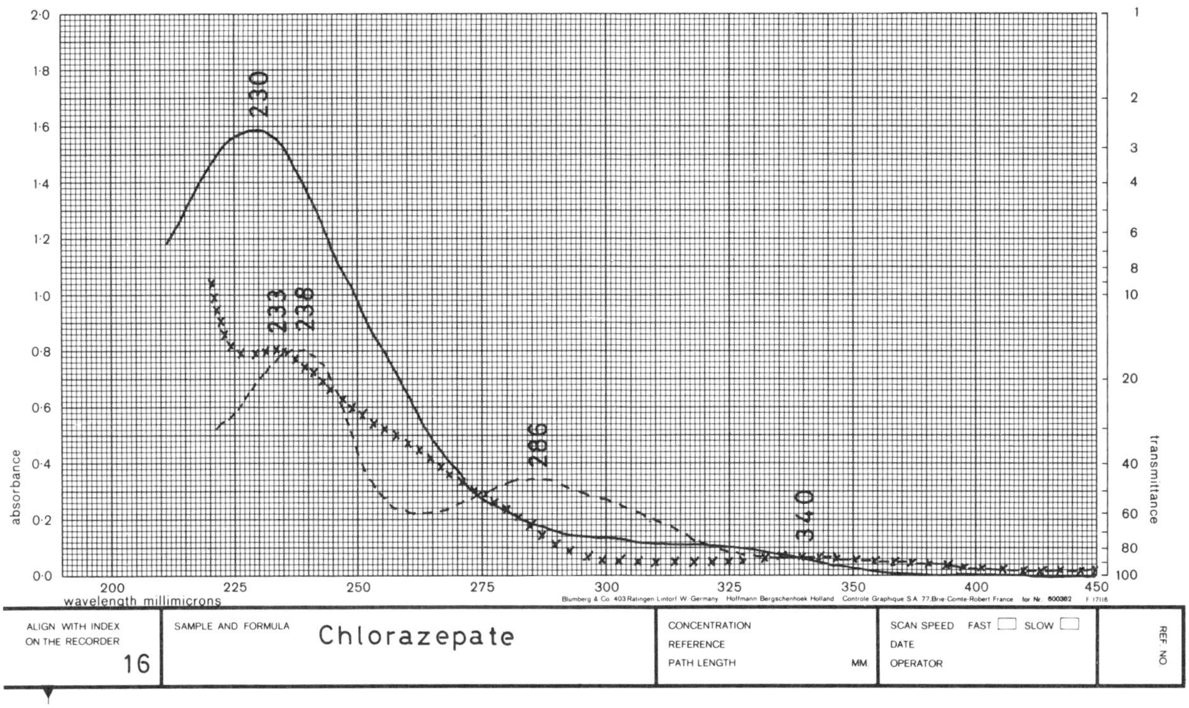

ULTRAVIOLET SPECTROPHOTOMETER

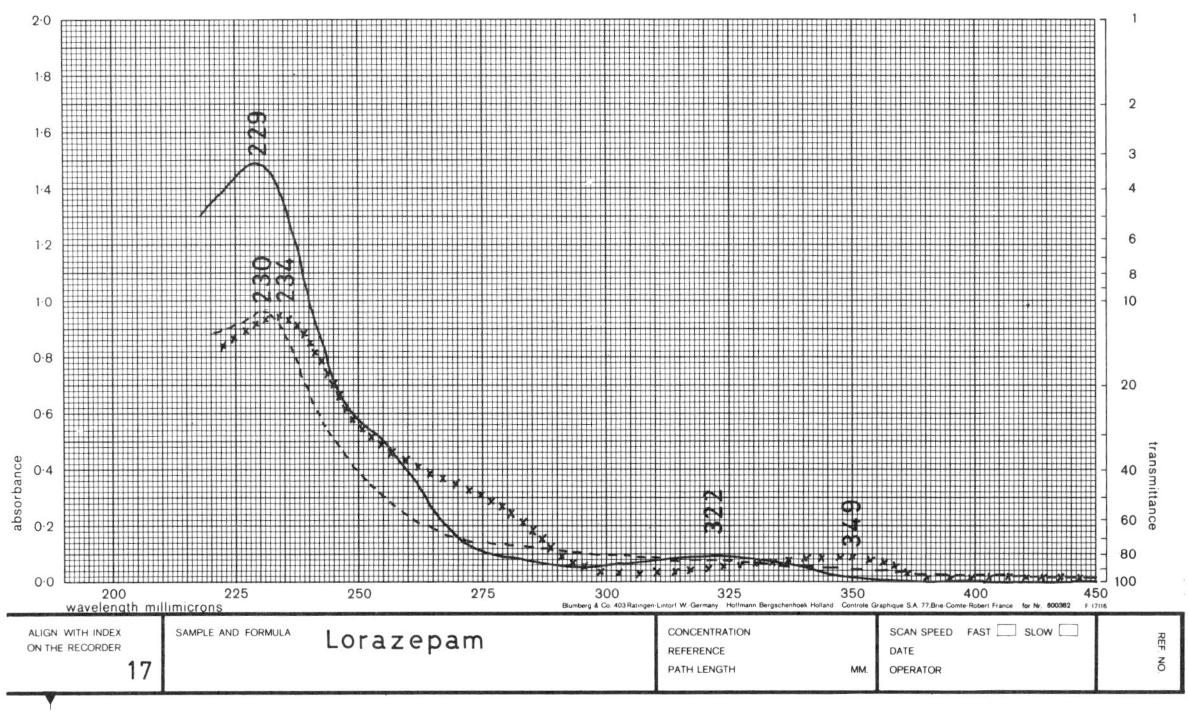

ULTRAVIOLET SPECTROPHOTOMETER

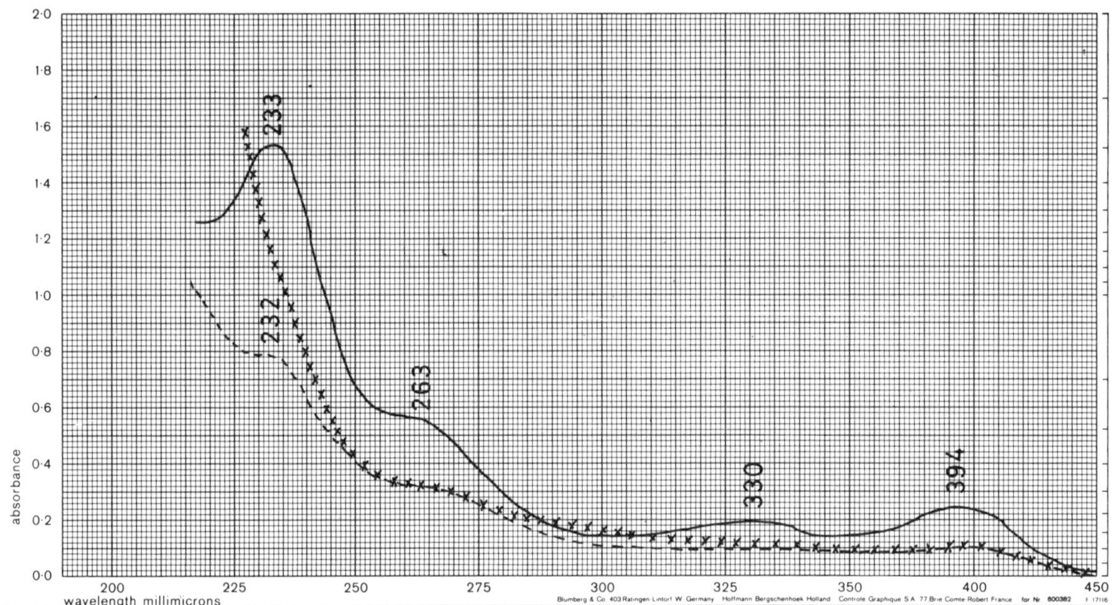

ALIGN WITH INDEX ON THE RECORDER 18	SAMPLE AND FORMULA 2-Amino-5,2'-dichlor-benzophenone	CONCENTRATION REFERENCE PATH LENGTH MM	SCAN SPEED FAST ☐ SLOW ☐ DATE OPERATOR	REF NO

ULTRAVIOLET SPECTROPHOTOMETER

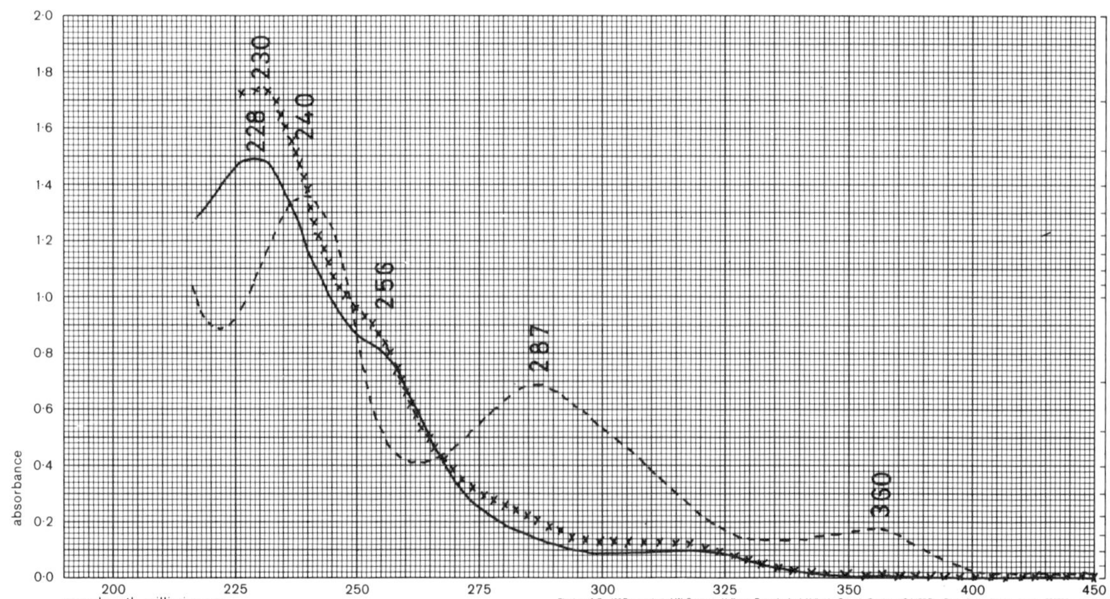

ALIGN WITH INDEX ON THE RECORDER 19	SAMPLE AND FORMULA Prazepam	CONCENTRATION REFERENCE PATH LENGTH MM	SCAN SPEED FAST ☐ SLOW ☐ DATE OPERATOR	REF NO

ULTRAVIOLET SPECTROPHOTOMETER

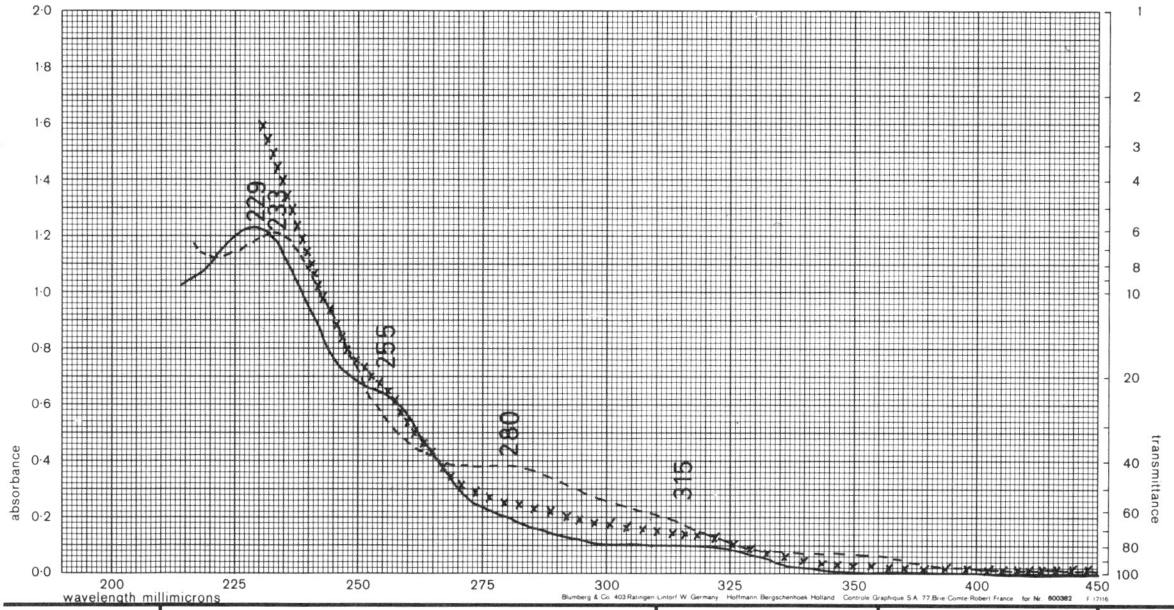

ALIGN WITH INDEX ON THE RECORDER 20	SAMPLE AND FORMULA 3-Hydroxy-Prazepam	CONCENTRATION REFERENCE PATH LENGTH MM	SCAN SPEED FAST ☐ SLOW ☐ DATE OPERATOR	REF NO

ULTRAVIOLET SPECTROPHOTOMETER

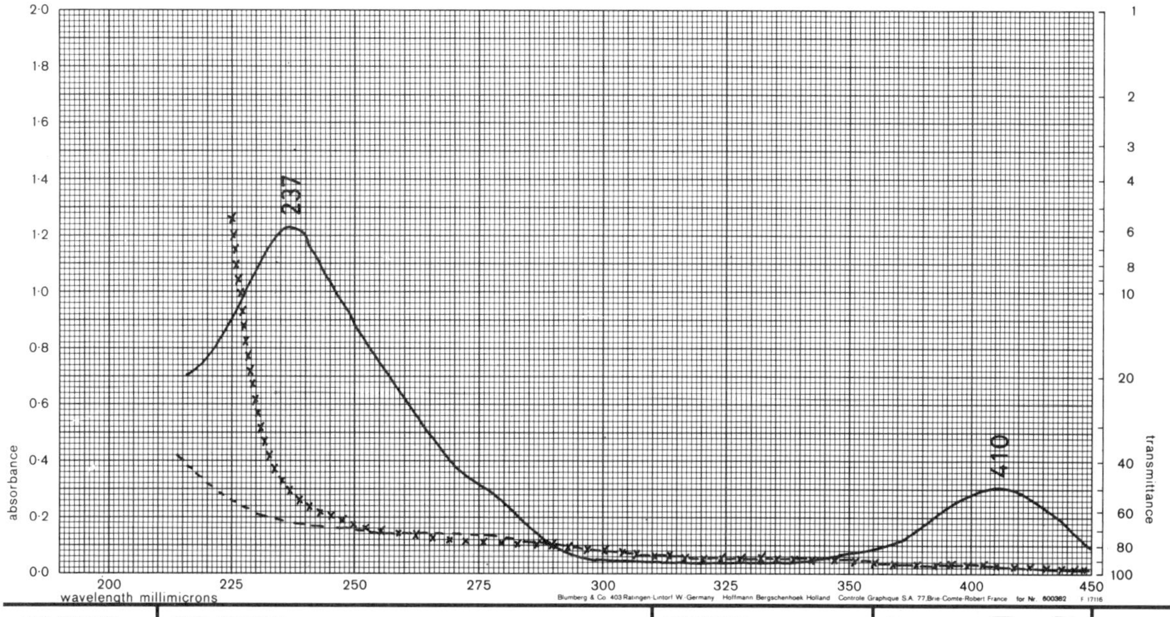

ALIGN WITH INDEX ON THE RECORDER 21	SAMPLE AND FORMULA 2-Cyclopropyl-methylamino-5-chlor-benzoph.	CONCENTRATION REFERENCE PATH LENGTH MM	SCAN SPEED FAST ☐ SLOW ☐ DATE OPERATOR	REF NO

ULTRAVIOLET SPECTROPHOTOMETER

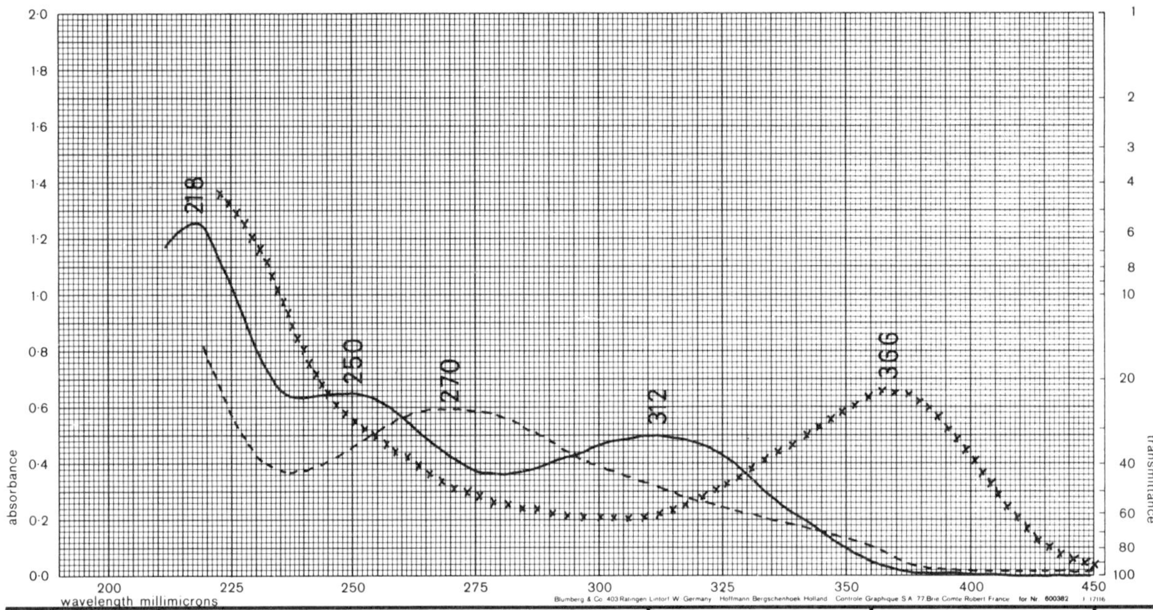

ALIGN WITH INDEX ON THE RECORDER	SAMPLE AND FORMULA	CONCENTRATION	SCAN SPEED FAST ☐ SLOW ☐	REF. NO.
22	Clonazepam	REFERENCE	DATE	
		PATH LENGTH MM	OPERATOR	

ULTRAVIOLET SPECTROPHOTOMETER

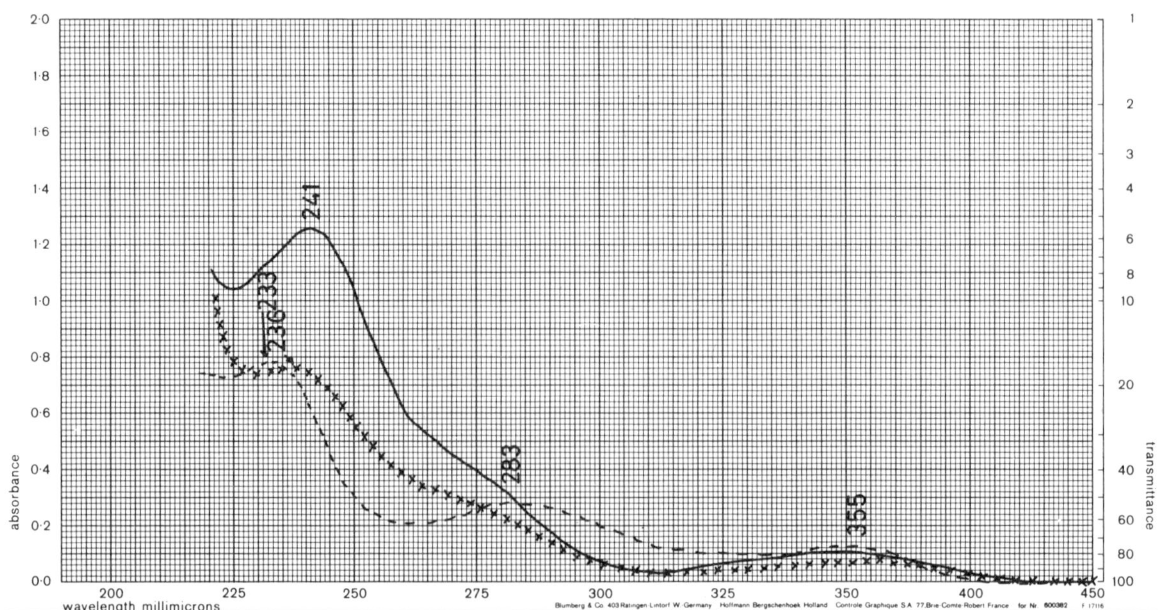

ALIGN WITH INDEX ON THE RECORDER	SAMPLE AND FORMULA	CONCENTRATION	SCAN SPEED FAST ☐ SLOW ☐	REF. NO.
23	7-Amino-Clonazepam	REFERENCE	DATE	
		PATH LENGTH MM	OPERATOR	

ULTRAVIOLET SPECTROPHOTOMETER

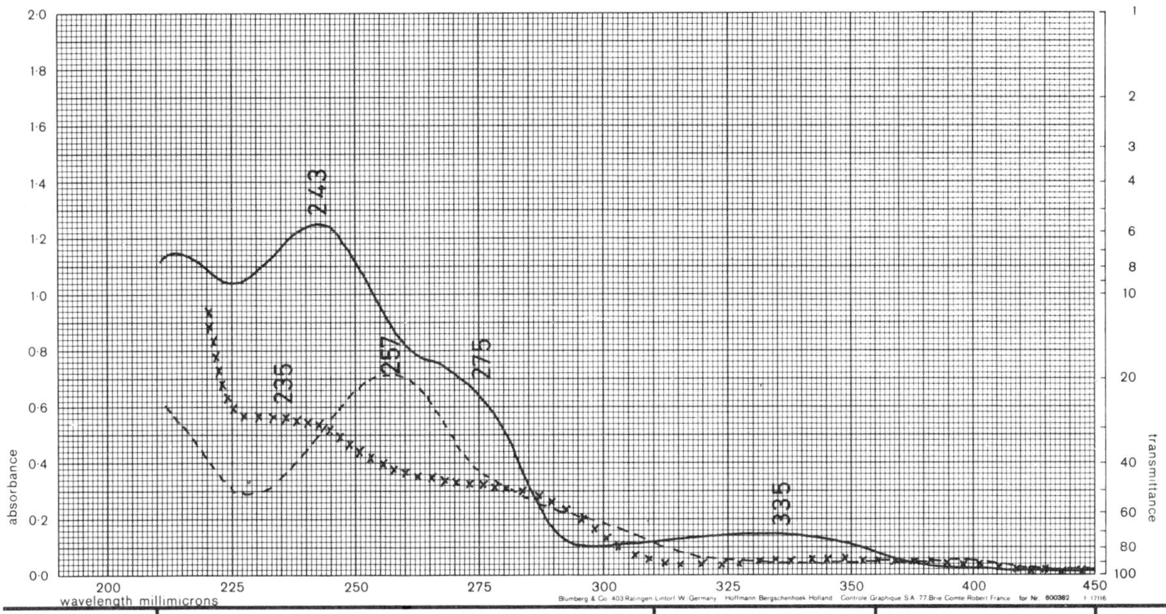

ALIGN WITH INDEX ON THE RECORDER	SAMPLE AND FORMULA	CONCENTRATION	SCAN SPEED FAST ☐ SLOW ☐	REF NO
24	7-Acetamido-Clonazepam	REFERENCE	DATE	
		PATH LENGTH MM	OPERATOR	

ULTRAVIOLET SPECTROPHOTOMETER

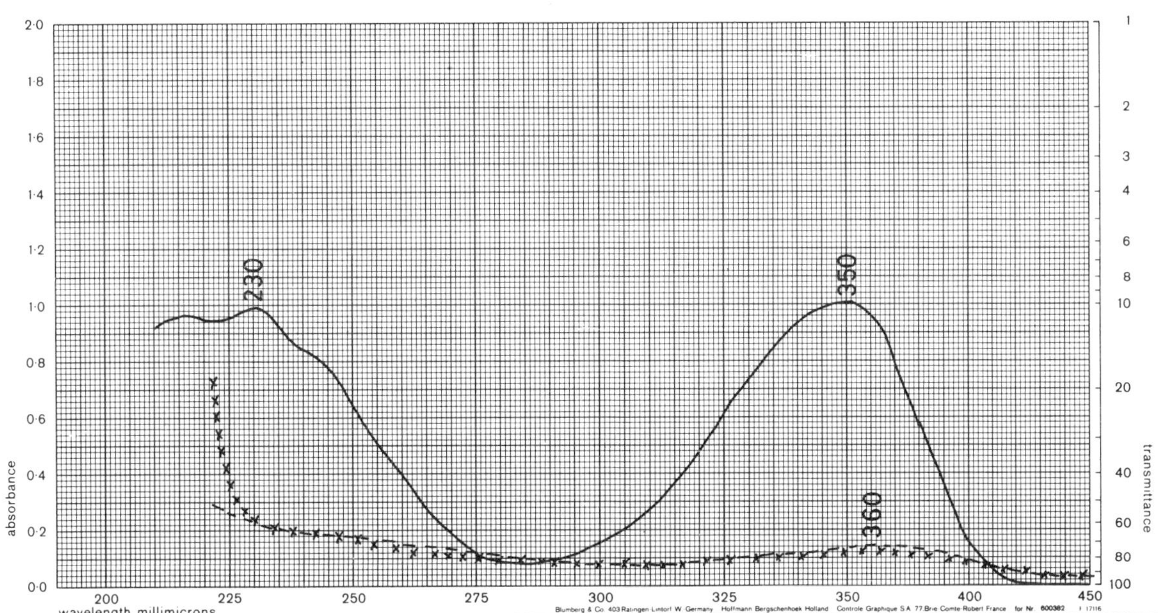

ALIGN WITH INDEX ON THE RECORDER	SAMPLE AND FORMULA	CONCENTRATION	SCAN SPEED FAST ☐ SLOW ☐	REF NO
25	2-Amino-5-nitro-2'-chlor-benzophenone	REFERENCE	DATE	
		PATH LENGTH MM	OPERATOR	

ULTRAVIOLET SPECTROPHOTOMETER

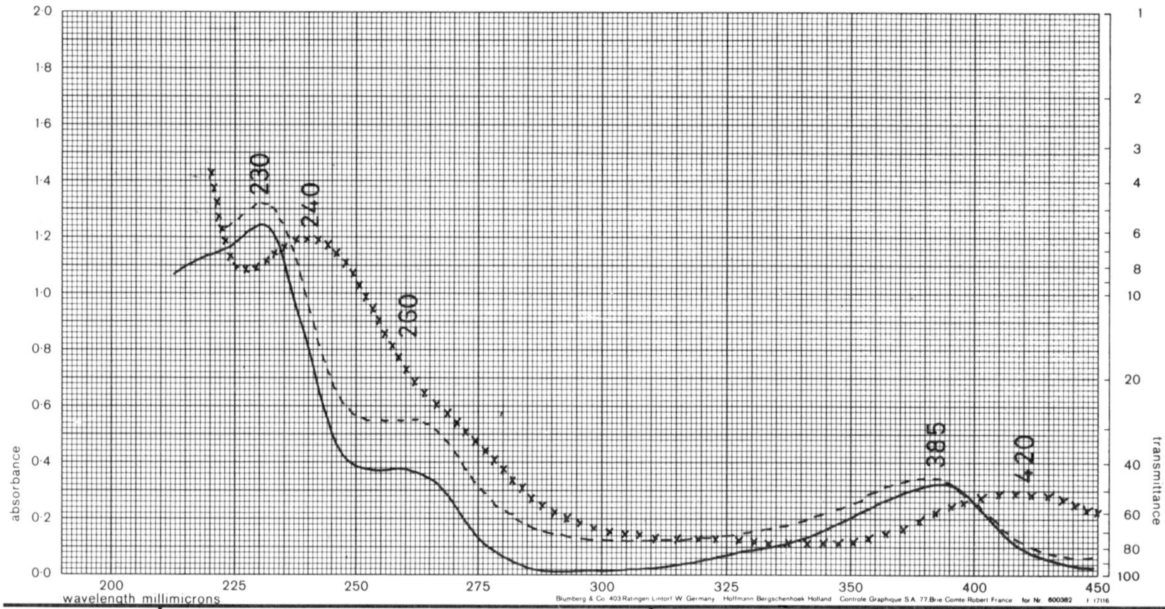

ALIGN WITH INDEX ON THE RECORDER	SAMPLE AND FORMULA	CONCENTRATION / REFERENCE / PATH LENGTH MM	SCAN SPEED FAST ☐ SLOW ☐ / DATE / OPERATOR	REF. NO.
26	2,5 - Diamino - 2'- chlor - benzophenone x HCl			

ULTRAVIOLET SPECTROPHOTOMETER

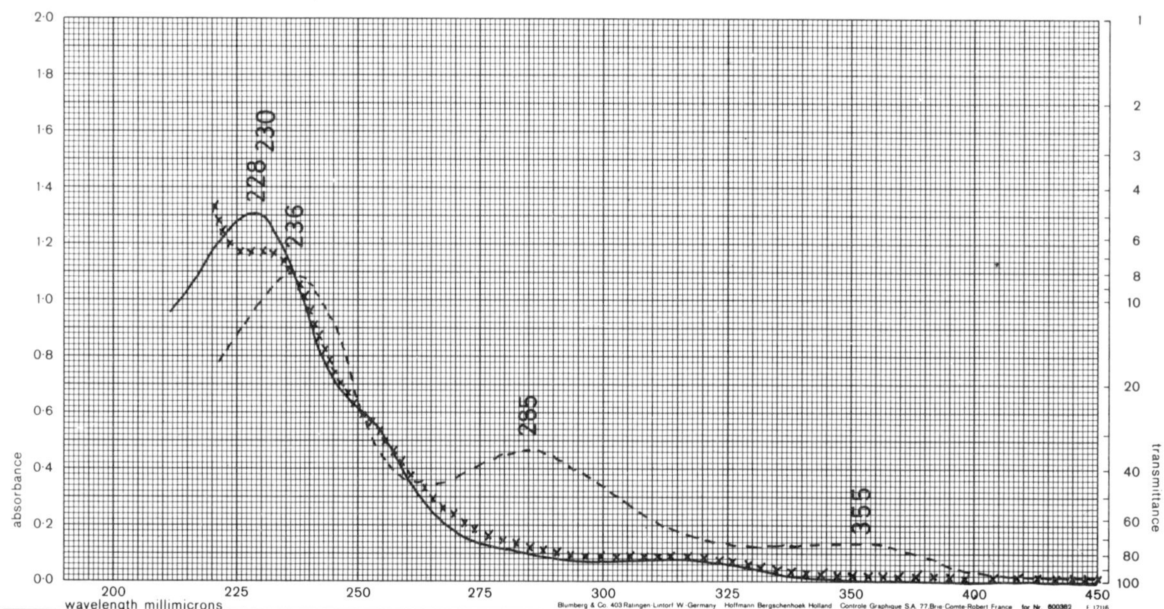

ALIGN WITH INDEX ON THE RECORDER	SAMPLE AND FORMULA	CONCENTRATION / REFERENCE / PATH LENGTH MM	SCAN SPEED FAST ☐ SLOW ☐ / DATE / OPERATOR	REF. NO.
27	Flurazepam x HCl			

ULTRAVIOLET SPECTROPHOTOMETER

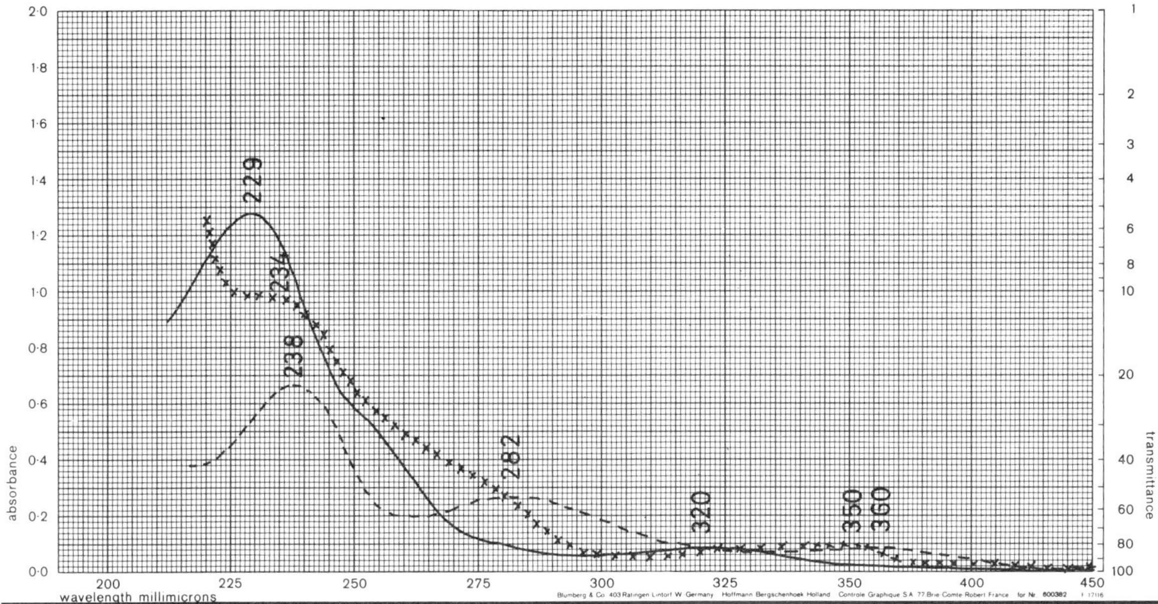

ALIGN WITH INDEX ON THE RECORDER	SAMPLE AND FORMULA	CONCENTRATION	SCAN SPEED FAST ☐ SLOW ☐	REF NO
28	N-1-Desalkyl-Flurazepam	REFERENCE	DATE	
		PATH LENGTH MM	OPERATOR	

ULTRAVIOLET SPECTROPHOTOMETER

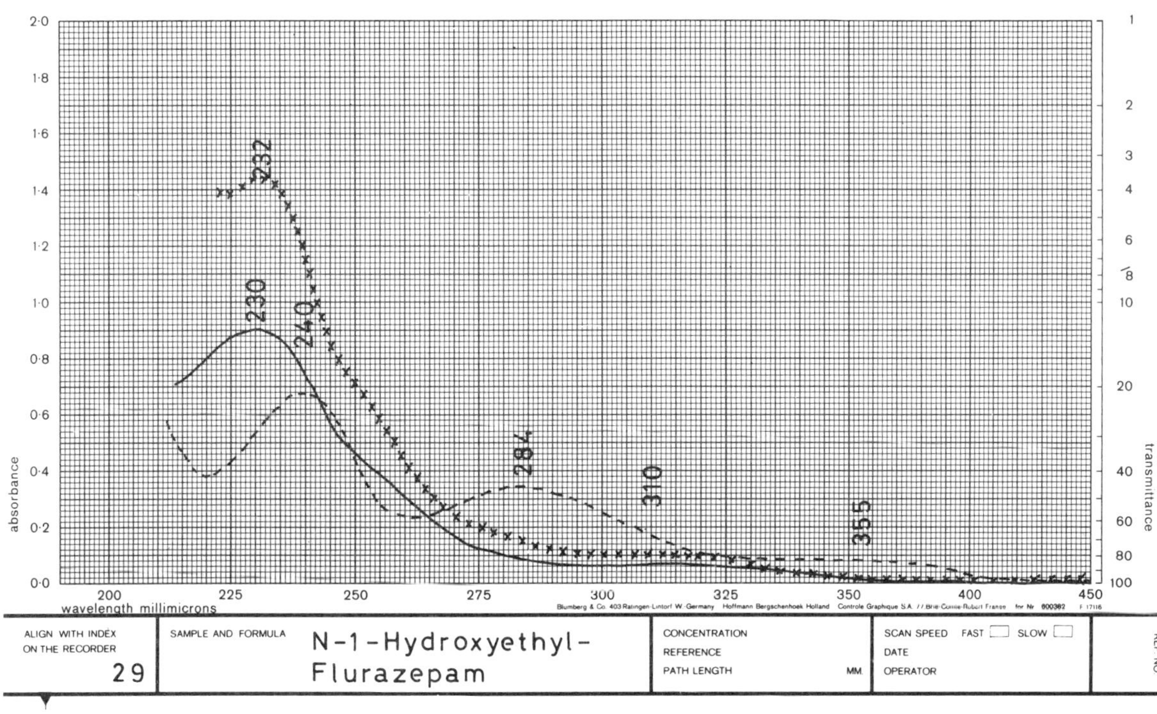

ALIGN WITH INDEX ON THE RECORDER	SAMPLE AND FORMULA	CONCENTRATION	SCAN SPEED FAST ☐ SLOW ☐	REF NO
29	N-1-Hydroxyethyl-Flurazepam	REFERENCE	DATE	
		PATH LENGTH MM	OPERATOR	

ULTRAVIOLET SPECTROPHOTOMETER

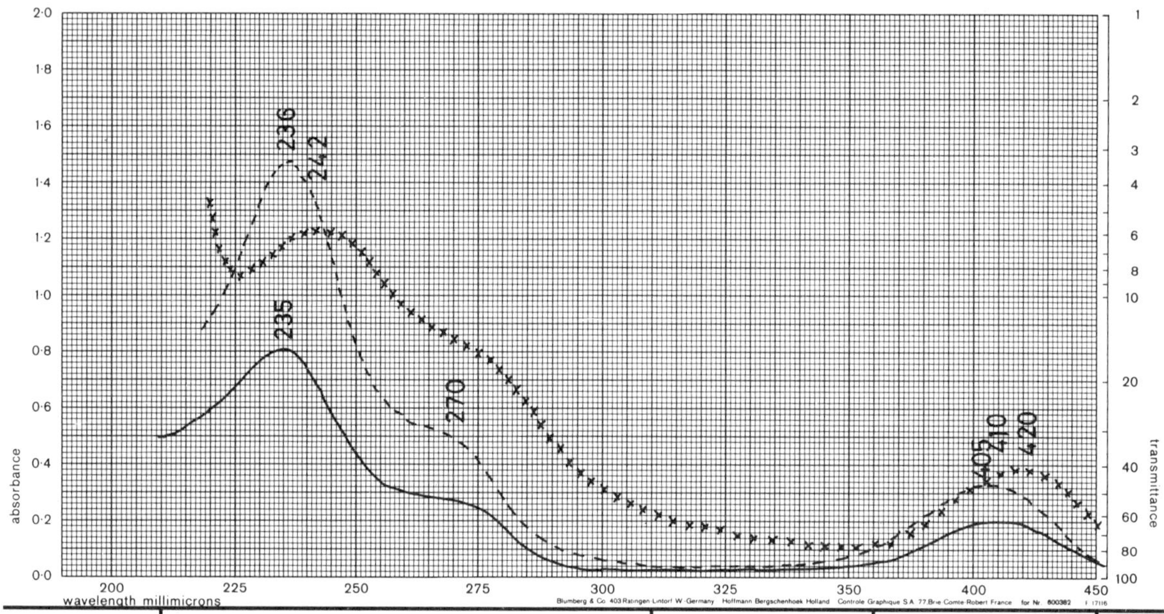

ALIGN WITH INDEX ON THE RECORDER	SAMPLE AND FORMULA	CONCENTRATION / REFERENCE / PATH LENGTH MM	SCAN SPEED FAST SLOW / DATE / OPERATOR	REF NO
30	2-Diethylamino-ethyl-amino-5-chlor-2'-fluor-benzoph			

ULTRAVIOLET SPECTROPHOTOMETER

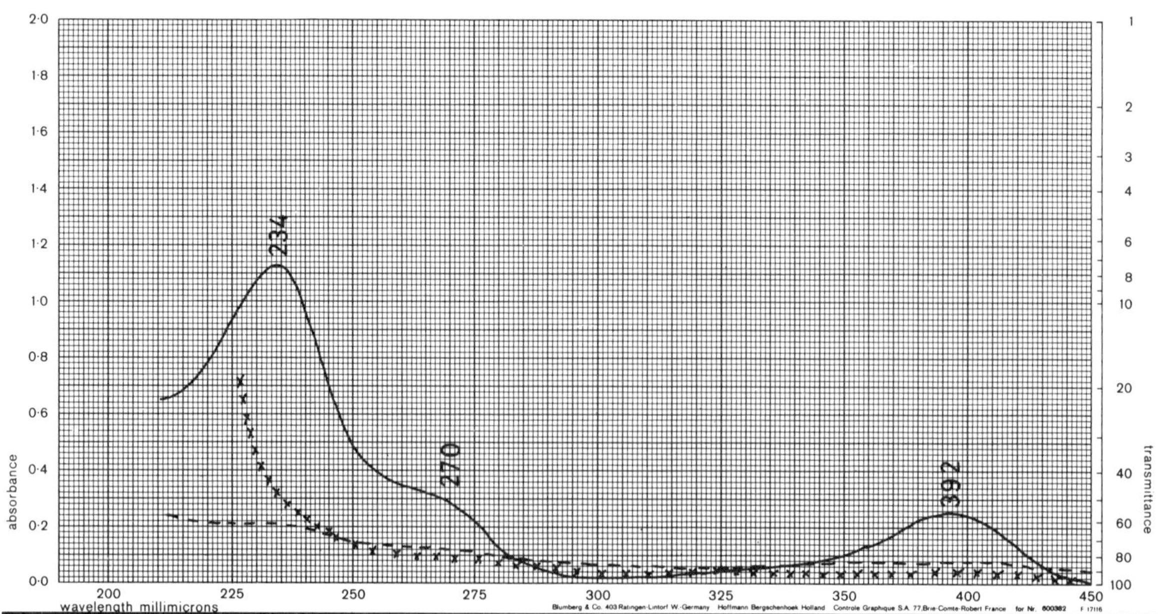

ALIGN WITH INDEX ON THE RECORDER	SAMPLE AND FORMULA	CONCENTRATION / REFERENCE / PATH LENGTH MM	SCAN SPEED FAST SLOW / DATE / OPERATOR	REF NO
31	2-Amino-5-chlor-2'-fluor-benzophenone			

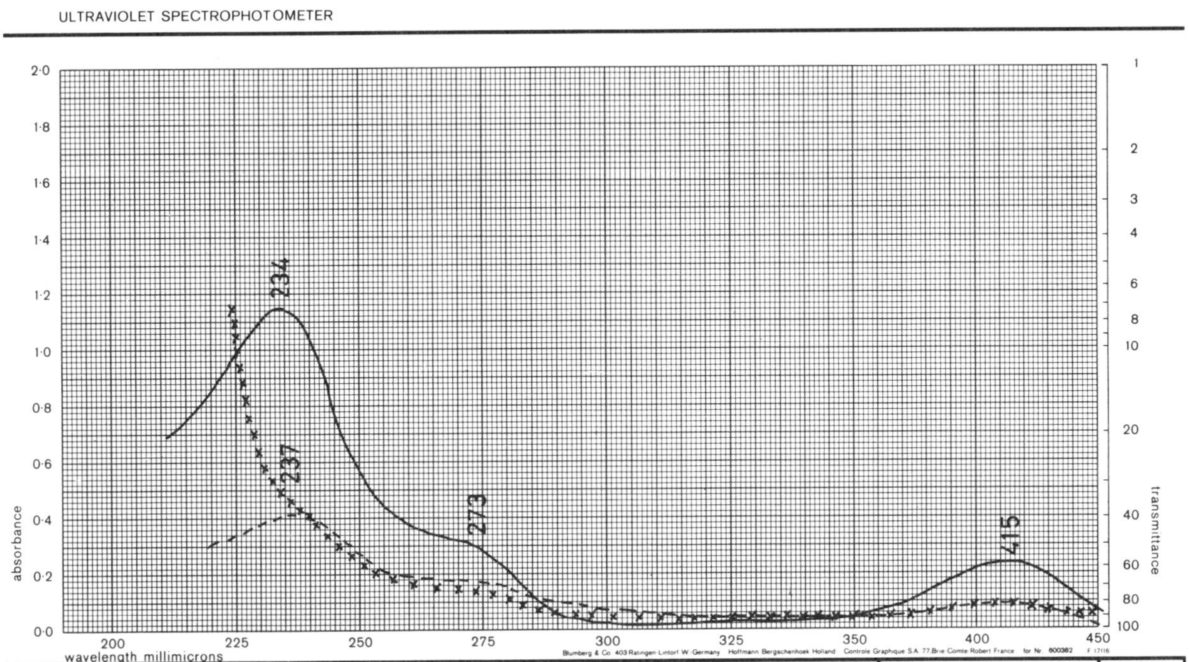

ALIGN WITH INDEX ON THE RECORDER 32	SAMPLE AND FORMULA 2-Hydroxyethylamino-5-chlor-2'-fluor-benzophenone	CONCENTRATION REFERENCE PATH LENGTH MM.	SCAN SPEED FAST ☐ SLOW ☐ DATE OPERATOR	REF. NO.

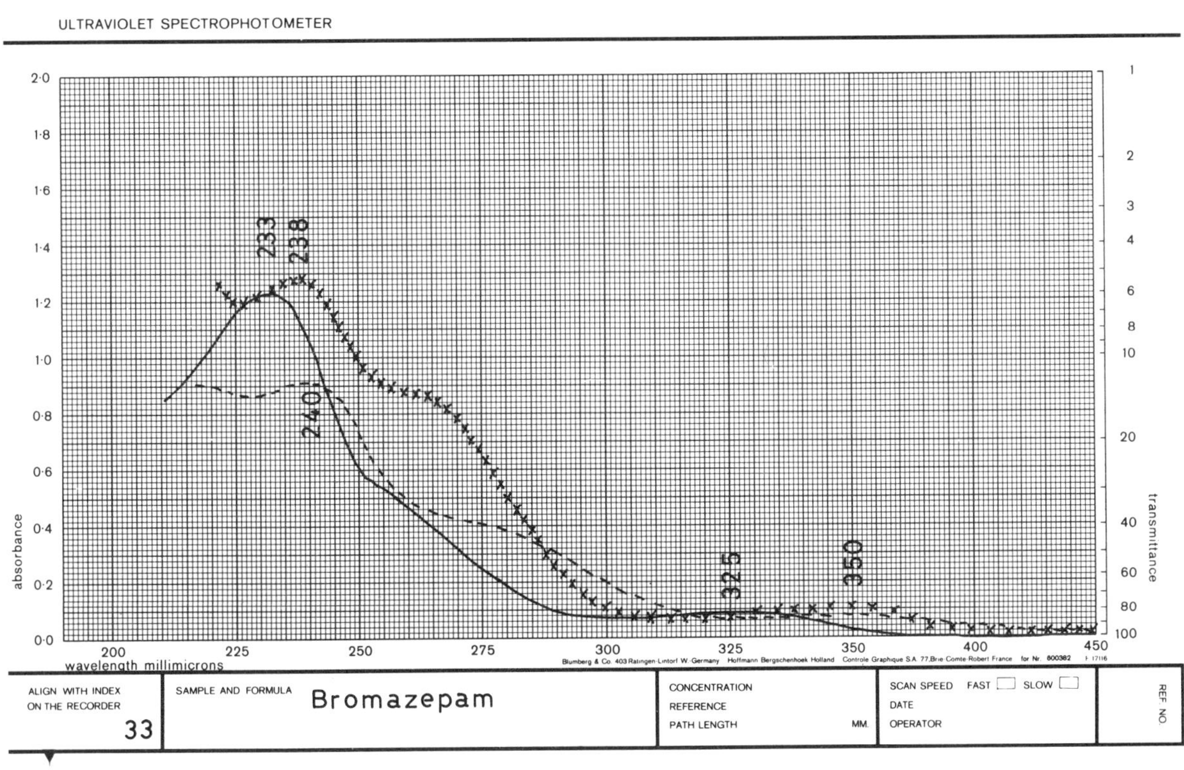

ALIGN WITH INDEX ON THE RECORDER 33	SAMPLE AND FORMULA Bromazepam	CONCENTRATION REFERENCE PATH LENGTH MM.	SCAN SPEED FAST ☐ SLOW ☐ DATE OPERATOR	REF. NO.

ULTRAVIOLET SPECTROPHOTOMETER

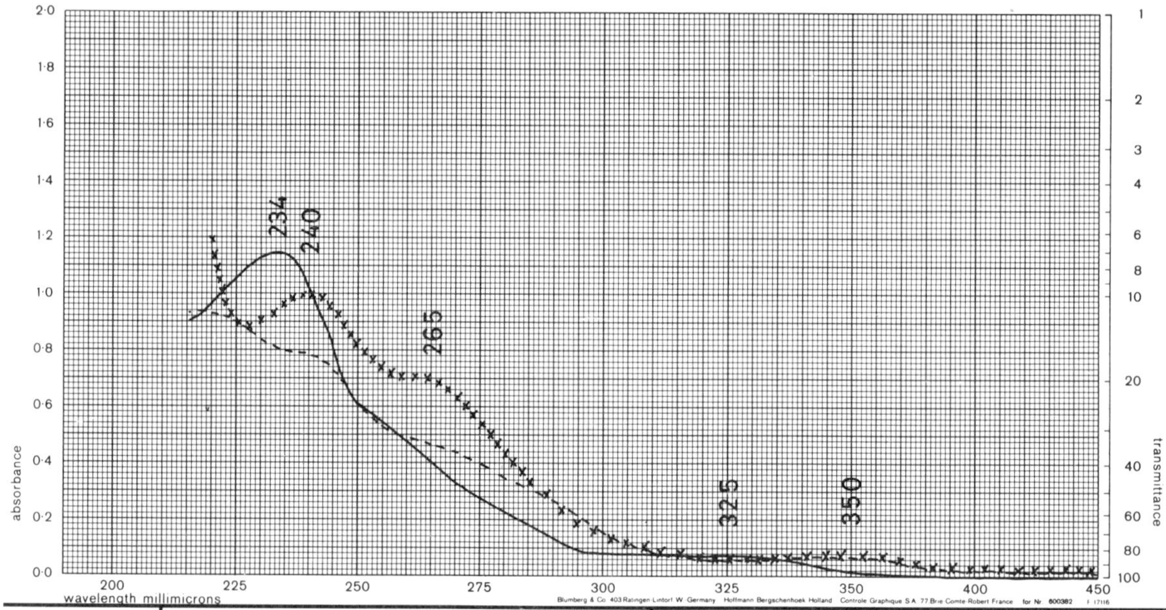

ALIGN WITH INDEX ON THE RECORDER	SAMPLE AND FORMULA	CONCENTRATION	SCAN SPEED FAST ☐ SLOW ☐	REF. NO.
34	3-Hydroxy-Bromazepam	REFERENCE PATH LENGTH MM	DATE OPERATOR	

ULTRAVIOLET SPECTROPHOTOMETER

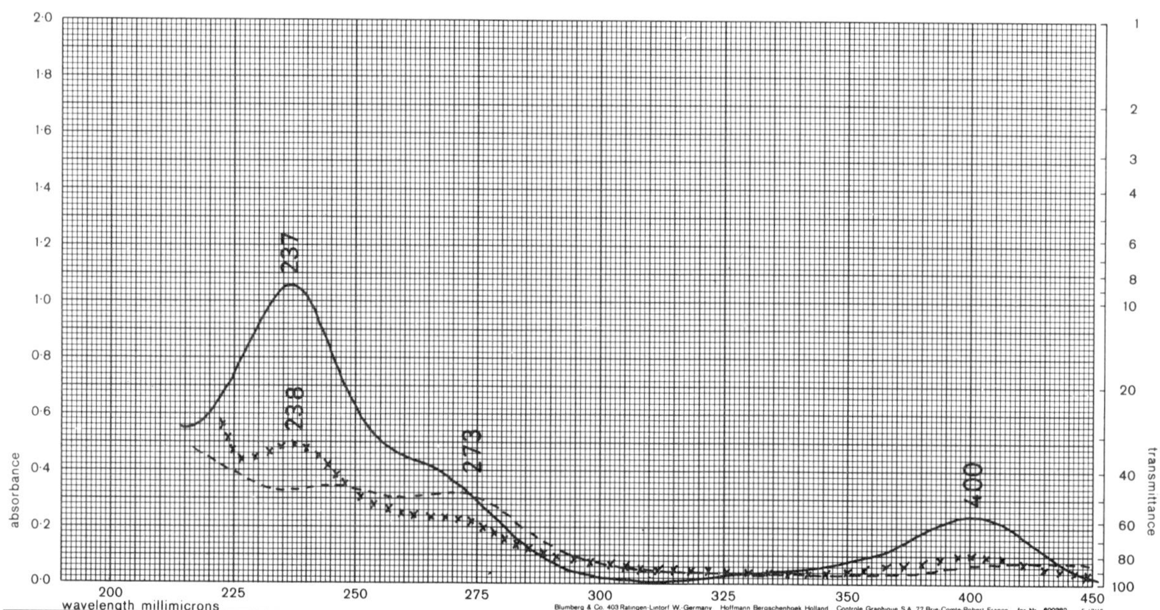

ALIGN WITH INDEX ON THE RECORDER	SAMPLE AND FORMULA	CONCENTRATION	SCAN SPEED FAST ☐ SLOW ☐	REF. NO.
35	2-(2-Amino-5-brom-benzoyl)-pyridine	REFERENCE PATH LENGTH MM.	DATE OPERATOR	

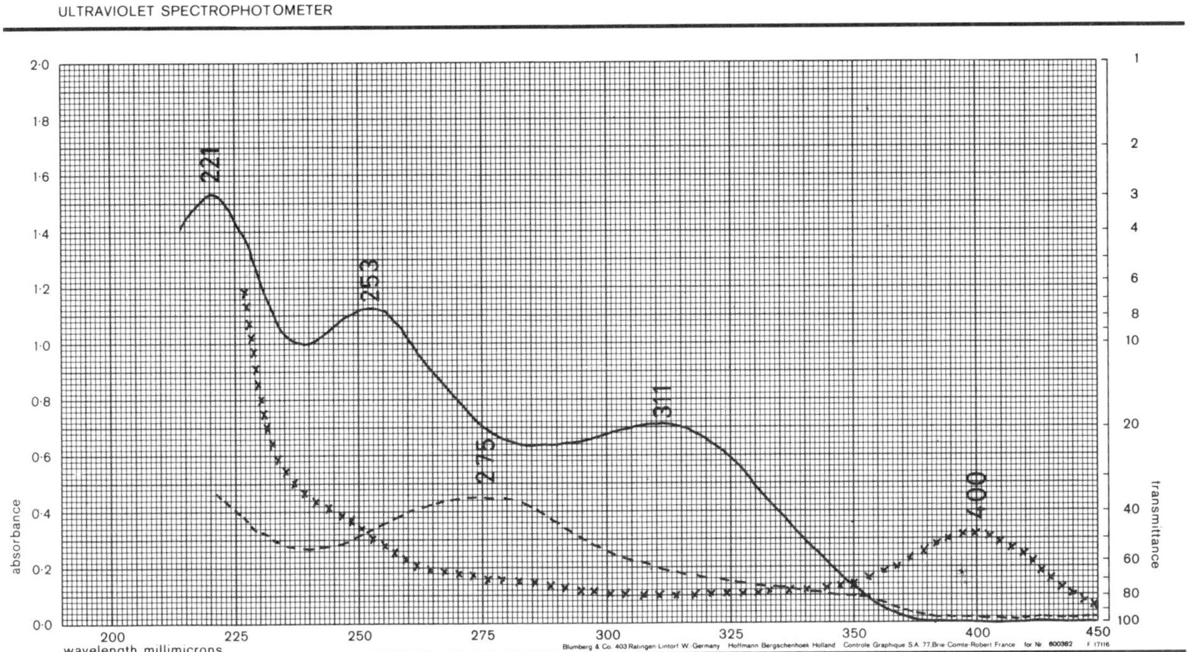

ALIGN WITH INDEX ON THE RECORDER	SAMPLE AND FORMULA	CONCENTRATION	SCAN SPEED FAST ☐ SLOW ☐	REF NO
36	Flunitrazepam	REFERENCE	DATE	
		PATH LENGTH MM.	OPERATOR	

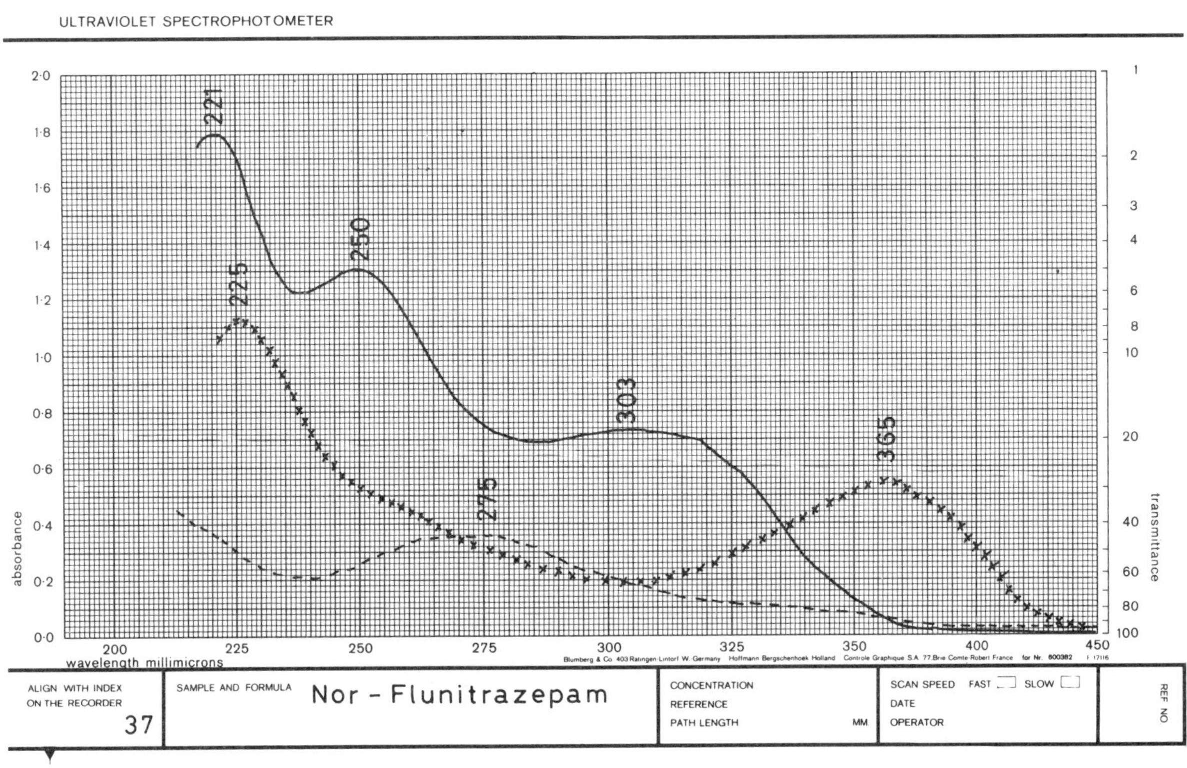

ALIGN WITH INDEX ON THE RECORDER	SAMPLE AND FORMULA	CONCENTRATION	SCAN SPEED FAST ☐ SLOW ☐	REF NO
37	Nor - Flunitrazepam	REFERENCE	DATE	
		PATH LENGTH MM.	OPERATOR	

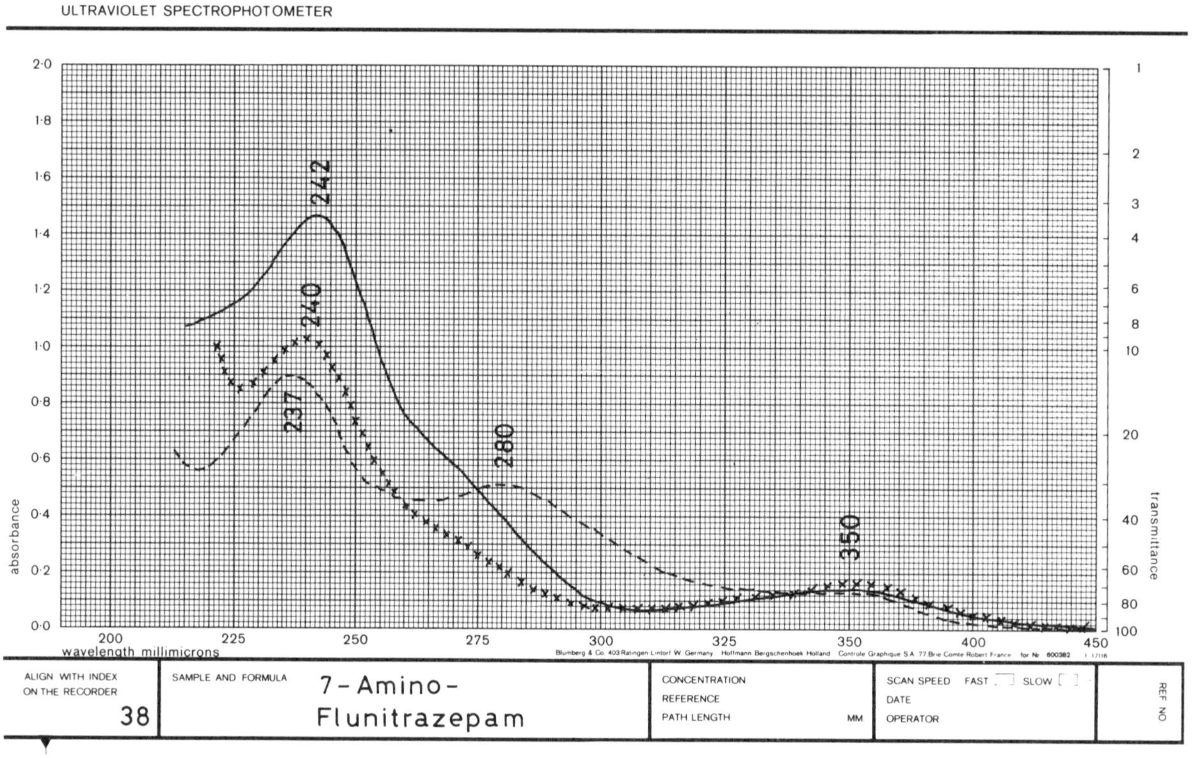
ULTRAVIOLET SPECTROPHOTOMETER
absorbance
transmittance
wavelength millimicrons
242
240
237
280
350
ALIGN WITH INDEX ON THE RECORDER
38
SAMPLE AND FORMULA
7-Amino-Flunitrazepam
CONCENTRATION
REFERENCE
PATH LENGTH MM
SCAN SPEED FAST SLOW
DATE
OPERATOR
REF NO

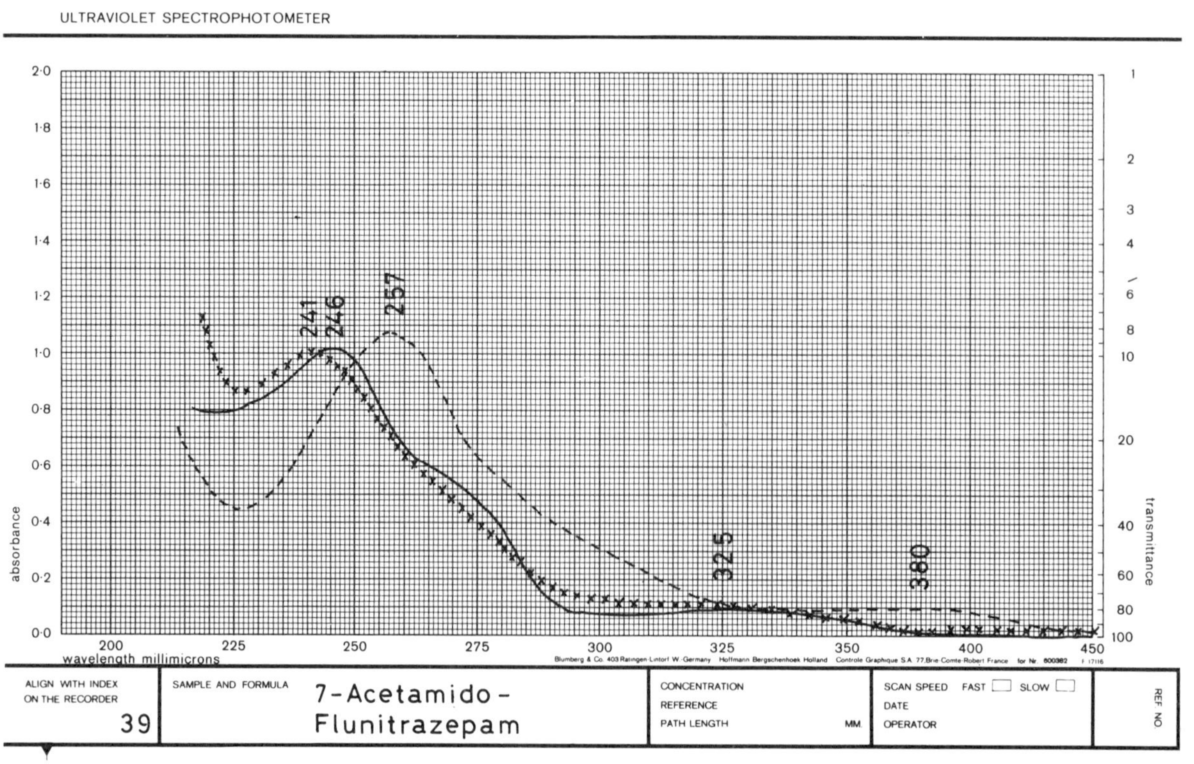
ULTRAVIOLET SPECTROPHOTOMETER
absorbance
transmittance
wavelength millimicrons
241
246
257
325
380
ALIGN WITH INDEX ON THE RECORDER
39
SAMPLE AND FORMULA
7-Acetamido-Flunitrazepam
CONCENTRATION
REFERENCE
PATH LENGTH MM
SCAN SPEED FAST SLOW
DATE
OPERATOR
REF NO

ULTRAVIOLET SPECTROPHOTOMETER

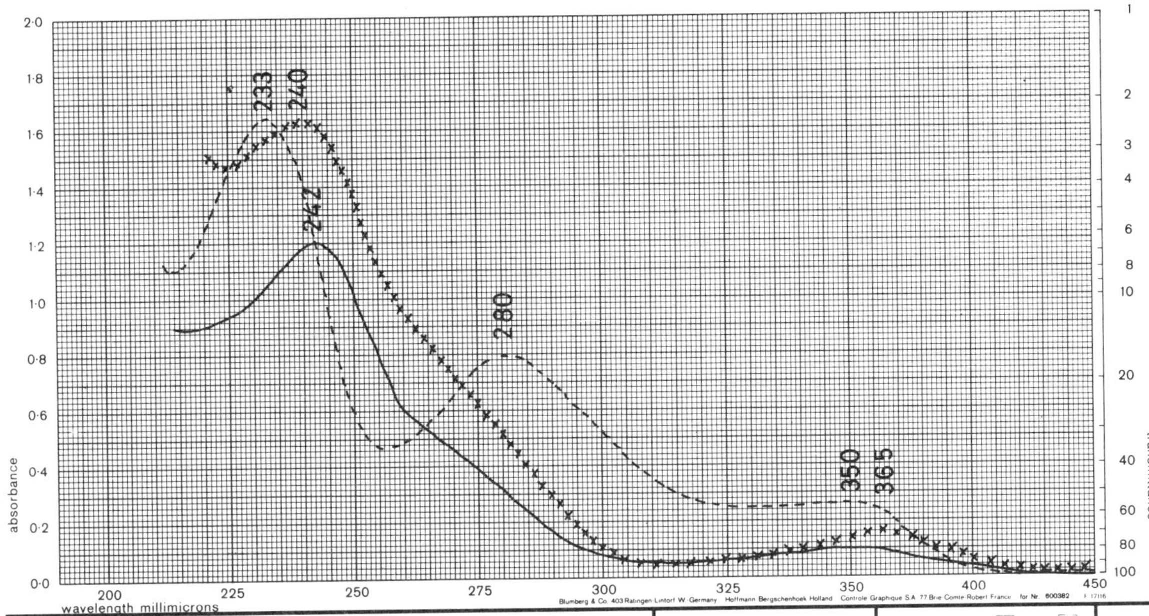

ALIGN WITH INDEX ON THE RECORDER	SAMPLE AND FORMULA	CONCENTRATION / REFERENCE / PATH LENGTH MM	SCAN SPEED FAST ☐ SLOW ☐ / DATE / OPERATOR	REF NO
40	7-Amino-Nor-Flunitrazepam			

ULTRAVIOLET SPECTROPHOTOMETER

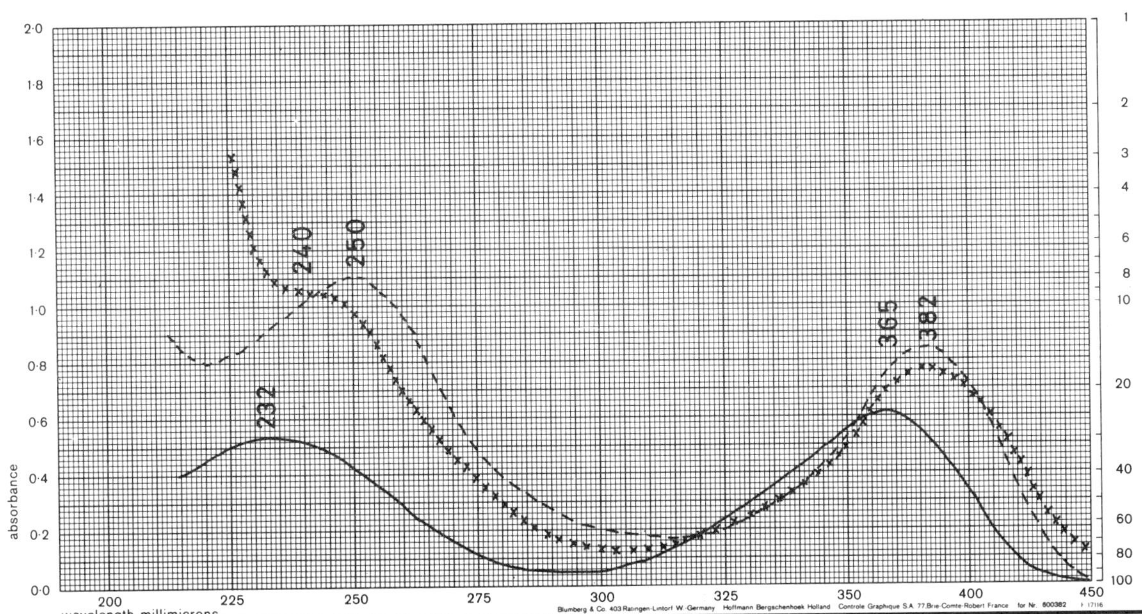

ALIGN WITH INDEX ON THE RECORDER	SAMPLE AND FORMULA	CONCENTRATION / REFERENCE / PATH LENGTH MM	SCAN SPEED FAST ☐ SLOW ☐ / DATE / OPERATOR	REF NO
41	2-Methylamino-5-nitro-2'-fluor-benzophenone			

ULTRAVIOLET SPECTROPHOTOMETER

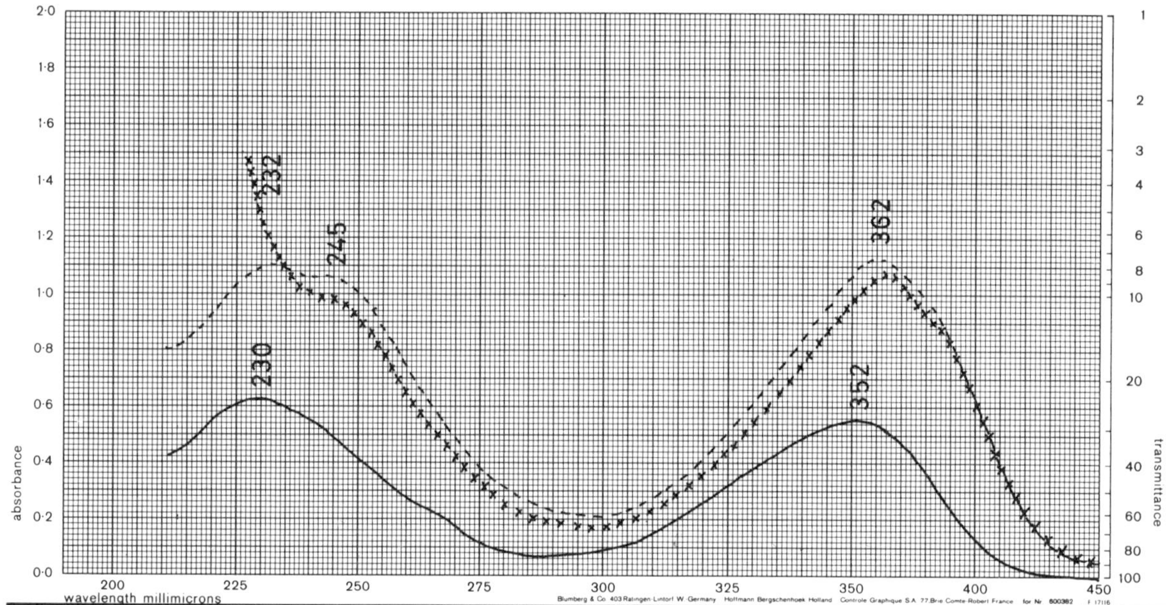

ALIGN WITH INDEX ON THE RECORDER	SAMPLE AND FORMULA	CONCENTRATION	SCAN SPEED FAST ☐ SLOW ☐	REF NO
42	2-Amino-5-nitro-2'-fluor-benzophenone	REFERENCE	DATE	
		PATH LENGTH MM	OPERATOR	

ULTRAVIOLET SPECTROPHOTOMETER

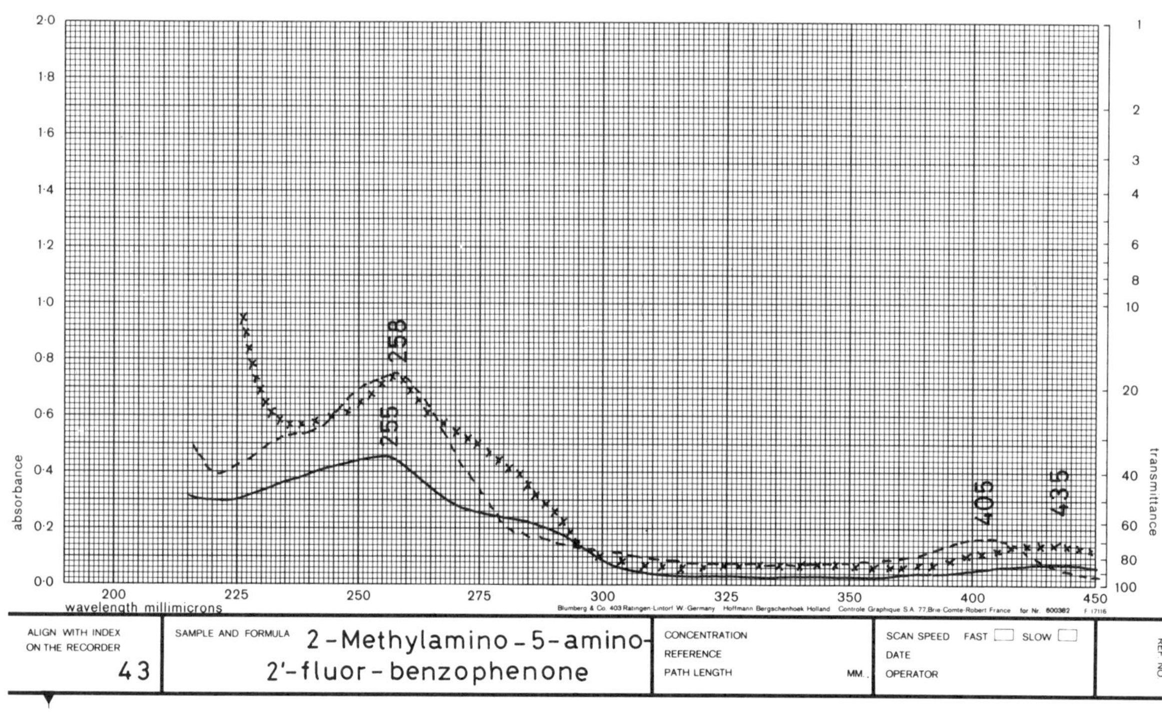

ALIGN WITH INDEX ON THE RECORDER	SAMPLE AND FORMULA	CONCENTRATION	SCAN SPEED FAST ☐ SLOW ☐	REF NO
43	2-Methylamino-5-amino-2'-fluor-benzophenone	REFERENCE	DATE	
		PATH LENGTH MM.	OPERATOR	

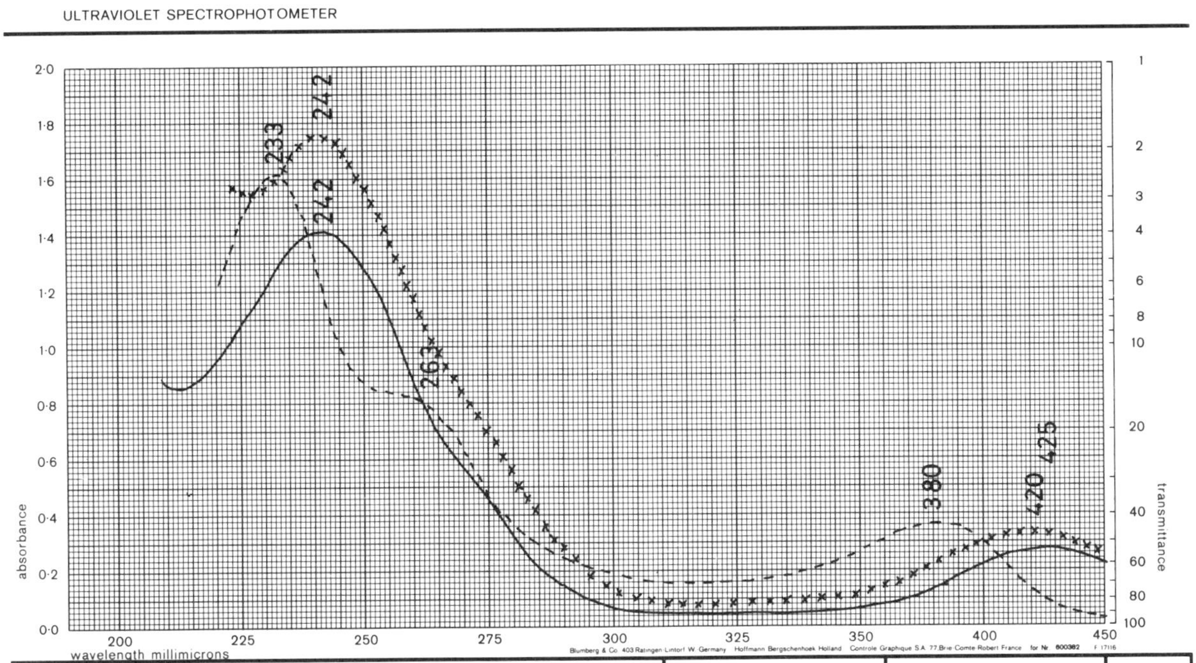

ALIGN WITH INDEX ON THE RECORDER	SAMPLE AND FORMULA	CONCENTRATION	SCAN SPEED FAST ☐ SLOW ☐	REF NO
44	2,5-Diamino-2'-fluor-benzophenone	REFERENCE	DATE	
		PATH LENGTH MM	OPERATOR	

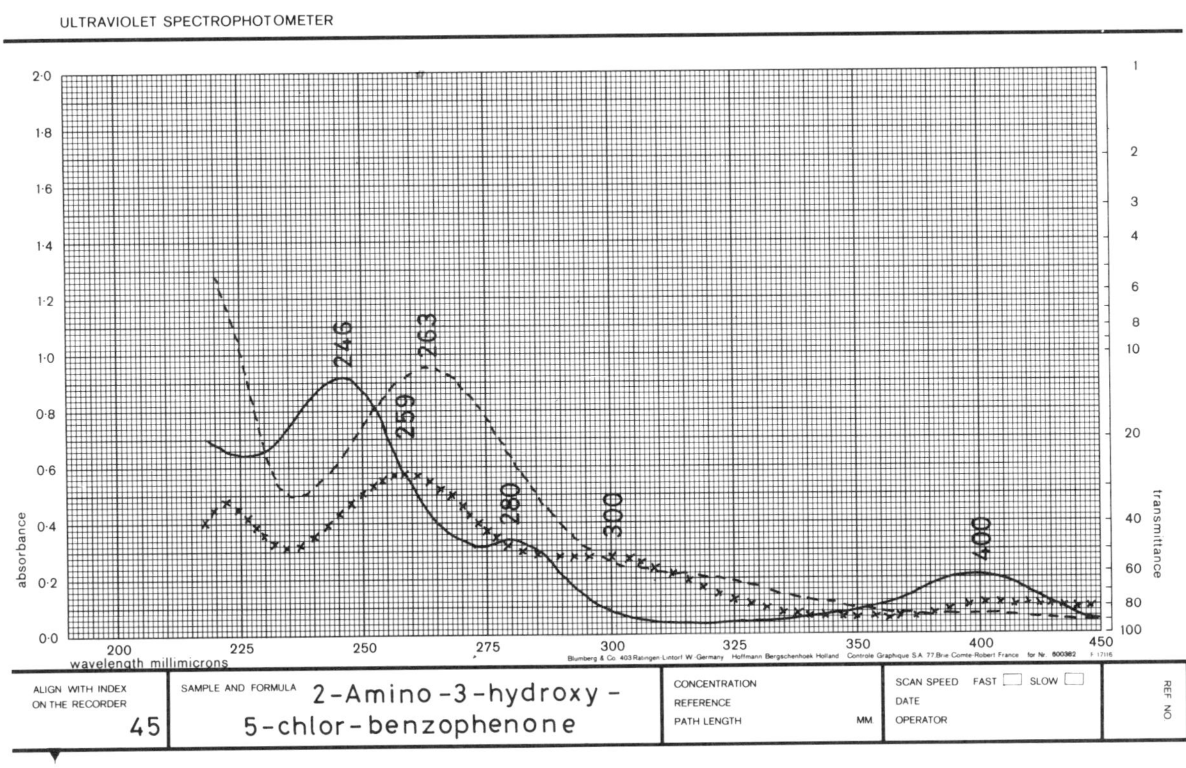

ALIGN WITH INDEX ON THE RECORDER	SAMPLE AND FORMULA	CONCENTRATION	SCAN SPEED FAST ☐ SLOW ☐	REF NO
45	2-Amino-3-hydroxy-5-chlor-benzophenone	REFERENCE	DATE	
		PATH LENGTH MM	OPERATOR	

ULTRAVIOLET SPECTROPHOTOMETER

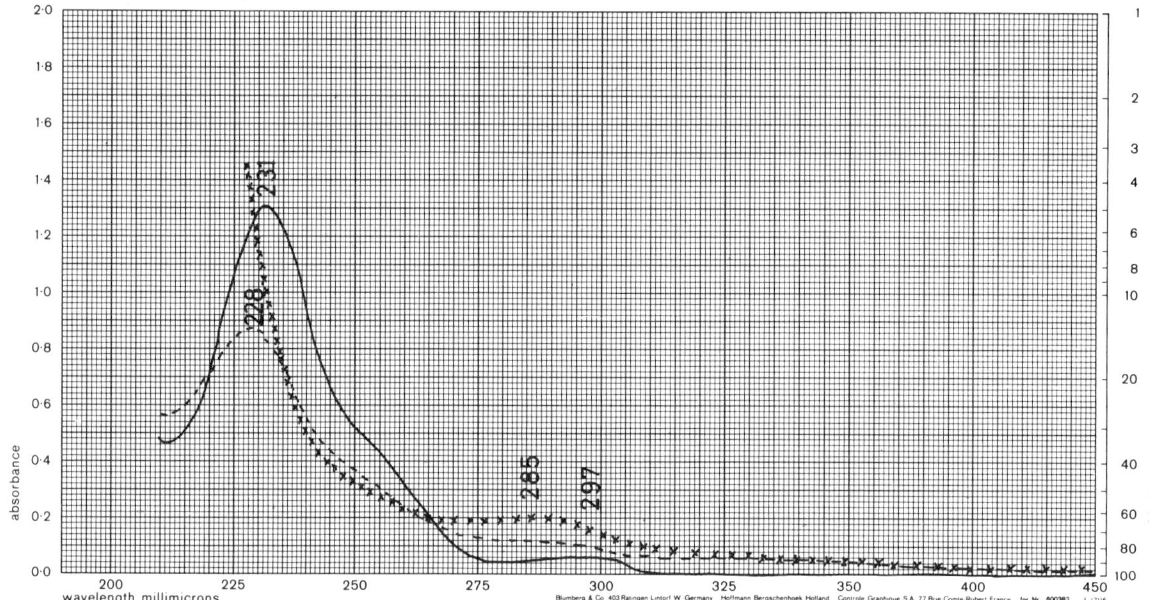

ALIGN WITH INDEX ON THE RECORDER 46	SAMPLE AND FORMULA Clobazam	CONCENTRATION REFERENCE PATH LENGTH MM	SCAN SPEED FAST ☐ SLOW ☐ DATE OPERATOR	REF NO

ULTRAVIOLET SPECTROPHOTOMETER

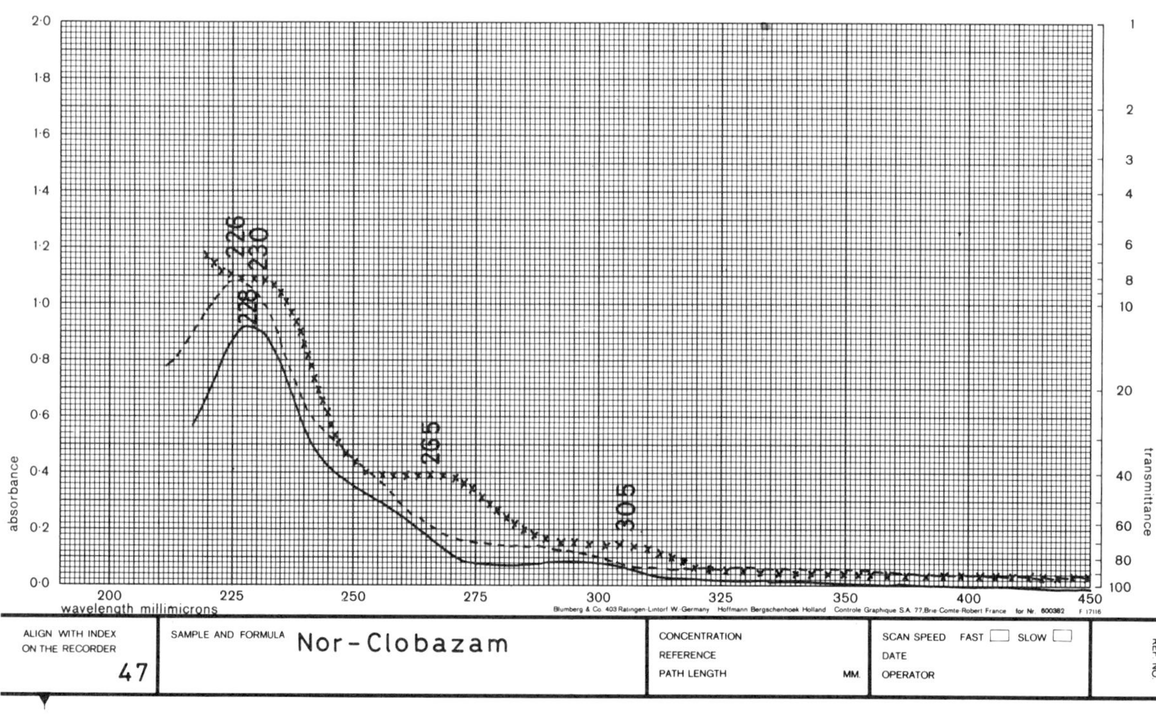

ALIGN WITH INDEX ON THE RECORDER 47	SAMPLE AND FORMULA Nor-Clobazam	CONCENTRATION REFERENCE PATH LENGTH MM.	SCAN SPEED FAST ☐ SLOW ☐ DATE OPERATOR	REF NO

ULTRAVIOLET SPECTROPHOTOMETER

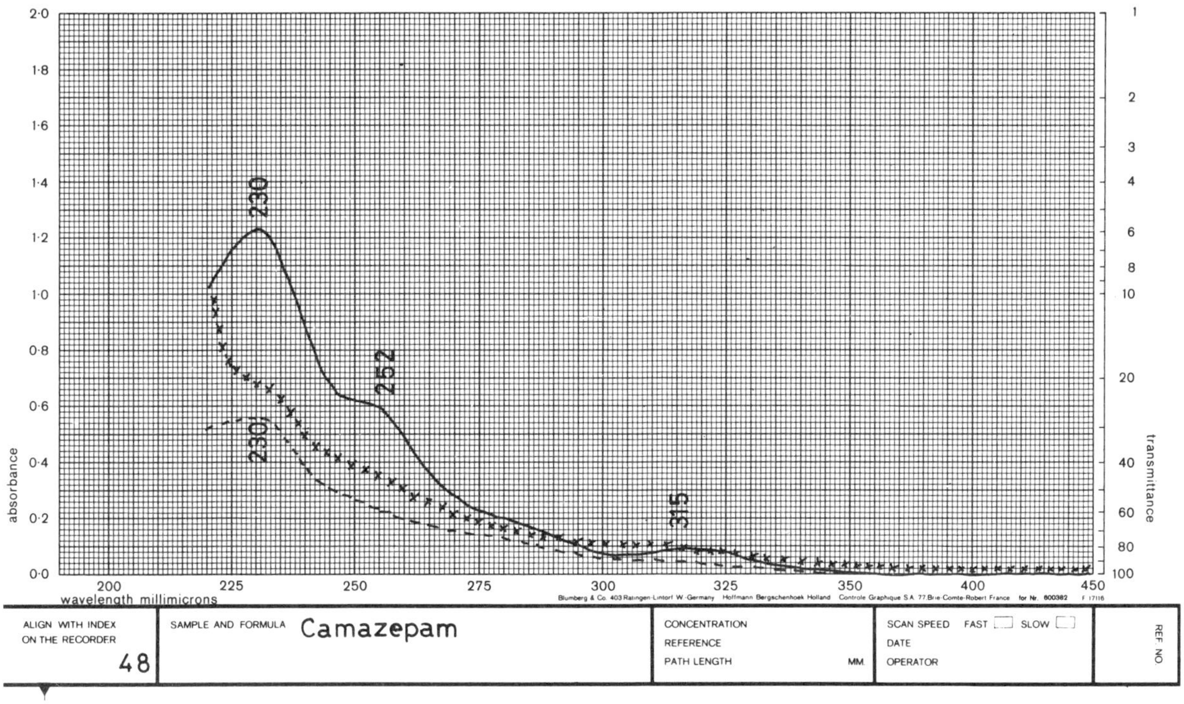

ULTRAVIOLET SPECTROPHOTOMETER

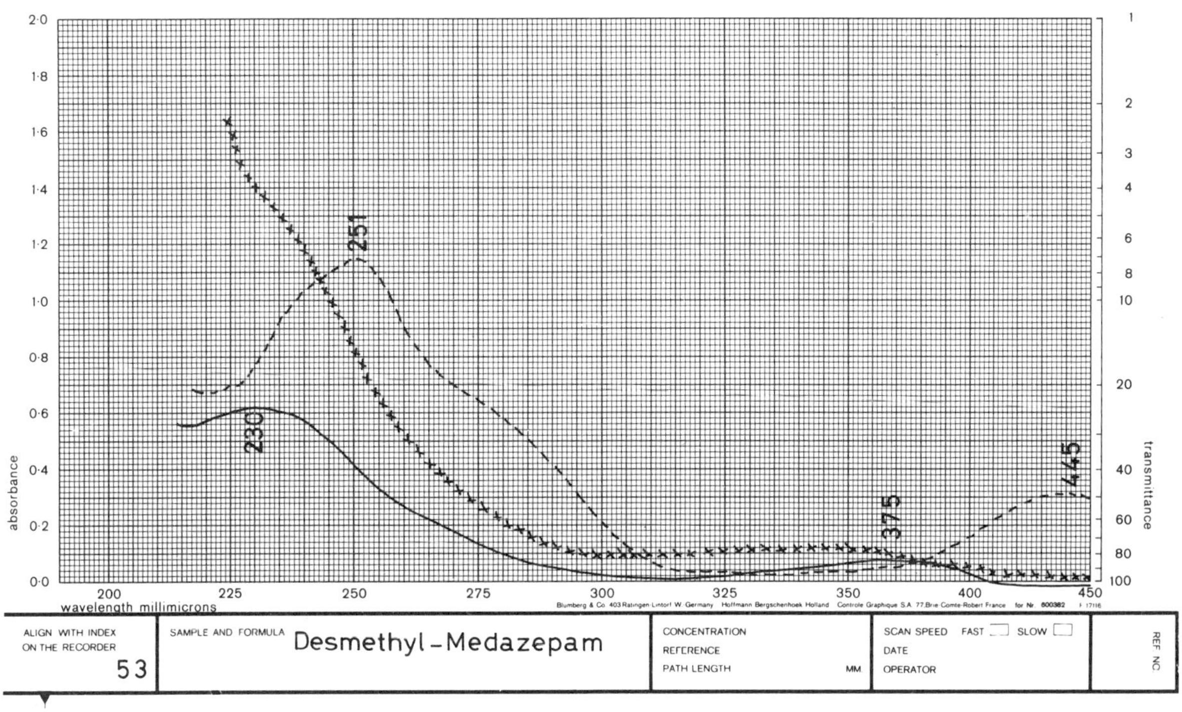

ULTRAVIOLET SPECTROPHOTOMETER

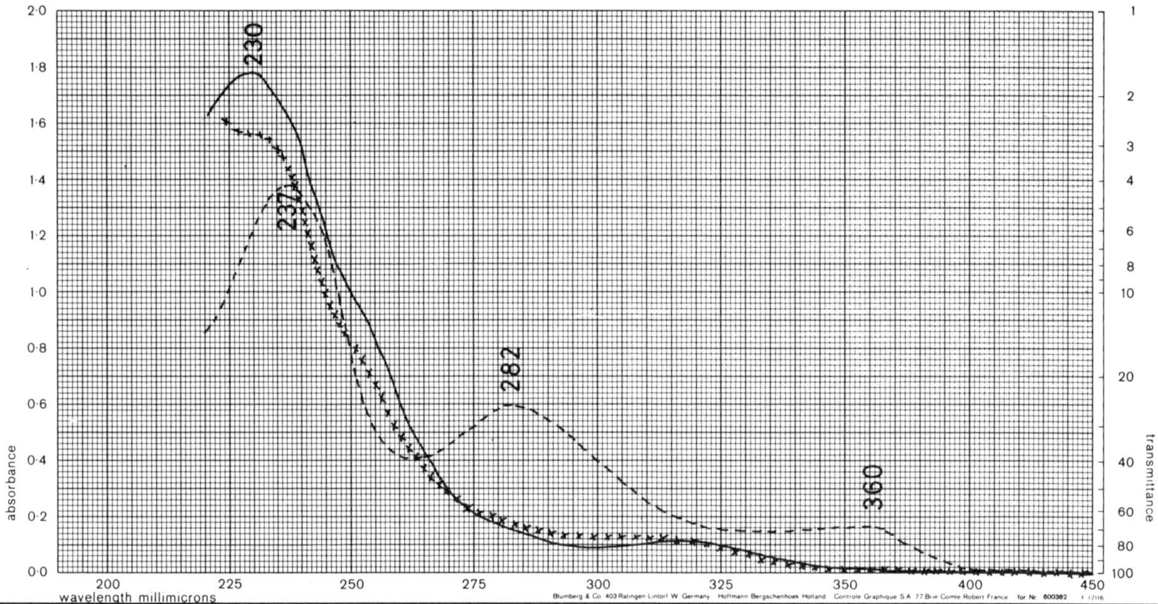

ALIGN WITH INDEX ON THE RECORDER 54	SAMPLE AND FORMULA Monodesethyl-Flurazepam	CONCENTRATION REFERENCE PATH LENGTH MM	SCAN SPEED FAST ☐ SLOW ☐ DATE OPERATOR	REF NO

ULTRAVIOLET SPECTROPHOTOMETER

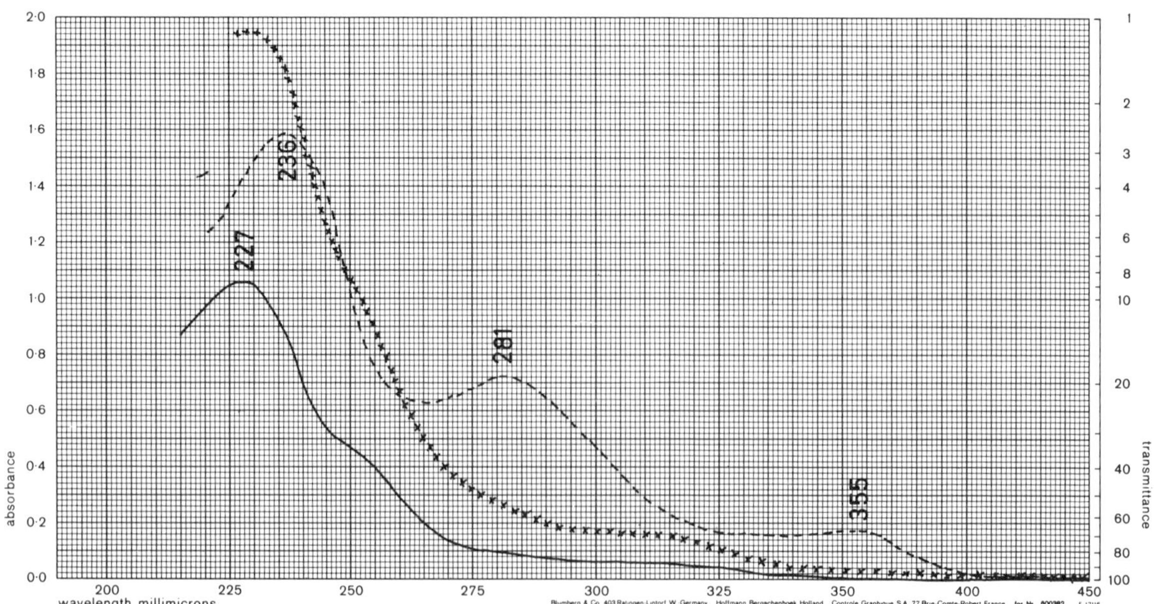

ALIGN WITH INDEX ON THE RECORDER 55	SAMPLE AND FORMULA Didesethyl-Flurazepam	CONCENTRATION REFERENCE PATH LENGTH MM	SCAN SPEED FAST ☐ SLOW ☐ DATE OPERATOR	REF NO

ULTRAVIOLET SPECTROPHOTOMETER

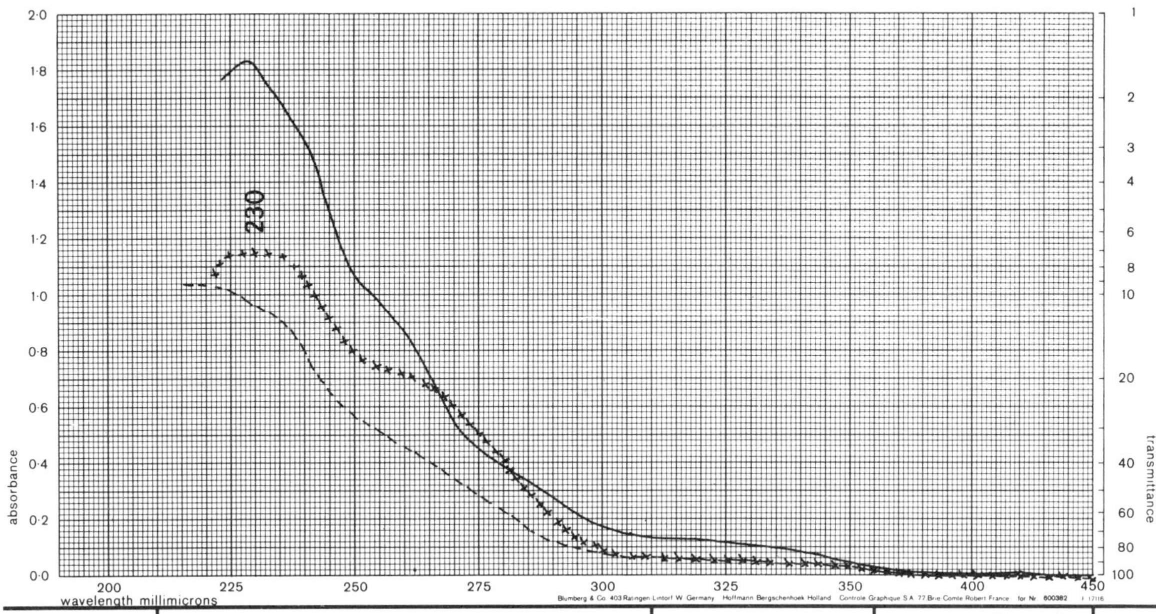

ALIGN WITH INDEX ON THE RECORDER 56	SAMPLE AND FORMULA Bromazepam-(pyr)N-Oxide	CONCENTRATION REFERENCE PATH LENGTH MM	SCAN SPEED FAST ☐ SLOW ☐ DATE OPERATOR	REF NO

ULTRAVIOLET SPECTROPHOTOMETER

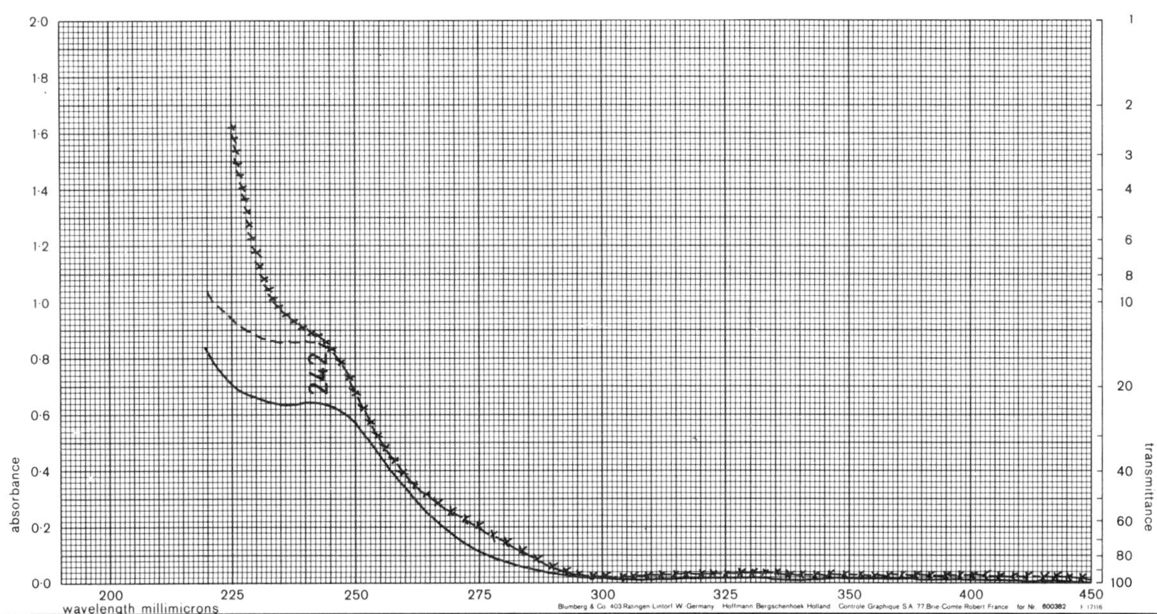

ALIGN WITH INDEX ON THE RECORDER 57	SAMPLE AND FORMULA Ketazolam	CONCENTRATION REFERENCE PATH LENGTH MM	SCAN SPEED FAST ☐ SLOW ☐ DATE OPERATOR	REF NO

ULTRAVIOLET SPECTROPHOTOMETER

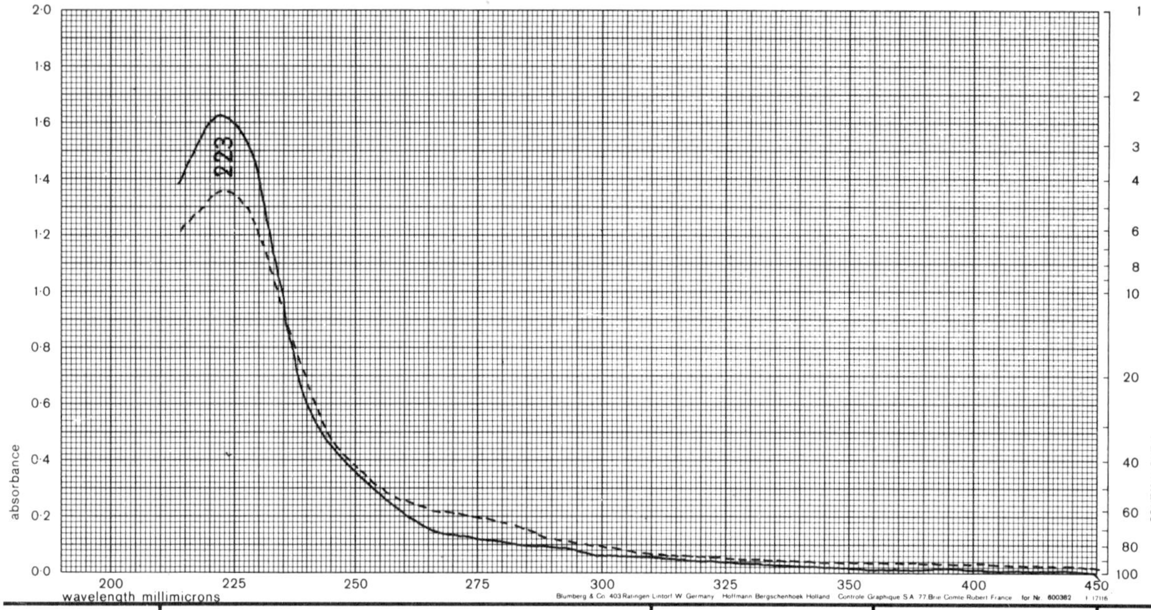

ALIGN WITH INDEX ON THE RECORDER 58	SAMPLE AND FORMULA Triazolam	CONCENTRATION REFERENCE PATH LENGTH MM	SCAN SPEED FAST ☐ SLOW ☐ DATE OPERATOR	REF NO

ULTRAVIOLET SPECTROPHOTOMETER

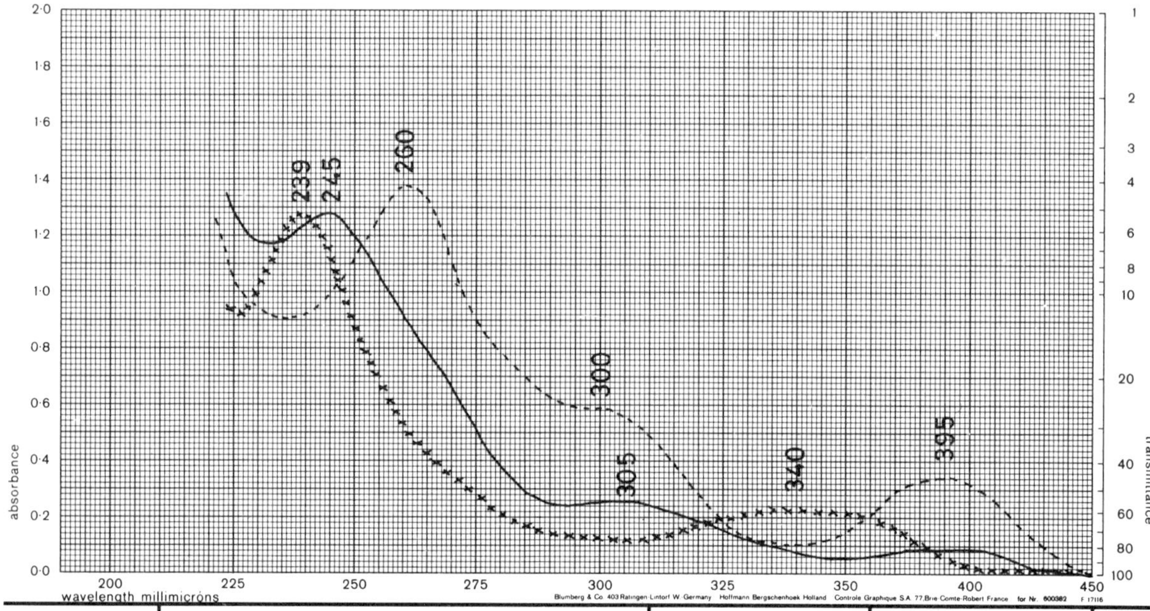

ALIGN WITH INDEX ON THE RECORDER 59	SAMPLE AND FORMULA Clotiazepam	CONCENTRATION REFERENCE PATH LENGTH MM	SCAN SPEED FAST ☐ SLOW ☐ DATE OPERATOR	REF NO

ULTRAVIOLET SPECTROPHOTOMETER

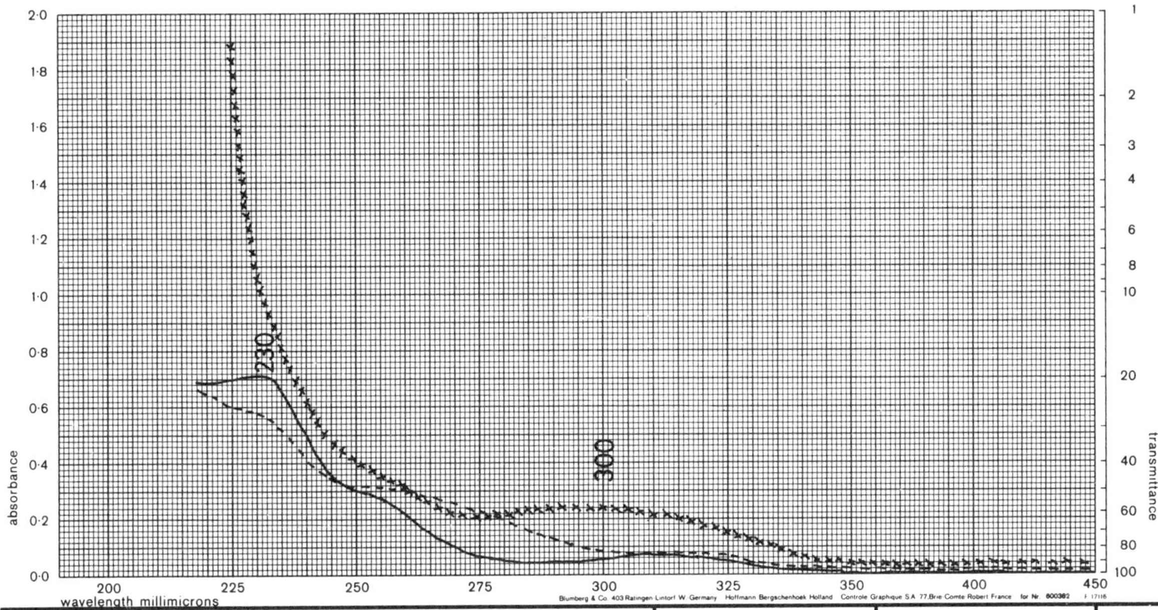

ALIGN WITH INDEX ON THE RECORDER 60	SAMPLE AND FORMULA Lormetazepam	CONCENTRATION REFERENCE PATH LENGTH MM	SCAN SPEED FAST ☐ SLOW ☐ DATE OPERATOR	REF. NO

ULTRAVIOLET SPECTROPHOTOMETER

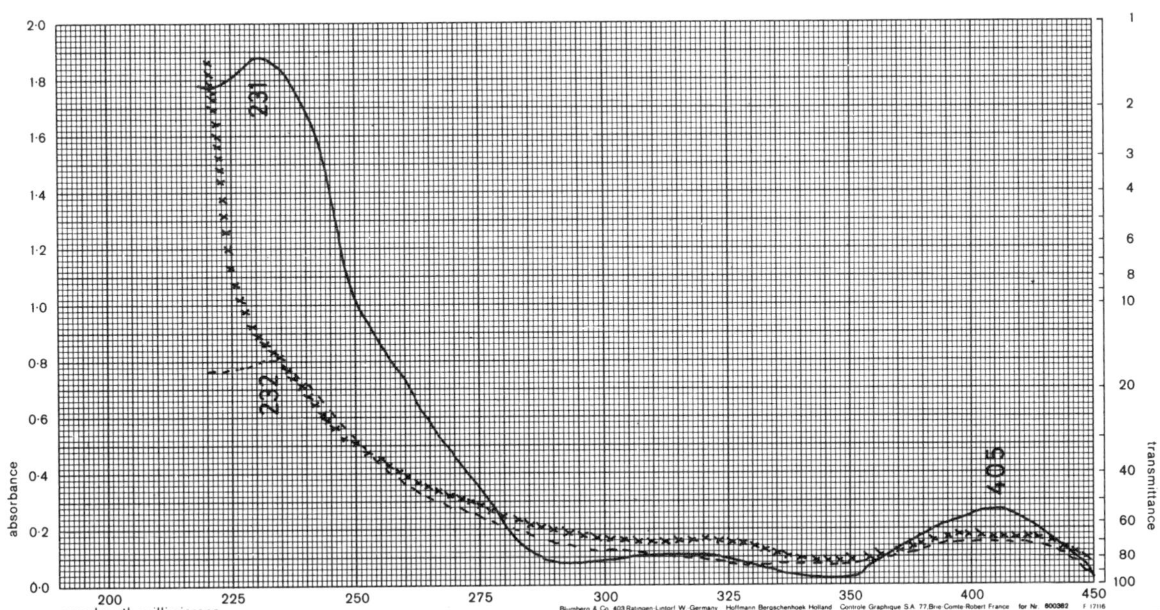

ALIGN WITH INDEX ON THE RECORDER 61	SAMPLE AND FORMULA 2-Methylamino-2',5-dichlor-benzophenon	CONCENTRATION REFERENCE PATH LENGTH MM	SCAN SPEED FAST ☐ SLOW ☐ DATE OPERATOR	REF. NO

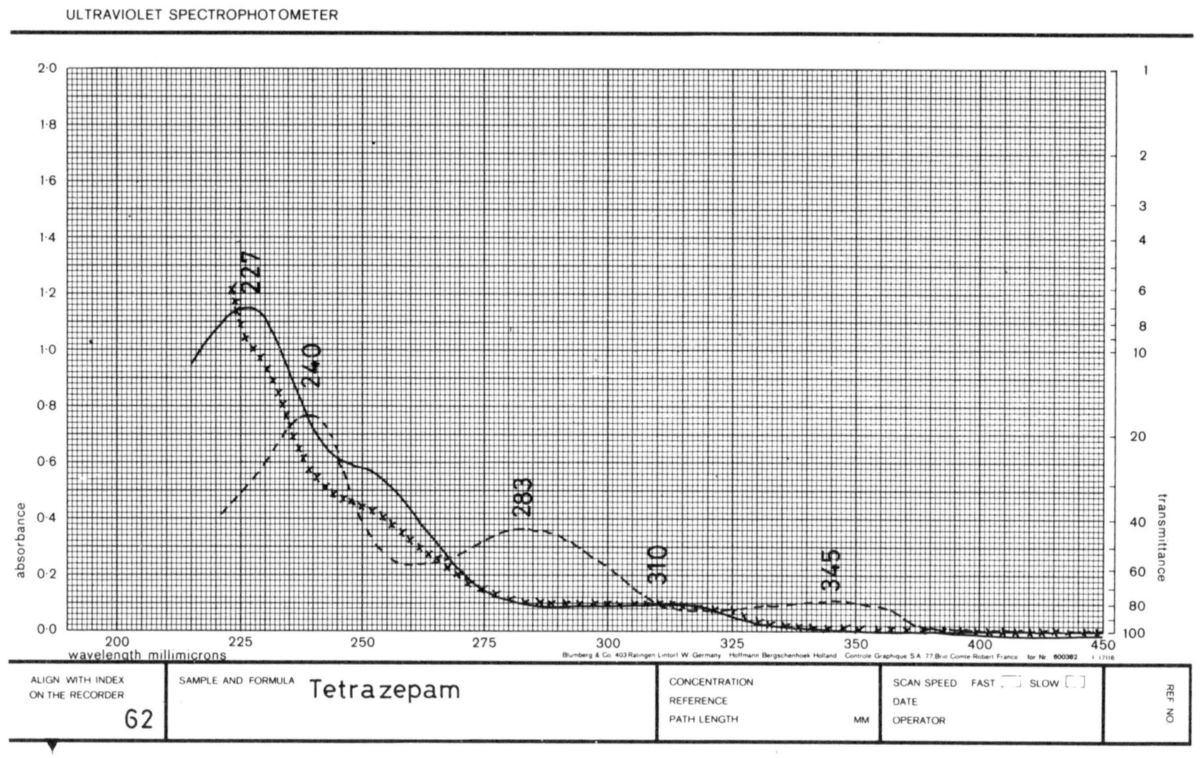
ULTRAVIOLET SPECTROPHOTOMETER
absorbance
transmittance
wavelength millimicrons
227
240
283
310
345
ALIGN WITH INDEX ON THE RECORDER
62
SAMPLE AND FORMULA
Tetrazepam
CONCENTRATION
REFERENCE
PATH LENGTH
MM
SCAN SPEED FAST SLOW
DATE
OPERATOR
REF NO

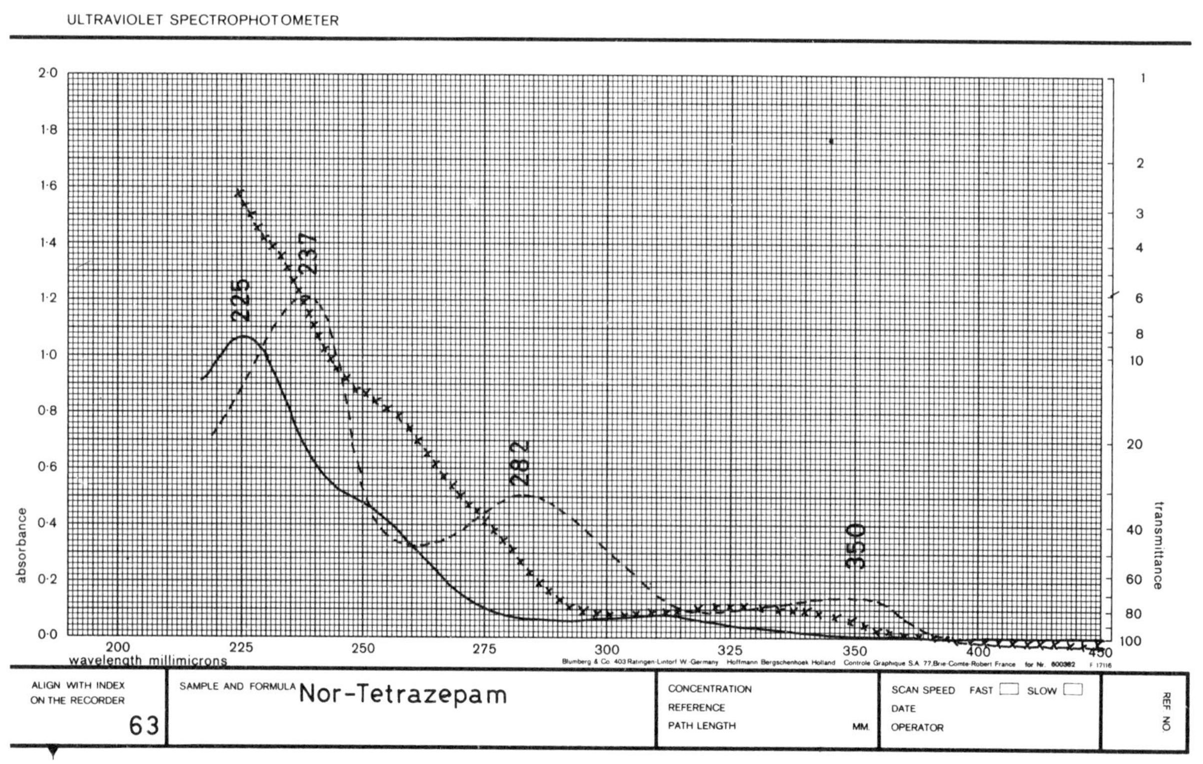
ULTRAVIOLET SPECTROPHOTOMETER
absorbance
transmittance
wavelength millimicrons
225
237
282
350
ALIGN WITH INDEX ON THE RECORDER
63
SAMPLE AND FORMULA
Nor-Tetrazepam
CONCENTRATION
REFERENCE
PATH LENGTH
MM
SCAN SPEED FAST SLOW
DATE
OPERATOR
REF NO

Presentation of Analytical Methods

Darstellung der Analysenmethoden

Methods for the Detection and Determination of Various Benzodiazepines (Simultaneous Methods)

Benzodiazepine(s)/ Benzodiazepin(e)	Chlordiazepoxide, Diazepam, Nitrazepam, Lorazepam, Flurazepam, Flunitrazepam and other Drugs which are not Benzodiazepines
Method / Methode	GLC - ECD (3 % OV-17 on Chromosorb W-HP (100 - 120 mesh)
Authors / Verfasser	MISSEN
Lit.Ref./ Lit.Zitat	(728)
Year of Publication/ Publikationsjahr	1977
Extraction Procedure/ Extraktionsverfahren	pH 3, chloroform, CELITE 545, oxidation with dichromate
Drug analyzed/ analysierte Substanz	Oxidation products
Drug calculated / berechnete Substanz	-----------
Metabolites included / Metabolite inbegriffen	yes
qual./quant./Screening Method (e)	Screening / qual.
Sample required/ benötigtes Untersuchungsmaterial	0.4 ml blood
Concentration Range/ Konzentrationsbereich	----------
Special Equipment/ Spezialausstattung	ECD-Detection
Hydrolysis / Hydrolyse	no
Some Other Data: Einige andere Daten:	minimum detectable quantity between 0.3 and 5.4 ng
Pharmacokinetic Data obtained by this Method described on pp. Mit der Methode erhaltene pharmakokinetische Daten sind beschrieben auf S.	-----------
Method is recommended for: Methode ist empfohlen für:	the mass-screening of blood samples for therapeutic and overdose levels of benzodiazepines and some other drugs (e.g. amitriptyline, nortriptyline, chlorprothixene, dothiepin and chlorcyclizine).

Benzodiazepine(s)/ Benzodiazepin(e)	Chlordiazepoxide, Diazepam, Oxazepam, Medazepam, Lorazepam, Clonazepam, Flurazepam, Bromazepam and Flunitrazepam
Method / Methode	GLC - ECD (incl. derivatization) (3 % OV-17 on Gas Chrom Q (60-80 mesh)
Authors / Verfasser	DE SILVA, BEKERSKY, PUGLISI, BROOKS and WEINFELD
Lit.Ref./ Lit.Zitat	(236)
Year of Publication/ Publikationsjahr	1976
Extraction Procedure/ Extraktionsverfahren	Benzene - methylene chloride (90 : 10), specified pH-values depending on structure
Drug analyzed/ analysierte Substanz	Benzodiazepine (derivative)
Drug calculated / berechnete Substanz	Benzodiazepine
Metabolites included / Metabolite inbegriffen	yes
qual./quant./Screening Method (e)	quant.
Sample required/ benötigtes Untersuchungsmaterial	1 ml blood
Concentration Range/ Konzentrationsbereich	ca. 0.4 - 10.0 ng/ml (Flunitrazepam), ca. 0.5 - 150 ng/ml (Diazepam), ca. 10 - 170 ng/ml (Bromazepam), ca. 50 ng/ml Clonazepam
Special Equipment/ Spezialausstattung	ECD - Detection
Hydrolysis / Hydrolyse	no
Some Other Data: Einige andere Daten:	Sensitivity limit of the order of 1.0 to 10.0 ng / ml of blood Overall Recoveries: Diazepam 95 ± 5 % (S.D.) Chlordiazepoxide 85 ± 5 % (S.D.) Oxazepam 80 ± 5 % (S.D.) Medazepam 90 ± 5 % (S.D.) Lorazepam 80 ± 5 % (S.D.) Clonazepam 85 ± 5 % (S.D.) Flurazepam 76 ± 5 % (S.D.) Bromazepam 94 ± 5 % (S.D.) (Methylbromazepam) Flunitrazepam 90 ± 5 % (S.D.)
Pharmacokinetic Data obtained by this Method described on pp. Mit der Methode erhaltene pharmakokinetische Daten sind beschrieben auf S.	See part: Blood-, Serum- and Plasma-Levels and Other Pharmacokinetic Data from Literature
Method is recommended for: Methode ist empfohlen für:	the sensitive monitoring of blood concentrations following single oral therapeutic doses of diazepam, clonazepam, bromazepam and flunitrazepam (as low as 1.0 mg).

Benzodiazepine(s)/ Benzodiazepin(e)	Chlordiazepoxide, Diazepam, Oxazepam, Clonazepam, Flurazepam.
Method / Methode	GLC - ECD (3 % OV-17 on Chromosorb W AW / DMCS, 100-120 mesh)
Authors / Verfasser	FERGUSON and COURI
Lit.Ref./ Lit.Zitat	(312)
Year of Publication/ Publikationsjahr	1977
Extraction Procedure/ Extraktionsverfahren	pH 9, 1.5 % Isoamylalcohol in toluene, then reextraction with 6 N HCl and second extraction with isoamylalcohol - toluene from alkaline sol.
Drug analyzed/ analysierte Substanz	Benzodiazepines
Drug calculated / berechnete Substanz	Benzodiazepines
Metabolites included / Metabolite inbegriffen	yes
qual./quant./Screening Method (e)	quant.
Sample required/ benötigtes Untersuchungsmaterial	1 ml plasma
Concentration Range/ Konzentrationsbereich	ca. 0.1 - 10.0 ng / ml
Special Equipment/ Spezialausstattung	ECD - Detection
Hydrolysis / Hydrolyse	no
Some Other Data: Einige andere Daten:	Sensitivity limit: 0.1 ng (Chlordiazepoxide); 0.5 ng (Diazepam); 0.1 ng (Oxazepam); 0.1 ng (Flurazepam) Recovery: Chlordiazepoxide 97.4 ± 4.6 % (S.D.) Diazepam 82.7 ± 1.2 % (S.D.) Oxazepam 32.6 ± 2.6 % (S.D.) Flurazepam 100.2 ± 5.3 % (S.D.) Desmethyl Diazepam 95.1 ± 2.4 % (S.D.) Methylclonazepam 89.4 ± 1.3 % (S.D.)
Pharmacokinetic Data obtained by this Method described on pp. Mit der Methode erhaltene pharmakokinetische Daten sind beschrieben auf S.	-----
Method is recommended for: Methode ist empfohlen für:	a rapid screening and quantitative determination of chlordiazepoxide, diazepam, N-desmethyldiazepam, oxazepam, flurazepam and methylclonazepam in 1 ml of plasma.

Benzodiazepine(s)/ Benzodiazepin(e)	Chlordiazepoxide, Diazepam, Oxazepam, Flurazepam
Method / Methode	GLC - ECD (3 % OV-17 on Chromosorb W (HP), 80-100 mesh)
Authors / Verfasser	KELLY, ANTHONY, KRENT, THOMPSON and SUNSHINE
Lit.Ref./ Lit.Zitat	(2482)
Year of Publication/ Publikationsjahr	1979
Extraction Procedure/ Extraktionsverfahren	pH 9.2, toluene - hexane - isoamylalcohol (78 : 20 : 2)
Drug analyzed/ analysierte Substanz	Benzodiazepine
Drug calculated / berechnete Substanz	Benzodiazepine
Metabolites included / Metabolite inbegriffen	yes
qual./quant./Screening Method (e)	quant.
Sample required/ benötigtes Untersuchungsmaterial	about 1 ml blood, serum or gastric fluid
Concentration Range/ Konzentrationsbereich	ca. 50 - 5.000 ng / ml
Special Equipment/ Spezialausstattung	ECD - Detection
Hydrolysis / Hydrolyse	no

Some Other Data:
Einige andere Daten:

Method Precision:	Within day (n = 10)	Day-to-day (n = 15)
Chlordiazepoxide	12.1 %	19.2 %
Diazepam	1.4 %	3.9 %
N-Desmethyldiazepam	1.6 %	8.8 %
Flurazepam	1.1 %	6.9 %

Detection limit: about 50 ng / ml

Pharmacokinetic Data obtained by this Method described on pp.
Mit der Methode erhaltene pharmakokinetische Daten sind beschrieben auf S.

Method is recommended for: Methode ist empfohlen für:	the rapid determination of chlordiazepoxide, diazepam, N-desmethyldiazepam and flurazepam in blood, serum or gastric fluid at concentrations of greater than 50 ng / ml.

Benzodiazepine(s)/ Benzodiazepin(e)	Chlordiazepoxide, Diazepam and Flurazepam
Method / Methode	GLC - ECD (3 % OV - 17 on Gas Chrom Q (100 - 120 mesh)
Authors / Verfasser	PEAT and KOPJAK
Lit.Ref./ Lit.Zitat	(3382)
Year of Publication/ Publikationsjahr	1980
Extraction Procedure/ Extraktionsverfahren	approx. pH 10, toluene - heptane - isoamylalcohol (76 : 20 : 4)
Drug analyzed/ analysierte Substanz	Benzodiazepine
Drug calculated / berechnete Substanz	Benzodiazepine
Metabolites included / Metabolite inbegriffen	yes
qual./quant./Screening Method (e)	quant.
Sample required/ benötigtes Untersuchungsmaterial	1 ml plasma or whole blood
Concentration Range/ Konzentrationsbereich	ca. 50 - 1,000 ng/ml (Diazepam, Flurazepam, Desmethyldiazepam, Desalkylflurazepam)
Special Equipment/ Spezialausstattung	ECD - Detection
Hydrolysis / Hydrolyse	no

Some Other Data: / Einige andere Daten:

Compound	Within-Run C.V.		Run-to-run C.V.	
Diazepam	1.4 % (500 ng/ml)		2.8 % (500 ng/ml)	n= 20
Desmethyldiazepam	2.2 % (500 ng/ml)	n = 10	2.5 % (500 ng/ml)	
Flurazepam	1.7 % (500 ng/ml)		2.6 % (500 ng/ml)	
Desalkylflurazepam	1.5 % (500 ng/ml)		3.0 % (500 ng/ml)	
Chlordiazepoxide	3.4 % (383 ng/ml)		7.2 % (750 ng/ml)	n= 5
Desmethylchlordiazepoxide	4,4 % (273 ng/ml)	n = 10	7.8 % (666 ng/ml)	
Demoxepam	6.3 % (307 ng/ml)		8.0 % (424 ng/ml)	
Chlordiazepoxide	6.8 % (221 ng/ml)		4.0 % (184 ng/ml)	n= 5
Desmethylchlordiazepoxide	7.4 % (132 ng/ml)	n = 10	5.2 % (103 ng/ml)	
Demoxepam	8.0 % (118 ng/ml)		4.5 % (78 ng/ml)	

Pharmacokinetic Data obtained by this Method described on pp.
Mit der Methode erhaltene pharmakokinetische Daten sind beschrieben auf S.

Method is recommended for: / Methode ist empfohlen für:	both clinical and forensic-toxicological cases (screening and quantitation)

Benzodiazepine(s)/ Benzodiazepin(e)	Chlordiazepoxide, Diazepam, Oxazepam, Nitrazepam, Medazepam, Clorazepate, Lorazepam, Prazepam, Clonazepam, Flurazepam, Bromazepam, Flunitrazepam and Temazepam
Method / Methode	GLC - ECD (10 % OV-1 on Chromosorb G-HP (80 - 100 mesh) (3 % OV-17 on Chromosorb W-HP (80 - 100 mesh)
Authors / Verfasser	PEEL and PERRIGO
Lit.Ref./ Lit.Zitat	(3384)
Year of Publication/ Publikationsjahr	1980
Extraction Procedure/ Extraktionsverfahren	pH 10, n-butylchloride
Drug analyzed/ analysierte Substanz	Benzodiazepine or Benzophenone
Drug calculated / berechnete Substanz	Benzodiazepine
Metabolites included / Metabolite inbegriffen	yes (many)
qual./quant./Screening Method (e)	qual./quant./Screening
Sample required/ benötigtes Untersuchungsmaterial	1 ml blood
Concentration Range/ Konzentrationsbereich	ca. 100 - 1,000 ng/ml
Special Equipment/ Spezialausstattung	ECD - Detection
Hydrolysis / Hydrolyse	no (yes)

Some Other Data:
Einige andere Daten:

Compound	Recovery (%) ± 5%	Sensitivity (ng/ml)
Chlordiazepoxide	83	Var.
Clonazepam	84	100 - 500
Desalkylflurazepam	95	100 - 500
Diazepam	94	100 - 500
Flurazepam	94	500 -1000
Lorazepam	70	500 -1000
Nordiazepam	95	500 -1000
Oxazepam	78	1000 -1500
Prazepam	93	---------

Pharmacokinetic Data obtained by this Method described on pp.
Mit der Methode erhaltene pharmakokinetische Daten sind beschrieben auf S.

Method is recommended for: Methode ist empfohlen für:	toxicological analysis in post-mortem samples

Benzodiazepine(s)/ Benzodiazepin(e)	Chlordiazepoxide, Diazepam, Oxazepam, N-Desmethyl-Diazepam, Nitrazepam, Medazepam, Prazepam, Clonazepam, Flurazepam, Flunitrazepam.
Method / Methode	GLC - FID (2 % OV-17 on Chromosorb G-HP, 100-120 mesh)
Authors / Verfasser	BASELT, STEWART and FRANCH
Lit.Ref./ Lit.Zitat	(56)
Year of Publication/ Publikationsjahr	1977
Extraction Procedure/ Extraktionsverfahren	with n-butylchloride from alkaline solution, reextraction with 1 N HCl, second extraction from alkaline solution with chloroform
Drug analyzed/ analysierte Substanz	Benzodiazepine
Drug calculated / berechnete Substanz	Benzodiazepine
Metabolites included / Metabolite inbegriffen	yes
qual./quant./Screening Method (e)	quant.
Sample required/ benötigtes Untersuchungsmaterial	about 4 ml biological fluids or tissues
Concentration Range/ Konzentrationsbereich	200 ng / ml or more (e.g. 200 ng - 2000 ng / ml)
Special Equipment/ Spezialausstattung	FID - Detection
Hydrolysis / Hydrolyse	no
Some Other Data: Einige andere Daten:	Recovery (1000 ng /ml blood added) Chlordiazepoxide 105 %; Diazepam 105 %; N-Desmethyldiazepam 96 %; Oxazepam 99 %; Flurazepam 92 %; Desalkylflurazepam 100 %. Day-to-day Reproducibility (1000 ng/ ml blood added) C.V. = Chlordiazepoxide 19.8 %; Diazepam 5.2 %; N-Desmethyldiazepam 11.7 %; Oxazepam 21.6 %; Flurazepam 12.7 %; Desalkylflurazepam 9.2 %.
Pharmacokinetic Data obtained by this Method described on pp. Mit der Methode erhaltene pharmakokinetische Daten sind beschrieben auf S.	
Method is recommended for: Methode ist empfohlen für:	the determination of concentrations of chlordiazepoxide, diazepam, N-desmethyl diazepam, oxazepam, flurazepam and desalkylflurazepam in biological fluids and tissues at concentrations of 200 ng/ml or more (between the high therapeutic range after a chronic daily dosage and the low toxic range).

Benzodiazepine(s)/ Benzodiazepin(e)	Chlordiazepoxide, Diazepam, Oxazepam, Nitrazepam, Medazepam, Clorazepate, Lorazepam, Prazepam, Clonazepam, Flurazepam, Bromazepam, Flunitrazepam, Camazepam.
Method / Methode	GLC - FID and TLC resp.
Authors / Verfasser	SCHUETZ and WESTENBERGER ; SCHUETZ
Lit.Ref./ Lit.Zitat	(989) GLC; (984) TLC
Year of Publication/ Publikationsjahr	1978 1978
Extraction Procedure/ Extraktionsverfahren	pH 9 and pH 11, chloroform- isopropanol (40 : 10) or ethylacetate
Drug analyzed/ analysierte Substanz	Benzophenone
Drug calculated / berechnete Substanz	(Benzodiazepine)
Metabolites included / Metabolite inbegriffen	yes
qual./quant./Screening Method (e)	qual. screening
Sample required/ benötigtes Untersuchungsmaterial	ca. 2 ml blood ca. 5 ml urine
Concentration Range/ Konzentrationsbereich	ca. 100 ng/ml or more
Special Equipment/ Spezialausstattung	FID - Detection
Hydrolysis / Hydrolyse	yes
Some Other Data: Einige andere Daten:	qual. method
Pharmacokinetic Data obtained by this Method described on pp. Mit der Methode erhaltene pharmakokinetische Daten sind beschrieben auf S.	
Method is recommended for: Methode ist empfohlen für:	a sensitive screening of 19 hydrolysis derivatives rised from 12 benzodiazepine trade-products and 17 metabolites.

Benzodiazepine(s)/ Benzodiazepin(e)	Chlordiazepoxide, Diazepam, Oxazepam, Nitrazepam, Medazepam, Clorazepate, Lorazepam, Prazepam, Clonazepam, Flurazepam, Bromazepam, Flunitrazepam, Clobazam and Camazepam.
Method / Methode	GLC - FID and TLC resp.
Authors / Verfasser	SCHUETZ and WESTENBERGER; SCHUETZ
Lit.Ref./ Lit.Zitat	(988) GLC; (983) TLC
Year of Publication/ Publikationsjahr	1979 1979
Extraction Procedure/ Extraktionsverfahren	pH 9 and pH 11, diethylether or ethylacetate
Drug analyzed/ analysierte Substanz	Benzodiazepine or rearrangement products
Drug calculated / berechnete Substanz	(Benzodiazepine)
Metabolites included / Metabolite inbegriffen	yes
qual./quant./Screening Method (e)	qual. screening
Sample required/ benötigtes Untersuchungsmaterial	ca. 2 ml blood ca. 5 ml urine
Concentration Range/ Konzentrationsbereich	ca. 100 ng/ml or more
Special Equipment/ Spezialausstattung	FID - Detection
Hydrolysis / Hydrolyse	no acid hydrolysis, but enzymatic cleavage of the 3-hydroxy- and other conjugates
Some Other Data: Einige andere Daten:	qual. Method
Pharmacokinetic Data obtained by this Method described on pp. Mit der Methode erhaltene pharmakokinetische Daten sind beschrieben auf S.	
Method is recommended for: Methode ist empfohlen für:	the screening of 31 benzodiazepine derivatives (trade-products and metabolites).

Benzodiazepine(s)/ Benzodiazepin(e)	Chlordiazepoxide, Diazepam, Oxazepam.
Method / Methode	GLC - NFID (3 % OV-25 on WHP, 100-120 mesh)
Authors / Verfasser	VANDEMARK and ADAMS
Lit.Ref./ Lit.Zitat	(2427)
Year of Publication/ Publikationsjahr	1977
Extraction Procedure/ Extraktionsverfahren	pH 9, Benzene - heptane - isoamylalcohol (80 : 18 : 1)
Drug analyzed/ analysierte Substanz	Benzodiazepine
Drug calculated / berechnete Substanz	Benzodiazepine
Metabolites included / Metabolite inbegriffen	yes
qual./quant./Screening Method (e)	quant.
Sample required/ benötigtes Untersuchungsmaterial	1 ml serum
Concentration Range/ Konzentrationsbereich	150 - 10,000 ng / ml
Special Equipment/ Spezialausstattung	NFID- Detection
Hydrolysis / Hydrolyse	no
Some Other Data: Einige andere Daten:	<u>Within-run precision</u> (n = 10, samples containing each 150 ng/ ml) Chlordiazepoxide $\bar{X}$ = 152 ng/ml, S.D. = 8.4 , CV = 5.5 % Diazepam $\bar{X}$ = 151 ng/ml, S.D. = 7.3 , CV = 4.8 % Oxazepam $\bar{X}$ = 153 ng/ml, S.D. = 9.4 , CV = 6.2 % <u>Sensitivity</u>: ca. 100 ng / ml
Pharmacokinetic Data obtained by this Method described on pp. Mit der Methode erhaltene pharmakokinetische Daten sind beschrieben auf S.	
Method is recommended for: Methode ist empfohlen für:	the rapid and routine determination of therapeutic levels of chlordiazepoxide, diazepam and oxazepam in 1 ml samples of serum. Total analysis time = 15 minutes.

Benzodiazepine(s)/ Benzodiazepin(e)	Chlordiazepoxide, Diazepam
Method / Methode	TLC
Authors / Verfasser	KAISTHA and TADRUS
Lit.Ref./ Lit.Zitat	(1618)
Year of Publication/ Publikationsjahr	1978
Extraction Procedure/ Extraktionsverfahren	pH 10, Chloroform - isopropanol (5 : 2) after acid hydrolysis
Drug analyzed/ analysierte Substanz	Benzophenone derivative
Drug calculated / berechnete Substanz	-------
Metabolites included / Metabolite inbegriffen	yes, also other drugs (e.g. opiates, amphetamines, barbiturates)
qual./quant./Screening Method (e)	qual. screening
Sample required/ benötigtes Untersuchungsmaterial	20 - 50 ml urine
Concentration Range/ Konzentrationsbereich	qual.
Special Equipment/ Spezialausstattung	no
Hydrolysis / Hydrolyse	yes (acid)
Some Other Data: Einige andere Daten:	
Pharmacokinetic Data obtained by this Method described on pp. Mit der Methode erhaltene pharmakokinetische Daten sind beschrieben auf S.	
Method is recommended for: Methode ist empfohlen für:	the TLC - screening of diazepam and / or chlordiazepoxide alone or in combination with other drugs.

Benzodiazepine(s)/ Benzodiazepin(e)	Chlordiazepoxide, Diazepam, Oxazepam, Nitrazepam, Medazepam, Clorazepate, Lorazepam, Prazepam, Clonazepam, Flurazepam, Bromazepam, Flunitrazepam, Clobazam and Temazepam.
Method / Methode	GLC, TLC, UV-, IR- and Mass-Spectra 3% OV-1 + 0.1% BTPPC and 2.5% OV-17 resp.
Authors / Verfasser	BATTISTA, UDERMANN, HENNING and VYCUDILIK
Lit.Ref./ Lit.Zitat	(2477)
Year of Publication/ Publikationsjahr	1979
Extraction Procedure/ Extraktionsverfahren	
Drug analyzed/ analysierte Substanz	Benzophenone / Benzodiazepine
Drug calculated / berechnete Substanz	Benzodiazepine
Metabolites included / Metabolite inbegriffen	(yes)
qual./quant./Screening Method (e)	qual.
Sample required/ benötigtes Untersuchungsmaterial	body fluids and tissues
Concentration Range/ Konzentrationsbereich	---------
Special Equipment/ Spezialausstattung	GLC-, UV-, IR- and / or MS equipment
Hydrolysis / Hydrolyse	yes
Some Other Data: Einige andere Daten:	-----------
Pharmacokinetic Data obtained by this Method described on pp. Mit der Methode erhaltene pharmakokinetische Daten sind beschrieben auf S.	
Method is recommended for: Methode ist empfohlen für:	the identification of unknown samples using the different methods.

Benzodiazepine(s)/ Benzodiazepin(e)	Chlordiazepoxide, Diazepam and Major Metabolites
Method / Methode	Spectrophotodensitometry
Authors / Verfasser	STROJNY, BRATIN, BROOKS and DE SILVA
Lit.Ref./ Lit.Zitat	(1106)
Year of Publication/ Publikationsjahr	1977
Extraction Procedure/ Extraktionsverfahren	pH 9, diethylether, reextraction of demoxepam with 0.1 N NaOH, (see 1106 for details)
Drug analyzed/ analysierte Substanz	Demoxepam as quinazoline derivative the other compounds as benzodiazepines
Drug calculated / berechnete Substanz	Benzodiazepine
Metabolites included / Metabolite inbegriffen	yes
qual./quant./Screening Method (e)	quant.
Sample required/ benötigtes Untersuchungsmaterial	1 - 2 ml blood or plasma
Concentration Range/ Konzentrationsbereich	50 ng / ml - ca. 1,500 ng / ml (chlordiazepoxide) 30 ng / ml - ca. 250 ng / ml (N-desmethylchlordiazepoxide) 350 ng / ml - ca. 2,000 ng / ml (diazepam, overdoses)
Special Equipment/ Spezialausstattung	Spectrophotodensitometer
Hydrolysis / Hydrolyse	no
Some Other Data: Einige andere Daten:	Recovery: Chlordiazepoxide 75 ± 10 % N-Desmethylchlordiazepoxide 72 ± 6 % Diazepam 92 ± 8 % Nordiazepam 95 ± 5 % Demoxepam 95 ± 5 % Sensitivity limits: 50 - 200 ng / ml (all except demoxepam) 100 - 200 ng / ml (demoxepam)
Pharmacokinetic Data obtained by this Method described on pp. Mit der Methode erhaltene pharmakokinetische Daten sind beschrieben auf S.	See part: Blood-, Serum- and Plasma-Levels and Other Pharmacokinetic Data from Literature
Method is recommended for: Methode ist empfohlen für:	monitoring plasma levels of chlordiazepoxide and its major metabolites following single or chronic oral administration of chlordiazepoxide and for measuring plasma levels resulting from high dosage of diazepam.

Benzodiazepine(s)/ Benzodiazepin(e)	Chlordiazepoxide, Diazepam, Oxazepam, Nitrazepam, Clorazepate, Lorazepam, Prazepam, Clonazepam, Flurazepam and N-Desmethyldiazepam.
Method / Methode	UV- and IR-Spectra, HPLC
Authors / Verfasser	NOGGLE, jr. and CLARK
Lit.Ref./ Lit.Zitat	(2487)
Year of Publication/ Publikationsjahr	1979
Extraction Procedure/ Extraktionsverfahren	approx. pH 11, Chloroform
Drug analyzed/ analysierte Substanz	Benzodiazepines
Drug calculated / berechnete Substanz	Benzodiazepines
Metabolites included / Metabolite inbegriffen	(yes)
qual./quant./Screening Method (e)	qual. (identification)
Sample required/ benötigtes Untersuchungsmaterial	solid dosage form
Concentration Range/ Konzentrationsbereich	usual solid samples
Special Equipment/ Spezialausstattung	UV- and IR-Spectrophotometer, HPLC
Hydrolysis / Hydrolyse	no
Some Other Data: Einige andere Daten:	------------
Pharmacokinetic Data obtained by this Method described on pp. Mit der Methode erhaltene pharmakokinetische Daten sind beschrieben auf S.	------------
Method is recommended for: Methode ist empfohlen für:	the identification of chlordiazepoxide, diazepam, oxazepam, nitrazepam, clorazepate, lorazepam, prazepam, clonazepam, flurazepam and N-desmethyldiazepam in solid dosage forms.

Benzodiazepine(s)/ Benzodiazepin(e)	Chlordiazepoxide, Diazepam, Oxazepam, Flurazepam.
Method / Methode	Polarography (Differential-Pulse Mode)
Authors / Verfasser	BROOKS, D'ARCONTE, HACKMAN and DE SILVA
Lit.Ref./ Lit.Zitat	(147)
Year of Publication/ Publikationsjahr	1977
Extraction Procedure/ Extraktionsverfahren	pH 12.8, benzene - methylene chloride (90 : 10)
Drug analyzed/ analysierte Substanz	Benzodiazepine
Drug calculated / berechnete Substanz	Benzodiazepine
Metabolites included / Metabolite inbegriffen	yes
qual./quant./Screening Method (e)	Screening / quant.
Sample required/ benötigtes Untersuchungsmaterial	1 ml blood 2 ml urine 2 ml gastric fluid
Concentration Range/ Konzentrationsbereich	sensitivity of 250 - 500 ng / ml
Special Equipment/ Spezialausstattung	Polarograph (DPP mode)
Hydrolysis / Hydrolyse	no
Some Other Data: Einige andere Daten:	<u>Recovery:</u> 75 - 85 % (except oxazepam) from blood or plasma 25 % (oxazepam) from blood or plasma <u>Sensitivity limit:</u> 250 - 500 ng/ml (blood, urine and gastric fluid)
Pharmacokinetic Data obtained by this Method described on pp. Mit der Methode erhaltene pharmakokinetische Daten sind beschrieben auf S.	
Method is recommended for: Methode ist empfohlen für:	a selective screening procedure to determine the "total" concentration of a particular 1,4-benzodiazepine and its metabolites prior to quantitation by more specific methods.

Benzodiazepine(s)/ Benzodiazepin(e)	Chlordiazepoxide, Diazepam, Oxazepam, Nitrazepam, Medazepam, Lorazepam, Prazepam, Flunitrazepam, Clobazam, Triazolam
Method / Methode	Radioimmunoassay
Authors / Verfasser	ROBINSON, RUTTERFORD and SMITH
Lit.Ref./ Lit.Zitat	(3439)
Year of Publication/ Publikationsjahr	1980
Extraction Procedure/ Extraktionsverfahren	pH 9, ethyl acetate
Drug analyzed/ analysierte Substanz	Benzodiazepine
Drug calculated / berechnete Substanz	Benzodiazepine
Metabolites included / Metabolite inbegriffen	yes (Demoxepam, Desalkylflurazepam, Desmethyldiazepam, Temazepam)
qual./quant./Screening Method (e)	quant. / Screening
Sample required/ benötigtes Untersuchungsmaterial	0,075 ml Blood
Concentration Range/ Konzentrationsbereich	0 - 2.5 ng/ml (Diazepam)
Special Equipment/ Spezialausstattung	RIA - equipment
Hydrolysis / Hydrolyse	no
Some Other Data: Einige andere Daten:	Standard Deviation about 4.9 %
Pharmacokinetic Data obtained by this Method described on pp. Mit der Methode erhaltene pharmakokinetische Daten sind beschrieben auf S.	
Method is recommended for: Methode ist empfohlen für:	the screening and determination of sub-therapeutic levels

Benzodiazepine(s)/ Benzodiazepin(e)	Diazepam, Oxazepam, Nitrazepam and Clobazam
Method / Methode	Radioreceptor Assay
Authors / Verfasser	HUNT, HUSSON and RAYNAUD
Lit.Ref./ Lit.Zitat	(2481)
Year of Publication/ Publikationsjahr	1978
Extraction Procedure/ Extraktionsverfahren	pH 9, diethylether
Drug analyzed/ analysierte Substanz	Benzodiazepine
Drug calculated / berechnete Substanz	Benzodiazepine
Metabolites included / Metabolite inbegriffen	yes
qual./quant./Screening Method (e)	quant.
Sample required/ benötigtes Untersuchungsmaterial	ca. 0.5 ml serum
Concentration Range/ Konzentrationsbereich	0.5 - 50 ng for Diazepam and Nitrazepam 10 - 1000 ng for Clobazam
Special Equipment/ Spezialausstattung	Radioreceptor Assay
Hydrolysis / Hydrolyse	no
Some Other Data: Einige andere Daten:	Within-assay precision: C.V. = 8 - 10 % (n = 6, 4, 4, 8 and 18 ng) Day-to-day precision: C.V. = 9 - 13 % (n = 6) Detection limit: ca. 0.5 ng
Pharmacokinetic Data obtained by this Method described on pp. Mit der Methode erhaltene pharmakokinetische Daten sind beschrieben auf S.	
Method is recommended for: Methode ist empfohlen für:	the high sensitive determination of diazepam, nitrazepam and clobazam in serum after single oral doses (e.g. in long term studies).

Benzodiazepine(s)/ Benzodiazepin(e)	Chlordiazepoxide, Oxazepam, Nitrazepam
Method / Methode	Radioreceptor Assay
Authors / Verfasser	ROSENBLATT, BRIDGE and WYATT
Lit.Ref./ Lit.Zitat	(2489)
Year of Publication/ Publikationsjahr	1979
Extraction Procedure/ Extraktionsverfahren	pH 7.7, without extraction
Drug analyzed/ analysierte Substanz	Benzodiazepine
Drug calculated / berechnete Substanz	Benzodiazepine
Metabolites included / Metabolite inbegriffen	yes
qual./quant./Screening Method (e)	quant.
Sample required/ benötigtes Untersuchungsmaterial	ca. 0,1 ml saliva
Concentration Range/ Konzentrationsbereich	10^{-6} - 10^{-9} molar concentration in saliva
Special Equipment/ Spezialausstattung	Radioreceptor Assay
Hydrolysis / Hydrolyse	no
Some Other Data: Einige andere Daten:	Recovery: quantitative Sensitivity: 1.50 ng/ml (chlordiazepoxide) 0.14 ng/ml (diazepam) 2.87 ng/ml (oxazepam) 0.28 ng/ml (nitrazepam)
Pharmacokinetic Data obtained by this Method described on pp. Mit der Methode erhaltene pharmakokinetische Daten sind beschrieben auf S.	
Method is recommended for: Methode ist empfohlen für:	routine analysis of saliva concentrations in large patient populations. 100 samples can be processed in a day. Saliva concentration may more closely reflect intracellular drug concentration, and thus correlate more closely with clinical efficacy.

Benzodiazepine(s)/ Benzodiazepin(e)	Chlordiazepoxide, Diazepam, Oxazepam, Nitrazepam, Medazepam, Clorazepate, Lorazepam, Prazepam and Flurazepam
Method / Methode	HPLC LiChrosorb Si-100 (reversed-phase mode) 10 µm
Authors / Verfasser	HARZER and BARCHET
Lit.Ref./ Lit.Zitat	(1549)
Year of Publication/ Publikationsjahr	1977
Extraction Procedure/ Extraktionsverfahren	pH 9.5, EXTRELUT[R], diethylether
Drug analyzed/ analysierte Substanz	Benzodiazepines or Benzophenones
Drug calculated / berechnete Substanz	Benzodiazepines
Metabolites included / Metabolite inbegriffen	yes
qual./quant./Screening Method (e)	qual. / quant./ Screening
Sample required/ benötigtes Untersuchungsmaterial	5 - 10 ml blood / urine
Concentration Range/ Konzentrationsbereich	ca. 100 - 1000 µg
Special Equipment/ Spezialausstattung	HPLC-equipment (reversed-phase mode)
Hydrolysis / Hydrolyse	yes (or not)
Some Other Data: Einige andere Daten:	Recovery: (n = 7) 79 % (nitrazepam) 86 % (oxazepam) 81 % (chlordiazepoxide) Within-run precision: S.D. = 1.7 % (n = 10) Sensitivity limit: 5000 ng/ml (1 µl injected) Recovery: (n = 10) 66 % (2-amino-5-chlor-benzophenone) Within-run precision: S.D. = 1.8 % (n = 10) Sensitivity limit: 5000 ng/ml (1 µl injected)
Pharmacokinetic Data obtained by this Method described on pp. Mit der Methode erhaltene pharmakokinetische Daten sind beschrieben auf S.	
Method is recommended for: Methode ist empfohlen für:	the determination of various benzodiazepines and aminobenzophenones in biological samples (especially in overdoses and chronic treatment cases).

Benzodiazepine(s)/ Benzodiazepin(e)	Chlordiazepoxide, Diazepam, Flurazepam
Method / Methode	HPLC (Bondapack-C 18, reversed-phase mode)
Authors / Verfasser	PEAT and KOPJAK
Lit.Ref./ Lit.Zitat	(3382)
Year of Publication/ Publikationsjahr	1980

Extraction Procedure/
Extraktionsverfahren

Drug analyzed/ analysierte Substanz	Benzodiazepines
Drug calculated / berechnete Substanz	Benzodiazepines
Metabolites included / Metabolite inbegriffen	yes
qual./quant./Screening Method (e)	quant.
Sample required/ benötigtes Untersuchungsmaterial	1 ml plasma or whole blood
Concentration Range/ Konzentrationsbereich	ca. 1,000 - 10,000 ng/ml (Chlordiazepoxide, Desmethylchlordiazepoxide
Special Equipment/ Spezialausstattung	UV - detection
Hydrolysis / Hydrolyse	no
Some Other Data: Einige andere Daten:	see data on the sheet PEAT and KOPJAK - ECD-GLC on page 127

Pharmacokinetic Data obtained by this Method described on pp.
Mit der Methode erhaltene pharmakokinetische Daten sind beschrieben auf S.

Method is recommended for: Methode ist empfohlen für:	both clinical and forensic-toxicology cases (screening and quantitation)

Benzodiazepine(s)/ Benzodiazepin(e)	Chlordiazepoxide, Diazepam, Oxazepam, Nitrazepam, Medazepam, Prazepam, Flurazepam, Clonazepam, Cyprazepam
Method / Methode	HPLC (Micro Porasil)
Authors / Verfasser	WITTWER
Lit.Ref./ Lit.Zitat	(3712)
Year of Publication/ Publikationsjahr	1980
Extraction Procedure/ Extraktionsverfahren	approx. pH 11, chloroform
Drug analyzed/ analysierte Substanz	Benzodiazepine
Drug calculated / berechnete Substanz	Benzodiazepine
Metabolites included / Metabolite inbegriffen	yes (Demoxepam, Desmethyldiazepam)
qual./quant./Screening Method (e)	quant.
Sample required/ benötigtes Untersuchungsmaterial	powder or other solid preparation
Concentration Range/ Konzentrationsbereich	ca. 50,000 - 100,000 ng/ml
Special Equipment/ Spezialausstattung	Dual wavelength detection (254 nm and 280 nm)
Hydrolysis / Hydrolyse	no
Some Other Data: Einige andere Daten:	Diazepam: rel.stand.dev. 1.9 % C.V. 1.7 %
Pharmacokinetic Data obtained by this Method described on pp. Mit der Methode erhaltene pharmakokinetische Daten sind beschrieben auf S.	
Method is recommended for: Methode ist empfohlen für:	the determination of benzodiazepines in solid formulations

Methods for the Detection and Determination of a Special Benzodiazepine (Mono Method)

Benzodiazepine(s)/ Benzodiazepin(e)	Chlordiazepoxide	Chlordiazepoxide
Method / Methode	GLC-ECD 2% OV-17 Chromosorb W HP 80 - 100 mesh	GLC-ECD 5% OV-225 Gas Chrom Q (60-80 mesh)
Authors / Verfasser	ZINGALES	SUN and HOFFMAN
Lit.Ref./ Lit.Zitat	(1226)	(1948)
Year of Publication/ Publikationsjahr	1971	1978
Extraction Procedure/ Extraktionsverfahren	pH 9-10, n-heptane - iso-amylalcohol (98.5 : 1.5)	0.1 M K_2PO_4, diethylether, then methylation
Drug analyzed/ analysierte Substanz	Benzodiazepine	Methyl derivative
Drug calculated / berechnete Substanz	Benzodiazepine	Benzodiazepine
Metabolites included / Metabolite inbegriffen	yes (N-desmethylchlordiazepoxide) and demoxepam)	yes (demoxepam)
qual./quant./Screening Method (e)	quant.	quant.
Sample required/ benötigtes Untersuchungsmaterial	1 ml plasma	0.4 ml serum
Concentration Range/ Konzentrationsbereich	Ca. 100 - 7000 ng / ml linearity 30 - 10 000 ng	Ca. 100 - 1500 ng / ml
Special Equipment/ Spezialausstattung	ECD-Detection	ECD-Detection
Hydrolysis / Hydrolyse	no	no
Some Other Data: Einige andere Daten:	Recovery: ca. 87 - 93 % (± 1.5 - 5.1 S.D.) (range 30 - 1000 ng/ml plasma) Detection limit: ca. 0.5 ng	Assay Reproducibility: between 1.7 and 27.2 % (rel.S.D.) Sensitivity: 45 ng / ml
Pharmacokinetic Data obtained by this Method described on pp. Mit der Methode erhaltene pharmakokinetische Daten sind beschrieben auf S.	See part: Blood-, Serum- and Plasma-Levels and Other Pharmacokinetic Data from Literature	
Method is recommended for: Methode ist empfohlen für:	the determination of serum concentrations after single oral chlordiazepoxide doses of 5mg and more.	the simple and sensitive determination of chlordiazepoxide plasma levels which can be automated for large-scale clinical analysis .

Benzodiazepine(s)/ Benzodiazepin(e)	Chlordiazepoxide	Chlordiazepoxide
Method / Methode	GLC-ECD 10% OV-1 Chromosorb G HP 80 - 100 mesh	TLC (Fluorescence Densitometry)
Authors / Verfasser	SUN	SUN
Lit.Ref./ Lit.Zitat	(1945)	(1946)
Year of Publication/ Publikationsjahr	1978	1978
Extraction Procedure/ Extraktionsverfahren	alkaline, heptane - iso-amylalcohol (98.5 : 1.5)	pH 7, diethylether (see (1946) for further procedure)
Drug analyzed/ analysierte Substanz	Benzodiazepine	Fluorescence derivative with sulphuric acid
Drug calculated / berechnete Substanz	Benzodiazepine	Benzodiazepine
Metabolites included / Metabolite inbegriffen	no	yes (N-desmethylchlordiazepoxide and demoxepam)
qual./quant./Screening Method (e)	quant.	quant.
Sample required/ benötigtes Untersuchungsmaterial	1 ml serum	1 ml serum
Concentration Range/ Konzentrationsbereich	100 - 1000 ng / ml	100 - 1100 ng / ml
Special Equipment/ Spezialausstattung	ECD-Detection	Fluorimeter
Hydrolysis / Hydrolyse	no	no
Some Other Data: Einige andere Daten:	Assay reproducibility: rel.S.D. — serum-conc. 6.6% — 100 ng/ml 10.8% — 250 ng/ml 10.6% — 500 ng/ml 3.3% — 1000 ng/ml	Recoveries (mean ± S.D.): 99.0 % ± 1.2 % (chlordiazepoxide) 78.6 % ± 4.5 % (demoxepam) 83.6 % ± 3.2 % (N-desmethylchlordiazepoxide) (1.500 ng/ml Chlordiazepoxide) (300 ng/ml metabolites) Reproducibility: rel.S.D. 1.5 - 13.1 (chlordiazepoxide) 5.5 - 7.7 (demoxepam) 1.8 - 6.8 (N-desmethylchlord.) Sensitivity limits: between 10 and 50 ng / ml
Pharmacokinetic Data obtained by this Method described on pp. Mit der Methode erhaltene pharmakokinetische Daten sind beschrieben auf S.	See part: Blood-, Serum- and Plasma-Levels and Other Pharmacokinetic Data from Literature	
Method is recommended for: Methode ist empfohlen für:	pharmacokinetic studies after single doses of chlordiazepoxide	the determination of chlordiazepoxide and its major metabolites in serum after single doses.

Benzodiazepine(s)/ Benzodiazepin(e)	Chlordiazepoxide	Chlordiazepoxide
Method / Methode	UV-Photometry	Spectrofluorometry
Authors / Verfasser	JATLOW	KOECHLIN and D'ARCONTE
Lit.Ref./ Lit.Zitat	(523)	(598)
Year of Publication/ Publikationsjahr	1972	1963
Extraction Procedure/ Extraktionsverfahren	pH 7.4, chloroform, reextraction into HCl	pH 7.2, diethylether (see (598) for details of the procedure)
Drug analyzed/ analysierte Substanz	Benzodiazepine	Lactam Derivative (Demoxepam)
Drug calculated / berechnete Substanz	Benzodiazepine	Benzodiazepine
Metabolites included / Metabolite inbegriffen	no	yes (demoxepam)
qual./quant./Screening Method (e)	quant.	quant.
Sample required/ benötigtes Untersuchungsmaterial	3 ml plasma	1 ml plasma
Concentration Range/ Konzentrationsbereich	2000 - 70,000 ng / ml	ca. 500 - 2,000 ng / ml
Special Equipment/ Spezialausstattung	Photometer	Spectrofluorometer
Hydrolysis / Hydrolyse	no	yes (acid)
Some Other Data: Einige andere Daten:	Recovery: Overall ca. 84 % Precision: C.V. = 3 % (n = 10, 17 mg/l) Sensitivity limit: ca. 2000 ng / ml	Recovery: Overall ca. 69.5 - 100 % Sensitivity limit: 250 ng / ml (either compounds)
Pharmacokinetic Data obtained by this Method described on pp. Mit der Methode erhaltene pharmakokinetische Daten sind beschrieben auf S.		See part: Blood-, Serum- and Plasma-Levels and Other Pharmacokinetic Data from Literature
Method is recommended for: Methode ist empfohlen für:	emergency spectrophotometric measurements in cases of poisoning.	the determination of chlordiazepoxide and demoxepam in plasma after normal therapeutic doses (10 - 30 mg chlordiazepoxide).

Benzodiazepine(s)/ Benzodiazepin(e)	Chlordiazepoxide	Chlordiazepoxide
Method / Methode	Polarography (DPP-mode)	Radioimmunoassay
Authors / Verfasser	HACKMAN, BROOKS, DE SILVA and MA	DIXON, EARLEY and POSTMA
Lit.Ref./ Lit.Zitat	(445)	(261)
Year of Publication/ Publikationsjahr	1974	1975
Extraction Procedure/ Extraktionsverfahren	pH 9.0, diethylether	
Drug analyzed/ analysierte Substanz	Benzodiazepine	Benzodiazepine
Drug calculated / berechnete Substanz	Benzodiazepine	Benzodiazepine
Metabolites included / Metabolite inbegriffen	yes (demoxepam and N-desmethyl-chlordiazepoxide)	no
qual./quant./Screening Method (e)	quant.	quant.
Sample required/ benötigtes Untersuchungsmaterial	2 ml plasma	0.02 - 0.1 ml plasma
Concentration Range/ Konzentrationsbereich	50 - 1000 ng / ml	ca. 100 - 3,000 ng / ml
Special Equipment/ Spezialausstattung	Polarograph (DPP-mode)	RIA - equipment
Hydrolysis / Hydrolyse	no	no
Some Other Data: Einige andere Daten:	Recovery: Overall ± S.D. 61.9 % ± 3.1 (chlordiazepoxide) 62.0 % ± 3.7 (N-desmethylchlordiazepoxide) 62.7 % ± 4.3 (demoxepam) Sensitivity limit: 50 ng/ml (chlordiazepoxide and N-desmethylchlordiazepoxide) 100ng/ml (demoxepam)	Recovery: about 100 % (no extraction steps) Reproducibility: C.V. = 4 % (n = 6) Sensitivity limit: 20 ng / ml using 0.1 ml samples
Pharmacokinetic Data obtained by this Method described on pp. Mit der Methode erhaltene pharmakokinetische Daten sind beschrieben auf S.	See part: Blood-, Serum- and Plasma-Levels and Other Pharmacokinetic Data from Literature	See part: Blood-, Serum- and Plasma-Levels and Other Pharmacokinetic Data from Literature
Method is recommended for: Methode ist empfohlen für:	the determination of chlordiazepoxide and its major metabolites in blood following single and chronic administration of chlordiazepoxide.	the rapid and sensitive screening of large numbers of plasma samples (without extraction steps) after single and chronic doses of chlordiazepoxide.

Benzodiazepine(s)/ Benzodiazepin(e)	Chlordiazepoxide	Chlordiazepoxide
Method / Methode	Radioimmunoassay	HPLC (Mikro-Bondapack C-18, reverse phase)
Authors / Verfasser	LUCEK and DIXON	STROJNY, PUGLISI and DE SILVA
Lit.Ref./ Lit.Zitat	(3211)	(1107)
Year of Publication/ Publikationsjahr	1980	1978
Extraction Procedure/ Extraktionsverfahren		pH 8.8-9.2, diethylether, reextraction (see (1107)
Drug analyzed/ analysierte Substanz	Benzodiazepine	Benzodiazepine
Drug calculated / berechnete Substanz	Benzodiazepine	Benzodiazepine
Metabolites included / Metabolite inbegriffen	no	yes (Desmethylchlordiazepoxide, demoxepam and nordiazepam)
qual./quant./Screening Method (e)	quant.	quant.
Sample required/ benötigtes Untersuchungsmaterial	0,025 ml plasma or saliva	0.1 - 2.0 ml plasma
Concentration Range/ Konzentrationsbereich	ca. 170 - 2,000 ng/ml	ca. 50 - 1,400 ng/ml (Chlordiazepoxide/ plasma)
Special Equipment/ Spezialausstattung	RIA - equipment	UV - detection (254 nm)
Hydrolysis / Hydrolyse	no	no
Some Other Data: Einige andere Daten:	Sensitivity-limit: about 2 ng/ml Intra-assay C.V. less 6% (range 170 - 2,000 ng/ml) Inter-assay C.V. less 10%	Recovery 80 ± 5% (Chlordiazepoxide) 80 ± 4% (Desmethyl-metabolite) 83 ± 5% (Demoxepam) 91 ± 2% (Nordiazepam) Sensitivity limits 50-100 ng/ml using 1 ml plasma
Pharmacokinetic Data obtained by this Method described on pp. Mit der Methode erhaltene pharmakokinetische Daten sind beschrieben auf S.		See part: Blood-, Serum- and Plasma-Levels and Other Pharmacokinetic Data from Literature
Method is recommended for: Methode ist empfohlen für:	the determination of Chlordiazepoxide in microsamples of plasma and saliva	the determination of chlordiazepoxide and metabolites in plasma following oral administration (drug monitoring, drug abuse screening)

Benzodiazepine(s)/ Benzodiazepin(e)	Diazepam	Diazepam
Method / Methode	GLC-ECD 2% Carbowax 20 M sil.Gas Chrom P (100-120 mesh)	GLC-ECD 3% E 350 Diatomite CQ sil. (100-120 mesh)
Authors / Verfasser	DE SILVA, SCHWARTZ, STEFANOVIC, KAPLAN and D'ARCONTE	ARNOLD
Lit.Ref./ Lit.Zitat	(243)	(22)
Year of Publication/ Publikationsjahr	1964	1975
Extraction Procedure/ Extraktionsverfahren	pH 6.9-7.1, diethylether, hydrolysis, neutralization, ether	serum/plasma: benzene, urine: pH 7.5, benzene
Drug analyzed/ analysierte Substanz	Benzophenone	Benzodiazepine
Drug calculated / berechnete Substanz	Benzodiazepine	Benzodiazepine
Metabolites included / Metabolite inbegriffen	yes (nordiazepam)	yes (nordiazepam, temazepam, oxazepam)
qual./quant./Screening Method (e)	quant.	quant.
Sample required/ benötigtes Untersuchungsmaterial	1 ml blood	0.2 - 1.0 ml serum 2.0 ml urine
Concentration Range/ Konzentrationsbereich	5.0 - 30.0 ng / ml (MABP) linear response of ECD	25 - 1300 ng/ml (diazepam) 30 - 230 ng/ml (nordiazepam)
Special Equipment/ Spezialausstattung	ECD-Detection	ECD-Detection
Hydrolysis / Hydrolyse	yes (Acid)	no
Some Other Data: Einige andere Daten:	Recovery: 94 % ± 5.0 (MABP) Sensitivity limit: 20 - 30 ng / ml	Recovery: 98 % ± 11 % (diazepam, range 400 - 50 ng / ml added) Standard Deviation: Diazepam ± 8.4 % Nordiazepam ± 9.7 % Sensitivity limit: Ca. 5 ng diazepam / ml serum
Pharmacokinetic Data obtained by this Method described on pp. Mit der Methode erhaltene pharmakokinetische Daten sind beschrieben auf S.	See part: Blood-, Serum- and Plasma-Levels and Other Pharmacokinetic Data from Literature	See part: Blood-, Serum- and Plasma-Levels and Other Pharmacokinetic Data from Literature
Method is recommended for: Methode ist empfohlen für:	the determination of diazepam in blood samples obtained from a variety of clinical studies.	the determination of diazepam and nordiazepam in serum following the administration of therapeutic doses of diazepam (with a simple extraction procedure).

Benzodiazepine(s)/ Benzodiazepin(e)	Diazepam	Diazepam
Method / Methode	GLC-ECD 3% OV-17 Chromosorb W HP (80-100 mesh)	GLC-ECD 3% OV-7 Varaport 30 (80-100 mesh)
Authors / Verfasser	LINNOILA and DORRITY	RUTHERFORD
Lit.Ref./ Lit.Zitat	(639)	(927)
Year of Publication/ Publikationsjahr	1977	1977
Extraction Procedure/ Extraktionsverfahren	pH 9, toluene - heptane (4 : 1), containing 1.6% isoamylalcohol	n-butylacetate
Drug analyzed/ analysierte Substanz	Benzodiazepine	Benzodiazepine
Drug calculated / berechnete Substanz	Benzodiazepine	Benzodiazepine
Metabolites included / Metabolite inbegriffen	yes (nordiazepam)	yes (nordiazepam)
qual./quant./Screening Method (e)	quant.	quant.
Sample required/ benötigtes Untersuchungsmaterial	1 ml serum	0.02 - 0.1 ml plasma
Concentration Range/ Konzentrationsbereich	ca. 50 - 500 ng / ml (extended range 5 x 10^2)	ca. 20 - 8000 ng / ml
Special Equipment/ Spezialausstattung	ECD-Detection	ECD-Detection
Hydrolysis / Hydrolyse	no	no
Some Other Data: Einige andere Daten:	Recovery: 98 % Diazepam, 100 % nordiazepam Within-run precision: (n=6) C.V. = 0.6 - 3.3 for diazepam C.V. = 0.8 - 4.8 nordiazepam (amount added: 100-500 ng/ml of both benzodiazepines) Between-run precision: (n=16) C.V. = 1.4 - 2.7 (diazepam) C.V. = 1.7 - 5.8 (nordiazepam) (100-500 ng/ml added)	Recovery: (n = 36 analyses) 100 % (S.D. = 4) diazepam 100 % (S.D. = 5 nordiazepam Sensitivity: 5 ng / ml plasma
Pharmacokinetic Data obtained by this Method described on pp. Mit der Methode erhaltene pharmakokinetische Daten sind beschrieben auf S.		
Method is recommended for: Methode ist empfohlen für:	the determination of serum diazepam, nordiazepam and N-desmethylflurazepam levels in clinical samples over a 5 x 10^2 concentration range (serial dilution unnecessary).	the determination of diazepam and nordiazepam in microsamples of blood plasma during therapy and after overdosage (micromethod with no serial dilution is necessary).

Benzodiazepine(s)/ Benzodiazepin(e)	Diazepam	Diazepam
Method / Methode	GLC-ECD 3% OV-17 Gas Chrom Q (60-80 mesh)	GLC-ECD GP 3% SP 2250-DB Supelcoport (100-120 mesh)
Authors / Verfasser	WEINFELD, POSMANTER, KHOO and PUGLISI	WALLACE, SCHWERTNER and SHIMEK
Lit.Ref./ Lit.Zitat	(1195)	(2493)
Year of Publication/ Publikationsjahr	1977	1979
Extraction Procedure/ Extraktionsverfahren	saturated KCl, benzene	approx. pH 11, hexane - ethyl-acetate (70 : 30)
Drug analyzed/ analysierte Substanz	Benzodiazepine	Benzodiazepine
Drug calculated / berechnete Substanz	Benzodiazepine	Benzodiazepine
Metabolites included / Metabolite inbegriffen	yes (nordiazepam)	yes (nordiazepam)
qual./quant./Screening Method (e)	quant.	quant.
Sample required/ benötigtes Untersuchungsmaterial	0.5 ml plasma	1 ml serum
Concentration Range/ Konzentrationsbereich	ca. 5.0 - 500.0 ng / 0.5 ml plasma	ca. 100 - 1400 ng / ml
Special Equipment/ Spezialausstattung	ECD-Detection	ECD-Detection
Hydrolysis / Hydrolyse	no	no
Some Other Data: Einige andere Daten:	Recovery: (mean)± S.D. diazepam: 98.2 ± 3.3 nordiazepam: 94.8 ± 1.5 (5.0 - 500.0 ng diazepam or nordiazepam added to 0.5 ml plasma) Sensitivity limit: 5 ng diazepam / ml 10ng nordiazepam / ml	Recovery: (mean) ± S.D. diazepam: 102.6 ± 2.6 % nordiazepam: 100.3 ± 3.8 % Within-day precision: C.V. = 1.5 % (diazepam) C.V. = 4.7 % (nordiazepam) Day-to-day precision: C.V. = 2.4 % (diazepam) C.V. = 3.6 % (nordiazepam)
Pharmacokinetic Data obtained by this Method described on pp. Mit der Methode erhaltene pharmakokinetische Daten sind beschrieben auf S.	See part: Blood-, Serum- and Plasma-Levels and Other Pharmacokinetic Data from Literature	Sensitivity limit: 50 ng/ml
Method is recommended for: Methode ist empfohlen für:	the determination of diazepam and nordiazepam in plasma following first 5 mg-diazepam doses as well as during chronic oral administration of 5 mg diazepam three times daily and 15 mg diazepam once a day.	the determination of diazepam and nordiazepam in serum in therapeutic concentrations with special regard to steady-state levels.

Benzodiazepine(s)/ Benzodiazepin(e)	Diazepam	Diazepam
Method / Methode	GLC-FID 3% SE-30 Chromosorb W AW (80-100 mesh)	GLC-FID 3% SE-30 Chromosorb W (80-100 mesh)
Authors / Verfasser	FOSTER and FRINGS	STEYN and HUNDT
Lit.Ref./ Lit.Zitat	(329)	(1100)
Year of Publication/ Publikationsjahr	1970	1975
Extraction Procedure/ Extraktionsverfahren	pH 7, chloroform	pH 6.9, diethylether
Drug analyzed/ analysierte Substanz	Benzodiazepine	Benzophenone
Drug calculated / berechnete Substanz	Benzodiazepine	Benzodiazepine
Metabolites included / Metabolite inbegriffen	yes (qual.)	yes (nordiazepam)
qual./quant./Screening Method (e)	quant.	quant.
Sample required/ benötigtes Untersuchungsmaterial	2 ml serum	3 ml serum
Concentration Range/ Konzentrationsbereich	5000 - 30 000 ng / ml	100 - 4000 ng / ml
Special Equipment/ Spezialausstattung	FID-Detection	FID-Detection
Hydrolysis / Hydrolyse	no	yes (acid)
Some Other Data: Einige andere Daten:	Recovery: 85 - 97 % (0.5 - 3.0 mg /100 ml added) C.V. = 5 % Detection limit: 1000 ng / ml	Recovery: Mean ± S.D. Diazepam added / Amount recovered 100 ng / ml — 104.4 ± 0.8 330 ng / ml — 338.2 ± 10 1000 ng / ml — 999.8 ± 23 Sensitivity limit: ca. 50 ng / ml
Pharmacokinetic Data obtained by this Method described on pp. Mit der Methode erhaltene pharmakokinetische Daten sind beschrieben auf S.		
Method is recommended for: Methode ist empfohlen für:	the simple, rapid and precise determination of diazepam concentrations in serum especially in cases of overdoses.	the determination of diazepam and nordiazepam in serum at both therapeutic and toxic levels via the benzophenones.

Benzodiazepine(s)/ Benzodiazepin(e)	Diazepam	Diazepam
Method / Methode	GLC - MS 2% SP-2250 Chromosorb W-HP (100 - 120 mesh)	GLC - MS 3% OV-17 Gas Chrom Q (100 - 120 mesh)
Authors / Verfasser	RODGERS, POWEL and VASILIADES	YEHIA, OLIVER and MACKEY
Lit.Ref./ Lit.Zitat	(3444)	(3725)
Year of Publication/ Publikationsjahr	1980	(1979)
Extraction Procedure/ Extraktionsverfahren	pH 7.4, chloroform - isopropanol (20 : 1)	pH 9, diethylether
Drug analyzed/ analysierte Substanz	Benzodiazepine	Diazepam
Drug calculated / berechnete Substanz	Benzodiazepine	Diazepam
Metabolites included / Metabolite inbegriffen	yes (Nordiazepam)	no
qual./quant./Screening Method (e)	qual./quant.	qual./quant.
Sample required/ benötigtes Untersuchungsmaterial	2 ml serum	1 ml plasma
Concentration Range/ Konzentrationsbereich	ca. 500 - 10,000 ng/ml	ca. 20 - 200 ng/ml
Special Equipment/ Spezialausstattung	(N-FID) MS	MS (peak selection)
Hydrolysis / Hydrolyse	no	no
Some Other Data: Einige andere Daten:	rel. percent recovery of serum extracts: 100 ± 8% (n=24) diazepam 102 ±12% (n=24) nordiazepam Within-run precision: (5 mg/l) GLC-N-FID: (n = 3) 4 % diazepam 9 % nordiazepam GLC-MS: (n = 3) 6 % diazepam 4 % nordiazepam Between-run precision: (5 mg/l) GLC-N-FID: 8% diazepam (n= 23) 11% nordiazepam (n=10) GLC-MS: 9% diazepam (n= 8) 12% nordiazepam (n= 4) Sensitivity: less than 25 ng/ml for diazepam	
Pharmacokinetic Data obtained by this Method described on pp. Mit der Methode erhaltene pharmakokinetische Daten sind beschrieben auf S.		
Method is recommended for: Methode ist empfohlen für:	the selected ion-monitoring of diazepam (m/e: 258,283), nordiazepam (m/e: 269,270) and prazepam (m/e:269,295) in serum	monitoring plasma levels of diazepam (m/e: 256,283) after therapeutic i.v. doses

Benzodiazepine(s)/ Benzodiazepin(e)	Diazepam	Diazepam
Method / Methode	GLC-NPD 3% OV-1 Chromosorb W HP (80 - 100 mesh)	TLC
Authors / Verfasser	McCURDY, SLIGHTOM and HARRILL	WAD, ROSENMUND and HANIFL
Lit.Ref./ Lit.Zitat	(2485)	(1189)
Year of Publication/ Publikationsjahr	1979	1976
Extraction Procedure/ Extraktionsverfahren	pH 10, diethylether, reextraction with 1 N HCl, another extraction with CH_2Cl_2 from alk.	pH 10.5, toluene
Drug analyzed/ analysierte Substanz	Benzodiazepine-N-propyl-derivative	Benzodiazepine
Drug calculated / berechnete Substanz	Benzodiazepine	Benzodiazepine
Metabolites included / Metabolite inbegriffen	yes (nordiazepam)	yes (nordiazepam, temazepam and oxazepam)
qual./quant./Screening Method (e)	quant.	quant.
Sample required/ benötigtes Untersuchungsmaterial	2 ml blood	1 ml serum
Concentration Range/ Konzentrationsbereich	ca. 250 - 1500 ng / ml	ca. 200 - 1000 ng / ml
Special Equipment/ Spezialausstattung	Nitrogen sensitive detector - Detection	TLC - Scanner
Hydrolysis / Hydrolyse	no	no
Some Other Data: Einige andere Daten:	Within-run precision: C.V. = 3 - 8 % (250 - 1500 ng/ml) Day-to-day precision: C.V. = 5 - 7 % (125 ng- 750 ng/ml) Detection limit: ca. 10 ng / ml	Recovery: from serum 92.7 % (diazepam) 93.9 % (nordiazepam) 99.0 % (temazepam) 86.8 % (oxazepam) Reproducibility (n = 30) C.V. = 5.4 % (diazepam) C.V. = 4.7 % (nordiazepam) C.V. = 2.4 % (temazepam) C.V. = 8.5 % (oxazepam)
Pharmacokinetic Data obtained by this Method described on pp. Mit der Methode erhaltene pharmakokinetische Daten sind beschrieben auf S.		
Method is recommended for: Methode ist empfohlen für:	the quantitation of diazepam and nordiazepam in clinical and forensic cases. The derivatization step provides symmetrical peaks.	the determination of diazepam and its main metabolites in serum.

Benzodiazepine(s)/ Benzodiazepin(e)	Diazepam and Clonazepam	Diazepam
Method / Methode	TLC	TLC-Fluorometry
Authors / Verfasser	WAD and HANIFL	VAN DER MERWE and STEYN
Lit.Ref./ Lit.Zitat	(1188)	(1160)
Year of Publication/ Publikationsjahr	1977	1978
Extraction Procedure/ Extraktionsverfahren	pH 10.5, toluene	pH 8, n-hexane - isobutanol (90 : 10)
Drug analyzed/ analysierte Substanz	Benzodiazepine	Benzodiazepine-fluorescence-product
Drug calculated / berechnete Substanz	Benzodiazepine	Benzodiazepine
Metabolites included / Metabolite inbegriffen	yes (nordiazepam, temazepam and oxazepam)	Nordiazepam
qual./quant./Screening Method (e)	quant.	quant.
Sample required/ benötigtes Untersuchungsmaterial	1 ml serum	1 ml serum
Concentration Range/ Konzentrationsbereich	200 - 1000 ng / ml	50 - 500 ng / ml diazepam 50 - 300 ng / ml nordiazepam
Special Equipment/ Spezialausstattung	TLC - Scanner	TLC - Scanner with spectrofluorimeter
Hydrolysis / Hydrolyse	no	no
Some Other Data: Einige andere Daten:	Recovery (from serum) C.V. Diazepam 92.7 % 5.4 % Nordiazepam 93.9 % 4.7 % Temazepam 99.0 % 2.4 % Oxazepam 86.8 % 8.5 % Clonazepam 98.6 % 5.2 % 7-Amino-clonazepam 77.1 % 6.8 % 7-Acetamido-clonazepam 40.3 % 4.8 %	Recovery: over 100 % (fluorimetric method) mean ± S.D. 80 ng / ml added: diazepam 82.7 ± 3.4 nordiazepam 82.5 ± 5.8 150 ng / ml added: diazepam 157.2 ± 6.9 nordiazepam 151,6 ± 8.3 200 ng / ml added: diazepam 205.4 ± 8.2 nordiazepam 200.7 ± 9.0 Sensitivity limit: ca. 10 ng/ml
Pharmacokinetic Data obtained by this Method described on pp. Mit der Methode erhaltene pharmakokinetische Daten sind beschrieben auf S.		
Method is recommended for: Methode ist empfohlen für:	the drug-monitoring of diazepam, clonazepam and their metabolites in epileptic cases.	the determination of diazepam and nordiazepam in serum.

Benzodiazepine(s)/ Benzodiazepin(e)	Diazepam	Diazepam
Method / Methode	TLC - Fluorometry	Polarography (DPP-mode)
Authors / Verfasser	SUN	JACOBSEN, JACOBSEN and ROJAHN
Lit.Ref./ Lit.Zitat	(1947)	(521)
Year of Publication/ Publikationsjahr	1978	1973
Extraction Procedure/ Extraktionsverfahren	0.1 M K_2HPO_4, benzene	saturated KCl, benzene
Drug analyzed/ analysierte Substanz	Benzodiazepine-fluorescence-product	Benzodiazepine
Drug calculated / berechnete Substanz	Benzodiazepine	Benzodiazepine
Metabolites included / Metabolite inbegriffen	yes (nordiazepam and oxazepam)	yes (qual.)
qual./quant./Screening Method (e)	quant.	quant.
Sample required/ benötigtes Untersuchungsmaterial	2 ml serum	5 ml serum (2 ml)
Concentration Range/ Konzentrationsbereich	ca.25 - 600 ng / ml	50 - 1000 ng / ml
Special Equipment/ Spezialausstattung	Fluorimeter	Polarograph (Differential-Pulse-Mode)
Hydrolysis / Hydrolyse	no	no
Some Other Data: Einige andere Daten:	Recovery: (mean ± S.D.) 96.4 ± 0.7% (diazepam) 87.8 ± 4.3% (nordiazepam) 87.3 ± 3.9% (oxazepam) Reproducibility (n = 3) C.V. = 1.1 - 15.1 (diazepam) C.V. = 2.0 - 6.3 (nordiazepam) C.V. = 9.1 - 12.2 (oxazepam) (range: 50 - 600 ng/ml) Sensitivity limit: 18 ng/ml diazepam, 6 ng/ml nordiazepam and 5 ng/ml oxazepam.	Reproducibility: Error between -5.2 and + 7.0 % (concentrations lower than 100 ng/ml) and between - 0.4 and + 0.9 % (concentrations between 100 and 230 ng/ml). Detection limit: ca. 10 ng/ml serum
Pharmacokinetic Data obtained by this Method described on pp. Mit der Methode erhaltene pharmakokinetische Daten sind beschrieben auf S.	See part: Blood-, Serum- and Plasma-Levels and Other Pharmacokinetic Data from Literature	
Method is recommended for: Methode ist empfohlen für:	the TLC-fluorometric determination of diazepam, nordiazepam and oxazepam in single-dose availability studies.	the rapid determination of diazepam in the concentration range 50 - 1000 ng/ml of serum.

Benzodiazepine(s)/ Benzodiazepin(e)	Diazepam	Diazepam
Method / Methode	Radioimmunoassay	Radioimmunoassay
Authors / Verfasser	PESCAR and SPECTOR	GELBKE, SCHLICHT and SCHMIDT
Lit.Ref./ Lit.Zitat	(845)	(373)
Year of Publication/ Publikationsjahr	1973	1977
Extraction Procedure/ Extraktionsverfahren		XAD 2
Drug analyzed/ analysierte Substanz	Benzodiazepine	Benzodiazepine
Drug calculated / berechnete Substanz	Benzodiazepine	Benzodiazepine
Metabolites included / Metabolite inbegriffen	no	no
qual./quant./Screening Method (e)	quant.	quant.
Sample required/ benötigtes Untersuchungsmaterial	1 ml blood or less	0.5 ml blood (GLC and RIA)
Concentration Range/ Konzentrationsbereich	ca.10ng - 100 ng (linear range)	10 ng - 200 ng / ml
Special Equipment/ Spezialausstattung	RIA - equipment	RIA - equipment XAD-2 resin
Hydrolysis / Hydrolyse	no	no
Some Other Data: Einige andere Daten:	Sensitivity limit: ca. 1 ng Diazepam	Precision of the Standard Curve: C.V. = 5 - 12.5% (n = 20, range 10-160 ng / ml) Intra-Assay Precision: (serum) C.V. = 12% (mean 23.6 ng/ml) C.V. = 7.8%(mean 69 ng/ml) Intra-Assay Precision: (blood) C.V. = 6.6% (mean 61.3 ng/ml) C.V. =12.3% (mean124.5 ng/ml) Detection limit: ca. 5 ng/ml
Pharmacokinetic Data obtained by this Method described on pp. Mit der Methode erhaltene pharmakokinetische Daten sind beschrieben auf S.	See part: Blood-, Serum- and Plasma-Levels and Other Pharmacokinetic Data from Literature	
Method is recommended for: Methode ist empfohlen für:	the screening of diazepam if only small amounts of blood or plasma are available (one person can do up to 250 determinations a day).	the screening of more than 200 samples for diazepam by one technician within two working days.

Benzodiazepine(s)/ Benzodiazepin(e)	Diazepam	Diazepam
Method / Methode	Radioimmunoassay	Radioreceptor Assay
Authors / Verfasser	DIXON and CREWS	OWEN, LOFTHOUSE and BOURNE
Lit.Ref./ Lit.Zitat	(1396)	(2488)
Year of Publication/ Publikationsjahr	1978	1979
Extraction Procedure/ Extraktionsverfahren		
Drug analyzed/ analysierte Substanz	Benzodiazepine	Benzodiazepine
Drug calculated / berechnete Substanz	Benzodiazepine	Benzodiazepine
Metabolites included / Metabolite inbegriffen	no	yes (nordiazepam, temazepam, oxazepam)
qual./quant./Screening Method (e)	quant.	quant.
Sample required/ benötigtes Untersuchungsmaterial	0.01 ml blood or plasma 0.1 ml saliva	0.15 ml serum
Concentration Range/ Konzentrationsbereich	ca. 40 - 2000 ng/ml	ca. 100 - 6000 ng / ml
Special Equipment/ Spezialausstattung	RIA - equipment	Radioreceptor- equipment
Hydrolysis / Hydrolyse	no	no
Some Other Data: Einige andere Daten:	Intra-Assay Precision: C.V. = less than 7 % (n=5) recovery 103 - 109 % Inter-Assay Precision: C.V. = less than 10% (n=6) recovery 103 - 110 % Sensitivity limit: 3.0 ng/ml using 0.01 ml samples	Sensitivity limit: 10 ng/ml
Pharmacokinetic Data obtained by this Method described on pp. Mit der Methode erhaltene pharmakokinetische Daten sind beschrieben auf S.	See part: Blood-, Serum- and Plasma-Levels and Other Pharmacokinetic Data from Literature	
Method is recommended for: Methode ist empfohlen für:	the determination of diazepam in microsamples of blood or plasma (0.01 ml) and saliva (0.1 ml).	the estimation of serum concentrations of diazepam and its metabolites (simple, rapid and suitable for batch analysis).

Benzodiazepine(s)/ Benzodiazepin(e)	Diazepam	Diazepam
Method / Methode	Radioimmunoassay	Radioreceptor Assay
Authors / Verfasser	RUTTERFORD and SMITH	SKOLNICK, GOODWIN and PAUL
Lit.Ref./ Lit.Zitat	(3470)	(1911)
Year of Publication/ Publikationsjahr	1980	1979
Extraction Procedure/ Extraktionsverfahren	pH 9, ethylacetate	pH 7.4
Drug analyzed/ analysierte Substanz	Benzodiazepine	Benzodiazepine
Drug calculated / berechnete Substanz	Benzodiazepine	Benzodiazepine
Metabolites included / Metabolite inbegriffen	no	yes (nordiazepam)
qual./quant./Screening Method (e)	qual./quant./Screening	qual./quant./Screening
Sample required/ benötigtes Untersuchungsmaterial	0,05 ml blood	0,2 ml plasma
Concentration Range/ Konzentrationsbereich	ca. 1 - 50 ng/ml	ca. 50 - 2,000 ng/ml
Special Equipment/ Spezialausstattung	RIA - equipment	Radioreceptor-Assay-Equipment
Hydrolysis / Hydrolyse	no	no
Some Other Data: Einige andere Daten:	Inter-assay C.V.: 11.5 % (50 ng/ml) 120 % (1 ng/ml) Sensitivity: about 0.3 ng/ml	Recovery: 98.5 % ± 3% (range 50-800 ng/ml) Inter-assay C.V.: less than 5 % Intra-assay C.V.: less than 5 %
Pharmacokinetic Data obtained by this Method described on pp. Mit der Methode erhaltene pharmakokinetische Daten sind beschrieben auf S.		
Method is recommended for: Methode ist empfohlen für:	samples in forensic toxicology that may be haemolyzed, decomposed and of small volume	monitoring blood levels for both therapeutic and toxicologic purposes

Benzodiazepine(s)/ Benzodiazepin(e)	Diazepam	Diazepam
Method / Methode	EMIT^R -TLC	HPLC (Mikro-Bondapack C-18, reversed phase mode)
Authors / Verfasser	BUDD and WALKIN	RAISYS, FRIEL, GRAAFF, OPHEIM and WILENSKY
Lit.Ref./ Lit.Zitat	(2691)	(3407)
Year of Publication/ Publikationsjahr	1980	1980
Extraction Procedure/ Extraktionsverfahren	alkaline, hexane	pH 9, toluene
Drug analyzed/ analysierte Substanz	Benzodiazepine Benzophenone (TLC)	Benzodiazepine
Drug calculated / berechnete Substanz	Benzodiazepine	Benzodiazepine
Metabolites included / Metabolite inbegriffen	yes	yes (nordiazepam)
qual./quant./Screening Method (e)	qual./quant./Screening	qual./quant.
Sample required/ benötigtes Untersuchungsmaterial	urine	1 ml plasma
Concentration Range/ Konzentrationsbereich	ca. 500 - 1,000 ng/ml	ca. 20 - 1,400 ng/ml
Special Equipment/ Spezialausstattung	EMIT^R automatic analysis system	Dual wavelength detection (230nm and 254nm)
Hydrolysis / Hydrolyse	yes	no
Some Other Data: Einige andere Daten:		Within-run C.V. (n=10, 2500ng/ml) 1.6 % (diazepam) 1.6 % (nordiazepam) (n=6, 700ng/ml) 1.5 % (diazepam) 7.1 % (nordiazepam) Between-run C.V. (n= 21, 2,500 ng/ml) 3.6% (diazepam) 2.6% (nordiazepam) (n=15, 700 ng/ml) 4.3% (diazepam) 4.3% (nordiazepam)
Pharmacokinetic Data obtained by this Method described on pp. Mit der Methode erhaltene pharmakokinetische Daten sind beschrieben auf S.		
Method is recommended for: Methode ist empfohlen für:	the mass-screening of urine samples for diazepam and metabolites	the determination of subtherapeutic, therapeutic and toxic plasma levels

Benzodiazepine(s)/ Benzodiazepin(e)	Diazepam	Diazepam
Method / Methode	HPLC Partisil 10 10 µm	HPLC Micro-Bondapack C 18 reversed-phase mode
Authors / Verfasser	BUGGE	BRODIE, CHASSEAUD and TAYLOR
Lit.Ref./ Lit.Zitat	(1318)	(1306)
Year of Publication/ Publikationsjahr	1976	1978
Extraction Procedure/ Extraktionsverfahren	saturated KCl, benzene	pH 9.0, diethylether
Drug analyzed/ analysierte Substanz	Benzodiazepine	Benzodiazepine
Drug calculated / berechnete Substanz	Benzodiazepine	Benzodiazepine
Metabolites included / Metabolite inbegriffen	yes (nordiazepam)	yes (nordiazepam)
qual./quant./Screening Method (e)	quant.	quant.
Sample required/ benötigtes Untersuchungsmaterial	1 ml blood	2 ml plasma
Concentration Range/ Konzentrationsbereich	ca. 25 - 1500 ng/ml	ca. 10 - 400 ng/ml
Special Equipment/ Spezialausstattung	HPLC-equipment	HPLC-equipment reverse-phase mode
Hydrolysis / Hydrolyse	no	no
Some Other Data: Einige andere Daten:	Recovery: 92 ± 7% (mean ± S.D.) in the range 100 ng/ml - 500 ng/ml for diazepam and nordiazepam Sensitivity limit: Ca. 25 ng/ml (using 2 ml blood)	Recovery: overall 96 ± 3% (diazepam) 94 ± 4% (nordiazepam) range: 10 - 400 ng/ml C.V. less than ± 1% Detection limit: ca. 10 ng/ml (diazepam) ca. 2 ng/ml (nordiazepam)
Pharmacokinetic Data obtained by this Method described on pp. Mit der Methode erhaltene pharmakokinetische Daten sind beschrieben auf S.		See part: Blood-, Serum- and Plasma-Levels and Other Pharmacokinetic Data from Literature
Method is recommended for: Methode ist empfohlen für:	the determination of diazepam and nordiazepam in blood.	the determination of diazepam and nordiazepam in plasma at concentrations which would be encountered during therapy.

Benzodiazepine(s)/ Benzodiazepin(e)	Diazepam	Diazepam
Method / Methode	HPLC Partisil 10 ODS reversed-phase mode	HPLC Mikro-Bondapack C_{18} reversed-phase mode
Authors / Verfasser	KABRA, STEVENS and MARTON	EMERY and KOWTKO
Lit.Ref./ Lit.Zitat	(1614)	(2479)
Year of Publication/ Publikationsjahr	1978	1979
Extraction Procedure/ Extraktionsverfahren	pH 7.0, diethylether	no extraction
Drug analyzed/ analysierte Substanz	Benzodiazepine	Benzodiazepine
Drug calculated / berechnete Substanz	Benzodiazepine	Benzodiazepine
Metabolites included / Metabolite inbegriffen	yes (nordiazepam and oxazepam)	no
qual./quant./Screening Method (e)	quant.	quant.
Sample required/ benötigtes Untersuchungsmaterial	2 ml blood	tablets
Concentration Range/ Konzentrationsbereich	50 - 10 000 ng/ml	usual doses (e.g. 2 - 10 mg)
Special Equipment/ Spezialausstattung	HPLC - equipment reversed-phase mode	HPLC - equipment reversed-phase mode
Hydrolysis / Hydrolyse	no	no
Some Other Data: Einige andere Daten:	Recovery: mean values (n = 5) 98 - 116 % (diazepam) 94 - 114 % (nordiazepam) 91 - 110 % (oxazepam) (range: 50 - 2000 ng/ml) Day-to-day precision: (n = 10) C.V. = 6.0 - 9.5 % (diazepam) C.V. = 6.7 - 9.6 % (nordiazepam) C.V. = 2.8 - 6.5 % (oxazepam) Within-run precision: (n = 10) C.V. = 3.7 - 5.3 % (diazepam) C.V. = 5.1 - 6.0 % (nordiazepam) C.V. = 5.6 - 6.3 % (oxazepam) (range: 200 - 1000 ng/ml) Sensitivity limits: 30-40 ng/ml	0.1 % of decomposition products are detectable. Second-Day reproducibility data: C.V. = 1.3 % (2-mg tablets) C.V. = 0.7 - 0.9 % (5-mg tablets) C.V. = 0.3 - 1.0 % (10mg tablets)
Pharmacokinetic Data obtained by this Method described on pp. Mit der Methode erhaltene pharmakokinetische Daten sind beschrieben auf S.		
Method is recommended for: Methode ist empfohlen für:	monitoring diazepam, nordiazepam and oxazepam at the lower concentrations normally found in blood.	the stability-indicating assays of diazepam tablets.

Benzodiazepine(s)/ Benzodiazepin(e)	Diazepam	Diazepam
Method / Methode	HPLC Micro-Bondapak CN reversed-phase mode	HPLC LiChrosorb RP 8 5 µm
Authors / Verfasser	MacKICHAN, JUSKO, DUFFNER and COHEN	VREE, BAARS, HEKSTER and VAN DER KLEIJN
Lit.Ref./ Lit.Zitat	(2484)	(2492)
Year of Publication/ Publikationsjahr	1979	1979
Extraction Procedure/ Extraktionsverfahren	alkaline, chloroform	diethylether
Drug analyzed/ analysierte Substanz	Benzodiazepine	Benzodiazepine
Drug calculated / berechnete Substanz	Benzodiazepine	Benzodiazepine
Metabolites included / Metabolite inbegriffen	yes (nordiazepam and oxazepam)	yes (nordiazepam, temazepam and oxazepam)
qual./quant./Screening Method (e)	quant.	quant.
Sample required/ benötigtes Untersuchungsmaterial	0.25 ml plasma	0.2 ml plasma or urine
Concentration Range/ Konzentrationsbereich	ca. 30 - 2000 ng / ml	ca. 30 - 10 000 ng / ml
Special Equipment/ Spezialausstattung	HPLC-equipment reversed-phase mode	HPLC-equipment
Hydrolysis / Hydrolyse	no	enzymatic cleavage of the conjugates
Some Other Data: Einige andere Daten:	Recovery: (100 - 500 ng / ml) 94.6 - 98.9 % (oxazepam) 95.9 -106.0 % (nordiazepam) 89.4 - 97.4 % (oxazepam) 93.6 -103 % (chlordiazepoxide) Within-day precision: n = 10 C.V. = 1.7 - 8.0 % (oxazepam) C.V. = 3.2 - 5.3 % (nordiazepam) C.V. = 2.6 - 5.4 % (diazepam) Day-to-day precision: n = 10-17 C.V. = 4.0 - 8.7 % (nordiazepam) C.V. = 5.6 -10.3 % (diazepam) range: ca. 45 - 1100 ng/ml	Recovery: (mean ± S.D.) 96 ± 7% (diazepam 91 ± 7% (nordiazepam) 94 ± 7% (temazepam) 89 ± 6% (oxazepam) Sensitivity limit: 30 ng/ml
Pharmacokinetic Data obtained by this Method described on pp. Mit der Methode erhaltene pharmakokinetische Daten sind beschrieben auf S.		
Method is recommended for: Methode ist empfohlen für:	monitoring plasma levels of diazepam, nordiazepam and oxazepam in cases of epilepsy (micromethod in pediatry).	the study of pharmacokinetics of diazepam and its metabolites nordiazepam, temazepam and oxazepam in man.

Benzodiazepine(s)/ Benzodiazepin(e)	Diazepam	
Method / Methode	HPLC Micro Pak MCH-10 reversed-phase mode	
Authors / Verfasser	WALLACE, SCHWERTNER and SHIMEK jr.	
Lit.Ref./ Lit.Zitat	(2493)	
Year of Publication/ Publikationsjahr	1979	
Extraction Procedure/ Extraktionsverfahren	hexane - ethylacetate (70 : 30)	
Drug analyzed/ analysierte Substanz	Benzodiazepine	
Drug calculated / berechnete Substanz	Benzodiazepine	
Metabolites included / Metabolite inbegriffen	yes (nordiazepam)	
qual./quant./Screening Method (e)	quant.	
Sample required/ benötigtes Untersuchungsmaterial	1 ml plasma	
Concentration Range/ Konzentrationsbereich	ca. 50 - 1400 ng / ml	
Special Equipment/ Spezialausstattung	HPLC-equipment reversed-phase mode	
Hydrolysis / Hydrolyse	no	
Some Other Data: Einige andere Daten:	Recovery: mean ± S.D. 102.6 ± 2.6% (diazepam) 100.3 ± 3.8% (nordiazepam) Within-day precision: C.V. = 1.7 % (diazepam) C.V. = 2.4 % (nordiazepam) Day-to-day precision: C.V. = 2.5 % (diazepam) C.V. = 3.3 % (nordiazepam) Detection limit: ca. 50 ng/ml	
Pharmacokinetic Data obtained by this Method described on pp. Mit der Methode erhaltene pharmakokinetische Daten sind beschrieben auf S.		
Method is recommended for: Methode ist empfohlen für:	the determination of diazepam and nordiazepam in serum in therapeutic concentrations.	

Benzodiazepine(s)/ Benzodiazepin(e)	Oxazepam	Oxazepam
Method / Methode	GLC-ECD 2% XE-60 Chromosorb W (HP) 80-100 mesh	GLC-ECD 6% OV-17
Authors / Verfasser	KNOWLES and RUELIUS	VESSMAN, FREIJ and STRÖMBERG
Lit.Ref./ Lit.Zitat	(595)	(1165)
Year of Publication/ Publikationsjahr	1972	1972
Extraction Procedure/ Extraktionsverfahren	pH 7, diethylether, acid hydrolysis	pH 7.4, methylene chloride
Drug analyzed/ analysierte Substanz	Benzophenone	Benzophenone
Drug calculated / berechnete Substanz	Benzodiazepine	Benzodiazepine
Metabolites included / Metabolite inbegriffen	yes (glucuronide)	yes (glucuronide)
qual./quant./Screening Method (e)	quant.	quant.
Sample required/ benötigtes Untersuchungsmaterial	1 ml plasma, serum or urine	1 - 2 ml serum and urine
Concentration Range/ Konzentrationsbereich	ca. 200 - 2000 ng / ml	ca. 1 - 500 ng / ml
Special Equipment/ Spezialausstattung	ECD-detection	ECD-detection
Hydrolysis / Hydrolyse	yes (acid and enzymatic)	yes (acid)
Some Other Data: Einige andere Daten:	Recovery: 75 - 89 % Sensitivity limit: ca. 20 ng/ml	Recovery: mean ± S.D. 100 ± 2.6 % (conc. 30 ng/ ml) 100 ± 7.0 % (conc. 1 ng/ ml) Detection limit: ca. 0.8 ng/ml
Pharmacokinetic Data obtained by this Method described on pp. Mit der Methode erhaltene pharmakokinetische Daten sind beschrieben auf S.	See part: Blood-, Serum- and Plasma-Levels and Other Pharmacokinetic Data from Literature	See part: Blood-, Serum- and Plasma-Levels and Other Pharmacokinetic Data from Literature
Method is recommended for: Methode ist empfohlen für:	the determination of free and conjugated oxazepam in blood, serum, plasma and urine after single and multiple oral administration of oxazepam (via hydrolysis product).	the determination of oxazepam and its glucuronide in biological samples after therapeutic single and multiple dosage of oxazepam (via its hydrolysis product).

Benzodiazepine(s)/ Benzodiazepin(e)	Oxazepam	Oxazepam
Method / Methode	GLC-ECD 3% OV-225 Chromosorb G AW 100-120 mesh	GLC-ECD 3% OV-17 Chromosorb W (HP) 80-100 mesh
Authors / Verfasser	VESSMAN, JOHANNSSON, MAGNUSSON and STRÖMBERG	GILES, FAN, NARANJO and SELLERS
Lit.Ref./ Lit.Zitat	(1166)	(1481)
Year of Publication/ Publikationsjahr	1977	1978
Extraction Procedure/ Extraktionsverfahren	pH 7.4, methylene chloride, extractive alkylation	benzene - diethylether (5 : 1)
Drug analyzed/ analysierte Substanz	Methylderivative	Thermal degradation product
Drug calculated / berechnete Substanz	Oxazepam	Oxazepam
Metabolites included / Metabolite inbegriffen	no	no
qual./quant./Screening Method (e)	quant.	quant.
Sample required/ benötigtes Untersuchungsmaterial	ca. 2 ml serum	1 ml plasma
Concentration Range/ Konzentrationsbereich	ca. 5 - 200 ng / ml	10 - 600 ng / ml
Special Equipment/ Spezialausstattung	ECD-detection	ECD-detection
Hydrolysis / Hydrolyse	no (but derivatization)	no
Some Other Data: Einige andere Daten:	<u>Recovery:</u> mean ± S.D. 98.4 ± 3.2 % (at 25 ng/ml level) <u>Sensitivity limit:</u> 1 ng/ml	<u>Recovery:</u> mean ± S.D. 94.7 ± 3.3 % (at 600 ng/ml level) C.V. = 4 % <u>Sensitivity limit:</u> 10 ng/ml
Pharmacokinetic Data obtained by this Method described on pp. Mit der Methode erhaltene pharmakokinetische Daten sind beschrieben auf S.		See part: Blood-, Serum- and Plasma-Levels and Other Pharmacokinetic Data from Literature
Method is recommended for: Methode ist empfohlen für:	the rapid determination of oxazepam without hydrolysis procedure after the administration of oxazepam, diazepam and clorazepate. For monitoring blood levels of oxazepam hydrolysis methods are recommended.	the determination of oxazepam in plasma via its thermal degradation product after typical oral doses.

Benzodiazepine(s)/ Benzodiazepin(e)	Oxazepam / Lorazepam	Oxazepam / Lorazepam
Method / Methode	GLC-FID MS 3% OV-17 Gas Chrom Q 100-120 mesh	GLC MS 3% OV-1 Chromosorb W -AW (DMCS) 80-100 mesh
Authors / Verfasser	MARCUCCI, BIANCHI, AIROLDI, SALMONA, FANELLI, CHIABRANDO, FRIGERIO, MUSSINI and GARATTINI	HIGUCHI, URABE and SHIOBARA
Lit.Ref./ Lit.Zitat	(680)	(2480)
Year of Publication/ Publikationsjahr	1975	1979
Extraction Procedure/ Extraktionsverfahren	special procedure (see 680)	acid and alkaline medium, n-hexane
Drug analyzed/ analysierte Substanz	as derivatives (methylesters and trimethylsilyl derivative)	as N_1,O_3 bistrimethylsilylderivat.
Drug calculated / berechnete Substanz	Benzodiazepine	Benzodiazepine
Metabolites included / Metabolite inbegriffen	not for N-methyl-glucuronides	yes (glucuronide)
qual./quant./Screening Method (e)	quant.	quant.
Sample required/ benötigtes Untersuchungsmaterial	1 - 5 ml urine	1 ml plasma or urine
Concentration Range/ Konzentrationsbereich	ca. 50 - 1000 ng/ml	ca. 5 - 50 ng/ml (lorazepam) ca. 20 - 600 ng/ml (oxazepam)
Special Equipment/ Spezialausstattung	GLC-MS	GLC-MS
Hydrolysis / Hydrolyse	no, but derivatization	yes (enzymatic)
Some Other Data: Einige andere Daten:	Recovery: ca. 80 % Sensitivity limit: ca. 30 ng/ml	Recovery: mean ± S.D. 87.8 ± 0.6 % (conc. 30 ng/ml) 76.8 ± 1.8 % (conc.300 ng/ml) (lorazepam and oxazepam) Sensitivity limit: 2 ng / ml
Pharmacokinetic Data obtained by this Method described on pp. Mit der Methode erhaltene pharmakokinetische Daten sind beschrieben auf S.	See part: Blood-, Serum- and Plasma-Levels and Other Pharmacokinetic Data from Literature	See part: Blood-, Serum- and Plasma-Levels and Other Pharmacokinetic Data from Literature
Method is recommended for: Methode ist empfohlen für:	the determination of intact oxazepam- and lorazepam-glucuronides in urine.	the determination of plasma and urine concentrations of lorazepam and oxazepam after therapeutic doses.

Benzodiazepine(s)/ Benzodiazepin(e)	Nitrazepam	Nitrazepam
Method / Methode	GLC-ECD 3% OV-17 Gas Chrom Q 60-80 mesh	GLC-ECD 5% OV-17 Gas Chrom Q 80-100 mesh
Authors / Verfasser	BEHARRELL, HAILEY and McLAURIN	EHRSSON and TILLY
Lit.Ref./ Lit.Zitat	(61)	(291)
Year of Publication/ Publikationsjahr	1972	1973
Extraction Procedure/ Extraktionsverfahren	pH 9.0, diethylether, hydrolysis, diethylether	pH 6.5, benzene, methylation
Drug analyzed/ analysierte Substanz	Benzophenone	Methyl-derivative
Drug calculated / berechnete Substanz	Benzodiazepine	Benzodiazepine
Metabolites included / Metabolite inbegriffen	no	no
qual./quant./Screening Method (e)	quant.	quant.
Sample required/ benötigtes Untersuchungsmaterial	1 ml plasma	0.5 ml plasma
Concentration Range/ Konzentrationsbereich	ca. 25 - 200 ng/ml	ca. 5 - 100 ng/ml
Special Equipment/ Spezialausstattung	ECD-detection	ECD-detection
Hydrolysis / Hydrolyse	yes	no, but derivatization
Some Other Data: Einige andere Daten:	Recovery: more than 95 % Sensitivity limit: 0.1 ng / ml plasma	Recovery: mean ± S.D. 103 ± 3% (n = 10) rel. standard deviation: 3 % (n = 10, level 50 ng/ml) Sensitivity limit: ca. 1 ng / ml
Pharmacokinetic Data obtained by this Method described on pp. Mit der Methode erhaltene pharmakokinetische Daten sind beschrieben auf S.	See part: Blood-, Serum- and Plasma-Levels and Other Pharmacokinetic Data from Literature	
Method is recommended for: Methode ist empfohlen für:	the determination of nitrazepam in plasma in clinical situation with a high recovery via benzophenone derivative after hydrolysis.	the determination of nitrazepam in plasma as methyl-derivative which provides a good peak-symmetry.

Benzodiazepine(s)/ Benzodiazepin(e)	Nitrazepam	Nitrazepam
Method / Methode	GLC-ECD 3% OV-17 Diatomite CQ 80-100 mesh	GLC-ECD 3% OV-17 or 3% SP-2250 Chromosorb W Supelcoport 100-120 mesh 100-120 mesh
Authors / Verfasser	MØLLER JENSEN	KANGAS
Lit.Ref./ Lit.Zitat	(738)	(542)
Year of Publication/ Publikationsjahr	1975	1977
Extraction Procedure/ Extraktionsverfahren	benzene, hydrolysis, benzene	hydrolysis, toluene - n-heptane - ethylacetate (80 : 20 : 5)
Drug analyzed/ analysierte Substanz	Benzophenone	Benzophenone
Drug calculated / berechnete Substanz	Benzodiazepine	Benzodiazepine
Metabolites included / Metabolite inbegriffen	no	no
qual./quant./Screening Method (e)	quant.	quant.
Sample required/ benötigtes Untersuchungsmaterial	1 ml serum	0.5 ml plasma
Concentration Range/ Konzentrationsbereich	10 - 50 ng/ml	10 - 200 ng/ml
Special Equipment/ Spezialausstattung	ECD-detection	ECD-detection
Hydrolysis / Hydrolyse	yes (acid)	yes (acid)
Some Other Data: Einige andere Daten:	Recovery: mean ± S.D. 105 ± 15 % (conc. range 10-40 ng/ml) C.V. = 13 % (day-to day) Detection limit: 5 ng / ml	Recovery: more than 96 % (range 5 - 150 ng/ml) Sensitivity: 0.2 - 0.5 ng / ml
Pharmacokinetic Data obtained by this Method described on pp. Mit der Methode erhaltene pharmakokinetische Daten sind beschrieben auf S.	See part: Blood-, Serum- and Plasma-Levels and Other Pharmacokinetic Data from Literature	
Method is recommended for: Methode ist empfohlen für:	measuring serum concentrations of nitrazepam in bioavailability studies on subjects given a single dose of nitrazepam.	the analysis of samples with many impurities (e.g. tissue samples) or extremely low concentrations of nitrazepam.

Benzodiazepine(s)/ Benzodiazepin(e)	Nitrazepam	Nitrazepam, Clonazepam
Method / Methode	GLC-ECD 3% OV-17 Chromosorb W 100-120 mesh; 3% SP-2250 Supelcoport 100-120 mesh	GLC-ECD capill. 3% OV-17 CARBOWAX 20 M
Authors / Verfasser	KANGAS	DE BOER, RÖST-KAISER, BRACHT and BREIMER
Lit.Ref./ Lit.Zitat	(542)	(224)
Year of Publication/ Publikationsjahr	1977	1978
Extraction Procedure/ Extraktionsverfahren	benzene - dichlormethane (90 : 10)	pH 9.0, light petroleum (b.p. 40-60°C - dichlormethane (1 : 1)
Drug analyzed/ analysierte Substanz	Benzodiazepine	Benzodiazepine
Drug calculated / berechnete Substanz	Benzodiazepine	Benzodiazepine
Metabolites included / Metabolite inbegriffen	no	no
qual./quant./Screening Method (e)	quant.	quant.
Sample required/ benötigtes Untersuchungsmaterial	0.5 ml plasma	1.0 ml plasma
Concentration Range/ Konzentrationsbereich	10 - 200 ng/ml	10 - 100 ng/ml
Special Equipment/ Spezialausstattung	ECD-detection	ECD-detection capillary mode
Hydrolysis / Hydrolyse	no	no
Some Other Data: Einige andere Daten:	Recovery: more than 96% (range 5 - 150 ng/ml) Sensitivity: 1 ng/ml	Recovery: ca. 92% for nitrazepam ca. 75% for clonazepam Sensitivity limit: 1 ng/ml
Pharmacokinetic Data obtained by this Method described on pp. Mit der Methode erhaltene pharmakokinetische Daten sind beschrieben auf S.		See part: Blood-, Serum- and Plasma-Levels and Other Pharmacokinetic Data from Literature
Method is recommended for: Methode ist empfohlen für:	the clinical monitoring of nitrazepam in plasma and when rapid analysis is required (e.g. toxicological analysis).	the determination of nitrazepam and/or clonazepam in plasma following single therapeutic doses of nitrazepam and/or clonazepam.

Benzodiazepine(s)/ Benzodiazepin(e)	Nitrazepam	Nitrazepam, Clonazepam, Flunitrazepam
Method / Methode	GLC-FID 1.5% SE-30 Chromosorb W 60 - 80 mesh	TLC
Authors / Verfasser	MASUDA	HAEFELFINGER
Lit.Ref./ Lit.Zitat	(703)	(2199)
Year of Publication/ Publikationsjahr	1971	1979
Extraction Procedure/ Extraktionsverfahren	pH 9 - 10, diethylether, hydrolysis, diethylether	pH 9, diethylether, pH 9, dichlormethane - toluene (100:1)
Drug analyzed/ analysierte Substanz	Benzophenone	7-Aminometabolites
Drug calculated / berechnete Substanz	Benzodiazepine	7-Aminometabolites
Metabolites included / Metabolite inbegriffen	no	yes (7-Aminometabolites)
qual./quant./Screening Method (e)	quant.	quant.
Sample required/ benötigtes Untersuchungsmaterial	5 - 10 ml blood or urine	1 ml plasma
Concentration Range/ Konzentrationsbereich	200 - 1000 µg / ml	0.5 - 10 ng/ml
Special Equipment/ Spezialausstattung	FID-detection	densitometer
Hydrolysis / Hydrolyse	yes	no
Some Other Data: Einige andere Daten:	Recovery: mean ± S.D. 94.6 ± 0.90 % (from blood) 95.5 ± 0.77 % (from urine) Sensitivity limit: 5 - 10 µg / ml	Recovery: 85% or more S.D. rel.: less than ± 15 % Detection limit: 0.5 - 1 ng/ml
Pharmacokinetic Data obtained by this Method described on pp. Mit der Methode erhaltene pharmakokinetische Daten sind beschrieben auf S.		See part: Blood-, Serum- and Plasma-Levels and Other Pharmacokinetic Data from Literature
Method is recommended for: Methode ist empfohlen für:	the determination of toxic levels of nitrazepam in poisoning and forensic cases.	the determination of the 7-amino-metabolites of 7-nitrobenzodiazepines after single and multiple doses.

Benzodiazepine(s)/ Benzodiazepin(e)	Nitrazepam	Nitrazepam
Method / Methode	UV-photometry, colorimetry	Colorimetry
Authors / Verfasser	OLIVER and SMITH	SAWADA and SHINOHARA
Lit.Ref./ Lit.Zitat	(820)	(953)
Year of Publication/ Publikationsjahr	1974	1970
Extraction Procedure/ Extraktionsverfahren	alkaline, chloroform pH 10, methylenechloride - ethylacetate (2 : 1)	pH 9-11, ethylacetate, hydrolysis
Drug analyzed/ analysierte Substanz	Benzodiazepine or reduction-product	Benzophenone
Drug calculated / berechnete Substanz	Benzodiazepine	Benzodiazepine
Metabolites included / Metabolite inbegriffen	no	no
qual./quant./Screening Method (e)	quant.	quant.
Sample required/ benötigtes Untersuchungsmaterial	5 - 25 ml blood, serum or urine	ca. 10 ml urine
Concentration Range/ Konzentrationsbereich	6 - 100 µg / ml	2 - 20 µg / ml
Special Equipment/ Spezialausstattung	Photometer	Photometer
Hydrolysis / Hydrolyse	yes (acid)	yes (acid)
Some Other Data: Einige andere Daten:	Recovery: ca. 75 % Sensitivity limit: ca. 100 ng / ml	Recovery: mean ± S.D. 91 ± 4% Sensitivity limit: ca. 500 ng / ml
Pharmacokinetic Data obtained by this Method described on pp. Mit der Methode erhaltene pharmakokinetische Daten sind beschrieben auf S.	See part: Blood-, Serum- and Plasma-Levels and Other Pharmacokinetic Data from Literature	
Method is recommended for: Methode ist empfohlen für:	the determination of nitrazepam in blood, serum or urine in poisoning cases.	the determination of toxic levels of nitrazepam in urine in forensic chemistry.

Benzodiazepine(s)/ Benzodiazepin(e)	Nitrazepam	Nitrazepam
Method / Methode	Fluorometry	Polarography
Authors / Verfasser	RIEDER	HALVORSEN and JACOBSEN
Lit.Ref./ Lit.Zitat	(909)	(458)
Year of Publication/ Publikationsjahr	1973	1972
Extraction Procedure/ Extraktionsverfahren	see (909) for the detailed extraction procedure	pH 6.9 as medium
Drug analyzed/ analysierte Substanz	fluorescence product with o-phthalaldehyde	Benzodiazepine
Drug calculated / berechnete Substanz	Benzodiazepine	Benzodiazepine
Metabolites included / Metabolite inbegriffen	yes (sum of main metabolites)	no
qual./quant./Screening Method (e)	quant.	quant.
Sample required/ benötigtes Untersuchungsmaterial	2 ml plasma 5 ml urine	5 ml serum
Concentration Range/ Konzentrationsbereich	200 - 2000 ng/ml	500 - 80000 ng/ml
Special Equipment/ Spezialausstattung	Fluorometer	Polarograph
Hydrolysis / Hydrolyse	yes (acid)	no
Some Other Data: Einige andere Daten:	Recovery: between 72 and 92 % Sensitivity limits: in human plasma: 6 ng/ml (unchanged nitrazepam) 15ng/ml (metabolites) in human urine: 9 ng/ml (unchanged nitrazepam) 25ng/ml (metabolites)	Detection limit: lower than 1000 ng/ml serum
Pharmacokinetic Data obtained by this Method described on pp. Mit der Methode erhaltene pharmakokinetische Daten sind beschrieben auf S.	See part: Blood-, Serum- and Plasma-Levels and Other Pharmacokinetic Data from Literature	
Method is recommended for: Methode ist empfohlen für:	pharmacokinetic studies (including the main metabolites) with the therapeutic doses of nitrazepam used in man.	the rapid screening of toxic levels of nitrazepam in serum (cases of poisoning).

Benzodiazepine(s)/ Benzodiazepin(e)	Nitrazepam	Nitrazepam
Method / Methode	HPLC (Zipax SAX (30 µm)	HPLC (LiChrosorb RP8 (10 µm)
Authors / Verfasser	MOORE, NICKLESS, HALLETT and HOWARD	HANEKAMP, VOOGT, BOS and FREI
Lit.Ref./ Lit.Zitat	(740)	(3004)
Year of Publication/ Publikationsjahr	1977	1980
Extraction Procedure/ Extraktionsverfahren	pH 7, ethylacetate	direct method after precipitation of proteins
Drug analyzed/ analysierte Substanz	Benzodiazepine	Benzodiazepine
Drug calculated / berechnete Substanz	Benzodiazepine	Benzodiazepine
Metabolites included / Metabolite inbegriffen	yes (7-amino- and 7-acetamidometabolites)	no
qual./quant./Screening Method (e)	quant.	qual./quant.
Sample required/ benötigtes Untersuchungsmaterial	10 ml urine	1 ml serum
Concentration Range/ Konzentrationsbereich	20 - 700 ng/ml 400-1400 ng/ml	7-70 ng/injection 70-700 ng/injection
Special Equipment/ Spezialausstattung	UV-detection (260 nm)	Pulse DME-detection
Hydrolysis / Hydrolyse	no	no
Some Other Data: Einige andere Daten:	Recovery: mean ± S.D. 80 ± 4% (range 10 µg/ml) Detection limit: 400 - 2000 ng/ml urine	Recovery: 67 % rel.Stand.Dev.: 1.8 % (n = 15)
Pharmacokinetic Data obtained by this Method described on pp. Mit der Methode erhaltene pharmakokinetische Daten sind beschrieben auf S.		
Method is recommended for: Methode ist empfohlen für:	the determination of nitrazepam and its main metabolites in urine without the necessity for an hydrolysis stage	the sensitive polarographic detection and determination of nitrazepam after HPLC-separation

Benzodiazepine(s)/ Benzodiazepin(e)	Medazepam	Medazepam
Method / Methode	GLC-ECD 3% OV-17 Gas Chrom Q (60/80mesh)	GLC-NFID 3% OV-25 Chromosorb W/AW DMCS (80-100 mesh)
Authors / Verfasser	DE SILVA and PUGLISI	MALLACH, MOOSMAYER and RUPP
Lit.Ref./ Lit.Zitat	(240)	(672)
Year of Publication/ Publikationsjahr	1970	1973
Extraction Procedure/ Extraktionsverfahren	pH 9.0, diethylether (see (240) for details)	pH 9, diethylether, reextraction with 2 N and 6 N HCl resp.
Drug analyzed/ analysierte Substanz	Benzodiazepine	Benzodiazepine
Drug calculated / berechnete Substanz	Benzodiazepine	Benzodiazepine
Metabolites included / Metabolite inbegriffen	yes (diazepam, nordiazepam, temazepam and oxazepam)	yes (normedazepam, diazepam, nordiazepam, temazepam, oxazepam)
qual./quant./Screening Method (e)	quant.	quant.
Sample required/ benötigtes Untersuchungsmaterial	1 ml blood 5 ml urine	4 ml serum / urine
Concentration Range/ Konzentrationsbereich	ca. 10 - 1000 ng / ml (medazepam)	ca. 10 - 1000 ng / ml (medazepam)
Special Equipment/ Spezialausstattung	ECD-detection	N-FID-detection
Hydrolysis / Hydrolyse	no	no
Some Other Data: Einige andere Daten:	Recovery: overall medazepam 94.5% ± 5.2 (blood) 80.0% ± 4.5 (urine) diazepam 86.0% ± 5.8 (blood) nordiazepam: 94.0% ± 6.0 (blood) oxazepam, nordiazepam and temazepam from urine: 80 - 85 % Sensitivity limits: 40-50 ng medazepam/ ml blood or urine	Recovery: extraction medazepam 70 % (serum) 74 % (urine) diazepam 83 % (serum) 85 % (urine) nordiazepam 76% (serum) 78% (urine) oxazepam 79% (serum) 67% (urine) normedazepam 66% (serum) 74% (urine) Detection limit: 2.5 - 20 ng/ml (medazepam)
Pharmacokinetic Data obtained by this Method described on pp. Mit der Methode erhaltene pharmakokinetische Daten sind beschrieben auf S.	See part: Blood-, Serum- and Plasma-Levels and Other Pharmacokinetic Data from Literature	
Method is recommended for: Methode ist empfohlen für:	the determination of blood levels and/or the urinary excretion pattern following single and multiple doses of 50 mg oral doses of medazepam.	the determination of medazepam and its major metabolites in serum and/or urine after administration of therapeutic doses to man.

Benzodiazepine(s)/ Benzodiazepin(e)	Clorazepate	Clorazepate
Method / Methode	GLC-ECD 3% Poly A-103 Gas Chrom Q	GLC-ECD 3% OV-17 Gas Chrom Q (60-80 mesh)
Authors / Verfasser	HOFFMAN and CHUN	BROOKS, HACKMAN, WEINFELD and MACASIEB
Lit.Ref./ Lit.Zitat	(489)	(153)
Year of Publication/ Publikationsjahr	1975	1977
Extraction Procedure/ Extraktionsverfahren	pH 9.2, diethylether	alkaline, benzene - methylene chloride (90 : 10)
Drug analyzed/ analysierte Substanz	Benzophenone	Nordiazepam
Drug calculated / berechnete Substanz	Benzodiazepine	Clorazepate
Metabolites included / Metabolite inbegriffen	yes (nordiazepam)	yes (nordiazepam)
qual./quant./Screening Method (e)	quant.	quant.
Sample required/ benötigtes Untersuchungsmaterial	0.5 ml plasma	1 ml blood or urine
Concentration Range/ Konzentrationsbereich	ca. 10 - 800 ng / ml	ca. 5 - 150 ng / ml
Special Equipment/ Spezialausstattung	ECD-detection	ECD-detection
Hydrolysis / Hydrolyse	yes	no (but decarboxylation)
Some Other Data: Einige andere Daten:	Assay Reproducibility (n = 8) C.V. = 4.31 % (range 150 ng/ml) Detection limit: 10 ng / ml plasma	Recovery: overall (mean ± S.D.) 60 ± 5 % (clorazepate) from blood 95 ± 5 % (nordiazepam) from blood Sensitivity limits: 4.0 ng / ml blood (both compounds)
Pharmacokinetic Data obtained by this Method described on pp. Mit der Methode erhaltene pharmakokinetische Daten sind beschrieben auf S.		See part: Blood-, Serum- and Plasma-Levels and Other Pharmacokinetic Data from Literature
Method is recommended for: Methode ist empfohlen für:	monitoring nordiazepam levels in plasma after the administration of therapeutic clorazepate doses.	the determination of clorazepate and nordiazepam in blood and urine following single therapeutic doses of clorazepate dipotassium.

Benzodiazepine(s)/ Benzodiazepin(e)	Clorazepate	Clorazepate
Method / Methode	GLC-ECD 3% OV-17 Gas-Chrom Q (60 - 80 mesh)	Polarography (DPP-mode)
Authors / Verfasser	HAIDUKEWYCH, RODIN and DAVENPORT	ABRUZZO, BROOKS, COTLER and KAPLAN
Lit.Ref./ Lit.Zitat	(2995)	(1)
Year of Publication/ Publikationsjahr	1980	1976
Extraction Procedure/ Extraktionsverfahren	saturated KCl solution, benzene	
Drug analyzed/ analysierte Substanz	Desmethyldiazepam	Desmethyldiazepam
Drug calculated / berechnete Substanz	Clorazepate	Clorazepate
Metabolites included / Metabolite inbegriffen	yes	yes
qual./quant./Screening Method (e)	qual./quant.	quant.
Sample required/ benötigtes Untersuchungsmaterial	0.1 ml plasma	1 ml blood
Concentration Range/ Konzentrationsbereich	ca. 100 - 500 ng / 0.1 ml	ca. 500 - 20,000 ng/ml
Special Equipment/ Spezialausstattung	ECD - detection	DPP-Polarograph
Hydrolysis / Hydrolyse	no	no (decarboxylation)
Some Other Data: Einige andere Daten:	Sensitivity limit: 20 ng / ml Within-run precision: 2.9 % (3.5 mg/L) 3.9 % (1.5 mg/L) 4.3 % (1.0 mg/L) Between-run precision: 3.5 % (3.5 mg/L)	Sensitivity limit: 500 ng/ml Recovery: (overall, mean ± S.D.) 100 ± 5% (from aqu. stand.) 95 ± 5% (from blood)
Pharmacokinetic Data obtained by this Method described on pp. Mit der Methode erhaltene pharmakokinetische Daten sind beschrieben auf S.		
Method is recommended for: Methode ist empfohlen für:	monitoring desmethyldiazepam levels after administration of clorazepate	the polarographic determination of clorazepate and nordiazepam following the administration of clorazepate dipotassium

Benzodiazepine(s)/ Benzodiazepin(e)	Lorazepam	Lorazepam
Method / Methode	GLC-ECD 3% OV-17 Chromosorb W (HP) (80-100 mesh)	GLC-ECD 3% OV-17 GAS Chrom Q (60-80 mesh)
Authors / Verfasser	KNOWLES, COMER and RUELIUS	DE SILVA, BEKERSKY and PUGLISI
Lit.Ref./ Lit.Zitat	(594)	(234)
Year of Publication/ Publikationsjahr	1971	1973
Extraction Procedure/ Extraktionsverfahren	pH 7, diethylether	pH 9.0, diethylether (see (234) for details)
Drug analyzed/ analysierte Substanz	Benzophenone	Thermal rearrangement product
Drug calculated / berechnete Substanz	Benzodiazepine	Benzodiazepine
Metabolites included / Metabolite inbegriffen	yes (glucuronide)	Ro - 5-3027
qual./quant./Screening Method (e)	quant.	quant.
Sample required/ benötigtes Untersuchungsmaterial	1 ml serum / urine feces	1 ml blood 5 ml urine
Concentration Range/ Konzentrationsbereich	ca. 10 ng - 100 ng / ml	ca. 30 ng - 3000 ng/ml
Special Equipment/ Spezialausstattung	ECD-detection	ECD-detection
Hydrolysis / Hydrolyse	yes	no
Some Other Data: Einige andere Daten:	Recovery: overall 50 - 60 % Sensitivity limit: 10 ng / ml	Recovery: overall more than 95 % (Ro 5-3027) 40 % (lorazepam) Sensitivity limit: 2 - 3 ng/ml (Ro 5-3027) 4 - 5 ng/ml (lorazepam)
Pharmacokinetic Data obtained by this Method described on pp. Mit der Methode erhaltene pharmakokinetische Daten sind beschrieben auf S.	See part: Blood-, Serum- and Plasma-Levels and Other Pharmacokinetic Data from Literature	
Method is recommended for: Methode ist empfohlen für:	the determination of conjugated lorazepam (glucuronide) as well as free drug in biological samples (blood, serum, urine and feces resp.).	the determination of Ro 5-3027, a lorazepam derivative.

Benzodiazepine(s)/ Benzodiazepin(e)	Lorazepam	Lorazepam
Method / Methode	GLC-ECD	GLC-ECD
Authors / Verfasser	DE GROOT, MAES and LEMMENS	HOWARD, LILBURN, DUNDEE, TONER and McILROY
Lit.Ref./ Lit.Zitat	(437)	(498, 499)
Year of Publication/ Publikationsjahr	1976	1977 / 1978
Extraction Procedure/ Extraktionsverfahren	ethylacetate	KCl solution, benzene
Drug analyzed/ analysierte Substanz	Thermal rearrangement product	Thermal rearrangement product
Drug calculated / berechnete Substanz	Benzodiazepine	Benzodiazepine
Metabolites included / Metabolite inbegriffen	no	no
qual./quant./Screening Method (e)	quant.	quant.
Sample required/ benötigtes Untersuchungsmaterial	1 ml plasma	0.5 ml plasma (498) 0.1 ml plasma (499)
Concentration Range/ Konzentrationsbereich	10 - 800 ng / ml (linear range)	ca. 20 - 400 ng / ml
Special Equipment/ Spezialausstattung	ECD-detection	ECD-detection
Hydrolysis / Hydrolyse	no	no
Some Other Data: Einige andere Daten:	Recovery: mean ± S.D. 86 ± 2 % Day-to-day precision: C.V. = ± 3 % Detection limit: 10 ng / ml	Within-run precision: C.V. = 10 - 15 % Sensitivity limit: ca. 10 ng / ml
Pharmacokinetic Data obtained by this Method described on pp. Mit der Methode erhaltene pharmakokinetische Daten sind beschrieben auf S.		
Method is recommended for: Methode ist empfohlen für:	the determination of very low plasma levels as appearing in the placental transfer of lorazepam but also in samples of patients who have taken overdoses of lorazepam.	the determination of lorazepam in small samples of plasma (neonates) within the clinical range.

Benzodiazepine(s)/ Benzodiazepin(e)	Lorazepam	Lorazepam
Method / Methode	GLC-ECD 3% OV-17 Chromosorb W HP 80 - 100 mesh	Polarography (DPP-mode)
Authors / Verfasser	GREENBLATT, FRANKE and SHADER	DE SILVA, BEKERSKY and BROOKS
Lit.Ref./ Lit.Zitat	(1506)	(232)
Year of Publication/ Publikationsjahr	1978	1974
Extraction Procedure/ Extraktionsverfahren	benzene - isoamylalcohol (98.5 : 1.5)	pH 9, ether
Drug analyzed/ analysierte Substanz	Thermal rearrangement product	Benzodiazepine
Drug calculated / berechnete Substanz	Benzodiazepine	Benzodiazepine
Metabolites included / Metabolite inbegriffen	yes (glucuronide and oxazepam)	no (but Ro 5-3027)
qual./quant./Screening Method (e)	quant.	quant.
Sample required/ benötigtes Untersuchungsmaterial	1 ml plasma and urine	2 ml urine
Concentration Range/ Konzentrationsbereich	5 - 50 ng / ml	200 - 1000 ng / ml
Special Equipment/ Spezialausstattung	ECD-detection	Polarograph (DPP - mode)
Hydrolysis / Hydrolyse	yes (enzymatic cleavage of the glucuronide)	yes (enzymatic cleavage of the glucuronide)
Some Other Data: Einige andere Daten:	Recovery: ca. 95 % C.V. = 2.8 % (level 25 ng/ml) 4.5 % (level 12.5 ng/ml) 4.3 % (level 6.2 ng/ml) 5.1 % (level 2.5 ng/ml) Day-to-day precision: C.V. = 8.6 % (level 50 ng/ml) Sensitivity limit: 1-3 ng/ml	Recovery: overall over 85 % (ethylacetate)
Pharmacokinetic Data obtained by this Method described on pp. Mit der Methode erhaltene pharmakokinetische Daten sind beschrieben auf S.	See part: Blood-, Serum- and Plasma-Levels and Other Pharmacokinetic Data from Literature	See part: Blood-, Serum- and Plasma-Levels and Other Pharmacokinetic Data from Literature
Method is recommended for: Methode ist empfohlen für:	studies on the pharmacokinetics and bioavailability of lorazepam in humans following oral, i.v. and i.m. administration .	the determination of lorazepam concentrations in urine following administration of single oral 4-mg doses.

Benzodiazepine(s)/ Benzodiazepin(e)	Prazepam	Prazepam
Method / Methode	GLC-EDC 3% SP-2250 Supelcoport (100-120 mesh)	GLC-ECD 3% OV-225 Gas Chrom Q (80-100 mesh)
Authors / Verfasser	NAU, LIDDIARD, JESDINSKY and WITTFOHT	SMITH, EVANS, EADIE and TYRER
Lit.Ref./ Lit.Zitat	(1773)	(2490)
Year of Publication/ Publikationsjahr	1978	1979
Extraction Procedure/ Extraktionsverfahren	ethylacetate, EXTRELUT[R]	pH 9, diethylether
Drug analyzed/ analysierte Substanz	Benzodiazepine	Benzodiazepine
Drug calculated / berechnete Substanz	Benzodiazepine	Benzodiazepine
Metabolites included / Metabolite inbegriffen	yes (nordiazepam = norprazepam, 3-hydroxyprazepam, oxazepam)	yes (nordiazepam = norprazepam)
qual./quant./Screening Method (e)	quant.	quant.
Sample required/ benötigtes Untersuchungsmaterial	0.05 - 0.2 ml serum	0.1 - 2 ml plasma
Concentration Range/ Konzentrationsbereich	50 - 330 ng / ml	ca. 50 - 400 ng / ml
Special Equipment/ Spezialausstattung	ECD-detection	ECD-detection
Hydrolysis / Hydrolyse	no	no
Some Other Data: Einige andere Daten:	Recovery: Ethylacetate extraction: / Extrelut column: 93.5 % / 80 % (prazepam) 99.6 % / 85 % (nordiazepam) 83 % / 93 % (3-OH-prazepam) 75 % / 69 % (oxazepam) Day-to-Day variation: / Within-run variation: 5.9 / 3.7 (prazepam) 4.2 / 2.8 (nordiazepam) 9.1 / 4.9 (oxazepam) 7.5 / 5.9 (3-OH-prazepam)	Recovery: 101.9 ± 5.1 % (prazepam) 101.6 ± 6.5 % (nordiazepam) (range 100 ng/ ml) Detection limit: 2.5 ng / ml for both prazepam and nordiazepam.
Pharmacokinetic Data obtained by this Method described on pp. Mit der Methode erhaltene pharmakokinetische Daten sind beschrieben auf S.	Detection limit: (pg) 1.8 (diazepam), 7.2 (prazepam), 4.1 (nordiazepam), 5.7 (oxazepam) 29 (3-OH-prazepam),	See part: Blood-, Serum- and Plasma-Levels and Other Pharmacokinetic Data from Literature
Method is recommended for: Methode ist empfohlen für:	the determination of prazepam and its metabolites nordiazepam, 3-hydroxy-prazepam and oxazepam in small blood samples (micromethod).	the simultaneous measurement of prazepam and nordiazepam levels in plasma after therapeutic doses.

Benzodiazepine(s)/ Benzodiazepin(e)	Clonazepam	Clonazepam
Method / Methode	GLC-ECD 3% OV-17 Gas Chrom Q (60-80 mesh)	GLC-ECD 3% OV-17 Gas Chrom Q (60-80 mesh)
Authors / Verfasser	DE SILVA and BEKERSKY	DE SILVA, PUGLISI and MUNNO
Lit.Ref./ Lit.Zitat	(231)	(242)
Year of Publication/ Publikationsjahr	1974	1974
Extraction Procedure/ Extraktionsverfahren	pH 9.0, benzene - methylene chloride (90 : 10)	pH 9.0, diethylether
Drug analyzed/ analysierte Substanz	Methyl derivative	Benzophenone
Drug calculated / berechnete Substanz	Benzodiazepine	Benzodiazepine
Metabolites included / Metabolite inbegriffen	no (no metabolites but flunitrazepam via nor-flunitrazepam)	no (no metabolites but flunitrazepam via nor-flunitrazepam)
qual./quant./Screening Method (e)	quant.	quant.
Sample required/ benötigtes Untersuchungsmaterial	1 ml blood	2 ml blood 5 ml urine
Concentration Range/ Konzentrationsbereich	ca. 0.5 - 100ng / ml	2.0 - 50 ng / ml
Special Equipment/ Spezialausstattung	ECD-detection	ECD-detection
Hydrolysis / Hydrolyse	no	yes (acid)
Some Other Data: Einige andere Daten:	Recovery: overall 85 ± 5% (range 2.0 -50 ng/ml) Sensitivity limit: 0.5 - 1.0 ng / ml	Recovery: overall 86 ± 6.5% (range 2.0-50 ng/ml) Sensitivity limit: 0.5 - 1.0 ng / ml
Pharmacokinetic Data obtained by this Method described on pp. Mit der Methode erhaltene pharmakokinetische Daten sind beschrieben auf S.	See part: Blood-, Serum- and Plasma-Levels and Other Pharmacokinetic Data from Literature	See part: Blood-, Serum- and Plasma-Levels and Other Pharmacokinetic Data from Literature
Method is recommended for: Methode ist empfohlen für:	the rapid determination of blood levels of clonazepam following single oral 2-mg doses of clonazepam.	the determination of clonazepam in blood after administration of single 2-mg doses of clonazepam (suitable for batch samples).

Benzodiazepine(s)/ Benzodiazepin(e)	Clonazepam	Clonazepam
Method / Methode	GLC-ECD 1 % OV-17 Celite J.J. CQ (100-120 mesh)	GLC-ECD 3% OV-17 GAS CHROM Q (100-120 mesh)
Authors / Verfasser	NAESTOFT and LARSEN	KNOP, VAN DER KLEIJN and EDMUNDS
Lit.Ref./ Lit.Zitat	(771)	(591)
Year of Publication/ Publikationsjahr	1974	1975
Extraction Procedure/ Extraktionsverfahren	ethylacetate	diethylether or n-hexane
Drug analyzed/ analysierte Substanz	Benzodiazepine / Benzophenone	Benzophenone
Drug calculated / berechnete Substanz	Benzodiazepine	Benzodiazepine
Metabolites included / Metabolite inbegriffen	yes (7-amino- and 7-acetamido-clonazepam)	no
qual./quant./Screening Method (e)	quant.	quant.
Sample required/ benötigtes Untersuchungsmaterial	2 ml plasma	0.5 ml plasma
Concentration Range/ Konzentrationsbereich	ca. 20 - 100 ng / ml	ca. 5 - 50 ng / ml
Special Equipment/ Spezialausstattung	ECD-detection	ECD-detection
Hydrolysis / Hydrolyse	no (yes)	yes (acid)
Some Other Data: Einige andere Daten:	Recovery: extractions with ethylacetate ca. 100 % (clonazepam) ca. 100 % (7-aminoclonazepam) ca. 93 % (7-acetamidoclonaz.) rel.stand. deviation 4 % (clonazepam) 10 % (metabolites) n = 20 Sensitivity limits: 3 ng/ml (clonazepam), 5 ng/ml (7-aminoclonazepam)	Recovery: 72.1 % ± 0.78 (n = 10) Within-run precision: 2.17 % (5 ng / ml) 1.39 % (50 ng / ml) Detection limit: ca. 5 ng / ml
Pharmacokinetic Data obtained by this Method described on pp. Mit der Methode erhaltene pharmakokinetische Daten sind beschrieben auf S.	See part: Blood-, Serum- and Plasma-Levels and Other Pharmacokinetic Data from Literature	See part: Blood-, Serum- and Plasma-Levels and Other Pharmacokinetic Data from Literature
Method is recommended for: Methode ist empfohlen für:	the determination of clonazepam, 7-aminoclonazepam and 7-acetamidoclonazepam in plasma after single and multiple doses of clonazepam (with and without hydrolysis).	drug monitoring in the treatment of epilepsy.

Benzodiazepine(s)/ Benzodiazepin(e)	Clonazepam	Clonazepam
Method / Methode	GLC-ECD 3% OV-17 Chromosorb Q (100-120 mesh)	GLC-ECD 3% OV-225 GAS CHROM Q (60-80 mesh)
Authors / Verfasser	GERNA and MORSELLI	CANO, GUINTRAND, AUBERT and VIALA
Lit.Ref./ Lit.Zitat	(381)	(163)
Year of Publication/ Publikationsjahr	1976	1977
Extraction Procedure/ Extraktionsverfahren	pH 9, diethylether	pH 9, diethylether
Drug analyzed/ analysierte Substanz	Benzodiazepine	Benzophenone
Drug calculated / berechnete Substanz	Benzodiazepine	Benzodiazepine
Metabolites included / Metabolite inbegriffen	no	no
qual./quant./Screening Method (e)	quant.	quant.
Sample required/ benötigtes Untersuchungsmaterial	0.5 ml plasma (0.2 ml)	0.5 - 1.0 ml plasma
Concentration Range/ Konzentrationsbereich	ca. 5 - 120 ng / ml	ca. 2 - 100 ng / ml
Special Equipment/ Spezialausstattung	ECD-detection	ECD-detection
Hydrolysis / Hydrolyse	no	yes (acid)
Some Other Data: Einige andere Daten:	Recovery: mean ± S.D. 82.6 ± 1.18 % (range 20 - 80 ng/ml) Detection limit: 4 ng / ml	Sensitivity limit: ca. 0.5 - 1.0 ng/ml
Pharmacokinetic Data obtained by this Method described on pp. Mit der Methode erhaltene pharmakokinetische Daten sind beschrieben auf S.	See part: Blood-, Serum- and Plasma-Levels and Other Pharmacokinetic Data from Literature	See part: Blood-, Serum- and Plasma-Levels and Other Pharmacokinetic Data from Literature
Method is recommended for: Methode ist empfohlen für:	the routine analysis (drug monitoring) of clonazepam levels in the treatment of epilepsy).	pharmacokinetic studies after administration of therapeutic doses of clonazepam (incl. drug-monitoring).

Benzodiazepine(s)/ Benzodiazepin(e)	Clonazepam	Clonazepam
Method / Methode	GLC-ECD 5% OV-17 Gas Chrom Q (100-120 mesh)	GLC-ECD 3% OV-17 Supelcoport (60-70 mesh)
Authors / Verfasser	SOLOW and KENFIELD	EDELBROEK and DE WOLFF
Lit.Ref./ Lit.Zitat	(1068)	(1416)
Year of Publication/ Publikationsjahr	1977	1978
Extraction Procedure/ Extraktionsverfahren	Na_3PO_4 sol., benzene	pH 9, cyclohexane -dichloro-methane (40 : 60)
Drug analyzed/ analysierte Substanz	Methyl-derivative	Benzodiazepine
Drug calculated / berechnete Substanz	Benzodiazepine	Benzodiazepine
Metabolites included / Metabolite inbegriffen	no	no
qual./quant./Screening Method (e)	quant.	quant.
Sample required/ benötigtes Unter-suchungsmaterial	0.1 ml serum	0.1 ml serum
Concentration Range/ Konzentrationsbereich	10 - 100 ng / ml serum	5 - 150 ng / ml serum
Special Equipment/ Spezialausstattung	ECD-detection	ECD-detection
Hydrolysis / Hydrolyse	no	no
Some Other Data: Einige andere Daten:	Recovery: ca. 93 % Day-to-day reproducibility: C.V. = 4.3 % (n = 10, range 23ng) Within-run reproducibility: C.V. = 6.7 % (n = 2, range 19.6ng) Sensitivity limit: 2-3 ng/ml	Recovery: ca. 86 % Within-run precision: C.V. = 4.3 - 8.7 % (range 10-100 ng / ml) n=20 Day-to day reproducibility: C.V. = 5.7 % (range ca. 50 ng/ml) n = 11 Detection limit: 1 ng / ml
Pharmacokinetic Data obtained by this Method described on pp. Mit der Methode erhaltene pharmakokinetische Daten sind beschrieben auf S.		
Method is recommended for: Methode ist empfohlen für:	monitoring clonazepam levels as a micromethod.	the clinical routine determination of clonazepam in serum in therapeutic concentrations.

Benzodiazepine(s)/ Benzodiazepin(e)	Clonazepam	
Method / Methode	GLC-ECD 3% OV-17 Gas Chrom Q (80 - 100 mesh)	
Authors / Verfasser	CANO, GOUEZO, LINDOULSI and VIALA	
Lit.Ref./ Lit.Zitat	(2708)	
Year of Publication/ Publikationsjahr	1979	
Extraction Procedure/ Extraktionsverfahren	different pH-values, diethylether	
Drug analyzed/ analysierte Substanz	Benzodiazepines	
Drug calculated / berechnete Substanz	Benzodiazepines	
Metabolites included / Metabolite inbegriffen	yes (7-Aminoclonazepam)	
qual./quant./Screening Method (e)	quant.	
Sample required/ benötigtes Untersuchungsmaterial	0.5 - 1 ml plasma	
Concentration Range/ Konzentrationsbereich	ca. 10 - 100 ng/ml	
Special Equipment/ Spezialausstattung	ECD-detection	
Hydrolysis / Hydrolyse	no	
Some Other Data: Einige andere Daten:	Sensitivity: 5 ng/ml Recovery: 94% (clonazepam) 80% (7-aminoclonazepam) C.V.: 2.13 % (clonazepam) 6.25 % (7-aminoclonazepam)	
Pharmacokinetic Data obtained by this Method described on pp. Mit der Methode erhaltene pharmakokinetische Daten sind beschrieben auf S.		
Method is recommended for: Methode ist empfohlen für:	monitoring plasma levels of clonazepam and 7-aminoclonazepam	

Benzodiazepine(s)/ Benzodiazepin(e)	Clonazepam	Clonazepam (and Diazepam)
Method / Methode	GLC-MS Gas Chrom Q 1% OV-25 (100-120 mesh)	TLC
Authors / Verfasser	MIN, GARLAND, KHOO and TORRES	WAD and HANIFL
Lit.Ref./ Lit.Zitat	(2486)	(1188)
Year of Publication/ Publikationsjahr	1978	1977
Extraction Procedure/ Extraktionsverfahren	pH 10, benzene - dichloroethane (80 : 20)	pH 10.5, toluene
Drug analyzed/ analysierte Substanz	Benzodiazepine	Benzodiazepine
Drug calculated / berechnete Substanz	Benzodiazepine	Benzodiazepine
Metabolites included / Metabolite inbegriffen	yes (7-aminoclonazepam and 7-acetamidoclonazepam)	yes (7-aminoclonazepam and 7-acetamidoclonazepam)
qual./quant./Screening Method (e)	quant.	quant.
Sample required/ benötigtes Untersuchungsmaterial	0.5 - 1 ml plasma	1 ml serum
Concentration Range/ Konzentrationsbereich	ca. 10 - 600 ng / ml	200 - 1000 ng / ml
Special Equipment/ Spezialausstattung	GLC-MS (chemical ionization)	scanner
Hydrolysis / Hydrolyse	no	no
Some Other Data: Einige andere Daten:	Recovery: mean ± S.D. 100 ± 4% (clonazepam) 89 ± 12% (7-aminoclonazepam) 100 ± 5% (7-acetamidoclonazep.) Sensitivity limit: 0.5 ng / ml	Recovery: 98.6 % (clonazepam) 77.1 % (7-aminoclonazepam) 40.3 % (7-acetamidoclon.) Within-run reproducibility: C.V. = 5.2 % (clonazepam) C.V. = 6.8 % (7-aminoclonaz.) C.V. = 4.8 % (7-acetamidocl.) (range ca. 500- 600 ng/ml)
Pharmacokinetic Data obtained by this Method described on pp. Mit der Methode erhaltene pharmakokinetische Daten sind beschrieben auf S.	See part: Blood-, Serum- and Plasma-Levels and Other Pharmacokinetic Data from Literature	
Method is recommended for: Methode ist empfohlen für:	the determination of serum levels of clonazepam with special regard to the 7-amino- and 7-acetamido-metabolites.	the drug monitoring of diazepam, clonazepam and their metabolites in epileptic patients.

Benzodiazepine(s)/ Benzodiazepin(e)	Clonazepam	Clonazepam
Method / Methode	Polarography (DPP-mode)	Radioimmunoassay
Authors / Verfasser	DE SILVA, PUGLISI and MUNNO	DIXON and CREWS
Lit.Ref./ Lit.Zitat	(242)	(260)
Year of Publication/ Publikationsjahr	1974	1977
Extraction Procedure/ Extraktionsverfahren	pH 9, ethylacetate	
Drug analyzed/ analysierte Substanz	Benzodiazepine	Benzodiazepine
Drug calculated / berechnete Substanz	Benzodiazepine	Benzodiazepine
Metabolites included / Metabolite inbegriffen	yes (7-aminoclonazepam and 7-acetamidoclonazepam)	no
qual./quant./Screening Method (e)	quant.	quant.
Sample required/ benötigtes Untersuchungsmaterial	5 ml urine	ca. 0.01 ml blood or serum
Concentration Range/ Konzentrationsbereich	variable by dilution	5 - 100 ng / ml
Special Equipment/ Spezialausstattung	Polarograph (differential-pulse mode)	(RIA-equipment)
Hydrolysis / Hydrolyse	no	no
Some Other Data: Einige andere Daten:	Recovery: 65 - 93 % (incl. TLC-procedure) Sensitivity limit: 500 - 750 ng / 5 ml urine	Recovery: quantitative (RIA) Within-run precision: C.V. = less than 3 % Day-to-day precision: C.V. = less than 9 % Sensitivity limit: 2.5 ng / ml
Pharmacokinetic Data obtained by this Method described on pp. Mit der Methode erhaltene pharmakokinetische Daten sind beschrieben auf S.	See part: Blood-, Serum- and Plasma-Levels and Other Pharmacokinetic Data from Literature	
Method is recommended for: Methode ist empfohlen für:	the determination of the major urinary metabolites of clonazepam following chronic administration.	the routine clinical monitoring of clonazepam levels in serum.

Benzodiazepine(s)/ Benzodiazepin(e)	Clonazepam	Clonazepam
Method / Methode	HPLC (LiChrosorb SI 100-10)	HPLC (Spherisorb C_6, reversed phase)
Authors / Verfasser	UGES and BOUMA	ROVEI and SANJUAN
Lit.Ref./ Lit.Zitat	(1983)	(3461)
Year of Publication/ Publikationsjahr	1976	1980
Extraction Procedure/ Extraktionsverfahren	pH 9, dichloromethane	pH 9.1, chloroform
Drug analyzed/ analysierte Substanz	Benzodiazepine	Benzodiazepine
Drug calculated / berechnete Substanz	Benzodiazepine	Benzodiazepine
Metabolites included / Metabolite inbegriffen	no metabolites but many other antiepileptics	no
qual./quant./Screening Method (e)	quant.	quant.
Sample required/ benötigtes Untersuchungsmaterial	0.5 ml serum	1 ml plasma
Concentration Range/ Konzentrationsbereich	ca. 10 - 120 ng/ml	ca. 2 - 200 ng/ml
Special Equipment/ Spezialausstattung	UV-detection	UV-detection
Hydrolysis / Hydrolyse	no	no
Some Other Data: Einige andere Daten:	Recovery: more than 95% Detection limit: 2 ng/ml Standard Dev. (n=10) 3.3 % (range 10 ng/ml) 1.3 % (range 90 ng/ml)	C.V. (range 2 ng/ml): 14 %
Pharmacokinetic Data obtained by this Method described on pp. Mit der Methode erhaltene pharmakokinetische Daten sind beschrieben auf S.		
Method is recommended for: Methode ist empfohlen für:	the determination of clonazepam in serum following clinical dosages	routine monitoring of clonazepam in plasma

Benzodiazepine(s)/ Benzodiazepin(e)	Flurazepam	Flurazepam
Method / Methode	GLC-ECD 3% QF - 1 Gas Chrom Q (60-80 mesh)	GLC-ECD 2% OV-17 Chromosorb W (100-120 mesh)
Authors / Verfasser	DE SILVA, PUGLISI, BROOKS and HACKMAN	HASEGAWA and MATSUBARA
Lit.Ref./ Lit.Zitat	(241)	(468)
Year of Publication/ Publikationsjahr	1974	1975
Extraction Procedure/ Extraktionsverfahren	pH 9, benzene - methylene chloride (90 : 10)	pH 9, ethylacetate
Drug analyzed/ analysierte Substanz	Benzodiazepine	Methyl-derivatives
Drug calculated / berechnete Substanz	Benzodiazepine	Benzodiazepine
Metabolites included / Metabolite inbegriffen	yes (N-1-hydroxyethylflurazepam, N-1-desalkylflurazepam, N-1-desalkyl-3-hydroxyflurazepam	yes (N-1-hydroxyethylflurazepam, N-1-desalkylflurazepam, N-1-desalkyl-3-hydroxyflurazepam)
qual./quant./Screening Method (e)	quant.	quant.
Sample required/ benötigtes Untersuchungsmaterial	1 ml (toxicological analysis) 2 ml (therapeutic level analysis)	2-4 ml plasma / 5 ml urine
Concentration Range/ Konzentrationsbereich	ca. 100 - 3000 ng / ml	ca. 100 - 4000 ng / ml
Special Equipment/ Spezialausstattung	ECD-detection	ECD-detection
Hydrolysis / Hydrolyse	no	no
Some Other Data: Einige andere Daten:	Recovery: overall 76% ± 6.0 (flurazepam) 96% ± 8.0 (hydroxyethylflurazep.) 94% ± 6.0 (N-desalkylflurazepam) 42% ± 9.0 (N-desalkyl-3-OH-flur.) Detection limits: 5-10 ng (flurazepam and N-desalkylflurazepam) 20-40ng (hydroxyethylflurazepam and N-desalkyl-3-OH-fluraz.) per ml of blood using 2ml sample	Recovery: overall urine level 99% ± 3.0 (1000ng/ml) flurazepam 98% ± 5.0 (20000ng/ml) hydroxyethylflurazepam 95% ± 4.0 (2000ng/ml) N-desalkylflurazepam 93% ± 6.0 (2000ng/ml) N-desalkyl-3-OH-flurazepam 93% ± 2.0 (1000ng/ml) flurazepam-N-1-yl-acetic acid serum level 94% ± 6.0 (4000ng/ml) flurazepam 100% ± 7.0 (10000ng/ml) hydroxyethylfl 93% ± 5.0 (10000ng/ml) N-desalkylfl. 96% ± 6.0 (10000ng/ml) N-desalkyl-3-OH-flurazepam 88% ± 5.0 (5000ng/ml) flurazepam-N-1-yl-acetic acid
Pharmacokinetic Data obtained by this Method described on pp. Mit der Methode erhaltene pharmakokinetische Daten sind beschrieben auf S.	See part: Blood-, Serum- and Plasma-Levels and Other Pharmacokinetic Data from Literature	Lower detection limit: between 0.3 and 2.0 ng / ml sample
Method is recommended for: Methode ist empfohlen für:	the determination of blood levels of flurazepam, N-1-hydroxyethylflurazepam, N-1-desalkylflurazepam and N-1-desalkyl-3-hydroxyflurazepam following single and multiple 30-mg doses of Dalmane (also for toxic levels).	the determination of flurazepam and its metabolites N-1-hydroxyethylflurazepam, N-1-desalkylflurazepam, N-1-desalkyl-3-hydroxyflurazepam and flurazepam-N-1-yl-acetic acid in urine and serum following single or chronic dose of 30-mg.

Benzodiazepine(s)/ Benzodiazepin(e)	Flurazepam	Flurazepam
Method / Methode	Spectrofluorometry Spectrophotometry	Spectrofluorodensitometry
Authors / Verfasser	DE SILVA and STROJNY	DE SILVA, BEKERSKY and PUGLISI
Lit.Ref./ Lit.Zitat	(244)	(235)
Year of Publication/ Publikationsjahr	1971	1974
Extraction Procedure/ Extraktionsverfahren	pH 9, diethylether, derivatization	pH 9, diethylether, derivatization
Drug analyzed/ analysierte Substanz	benzophenone-9-acridanone-derivative	benzophenone-9-acridanone-derivative
Drug calculated / berechnete Substanz	Benzodiazepine	Benzodiazepine
Metabolites included / Metabolite inbegriffen	yes (N-1-hydroxyethylflurazepam, N-1-desalkylflurazepam, N-1-desalkyl-3-OH-flurazepam a.o.)	yes (N-1-hydroxyethylflurazepam, N-1-desalkylflurazepam, N-1-desalkyl-3-OH-flurazepam a.o.)
qual./quant./Screening Method (e)	quant.	quant.
Sample required/ benötigtes Untersuchungsmaterial	1 ml blood / 5 ml urine	4 ml blood
Concentration Range/ Konzentrationsbereich	2.5 - 2000 ng/ml (fluorometry) over 1000-2000 ng/ml (photometry	ca. 200 - 10000 ng/ml
Special Equipment/ Spezialausstattung	Fluorimeter / TLC / photometer	TLC-scanner - fluorimeter
Hydrolysis / Hydrolyse	yes (acid)	yes (acid)
Some Other Data: Einige andere Daten:	Recovery: overall from blood: 50% ± 9.0 (flurazepam) 71% ± 4.0 (N-1-hydroxyethylflur from urine: 64% ± 5.0 (N-1-hydroxyethylflur (spectrofluorimetric assay) from urine: 85 % (N-1-hydroxyethylflurazepam 35 % (N-1-desalkyl-3-hydroxy-flurazepam) 78 % (flurazepam-N-1-yl-acetic acid) (photometric assay) Sensitivity limits: 2000 - 3000 ng/ml (photometry) 3-5 ng/ml (spectrofluorometry)	Reproducibility: see table (235) Detection limit: 0.5 - 1.0 ng/ ml of blood each of flurazepam, N-1-hydroxy-ethylflurazepam and N-1-desalkyl-flurazepam (using 4 ml samples).
Pharmacokinetic Data obtained by this Method described on pp. Mit der Methode erhaltene pharmakokinetische Daten sind beschrieben auf S.		See part: Blood-, Serum- and Plasma-Levels and Other Pharmacokinetic Data from Literature
Method is recommended for: Methode ist empfohlen für:	the determination of flurazepam and its main metabolites in blood and urine following therapeutic doses of flurazepam.	the spectrofluorimetric determination of flurazepam and its main metabolites in blood with more precision after therapeutic doses of 30-mg Dalmane.

Benzodiazepine(s)/ Benzodiazepin(e)	Flurazepam	Flurazepam
Method / Methode	Polarography (DPP-mode)	Polarography (DPP-mode)
Authors / Verfasser	CLIFFORD, SMYTH and SMYTH	DE SILVA, PUGLISI, BROOKS and HACKMAN
Lit.Ref./ Lit.Zitat	(194)	(241)
Year of Publication/ Publikationsjahr	1974	1974
Extraction Procedure/ Extraktionsverfahren		pH 11, diethylether (see (241) for details)
Drug analyzed/ analysierte Substanz	Benzodiazepine	Benzodiazepine
Drug calculated / berechnete Substanz	Benzodiazepine	Benzodiazepine
Metabolites included / Metabolite inbegriffen	yes (N-1-hydroxyethylflurazepam, N-1-desalkylflurazepam).	yes (N-1-hydroxyethylflurazepam, and others)
qual./quant./Screening Method (e)	quant.	quant.
Sample required/ benötigtes Untersuchungsmaterial	2 ml plasma	0.1 ml urine (toxicological anal.) 5.0 ml urine (individual metabolites analysis)
Concentration Range/ Konzentrationsbereich	ca. 100 - 5000 ng/ml	ca. 500 - 10000 ng/ ml (mono- and didesethylflurazepam resp.) ca. 5 - 500 µg / ml urine (N-1-hydroxyethylflurazepam)
Special Equipment/ Spezialausstattung	Polarograph (differential-pulse mode)	Polarograph (differential-pulse mode)
Hydrolysis / Hydrolyse	no	yes (enzymatic)
Some Other Data: Einige andere Daten:	Recovery: nearly quant. with ethylacetate Sensitivity limit: 30 ng/ml Detection limit: 10 - 20 ng/ml	Recovery: overall 75.0 % ± 5.0 (flurazepam, N-1-hydroxyethylflurazepam, N-1-desalkylflurazepam, N-1-desalkyl-3-hydroxyflurazepam) 71.2 % ± 4.6 (monodesethylfluraz.) 28.6 % ± 2.7 (didesethylfluraz.) Sensitivity limit: 250 - 500 ng / ml for monodesethylflurazepam, didesethylflurazepam or N-1-hydroxaethylflurazepam.
Pharmacokinetic Data obtained by this Method described on pp. Mit der Methode erhaltene pharmakokinetische Daten sind beschrieben auf S.		See part: Blood-, Serum- and Plasma-Levels and Other Pharmacokinetic Data from Literature
Method is recommended for: Methode ist empfohlen für:	monitoring plasma levels of flurazepam and its main metabolites following i.v. administration of Dalmane.	the quantitation of the major urinary metabolites in subjects who received a single 90-mg dose of Dalmane.

Benzodiazepine(s)/ Benzodiazepin(e)	Flurazepam	
Method / Methode	Radioimmunoassay	
Authors / Verfasser	GLOVER, EARLEY, DELANEY and DIXON	
Lit.Ref./ Lit.Zitat	(2948)	
Year of Publication/ Publikationsjahr	1980	
Extraction Procedure/ Extraktionsverfahren		
Drug analyzed/ analysierte Substanz	Benzodiazepine	
Drug calculated / berechnete Substanz	Benzodiazepine	
Metabolites included / Metabolite inbegriffen	no	
qual./quant./Screening Method (e)	quant. / Screening	
Sample required/ benötigtes Untersuchungsmaterial	1 ml plasma	
Concentration Range/ Konzentrationsbereich	0.1 - 5 ng/ml	
Special Equipment/ Spezialausstattung	RIA	
Hydrolysis / Hydrolyse	no	
Some Other Data: Einige andere Daten:	Sensitivity limit: 0.1 ng/ml C.V. (n = 6) less than 9 % (range 0.1 - 1.6 ng/ml)	
Pharmacokinetic Data obtained by this Method described on pp. Mit der Methode erhaltene pharmakokinetische Daten sind beschrieben auf S.		
Method is recommended for: Methode ist empfohlen für:	monitoring and screening plasma levels of flurazepam	

Benzodiazepine(s)/ Benzodiazepin(e)	Bromazepam	Bromazepam
Method / Methode	GLC-ECD 2% Carbowax 20M-TPA Gas Chrom P (100-120 mesh)	GLC-ECD 3% OV-17 Gas Chrom Q (60-80 mesh)
Authors / Verfasser	DE SILVA and KAPLAN	DE SILVA, BEKERSKY, BROOKS, WEINFELD, GLOVER and PUGLISI
Lit.Ref./ Lit.Zitat	(237)	(233)
Year of Publication/ Publikationsjahr	1966	1974
Extraction Procedure/ Extraktionsverfahren	pH 9, diethylether, hydrolysis (see (237)	pH 9, diethylether, (see 233 for details)
Drug analyzed/ analysierte Substanz	Hydrolysis product	Benzodiazepine
Drug calculated / berechnete Substanz	Benzodiazepine	Benzodiazepine
Metabolites included / Metabolite inbegriffen	(yes) (metabolites which also yield 2-amino-5-bromo-benzoylpyridine)	no
qual./quant./Screening Method (e)	quant.	quant.
Sample required/ benötigtes Untersuchungsmaterial	1 ml blood	2 ml blood
Concentration Range/ Konzentrationsbereich	ca. 100- 500 ng / ml	ca. 10 - 500 ng / ml
Special Equipment/ Spezialausstattung	ECD-detection	ECD-detection
Hydrolysis / Hydrolyse	yes (acid)	no
Some Other Data: Einige andere Daten:	Recovery: ca. 61.0 % ± 3 Sensitivity limit: 70 - 100 ng / ml	Recovery: overall from blood 85 % ± 5 (bromazepam) Sensitivity limit: 5 - 10 ng / ml (bromazepam)
Pharmacokinetic Data obtained by this Method described on pp. Mit der Methode erhaltene pharmakokinetische Daten sind beschrieben auf S.	See part: Blood-, Serum- and Plasma-Levels and Other Pharmacokinetic Data from Literature	See part: Blood-, Serum- and Plasma-Levels and Other Pharmacokinetic Data from Literature
Method is recommended for: Methode ist empfohlen für:	the determination of bromazepam levels in blood after blood-level fall-off studies (via hydrolysis product).	the determination of blood levels of bromazepam after single oral 12-mg doses.

Benzodiazepine(s)/ Benzodiazepin(e)	Bromazepam	Bromazepam
Method / Methode	GLC-ECD 3% OV-225 Gas Chrom Q (60-80 mesh)	TLC
Authors / Verfasser	CANO, BAILLE and VIALA	HAEFELFINGER
Lit.Ref./ Lit.Zitat	(161)	(448)
Year of Publication/ Publikationsjahr	1975	1977
Extraction Procedure/ Extraktionsverfahren	pH 9, diethylether	Na_3PO_4-sol., chloromethane - toluene (99 : 1)
Drug analyzed/ analysierte Substanz	Hydrolysis product	Benzodiazepine Hydrolysis product
Drug calculated / berechnete Substanz	Benzodiazepine	Benzodiazepine
Metabolites included / Metabolite inbegriffen	no	no
qual./quant./Screening Method (e)	quant.	quant.
Sample required/ benötigtes Untersuchungsmaterial	1 ml plasma	0.5 ml plasma
Concentration Range/ Konzentrationsbereich	ca. 10 - 100 ng / ml	ca. 5 - 120 ng/ml
Special Equipment/ Spezialausstattung	ECD-detection	Scanner for TLC
Hydrolysis / Hydrolyse	yes (acid)	without and with hydrolysis
Some Other Data: Einige andere Daten:	Recovery: 86 % ± 2.35 (range 50-100 ng/ml plasma) Sensitivity limit: 5 ng / ml	Recovery: more than 90 % (down to 5 ng/ml) Reproducibility: C.V. = 6 % (5 - 150 ng/ml) (both methods) Sensitivity limits: 5 ng / ml using 0.5 ml plasma (both methods)
Pharmacokinetic Data obtained by this Method described on pp. Mit der Methode erhaltene pharmakokinetische Daten sind beschrieben auf S.		
Method is recommended for: Methode ist empfohlen für:	measuring the blood kinetics of bromazepam up to the 72nd hour following the oral administration of a single dose of between 3 and 12 mg.	the determination of bromazepam levels in plasma after single therapeutic doses of bromazepam.

Benzodiazepine(s)/ Benzodiazepin(e)	Bromazepam	
Method / Methode	Polarography (DPP-mode)	
Authors / Verfasser	DE SILVA, BEKERSKY, BROOKS, WEINFELD, GLOVER and PUGLISI	
Lit.Ref./ Lit.Zitat	(233)	
Year of Publication/ Publikationsjahr	1974	
Extraction Procedure/ Extraktionsverfahren	pH 9, diethylether (see (233)for details)	
Drug analyzed/ analysierte Substanz	Benzodiazepine	
Drug calculated / berechnete Substanz	Benzodiazepine	
Metabolites included / Metabolite inbegriffen	yes (3-hydroxybromazepam, bromazepam-N-oxide, hydrolysis products)	
qual./quant./Screening Method (e)	quant.	
Sample required/ benötigtes Untersuchungsmaterial	5 ml urine	
Concentration Range/ Konzentrationsbereich	ca. 100 - 500 ng/ml (bromazepam and 2-amino-5-bromobenzoylpyridine)	ca. 500 - 3000 ng/ ml (3-hydroxybromazepam and 2-amino-3-hydroxy-5-bromobenzoylpyridine)
Special Equipment/ Spezialausstattung	Polarograph (DPP-mode)	
Hydrolysis / Hydrolyse	yes (enzymatic)	
Some Other Data: Einige andere Daten:	Recovery: overall 80 % ± 5 (bromazepam and 2-amino-5-bromobenzoylpyridine) Sensitivity limits: 100 ng/ 5 ml urine (bromazepam) 50 ng/ 5ml urine (2-amino-5-bromobenzoylpyridine)	45 % ± 5 (3-hydroxybromazepam and 2-amino-3-hydroxy-5-bromobenzoylpyridine) Sensitivity limits: 100 ng / 5 ml urine (3-hydroxybromazepam and 2-amino-3-hydroxy-5-bromobenzoylpyridine resp.)
Pharmacokinetic Data obtained by this Method described on pp. Mit der Methode erhaltene pharmakokinetische Daten sind beschrieben auf S.	See part: Blood-, Serum- and Plasma-Levels and Other Pharmacokinetic Data from Literature	
Method is recommended for: Methode ist empfohlen für:	the determination of the urinary excretion of bromazepam and its major urinary metabolites after single oral 12-mg doses.	

Benzodiazepine(s)/ Benzodiazepin(e)	Flunitrazepam	Flunitrazepam
Method / Methode	GLC-ECD 3% OV-17 Gas Chrom Q (60-80 mesh)	GLC-ECD 3% OV-225 Gas Chrom Q (60-80 mesh)
Authors / Verfasser	DE SILVA and BEKERSKY	DE SILVA, PUGLISI and MUNNO
Lit.Ref./ Lit.Zitat	(231)	(242)
Year of Publication/ Publikationsjahr	1974	1974
Extraction Procedure/ Extraktionsverfahren	pH 9, benzene - methylene chloride (90 : 10)	pH 9, benzene - methylene chloride (90 : 10)
Drug analyzed/ analysierte Substanz	Benzodiazepine	Benzophenone
Drug calculated / berechnete Substanz	Benzodiazepine	Benzodiazepine
Metabolites included / Metabolite inbegriffen	yes (N-desmethylflunitrazepam	no
qual./quant./Screening Method (e)	quant.	quant.
Sample required/ benötigtes Untersuchungsmaterial	1 ml blood	2 ml blood 5 ml urine
Concentration Range/ Konzentrationsbereich	ca. 1 - 10 ng / ml	ca. 50 - 250 ng / ml
Special Equipment/ Spezialausstattung	ECD-detection	ECD-detection
Hydrolysis / Hydrolyse	no	yes (acid)
Some Other Data: Einige andere Daten:	Recovery: overall 90 % ± 5.0 (flunitrazepam) 80 % ± 5.0 (norflunitrazepam) (range 2 - 10 ng / ml) Sensitivity limit: 0.5 - 1.0 ng / ml	Recovery: overall 108.7 % ± 8.0 (flunitrazepam) 110.6 % ± 8.3 (norflunitrazepam) (range 50-250 ng / ml) Sensitivity limit: 0.5 - 1.0 ng / ml
Pharmacokinetic Data obtained by this Method described on pp. Mit der Methode erhaltene pharmakokinetische Daten sind beschrieben auf S.	See part: Blood-, Serum- and Plasma-Levels and Other Pharmacokinetic Data from Literature	See part: Blood-, Serum- and Plasma-Levels and Other Pharmacokinetic Data from Literature
Method is recommended for: Methode ist empfohlen für:	the determination of blood levels of flunitrazepam and norflunitrazepam following single oral 2-mg doses of flunitrazepam (rapid method).	the determination of flunitrazepam (and clonazepam) in blood after administration of single doses.

Benzodiazepine(s)/ Benzodiazepin(e)	Flunitrazepam	Flunitrazepam
Method / Methode	GLC-ECD 3% OV-225 Gas Chrom Q (60-80 mesh)	GLC-ECD 8% SE-30 Chromosorb W AW DMCS (80-100 mesh)
Authors / Verfasser	CANO, GUINTRAND, AUBERT and VIALA	FABER, KOK and REMPT-VAN DIJK
Lit.Ref./ Lit.Zitat	(163)	(301)
Year of Publication/ Publikationsjahr	1977	1977
Extraction Procedure/ Extraktionsverfahren	pH 9, diethylether	benzene
Drug analyzed/ analysierte Substanz	Benzophenone	Benzodiazepine
Drug calculated / berechnete Substanz	Benzodiazepine	Benzodiazepine
Metabolites included / Metabolite inbegriffen	yes (norflunitrazepam)	yes (norflunitrazepam)
qual./quant./Screening Method (e)	quant.	quant.
Sample required/ benötigtes Untersuchungsmaterial	0.5 - 1 ml plasma	1 ml serum
Concentration Range/ Konzentrationsbereich	ca. 2.5 - 15 ng / ml	10 - 300 ng / ml
Special Equipment/ Spezialausstattung	ECD-detection	ECD-detection
Hydrolysis / Hydrolyse	yes (acid)	no
Some Other Data: Einige andere Daten:	Sensitivity limit: 0.5 ng / ml plasma	Recovery: overall 99.7 % ± 4.9 (flunitrazepam) 98.6 % ± 7.8 (norflunitrazepam) (from serum) Detection limit: ca. 1 ng / ml serum
Pharmacokinetic Data obtained by this Method described on pp. Mit der Methode erhaltene pharmakokinetische Daten sind beschrieben auf S.	See part: Blood-, Serum- and Plasma-Levels and Other Pharmacokinetic Data from Literature	
Method is recommended for: Methode ist empfohlen für:	pharmacokinetic studies after administration of therapeutic doses of flunitrazepam (also drug monitoring).	single dose experiments and interaction studies with some other benzodiazepines and their metabolites and non-related drugs.

Benzodiazepine(s)/ Benzodiazepin(e)	Flunitrazepam Bromazepam	Flunitrazepam
Method / Methode	GLC N-FID (bromazepam) ECD (flunitrazepam)	Radioimmunoassay
Authors / Verfasser	KANIEWSKA and WEJMAN	GLOVER and DIXON
Lit.Ref./ Lit.Zitat	(3100)	(2947)
Year of Publication/ Publikationsjahr	1980	1980
Extraction Procedure/ Extraktionsverfahren	pH 7, diethylether	pH 9, hexane
Drug analyzed/ analysierte Substanz	Benzodiazepine	Benzodiazepine
Drug calculated / berechnete Substanz	Benzodiazepine	Benzodiazepine
Metabolites included / Metabolite inbegriffen	no	no
qual./quant./Screening Method (e)	quant.	quant./Screening
Sample required/ benötigtes Untersuchungsmaterial	1 - 4 ml plasma 1 ml urine	0.1 ml plasma 0.1 ml whole blood
Concentration Range/ Konzentrationsbereich	2,500 - 10,000 ng/ml (bromazepam) 12.5 - 50 ng/ml (flunitrazepam)	1.65 - 10 ng/ml
Special Equipment/ Spezialausstattung	N-FID or ECD resp.	RIA
Hydrolysis / Hydrolyse	no	no
Some Other Data: Einige andere Daten:	Bromazepam Recovery (n=10) 94.7 ± 7.5% (from plasma) 93.4 ± 8 % (from urine) Sensitivity limit: 600 ng/ml Flunitrazepam Recovery (n=15 and 6 resp.) 92.7 ± 8 % (from plasma) 94.8 ± 6.5% (from urine) Sensitivity limit: 3 ng/ml	Intra-Assay C.V.: less than 10% Inter-Assay C.V.: less than 10% Sensitivity limit: 0.15 ng/ml
Pharmacokinetic Data obtained by this Method described on pp. Mit der Methode erhaltene pharmakokinetische Daten sind beschrieben auf S.		
Method is recommended for: Methode ist empfohlen für:	monitoring flunitrazepam and bromazepam levels in plasma and urine	the screening and quantitation of therapeutic concentrations of flunitrazepam in plasma and whole blood

Benzodiazepine(s)/ Benzodiazepin(e)	Flunitrazepam	
Method / Methode	HPLC	
Authors / Verfasser	VREE, LENSELINK and VAN DER KLEIJN	
Lit.Ref./ Lit.Zitat	(1185)	
Year of Publication/ Publikationsjahr	1977	
Extraction Procedure/ Extraktionsverfahren	pH 7.4, n-hexane	
Drug analyzed/ analysierte Substanz	Benzodiazepine	
Drug calculated / berechnete Substanz	Benzodiazepine	
Metabolites included / Metabolite inbegriffen	yes (norflunitrazepam and 7-aminoflunitrazepam)	
qual./quant./Screening Method (e)	quant.	
Sample required/ benötigtes Untersuchungsmaterial	1 ml blood or plasma	
Concentration Range/ Konzentrationsbereich	more than 1 ng / ml	
Special Equipment/ Spezialausstattung	HPLC-equipment (detection 230 nm)	
Hydrolysis / Hydrolyse	no	
Some Other Data: Einige andere Daten:	Recovery: overall 75 % ± 3 (flunitrazepam) Detection limit: 1 ng / ml	
Pharmacokinetic Data obtained by this Method described on pp. Mit der Methode erhaltene pharmakokinetische Daten sind beschrieben auf S.		
Method is recommended for: Methode ist empfohlen für:	pharmacokinetic studies and routine determination of plasma concentrations associated with anesthesia.	

Benzodiazepine(s)/ Benzodiazepin(e)	Clobazam	Clobazam
Method / Methode	GLC-NFID 2% OV-101 Chromosorb W 120-150 um	GLC-ECD OV-101 Chromosorb WHP 80 - 100 mesh
Authors / Verfasser	HAJDU, UIHLEIN and DAMM	GREENBLATT
Lit.Ref./ Lit.Zitat	(2996)	(2958)
Year of Publication/ Publikationsjahr	1980	1980
Extraction Procedure/ Extraktionsverfahren	diethylether	benzene - isopentanol (98.5 : 1.5)
Drug analyzed/ analysierte Substanz	Benzodiazepine	Benzodiazepine
Drug calculated / berechnete Substanz	Benzodiazepine	Benzodiazepine
Metabolites included / Metabolite inbegriffen	yes (norclobazam)	yes (norclobazam)
qual./quant./Screening Method (e)	quant.	quant.
Sample required/ benötigtes Untersuchungsmaterial	1 ml serum	0.5 - 1ml plasma or serum
Concentration Range/ Konzentrationsbereich	1 - 25 ng/injection	10 - 300 ng/ml
Special Equipment/ Spezialausstattung	NFID	ECD
Hydrolysis / Hydrolyse	no	no
Some Other Data: Einige andere Daten:	Detection limit: 5 ng/ml (clobazam) 15 ng/ml (norclobazam)	Detection limit: 3-5 ng/ml (clobazam) 5-10ng/ml (norclobazam) rel.S.D.: less than 6 %
Pharmacokinetic Data obtained by this Method described on pp. Mit der Methode erhaltene pharmakokinetische Daten sind beschrieben auf S.		
Method is recommended for: Methode ist empfohlen für:	monitoring of clobazam and norclobazam levels after therapeutic doses	pharmacokinetic studies of clobazam and norclobazam following single therapeutic doses

Benzodiazepine(s)/ Benzodiazepin(e)	Clobazam	Clobazam
Method / Methode	GLC-ECD 5% OV-25 Chromosorb G AW DMCS (80-100 mesh)	Fluorimetry
Authors / Verfasser	CACCIA, BALLABIO, GUISO and ZANINI	STEWART, HONIGBERG, TSAI and HAJDU
Lit.Ref./ Lit.Zitat	(2478)	(2491)
Year of Publication/ Publikationsjahr	1979	1979
Extraction Procedure/ Extraktionsverfahren	pH 9.5, benzene	hexane
Drug analyzed/ analysierte Substanz	Benzodiazepine	Benzodiazepine
Drug calculated / berechnete Substanz	Benzodiazepine	Benzodiazepine
Metabolites included / Metabolite inbegriffen	yes (norclobazam)	no
qual./quant./Screening Method (e)	quant.	quant.
Sample required/ benötigtes Untersuchungsmaterial	0.1 - 0.5 ml plasma	1ml plasma
Concentration Range/ Konzentrationsbereich	10 - 200 ng / ml	100 - 6400 ng / ml
Special Equipment/ Spezialausstattung	ECD-detection	Fluorimeter
Hydrolysis / Hydrolyse	no	no
Some Other Data: Einige andere Daten:	Recovery: mean ± S.D. (n = 8) 94 ± 0.6 (10 ng added) clobazam 98 ± 5.6 (200ng added) clobazam 90 ± 0.7 (10 ng added) norclobaz. 94 ± 8.8 (200ng added) norclobaz. Reproducibility: C.V. = 4.26 - 6.32 (clobazam) C.V. = 4.8 - 9.8 (norclobazam) Detection limit: 0.1 ng	Recovery: (extraction with hexane) 51.27 % ± 2.00 (clobazam) Accuracy: 0.5 - 7.8 % Detection limit: 50 ng / ml
Pharmacokinetic Data obtained by this Method described on pp. Mit der Methode erhaltene pharmakokinetische Daten sind beschrieben auf S.		See part: Blood-, Serum- and Plasma-Levels and Other Pharmacokinetic Data from Literature
Method is recommended for: Methode ist empfohlen für:	the determination of clobazam and N-desmethylclobazam in plasma.	the determination of clobazam in plasma especially in the range 100 - 1000 ng / ml.

Benzodiazepine(s)/ Benzodiazepin(e)	Clobazam	Clobazam
Method / Methode	Fluorometry	TLC
Authors / Verfasser	HAJDU, UIHLEIN and DAMM	HAJDU, UIHLEIN and DAMM
Lit.Ref./ Lit.Zitat	(2996)	(2996)
Year of Publication/ Publikationsjahr	1980	1980
Extraction Procedure/ Extraktionsverfahren	diethylether	pH 7.5, ethylacetate
Drug analyzed/ analysierte Substanz	Fluorophore	Benzodiazepine
Drug calculated / berechnete Substanz	Benzodiazepine	Benzodiazepine
Metabolites included / Metabolite inbegriffen	yes	yes (desmethyl- and hydroxy-metabolites)
qual./quant./Screening Method (e)	quant.	qual./quant./Screening
Sample required/ benötigtes Untersuchungsmaterial	1 ml serum	1 ml urine
Concentration Range/ Konzentrationsbereich	100 - 1000 ng/ml	ca. 100 - 1000 ng/ml
Special Equipment/ Spezialausstattung		
Hydrolysis / Hydrolyse	no	no
Some Other Data: Einige andere Daten:	Detection limit: 40 ng/ml	Detection limit: 50 ng/ml (clobazam) 35 ng/ml (norclobazam) 65 ng/ml (4'-hydroxyclobazam) 25 ng/ml (4'-hydroxynorclobazam)
Pharmacokinetic Data obtained by this Method described on pp. Mit der Methode erhaltene pharmakokinetische Daten sind beschrieben auf S.		
Method is recommended for: Methode ist empfohlen für:	therapeutic drug monitoring of clobazam levels	determination of clobazam and metabolites in urine

Benzodiazepine(s)/ Benzodiazepin(e)	Camazepam	
Method / Methode	GLC-ECD 3% OV-17 Chromosorb W (HP) (80-100 mesh)	
Authors / Verfasser	CUISINAUD, PEILLON, FERRY, DERUAZ and SASSARD	
Lit.Ref./ Lit.Zitat	(2494)	
Year of Publication/ Publikationsjahr	1979	
Extraction Procedure/ Extraktionsverfahren	pH 7.2, diethylether	
Drug analyzed/ analysierte Substanz	Benzodiazepine	
Drug calculated / berechnete Substanz	Benzodiazepine	
Metabolites included / Metabolite inbegriffen	no	
qual./quant./Screening Method (e)	quant.	
Sample required/ benötigtes Untersuchungsmaterial	1 ml plasma	
Concentration Range/ Konzentrationsbereich	10 - 200 ng / ml	
Special Equipment/ Spezialausstattung	ECD-detection	
Hydrolysis / Hydrolyse	no	
Some Other Data: Einige andere Daten:	Recovery: mean ± S.D. n = 7-8 9.1 ± 0.19 ng/ml (10ng/ml added) 19.0 ± 1.16 ng/ml (20ng/ml added) 36.9 ± 0.54 ng/ml (40ng/ml added) 98.1 ± 2.51 ng/ml (100ng/ml added) Sensitivity limit: about 5 ng/ml	
Pharmacokinetic Data obtained by this Method described on pp. Mit der Methode erhaltene pharmakokinetische Daten sind beschrieben auf S.	See part: Blood-, Serum- and Plasma-Levels and Other Pharmacokinetic Data from Literature	
Method is recommended for: Methode ist empfohlen für:	the determination of camazepam concentrations in plasma following single and multiple oral doses of camazepam.	

Blood-, Serum- and Plasma-Levels and Other Pharmacokinetic Data from Literature

Blut-, Serum und Plasma-Spiegel und andere pharmakokinetische Daten aus der Literatur

Scheme of the Compilation

Single Oral Administration
Single i.v. Administration
Single i.m. Administration
Single Rectal Administration
Multiple Oral Administration
Other Pharmacokinetic Data

CHLORDIAZEPOXIDE — Single Dose Studies - Oral Administration

Dose	Body fluid sampled	Peak concentration C = Chlordiazepoxide	(Lit.Ref.)	Time of peak concentration (hr after dose)	Subjects Characteristics
5 mg	plasma	C = 170 - 190 ng/ml	(1226)		2 Subjects
10 mg	plasma	C = 390 - 420 ng/ml	(1226)		2 Subjects
10 mg	plasma	C = 320 - 540 ng/ml	(134)	approx. after 2 hr.	3 Subjects
20 mg	plasma	C approx. 1000 ng/ml N-Desmethylchlordiazepoxide: 140 - 460 ng/ml	(1003)		6 Subjects[a]
20 mg	serum	C approx. 1000 ng/ml	(1945)	approx. after 1 hr.	
20 mg	serum	C= 1100 - 1160 ng/ml N-Desmethylchlordiazepoxide: 100 - 300 ng/ml Demoxepam: approx. 50 ng/ml	(1946)	approx. after 40 min. approx. after 6 hr. approx. after 24 hr.	2 Subjects
20 mg	plasma	C= 800 - 2200 ng/ml	(1063)	0.33 hr.- 8 hr.	12 Subjects
25 mg	blood	C= 760 - 2050 ng/ml N-Desmethylchlordiazepoxide: approx. 510 ng/ml	(426)	after 1 - 12 hr.	9 Subjects[b]
25 mg	serum	C= 1320 ± 230 ng/ml C= 1420 ± 230 ng/ml	(402)	after 1 hr. after 2 hr.	8 Subjects
25 mg	plasma	C= 260 - 1630 ng/ml	(1497)		18 Subjects
25 mg	blood	C= 480 - 1250 ng/ml	(1027)	after 0.48 - 1.25 hr.	28 Subjects[c]

[a] 25 - 43 years, [b] 18 - 38 years, [c] 21 - 30 years (another study: 8 male between 63 and 74 years, results: peak blood conc. between 370 and 980 ng/ml after 1.0-8.0 hr. $t_{1/2\alpha}$ = 19.6 min)

CHLORDIAZEPOXIDE	Single Dose Studies - Oral Administration (continued)				
Dose	Body fluid sampled	Peak concentration C= Chlordiazepoxide	(Lit.Ref.)	Time of peak concentration (hr after dose)	Subjects Characteristics
30 mg	plasma	C= 1300 - 2000 ng/ml	(598)	after 2 - 4 hr.	3 Subjects
(3 x 10mg) (0,3,6 hr.)	plasma	C= 1000 - 2000 ng/ml			
30 mg	plasma	C= 2390 ng/ml	(445)	after 1.5 hr.	1 Subject
		N-Desmethylchlordiazepoxide: 560 ng/ml		after 8 hr.	
		Demoxepam: 80 ng/ml		after 72 hr.	
30 mg	plasma	C= 2300 ng/ml	(261)	after 1 hr.	1 Subject
30 mg	plasma	C= 1380 ng/ml	(1106)	after 1 - 1.5 hr	1 Subject
		N-Desmethylchlordiazepoxide: 500 ng/ml		after 24 hr.	
30 mg	plasma	C = 860 ng/ml	(1107)	after 5.5 hr.	1 Subject
		N-Desmethylchlordiazepoxide: 450 ng/ml		after 15 - 30 hr.	
		Demoxepam: 130 ng/ml		after 48 hr	
30 mg	plasma	C = 950 - 1600 ng/ml	(134)	approx. after 2 hr.	6 Subjects[d)]
50 mg	blood	C =1150 - 2070 ng/ml	(1524)	after 1.0 - 6.0 hr.	14 Subjects[e)]
50 mg	blood	C =1750 ± 180 ng/ml	(428)	after 1.0 - 1.5 hr.	8 Subjects
50 mg	blood	C =1000 - 2000 ng/ml	(1517)	approx. 1 - 7 hr.	3 Subjects
		N-Desmethylchlordiazepoxide: 500 - 700 ng/ml		approx. 8 - 12 hr.	
100 mg	plasma	C =2320 -13340 ng/ml	(1080)		30 Subjects (14 received also 100 mg night before surgery)
		N-Desmethylchlordiazepoxide: 200 - 4090 ng/ml			

d) 25 - 29 years, e) 21 - 38 years

CHLORDIAZEPOXIDE	Single Dose Studies - Intravenous Administration				
Dose	Body fluid sampled	Peak concentration C= Chlordiazepoxide	(Lit.Ref.)	Time of peak concentration (after dose)	Subjects Characteristics
30 mg	plasma	C = 1350 ng/ml	(445)	(after 1 hr.)	1 Subject
		N-Desmethylchlordiazepoxide: 320 ng/ml		after 8 - 12 hr.	
		Demoxepam: 70 ng/ml		after 24 -72 hr.	
30 mg	plasma	C= 1500 - 2000 ng/ml approx.	(134)	after some min.	6 Subjects[a)]
50 mg	blood	C= 1490 - 2390 ng/ml	(2196)	after some min.	11 Subjects
		N-Desmethylchlordiazepoxide: 230 - 830 ng/ml		after 8 - 36 hr.	
50 mg	blood	C= approx. 2100ng/ml	(424)	after some min.	14 Subjects[b)]
		N-Desmethylchlordiazepoxide: approx. 500ng/ml		after approx. 10 hr.	
100 mg	plasma	C= 6000 - 9000 ng/ml	(999)	after some min.	2 Subjects
		N-Desmethylchlordiazepoxide: 600 - 1800 ng/ml		after approx. 24 hr.	
		Demoxepam: 250 - 500 ng/ml		after 23 - 50 hr	

a) 25 - 29 years, b) 24 - 30 years

CHLORDIAZEPOXIDE	Single Dose Studies - Intramuscular Administration				
Dose	Body fluid sampled	Peak concentration C= Chlordiazepoxide	(Lit.Ref.)	Time of peak concentration (after dose)	Subjects Characteristics
25 mg	serum	C= 560 ± 220 ng/ml C= 640 ± 280 ng/ml	(402)	after 1 hr. after 2 hr.	10 Subjects
30 mg	plasma	C= 400-900 ng/ml	(134)	after 4 - 6 hr	6 Subjects
50 mg	blood	C= 1000 ± 240 ng/ml	(428)	after 1.5-10.5 hr	8 Subjects
50 mg	blood	C= 870 ng/ml (mean)	(1525)	after 7.6 hr (mean)	14 Subjects

CHLORDIAZEPOXIDE	Multiple Dose Studies - Oral Administration			
Dose per day	Body fluid sampled	Steady state concentrations C = Chlordiazepoxide	(Lit.Ref.)	Subjects Characteristics
20 mg (10 mg b.i.d.)	plasma	C = 890 ng/ml	(1226)	1 Subject 2 weeks therapy
28 mg (mean)	plasma	C= 460 - 3210 ng/ml N-Desmethylchlordiazepoxide: 850 - 3540 ng/ml Demoxepam: 670 - 3800 ng/ml	(126)	19 Subjects
30 mg	plasma	C= 1230 - 1650 ng/ml N-Desmethylchlordiazepoxide: 330 - 410 ng/ml Demoxepam: 400 - 530 ng/ml	(445)	1 Subject
30 mg (10 mg t.i.d.) (30 mg q.d.)	plasma	C= 376 - 1310 ng/ml N-Desmethylchlordiazepoxide: 311 - 851 ng/ml Demoxepam: ND - 550 ng/ml	(133)	8 Subjects
30 mg (10 mg t.i.d.)	plasma	C= 1210 ng/ml (after 11 hr.) N-Desmethylchlordiazepoxide: 760 ng/ml (after 15 hr.) Demoxepam: 230 ng/ml (after 24-36 hr.)	(1107)	1 Subject
30 mg (10 mg t.i.d.)	plasma	C= 670 ng/ml (after 15 hr.) N-Desmethylchlordiazepoxide: 340 ng/ml (after 30 hr.)	(1106)	1 Subject
40 mg (10 mg q.i.d.)	plasma	C= 3420 ng/ml (after 14 days) N-Desmethylchlordiazepoxide: 1270 ng/ml (after 6 - 12 days) Demoxepam: 1410 ng/ml (after 10-12 days)	(999)	1 Subject (14 days therapy)
50 mg	blood	C= 1200 - 2100 ng / ml N-Desmethylchlordiazepoxide: 580 - 860 ng / ml Demoxepam: 490 - 560 ng / ml	(1517)	3 Subjects
55 mg	plasma	C= 0 - 4500 ng / ml N-Desmethylchlordiazepoxide: 700 - 2200 ng / ml Demoxepam: 0 - 130 ng / ml	(1687)	15 Subjects
75 mg (25 mg t.i.d.)	plasma	C= 3240 ng/ml	(1226)	1 Subject (39 week therapy)
100 mg (25 mg q.i.d.)	plasma	C= 2010 - 4110 ng/ml	(1226)	2 Subjects (6-7 weeks therapy)
150 mg (50 mg t.i.d.)	plasma	C= 6890 ng/ml	(1226)	1 Subject (1 week therapy)

Single Dose - Oral Administration

Absorption Half-Life $t_{1/2\,a}$

blood

19.2 - 193 min (1524)
0.71 hr. (428)
5.5 min (1027)
(21 - 30 years)
19.6 min (1027)
(63 - 74 years)

plasma

15.5 - 57.4 min (134)

Elimination Half-Life $t_{1/2\beta}$

blood

5 - 30 hr. (1524)

plasma

22 - 24 hr. (^{14}C) (600)
20 - 24 hr. (598)
6.6 - 28 hr. (1003)
9.5 - 10.3hr. (1946)

Single Dose - Intravenous Administration

Distribution Half-Life $t_{1/2\alpha}$

blood

0.75 - 3.36 hr.(424)

plasma

0.15 - 0.61 hr.(134)
0.06 hr. (1003)
0.2 hr. (1509)

Elimination Half-Life $t_{1/2\beta}$

blood

5 - 26 hr. (2196)
9.1 - 34.1hr. (424)

plasma

6.6 - 13.6hr. (134)
14.2 hr. (1003)
12.0 hr. (1509)
9.5 hr. (1849)
4.1 - 16.4 hr.(1704)

Single Dose - Intramuscular Administration

Distribution Half-Life $t_{1/2\alpha}$

blood

3.39 hr. ± 0.66 SE (1525)

Absorption Half-Life $t_{1/2\,a}$

9.0 min ± 3.2 min (1525)

Remarks: Elimination Half-Life of chlordiazepoxide is prolonged in elderly, in those with cirrhosis and in subjects receiving concurrent disulfiram therapy, (1524).
Volumes of Distribution between 0.25 and 0.50 ltrs/kg (1524), (following oral administration).
Differences in peak levels after single i.v. administration are only partially explained by body weight (2196).
Elimination Half-Life of chlordiazepoxide and Clearance did not differ significantly between sexes (424).
Volumes of Distribution between 0.22 and 0.75 ltrs/kg following single i.v. administration (134, 424, 1003, 1509, 1704, 1849).

Clearance between 11.0 and 127.8 ml/min after i.v. administration (134, 424, 1003, 1509, 1704, 1849) (= 0.17 - 2.16 ml/min/kg).

No correlations were found between anxiety reduction and Chlordiazepoxide levels but between anxiety reduction and N-Desmethylchlordiazepoxide and Demoxepam levels (1687).
For other influences see: disease (1850), age (1027, 1849, 1524), sex (424, 1389), alcohol (1810), antacids (425).

Overdose-Levels: Serum concentrations in 60 cases of poisoning between 1000 and 66 000 ng/ml (174).

DIAZEPAM	Single Dose Studies - Oral Administration

Dose	Body-fluid sampled	Peak concentration observed D = Diazepam, DD = Desmethyl-diazepam (= Nordiazepam)	Lit.Ref.	Time of peak conc. after dose	Subjects Characteristics/ Remarks
2-mg	serum	60 - 159 ng/ml (D)	(115)	30 - 90 min.	6 healthy Subj.
2.5-mg	plasma	mean levels of D: 22.7 (± 2.9 S.E.) ng/ml after 3 hr; 19.6 (± 2.9 S.E.) ng/ml after 6 hr	(2208)		12 healthy Subj.
5-mg	blood saliva	72 ng/ml (D) 1.45 ng/ml (D)	(1396)	2 hr. 2 hr.	1 healthy Subj.
5-mg	plasma	ca. 160 - 220 ng/ml (D)	(548)	0.5 - 1 hr.	10 healthy Subj. free plasma oxazepam was found only in one subject
5-mg	plasma	165 (± 53.5 S.D.) (D) 206 (± 47.5 S.D.) (D)	(1473)	1 hr. 1 hr.	13 healthy Subj. without alcohol 8 healthy Subj. with alcohol (0.45 g/kg)
5-mg	plasma	199.3 (± 18.0 S.E.) ng/ml (D) 130.8 (± 9.0 S.E.) ng/ml (D) 143.6 (± 14.1 S.E.) ng/ml (D)	(1504)	1(± 0.3 S.E.)hr. 1.4(± 0.2 S.E.)hr. 1.3(± 0.2 S.E.)hr.	9 healthy Subj. (with water) 9 healthy Subj. (with Maalox) 9 healthy Subj. (with Gelusil)
5-mg	plasma	221.1 (± 17.9 S.E.) ng/ml (D) 207.5 (± 29.7 S.E.) ng/ml (D)	(1526)	0.79(±0.10S.E.)hr. 1.79(±0.48S.E.)hr.	6 healthy Subj. (25-42 years) without alcohol with alcohol
5-mg	plasma urine	ca. 170 - 220 ng/ml (D) ca. 30 ng/ml (DD) ca. 300 - 450 ng/ml (conj. DD)	(1630)	ca. 1 hr. ca. 24 hr. 0 - 6 hr.	6 healthy Subj. (31 ± 4 years)
5-mg	plasma	mean levels of D: 35.2 (± 4.6 S.E.) ng/ml after 3 hr; 39.3 (± 7.4 S.E.) ng/ml after 6 hr	(2208)		12 healthy Subj.
5-mg	plasma	ca. 105 ng/ml (D)	(2415)	45 min	10 pregnant women (normal)
5-mg	serum	168 - 240 ng/ml (D)	(115)	30 - 90 min.	6 healthy Subjects
5-mg	serum	150 - 274 ng/ml (D)	(1211)	0.5 - 1.0 hr.	7 healthy Subj.
10-mg	blood	110 - 186 ng/ml (D) 0 - 44 ng/ml (DD)	(236)	0.5 - 2.0 hr. 24 hr.	9 healthy Subj. 3 healthy Subj.
10-mg	blood	ca. 180 - 230 ng/ml (D)	(238)	ca. 1 hr.	
10-mg	blood	160 - 200 ng/ml (D)	(243)	ca. 1 hr.	2 healthy Subj.
10-mg	blood	137 - 189 ng/ml (D) 26 - 37 ng/ml (DD)	(556)	1 - 1.5 hr. 30 - 48 hr.	4 healthy Subj.
10-mg	blood	ca. 130 - 150 ng/ml (D) ca. 20 - 40 ng/ml (DD)	(845)	ca. 1 - 2 hr. ca. 24 hr.	2 healthy Subj.
10-mg	blood	54 - 186 ng/ml (D)	(2171)	0.5 - 2.0 hr.	12 healthy Subj.
10-mg	plasma	250 - 460 ng/ml (D)	(81)	1.0 - 4.0 hr.	5 healthy Subj.
10-mg	plasma	ca. 180 - 225 ng/ml (D) ca. 60 - 380 ng/ml (D)	(351)	1.0 - 1.5 hr. 1.5 hr.	10 healthy Subj. 40 healthy Subj.
10-mg	plasma	205 (± 22.9 SEM) ng/ml (D)	(352)	1.0 hr.	15 healthy Subj.

DIAZEPAM	Single Dose Studies - Oral Administration (continued)				
Dose	Body-fluid sampled	Peak concentration observed D = Diazepam, DD = Desmethyl-diazepam (= Nordiazepam)	Lit.Ref.	Time of peak conc. after dose	Subjects Characteristics/ Remarks
10-mg	plasma	ca. 50 - 270 ng/ml (D)	(353)	1.5 hr	22 Subjects (prior to minor Gynaecol.Oper.)
ca. 10-mg	plasma	ca. 250 -400 ng/ml (D) ca. 20 - 30 ng/ml (DD)	(383)	ca. 1 hr ca. 25 hr.	5 healthy Subj.
	saliva	ca. 3.8 -4.5 ng/ml (D) ca. 0.5 -1.0 ng/ml (DD)		ca. 2 hr. ca. 24 hr.	
10-mg	plasma	150 - 300 ng/ml (D)	(451)	ca. 1.75 hr.	8 healthy Subj.
10-mg	plasma	130 (± 20.5 SEM) ng/ml (D)	(547)	2 hr.	10 Subjects
10-mg	plasma	221 - 440 ng/ml (D)	(587)	1 hr.	33 healthy Subj.
10-mg	plasma	ca. 170 - 410 ng/ml (D)	(742)	ca.1 hr	8 healthy Subj.
10-mg	plasma	ca. 130 - 155 ng/ml (D)	(1017)	ca.2 hr.	14 healthy Subj.
10-mg	plasma	ca. 40 - 80 ng/ml (D)	(1017)	ca.2 hr.	12 alcoholics
10-mg	plasma	ca. 220 - 370 ng/ml (D)	(1253)	ca. 1.5 hr.	7 healthy Subj.
10-mg	plasma	196 (± 16.4 SE) ng/ml (D)	(1393)	0.75 hr.	9 healthy Subj.
	parotid saliva	6.3 (± 0.77 SE) ng/ml (D)		0.75 hr.	
	mixed saliva	6.0 (± 0.80 SE) ng/ml (D)		0.75 hr.	
10-mg	plasma	<u>mean</u> 261 (± 88 S.D.) ng/ml (D)	(1473)	1.0 hr.	30 healthy Subj. without alcohol
		<u>mean</u> 338 (±124 S.D.) ng/ml (D)		1.0 hr.	14 healthy Subj. with 0.45g/kg alcohol
10-mg	plasma	ca. 530 ng/ml (D)		1.0 hr.	8 subjects with 0.5 g/kg alcohol
10-mg	plasma	ca. 250 (± ca. 40 S.A.) ng/ml (D)	(1791)	ca.1.0 hr.	10 healthy Subj.
10-mg	plasma	ca. 200 ng/ml (D)	(2313)	ca.1.0 hr.	17 healthy Subj. without antacids
		ca. 200 ng/ml (D)		ca. 45 min.	20 Subj. with Alum.Hydrox.Gel
		ca. 180 ng/ml (D)		ca.1.0 hr.	15 Subj. with Sodium Citrate
		ca. 160 ng/ml (D)		ca. 90 min.	15 Subj. with Magnes.Trisilicate
10-mg	serum	ca. 290 - 400 ng/ml (D)	(22)	1 - 2 hr.	16 healthy Subj. (two different brands of tablets)
10-mg	serum	265 - 566 ng/ml (D)	(115)	30-90 min.	6 healthy Subj.
10-mg	serum	232 - 311 ng/ml (D)	(607)	40-90 min.	7 healthy Subj.
10-mg	serum	ca. 200 - 600 ng/ml (D)	(641)	60-120min.	5 healthy Subj.
10-mg	serum	209 (± 49 S.D.) ng/ml (D)	(1656)	90 min.	8 healthy Subj.
10-mg	serum	299 (± 64 S.D.) ng/ml (D) ca. 20 ng/ml (DD)	(1894)	1 hr. 1 hr.	6 healthy Subj.
10-mg	serum	ca. 470 ng/ml (D)	(1947)	20 min.	1 healthy Subj. (fasted before)
10-mg	serum	164 (± 95 S.D.) ng/ml (D)	(2282)	90 min.	5 healthy Subj. without alcohol
		285 (± 54 S.D.) ng/ml (D)		150 min.	with 0.8g/kg alc.
20-mg	blood	ca. 190± ca. 25 SEM ng/ml (D)	(991)	1 - 2 hr.	9 healthy Subj.
20-mg	blood	ca. 230 - 320 ng/ml (D)	(1167)	1 hr.	4 healthy fem. S.
20-mg	plasma	290 - 890 ng/ml (D)	(81)	1 - 4 hr.	3 healthy Subj.

DIAZEPAM	Single Dose Studies - Oral Administration (continued)				
Dose	Body-fluid sampled	Peak concentration observed D = Diazepam, DD = Desmethyl-diazepam (= Nordiazepam)	Lit.Ref.	Time of peak conc. after dose	Subjects Characteristics/ Remarks
20-mg	plasma	ca. 300 - 800 ng/ml (D)	(451)	ca. 1.75 hr.	8 healthy Subj.
20-mg	plasma	574 (± 127.3 S.D.) ng/ml (D)	(1473)	1 hr.	15 healthy Subj.
20-mg	plasma	ca. 400 (± ca. 40 S.D.) ng/ml (D)	(1791)	1 hr.	10 healthy Subj.
20-mg	serum	ca. 300 - 500 ng/ml (D) ca. 50 ng/ml (DD)	(485)	1 hr. 4 - 24 hr.	6 healthy Subj.
30-mg	plasma	ca. 600 - 900 ng/ml (D) ca. 40 - 100 ng/ml (DD)	(1155)	1 hr. ca. 8 hr.	5 Subjects
30-mg	plasma	ca. 700 ng/ml (D)	(1156)	ca. 1 hr.	1 Subject
30-mg	plasma	ca. 700 ng/ml (D)	(1158)	ca. 1 hr.	1 Subject
30-mg	plasma	ca. 600 (± ca.40 S.A.) ng/ml (D)	(1791)	1.5 hr.	10 healthy Subj.
Forensic Cases:					
250-mg	plasma	ca. 1700 ng/ml (D) ca. 800 ng/ml (DD) ca. 3000 ng/ml (Oxazepam unconjugated)	(1630)	after 1 day	14 year-old girl (abuse)
	urine	ca. 2000 ng/ml (DD conjug.) ca. 6000 ng/ml (Oxazepam conjug.)		after 3 days	
?	blood	ca. 1300 ng/ml (D)	(1048)		death in combin. with alcohol
?	blood	7000 - 17 000 ng/ml (total D + DD)	(1205)		18 year old male driving under the influence of D
?	blood (heart)	30 000 ng/ml (D) 4 000 ng/ml (DD)	(167)		young drug addict
1000-mg suggested	blood	7 000 ng/ml (D) 3 100 ng/ml (DD)	(150)	after 1 day after 5 days	

DIAZEPAM	Single Dose Studies - Intravenous Administration				
Dose	Body-fluid sampled	Peak concentration observed D = Diazepam, DD = Desmethyl-diazepam (= Nordiazepam)	Lit.Ref.	Time of peak conc.after dose	Subjects Characteristics Remarks
0.2-mg	plasma	ca. 410 - 520 ng/ml (D)	(554)	ca. 15 min.	12 children
5-mg	plasma	ca. 300 ng/ml (D) ca. 20 ng/ml (DD)	(1502)	few minutes ca. 50-70 hr.	1 healthy S. (29-year-old woman)
8-mg	plasma	ca. 1000 ng/ml (D) ca. 100 ng/ml (DD)	(2484)	few minutes ca. 20 hr.	8-year-old epileptic child
10-mg	blood	ca. 70 - 290 ng/ml (D)	(238)	15 min.	3 healthy S.
10-mg	blood	294 - 574 ng/ml (D)	(556)	1 - 5 min.	4 healthy S.
10-mg	blood	19 - 39 ng/ml (DD)	(556)	30 - 48 hr.	4 healthy S.
10-mg	blood	ca. 300 ng/ml (D) ca. 20 ng/ml (DD)	(845)	few minutes ca. 30 hr.	2 healthy S.
10-mg	plasma	54.7 - 95 ng/ml (DD)	(16)	few minutes (D) mean 43 hr. (DD)	4 healthy S.
10-mg	plasma	490 - 1010 ng/ml (D)	(81)	15 min.	6 healthy S.

DIAZEPAM		Single Dose Studies - Intravenous Administration (continued)			
Dose	Body-fluid sampled	Peak concentration observed D = Diazepam, DD = Desmethyl-diazepam (= Nordiazepam)	Lit.Ref.	Time of peak conc. after dose	Subjects Characteristics Remarks
10-mg	plasma	420 - 630 ng/ml (D) 10 - 40 ng/ml (DD)	(387)	few minutes ca. 8 hr.	5 healthy S.
10-mg	plasma	10 - 40 ng/ml (DD)	(552)	ca. 3 hr.	2 healthy S.
10-mg	plasma	ca. 560 - 620 ng/ml (D) ca. 40 - 50 ng/ml(DD)	(1016)	15 min. 24 hr.	13 healthy S.
10-mg	plasma	ca. 280 - 320 ng/ml (D) 30 - 40 ng/ml(DD)	(1016)	15 min. 24 hr.	14 alcoholics
10-mg	plasma	ca. 570 - 620 ng/ml (D)	(1018)	15 min.	13 healthy S.
10-mg	plasma	ca. 700 -1050 ng/ml (D)	(1253)	few minutes	12 healthy S.
10-mg	plasma	600-1232 ng/ml (D) 16- 90 ng/ml(DD)	(2215)	10 min. 24 hr.	3 Subjects (no liver disease)
10-mg	serum	ca. 400 ng/ml (D) ca. 80 ng/ml(DD)	(485)	few minutes 24-48 hr.	1 healthy S.
0.15-mg/kg	serum	190 (± 36 S.D.) ng/ml (D) 25 (± 7 S.D.) ng/ml(DD)	(605)	4 hr. (!) 8 hr.	12 healthy S.
0.15-mg/kg	serum	204 (± 34 S.D.) ng/ml (D) 41 (± 18 S.D.) ng/ml(DD)	(1655)	4 hr.(!) 10 hr	10 healthy S.
0.2-mg/kg	plasma	176 (± 37 SEM) ng/ml (D) 3 (± 3 SEM ng/ml (DD)	(550)	17 - 265 min.	6 fem. Subj.
20-mg	plasma	970-2060 ng/ml (D) 40- 90 ng/ml (DD)	(387)	30 min. 8 hr.	5 healthy S.
20-mg	plasma	ca. 950 - 1300 ng/ml (D) ca. 80 ng/ml (DD)	(1253)	few minutes 24 hr.	10 healthy S.
20-mg	serum	ca. 630 - 1600 ng/ml (D) ca. 100 ng/ml (DD)	(485)	few minutes 24 - 72 hr.	6 healthy S.
0.3-mg/kg	serum	ca. 290 - 350 ng/ml (D) ca. 50 - 60 ng/ml (DD)	(604)	ca. 2 min. ca. 6 hr.	7 healthy S.
0.30-mg/kg	serum	ca. 339 (± 79 S.D.) ng/ml (D) ca. 48 (± 15 S.D.) ng/ml (DD)	(605)	4 hr. (!) 10 hr.	11 healthy S.
0.30-mg/kg	serum	ca. 320 - 450 ng/ml (D) ca. 90 - 100 ng/ml (DD)	(638)	4 - 8 hr. 4 - 8 hr.	7 healthy S.
0.30-mg/kg	serum	ca. 336 (± 89 S.D.) ng/ml (D) ca. 48 (± 19 S.D.) ng/ml (DD)	(1655)	4 hr. (!) 10 hr.	11 healthy S.
0.30-mg/kg	serum	ca. 470 - 550 ng/ml (D)	(1660)	2 hr. (!)	6 healthy S.
0.45-mg/kg	serum	ca. 446 (± 71 S.D.) ng/ml (D) ca. 105 (± 67 S.D.) ng/ml (DD)	(605)	6 hr. (!) 10 hr.	11 healthy S.

DIAZEPAM	Single Dose Studies - Intramuscular Administration				
Dose	Body-fluid sampled	Peak concentration observed (D = Diazepam, DD = Desmethyl-diazepam (= Nordiazepam)	Lit.Ref.	Time of peak conc. after dose	Subjects Characteristics Remarks
5-mg	blood	ca. 31 - 45 ng/ml (D)	(508)	30 min.	5 women (pregnant)
5-mg	plasma	ca. 70 ng/ml (D)	(548)	3 hr.	10 healthy S.
5-mg	plasma	ca. 12 (± 4 SEM) ng/ml (D)	(548)	24 hr.	10 healthy S.
5-mg	plasma	ca. 70 - 90 ng/ml (D)	(1627)	1 - 2 hr.	10 healthy S.
5-mg	plasma	ca. 60 ng/ml (D)	(2415)	45 min.	10 women normal pregnancy
10-mg	blood	ca. 80 -220 ng/ml (D)	(238)	15 - 60 min.	3 healthy S.
10-mg	plasma	ca. 180 -270 ng/ml (D)	(41)	ca. 1 - 10 hr.	4 healthy S.
10-mg	plasma	ca. 30 - 70 ng/ml (DD)	(41)	ca. 10 - 70 hr.	4 healthy S.
10-mg	plasma	ca. 28 -133 ng/ml (D)	(269)	ca. 60 min.	31 healthy S.
10-mg	plasma	<u>mean</u> concentrations: (D) 151 (± 90 SEM) ng/ml (D) 51 (± 24 SEM) ng/ml (D) 30 (± 15 SEM) ng/ml (D) 47 (± 18 SEM) ng/ml (D) 53 (± 31 SEM) ng/ml (D) 21 (± 7 SEM) ng/ml (D) 43 (± 13 SEM) ng/ml (D) 34 (± 6 SEM) ng/ml (D)	(296) (1473)	 0 - 15 min. 16 - 45 min. 46 - 75 min. 76 -105 min. 106 -135 min. 136 -165 min. 166 -195 min. 196 -401 min.	 5 pregnant 4 women 5 during 5 labour 5 5 4 4
10-mg	plasma	ca. 10 -320 ng/ml (D)	(351)	90 min.	74 Subjects
10-mg	plasma	ca. 10 -160 ng/ml (D)	(353)	90 min.	14 Subjects
10-mg	plasma	80 (± 14 SEM) ng/ml (D)	(549)	40 - 120 min.	14 women (10 - 14 weeks duration of pregnancy)
10-mg	plasma	41 (± 6 SEM) ng/ml (D) 4 (± 1 SEM) ng/ml(DD)	(550)	30 - 140 min. 30 - 140 min.	16 women during labour
10-mg	plasma saliva	ca. 90 -140 ng/ml (D) ca. 15 - 35 ng/ml (D)	(553)	30 - 60 min. 60 min.	42 S. suffering from neurological diseases
10-mg	plasma	80 (± 13 SEM) ng/ml (D)	(1430)	40 - 120 min.	12 women (pregn.)
10-mg	serum	ca. 180 - 320 ng/ml (D)	(607)	20 - 90 min.	7 healthy S.
10.mg	serum	152 (± 60 SD) ng/ml (D) 143 (± 62 SD) ng/ml (D)	(1656)	60 min. 60 min.	shoulder admin. thigh admin.
10-mg	serum	ca. 295 (± 82 SD) ng/ml (D) ca. 20 ng/ml(DD)	(1657)	ca. 60 min. ca. 7 hr.	11 Subjects
20-mg (within 12 hr)	plasma	56 - 262 ng/ml (D) 16 - 32 ng/ml (DD)	(477)		8 Subjects
20-mg	serum	ca. 200 - 400 ng/ml (D)	(485)	1 hr.	6 healthy S.
1-mg/kg	plasma	ca.400 - 1400 ng/ml (D)	(1736)	10 - 60 min.	3 children (3-12 years)
0.3-mg/kg	plasma	84 - 171 ng/ml (D) 75 - 127 ng/ml (DD)	(745)	1 - 4 hr. 8 -48 hr.	4 children (3-8 years)
0.2-0.9-mg/kg	plasma	383 - 1152 ng/ml (D)	(7)	10min.-4 hr.	7 children (2-5 years)

DIAZEPAM		Single Dose Studies - Rectal Administration			
Dose	Body-fluid sampled	Peak concentration observed (D = Diazepam, DD = Desmethyl-diazepam (= Nordiazepam)	Lit.Ref.	Time of peak conc. after dose	Subjects Characteristics Remarks
5-mg	plasma	ca. 50 - 150 ng/ml (D) e.g. 28 (± 5 SEM) ng/ml (DD)	(548)	1 - 3 hr. 24 hr.	10 healthy S. 3 diff.supp.
10-mg	serum	ca. 200- 280 ng/ml (D)	(607)	90 min.	8 women with normal pregn.
20-mg	blood	ca. 80- 120 ng/ml (D)	(991)	ca. 4 hr.	9 fem. patients
0.5 -mg/kg	blood	353 - 1506 ng/ml (D)	(1407)	4 - 15 min.	11 children (0.5-11 years)
0.5-1.0-mg/kg	plasma	600 - 1300 ng/ml (D)	(1736)	10 - 60 min.	9 children (3-12 years)
0.4-0.6-mg/kg	plasma	mean: 564 ng/ml (D)	(1649)	1 hr.	10 children (10-22 months)
0.7-mg/kg	plasma	1100 - 2610 ng/ml (D)	(1649)	10 - 60 min.	10 children (12-24 months)
0.3-0.8-mg/kg	plasma	214 - 687 ng/ml (D)	(7)	20 - 60 min.	7 children (0.75-4.5 yrs.)
0.1-0.3-mg/kg	plasma	335 - 591 ng/ml (D)	(7)	10 - 60 min.	5 children (11-15 years)

DIAZEPAM		Multiple Dose Studies - Oral Administration		
Dose per day Duration of Therapy	Body-fluid sampled	Steady-state concentrations D = Diazepam, DD = Desmethyl-diazepam (= Nordiazepam)	Lit.Ref.	Subjects Characteristics and Remarks
4-mg (2-mg b.i.d.) 8 - 32 weeks	plasma	93 - 125 ng/ml (D) 68 - 173 ng/ml (DD) 16 ng/ml (3-Hydroxy-D)	(1227)	3 Subjects, 3-Hydroxy-D was found only in 1 case
5-mg (5-mg o.d.) 2 - 60 weeks	plasma	101 - 176 ng/ml (D) 83 - 172 ng/ml (DD) 18 - 29 ng/ml (3-Hydroxy-D)	(1227)	6 Subjects, 3-Hydroxy-D was found in 4 cases
5-mg (5-mg o.d.) 10 days	plasma	116 (± 35 S.D.) ng/ml (D) 143 (± 33 S.D.) ng/ml (DD)	(1306)	5 Subjects (after day 9)
5-mg (5-mg h.s.) 5 - 13 days	serum	70 - 208 ng/ml (D) 84 - 315 ng/ml (DD)	(1119)	7 Subjects
6-mg (3 x 2-mg) daily	plasma	100 - 180 ng/ml (D)	(81)	1 Subject (determined 2 and 4 hours after morning dose)
6-mg (2-mg t.i.d.) 1 - 60 weeks	plasma	114 - 251 ng/ml (D) 89 - 461 ng/ml (DD) 30 ng/ml (3-Hydroxy-D) (in 1 case)	(1227)	4 Subjects (urine analysis: 8 - 22 ng/ml (D) 25- 92 ng/ml(DD)
6-mg (2-mg t.i.d.) 5 - 10 days	serum	31 - 212 ng/ml (D) 0 - 213 ng/ml (DD)	(1119)	5 Subjects
8-mg (2-mg q.6.h.) 6 - 7 days	serum	110 - 210 ng/ml (D) 0 - 200 ng/ml (DD)	(1119)	2 Subjects
10-mg 15 days	blood	ca. 60 - 300 ng/ml (D) ca.100 - 150 ng/ml (DD)	(556)	4 Subjects levels after 1 week administr.

DIAZEPAM — Multiple Dose Studies - Oral Administration (continued)

Dose per day Duration of therapy	Body-fluid sampled	Steady-state concentrations D = Diazepam, DD = Desmethyl-diazepam (= Nordiazepam)	Lit.Ref.	Subjects Characteristics and Remarks
10-mg (2 x 5-mg) 5 - 41 days	serum	106 - 275 ng/ml (D) 78 - 594 ng/ml (DD)	(1119)	2 Subjects
10-mg (5-mg b.i.d.) 2 - 106 weeks	plasma	93 - 371 ng/ml (D) 130 - 464 ng/ml (DD) 13 - 48 ng/ml (3-Hydroxy-D) 15 - 31 ng/ml (Oxazepam)	(1227)	15 Subjects
10-mg (5-mg b.i.d.) 53 - 84 weeks	plasma	17 - 21 ng/ml (D) 32 - 53 ng/ml (DD)	(1227)	2 Subjects (sample obtained 6 days after the drug had been discontinued).
10-mg (10-mg o.d.) 5 - 6 days	plasma	117 - 158 ng/ml (D) 86 - 186 ng/ml (DD)	(138)	4 healthy mothers during lactation period
10-mg (10-mg o.d.) 3 weeks	plasma	233 ng/ml (D) 424 ng/ml (DD) 21 ng/ml (3-Hydroxy-D) 21 ng/ml (Oxazepam)	(1227)	1 Subject
10-mg 6 days	plasma	82 - 143 ng/ml (DD)	(585)	11 Subjects with liver disease
11-mg (mean) (range 2 -20-mg) 2 - 4 weeks	plasma	170 (± 20 SEM) ng/ml (D) 317 (± 62 SEM) ng/ml (DD)	(126)	19 Subjects
15-mg see Remarks	plasma	ca. 200 - 800 ng/ml (D) 381 - 608 ng/ml (DD)	(275)	6 Subjects (5-mg t.i.d. from day 1 - 13, 25-mg on day 14, 15-mg o.d. from day 15-24)
15-mg 5-mg t.i.d. 30 days	plasma	170 - 341 ng/ml (D) 260 - 644 ng/ml (DD)	(77)	7 Subjects
15-mg 5-mg t.i.d. regular daily	plasma	600 ng/ml (D) 430 ng/ml (D)	(81)	1 Subject after 2 hr. after 4 hr.
15-mg Day 5	plasma	325 - 635 ng/ml (D) 135 - 295 ng/ml (DD)	(218)	6 Subjects
15-mg 5-mg t.i.d. 14 days	plasma	240 ng/ml (D) 350 ng/ml (DD)	(917)	11 Subjects
15-mg 5-mg t.i.d. 4 - 16 days	serum	60 - 328 ng/ml (D) 115 - 452 ng/ml (DD)	(1119)	6 Subjects
15-mg see Remarks	plasma	ca. 200 - 800 ng/ml (D) ca. 300 - 600 ng/ml (DD)	(1195)	1 Subject (5-mg t.i.d. from day 1-13, 25-mg on day 14, 15-mg o.d. from day 15-24).
15-mg 5-mg t.i.d. 1 - 56 weeks	plasma	165 - 556 ng/ml (D) 96 - 482 ng/ml (DD) 19 - 52 ng/ml (3-Hydroxy-D) 15 - 31 ng/ml (Oxazepam)	(1227)	11 Subjects
15-mg 5-mg t.i.d. 9 - 30 days	plasma	117 - 240 ng/ml (D) 170 - 468 ng/ml (DD)	(1430)	7 women in early human pregnancy (12.-15-week)
15-mg 5-mg t.i.d. 14 days	plasma	524 (± 174 S.D.) ng/ml (D) 401 (± 185 S.D.) ng/ml (DD) 561 (± 185 S.D.) ng/ml (D) 589 (± 187 S.D.) ng/ml (DD)	(1693)	20 Subjects after 7 days after 14 days
15-mg 5-mg t.i.d. 14 days	plasma	373 (± 163 S.D.) ng/ml (D) 412 (± 241 S.D.) ng/ml (DD) 504 (± 305 S.D.) ng/ml (D) 498 (± 298 S.D.) ng/ml (DD)	(2360)	15 Subjects after 7 days after 14 days
15-mg 14 days	plasma	ca. 200 - 400 ng/ml (D) ca. 200 - 500 ng/ml (DD)	(552)	12 Subjects

DIAZEPAM	Multiple Dose Studies - Oral Administration (continued)			
Dose per day Duration of therapy	Body-fluid sampled	Steady-state concentrations D = Diazepam, DD = Desmethyl-diazepam (= Nordiazepam)	Lit.Ref.	Subjects Characteristics Remarks
15-mg 2 - 4 years	plasma	ca. 42 - 207 ng/ml (D) ca. 182 - 920 ng/ml (DD)	(552)	5 Subjects
15-mg 5-mg t.i.d. 14 days	serum	ca. 250 ng/ml (D) ca. 330 - 350 ng/ml (DD)	(486)	3 Subjects
15-mg 5-mg t.i.d. 14 days	serum	561 (± 160 S.D.) ng/ml (D) 589 (± 187 S.D.) ng/ml (DD)	(2280)	40 Subjects
20-mg 5-mg t.i.d. & hs 5 days	serum	495 - 500 ng/ml (D) 278 - 331 ng/ml (DD)	(1119)	2 Subjects
20-mg 5-mg ac & hs 5 - 7 days	serum	275 - 356 ng/ml (D) 269 - 389 ng/ml (DD)	(1119)	1 Subject
20-mg 5-mg q.i.d. 7 -23 days	serum	284 - 500 ng/ml (D) 211 - 756 ng/ml (DD)	(1119)	2 Subjects
20-mg 5-mg q.6.h. 7-31 days	serum	115 - 206 ng/ml (D) 131 - 194 ng/ml (DD)	(1119)	2 Subjects
20-mg 10-mg b.i.d. regular	plasma	520 ng/ml (D) 490 ng/ml (D)	(81)	1 Subject
20-mg 10-mg b.i.d. 3 - 61 weeks	plasma	252 - 378 ng/ml (D) 319 - 552 ng/ml (DD) 23 - 42 ng/ml (3-Hydroxy-D)	(1227) 15 - 80 ng/ml (Oxazepam)	3 Subjects
20-mg 20-mg od 5 days	plasma	433.8 (± 146.4 S.D.) ng/ml (D) 350.3 (± 219.2 S.D.) ng/ml (DD)	(219)	14 Subjects
20-25-mg 5 days	blood	164 - 402 ng/ml (D) 118 - 413 ng/ml (DD)	(243)	2 Subjects
30-mg 10-mg t.i.d. 10 days	blood	ca. 800 ng/ml (D) ca. 400 ng/ml (DD)	(238)	1 Subject
30-mg 15-mg b.i.d. 15 days	blood	ca. 500 ng/ml (D) ca. 200 ng/ml (DD)	(238)	1 Subject
30-mg 10-mg t.i.d.	plasma	850 - 1250 ng/ml (D) 620 - 1210 ng/ml (D)	(81)	3 Subjects after 2 hr. after 4 hr.
30-mg 10-mg t.i.d. 14 days	plasma	ca.250 - 1900 ng/ml (D) ca.200 - 1100 ng/ml (DD) ca.600 - 1200 ng/ml (D) ca.300 - 1800 ng/ml (DD)	(1155)	5 Subjects after 7 days after 14 days
30-mg 10-mg t.i.d. 14 days	plasma	ca. 1900 ng/ml (D) ca. 500 ng/ml (DD)	(1156)	1 Subject after 14 days
30-mg 10-mg t.i.d. 14 days	plasma	ca. 1000 ng/ml (D) ca. 300 ng/ml (DD)	(1156)	1 Subject after 14.5 days
30-mg 10-mg t.i.d. 14 days	plasma	ca. 600 - 2000 ng/ml (D) ca. 200 - 500 ng/ml (DD)	(1158)	5 Subjects after 14 days
30-mg 10-mg t.i.d.	plasma	445 - 520 ng/ml (D) 471 - 509 ng/ml (DD) 11 - 23 ng/ml (3-Hydroxy-D) 24 - 31 ng/ml (Oxazepam)	(1227)	3 Subjects
30-mg 10-mg t.i.d. 14 days	plasma	ca. 400 - 800 ng/ml (D)	(1374)	7 Subjects
30-mg 10-mg t.i.d. 7 days	serum	ca. 700 ng/ml (D) ca. 800 ng/ml (DD)	(486)	2 Subjects

DIAZEPAM	Multiple Dose Studies - Oral Administration (continued)			
Dose per day Duration of therapy	**Body-fluid sampled**	**Steady-state concentrations D = Diazepam, DD = Desmethyl-diazepam (= Nordiazepam)**	**Lit.Ref.**	**Subjects Characteristics Remarks**
30-40-mg 2 - 5 years	plasma	85 - 400 ng/ml (D) 170 -1089 ng/ml (DD)	(552)	9 Subjects
40-mg 20-mg b.i.d. 60-106 weeks	plasma	792 - 969 ng/ml (D) 1025 -1092 ng/ml (DD) 42 - 56 ng/ml (3 Hydroxy-D) 59 - 121 ng/ml (Oxazepam)	(1227)	3 Subjects
60-mg 20-mg t.i.d. 10-40 weeks	plasma	845 -1942 ng/ml (D) 1465 -2749 ng/ml (DD) 111 - 185 ng/ml (3-Hydroxy-D) 99 - 292 ng/ml (Oxazepam)	(1227)	4 Subjects
60-80-mg many years	plasma	422 ng/ml (D) 630 ng/ml (DD)	(552)	1 Subject
200-mg 8 weeks	blood	1700 ng/ml (D) 4000 ng/ml (DD) 600 ng/ml (D) 2500 ng/ml (DD)	(238)	1 Subject after 8 weeks after 9 weeks

DIAZEPAM	Pharmacokinetic Data derived from the different Studies

D = Diazepam
DD = Desmethyldiazepam

Oral Administration

Distribution Half-Life $t_{1/2\alpha}$

plasma

1.14 - 13.8 hr. (275)

Absorption Half-Life $t_{1/2a}$

plasma

32 min. (275)

18.5 ± 7.1 - 24.4 ± 5.0 min.
(= mean ± S.E.) (1504)

8.8 - 29.1 min. (1526)
(without EtOH)

13.1 - 77.9 min. (1526)
(with EtOH)

Elimination Half-Life $t_{1/2\beta}$

blood

D: 2 - 3 hr. (during first 2-3 hr.) (238)
D: 27 -48 hr. (after 24 hr.) (238)

D: 21.0 - 46.2 hr. (556)
DD: 50 - 99 hr. (556)

plasma or serum:

D: 52.8 (± 23.6 S.D.) 2 different (22)
D: 44.4 (± 17.5 S.D.) brands of tablets (22)

D: 26 - 53 hr. (77)

D: 34.6 - 87.2 hr. (275)

D: mean 54 hr. (486)
DD: mean 92 hr. (486)

D: 18.2 - 44.7 hr. (age 15 - 34 years) (586)
D: 32.8 - 67.1 hr. (age 35 - 54 years) (586)
D: 47.5 -112.4 hr. (age 55 - 82 years) (586)

D: 8.7 - 42 hr. (1155)
DD: 42 - 96 hr. (1155)

D: 20 - 42 hr. (1158)
DD: 44 - 96 hr. (1158)

D: 23 - 78 hr. (1211)
DD: 32 -146 hr. (1211)

D: 36 -160 hr. (1957)
DD: 57 -260 hr. (1957)

Intravenous Administration

Distribution Half-Life $t_{1/2\alpha}$

blood

D:0.94 - 3.3 hr (556)

Elimination Half-Life $t_{1/2\beta}$

blood

D: 26.7 - 36.5 hr. (556)

DIAZEPAM	Pharmacokinetic Data derived from the different Studies (continued)

plasma

D:0.96 (±0.34 hr.) (583)
(mean ± S.D.)

plasma

D: 14.3 - 61.2 hr. (normal subjects) (16)
D: 28.6 -517.2 hr. (patients with liver disease) (16)

D: 32.9 ± 8.8 hr. (mean ± S.D.) (583)

D: 46.6 ± 14.2 hr. (mean ± S.D.) (normal subjects) (585)
D: 99.2 ± 23.2 hr. (mean ± S.D.) (patients with liver disease, single dose) (585)
D: 107.6 ± 25.1 hr. (mean ± S.D.) (patients with liver disease, subchronic dose) (585)

DD: 50.9 ± 6.2 hr. (mean ± S.D.) (normal subjects, DD administered) (585)

DD: 108 ± 40.3 hr. (mean ± S.D.) (patients with liver disease, DD administered) (585)

D: 23 - 61 hr. (normal subjects) (2215)
38 -194 hr. (patients with liver disease) (2215)

Intramuscular Administration

Elimination Half-Life $t_{1/2\beta}$

D: 58 hr. (premature infants) (745)
D: 18 hr. (children) (745)

rate of formation of DD was slower in prematures than in children (745)

Rectal Administration

Elimination Half-Life $t_{1/2\beta}$

D: 56.6 ± 13.5 (mean ± S.D.) (22)

D: 56.8 ± 29.1 (mean ± S.D.) (22)

two different kinds of Supp.

---

relative Clearance(ml/hr/kg):	37.5 (range 19 - 46) (D)	(219)
	54.2 (range 19 -110) (DD)	(219)
apparent oral total drug plasma Clearance (ml/h/kg):	13.9 - 26.5	(275)
apparent volume of central compartment: (l/kg)	0.353 - 0.642	(275)
Proteinbinding:	D: 97.5 % (586), 98.0 % (553), 96 % (1153), DD: 97 % (553)	
ratio Diazepam / Nordiazepam :	0.72 (2 - 20-mg/d, 2 - 4 weeks)	(126)
	1.14 (range 0.60 - 2.05 after 7 days)	(1957)
	0.25 (range 0.62 - 0.86 after 48 days)	(1468)
	0.72 (range 0.20 - 1.70 after)	(126)
ratio feto/maternal:	D: 1.8 - 3.0 (550)	
ratio D in blood / D in plasma :	0.5 (586), 0.5 - 0.6	(2495)

Remarks

Patients taking D for 2 - 5 years in doses of 15-mg or 20-40-mg daily had much lower plasma concentrations of D and DD than patients of acute experiments. It is assumed, that hepatic enzyme induction is the reason for this phenomenon. (552).

The increases in serum concentrations of D after the intake of food support the concept of an enterohepatic cycle for D.

OXAZEPAM	Single Dose Studies - Oral Administration				
Dose	Body fluid sampled	Peak concentration (f = free oxazepam, c = conjug.oxazepam)	Lit.Ref.	Time of peak conc. after dose	Subjects Character.
10-mg	plasma	ca. 170 - 240 ng/ml (f)	(2480)	ca. 3 hr.	3 Subj.
10-mg	plasma	ca. 150 - 190 ng/ml (c)	(2480)	ca. 5 hr.	3 Subj.
10-mg	urine	7.7 % 1-24 hr. (f) 67 % 1-24 hr. (c)	(2480)		3 Subj.
10-mg	serum	ca. 160 - 220 ng/ml (f)	(1813)	2 hr.	12 Subj.
15-mg	plasma	ca. 150 - 380 ng/ml (f) ca. 100 - 200 ng/ml (c)	(13)	1 - 4 hr. 1 - 4 hr.	4 Subj.
15-mg	serum	202 - 316 ng/ml (f)	(115)	1.5-4 hr.	6 Subj.
15-mg	serum	ca. 200 ng/ml (f)	(1165)	2 hr.	1 Subj.
15-mg	serum	301 - 399 ng/ml (f)	(1211)	1 - 4 hr.	7 Subj.
15-mg	serum	315 ± 69 ng/ml (f) (mean ± S.D.) urinary excretion 82.7% of dose	(1813)	2 hr.	18 Subj.
20-mg	plasma	ca. 220 - 350 ng/ml (f)	(842)	1 - 2 hr.	3 Subj.
23.6-mg	plasma	ca. 420 ng/ml (f)	(2492)	ca. 3 - 4 hr.	1 Subj.
25-mg	plasma	188 - 539 ng/ml (f)	(1975)	1 - 3 hr.	8 Subj. women prior to delivery
25-mg	serum	186 - 375 ng/ml (f)	(115)	1.5 - 6 hr.	6 Subj.
25-mg	serum	184 - 392 ng/ml (f)	(715)	1 - 5 hr.	8 Subj.
25-mg	serum	ca. 500 - 600 ng/ml (f)	(1813)	ca. 2 hr.	6 Subj.
30-mg	plasma	ca. 460 - 750 ng/ml (f) + (c)	(541)	1 - 7 hr.	5 Subj.
30-mg	plasma	ca. 460 ng/ml (f)	(1481)	ca. 3 hr.	1 Subj.
30-mg	serum	351 -1114 ng/ml (f) 648 -1659 ng/ml (total !)	(671)	1 - 6 hr. 2 - 3 hr.	4 Subj.
45-mg	serum	880 -1440 ng/ml (f) 710 -1410 ng/ml (c)	(595)	1 - 4 hr. 2 - 5 hr.	8 Subj.
45-mg 15-mg t.i.d. 1 day	serum	400 -1110 ng/ml (f) 440 -1120 ng/ml (c)	(595)	6 -10 hr. 6 -12 hr.	8 Subj.
50-mg	serum	284 - 774 ng/ml (f)	(115)	1.5 - 6 hr.	6 Subj.

OXAZEPAM		Single Dose Studies - Rectal Administration			
Dose	Body-fluid sampled	Peak concentration (f = free oxazepam, c = conjugated oxazepam)	Lit.Ref.	Time of peak conc. after dose	Subjects Characteristics
20-mg	plasma	ca. 130 - 260 ng/ml (f)	(842)	3 - 4 hr.	3 Subj.
30-mg	plasma	ca. 300 - 400 ng/ml (total !)	(541)	4 - 6 hr.	5 Subj.

OXAZEPAM		Multiple Dose Studies - Oral Administration		
Dose per day Duration of therapy	Body-fluid sampled	Steady-state concentrations (f = free oxazepam, c = conjugated oxazepam)	Lit.Ref.	Subjects Characteristics / Remarks
15-mg/d 5-mg t.i.d. 10 days	plasma	ca. 20 - 130 ng/ml (f) ca. 27 - 85 ng/ml (c)	(13)	8 Subjects (after 2 days)
30-mg/d 10-mg t.i.d. 14 days	serum	100 - 350 ng/ml (f) 130 - 300 ng/ml (c)	(595)	6 healthy Subjects
30-mg/d 30-mg h.s. 14 days	plasma	ca. 200 - 400 ng/ml (total !)	(541)	2 Subjects
60-mg/d 15-mg q.i.d. 5 days	serum	300 - 650 ng/ml (f)	(595)	6 healthy Subjects
90-mg/d 30-mg t.i.d. 14 days	serum	270 - 950 ng/ml (f) 340 - 980 ng/ml (c)	(595)	3 healthy Subjects
100-mg/d 25-mg q.i.d. 4-6 weeks	serum	159 - 808 ng/ml (f)	(115)	4 patients

OXAZEPAM	Pharmacokinetic Data derived from the different Studies

Oral Administration

Plasma Clearance

0.071 - 0.212	l/kg/hr	(1975)
0.050 - 0.171	l/kg/hr	(13)
0.0358 - P.0919	l/kg/hr	(1211)

Volume of Distribution

0.52 - 2.35	l/kg	(1211)
0.59 - 1.44	l/kg	(1975)

Elimination Half-Life $t_{1/2\beta}$

plasma

5.9 - 24.9	hr.	(13)	
7.7	hr.	(1481)	
5.3 - 7.8	hr.	(1975)	(mother)
21.9	hr.	(1975)	(newborn)
5.5	hr.	(1645)	
4.0	hr.	(2480)	
7.5 ± 2.1	hr.	(2492)	

serum

5.7 - 9.8	hr.	(715)
8.4 - 17.9	hr.	(1211)

NITRAZEPAM

Single Dose Studies - Oral Administration

Dose	Body-fluid sampled	Peak concentration N = Nitrazepam	observed	Lit.Ref.	Time of peak-conc. after dose	Subjects Characteristics
4-mg	plasma	total ^{14}C-activity: 40 - 50 ng/ml		(908)	7 - 10 hr.	2 women
5-mg	plasma	40 - 50 ng/ml	(N)	(224)	0.5 - 4 hr.	7 Subjects
5-mg	plasma	12 - 38 ng/ml	(N)	(543)	ca. 12 hr.	6 women pregn. 14-17 weeks
5-mg	plasma	16 - 36 ng/ml	(N)	(543)	ca. 12 hr.	12 women late pregn.
5-mg	plasma	mean: 36.7 ± 5.7 ng/ml	(N)	(545)	2 hr.	7 patients
		33.3 ± 3.1 ng/ml	(N)		4 hr.	4 patients
		23.0 ± 1.5 ng/ml	(N)		6 hr.	4 patients
		24.5 ± 1.3 ng/ml	(N)		8 hr.	6 patients
		21.8 ± 3.1 ng/ml	(N)		12 hr.	5 patients
		19.7 ± 1.5 ng/ml	(N)		18 hr.	3 patients
		14.8 ± 2.1 ng/ml	(N)		24 hr.	5 patients
		15.3 ± 3.8 ng/ml (mean ± SEM)	(N)		36 hr.	4 patients
5-mg	plasma	46.9 ± 3.2 ng/ml (mean ± SEM)	(N)	(546)	2 hr.	10 Subjects
5-mg	plasma	ca. 40 - 53 ng/ml	(N)	(2514)	ca. 1 - 2 hr.	25 Subjects (young)
5-mg	plasma	ca. 13 - 22 ng/ml	(N)	(2514)	ca. 1 - 2 hr.	12 Subjects (older)
5-mg	serum	39.9 ± 12.7 ng/ml	(N)	(510)		25 young S.
5-mg	serum	21.8 ± 9.2 ng/ml	(N)	(510)		12 older S.
5-mg	serum	ca. 30 - 42 ng/ml	(N)	(738)	2 hr.	15 Subjects
5-mg	serum	mean: 40.7 ng/ml	(N)	(2513)	2.4 hr.	12 Subjects
	saliva	1.9 ng/ml	(N)	(2513)	2.5 hr.	12 Subjects
10-mg	plasma	82.8 ± 10.5 ng/ml	(N)	(546)	3 hr.	10 Subjects
10-mg	plasma	68 - 108 ng/ml	(N)	(910)	2 hr.	6 Subjects

NITRAZEPAM

Single Dose Studies - Intravenous Administration

Dose	Body-fluid sampled	Peak concentration N = Nitrazepam	observed	Lit.Ref.	Time of peak-conc. after dose	Subjects Characteristics
4-mg	plasma	39 - 56 ng/ml	(N)	(908)	1 - 6 hr.	2 women
		2.6 - 5.7 ng/ml	(7-Amino-N)		7 - 12 hr.	
10-mg	plasma	61 - 124 ng/ml	(N)	(910)	2 hr.	6 Subjects
30-mg	plasma	310 - 750 ng/ml	(N)	(908)	2 hr.	4 Subjects
		100 - 220 ng/ml	(7-Amino-N)		8 - 12 hr.	
		120 - 370 ng/ml	(7-Acetamido-N)		2 - 12 hr.	

NITRAZEPAM	Multiple Dose Studies - Oral Administration			
Dose per day Duration of Therapy	Body-fluid sampled	Steady-state concentrations N = Nitrazepam	Lit.Ref.	Subjects Characteristics Remarks
3.75-mg/d over 1.5 year	plasma	62 ng/ml (N)	(2514)	1 Child
5-mg/d 2 months	serum	59.8 ± 30.3 ng/ml (N)	(510)	12 aged Patients (reached after 7.5 days)
5-mg/d 14 days	serum	59.7 ± 21.0 ng/ml (N)	(510)	25 young Volunteers (reached after 3.5 days)
10-mg/d 4 days - several weeks	plasma	20 - 46 ng/ml (N)	(81)	7 Subjects
12.5-mg/d over 1.5 year	plasma	88 ng/ml (N)	(2514)	1 epileptic Child
75.3 ± 2.1 µg/kg 2 weeks	plasma	57 ± 17 ng/ml (N)	(2514)	11 Subjects
86.6 ± 9.0 µg/kg	plasma	45 ± 12 ng/ml (N)	(2514)	26 psychiatric older S.
280 ± 110 µg/kg	plasma	40 - 180 ng/ml (N)	(2514)	44 epileptic Children

NITRAZEPAM	Forensic Cases			
Nitrazepam-concentrations:	Liver	700 1500	ng/g	(2509)
	Urine	10 000	ng/ml	
	Blood	1 200	ng/ml	
	Liver	4 000	ng/g	(648)
	Blood	9 000	ng/ml	
	Urine	1 000	ng/ml	(1138)
	Urine	5 800 - 6 000	ng/ml	(820)

NITRAZEPAM	Pharmacokinetic Data derived from the different Studies

Oral Administration

Distribution Half-Life $t_{1/2\alpha}$

0.7 - 5.3 hr. (2513)

Absorption Half-Life $t_{1/2\,a}$

0.4 - 6.0 hr. (2513)

Elimination Half-Life $t_{1/2\beta}$

13 - 34 hr.	(224)	
28.9 ± 7.4 hr.	(510)	young volunteers
40.4 ±16.2 hr.	(510)	older patients
16.5 - 48.3 hr.	(546)	
28 ± 11 hr.	(738)	Brand I
25 ± 6 hr.	(738)	Brand II
21.2 - 28.1 hr.	(910)	
21 - 57 hr.	(2513)	
24.2 ± 4.9 hr.	(2514)	young volunteers
39.6 ±13.8 hr.	(2514)	older patients

Intravenous Administration

Distribution Half-Life $t_{1/2\alpha}$		Elimination Half-Life $t_{1/2\beta}$	
2.4 - 5.0 hr.	(910)	6.87 hr.	(908)
		17.8 - 24.0 hr.	(910)

Volume of Distribution:	(l/kg)	2.4 ± 0.8 young volunteers	(510)
		4.8 ± 1.7 older patients	(510)
		1.95± 0.52 (5-mg)	(546)
		2.55± 0.54 (10mg)	(546)
		0.71 - 1.7	(2513)
Clearance (tot):	(l/h)	4.1 ± 2.0 young volunteers	(510)
		4.7 ± 1.5 older patients	(510)
	(ml/min/kg)	0.94 ± 0.35	(546)
	(ml/min)	52 - 107	(2513)

MEDAZEPAM — Single Dose Studies - Oral Administration

Dose	Body-fluid sampled	Peak concentration observed M = Medazepam, DM = Desmethyl-Medazepam, D = Diazepam, DD = Desmethyldiazepam		Lit.Ref.	Time of peak conc. after dose	Subjects Characterist.
10-mg	plasma	ca. 140 - 200 ng/ml	(M)	(2510)	ca. 1 hr.	4 Subjects
		ca. 10 ng/ml	(D)		ca. 1 - 2 hr.	
		ca. 100 - 200 ng/ml	(DD)		ca. 30 - 70 hr.	
10-mg	plasma	310 - 510 ng/ml	(M)	(2510)	30 - 50 min.	3 Subjects
		ca. 3 ng/ml	(D)		10 - 60 min.	
		ca. 2-5 ng/ml	(DD)			
30-mg	blood	656 ng/ml (without EtOH)	(M)	(672)	40 min.	1 Subj.
		1037ng/ml (with EtOH)	(M)		100min.	
		ca. 170 ng/ml	(DM)		ca. 1 hr.	
		ca. 180 ng/ml	(D)		ca. 1 hr.	
		ca. 150 ng/ml	(DD)		ca.24 hr.	
30-mg	blood	116 - 165 ng/ml	(M)	(911)	1 - 2 hr.	2 Subjects
		60 - 97 ng/ml	(DM)		1 - 2 hr.	
		12.5- 33 ng/ml	(D)		1 -24 hr.	
		28.3- 195 ng/ml	(DD)		72-96 hr.	
30-mg	serum	ca. 800 ng/ml	(M)	(93)	ca. 1 hr.	1 Subject
50-mg	blood	980 ng/ml	(M)	(240)	ca. 1 hr.	1 Subject
		20 - 40 ng/ml	(D)		ca. 1-24 hr.	
50-mg	serum	ca. 1100 ng/ml	(M)	(93)	ca. 5 hr.	1 Subject
100-mg	serum	ca. 3500 ng/ml	(M)	(93)	ca. 2 hr.	1 Subject

MEDAZEPAM — Multiple Dose Studies - Oral Administration

Dose per day Duration of Therapy	Body-fluid sampled	Steady-state concentrations (Abbreviations see Single Studies -Oral Administration)		Lit.Ref.	Subjects Characteristics and Remarks
27-mg/d 2-4 weeks	plasma	10 - 160 ng/ml	(M)	(126)	20 patients
		0 - 120 ng/ml	(D)		
		210 - 1680 ng/ml	(DD)		
50-mg/d o.d. 4 days	blood	no steady-state levels Maximum levels were: 380, 500, 400, 600 ng/ml	(M)	(240)	1 Subject
		ca. 50 - 80 ng/ml	(D)		

Half-Life of Elimination (total radioactivity): 20.3 - 176 hr. (911) 11 Subjects

CLORAZEPATE

Single Dose Studies - Oral Administration

Dose	Body-fluid sampled	Peak concentration observed C = Clorazepate DD = Desmethyldiazepam		Lit.Ref.	Time of peak conc. after dose	Subjects Characteristics Remarks
10-mg	serum	191 - 382 ng/ml	(DD)	(1211)	0.75-2.5 hr.	7 Subjects
15-mg	blood	29 - 110 ng/ml	(C)	(2)	0.5 - 2 hr.	4 Subjects
		138 - 181 ng/ml	(DD)		0.5 - 1 hr.	
		pH of stomach < 3				
		20 - 121 ng/ml	(C)		1 - 2 hr.	
		20 - 64 ng/ml	(DD)		2 - 12 hr.	
		pH of stomach > 6				
15-mg	blood	19.0 - 22.5 ng/ml	(C)	(153)	0.5 -2 hr.	2 Subjects
		139 - 175 ng/ml	(DD)		1 hr.	
15-mg	plasma	257 ± 49 (mean ± S.D.) ng/ml (DD)		(181)	ca. 1 - 2 hr.	15 Subjects
		99 - 113 ng/ml	(C)		1 - 2 hr.	
15-mg	plasma	379 ng/ml	(DD)	(1501)	0.75 hr.	1 Subject
15-mg	plasma	188 (± 17.7) - 273 (± 21.9) (mean ± SEM) ng/ml	(DD)	(1899)	1.8 - 2.8 hr.	10 Subjects
20-mg	serum	127 - 345 ng/ml	(DD)	(1926)	1 - 13 hr.	14 Subjects
22.5-mg	plasma	ca. 510 ng/ml	(C)	(1170)	ca. 2 hr.	1 Subject
		ca. 430 ng/ml	(DD)		ca. 4 hr.	
22.5-mg	serum	230 - 320 ng/ml	(DD)	(1328)	2 - 12 hr.	30 Subjects

CLORAZEPATE

Multiple Dose Studies - Oral Administration

Dose per day Duration of Therapy	Body-fluid sampled	Steady-state concentrations C = Clorazepate DD= Desmethyldiazepam		Lit.Ref.	Subjects Characteristics and Remarks
20-mg 14 days	plasma	540 - 1347 ng/ml	(DD)	(1822)	12 Subjects
22.5-mg/d 8 days	plasma	100 - 290 ng/ml	(C)	(1170)	2 patients
		470 - 710 ng/ml	(DD)		
50-mg/d	plasma	1214 - 2640 ng/ml	(DD)	(2627)	10 patients

C = Clorazepate
DD= Desmethyldiazepam

Oral Administration

Absorption Half-Life $t_{1/2\,a}$

plasma

9.9 min.	(1501)	(DD)
14.8 - 30.7 min.	(1899)	(DD)

Elimination Half-Life $t_{1/2_\beta}$

blood

40 - 60 hr.	(2)	(DD)

plasma

1.65 - 2.66 hr.	(181)	(C)
64.8 - 70.0 hr.	(181)	(DD)
27.0 hr.	(1501)	(DD)
53 ± 6 hr.	(1822)	(DD)

serum

48 hr.	(1324)	(DD)

Apparent Volume of Distribution: (l/kg) 1.13 ± 0.08 (mean ± SEM) (1822)

LORAZEPAM

Single Dose Studies - Oral Administration

Dose	Body fluid sampled	Peak concentration observed (f = free lorazepam, c = conjugated lorazepam)		Lit.Ref.	Time of peak conc. after dose	Subjects Characterist.
2-mg	plasma	ca. 20 - 30 ng/ml	(f)	(271)	ca. 90 min.	20 Subj.
2-mg	plasma	9.1 - 18.3 ng/ml 8.6 - 29.4 ng/ml	(f) (c)	(432)	2 hr. ca. 4 hr.	8 Subj.
2-mg	plasma	21.5 - 36.2 ng/ml	(f)	(1518)	1 - 6 hr.	6 Subj.
2-mg	plasma	21 ng/ml	(f)	(2355)	2 hr.	1 Subj.
2.5-mg	serum	30 ng/ml 30 ng/ml	(f) (c)	(594)	2 hr. 4-6 hr.	4 Subj.
2.5-mg	plasma	22.0 - 46.0 ng/ml	(f)	(1996)	1-3 hr.	6 Subj.
4-mg	blood	5.9 - 15.5 ng/ml	(f)	(232)	2-4 hr.	3 Subj.
4-mg	plasma	ca. 15 - 20 ng/ml	(f)	(271)	90 min.	20 Subj.
4-mg	plasma	44.4 ng/ml	(f)	(1506)	1 hr.	1 Subj.
4-mg	plasma	38.8 - 68.1 ng/ml	(f)	(1518)	1-2.5 hr.	6 Subj.
5-mg	plasma	ca. 45 ng/ml	(f)	(1426)	2-4 hr.	4 Subj.
5-mg	serum	45 ng/ml 55 ng/ml	(f) (c)	(594)	2-4 hr. 2-6 hr.	4 Subj.
7.5-mg	serum	80 ng/ml 108 ng/ml	(f) (c)	(594)	6 hr. 12 hr.	4 Subj.

LORAZEPAM

Single Dose Studies - Intravenous Administration

Dose	Body fluid sampled	Peak concentration observed (f = free lorazepam, c = conjugated lorazepam)		Lit.Ref.	Time of peak conc. after dose	Subjects Characterist.
2-mg	plasma	ca. 50 - 60 ng/ml	(f)	(1518)	few min.	2 Subj.
2-mg	plasma	ca. 40 - 50 ng/ml	(f)	(1666)	few min.	1 Subj.
2.5-mg	plasma	ca. 100 - 115 ng/ml	(f)	(2529)	few min.	10 Subj.
4-mg	plasma	ca. 50 ng/ml	(f)	(1506)	few min.	1 Subj.
4-mg	plasma	ca. 100 - 110 ng/ml	(f)	(1518)	few min.	2 Subj.
5-mg	plasma	ca. 92 - 112 ng/ml	(f)	(271)	few min.	? Subj.
5-mg	plasma	ca. 140 ng/ml	(f)	(1426)	few min.	4 Subj.

LORAZEPAM

Single Dose Studies - Intramuscular Administration

Dose	Body fluid sampled	Peak concentration observed (f = free lorazepam, c = conjugated lorazepam)		Lit.Ref.	Time of peak conc. after dose	Subjects Characterist.
2-mg	plasma	ca. 35 - 42 ng/ml	(f)	(271)	90 min.	20 Subj.
2-mg	plasma	23.3 - 29.4 ng/ml	(f)	(1518)	0.75 - 2.0 hr.	6 Subj.
4-mg	plasma	ca. 30 - 55 ng/ml	(f)	(271)	90 min.	20 Subj.
4-mg	plasma	49.6 - 82.7 ng/ml 50.4 - 99.9 ng/ml	(f) (c)	(419)	1 - 3 hr. 5 -12 hr.	6 Subj.
4-mg	plasma	36.2 ng/ml	(f)	(1506)	2.5 hr.	1 Subj.
4-mg	plasma	34.3 - 62.9 ng/ml	(f)	(1518)	0.75 - 2.5 hr.	6 Subj.
5-mg	plasma	ca. 83 ng/ml ca. 90 ng/ml	(f) (c)	(1426)	2 hr. 4 - 12 hr.	4 Subj.

LORAZEPAM	Multiple Dose Studies - Oral Administration			
Dose per day Duration of therapy	Body fluid sampled	Steady-state concentrations (f = free lorazepam, c = conjugated lorazepam)	Lit.Ref.	Subjects Characteristics Remarks
6-mg/d (2-mg morning, 4-mg h.s.)	plasma	mean: 88 ng/ml (f) 170 ng/ml (c)	(420)	15 Subjects
10-mg/d ca. 12 weeks	plasma	mean: 164 ng/ml (f) 266 ng/ml (c)	(420)	15 Subjects

LORAZEPAM	Multiple Dose Studies - Intramuscular Administration			
5-mg/d 4 days	plasma	60 - 70 ng/ml (f) ca. 100 - 110 ng/ml (c)	(1426)	8 Subjects

LORAZEPAM	Pharmacokinetic Data derived from the different Studies

f = free lorazepam
c = conjugated lorazepam

Oral Administration

Absorption Half-Life $t_{1/2\,a}$

plasma

15.1 min	(432)	(f)
38.9 min	(432)	(c)
14.3 min	(1506)	(f)
8.5 - 60.2 min	(1518)	(f)

Elimination Half-Life $t_{1/2\beta}$

blood

10 - 15 hr.	(1026)	(f)

plasma

11.7 hr.	(432)	(f)
16.2 hr.	(432)	(c)
10.8 hr.	(1506)	(f)
9.0 - 25.9 hr.	(1518)	(f)
12.8 - 38.3 hr.	(1518)	(c)
8.7 - 14.0 hr.	(1996)	(f)

Intravenous Administration

Distribution Half-Life $t_{1/2\alpha}$

plasma

0.00 - 10.4 min.	(1518)	(f)

plasma

10.6 hr.	(1506)	(f)
8.4 - 24.9 hr.	(1518)	(f)
10.4 - 24.6 hr.	(1518)	(c)
22.1 ± 5.4 hr.	(1666)	(f) normal subj.
31.9 ± 9.6 hr.	(1666)	(f) cirrhotics

Intramuscular Administration

plasma

Distribution Half-Life $t_{1/2\alpha}$

1.75 - 5.87 hr.	(419)	(c)

Absorption Half-Life $t_{1/2\,a}$

15.5 - 29.2 min.	(419)	(f)
5.4 - 50.6 min.	(1518)	(f)

plasma

10.45 - 16.87 hr.	(419)	(f)
8.6 - 22.2 hr.	(419)	(c)
13.9 hr	(1506)	(f)
10.5 - 25.6 hr.	(1518)	(f)
11.3 - 31.7 hr.	(1518)	(c)

Total apparent volume of Distribution (l/kg)

0.69 - 1.00	(419)	after i.m. administration
1.05 - 1.62	(1518)	after i.v. administration

Clearance

(ml/min)	44.2 - 78.4	(419)	after i.m. administration
(ml/min/kg)	0.52 - 1.77	(1518)	after i.v. administration

PRAZEPAM	Single Dose Studies - Oral Administration				
Dose	Body fluid sampled	Peak concentration observed (P = Prazepam, DD = Desmethyldiazepam)	Lit.Ref.	Time of peak conc. after dose	Subjects Characterist.
25-mg	blood	ca. 900 ng/ml (unconj. ^{14}C-activity) ca. 400 ng/ml (gluc. ^{14}C-activity)	(253)	ca. 6 - 8 hr. ca. 6 -10 hr.	5 Subj.
30-mg as solution	plasma	ca. 23 - 42 ng/ml (P) 405 ± 56 ng/ml (Mean ± SD(DD)	(2490)	30 min. ca. 2 hr.	9 Subj.
30-mg as tablets	plasma	8 - 32 ng/ml (P) 321 ± 76 ng/ml (Mean ± SD(DD)	(2490)	1 hr. ca. 4 hr.	9 Subj.

PRAZEPAM	Pharmacokinetic Data derived from the different Studies

P = Prazepam
DD = Desmethyldiazepam

Oral Administration

Distribution Half-Life $t_{1/2\alpha}$

Elimination Half-Life $t_{1/2\beta}$

plasma

after 30-mg in solution

1.17 ± 0.38 hr. (P) (2490)
139 ± 162 hr. (DD)

after 30-mg as tablets

1.31 ± 0.65 hr. (P) (2490)
96 ± 34 hr. (DD)

Apparent volume of Distribution: (l/kg)

14.4 ± 5.1 (P) tablets	1.43 ± 0.33 (DD) tablets
11.7 ± 7.2 (P) solution	1.40 ± 0.71 (DD) solution

Clearance: (l/kg/h)

0.143 ± 0.103 (P)tablets	0.00017 ± 0.00012 (DD) tablets
0.113 ± 0.068 (P)solution	0.00019 ± 0.00013 (DD) tablets

CLONAZEPAM	Single Dose Studies - Oral Administration				
Dose	Body-fluid sampled	Peak concentration observed C = Clonazepam A = 7-Aminoclonazepam AA= 7-Acetamidoclonazepam	Lit.Ref.	Time of peak conc. after dose	Subjects Characteristics Remarks
1,5-mg	plasma	8.7 - 10.8 ng/ml (C)	(298)	1 - 3 hr.	4 Subjects
2-mg	blood	ca. 6 - 9 ng/ml (C)	(231)	1.5 - 2 hr.	3 Subjects
2-mg	blood	ca. 12 ng/ml (C)	(242)	ca. 1 hr.	1 Subject
2-mg	blood	6.5 - 13.5 ng/ml (C)	(555)	1 - 8 hr.	10 Subjects
2-mg	blood	13.6 ng/ml (C) ca. 5 ng/ml (A)	(725)	2 hr. 2 hr.	1 Subject
2-mg	plasma	7.1 - 23.6 ng/ml (C)	(76)	1 - 4 hr.	8 Subjects
2-mg	plasma	ca. 10 ng/ml (C)	(242)	ca. 1 hr.	1 Subject
9-mg	plasma	28.3 - 51.9 ng/ml (C)	(298)	6 - 10 hr.	4 Subjects

CLONAZEPAM	Single Dose Studies - Intravenous Administration				
Dose	Body-fluid sampled	Peak concentration observed C = Clonazepam A = 7-Aminoclonazepam AA= 7-Acetamidoclonazepam	Lit Ref.	Time of peak conc. after dose	Subjects Characteristics Remarks
1.5-mg	plasma	11.8 - 15.3 ng/ml (C)	(298)	1 - 3 hr.	4 Subjects
2-mg	plasma	mean: 36.8 ng/ml (C)	(76)	10 min.	8 Subjects
2-mg	plasma	ca. 13 ng/ml (C)	(591)	few min.	1 Subject

CLONAZEPAM	Multiple Dose Studies - Oral Administration			
Dose per day Duration of Therapy	Body-fluid sampled	Steady-state concentrations C = Clonazepam A = 7-Aminoclonazepam AA= 7-Acetamidoclonazepam	Lit.Ref.	Subjects Characteristics and Remarks
1-mg/d 0.5-mg b.i.d. 15 days	plasma	4.6 - 12 ng/ml (C)	(76)	5 Subjects 49 - 80 kg
1-mg/d	plasma	72 ng/ml (C) 89 ng/ml (A)	(725)	1 Subject 24.4 kg
2-mg/d 1-mg b.i.d.	plasma	13 ng/ml (C)	(591)	1 Subject 20 years old
2-mg/d 1-mg b.i.d.	plasma	13 ng/ml (C)	(591)	1 Subject 24 years old
3-mg/d	plasma	11 - 26 ng/ml (C) 22 - 55 ng/ml (A)	(725)	3 Subjects 45.0 - 58.5 kg
4.5-mg/d	plasma	72 - 112 ng/ml (C) 89 - 145 ng/ml	(725)	2 Subjects 27.3 and 29.9 kg

CLONAZEPAM		Multiple Dose Studies - Oral Administration (continued)		
Dose per day Duration of Therapy	Body-fluid sampled	Steady-state concentrations C = Clonazepam A = 7-Aminoclonazepam AA= 7-Acetamidoclonazepam	Lit.Ref.	Subjects Characteristics and Remarks
5-mg/d	plasma	10 - 35 ng/ml 18 - 43 ng/ml	(C) (725) (A)	3 Subjects 18.5 - 51.7 kg
6-mg/d 2-mg t.i.d.	blood	19.8 - 49.6 ng/ml	(C) (242)	1 Subject
6-mg/d 2-mg t.i.d.	plasma	80 ng/ml	(C) (591)	1 Child (2 years-old)
6-mg/d	plasma	48 ng/ml 108 ng/ml	(C) (725) (A)	1 Subject 63 kg
6-mg/d	plasma	29 - 75 ng/ml 23 -137 ng/ml 3 - 13 ng/ml	(C) (771) (A) (AA)	25 Subjects
6-mg/d	plasma	ca. 30 - 80 ng/ml	(C) (1054)	27 Subjects (epileptics) 12 - 71 years
6-8-mg/d	plasma	42 - 112 ng/ml 35 - 169 ng/ml 0 - 7 ng/ml	(C) (2486) (A) (AA)	6 Subjects 14.0 - 34.0 kg
10-mg/d	plasma	56 ng/ml 79 ng/ml	(C) (725) (A)	1 Subject 57.7 kg
12-mg/d one month	plasma	39.6 - 77.1 ng/ml	(C) (231)	1 Subject 22 kg
12-mg/d	plasma	68 ng/ml 70 ng/ml	(C) (725) (A)	1 Subject 18.1 kg
12-mg/d	plasma	50 - 102 ng/ml 58 - 112 ng/ml 0 - 1.8 ng/ml	(C) (2486) (A) (AA)	3 Subjects 19.0 - 95.4 kg
12-15-mg/d	plasma	24 - 50 ng/ml	(C) (236)	1 Subject 24 kg
15-mg/d	plasma	122 ng/ml 148 ng/ml	(C) (725) (A)	1 Subject 20 kg
30-mg/d	plasma	33 - 440 ng/ml 36 - 233 ng/ml 0 - 52 ng/ml	(C) (2486) (A) (AA)	2 Subjects 40.9 and 81.8 kg
121-mg/d (!)	plasma	44 ng/ml 43 ng/ml 1.6 ng/ml	(C) (2486) (A) (AA)	1 Subject 90.9 kg
0.028 - 0.111 mg/kg	serum	13 - 72 ng/ml	(C) (266)	10 Children with absence seizures
0.05-mg/kg 2 months	plasma	ca. 8 - 13 ng/ml	(C) (163)	20 Subjects
0.10-mg/kg 80 days	plasma	ca. 30 - 50 ng/ml	(C) (381)	1 Subject (epileptic)

CLONAZEPAM	Multiple Dose Studies - Oral Administration (continued)			
Dose per day Duration of Therapy	Body-fluid sampled	Steady-state concentrations C = Clonazepam A = 7-Aminoclonazepam AA= 7-Acetamidoclonazepam	Lit.Ref.	Subjects Characteristics and Remarks
0.10-mg/kg	plasma	ca. 18 ng/ml (C)	(163)	20 Subjects
0.12-mg/kg 80 days - 5 months	plasma	ca. 15 - 60 ng/ml (C)	(381)	2 Subjects (epileptics)
0.15-mg/d	plasma	ca. 25 ng/ml (C)	(163)	20 Subjects
0.20-mg/d	plasma	ca. 30 ng/ml (C)	(163)	20 Subjects
0.3 - 10-mg/d	serum	5 - 97 ng/ml (C)	(1416)	28 Subjects

CLONAZEPAM	Pharmacokinetic Data derived from the different Studies

Oral Administration

Distribution Half-Life $t_{1/2\alpha}$

Elimination Half-Life $t_{1/2\beta}$

plasma

19 - 60 hr.	(C)	(76)
47 hr.	(C)	(242)
26.5 - 49.2 hr.	(C)	(298)
18.7 - 39 hr.	(C)	(555)
19.1 hr.	(C)	(591)
31 hr.	(C)	(725)

Intravenous Administration

0.65 - 3.4 hr. (76)

plasma

28.3 - 56.4 hr.(C) (298)

Apparent volume of Distribution: (l/kg)

1.5 - 4.4	(76)
5.1	(231, 591)
6.2	(242, 591)
2.8	(555, 591)
2.5	(591)

Relative Clearance: (ml/kg/hr)

164	(231, 591)	
95	(242, 591)	
75	(555, 591)	
89	(591)	
103 - 208	(591)	co-medication (carbamazepin, phenobarbital, valproate-Na, amphetamine)

FLURAZEPAM	Single Dose Studies - Oral Administration					
Dose	Body-fluid sampled	Peak concentration observed F = Flurazepam H = N-1-Hydroxyethylflurazepam N = N-Desalkylflurazepam		Lit.Ref.	Time of peak conc. after dose	Subjects Character.
30-mg	blood	ca. 6 ng/ml	(F)	(235)	ca. 3 - 6 hr.	2 Subj.
		ca. 5 - 11 ng/ml	(H)		ca. 3 hr.	
		ca. 10- 14 ng/ml	(N)		12 - 24 hr.	
30-mg	blood	5.0 ng/ml	(F)	(241)	1 hr.	1 Subj.
30-mg	blood	1 - 2 ng/ml	(F)	(468)	1 hr.	2 Subj.
		38 - 50 ng/ml (free)	(H)		1 hr.	
		17 ng/ml	(N)		1 - 3 hr.	
30-mg	blood	non detected	(F)	(559)		4 Subj.
		4.3 - 14.8 ng/ml	(H)		ca. 1 - 6 hr.	
		10 - 22 ng/ml	(N)		6 - 24 hr.	
90-mg	blood	7 ng/ml	(F)	(244)	ca. 0.5 - 1.5 hr.	1 S.
		ca. 60 - 70 ng/ml	(H)		ca. 1 hr.	
		ca. 50 ng/ml	(N)		ca. 1 - 2 hr.	
90-mg	blood	20 ng/ml	(F)	(244)	1 hr.	1 Subj.
		72 ng/ml	(H)		40 min.	
		56 ng/ml	(N)		1 hr.	
60-mg	plasma	1 - 5 ng/ml	(F)	(2496)	0.5 - 1 hr.	10 Subj.
		150 - 250 ng/ml	(H)		1 - 4 hr.	
		30 - 50 ng/ml	(N)		3 hr.	
Autopsy Cases						
	blood	510 ng/ml	(F)	(2497)		1 Subj.
		9000 ng/ml	(H)			
		140 ng/ml	(N)			
	plasma	500 - 3200 ng/ml	(F)	(2167)		5 Subj.
		650 - 2500 ng/ml	(H)			
		400 - 1900 ng/ml	(N)			

FLURAZEPAM	Multiple Dose Studies - Oral Administration			
Dose per day Duration of Therapy	Body-fluid sampled	Steady-state concentrations F = Flurazepam H = N-1-Hydroxyethylflurazepam N = N-Desalkylflurazepam	Lit.Ref.	Subjects Characteristics and Remarks
30-mg/d o.d. 14 days	blood	35.1 - 48.0 ng/ml (N)	(241)	3 Subjects
30-mg/d	blood	0.2 - 1.3 ng/ml (F)	(468)	1 Subject
		ca. 40 ng/ml (free) (H)		
		ca. 120 - 200 ng/ml (conj.)(H)		
		ca. 30 - 60 ng/ml (N)		
30-mg/d o.d. 2 weeks	blood	below 3 - 4 ng/ml (F)	(559)	4 Subjects
		detectable in the early hours following administration (H)		
		28 - 88 ng/ml (N)		= calculated minimum steady-state level

FLURAZEPAM	Pharmacokinetic Data derived from the different Studies

F = Flurazepam
H = N-1-hydroxyethylflurazepam
N = N-Desalkylflurazepam

Oral Administration

Distribution Half-Life $t_{1/2\alpha}$

plasma

few minutes	(H)	(2496)
0.7 - 3 hr.	(N)	(2496)

Elimination Half-Life $t_{1/2\beta}$

blood

3.2 - 3.4 hr.	$(H)_{free}$	(468)
32 - 42 hr.	(N)	(468)
2 hr.	(H)	(244)
19 hr.	(N)	(244)
rapid	(H)	(559)
47 - 100 hr.	(N)	(559)

plasma

0.9 - 4.7 hr.	(H)	(2496)
1.6 - 5.3 hr.	(F)	(2496)

BROMAZEPAM — Single Dose Studies - Oral Administration

Dose	Body-fluid sampled	Peak concentrations observed	Lit.Ref.	Time of peak conc. after dose	Subjects Characterist.
6-mg	plasma	70 - 99 ng/ml	(872)	1 - 2 hr.	4 Subj.
9-mg	blood	70 - 164 ng/ml	(236)	2 hr.	5 Subj.
9-mg	blood	32 - 164 ng/ml	(2171)	1 - 2 hr.	12 Subj.
12-mg	blood	110 - 130 ng/ml	(233)	0.5 - 4 hr.	3 Subj.
12-mg	blood	107 - 172 ng/ml	(557)	0.5 - 12 hr.	10 Subj.
15-mg	blood	270 - 360 ng/ml	(237)	ca. 1 hr.	2 Subj.

BROMAZEPAM — Single Dose Studies - Intravenous Administration

6-mg	plasma	95 - 120 ng/ml	(872)	1 - 2 hr.	4 Subj.

BROMAZEPAM — Multiple Dose Studies - Oral Administration

Dose per day Duration of Therapy	Body-fluid sampled	Steady-state concentrations	Lit.Ref.	Subjects Characteristics Remarks
9-mg / d 3-mg t.i.d. 19 days	blood	81 - 154 ng/ml	(557)	7 Subjects

BROMAZEPAM — Pharmacokinetic Data derived from the different Studies

<u>Oral Administration</u>

Distribution Half-Life $t_{1/2\alpha}$	Elimination Half-Life $t_{1/2\beta}$	
	blood	
	18 - 19 hr.	(237)
	11.4 - 27.7 hr.	(557) single dose
	14.1 - 23.8 hr.	(557) chronic doses
	14.7 - 24.1 hr.	(872)

<u>Intravenous Administration</u>

	15 - 24 hr.	(872)

FLUNITRAZEPAM	Single Dose Studies - Oral Administration				
Dose	Body-fluid sampled	Peak concentrations observed F = Flunitrazepam N = Norflunitrazepam A = 7-Aminoflunitrazepam NA= 7-Aminonorflunitrazepam	Lit.Ref.	Time of peak conc. after dose	Subjects Characterist.
1-mg	blood	ca. 2.8 ng/ml (F)	(236)	1 - 2 hr.	1 Subject
1-mg	plasma	ca. 6 - 7 ng/ml (F)	(2501)	ca. 2 hr.	1 Subject
1-mg	plasma	1.8 - 10.7 ng/ml (F) (no max. levels)	(2515)	ca. 12 hr. (no max.lev.)	12 women (late pregnancy)
2-mg	blood	ca. 28 ng/ml (F)	(163)	ca. 1 hr.	1 Subject
2-mg	blood	ca. 6 ng/ml (F)	(231)	ca. 2 hr.	1 Subject
2-mg	blood	ca. 6 ng/ml (F)	(236)	ca. 2 hr.	1 Subject
2-mg	plasma	9 - 15 ng/ml (F)	(164)	ca. 1 hr.	4 Subjects
2-mg	plasma	ca. 10 - 20 ng/ml (F)	(1292)	ca. 1 - 4 hr.	4 Subjects
2-mg	plasma	ca. 10 - 11 ng/ml (F)	(2047)	ca. 2 hr.	1 Subject
2-mg	plasma	ca. 12 ng/ml (F)	(2501)	ca. 2 hr.	1 Subject
2-mg	plasma	no maximum concentrations ! 5.1 ng/ml (F) 2.8 ng/ml (N) 4.6 ng/ml (A) 1.8 ng/ml (NA)	(2501)	 9 hr. 9 hr. 9 hr. 24 hr.	1 Subject
2-mg	plasma	10 - 20 ng/ml (F)	(2502)	3 hr.	8 Subjects
2-mg	plasma	ca. 3.2 - 4.0 ng/ml no max. levels (!) (F) ca. 1 - 2 ng/ml (N)	(2515)	11 hr. 39 hr.	5 Subjects
2-mg	plasma	ca. 12 ng/ml (F)	(2525)	ca. 2 hr.	1 Subject
4-mg	plasma	ca. 20 ng/ml (F)	(2501)	ca. 2 - 3 hr.	1 Subject

FLUNITRAZEPAM	Single Dose Studies - Intravenous Administration				
Dose	Body-fluid sampled	Peak concentrations observed F = Flunitrazepam N = Norflunitrazepam A = 7-Aminoflunitrazepam NA= 7-Amino-norflunitrazepam	Lit.Ref.	Time of peak conc. after dose	Subjects Characterist. Remarks
1-mg	serum	6.0 ± 1.5 ng/ml (mean ± S.D.) (F) 2.2 ± 0.6 ng/ml (mean ± S.D.) (A)	(1655)	4 hr. 4 hr.	no maximum levels (!)
2-mg	blood	30 - 66 ng/ml (F)	(163)	few min.	2 Subjects
2-mg	blood	65 - 76 ng/ml (F)	(2500)	few min.	3 Subjects
2-mg	plasma	30 - 40 ng/ml (F)	(164)	few min.	3 Subjects
2-mg	plasma	ca. 35 ng/ml (F) ca. 2 - 3 ng/ml (N) ca. 6 ng/ml (A)	(2436)	few min. ca. 12 hr. ca. 12 hr.	1 Subject

FLUNITRAZEPAM	Single Dose Studies - Intravenous Administration (continued)				
Dose	Body-fluid sampled	Peak concentrations observed F = Flunitrazepam N = Norflunitrazepam A = 7-Aminoflunitrazepam NA= 7-Amino-norflunitrazepam	Lit.Ref.	Time of peak conc. after dose	Subjects Characterist. Remarks
2-mg	plasma	ca. 35 ng/ml (F)	(2501)	few min.	1 Subject
2-mg	plasma	65 ng/ml (F)	(2501)	few min.	1 Subject
2-mg	plasma	ca. 38 ng/ml (F)	(2525)	few min.	1 Subject
2-mg	serum	10.4 ± 3.0 ng/ml (mean ± S.D.) (F) 4.5 ± 1.6 ng/ml (mean ± S.D.) (A)	(1655)	4 hr. 4 hr.	no maximum levels (!)

FLUNITRAZEPAM	Single Dose Studies - Intramuscular Administration				
2-mg	blood	ca. 23 ng/ml (F)	(163)	ca. 2 hr.	1 Subject
2-mg	blood	ca. 14 - 23 ng/ml (F)	(2500)	ca. 1 - 2 hr.	3 Subjects

FLUNITRAZEPAM	Single Dose Studies - Rectal Administration				
2-mg	plasma	5 - 12 ng/ml (F)	(164)	ca. 1 - 2 hr.	6 Subjects

FLUNITRAZEPAM	Multiple Dose Studies - Oral Administration			
Dose per day Duration of Therapy	Body-fluid sampled	Steady-state concentrations F = Flunitrazepam A = 7-Aminoflunitrazepam	Lit. Ref.	Subjects Characteristics Remarks
2-mg/d day 15-19	blood	ca. 10 ng/ml (F)	(1292)	2 Subjects
2-mg/d 24 days	plasma	2.4 - 2.8 ng/ml (F) 5.6 - 12.0 ng/ml (A)	(2199)	2 Subjects
2-mg/d 28 days	plasma	ca. 2.5 ng/ml (F) < 8 ng/ml (metabolites)	(2502)	8 Subjects

FLUNITRAZEPAM	Pharmacokinetic Data derived from the different Studies

Oral Administration

Distribution Half-Life $t_{1/2\alpha}$

blood

0.48 - 5.6 hr. (single doses) (1292)

1.22 - 5.22 hr. (multiple doses) (1292)

Absorption Half-Life $t_{1/2\,a}$

0.009 - 1.22 hr. (1292)

Elimination Half-Life $t_{1/2\beta}$

blood

10.1 - 17.8 hr. (single doses) (1292)

15.5 - 22.0 hr. (multiple doses) (1292)

plasma

19.3 - 36.5 hr. (2502)

Clearance (l/hr/kg) 0.167 - 0.399 (multiple doses) (1292)

0.242 - 0.336 (single doses) (1292)

Volume of Distribution (l/kg) 4.51 - 7.75 (multiple doses) (1292)

3.44 - 5.51 (single doses) (1292)

CLOBAZAM	Single Dose Studies - Oral Administration					
Dose	Body-fluid sampled	Peak concentration observed C = Clobazam N = Norclobazam		Lit.Ref.	Time of peak conc. after dose	Subjects Characteristics
10-mg	serum	170 - 230 ng/ml	(C)	(1101)	2 hr.	2 Subjects
20-mg	serum	340 - 380 ng/ml	(C)	(1101)	1 - 2 hr.	3 Subjects
20-mg	serum	244 ± 31 (mean ± S.E.M.)	(C)	(2466)	1 - 4 hr.	8 Subjects
30-mg	serum	430 ± 26 (mean ± S.E.M.)	(C)	(2466)	1 - 4 hr.	10 Subjects
40-mg	plasma	ca. 500 ng/ml	(C)	(2491)	ca. 2 hr.	1 Subject
40-mg	serum	527 ± 78 (mean ± S.E.M.)	(C)	(2466)	1 - 4 hr.	3 Subjects

CLOBAZAM	Multiple Dose Studies - Oral Administration			
Dose per Day Duration of Therapy	Body-fluid sampled	Steady-state concentrations C = Clobazam N = Norclobazam	Lit.Ref.	Subjects Characteristics Remarks
30-mg/d 10 days	serum	333 ± 61 (mean ± S.E.M.) (C) 2811 ±540 (mean ± S.E.M.) (N)	(2466)	7 Subjects
30-mg/d 10 days	serum	900 ±230 (mean ± S.E.M.) (C) 3600 ±1300(mean ± S.E.M.) (N)	(1542)	7 Subjects

CLOBAZAM	Pharmacokinetic Data derived from the different Studies

Oral Administration

Distribution Half-Life $t_{1/2\alpha}$

Elimination Half-Life $t_{1/2\beta}$

serum

9.7 - 30.3 hr. (2466)

CAMAZEPAM	Single Dose Studies - Oral Administration				
Dose	Body-fluid sampled	Peak concentration observed	Lit.Ref.	Time of peak conc. after dose	Subjects Characteristics
20-mg	blood	140 - 190 ng/ml	(2458)	1 - 2 hr.	4 Subjects
20-mg	plasma	ca. 70 ng/ml	(2494)	ca. 6 hr.	1 Subject

CAMAZEPAM	Single Dose Studies - Intravenous Administration				
20-mg	blood	210 - 270 ng/ml	(2458)	20 min.	3 Subjects

CAMAZEPAM	Pharmacokinetic Data derived from the different Studies

Oral Administration

Distribution Half-Life $t_{1/2\alpha}$

Elimination Half-Life $t_{1/2\beta}$

blood

21 hr. (2458)

KETAZOLAM	Single Dose Studies - Oral Administration				
Dose	Body-fluid sampled	Peak concentration observed	Lit.Ref.	Time of peak conc. after dose	Subjects Characteristics
30-mg	serum	4.69 ng/ml (Ketazolam) 19.45 ng/ml (Diazepam)	(3769)	3.2 hr. 6 hr.	

KETAZOLAM	Pharmacokinetic Data derived from the different studies

Oral Administration

Elimination Half-Life $t_{1/2\beta}$

serum

2 hr (3769)

Proteinbinding: serum 92.9 % (3769)

serumalbumin 79.9 % (3769)

TRIAZOLAM	Single Dose Studies - Oral Administration				
Dose	Body-fluid sampled	Peak concentration observed	Lit.Ref.	Time of peak conc. after dose	Subjects Characteristics
0.88-mg	plasma	ca. 7.6 ng/ml	(3775)	0.75 - 2.5 hr.	
1.00-mg	plasma	ca. 11.5 ng/ml	(3775)	ca. 1.5 hr.	
0.88-mg	blood	ca. 4.8 ng/ml	(3775)	0.75 - 2.5 hr.	

TRIAZOLAM	Multiple Dose Studies - Oral Administration			
Dose per day Duration of Therapy	Body-fluid sampled	Concentrations observed	Lit.Ref.	Subjects Characteristics and Remarks
1.0-mg/d. o.d. 7 days	plasma	mean 0.44 - 0.66 ng/ml (24 hr. after dose) no steady state levels	(3775)	12 Subjects

TRIAZOLAM	Pharmacokinetic Data derived from the different studies

Oral Administration

Elimination Half-Life $t_{1/2\beta}$
plasma
2.7 hr. (± 0.5 hr.) S.D. (3775)

Proteinbinding: 89 % (3775)

LORMETAZEPAM	Single Dose Studies - Oral Administration				
Dose	**Body-fluid sampled**	**Peak concentration observed**	**Lit.Ref.**	**Time of peak conc. after dose**	**Subjects Characteristics**
1.0-mg	plasma	5.6 ± 0.7 ng/ml	(3047, 3048)	2 hr.	

LORMETAZEPAM	Pharmacokinetic Data derived from the different studies

Oral Administration

Distribution Half-Life $t_{1/2\alpha}$

ca. 2 hr. (3047, 3048)

Elimination Half-Life $t_{1/2\beta}$

ca. 10 hr. (3047, 3048)

Proteinbinding: more than 85 % (3047, 3048)

Ranges of Maximum Concentrations After Oral Administration

Bereiche maximaler Konzentration nach oraler Verabreichung

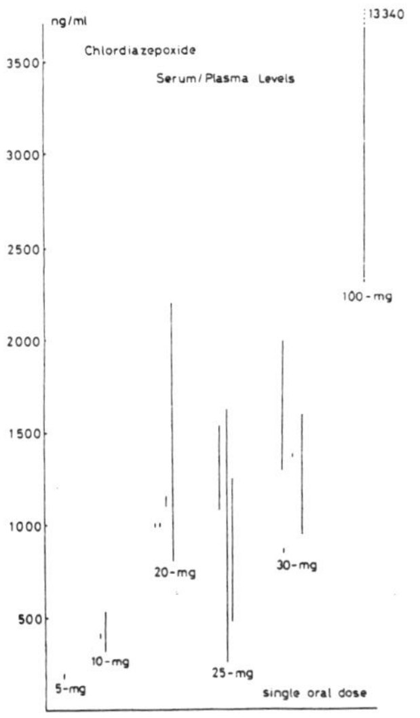

Ranges of maximum concentrations in serum and plasma after a single oral administration of 5, 10, 20, 25, 30 and 100 mg chlordiazepoxide

Bereiche maximaler Serum- bzw. Plasmakonzentrationen nach der einmaligen oralen Verabreichung von 5, 10, 20, 25, 30 und 100 mg Chlordiazepoxid

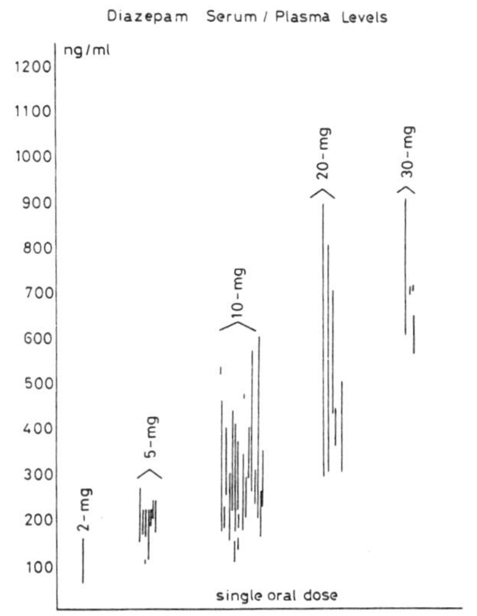

Ranges of maximum concentrations in serum and plasma after a single oral administration of 2, 5, 10, 20 and 30 mg diazepam

Bereiche maximaler Serum- bzw. Plasmakonzentrationen nach der einmaligen oralen Verabreichung von 2, 5, 10, 20 und 30 mg Diazepam

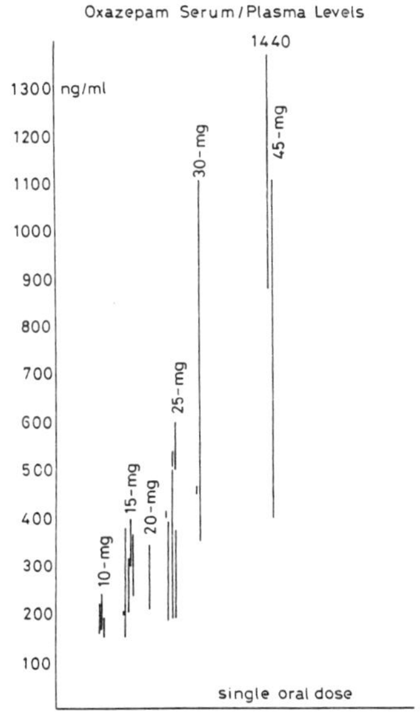

Ranges of maximum concentrations in serum and plasma after a single oral administration of 10, 15, 20, 30 and 45 mg oxazepam

Bereiche maximaler Serum- bzw. Plasmakonzentrationen nach der einmaligen oralen Verabreichung von 10, 15, 20, 30 und 45 mg Oxazepam

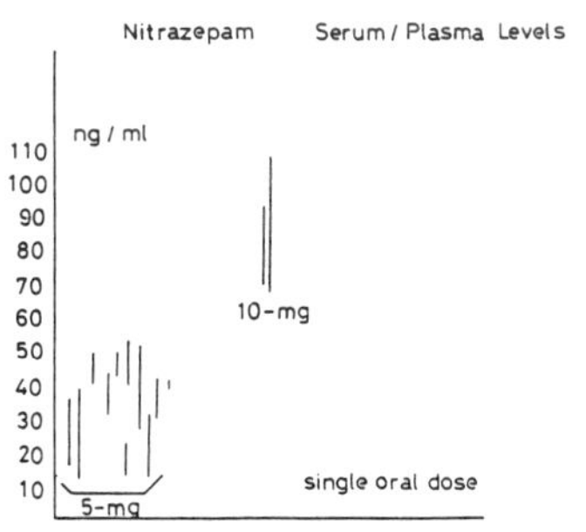

Ranges of maximum concentrations in serum and plasma after a single oral administration of 5 and 10 mg nitrazepam

Bereiche maximaler Serum- bzw. Plasmakonzentrationen nach der einmaligen oralen Verabreichung von 5 bzw. 10 mg Nitrazepam

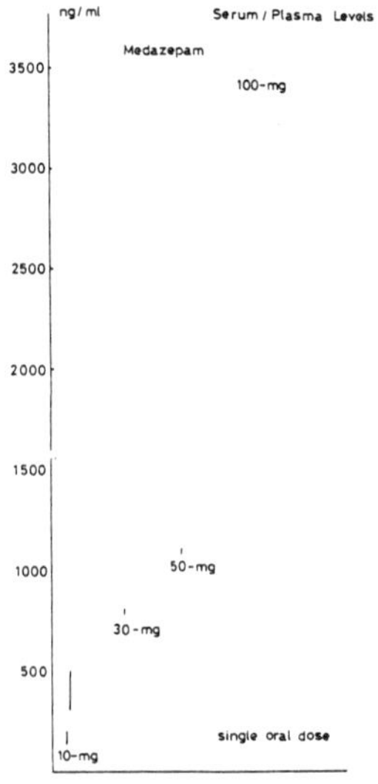

Ranges of maximum concentrations in serum and plasma after a single oral administration of 10, 30, 50 and 100 mg medazepam

Bereiche maximaler Serum- bzw. Plasmakonzentrationen nach der einmaligen oralen Verabreichung von 10, 30, 50 und 100 mg Medazepam

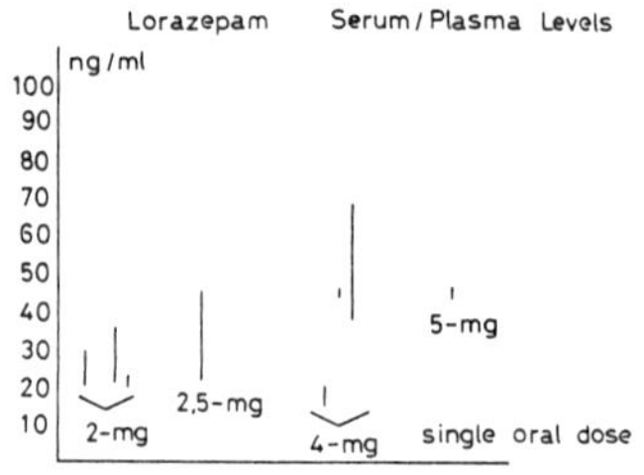

Ranges of maximum concentrations in serum and plasma after a single oral administration of 2, 2,5, 4 and 5 mg lorazepam

Bereiche maximaler Serum- bzw. Plasmakonzentrationen nach der einmaligen oralen Verabreichung von 2, 2,5, 4 und 5 mg Lorazepam

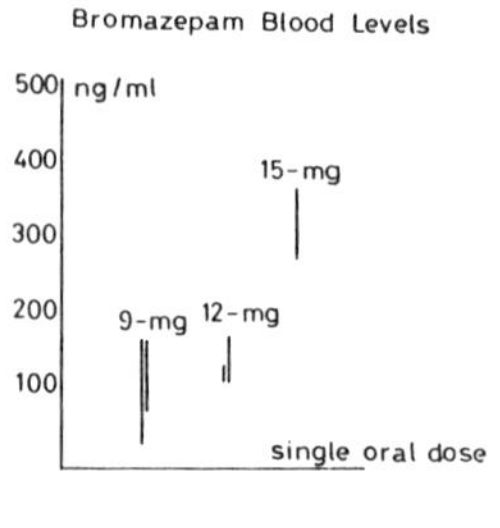

Ranges of maximum blood concentrations after a single oral administration of 9, 12 and 15 mg bromazepam

Bereiche maximaler Blutkonzentrationen nach der einmaligen oralen Verabreichung von 9, 12 und 15 mg Bromazepam

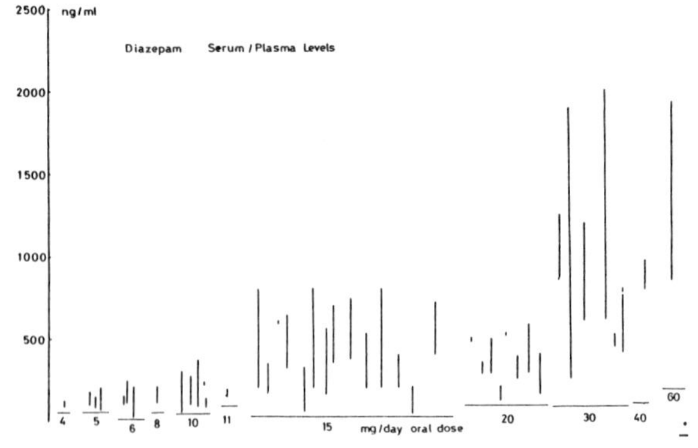

Steady-state concentrations of diazepam in serum and plasma after daily oral administration of 4, 5, 6, 8, 10, 11, 15, 20, 30, 40 and 60 mg diazepam

Steady-State Serum- bzw. Plasmakonzentrationen von Diazepam nach einer täglichen oralen Verabreichung von 4, 5, 6, 8, 10, 11, 15, 20, 30, 40 und 60 mg Diazepam

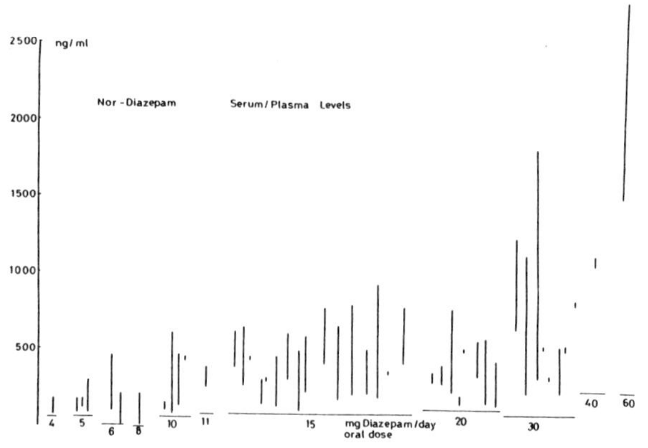

Steady-state concentrations of nordiazepam in serum and plasma after daily oral administration of 4, 5, 6, 8, 10, 11, 15, 20, 30, 40 and 60 mg diazepam

Steady-State Serum- bzw. Plasmakonzentrationen von Nor-Diazepam nach einer täglichen oralen Verabreichung von 4, 5, 6, 8, 10, 11, 15, 20, 30, 40 und 60 mg Diazepam

Survey of Benzodiazepine Literature

Übersicht zur Benzodiazepinliteratur

Scheme of the Compilation/ Schema der Zusammenstellung

Example

Gas-Liquid-Chromatography / Gaschromatographie

240. Medazepam, diazepam and major metabolites
(blood and urine, ECD, man)

indicates the method
indicates reference number (see References)
indicates treated substances
indicates special mode of the method
indicates the subject
indicates the kind of sample

Survey of Literature/Literaturübersicht

1. Absorption / Resorption
2. Benzodiazepines in Relation to Mother and Child / Benzodiazepine -Zusammenhänge zwischen Mutter und Kind.
3. Bioavailability Studies / Bioverfügbarkeitsstudien
4. Biotransformation-Metabolism / Biotransformation - Metabolismus-Stoffwechsel
5. Disposition / Disposition (see also 4. 16. 19.)
6. Effects with other Compounds / Wirkungen mit anderen Stoffen
7. Emergency-Drug-Analysis / Notfalluntersuchung
8. Extraction from Biological Samples / Extraktion aus biologischem Material
9. Fluorescence - Fluorometry / Fluoreszenz -Fluorometrie
10. Gas-Liquid-Chromatography / Gaschromatographie
11. General Analytical Data / Allgemeine analytische Daten
12. General Treatment (Books, Great Reviews) / Allgemeine Abhandlung (Bücher, große Übersichten)
13. High-Pressure-Liquid-Chromatography / Hochdruckflüssigkeitschromatographie (HPLC)
14. Hydrolysis of Benzodiazepines (special investigations)/ Benzodiazepinhydrolyse (spezielle Untersuchungen)
15. IR-Spectra / Infrarot-Spektren
16. Levels (Blood-, Plasma-, Serum-, Others) / Spiegel (Blut-, Plasma-, Serum-, Andere)
17. Mass-Spectra (also GLC / MS) / Massenspektren (auch GLC / MS)
18. NMR - Investigations / NMR - Untersuchungen
19. Pharmacokinetic / Pharmakokinetik
20. Pharmacology and Clinical Investigations (Selection) / Pharmakologie und klinische Untersuchungen (Auswahl)
21. Poisoning / Vergiftungen (Reports and Treatment) /(Berichte und Behandlung)
22. Polarography / Polarographie
23. Protein-Binding / Proteinbindung
24. Radioactive-Labelled-Compounds / Radioaktiv markierte Verbindungen
25. Radioimmunoassay / Radioimmunoassay
26. Screening / Suchanalyse
27. Side-, Adverse-, Withdrawal- and Residual-Effects / Nebenwirkungen und Entzugserscheinungen
28. Sleep-Effects / Schlafwirkungen
29. Synthesis / Synthesen
30. Theory of Action / Wirkungstheorie
31. Thin-Layer-Chromatography / Dünnschichtchromatographie
32. Toxicity - Toxicology / Toxizität - Toxikologie
33. Traffic-Medicine / Verkehrsmedizin
34. UV-Spectroscopy (also Visible) - Colorimetry / UV-Spektroskopie (auch im Sichtbaren) - Kolorimetrie
35. Other Themes / Andere Themen

Absorption / Resorption

2. Chlorazepate (changes in absorption at normal and elevated gastric pH). 78. Diazepam (absorption of a new preparation). 115. Benzodiazepines (effects of different rates of absorption on clinical parameters). 181. Chlorazepate (effects of antacids on absorption). 348. Diazepam (factors influencing absorption). 349. Diazepam (factors influencing absorption). 352. Diazepam (factors influencing absorption after oral administration). 425. Chlordiazepoxide (influence of magnesium- and aluminium-hydroxyde). 428. Chlordiazepoxide (slow absorption after i.m. administration). 432. Lorazepam (absorption after oral administration). 471. Diazepam (alcohol and oral absorption). 547. Diazepam (absorption of tablets in man).

595. Oxazepam (absorption in humans). 671. Oxazepam (Resorption in Kombination mit Alkohol). 1191. Oxazepam (absorption and excretion).

1504. Diazepam (effect of antacids and food). 1510. ^{14}C-Lorazepam. 1519. Chlordiazepoxide (oral). 1525. Chlordiazepoxide (oral and i.m.). 1526. Diazepam (effect of a cocktail). 1656. Diazepam (after oral, and i.m. administration into vastus lateralis muscle and deltoid muscle). 1810. Chlordiazepoxide (oral and i.m., absorption by alcoholics). 1899. Desmethyldiazepam (from chlorazepate, impaired absorption by magnesium aluminium hydroxyde).

2313. Diazepam (oral, influence of three antacids). 2396. Drugs (effect of abdominal radiation therapy on absorption in humans). 2415. Diazepam (woman with preclampsia, routes of administration and rate of adsorption, study). 2536. Clotiazepam (man).

2574. Diazepam (alcohol does not enhance its absorption). 2945. ^{14}C-Lormetazepam (dogs, rabbits, rats, rhesus monkeys). 3047. 3048. ^{14}C-Lormetazepam (humans). 3132. Triazolam (rat, dog, monkey). 3225. Diazepam (man, following rectal and parenteral administration). 3314. Diazepam (influence of neuroticism on oral absorption). 3343. Desmethyldiazepam (from clorazepate, effect of age and billroth gastrectomy). 3721. Diazepam (absorption from a lipid-containing dosage form).

Benzodiazepines in Relation to Mother and Child
(Key Words: fetus, newborn, infant, child, placental passage, perinatal, prenatal, labour, breast-feeding, milk, pregnancy, lactation period).

Benzodiazepine, Zusammenhänge zwischen Mutter und Kind
(Schlüsselwörter: Fötus, Neugeborenes, Säugling, Kleinkind, Placentarpassage, perinatal, pränatal, Wehen, Stillen, Muttermilch, Schwangerschaft, Stillperiode).

5. Diazepam (effect of maternal intake on the bilirubin-binding of cord blood). 15. Diazepam (respiratory and neurologic depression in the premature newborn infant of a mother treated with diazepam). 27. Chlordiazepoxide (withdrawal in the neonate). 86. Oxazepam (ability of the placenta to metabolize oxazepam). 87. Oxazepam (patterns of drug metabolism in liver and some none-hepatic tissues of fetal and newborn rabbits). 138. Diazepam, Desmethyldiazepam (in breast milk). 208. Diazepam (effect on clinical condition and thermogenesis of the newborn). 223. Oxazepam (and aminopyrine, transformation in the rabbit placenta). 295. Diazepam (perinatal metabolism). 296. Diazepam (transfer across placenta). 297. Diazepam (and breast feeding). 355. Diazepam (mother and infant). 389. Diazepam (floppy infant syndrome). 390. Diazepam (during neonatal period). 436. Lorazepam (placental transfer). 455. Diazepam (perinatal metabolism). 464. Diazepam (floppy infant syndrome and maternal diazepam). 465. Diazepam (transplacental passage). 490. Oxazepam (maternal and fetal level in guinea-pigs). 508. Diazepam (placental transfer in early human pregnancy). 543. Nitrazepam (across human placenta). 549. Diazepam (feto-maternal distribution in early pregnancy). 550. Diazepam, Desmethyldiazepam (accumulation in fetal blood during labour). 551. Diazepam (perinatal metabolism). 622. Psychotropic agents (lactation).

655. Diazepam (use in early pregnancy). 674. Diazepam (placental transfer and disposition in newborns). 677. Drugs (metabolism in the rabbit lung during pregnancy and in the perinatal period). 678. Oxazepam (and luminal, effect on drug metabolizing processes of the rabbit placenta in various periods of pregnancy). 691. Diazepam (metabolism in newborn animals). 698. Oxazepam (studies on fetal pharmacology). 699. Oxazepam (organotropism and drug metabolizing activity in the fetus and the newborn). 714. Diazepam (distribution in pregnant and lactating rabbits). 722. Chlordiazepoxide (and meprobamate, effect on human embryonic and fetal development). 744. Drugs (drug interactions in the fetus and in the newborn infant). 745. Diazepam (elimination in premature infants and children). 781. Diazepam (effect on fertility and gestation of female rats). 800. Diazepam (in the newborn). 819. Benzodiazepine (médecine perinatale). 827. Diazepam (effect of diazepam administrated to mother during labour on temperature regulation of neonate). 839. Diazepam (and breast feeding). 915. Diazepam (and meprobamate, fetus). 920. Diazepam (prenat ally administered, effect on the premature infant). 945. Diazepam (placental penetration, foetal uptake). 956. Diazepam (neonatal pharmacology). 957. Benzodiazepines (neonates). 1012. Diazepam (and meperidine, permeability of human chorion). 1102. Chlordiazepoxide (transplacental passage). 1134. Diazepam (effect on uterine activity during labor). 1144. Medikamente (praenatal verabreicht, Bedeutung für Früh- und Neugeborene)

1233. Diazepam (metabolism in the human fetus). 1268. Diazepam (parenterally administered, relief of emotional factor in labor). 1270. Diazepam (Wirkungsqualität am Uterus). 1271. Diazepam (Anwendung bei 3000 Gebärenden). 1319. Diazepam (effect of maternal diazepam on newborn). 1333. Diazepam (pilot study, concentrations in maternal blood, amniotic fluid and cord blood). 1387. Diazepam (humans, blood levels and placental transfer). 1424. Diazepam (and pethidine, during labour, effect on the newborn). 1429. Diazepam (early pregnancy, concentrations in mother and foetus). 1430. Diazepam (early pregnancy). 1456. Diazepam (effect on labor). 1546. Diazepam (transplacental passage during labor). 1571. Diazepam (Frühschwangerschaft und Stillperiode). 1584. Lorazepam (plasma estimation in neonates). 1591. ^{14}C-Diazepam (placental transfer, mice, hamsters, monkeys). 1676. Diazepam, N-Desmethyldiazepam (newborn infants, after i.v., i.m., rectal and oral administration). 1698. Diazepam (use in early pregnancy). 1732. Diazepam (blood levels in infants of two mothers given large doses in labour). 1773. Prazepam and metabolites (diaplacental passage and fetal hepatic-metabolism in early human pregnancy). 1858. Diazepam (effect of maternal intake on the newborn). 1876. Diazepam (effect on the fetus). 1951. Diazepam (i.v., effect on fetal and maternal acid-base balance during and after delivery). 1975. Oxazepam (placental passage). 2026. Diazepam (and fenoterol, influence of a tocolytic treatment of pregnant-women on the bilirubin levels and apgar score of newborn). 2029. Diazepam (and ketamin, Placentarpassage). 2031. Diazepam (side-effects of maternal diazepam on newborn-infants).

2044. Diazepam (metabolism in human fetal and adult liver). 2061. Benzodiazepines (Behandlung des Abortus imminens und der drohenden Frühgeburt). 2087. Diazepam, chlordiazepoxide (Behandlung des Abortus imminens, der drohenden Frühgeburt und der Placenta praevia). 2111. Diazepam (in breast milk). 2120. Diazepam and metabolites (in breast milk, transfer to the neonate). 2148. Diazepam (hohe Dosen in der Schwangerschaft, Kasuistik). 2160. Diazepam and N-desmethyldiazepam (feto-maternal concentrations after intra amniotic injection). 2237. Diazepam (distribution and metabolism in early and late human pregnancy, postnatal metabolism). 2316. + 2319. Diazepam (during labor). 2376. Diazepam (Behandlung des Abortus imminens).

2515. Flunitrazepam (placental transfer and breast-milk levels). 2529. Lorazepam (plasma concentrations in mother and neonate).

2767. Diazepam (+ phenobarbital, effects on the EEG in newborn babies during the first 24 hrs.). 2768. (see 2767.). 2986. Benzodiazepines (transfer in vitro across human placenta). 3007. Diazepam (as induction agent, caesarean section, fetal drug exposure). 3008. Diazepam (i.v., before breech delivery, fetal drug exposure). 3010. Chlordiazepoxide (+ barbital, + ethanol, effect on the behavior of the offspring). 3098. Oxazepam (transfer across human placenta). 3101. Lorazepam (and conjugate, transfer across human placenta). 3193. Prazepam (placental transfer in humans during first half of pregnancy). 3248. Diazepam (biochemical and pharmacological aspects of fetal exposure). 3261. Diazepam (just before delivery, placental transfer and neonatal effects). 3262. Lorazepam (placental transfer). 3308. Benzodiazepines (+ phenothiazines, effects on fetus). 3424. Clorazepate (pharmacokinetics in pregnant women). 3425. Clorazepate (pharmacokinetics of placental transfer). 3589. Diazepam (to women in labour, effects on neonatal hyperbilirubinaemia). 3657. Diazepam (during pregnancy, or labor, effects on the heart rate variability of the newborn).

Bioavailability Studies / Bioverfügbarkeits-Studien

22. Diazepam. 77. Diazepam. 118. Nitrazepam, Clonazepam. 224.Clonazepam, Nitrazepam (humans). 607. Diazepam (after i.m. injection). 614. Lorazepam (humans). 715. Oxazepam (influence of food intake). 738. Nitrazepam. 934. Psychotropic drugs including benzodiazepines. 1063. Chlordiazepoxide (two preparations).

1328. Chlorazepate (after two dosage forms). 1518. Lorazepam (humans, after i.v., i.m. and oral administration). 1652. General (drugs). 1813. Oxazepam (oral dosage forms).

2175. Temazepam (humans, after administration in soft gelatine capsules). 2251. Diazepam (comparative study of two oral preparations).

2737. Diazepam (availability from plastic containers). 2901. Temazepam (from soft gelatine capsules). 3159. Chlordiazepoxide (in humans). 3401. Diazepam (from tablets).

Biotransformation / Metabolism

Biotransformation / Metabolismus / Verstoffwechselung

3. Diazepam (in human cortex kidney microsomes). 11. Triflubazam (man). 12. Triflubazam (rat, dog, monkey). 23. Oxazepam (glucurone-conjugation, in situ isolation, liver). 24. Oxazepam (glucurone-conjugation, in situ, brain). 25. Chlordiazepoxide (effect on glucose metabolism). 52. Nitrazepam (perfused isolated liver). 53. Nitrazepam (reduction by rat liver). 54. Nitrazepam (reduction in vitro). 59. Triflubazam (Mice, dogs). 73. Oxazepam (isolated perfused liver in situ). 74. Oxazepam (cerebral drug metabolism). 85. Oxazepam (pregnant guinea pig and rat). 87. Oxazepam (patterns of drug-metabolism of fetal and newborn rabbits). 91. Diazepam (biliary metabolites). 97. Chlordiazepoxide, Diazepam, Oxazepam, Chlorazepate, Lorazepam, Nitrazepam, Medazepam. 98. (wie 97.). 99. Nitrazepam, Diazepam, Oxazepam, Chlordiazepoxid. 101. Nitrazepam. 107. Diazepam (species and substrate differences of liver microsomal N-desalkylation and N-oxidation). 164. Flunitrazepam (after intake of various galenic formulations). 199. Diazepam and pinazepam (different animal species). 204. Diazepam (changes in metabolism). 205. Chlordiazepoxid. 208. Diazepam. 223. Oxazepam (in rabbit placenta at various periods of pregnancy). 251. Prazepam (dog). 252. Prazepam (dog). 253. Prazepam (man). 254. Prazepam (man). 259. Chlordiazepoxide (man). 267. Diazepam (man). 280. Clonazepam, Nitrazepam. 283. Flunitrazepam. 284. Benzodiazepine (Übersicht). 298. Clonazepam (rat, dog, man). 303. Diazepam (rat, mice). 309. Oxazepam (Ringverengung). 341. Bromazepam (rat). 361. Nitrazepam, Oxazepam, Diazepam (Speziesunterschiede). 396. Nitrazepam (in the intestines of white rats). 397. (see 396.). 455. Diazepam (perinatal metabolism). 469. Flurazepam (new metabolite by in vitro metabolizing enzymes). 485. Diazepam (normal man). 508. Diazepam (fetal metabolism).

517. Chlordiazepoxide, Diazepam, Oxazepam (stimulatory effects on the drug metabolizing systems). 530. Diazepam (in rabbits). 551. Diazepam (perinatal metabolism). 599. Chlordiazepoxide (metabolic fate). 600. Chlordiazepoxid (man, dog, rat). 613. Diazepam (in isolated liver of rat and mouse). 651. Medazepam (rat). 658. Chlordiazepoxide (other data). 659. Diazepam (other data). 662. Drugs (microsomal desalkylation). 665. Flurazepam (by the small intestine). 677. Drugs (in the rabbit lung). 683. Diazepam (by liver microsomal enzymes of rats and mice). 684. Diazepam (effect of phenobarbital on in vitro metabolism in several animal species). 685. Diazepam (species difference in metabolism). 687. Diazepam (in guinea pigs). 688. Diazepam (species difference). 692. Diazepam (species difference). 694. N-desmethyldiazepam. 765. Diazepam (guinea pigs). 766. Diazepam and metabolites (guinea pig liver microsomes). 792. Flurazepam (rat). 842. Oxazepam (Mensch). 854. Diazepam (cat, chronic treatment). 855. Chlordiazepoxide (mice). 864. Chlordiazepoxide (Mensch). 908. Nitrazepam (Mensch und Ratte). 909. Nitrazepam. 910. Nitrazepam (man). 911. Medazepam (Mensch). 916. Aminoacetaminobenzophenone (cyclization to corresponding benzodiazepine in the rat in vivo). 923. Diazepam (dog). 947. Bromazepam (urine). 948. Bromazepam (urine). 949. Bromazepam (hydroxylation). 950. Bromazepam (new urinary metabolite). 951. Nitrazepam-metabolite (rabbit). 955. Nitrazepam and metabolites. 961. Lorazepam (humans and four animal species). 962. Lorazepam (male rat). 963. lorazepam (glucuronide formation, rat). 994. Medazepam (rat, dog, man). 995. Diazepam (rat, dog, man). 996. Diazepam (rat, dog, man). 997. Medazepam (dog, rat). 999. Chlordiazepoxide (metabolic demethylation). 1000. Diazepam (in vitro). 1001. Flurazepam (man, dog). 1002. Demoxepam (man). 1003. Chlordiazepoxide, metabolites (man). 1004. Demoxepam (dog). 1005. Bromazepam (human, dog, rat, mouse). 1006. Chlordiazepoxide (rat). 1007. Flurazepam (man, dog). 1008. Flurazepam (urinary metabolites). 1016. Diazepam (after chronic alcohol intake, man and animals). 1052. Oxazepam (man, pig, rat). 1053. Oxazepam (man, miniature swine, rat). 1065. Chlordiazepoxide (mice, following hepatic irradiation). 1082. Oxazepam. 1103. Diazepam (and phenobarbital and diphenylhydantoine). 1124. Bromazepam (attachment of a methylthio group). 1152. Diazepam, chlordiazepoxide (mice). 1154. Diazepam (animals, humans). 1155. Ataractic drugs. 1171. Prazepam (humans, after chronic administration). 1172. Prazepam (in vitro). 1173. Prazepam (in vitro). 1174. Prazepam (rat). 1191. Oxazepam. 1215. Nimetazepame, nitrazepam (comparative study). 1216. s. 1215. 1217. Oxazolam (rats). 1227. Diazepam (chronic administration).

1233. Diazepam (effect on human fetus). 1238. Oxazepam (dogs, first pass conjugation, enterohepatic recycling). 1240. Flunitrazepam (pharmacokinetic and metabolism). 1285. Diazepam (mice, hypergravity). 1287. Clonazepam (and carbamazepine, metabolic drug interaction). 1426. Lorazepam. 1466. Diazepam (animals and man). 1469. Benzodiazepines (metabolic studies, various animal species). 1489. Nitrazepam (dependence of method of administration and animal species). 1490. 1,4-Benzodiazepines (hydroxylation in endoplasmic-reticulum of albino rats). 1562. Nitrazepam (importance of intestinal microflora). 1573. ^{14}C-Chlordiazepoxide (rat, metabolism tolerance studies). 1595. Prazepam (metabolic fate, rats). 1596. Prazepam (cyclopropylmethyl-group, metabolic fate, rats). 1615. Prazepam (monkeys). 1710. Diazepam (man). 1718. Diazepam and metabolites (species differences). 1728. Prazepam (metabolism by rat-liver microsomes, desalkylprazepam). 1793. 4,5-Dihydrodiazepam (levorotary, rat). 1846.

Nitrazepam (biotransformation and pharmacokinetics). 1873. Bromazepam (rabbit, rat, guinea pig). 1885. 1,4-Benzodiazepines (metabolic rearrangement). 1886. Benzodiazepines (pathways of metabolism). 1891. Diazepam (induction effect on its own metabolism). 1960. Bromazepam (rat, methyl-thio-bromazepam). 1975. Oxazepam (mother and newborn, placental-passage). 1996. Lorazepam (excretion and biotransformation, chronic renal failure). 2004. Flunitrazepam (metabolic changes). 2019. Chlordiazepoxide (effect of acute alcohol intoxication on metabolism).

2044. Diazepam (metabolism in human fetal and adult liver). 2086. Nitrazepam (enzymic induction). 2237. Diazepam (metabolism in early and late human pregnancy, postnatal metabolism). 2355. Lorazepam (comparative metabolism in man and four animal species). 2365. Nitrazepam (biotransformation and new urinary metabolite). 2377. 1,4-Benzodiazepines (effects of enzyme induction and inhibition on microsomal oxidation). 2382. Chlordiazepoxide (+ disulfiram, inhibition of biotransformation). 2429. Prazepam (man, rat, effect of chronic administration on metabolism). 2435. Flunitrazepam (Schicksal im menschlichen Organismus).

2469. Clobazam (animals and Man). 2496. Flurazepam (interpretation). 2504. Diazepam, oxazepam, temazepam, nitrazepam, flurazepam. 2536. Clotiazepam (man).

2647. Nitrazepam (reduction by rat-liver mitochondria). 2651. Benzodiazepines (conversion by immobilized animal liver microsomal fraction). 2652. Phenacepam + Metabolites (intrahepatic circulation, albino rats). 2704. Clobazam (species differences in metabolism). 2720. Prazepam (metabolism in female subjects). 2741. Clonazepam (rat, first-pass metabolism). 2845. Benzodiazepines (biotransformation, review). 2846. ^{14}C-Triazolam (disposition in man). 2862. Diazepam (cerebral metabolic study). 2977. Diazepam (+ digitoxin, reciprocal effect on metabolism). 3042. Lorazepam (effect of short-term ethanol administration on metabolism). 3047. ^{14}C-Lormetazepam (humans). 3048. Lormetazepam (man, first-pass effects). 3121. Oxazepam (+ antipyrine, regulation of metabolism in man). 3132. Triazolam (rat, dog, monkey). 3133. Triazolam (rat, dog). 3175. Clonazepam (kinetics of biotransformation to 7-amino-clonazepam). 3193. Prazepam (in vitro fetal hepatic-metabolism). 3215. Diazepam (i.v., in epileptic children). 3216. Diazepam (relation to age). 3258. ^{14}C-Lormetazepam (dogs, rabbits, cats and rhesus monkeys). 3320. Benzodiazepines (metabolism in cultures of isolated hepatocytes and liver fragments of human fetus). 3321. Diazepam (postnatal developtment of sex-dependent differences in the metabolism by rat liver). 3347. Diazepam (effect of enzyme-induction). 3374. Oxazepam, lorazepam (cimetidine spares glucuronidation). 3509. Lormetazepam (man). 3510. Triazolam (man). 3512. Temazepam (man and several animal species). 3562. Diazepam (effects of oral contraceptives on demethylation). 3702. 2'-Chloro-nordiazepam (dog).

3759. Lormetazepam (man). 3760. Triazolam (man). 3769. Ketazolam (man). 3775. Triazolam (man).

Disposition

62. Clonazepam, antipyrine (influence of phenobarbital, dog). 191. Clonazepam, chlordiazepoxide, diazepam, desmethyldiazepam, flurazepam, oxazepam (sub-human primates). 203. Diazepam (mice). 285. Triazolam (dog). 341. Bromazepam (rat). 432. Lorazepam (oral). 478. Diazepam (neben Aminopyrin und Antipyrin). 585. Diazepam (and major metabolites, patients with liver desease). 587. Diazepam (effect of age and liver desease in adult man). 594. Lorazepam (humans). 674. Diazepam (in the newborn). 801. Oxazepam (in uremic patients). 962. Lorazepam (rats). 1027. Chlordiazepoxide (in young and elderly male volunteers). 1043. Oxazepam (in acute viral hepatitis and cirrhosis). 1211. Benzodiazepines (after single oral administration in man).

1339. Prazepam (man, metabolic disposition). 1389. Chlordiazepoxide (effects of sex and oral-contraceptive steroids). 1510. ^{14}C-Lorazepam (after oral application). 1585. Diazepam (and pentobarbital, alterations in disposition after chronic morphine in rats). 1586. Minor tranquilizers (influence of age and liver disease on disposition).

1587. Benzodiazepines (dogs, effects of alcohol on disposition). 1666. Lorazepam (effects of aging and liver disease). 1719. Camazepam (rats and mice). 1754. Diazepam (disposition kinetics in pregnant woman at parturition). 1849. Chlordiazepoxide (effect of age and cirrhosis). 1850. Chlordiazepoxide (effect of age and parenchymal liver-disease). 2021. Diazepam, Chlordiazepoxide, Oxazepam, Lorazepam (man, effect of liver-disease and aging).

2190. Diazepam, prazepam (man, multiple-dose studies). 2370. Sedatives (effect of liver diseases and aging).

2383. Benzodiazepines (influence of disulfiram and disease). 2536. Clotiazepam (man).

2846. ^{14}C-Triazolam (man). 2960. Diazepam (disposition determinants). 2979. Diazepam (effects of solvents). 3041. Benzodiazepines (+ ethanol, effects on disposition in dogs). 3047. + 3048. Lormetazepam (man). 3128. Clonazepam (influence of phenytoin and phenobarbital on disposition of single oral doses). 3215. Diazepam (i.v., in epileptic children). 3338. Lorazepam (rabbits). 3434. Chlordiazepoxide (sex-differences and effects of oral-contraceptives). 3514. Benzodiazepines (effects of disulfiram and ethanol on disposition). 3515. Oxazepam, Chlordiazepoxide (disposition in cirrhotics). 3769. Ketazolam (man).

Effects with other compounds
Wirkungen mit anderen Verbindungen

92. Chlordiazepoxide (+d-amphetamine (man, interaction). 108. Nitrazepam (+ phenprocoumon, influence on anticoagulation). 299. Nitrazepam (+ Äthanol, + Carbamazepin, + Methaqualon, Prüfung der statistischen Wechselwirkung). 307. Diazepam (+ tubocurarine). 310. Benzodiazepines (mouse, effect on brain amines). 311. Benzodiazepines (+ morphine, + sodium salicylate, effect on analgesic effect). 319. Prazepam (+ Alkohol, interaction). 326. Chlordiazepoxide (+ chymotrypsin, coadministration). 335. Oxazepam (absence of interference with glucose-determination). 346. Diazepam (+ doxepine, evaluation in 100 chronic alcoholic patients). 503. Drugs (alcohol, combined effects). 573. Chlordiazepoxide (+ phenprocoumon, interactions, rats). 578. Benzodiazepines (+ 5-hydroxytryptamine, participation in anticonvulsive action). 615. Chlordiazepoxide (+ amylobarbitone, comparative bioassay). 620. Diazepam, Chlordiazepoxide (+ amphetamine, rat, effect on tissue amphetamine levels). 664. Chlordiazepoxide (+ propanidid, interaction). 669. Arzneimittel (+ Alkohol). 670. Arzneimittel (+ Alkohol). 671. Oxazepam (+ Alkohol). 684. Diazepam (+ phenobarbital, several animal species). 701. Diazepam (effect on dopamine and homovanillic acid levels, rat). 739. Diazepam (drug induced stimulation). 741. Oxazepam (+ alcohol, Pharmakokinetik). 742. Diazepam (+ alcohol, combined effects). 743. Benzodiazepines (+ drinking, + smoking). 746. Diazepam (+ alcohol, interaction). 769. Benzodiazepines (+ alcohol, interactions). 821. Benzodiazepines (+ warfarin). 832. Diazepam (+ acetylsalicylic-acid). 840. Diazepam (+ ethanol, mice, supra additive effect). 844. Diazepam (+ pentobarbital, effect on accumulation).

868. Chlordiazepoxide (+ pentobarbital, + ethanol, + THC, rats). 873. Chlordiazepoxide (+ alcohol, overdose). 925. Clobazam (+ nomifensine, interaction). 926. Chlordiazepoxide (+ dexamphetamine, rat, combined effects). 928. Drugs (+ alcohol, man). 967. Oxazepam (+ anticoagulants). 1013. Chlordiazepoxide (+ propanolol, + alcohol, comparative efficacy). 1019. Diazepam (+ pyrithioxin, rat). 1025. Chlordiazepoxide (+ d-amphetamine, combined therapy). 1115. Diazepam (i.v. and oral, man, serum growth hormone, blood glucose, serum immunoreactive insulin). 1126. Diazepam, Chlordiazepoxide, Nitrazepam (catecholamine metabolism). 1148. Benzodiazepines (+ phenytoin). 1183. Diazepam (+ ethanol, drug metabolizing enzymes, rat liver). 1184. Diazepam (inhibition of drug metabolizing enzymes in rat liver). 1206. Benzodiazepines (effect on cholinesterase in serum). 1218. Diazepam (+ regional levels of glucose and malate in the CNS). 1231. Chlordiazepoxide (+ meperidine, arterial blood gases).

1243. Diazepam (+ dixirazine, + opropramol,+ placebo, comparison). 1255. Lorazepam (+ glutethimide, comparison). 1275. Diazepam (+ doxepin, comparative trial). 1276. Benzodiazepines (effects on transport of sugar and ions in rat skeletal muscles in vitro). 1284. Chlordiazepoxide (attenuation of tetrabenazine "reversal"). 1287. Clonazepam (+ carbamazepine, metabolic drug interactions). 1288. Nitrazepam, Flurazepam x HCl (+ pentobarbitone, residual effects on human performance). 1290. Diazepam, Chlordiazepoxide (+ cigarette smoking, effects on clinical depression of the CNS). 1303. Benzodiazepines (interactions with oral anticoagulants). 1305. Diazepam (+ quabain, increase of cardiac toxicity, dogs). 1334. Benzodiazepines (+ halothane, mouse, modification of sleeping-time). 1336. Chlordiazepoxide (+ ethanol). 1353. Diazepam (+ meperidine, respiratory response to carbon dioxide). 1390. Chlordiazepoxide (no effect of smoking on metabolism). 1395. Diazepam (+ cyclic GMP-levels). 1424. Diazepam (+ pethidine, effect on newborn). 1522. Chlordiazepoxide (serum creatine phosphokinase concentrations after i.m. application). 1539. Diazepam (effect of spironolactone on metabolism). 1566. Temazepam (+ alcohol, effect on psychomotor performance). 1578. Chlordiazepoxide (+ benzquinamide,+ placebo, effect on performance in some psychological tests). 1579. + 1580. Benzodiazepines (effects on human cholinesterase in vitro). 1583. Flunitrazepam (+ ketamine, + muscle relaxants, i.v., general anesthesia). 1585. Diazepam (+ pentobarbital, alterations of effects after chronic morphine). 1587. Benzodiazepines (+ alcohol, effect on disposition in dogs). 1598. Diazepam (+ ketamine, haemodynamic studies). 1599. Diazepam (+ diphenhydramine, effects on healthy subjects). 1629. Diazepam (+ halothane, rats). 1642. Diazepam, Nitrazepam (+ phenprocoumon, interactions). 1674. Clonazepam (+ carbamazepine, time course of interaction, normal man). 1691. Diazepam, Chlordiazepoxide (+ thioridazine, + haloperidol, + flupenthixole, + alcohol, effects on psychomotor skills related to driving). 1692. Diazepam (+ alcohol, effects on skills related to driving). 1693. Diazepam, Chlordiazepoxide (+ lithium, + alcohol, effect on psychomotor skills related to driving). 1703. Diazepam (+ ethanol, effects on actions). 1705. Benzodiazepines (+ disulfiram, interactions). 1721. Benzodiazepines (interactions with some other drugs). 1729. Diazepam (+ GABA, + alcohol, + drugs, interactions on psychomotor skills). 1741. Diazepam (+ pethidine, analgesia for cytoscopy). 1749. Diazepam, Oxazepam (+ methylperone, alone and in combination with alcohol). 1758. Diazepam (+ terfenadine, + diphenhydramin, + alcohol, psychomotor performance and subjective feelings). 1761.Diazepam (+ paracetamol, interactions). 1764. Diazepam (+ alcohol). 1776. Diazepam (+ octatropine-methylbromide, synergistic interaction at the gastrointestinal level. 1785. Diazepam (effects on meperidine requirements during labor). 1832. Diazepam (+ chlorpromazine, + imipramine, effect on central action of alcohol). 1851. Benzodiazepines (+ warfarin, interactions in man). 1853. Nitrazepam (+ mandrax, + alcohol, influence on human performance). 1872. Chlordiazepoxide (+ amphetamine, effect on avoidance behavior of reserpiniced mice). 1874. Chlordiazepoxide (+ trimetadione, + diphenylhydantoin, effect on after-discharges in brain of cat). 1881. Oxazepam (+ phenprocoumon, interactions ?). 1897. Psychotropic drugs (interactions). 1922. Diazepam (+ picrotoxin, interaction). 1926. Chlorazepate (+ Alkohol, Wechselwirkung nach oraler Applikation). 1963. Chlordiazepoxide, Diazepam, Nitrazepam (interactions with catecholamines and histamine, rat brain). 1966. Benzodiazepines (influence on fluorescence of tryptophan). 2019. Chlordiazepoxide (+ alcohol, effect of acute alcohol intoxication on metabolism and plasma kinetics of chlordiazepoxide). 2036. Benzodiazepines (+ alcohol, influence on the effects in rats and mice).

2045. Diazepam, oxazepam (+ phenobarbital, dogs, multiple oral dose, correlation with antipyrine half-life). 2046. Diazepam (+ methohexital, drug modification of ECT). 2060. Diazepam (+ ethanol, pigeons, effects on performance). 2074. Chlordiazepoxide (+ ethanol, + oxypertine, effect on human-motor coordination). 2094. Clobazam (+ ethanol, acute and chronic effect on activity in mouse. 2105. Chlordiazepoxide (+ alcohol, Beeinflussung im Straßenverkehr). 2131. Psychotropic drugs (+ alcohol, mice, effects on muscular tonus). 2137. Diazepam (in lidocaine-induced cardiovascular changes). 2139. Benzodiazepines (+ heparin, effect on benzodiazepin binding in plasma). 2153. Chlordiazepoxide, diazepam (+ alcohol, i.v., interaction). 2154. Tranquilizer (+ alcohol, interaction after rapid infusion). 2155. + 2156. Tranquilizer (+ alcohol, i.v., interaction). 2159. Diazepam (+ chlorpromazine, + droperidol, emergence from ketamin). 2164. Chlordiazepoxide (+ fluoxetine, rats, interactions). 2178. Chlordiazepoxide (+ ethanol, + phenobarbital, + chlorpromazine, effects). 2186. Diazepam (+ physostigmine, + scopolamine, interactions, effects on human memory). 2198. Diazepam (+ naloxone, interaction, anti-metrazol-test). 2231. Clonazepam (+ diphenylhydantoin, + phenobarbital, + carbamazepine, lack of effect on serum levels). 2247. Tranquilizer (effect on metabolism of alcohol). 2258. Diazepam (+ ketamine, conduction anesthesia, untoward effect). 2267. Medazepam (+ alcohol, car driving). 2270. Diazepam (+ alcohol, effect on psychomotor performance).

2273. Lorazepam (+ ketamine, preliminary report). 2274. Bromazepam (+ alcohol, effect on learning and memory in man). 2280. Benzodiazepines (+ alcohol, effects on performance). 2281. Diazepam (+ alcohol, effect on psychomotor performance). 2288. Diazepam (+ Alkohol, Leistungsbeeinträchtigung). 2299. Chlordiazepoxide (+ pentobarbital, chronic interactions on punished and unpunished behavior). 2302. Chlordiazepoxide (+ alcohol, combined effects). 2304. Benzodiazepines (+ barbiturates, + alcohol, interactions). 2320. Benzodiazepines (+ alcohol, interactions on sleeping-times). 2348. Chlordiazepoxide (+ saline infusion, effect on renal secretion). 2381. Drugs (+ alcohol, interactions). 2382. Chlordiazepoxide (+ disulfiram, inhibition of biotransformation). 2391. Drugs of abuse (interactions with alcohol). 2400. Oxazepam (+ Alkohol, Wechselwirkungen, Einfluß auf psychomotorische Koordination und Reaktionsverhalten). 2401. Oxazepam (+ Alkohol, Kombinationswirkungen, Einfluß auf Reaktionsverhalten, subjektive Befindlichkeit). 2428. Psychotropic drugs (influence of ethanol on toxicity). 2432. Diazepam (+ alcohol, interactions).

2440. Diazepam (+ cocaine, interactions on morphine-treated rats). 2442. Drugs (+ alcohol, influence on human-eye movement).

2468. Clobazam (+ ethanol, kinetic and dynamic interactions). 2521. Diazepam (+ ethanol, interaction, psychomotor skills). 2539. Clotiazepam (effects on metabolism of biogenic amines).

2567. Diazepam (+ ketamine, antagonism). 2569. Diazepam (growth-hormone response in diabetics). 2570. Diazepam (growth-hormone response in diabetics, effect of glucose). 2582. Benzodiazepines (+ barbiturates, + cannabinoids, effect on food-intake in rats). 2661. Clonazepam (+ carbamazepine, influence on UDP-glucuronyltransferase activity). 2686. Clonazepam (+ sodium valproate, interaction). 2689. Benzodiazepines (+ plasma-ACTH and cortisol levels, rats). 2695. Diazepam (+ ethanol, enhancement of ^{3}H-diazepam-binding at the benzodiazepine-GABA-receptor-ionophor complex). 2701. Chlordiazepoxide (+ ethanol, effects on prenatal and postnatal development in rats). 2713. Diazepam (+ digoxin, levels). 2714. Chlordiazepoxide (+ ethanol, combined effects on brain cyclic-nucleotides). 2715. Chlordiazepoxide (+ ethanol, combined effects on brain GABA-levels). 2726. Diazepam (+ naloxone, no antagonism). 2729. Diazepam (+ ketamine, combination in minor gynecological surgery). 2730. Diazepam (+ adenosine, potentiation of effects on isolated and smooth muscle). 2731. Diazepam (+ adenosine, potentiation of coronary vasodilator action). 2749. Diazepam (effect on serum testosterone and the ventral prostate gland, male rats). 2752. + 2753. Chlordiazepoxide (+ amphetamine or fenfluramine, interactions, feeding parameters, rat). 2758. Diazepam (+ pentazocine, supplementation, dentistry). 2771. Diazepam (+ xylazin, + ketamine, short duration anesthesia in horses). 2772. Benzodiazepines (+ barbiturates, interactions with muscimol). 2776. Diazepam (+ ethanol, addition or potentiation, humans). 2778. Benzodiazepines (+ ethanol, withdrawal syndromes). 2782. Benzodiazepines (+ cholinesterase, effects in human fetal brain). 2785. Diazepam (+ cimetidine, interactions). 2786. Diazepam (+ dipyridamole, +-1-methylisoguanosine, displacement in rat-brain). 2802. Chlordiazepoxide (+ ethanol, impairment of elimination, man). 2803. (see 2802.). 2804. Chlordiazepoxide (+ cimetidine, impairment of elimination, man). 2805. Benzodiazepines (+ heparin, effects on plasma binding). 2821. Diazepam (enhancement of ketamine plasma levels, man). 2847. Diazepam (alone or with alcohol, effect on key-pecking, pigeon). 2855. Nitrazepam (+ phenobarbital, enzyme inducing effects, dog). 2861. Diazepam (+ ketamine, cardiovascular effects, antagonism). 2879. Medazepam (effect on adrenocortical function in the preoperative state). 2915. Benzodiazepines (+ diphenylhydantoine, interaction in the CNS). 2916. Benzodiazepines (+ GABA, interaction). 2924. Diazepam, N-desmethyldiazepam (effects on morphine glucuronidation, rat liver microsomes). 2926. Diazepam (+ ketamine, anesthesia in gynecological surgery). 2933. Diazepam (+ methohexital, + fentanyl, comparison of recovery tests). 2936. Diazepam (+ physostigmine, antagonism). 2938. Diazepam (+ local anesthetics, pharmacokinetic interaction). 2972. Diazepam (+ 5-hydroxyindoleacetic and homovanillic acids, effects in cisternal cerebrospinal fluid of cats). 2973. Diazepam (+ oxygen, effects on consumption). 2977. Diazepam (+ digitoxin, reciprocal effects on metabolism). 3019. Clonazepam (+ atropine, effects in the limbic system). 3031. Diazepam (+ l-tryptophan, increasing of uptake, rat-brain). 3041. Benzodiazepines (+ ethanol, effect on disposition in dogs). 3042. Lorazepam (+ ethanol, effect on metabolism). 3071. Benzodiazepines (+ ACTH, functional antagonism). 3072. Benzodiazepines (+ valproic acid, effects on brain aldehyde reductase). 3075. Clonazepam (altered serotoninergic activity in mouse brain). 3086. Nitrazepam (+ ethanol, enhancement of reductive metabolism, rat). 3089. Diazepam (+ naloxone, effects on respiratory changes). 3090. Diazepam (+ naloxone, reversal of respiratory depression). 3097. Benzodiazepines (+ cholinesterase, interaction). 3110. Diazepam (inhibition of prostaglandin-synthesis in macrophages). 3111. Diazepam (effects on tumor growth and plasma prostaglandin E_2, rats). 3128. Clonazepam (influence of phenytoin and phenobarbital on the disposition after single oral doses). 3139. Diazepam (+ cimetidine, interaction). 3142. Diazepam (+ cimetidine, delayed clearance). 3143. Benzodiazepines (+ cimetidine, effects on clearance). 3144. Oxazepam, N-desmethyldiazepam (influence of cimetidine on pharmacokinetics). 3165. Chlordiazepoxide (+ sodium valproate, interaction, nucleus accumbens, rat). 3166. Triazolam (+ desipramine, interaction). 3174. Clonazepam (+ carbamazepine, interaction). 3176. Diazepam (+ ethanol, pharmacokinetic interaction). 3187. Diazepam (+ meperidine, + normeperidine, reduction of behavior suppressing effects). 3190. Benzodiazepines (+ plasma corticosteroids, relationships in stress). 3195. Chlordiazepoxide, N-desmethyldiazepam, oxazepam, methyloxazepam (+ ethanol, effects on learning and memory). 3297. Benzodiazepines (+ GABA, interaction in the cerebellar cortex). 3374. Lorazepam, oxazepam (+ cimetidine, spares glucuronidation). 3375. Diazepam (+ blood glucose level, influences). 3388. Chlordiazepoxide (+ theophylline, alteration of calcium-levels in subcellular fractions of rat brain cortex). 3392. Benzodiazepines (+ methylxanthines, + adenosine, interaction). 3412. Diazepam (+ bilirubin, effects on pharmacokinetics). 3434. Chlordiazepoxide (sex-differences and effects of oral-contraceptives). 3459. Diazepam, N-desmethyldiazepam (+ heparin, redistribution). 3465. Benzodiazepines (+ cimetidine, effect on clearance). 3483. Diazepam (+ 5-hydroxytryptamine, effects on cerebral synthesis). 3514. Benzodiazepines (+ disulfiram, + ethanol, effects on disposition). 3519. + 3520. Diazepam (i.v., + ethanol, interaction). 3523. Tofisopam (+ ethanol, interaction). 3526. Diazepam (+ levo-methadone, effects on disposition in mice). 3547. Diazepam (effects on acetylcholine content in rat-brain). 3558. Diazepam (+ muscimol, effects on GABA-mediated neurotransmission, interactions with inosine and nicotinamide). 3562. Diazepam (+ oral contraceptives, effect on the demethylation). 3566. Benzodiazepines (+ cimetidine, inhibition). 3567. Benzodiazepines (+ antilirium, + benzyl alcohol, + physostigmine, antagonism of binding in brain). 3568. Benzodiazepines (+ antilirium, antagonism of binding in rat and human brain). 3579. Clorazepate (+ ethanol, combined effects). 3580. Clorazepate (+ ethanol, changes in mood). 3610. + 3611. Benzodiazepines (+ GABA, interaction). 3623. Diazepam (+ beta-carboline-3-carboxylic acid ethyl-esters, antagonism). 3639. Diazepam (effects on the nocturnal release of growth-hormone, prolactin, ACTH and cortisol). 3662. Benzodiazepines (+ ethanol, pharmacokinetic interactions). 3670. Diazepam (inhibition of myosin synthesis). 3673. Benzodiazepines (alterations in plasma-lipid and lipoprotein-levels). 3677. Diazepam (+ physostigmine, + naloxone, antagonists). 3683. Clonazepam (+ sodium valproate, interactions).

Emergency-Drug-Analysis / Notfall-Untersuchungsmethoden

82. Drugs, commonly taken in overdoses. 110. Acute drug intoxications. 377. Chlordiazepoxide, Diazepam, Oxazepam, Chlorazepate, Medazepam, Prazepam(+ Methaqualone). 479. Nitrazepam, Chlordiazepoxide, Diazepam, Oxazepam (and other drugs). 495. Diazepam, Metabolites (rapid GLC-method). 596. Nitrobenzodiazepines, Clonazepam, Nitrazepam, Nimetazepam (acute poisoning). 631. Diazepam (+ gluthethimide,

pethidine, ethchlorvynol, meprobamate a.o., overdose cases). 636. Diazepam, N-desmethyldiazepam, Desalkylflurazepam (rapid GLC-assay in serum). 652. Benzodiazepines (GLC, biological material, serum, urine, gastric content, acute poisoning). 820. Nitrazepam (poisoning cases). 837. Clonazepam (GLC, rapid method, serum). 843. Oxazepam, Nitrazepam, Diazepam, Lorazepam, Chlorazepate (rapid GLC-method). 896. Diazepam (rapidscreening). 902. Diazepam, Chlordiazepoxide (GLC, rapid, comatose patients). 927. Diazepam, N-desmethyldiazepam (blood, GLC). 972. Lorazepam, others (TLC). 1049. Diazepam, Chlordiazepoxide, others (GLC, emergency cases). 1064. Diazepam, Chlordiazepoxide, Oxazepam (others, GLC, TLC). 1105. Drugs (rapid methods).

1266. Methyloxazepam (GLC, rapid method, small samples of blood). 1293. Diazepam (use in intensive therapy). 1945. Chlordiazepoxide (GLC, serum). 1948. Chlordiazepoxid and metabolites (GLC, serum, on-column methylation). 2614. Bromazepam, chlordiazepoxide, clorazepate, diazepam, flunitrazepam, flurazepam, lorazepam, medazepam, nitrazepam, oxazepam, clonazepam (analytical procedures for therapeutic drug monitoring and emergency toxicology).

Extraction from biological samples (special reference)
Extraktion aus biologischem Material (Spezialartikel)

89. Diazepam and metabolites. 280. Clonazepam, Nitrazepam, Metaboliten. 290. Drugs (rapid extraction). 522. Chlordiazepoxid and many other drugs. 652. Benzodiazepines (serum, urine, gastric content, acute poisonings). 727. Benzodiazepines (blood, procedures compared). 822. Benzodiazepines (tissues, enzymic digestion). 982. Clobazam. 985. Camazepam.

1443. 1,4-Benzodiazepines (thermomicroextraction).

1542. Clobazam. 2545. Benzodiazepincs (column extraction).

3464. Oxazepam-glucuronides (isolation and stereoselective enzymic hydrolysis). 3700. Benzodiazepines (automated extraction from blood and serum, HPLC).
(for extraction procedures see also the different analytical methods).

Fluorescence / Fluorometry
Fluoreszenz / Fluorometrie

140. Diazepam, Chlordiazepoxide, Nitrazepam, Oxazepam. 229. Benzodiazepines. 235. Flurazepam, major metabolites (blood). 239. Indolyl-benzodiazepines (blood). 244. Flurazepam, major metabolites (blood and urine). 292. Chlordiazepoxide (on TLC-plates). 443. Diazepam (fluorescence quenching). 598. Chlordiazepoxide, metabolites (plasma, humans, dog, rat). 630. Diazepam, Chlordiazepoxide, Oxazepam, Nitrazepam. 675. Benzodiazepines (fluorescence characteristics in strong acids). 761. Diazepam, Chlordiazepoxide (urine). 909. Nitrazepam, metabolites (plasma, urine). 1099. Chlordiazepoxide (in dosage forms and biological fluids). 1149. Benzodiazepines (blood, urine, screening). 1228. Chlordiazepoxide, metabolites (TLC-densitometry).

1323. Oxazepam (derivates also). 1324. 1,4-Benzodiazepines (also polarographic investigations). 1388. Benzodiazepines and other drugs (fluorescamine derivatives). 1542. Clobazam. 1946. Chlordiazepoxide (quant, on TLC). 1947. Diazepam and other Benzodiazepines (quant, on TLC). 2491. Clobazam.

2996. Clobazam (quantitative determination in serum).

Gas-Liquid-Chromatography / Gaschromatographie

8. Diazepam (in kleinen Blutplasmaproben, 3% OV-17, ECD), 28. Nitrazepam, Medazepam, Oxazepam, Diazepam, Chlordiazepoxid, Lorazepam, Prazepam (doping, 3% OV-17, Retentionsdaten. 40. Triflubazam. 42. Medazepam and major metabolites (in plasma). 56. Medazepam, Oxazepam, Diazepam, Desalkylflurazepam, Nordiazepam, Chlordiazepoxide, Prazepam, Flunitrazepam, Flurazepam, Nitrazepam, Clonazepam, (2% OV-17, $260^{\circ}C$, FID-GLC. 61. Nitrazepam (plasma, ECD). 69. Diazepam and metabolites (in biological fluids). 79. Diazepam (Blut, Retentionsindizes). 80. Bromazepam, Chlordiazepoxid, Diazepam, Nitrazepam, Oxazepam, Prazepam (Retentionsindizes). 91. Diazepam and metabolites. 152. 1,4-benzodiazepines (ECD). 153. Chlorazepate and metabolites (ECD). 161. Bromazepam (in plasma). 162. Clonazepam (in plasma). 163. Flunitrazepam, desmethylflunitrazepam, clonazepam (in plasma). 165. Diazepam (in Blut und Urin). 228. General. 229. 1,4-benzodiazepines (ECD). 230. benzodiazepines (ECD). 231. Clonazepam and flunitrazepam (ECD). 232. Lorazepam (ECD, plasma). 233. Bromazepam and major metabolites (ECD). 234. Lorazepam and metabolite (ECD). 236. Benzodiazepines (blood, ECD). 237. Bromazepam (blood). 240. Medazepam, diazepam and major-metabolites (blood and urine, ECD). 241. Flurazepam and major metabolites (blood). 242. Clonazepam and Flunitrazepam (in blood and urine, ECD). 243. Diazepam (in blood). 283. Flunitrazepam und Metabolite (OV-17, SE-30, FID). 291. Nitrazepam (plasma, ECD, as methyl-derivative). 301. Flunitrazepam (serum, ECD)., 312. Benzodiazepines and metabolites, Oxazepam, diazepam, desalkyl-flurazepam, desmethyl-diazepam, flurazepam, methylnitrazepam, methylclonazepam, clonazepam, chlordiazepoxide (ECD). 325. Diazepam, Flurazepam, Oxazepam, Chlordiazepoxide, Desmethyl-diazepam (screening, blood or tissues). 327. Diazepam, Nitrazepam, Oxazepam, Temazepam, Nor-Diazepam (GLC/MS). 329. Diazepam (serum).

334. Benzodiazepine (degradation during GC). 350. Diazepam (plasma). 359. Benzodiazepines. 364. screening. 373. Diazepam (blood and serum). 381. Clonazepam (human plasma). 411. Medazepam, diazepam, nitrazepam (FID). 437. Lorazepam (plasma, ECD). 442. Benzodiazepines (quant.). 452. Benzodiazepines (great review). 453. Benzodiazepines (great review). 454. Medazepam (electrolytic conductivity detector). 468. Flurazepam and metabolites (urine, blood, ECD). 474. Diazepam und Metabolite. 489. Chlorazepate (plasma). 495. Diazepam and metabolites (in body fluids). 497. Diazepam (plasma). 498. Lorazepam (plasma). 499. Lorazepam (plasma). 535. Diazepam (serum). 542. Nitrazepam (comparison of two methods). 547. Diazepam (^{63}Ni-detector). 591. Clonazepam (plasma). 594. Lorazepam (ECD). 601. Medazepam (plasma). 636. Diazepam, N-desmethyldiazepam, desalkylflurazepam (serum, rapid method). 652. Benzodiazepines (biological materials, acute poisonings). 667. Prazepam und andere Benzodiazepine bzw. Benzophenone. 672. Medazepam und Metabolite. 680. C_3-hydroxylated benzodiazepines (MS, urine). 682. Diazepam, nitrazepam, oxazepam, N-desmethyldiazepam, temazepam. 703. Nitrazepam (blood and urine). 708. Diazepam (plasma, internal standard). 711. Chlordiazepoxide. 720. Benzodiazepine und Benzophenone (Blut, Harn). 733. Benzodiazepine und andere (Retentionsindizes). 734. Diazepam, Chlordiazepoxid, Nitrazepam. 736. Diazepam, Nitrazepam, Oxazepam (SE 30). 738. Nitrazepam (serum). 741. Diazepam, Chlordiazepoxide, Oxazepam. 771. Clonazepam and metabolites (human, plasma, quant.). 828. Pinazepam (human, plasma, urine, milk, ECD). 833. Medazepam, N-desmethyl-medazepam, diazepam, N-desmethyl-diazepam, oxazepam, flurazepam, N-1-desalkyl-flurazepam, N-1-hydroxyethyl-flurazepam, nitrazepam (electrolytic conductivity detection). 834. Medazepam, diazepam, metabolites (plasma, electrolytic conductivity detection). 837. Clonazepam (serum, cerebrospinal fluid). 843. Oxazepam, nitrazepam, diazepam, lorazepam, chlorazepate (other drugs).

852. Methylnitrazepam, diazepam, flurazepam, prazepam, N-desalkyl-diazepam, N-desalkyl-flurazepam (nitrogen-phosphorus detector). 857. Oxazepam, diazepam, chlordiazepoxide, medazepam, nitrazepam, lorazepam, chlorazepate, prazepam (literature review). 867. Benzodiazepines (serum). 870. water soluble imidazo-benzodiazepines (blood, ECD). 871. 7-iodo-benzodiazepines (blood, urine, ECD). 875. Chlorazepate. 900. Diazepam (ECD). 921. Diazepam, N-desmethyl-

diazepam. 922. Flurazepam, 927. Diazepam, N-desmethyldiazepam (blood, plasma). 929. Diazepam, oxazepam, N-desalkyl-diazepam, temazepam, medazepam (thermolysis during GC). 939. Benzodiazepine-esters (ECD, multiple ion detection). 956. Diazepam (blood). 964. Diazepam u.a. (XAD-2). 982. Clobazam (OV 17, SE 30, FID). 985. Camazepam and metabolites (OV 17, SE 30, FID). 988. 31 benzodiazepines and metabolites (OV 17, SE 30, retention-data, FID). 989. 19 benzophenones (OV 17, SE 30, retention-data, FID). 1030. Clonazepam (whole blood). 1034. Oxazepam. 1068. Clonazepam (serum, ECD). 1100. Diazepam and major metabolites (human, serum,quant., ECD). 1139. Pinazepam and metabolites (serum, urine, brain, GLC/MS). 1157. 7-chloro-1,4-benzodiazepines (biological fluids). 1165. Oxazepam, (serum, urine, ECD). 1166. Oxazepam (after extractive alkylation reaction, ECD). 1170. N-desmethyldiazepam (plasma, internal standard). 1195. Diazepam, N-desmethyldiazepam (plasma, ECD). 1201. Diazepam, N-desmethyldiazepam, chlorpromazine. 1214. Diazepam (blood). 1226. Diazepam (plasma, ECD).

1266. Methyloxazepam (blood, small samples). 1325. Diazepam (blood and urine). 1391. Diazepam and Desmethyldiazepam (plasma, nitrogen-sensitive detector). 1416. Clonazepam (micromethod, serum). 1444. General (detection in forensic toxicology). 1474. Chlordiazepoxide and main metabolites (formation of thermally stable derivatives). 1481. Oxazepam (ECD, thermal degradation-product). 1501. Desmethyldiazepam (plasma, ECD). 1502. Diazepam, Desmethyldiazepam (double internal standardization). 1506. Lorazepam (ECD). 1532. Benzodiazepines. 1542. Clobazam. 1602. Nitrazepam (serum).

1677. Lorazepam, Chlordesmethyldiazepam (rats, mice). 1773. Prazepam and metabolites (ECD, selected ion monitoring). 1779. General (derivative formation). 1945. Chlordiazepoxide (serum). 1948. Chlordiazepoxide and metabolites (serum, on column-methylation). 2005. Allgemein (Derivatisierung). 2018. Diazepam und Metaboliten (Simultanbestimmung neben Ketamin). 2029. Diazepam (+ Ketamin).

2140. Benzodiazepines (nitrogen sensitive detector). 2179. Diazepam (in Blut und Serum). 2276. Diazepam, clonazepam (temperature dependence of ECD-responses). 2328. Diazepam, chlordiazepoxide, flurazepam (in blood and plasma). 2427. Benzodiazepines (serum, nitrogen detector).

2477. Bromazepam, clobazam, clonazepam, chlordiazepoxide, diazepam, clorazepate, flunitrazepam, flurazepam, lorazepam, medazepam, nitrazepam, oxazepam, prazepam, temazepam (OV-1 and OV-17). 2478. Clobazam, desmethylclobazam (plasma, ECD). 2480. Oxazepam, lorazepam (GLC/MS). 2482. Diazepam, chlordiazepoxide, clorazepate, flurazepam, oxazepam, prazepam, metabolites (ECD). 2485. Diazepam, desmethyldiazepam (whole blood, derivatization, N-FID). 2486. Clonazepam, 7-aminoclonazepam, 7-acetamidoclonazepam (plasma, GLC/MS). 2493. Diazepam, desmethyldiazepam (ECD). 2494. Camazepam (human plasma). 2507. Diazepam, desmethyldiazepam (plasma, ECD). 2534. Clonazepam (human plasma, GLC / negative ion chemical ionization MS). 2535. Nitrazepam, + main metabolites (urine, ECD, N-FID). 2543. Benzodiazepines, others (drug monitoring, acetone extraction).

2708. Clonazepam, 7-aminoclonazepam (in plasma). 2794. Diazepam (+ meprobamate, + phenylbutazone, + thioridazine, N-FID, serum). 2939. Clobazam (serum). 2958. Clobazam, desmethylclobazam (plasma, ECD). 2995. Clorazepate as desmethyldiazepam (ECD). 2996. Clobazam (serum, ECD). 3045. Diazepam (GC/MS investigation of diazepam injectable precipitates). 3100. Bromo- and fluorobenzodiazepines (in human body fluids). 3239. 2-flurinated benzodiazepines. 3264. Diazepam, desmethyldiazepam (whole blood, derivatization, N-FID). 3382. Diazepam, chlordiazepoxide, + metabolites (screening and quantitation, ECD). 3384. Clorazepate, medazepam, desmethylmedazepam, chlordiazepoxide, desmethylchlordiazepoxide, demoxepam, diazepam, temazepam, desmethyldiazepam, oxazepam, lorazepam, flurazepam, hydroxyethylflurazepam, didesethylflurazepam, desalkylflurazepam, hydroxyflurazepam, nitrazepam, aminonitrazepam, acetamidonitrazepam, flunitrazepam, desmethylflunitrazepam, prazepam, hydroxyprazepam, clonazepam, aminoclonazepam, acetamidoclonazepam, bromazepam, hydroxybromazepam (in post-mortem blood, ECD). 3407. Diazepam, nordiazepam (in plasma, ECD). 3426. Clorazepate (plasma).

3444. Diazepam (serum, ECD). 3509. Lormetazepam (FID). 3510. Triazolam (FID). 3658. Midazolam (serum, N-FID). 3659. Midazolam (N-FID). 3706. Clonazepam (determination by GC/MS). 3725. Diazepam (plasma, GLC/MS).

3741. 11 Benzodiazepines (nitrogen specific detector). 3743. Clonazepam (nitrogen sensitive detection, plasma). 3744. Temazepam (ECD, plasma). 3752. Bromazepam (ECD). 3754. 1,4- and 1,5-Benzodiazepines (urine, GLC-MS, single ion monitoring). 3756. Flurazepam, N-desalkylflurazepam (plasma, ECD, rapid method). 3757. Benzodiazepines and benzophenones (FID, Screening). 3759. Lormetazepam (FID). 3760. Triazolam (FID). 3764. Flunitrazepam (plasma, ECD). 3773. Clotiazepam (ECD). 3774. Benzodiazepines and many other drugs (compilation of retention indices, critical description).

General analytical data / Allgemeine analytische Daten

102. Chlordiazepoxid, Diazepam, Oxazepam, Nitrazepam (chromatographische Daten, Spektren u.a. analytische Größen). 125. (Spectroscopic data). 192. (TLC, GLC, IR, NMR, Polarogr.). 276. (Chlordiazepoxid, Diazepam, Medazepam, Oxazepam, Chlorazepat, Lorazepam, Flurazepam, Nitrazepam, Prazepam, Temazepam, Clonazepam, Ketazolam (Schmelzpunkte, Derivate, Identitätsreaktionen, DC, GLC, UV-Spektren, Löslichkeit, quant.Best. Fluorometrie, Polarographie, Literatur). 322., 323., 324. (Description, IR-, NMR-, UV-, Raman-, Mass-Spectra, Optical Rotation, Melting Range, Differential Thermal Analysis, Solubility, Crystal Properties, Dissociation Constant, Fluorescence, Hygroscopic Behavior, Synthesis, Stability, Degradation, Drug Metabolic Products and Pharmacokinetics, Elemental Analysis, Phase Solubility Analysis, Chromatograhic Analysis, TLC, GLC, Spectrophotometric analysis, Colorimetric Analysis, Non-Aqueous Titration, References). Available for: Chlordiazepoxide, Chlordiazepoxide-Hydrochloride, Diazepam, (Vol. 1); Flurazepam Hydrochloride, Oxazepam,(Vol. 3); Chlorazepate Dipotassium, (Vol.4). 362. Some analytical data. 375. Analytische Eigenschaften, 376. Dünnschichtchromatographische Schnellprüfung, UV-Spektren der Benzophenone. 405. Hauptsächlich Mikroreaktionen, Schmelzpunkte, Löslichkeiten. 748. Chemische Toxikologie (Methodik und Daten). 862. Umfangreiche analytische Daten. 863. Einzelbehandlung der Wirkstoffe in Monographien (Chlorazepat, Clonazepam, Diazepam, Flunitrazepam, Lorazepam, Nitrazepam, Oxazepam, Prazepam, weitere in Vorbereitung). 979. s. 863.. 982. Clobazam. 985. Camazepam. 1034. Oxazepam. 1079. Dünnschichtchromatographie. 1109. Analytical Toxicology. 1110. Literature.

1349. Benzodiazepines and others (isolation and identification). 1542. Clobazam. 2477. Benzodiazepines (GLC, TLC, MS, UV). 2614. Bromazepam, chlordiazepoxide, clorazepate, diazepam, flunitrazepam, flurazepam, lorazepam, medazepam, nitrazepam, oxazepam, clonazepam (drug monitoring and emergency analysis). 2849. Clobazam, 3509. Lormetazepam. 3510. Triazolam.

General Treatment (Books, great reviews)
Allgemeine Behandlung (Bücher, große Übersichten)

30. Pharmaceutical chemistry. 31. Analytical investigation. 159. Pharmacology, effects, indications. 179. Synthesen. 187. Isolation and identification. 192. Determination in

body fluids. 225. Psychopharmakologie. 276. Analytische Daten. 322. Analytical Profiles (also 323., 324.). 328. Pharmakologie und Toxikologie. 343. Dünnschichtchromatographie. 362. Pharmacology, toxicology, clinical effects, chemistry, synthesis and more). 375. Forensische Toxikologie. 376. Nachweis im klinischen Laboratorium. 444. Pharmakologie und Toxikologie. 514. Handelspräparate. 768. Pharmakologie und Toxikologie. 779. Präparatenamen, Formeln, Synonyma. 780. Metabolismus. 835. Biochemistry. 848. Biotransformation (ebenso 849., 850.). 862. Chemische Toxikologie, Analytik (ebenso 863.). 875. Analytische Daten. 890. Dünnschichtchromatographie. 922. Analytische Daten. 979. Analytische Daten, chemische Toxikologie. 1034. Analytische Daten. 1079. Dünnschichtchromatographie. 1109. Chemical toxicology. 1199. Pharmakologie und Toxikologie.

1349. Benzodiazepines and other drugs. 1368. Benzodiazepines and other drugs (isolation from human organs). 1569. Diazepam (Hämodynamik). 1570. Diazepam (Pharmakokinetik). 1571. Diazepam (Frühschwangerschaft und Stillperiode). 1572. Diazepam (Leberverträglichkeit). 1896. Benzodiazepines and other drugs (routine identification).

2458. Camazepam. 2459. Clobazam. 2498. Benzodiazepines (sleep). 2531. Triazolam. 2547. Benzodiazepines, others (clinical pharmacokinetics). 2549. Clotiazepam.

2614. Bromazepam, chlordiazepoxide, clorazepate, diazepam, flunitrazepam, flurazepam, lorazepam, medazepam, nitrazepam, oxazepam, clonazepam (analytical procedures for therapeutic drug monitoring and emergency toxicology). 2678. Clobazam. 2697. Camazepam. 2845. Biotransformation. 3140. Clinical pharmacokinetics. 3472. Drug level monitoring. 3535. Clotiazepam. 3679. Benzodiazepine - allgemeine chemische Betrachtungen.

High-Pressure-liquid-Chromatography

Hochdruckflüssigkeitschromatographie

158. Chlordiazepoxide and major related impurities in pharmaceuticals. 410. Pinazepam (in blood and urine). 434. Chlordiazepoxide, N-desmethyl-chlordiazepoxide (blood). 502. Triflubazam, metabolites (human and animal blood and urine). 505. 1,4-benzodiazepines (determination of partition coefficients). 661. Psychotropic drugs (high-resolution liquid chromatography). 740. Nitrazepam and metabolites. 822. Benzodiazepines (tissues, enzymic digestion and high performance liquid chromatography). 918. Psychopharmacologic drugs (high efficiency liquid chromatography). 1011. Nitrazepam, Diazepam, Chlordiazepoxide, N-desmethyldiazepam, Temazepam. 1101. Clobazam (biol. Flüssigkeiten). 1107. Chlordiazepoxide, metabolites (plasma). 1120. Chlordiazepoxid, Nitrazepam, Diazepam, Oxazepam. 1145. Fosazepam, Clobazam. 1185. Flunitrazepam (body fluids). 1193. Ketazolam.

1306. Benzodiazepines (human plasma, high performance). 1318. Diazepam, N-Desmethyldiazepam (blood). 1549. Benzodiazepines and hydrolysis-products (reverse phase). 1614. Diazepam, N-Desmethyldiazepam, Oxazepam (human blood). 1809. Benzodiazepines (plasma). 1909. Benzodiazepines and metabolites (plasma). 1983. Clonazepam (serum). 2037. Chlordiazepoxide and metabolites (quant.).

2113. Benzodiazepines and others (drugs of abuse). 2328. Diazepam, flurazepam, chlordiazepoxide, metabolites (in blood and plasma).

2479. Benzodiazepines (in tablets, stability test). 2483. Diazepam, nitrazepam, chlordiazepoxide (evaluation of amperometric detectors). 2484. Diazepam, metabolites (plasma). 2487. Clorazepate, nitrazepam, clonazepam, oxazepam, lorazepam, chlordiazepexide, nordiazepam, diazepam, prazepam (in forensic cases). 2492. Diazepam, oxazepam, temazepam, nordiazepam (plasma, urine). 2493. Diazepam, desmethyldiazepam. 2503. Alprazolam, triazolam (specific and sensitive method). 2522. Chlordiazepoxide, metabolites (in biological fluids).

2563. Triazolam (serum). 2571. Chlordiazepoxide (and two of its decomposition products). 2593. Chlordiazepoxide, + metabolites (plasma, reversed-phase mode). 2645. Oxazepam (resolution of racemates). 2684. Benzophenones (hydrolysis studies). 2698. Chlordiazepoxide (+ amitriptyline, in tablet formulations). 2889. Diazepam, desmethyldiazepam, chlordiazepoxide, desmethylchlordiazepoxide (simultaneous assay in serum). 2903. Benzodiazepines (in rat brain). 2971. Chlordiazepoxide, desmethylchlordiazepoxide (in mouse brain). 3004. Nitrazepam (with differential-pulse-polarographic detection). 3382. Diazepam, chlordiazepoxide, + metabolites (screening and quantitation). 3407. Diazepam, nordiazepam (plasma). 3461. Clonazepam (plasma, routine monitoring). 3633. Benzodiazepines (serum, saliva). 3665. Benzodiazepines (via benzophenones, screening). 3700. Benzodiazepines, + metabolites (automated extraction, serum). 3701. Benzodiazepines (serum, automated sample processing). 3712. Benzodiazepines (in forensic analysis).

3742. Diazepam and major metabolites (man, cat). 3760. Triazolam (serum). 3767. Benzodiazepines and other tricyclic antidepressants.

Hydrolysis of Benzodiazepines (special investigations)

Hydrolyse der Benzodiazepine (spezielle Untersuchungen)

101. Nitrazepam. 139. Aminobenzophenone (Anfärbungsmöglichkeit, Bratton-Marshall Originalarbeit). 377. Chlordiazepoxid, Diazepam, Oxazepam, Chlorazepat, Medazepam, Prazepam. 459. Chlordiazepoxide, demoxepam (kinetics and mechanisms of hydrolysis). 460. Oxazepam, diazepam (kinetics and mechanisms of hydrolysis). 706. Chlordiazepoxide (kinetic of hydrolysis). 707. Diazepam, Nitrazepam (Hydrolyseverlauf, Ringverengung). 984. und 989. Hydrolyse von Diazepam, Chlordiazepoxid, Nitrazepam, Oxazepam, Chlorazepat, Clonazepam, Medazepam, Prazepam, Flurazepam, Bromazepam, Flunitrazepam, Clobazam, Fosazepam.

2436. Chlordiazepoxide, demoxepam (kinetics and mechanisms).

2684. Benzodiazepines (hydrolysis studies). 3059. 2'-fluorobenzodiazepines (reversible azomethine bond-cleavage in acidic solutions at body-temperature). 3060. Nitrazepam, nimetazepam (reversible ring opening in acidic media at body-temperature). 3061. Benzodiazepines (hydrolysis in acidic media, reversible ring-opening reactions). 3227. + 3228. Oxazepam-esters (correlation between hydrolysis rates, hydrophobicity and pharmacological properties). 3312. Diazepam (reversible ring-opening in acidic-media around body-temperature). 3326. 2-Methylamino-5-chlorobenzophenone (pk_a-value). 3464. Oxazepam-glucuronides (stereoselective enzymic hydrolysis). 3509. Lormetazepam (screening via hydrolysis products).

IR-Spectra / IR-Spektren

250. Benzodiazepine (zahlreiche andere Pharmaka). 280. Nitrazepam, Clonazepam, Metaboliten. 282. Flunitrazepam und Metaboliten. 658. Chlordiazepoxide, chlordiazepoxide-hydrochloride. 659. Diazepam. 875. Chlorazepate. 922. Flurazepam. 982. Clobazam. 985. Camazepam. 1034. Oxazepam.

2477. Benzodiazepines (see GLC). 2487. (see HPLC).

2849. Clobazam. 3328. Flurazepam (solvent effects). 3509. Lormetazepam. 3510. Triazolam.

Levels (Blood-, Plasma-, Serum-)
Spiegel (Blut-, Plasma-, Serum-)

7. Diazepam (children, after parenteral and rectal administration). 41. Diazepam, Nor-Diazepam (following intramuscular admistration). 55. Clonazepam (in epileptic patients). 59. Triflubazam (mice, dogs). 90. Diazepam, metabolites (in tetanus therapy). 93. Chlordiazepoxid, Medazepam. 104. Diazepam(plasma level and anxiety state). 126. Benzodiazepines (plasma concentrations). 128. Diazepam (serum concentrations, epilepsy). 143. Nitrazepam (oral administration). 174. Chlordiazepoxide (serum concentrations after overdose). 175. Diazepam (brain and derum concentrations). 201. Diazepam (plasma levels). 202. Chlordiazepoxide, major metabolites (mice, anticonvulsant propertiesand levels). 211. Benzodiazepines (macaca mulatta, intraperitoneal injection). 218. N-Desmethyldiazepam (normal volunteers, after oral administration). 219. Diazepam, N-desmethyldiazepam (plasma concentrations in relation to anxiolytic effect). 232. Lorazepam (humans). 238. Diazepam, metabolites(man, distribution patterns). 266. Clonazepam (in children with absence seizures). 268. Diazepam (after single and oral administration). 269. Diazepam (after i.m. injection). 271. Lorazepam (single dose administration of 2 and 4 mg by different routes, study). 316. Benzodiazepines(relation to EEG). 326. Chlordiazepoxide (different brands). 341. Bromazepam (chronic administration). 351. Diazepam (after single dosis oral and i.m.). 353. Diazepam (plasma levels). 354. Diazepam (blood levels). 355. Diazepam (study, mother and infant). 381. Diazepam (after single oral dose). 387. Diazepam (plasma levels and mood ratings). 402. Chlordiazepoxide (effect of oral and i.m. administration). 418. Chlordiazepoxide (factors influencing blood concentrations). 476. Diazepam (after parenteral and rectal administration in children). 485. Diazepam (normal man, after i.v. and oral administration). 486. Diazepam (normal man, after oral administration and cumulation). 489. Chlorazepate (after oral administration). 506. Clonazepam (plasma levels). 546. Nitrazepam (after acute intake). 548. Diazepam, metabolites (after oral, i.m. and rectal administration, correlation between plasma concentrations and sedatory effects). 552. Diazepam, metabolite (after acute and chronic administration). 556. Diazepam (man, following single oral and i.v., and chronic oral administration). 559. Flurazepam (chronic administration). 560. Flurazepam (chronic administration). 604. Diazepam (effect of food intake). 638. Diazepam (effect of food and repeated injections on serum levels). 641. Diazepam, Chlordiazepoxide (+ Thioridazine, after alcohol and placebo drinks). 835. Clonazepam (sheep). 867. Benzodiazepines (serum). 910. Nitrazepam (man). 991. Diazepam (after administration in various forms). 1017. Diazepam (reduced plasma levels in chronic alcoholic patients following oral administration). 1047. Nitrazepam, Chlordiazepoxide, Diazepam (plasma levels). 1051. Diazepam (and other drugs, drug serum levels). 1080. Chlordiazepoxide, metabolites (plasma and cerebrospinal fluid concentrations). 1119. Diazepam, N-desmethyldiazepam (serum levels in hospitalized patients). 1132. Diazepam (+ Tolbutamide, in chronic alcoholics). 1167. Diazepam (after administration in capsules). 1168. Diazepam (after administration in solution or syrup forms). 1169. Diazepam, N-desmethyldiazepam (in an epileptic child). 1179. Medazepam, Diazepam, N-desmethyldiazepam (after single and multiple oral doses of medazepam). 1205. Diazepam (unusual high level in a chronic user). 1208. Diazepam, Chlordiazepoxide and other drugs (tabulation of therapeutic, toxic and lethal concentrations of drugs and chemicals in blood).

1253. Diazepam (oral and i.v., plasma levels and clinical effects, correlation). 1256. Diazepam (serum, + serum-creatine-kinase, after i.v. administration in two different vehicles). 1264. Drugs including benzodiazepines (therapeutic and toxic concentrations in human biofluids).

1265. Drugs including benzodiazepines (blood, plasma, serum, therapeutic and toxic concentrations). 1291. Diazepam (man, plasma, single dose studies). 1333. Diazepam (pilot-study, maternal blood, amniotic fluid and cord blood). 1392. Lorazepam (serum). 1393. Diazepam (plasma, parotid saliva, mixed saliva). 1408. Diazepam (blood, after single rectal administration, infants, children). 1429. Diazepam (early pregnancy, concentrations in mother and foetus). 1470. Benzodiazepines (significance of measuring blood-levels). 1495. Diazepam and ketazolam (relationship of blood-levels to anxiety and hostility in chronic alcoholics). 1497. Chlordiazepoxide (plasma levels and clinical responses). 1498. Chlordiazepoxide (plasma levels, relationship to psychological and biochemical responses). 1519. Chlordiazepoxide (after oral application). 1584. Lorazepam (plasma estimation in neonates). 1626. Nitrazepam (plasma, correlation with subjective sedatory effects). 1627. Diazepam (plasma, after oral and i.m. administration). 1630. Diazepam and metabolites (plasma, urine, children, adults and intoxicated patients). 1649. Diazepam (plasma, infants, rectal administration in solution and by suppository). 1651. General (serum concentrations as therapeutic guides). 1671. General (tricyclic antidepressants, plasma concentrations). 1676. Diazepam and Desmethyldiazepam (plasma, after i.v., i.m., rectal and oral administration). 1687. Chlordiazepoxide (relationship of plasma-levels to clinical response). 1703. Diazepam (plasma concentrations after ethanol ingestion). 1732. Diazepam (blood levels, in infants mother given large doses). 1736. Diazepam and N-desmethyldiazepam (plasma concentrations after single rectal or i.m. administration, children). 1772. Diazepam and Desmethyldiazepam (plasma). 1791. Diazepam (man, plasma). 1817. Diazepam (human plasma, parotid saliva, mixed saliva, relationship to plasma protein-binding). 1837. Diazepam (plasma). 1863. Diazepam and Desmethyldiazepam (plasma levels during chronic diazepam therapy). 1867. Oxazepam (blood levels and quantitative EEG, psychometric analysis). 1891. Chlordiazepoxide (plasma decline during fixed-dose therapy of alcohol withdrawals). 1893. Diazepam (reduced plasma concentrations in chronic alcoholic patients following an oral absorption test). 1916. Diazepam (blood, man). 1956. N-Desmethyldiazepam (+ amylobarbitone-sodium, plasma levels). 1957. Diazepam and Desmethyldiazepam (+ amylobarbitone, plasma concentrations after short-term treatment). 1986. Clobazam (healthy subjects, plasma levels after three oral dosage forms).

2067. Diazepam (blood concentrations after Ro 03-7355, a new benzodiazepine prodrug). 2126. Diazepam, Nordiazepam (in normal and pentobarbital addicted cats, comparative blood-level profile during withdrawal). 2140. Benzodiazepines (blood level monitoring with nitrogen-sensitive detector). 2167. Flurazepam (+ metabolites, + phenobarbital, autopsy cases). 2171. Diazepam, bromazepam (blood levels and EEG-effects). 2416. N-desmethyldiazepam (+ amylobarbitone sodium, in anxious patients, comparison of plasma levels and behavioral test). 2437. Chlordiazepoxide (man, correlation of serum levels with EEG-effect).

2482. Diazepam, chlordiazepoxide, clorazepate, flurazepam, oxazepam, prazepam, metabolites (high-dose levels, i.v.). 2510. Medazepam, metabolites (plasma, oral administration). 2511. Diazepam (levels in overdose-cases). 2512. Nitrazepam + main metabolites (urinary excretion). 2513. Nitrazepam (saliva and serum). 2515. Flunitrazepam (breast-milk levels). 2529. Lorazepam (in plasma of mother and neonate). 2530. Benzodiazepines (application of blood levels in medicine and toxicology).

2553. Lorazepam and conjugate (cerebrospinal-fluid).

2616. Diazepam, desmethyldiazepam (newborn after i.m. administration). 2627. Clorazepate (man, after repeated 50-mg oral doses). 2734. Flunitrazepam (after oral and i.m. administration). 2780. Chlordesmethyldiazepam (in humans). 2940. Diazepam (comparison of plasma and saliva levels). 2942. Diazepam, desmethyldiazepam (saliva). 2969. Desmethyldiazepam (plasma, following single doses of chlorazepate). 2999. Diazepam, desmethyldiazepam (in saliva, plasma and CSF). 3032. Flurazepam (in plasma after 30-mg doses). 3102. Oxazepam (+ diazepam, relation between plasma level and effect). 3103. Diazepam (+ pentobarbital, small children, relation between plasma level and clinical effects, rectal administration). 3138. Diazepam (rats, effect of age on levels in plasma and brain). 3153. Clobazam (blood). 3154. Diazepam (+ barbital, plasma levels during treatment of delirium tremens). 3209. Diazepam, desmethyldiazepam (plasma). 3211. Diazepam (in saliva and plasma). 3267. Flunitrazepam (levels following oral and i.m. administration). 3345. Diazepam (+ barbital, humans, in saliva). 3353. + 3354. Benzodiazepines. 3355. Diazepam, desmethyldiazepam (infants treated p.o.). 3525. Benzodiazepines (+ others, clinical indications for plasma-level monitoring). 3553. ^{3}H-Diazepam (brain levels following i.v. administration). 3604. Nitrazepam (plasma, acetylator phenotype). 3653. Clobazam (plasma levels after 10, 20, and 40-mg doses as tablets). 3717. Diazepam (+ propanolol, free levels). 3722. Diazepam (correlation between the order of drug administration and plasma levels).

3744. Temazepam (plasma). 3746. Oxazepam, lorazepam. 3747. Desalkylflurazepam (elderly, single and multiple doses). 3748. Diazepam, desmethyldiazepam (plasma, long-term therapy). 3775. Triazolam (oral, normal subjects).

Mass-Spectra / Massenspektren

35. Allgemein (neben anderen spektroskopischen Methoden). 70. 4-substituted phenyl-1,3-dihydro-2H-1,5-benzodiazepine-2-thiones. 119. Chlordiazepoxide, Diazepam, Oxazepam. 177. Oxazepam, lorazepam (chemical ionization). 280. Nitrazepam, Clonazepam, Metaboliten. 282. 3-Hydroxy-benzodiazepine. 283. Flunitrazepam, Metaboliten. 327. Diazepam, Chlordiazepoxide, Nitrazepam, Oxazepam, N-desmethyldiazepam, temazepam. 658. Chlordiazepoxide. 659. Diazepam. 875. Chlorazepate. 922. Flurazepam. 929. Diazepam, Oxazepam, N-desalkyldiazepam, temazepam, medazepam (thermolysis during MS). 982. Clobazam, Metabolit. 985. Camazepam. 993. Diazepam-metabolites (high resolution MS). 1006. Chlordiazepoxide-metabolites (rat, high resolution MS). 1034. Oxazepam. 1146. Diazepam, Chlordiazepoxide (others).

1977. 1,5-Benzodiazepines (studies).
2347. 1,4-Benzodiazepines.
2477. Benzodiazepines (see GLC). 2480. Oxazepam, lorazepam (GLC/MS). 2486. Clonazepam, 7-aminoclonazepam, 7-acetamidoclonazepam (GLC/MS, human plasma, chemical ionization, selected ion monitoring). 2534. Clonazepam (human plasma, GLC / negative ion chemical ionization MS).

3509. Lormetazepam. 3510. Triazolam.

MS (chemical ionization) / MS (chemische Ionisation)

177. Oxazepam, lorazepam. 723. Diazepam, Chlordiazepoxide. 725. Clonazepam, metabolites (plasma, blood). 2486. Clonazepam, metabolites. 2534. Clonazepam (negative-ion CI).

GLC - MS / GC - MS

189. Flurazepam, metabolites. 320. Chlordiazepoxide, diazepam (other drugs). 327. Diazepam, Nitrazepam, Oxazepam, N-desmethyldiazepam, temazepam. 680. C_3-hydroxylated benzodiazepines. 725. Clonazepam, metabolites (plasma, blood). 1139. Pinazepam (metabolites, serum, urine, brain). 2939. Clobazam. 3444. Diazepam (serum). 3659. Midazolam. 3706. Clonazepam. 3725. Diazepam (plasma).
3754. 1,4-benzodiazepines, 1,5-benzodiazepines (urine).

NMR- Investigations / NMR- Untersuchungen

114. Diazepam, Nitrazepam, Chlordiazepoxide (Konformation und Ringinversion). 658. Chlordiazepoxide (other data). 659. Diazepam (other data). 798. Diazepam, Nitrazepam, Chlordiazepoxide (Konfiguration). 875. Chlorazepate (other data). 922. Flurazepam (other data). 993. Diazepam and metabolites. 1034. Oxazepam (other analytical data).

1804. Diazepam, Nitrazepam (^{1}H-NMR investigations on the hydrogen-bond formation between diazepam and nitrazepam and some nucleobases).

2599. 1-Substituted 2,3-dihydro-1H-1,4-benzodiazepines (spatial coupling). 2600. 1-Methyl-5-phenyl-2,3,4,5-tetrahydro-1H-1,5-benzodiazepine-2,4-diones (stereochemistry). 2629. Chlordiazepoxide-hydrochloride / amitriptyline-hydrochloride-combinations (study of proton transfer in dipolar aprotic solvents). 2680. Diazepam and its 1-1 complex with chloral hydrate (^{35}C-nuclear-quadrupole resonance spectra). 2849. Clobazam. 3009. 1,4-Benzodiazepines (^{13}C- and proton-studies). 3376. 1,4-Benzodiazepines (investigations of a hammet-type substituent effect on the hydrogen bond interaction). 3446. 1,3-Dihydro-2H-1,4-benzodiazepine-2-ones (stereochemistry by lanthanide shift-reagents). 3494. Flurazepam (NMR study of the interactions with human serum albumin, nature of the complexation site on the benzodiazepine-molecule). 3702. 2'-Chloronordiazepam (identification of its metabolites in the dog).

Pharmacokinetic / Pharmakokinetik

13. Oxazepam (man, healthy volunteers). 16. Diazepam (man, disordered liver function). 76. Clonazepam (single oral and intravenous and repeated oral doses). 83. Oxazepam-O-glucuronide (enterohepatic-circulation). 84. Oxazepam (biliary excretion, rat, guinea pigs, mice). 118. Nitrazepam, Clonazepam (humans). 130. Pinazepam (rat brain). 133. Chlordiazepoxide (in healthy subjects, multiple dose oral administration). 134. Chlordiazepoxide (in healthy subjects, single dose, i.v., i.m. and oral routes). 200. Diazepam (antagonisme by LSD). 212. Diazepam, Nor-Diazepam (monkey, macaca mulatta). 215. Benzodiazepines (accumulation and elimination). 224. Nitrazepam, Clonazepam (humans). 263. Grundlagen (Lehrbuch, Dost). 264. Allgemein. 275. Diazepam (after multiple dose, oral administration, healthy human subjects). 300. Diazepam (biliary excretion). 391. Clazepam. 399. Nitrazepam, metabolites (biliary excretion). 416. Lorazepam (after intravenous injection). 419. Lorazepam (after i.m. injection). 420. Lorazepam (after long term injection). 424. Chlordiazepoxide (i.v., sex-differences in distribution). 426. Chlordiazepoxide (after single doses). 429. Oxazepam (versus other benzodiazepines). 430. Chlordiazepoxide (clinical pharmacokinetics). 431. Chlordiazepoxide (clinical pharmacokinetics). 432. Lorazepam (clinical pharmacokinetics, after oral administration). 439. Chlorazepate (+ Metaboliten, Ausscheidung). 507. Clonazepam (clinical pharmacokinetics). 510. Nitrazepam (young volunteers and aged patients). 513. Diazepam (biliary excretion). 555. Clonazepam (dog, humans), Flunitrazepam (dog). 556. Diazepam (man, single i.v. and oral, chronic oral). 557. Bromazepam (clinical pharmacokinetics). 558. Chlordiazepoxide (in the dog). 580. Diazepam (in man and different species). 581. Diazepam, metabolites (hepatic elimination). 582. Diazepam (comparison, after single and subchronic doses). 583. Diazepam (man, dog, rabbit, guinea pig, rat). 586. Diazepam (man). 587. Diazepam (in adult man, effect of liver desease). 592. Clonazepam (man and laboratory animal). 595. Oxazepam (humans). 619. Clonazepam (rhesus monkey). 666. Diazepam (biliary elimination in man). 671. Oxazepam (+ alcohol). 741. Oxazepam (+ Alkohol). 767. Oxazepam (pharmacokinetic studies on the optic isomers). 770. Benzodiazepines (practical comments). 772. Lorazepam (in humans). 792. Flurazepam (rat).

796. Drugs (abnormal distribution in fatal intoxications). 842. Oxazepam (beim Menschen). 854. Diazepam (cat, after chronic treatment). 855. Chlordiazepoxide (mice). 872. Bromazepam (beim Menschen). 893. Chlorazepate (+ metabolites) 894. Chlorazepate (+ metabolites). 908. Nitrazepam (Mensch und Ratte). 910. Nitrazepam (man). 911. Medazepam (man). 925. Clobazam (+ nomifensine, kinetic interaction). 939. Benzodiazepine-Esters (pharmacokinetic studies). 1003. Chlordiazepoxide, metabolites (man). 1014. Diazepam, metabolites (man, biliary excretion, repeated oral doses). 1015. Diazepam, metabolites (man, biliary excretion). 1016. Diazepam (human and animal studies, elimination from plasma, chronic alcohol intake). 1016. Diazepam (human and animal study, elimination from plasma). 1018. Diazepam (induction effect on its own metabolism). 1026. Benzodiazepines (study, clinical implications of pharmacokinetics). 1027. Chlordiazepoxide (in young and elderly male volunteers). 1054. Clonazepam, 7-amino-metabolite (man). 1062. Drugs and other endogenous compounds (conjugation). 1116. Chlordiazepoxide (+ chlorpromazine, influence of protein defiency in rats). 1117. Nitrazepam (influence of cystamine). 1152. Diazepam, Chlordiazepoxide (mice). 1154. Diazepam (animals and humans). 1155. Ataractic Drugs. 1157. 7-Chlorobenzodiazepines (brain distribution). 1158. Diazepam (dog, mice, humans). 1159. Diazepam (newborn rhesus monkey). 1191. Oxazepam (and succinate half-ester). 1195. Diazepam, Nor-Diazepam (clinical pharmacokinetic studies). 1204. Diazepam (rat, effect of ethanol).

1238. Oxazepam (dogs, first-pass conjugation, enterohepatic recycling). 1239. Oxazepam (pharmacokinetic profile). 1240. Flunitrazepam (pharmacokinetic). 1248. Chlorazepate (chronobiologic changes in pharmacokinetics). 1285. Diazepam (mice, hypergravity). 1291. Diazepam (plasma, single dose studies in man). 1292. Flunitrazepam (human healthy subjects, oral single and multiple dose). 1484. Einführung/ Introduction. 1500. Lorazepam (humans, effect of dose and route of administration). 1501. Chlorazepate and Desmethyldiazepam. 1505. Lorazepam (i.v.). 1506. Lorazepam (+ glucuronide metabolism). 1507. Diazepam (influence of age, sex and liver disease). 1509. General. 1510. ^{14}C-Lorazepam (oral absorption and disposition). 1514. General. 1515. Benzodiazepines (pharmacokinetic considerations of dependence, tolerance and addiction). 1517. Chlordiazepoxide and metabolites (single and multiple oral doses). 1518. Lorazepam (humans, i.v., i.m., oral). 1523. Lorazepam (clinical pharmacokinetics). 1524. Chlordiazepoxide (clinical pharmacokinetics). 1552. Allgemein. 1570. Diazepam (Übersicht/Review). 1645. Diazepam and metabolites (clinical pharmacokinetics). 1646. Diazepam (elimination after single and subchronic dosage). 1656. Diazepam (oral, i.m., absorption and sedative effects). 1659. Diazepam (repeated administration, saturation of tissues with N-Desmethyldiazepam). 1660. Diazepam (i.v., influence of food, charcoal ingestion and injection rate). 1670. Lorazepam (clinical pharmacokinetics). 1702. Diazepam (effect of age and gender). 1704. Chlordiazepoxide (i.v., plasma versus blood). 1711. Oxazepam-esters (kinetic investigations with livermicrosomal esterases). 1712. Oxazepam-Acetate (stereospecifity of esterases). 1715. Diazepam (clinical pharmacokinetics). 1719. Camazepam (distribution in rats and mice). 1757. ^{14}C-Diazepam and metabolites (cat brain, kinetics of distribution). 1772. Diazepam (diurnal variations). 1822. N-Desmethyldiazepam (healthy volunteers, after single daily doses of chloracepate). 1846. Nitrazepam (pharmacokinetic and metabolism). 1849. Chlordiazepoxide (effect of age and cirrhosis). 1850. Chlordiazepoxide (effect of age and parenchymal liver-disease). 1892. Diazepam (induction effect on its own metabolism). 1893. Diazepam (reduced plasma concentrations in chronic alcoholic patients following oral absorption). 1926. Chlorazepate (+ alcohol, oral, Wechselwirkungen). 1973. N-Desmethyl-diazepam (in patients suffering from insomnia and treated with nortriptyline). 1974. Oxazepam (given during labour). 1989. Ataractic drugs (pharmacokinetics). 1990. Diazepam (dogs, mice, humans). 1991. Benzodiazepines (+ barbiturates, + short chain fatty-acids). 1998. Oxazepam (+ nortriptyline, man, single oral dose, comparative study). 2018. Diazepam (+ ketamin, Verlaufskontrolle). 2019. Chlordiazepoxide (effect of acute alcohol intoxication on plasma kinetics). 2020. Chlorazepate (kinetics in treated epileptics).

2047. Flunitrazepam (i.v., i.m., oral, pharmakokinetische Befunde). 2086. Nitrazepam (enzymic reduction). 2096. Chlordiazepoxide (healthy subjects, multiple oral dose, pharmacokinetic profile). 2121. Prazepam (pharmacokinetics in man). 2157. Benzodiazepines and others (in petit mal epilepsy). 2175. Temazepam (human, after administration in soft gelatine capsules). 2196. Chlordiazepoxide (i.v.). 2197. Diazepam (use in general anesthesia). 2377. 1,4-Benzodiazepines (effect of enzyme induction and inhibition on microsomal oxidation).

2458. Camazepam. 2459. Clobazam. 2466. Clobazam (humans, single and multiple doses). 2468. Clobazam (+ ethanol, kinetic and dynamic interaction). 2469. Clobazam (animals and man). 2490. Prazepam (man). 2496. Flurazepam (interpretation). 2502. Flunitrazepam (in prolonged administration). 2510. Medazepam (plasma concentrations after oral administration). 2511. Diazepam (in overdose-cases). 2512. Nitrazepam + main metabolites (urinary elimination). 2513. Nitrazepam (after single oral doses, pharmacokinetics in saliva and serum). 2514. Nitrazepam (man, effects of age and diseases). 2515. Flunitrazepam (placental transfer and breast-milk levels). 2525. Flunitrazepam. 2529. Lorazepam (plasma, mother and neonate). 2532. Temazepam. 2533. Clonazepam, clobazam (comparison). 2536. Clotiazepam (man). 2547. Benzodiazepines and others (clinical pharmacokinetics).

2556. Diazepam (in obesity). 2573. Desmethyldiazepam (following oral prazepam in elderly). 2575. Estazolam (single- and multiple-dose kinetics). 2576. Prazepam (single-dose). 2577. Desmethyldiazepam (oral, elderly). 2578. Lorazepam (after overdosage). 2580. Prazepam (single-dose). 2616. Diazepam, desmethyldiazepam (newborn, after i.m. administration). 2617. Benzodiazepines (+ others, in elderly). 2652. Phenazepam (intrahepatic circulation). 2668. Benzodiazepines (interspecies variations). 2677. Benzodiazepines (short-acting versus long-acting). 2683. Midazolam maleate. 2702. Diazepam, clobazam (pharmacological activities in relation to brain level, rat). 2703. Clobazam, desmethylclobazam (brain concentrations and antileptazol activity). 2712. Nordiazepam (elimination half-life). 2750. Benzodiazepines. 2777. Benzodiazepines (pharmacokinetics of closely related compounds). 2779. Diazepam (in normal and uremic humans). 2800. Diazepam (effects of solvents on distribution). 2802. Chlordiazepoxide (+ ethanol, impairment of elimination in man). 2803. (see 2802.). 2804. Chlordiazepoxide (+ cimetidine, impairment of elimination, man). 2846. ^{14}C-triazolam (disposition in man). 2855. Nitrazepam (dogs, enzyme induction effect of phenobarbital). 2858. Diazepam (i.v., kinetics in the presence or absence of its active metabolite desmethyldiazepam, man). 2893. Flunitrazepam (repeated i.v. administration). 2894. Diazepam (+ ethanol, differentiation of CNS-effects). 2895. Diazepam (plasma and saliva levels). 2938. Diazepam (pharmacokinetic interaction of local anesthetics). 2945. ^{14}C-Lormetazepam (in dogs, rabbits, rats and rhesus monkeys). 2960. Diazepam (disposition determinants). 2961. + 2962. Lorazepam (kinetics in the elderly). 2963. Diazepam (influence of age and sex on kinetics). 2964. Lorazepam (humans, oral single-dose and multiple-dose kinetics). 2965. Oxazepam (effects of age and sex). 2966. Diazepam, metabolites (entry in cerebrospinal-fluid). 2967. Benzodiazepines (effects of age and other drugs on kinetics). 2969. Desmethyldiazepam (plasma concentrations following single doses of clorazepate). 2979. Diazepam (effects of solvents). 3000. Pirenzepine (profile).

3032. Flurazepam (plasma concentrations after 30-mg Dalmane). 3047. + 3048. ^{14}C-Lormetazepam (absorption, distribution, elimination, first-pass effects, humans). 3086. Nitrazepam (enhancement of reductive metabolism by ethanol, rats). 3105. Diazepam (effect of age). 3138. Diazepam (rat, effect of age). 3140. Benzodiazepines (clinical pharmacokinetics). 3141. Desmethyldiazepam (altered elimination in the elderly). 3142. Diazepam (delayed clearance due to cimetidine). 3143. Benzodiazepines (effect of cimetidine on clearance). 3144. Oxazepam, desmethyldiazepam (influence of cimetidine). 3159. Chlordiazepoxide (in humans). 3174. Clonazepam (+ carbamazepine, interactions, monkeys). 3175. Clonazepam (kinetics to 7-amino-metabolite, monkey). 3176. Diazepam (+ ethanol, pharmacokinetic interactions). 3198. Diazepam (in an abuser). 3215. Diazepam (i.v., in epileptic children). 3216. Diazepam (relation to age). 3218. Diazepam (gender-related differences). 3225. Diazepam (man, following rectal and parenteral administration). 3227. + 3228. Oxazepam-esters (man, hydrolysis-rates, hydrophobicity, correlation with brain penetration and excretion). 3306. Oxazepam (man, effects of renal-disease and age). 3315. Diazepam (man, circadian effects). 3318. Diazepam (diurnal variations in plasma concentrations). 3338. Lorazepam (rabbit). 3342. Lorazepam (entry in cerebrospinal-fluid). 3343. Desmethyldiazepam from clorazepate (effect of age and billroth-gastrectomy on absorption). 3345. Diazepam (+ barbital, human, salivary excretion). 3347. Diazepam (effect of enzyme induction, man). 3374. Oxazepam, lorazepam (cimetidine spares glucuronidation). 3400. Diazepam (kinetics in acute alcohol withdrawal). 3412. Diazepam (rat, effect of hyperbilirubinemia). 3424. Clorazepate (in pregnant and non-pregnant women). 3425. Clorazepate, nordiazepam (placental transfer and distribution in the feto-placental unit and in the neonate). 3434. Chlordiazepoxide (sex-differences and effects of oral contraceptives on disposition). 3459. Diazepam, desmethyldiazepam (redistribution after heparin). 3465. Benzodiazepines (effect of cimetidine on clearance). 3492. Midazolam maleate (steady-state concentrations). 3511. Benzodiazepines (survey). 3512. Temazepam (in man and several animal species). 3514. Benzodiazepines (effects of disulfiram and ethanol on disposition). 3515. Chlordiazepoxide, oxazepam (disposition in cirrhotics). 3559. Midazolam (man). 3662. Benzodiazepines (+ ethanol, pharmacokinetic interactions). 3691. Diazepam (humans, rabbits, influence of elevated serum-lipid levels on pharmacokinetics). 3722. Diazepam (correlations between the order of administration and the plasma levels). 3724. Diazepam (+ morphine, pharmacokinetics). 3746. Oxazepam, lorazepam (clinical pharmacokinetics). 3747. Desalkylflurazepam (single and multiple doses, elderly). 3748. Diazepam, desmethyldiazepam (long-term therapy). 3749. Benzodiazepines (summary of pharmacokinetic properties). 3752. Bromazepam (man). 3755. Chlordiazepoxide (in patients with alcoholic hepatitis). 3758. Benzodiazepines (influences of different parameters on pharmacokinetics). 3762. Midazolam (man). 3766. Benzodiazepines (factors influencing the activity and fate in body). 3773. Clotiazepam (man). 3775. Triazolam (normal subjects, oral).

Pharmacology and Clinical Investigations (selection)
Pharmakologie und klinische Untersuchungen (Auswahl)

17. Lorazepam (bei Angstneurose). 32. Benzodiazepine (effect on amphetamine-induced behavior). 46. Diazepam, Chlordiazepoxide and some other 1,4-benzodiazepines (anticonvulsant properties). 49. Chlordiazepoxide (+ d-amphetamine and promazine). 58. Lorazepam (clinical trial). 71. Diazepam (frog, synaptic transmission). 105. N-Oxides(pharmacology and biochemistry). 106. Antidepressiva (biochemical aspects). 116. Clonazepam (Pharmakologie und Toxikologie). 129. Clobazam, Diazepam, Chlordiazepoxide (immediate effects on human performance). 154. Oxazepam (effect on physiological responses to stress). 155. Chlorazepate (pharmacological, toxicological and teratological studies). 156. Benzodiazepines (influence on serum lipids in rabbits). 157. Chlordiazepoxide (changes in plasma cortisol). 166. Anticonvulsant Drugs (increased sulfobromophthalein clearance). 171. Nitrazepam (anxiety states). 173. Medazepam . 178. Diazepam (effect on serotonin). 180. Benzodiazepines (effect on aggressive behavior, mice, rats). 183. Chlordiazepoxide (persistent EEG changes). 185. Nor-Diazepam (activity). 197. Chlordiazepoxide (psychiatric disorders). 203. Diazepam (anticonvulsant activity). 227. Diazepam (effect on pancreatic secretion). 246. Oxazepam (+ meprobamate, anxious neurotic outpatients). 256. Oxazepam (anxious students). 257. Chlordiazepoxide (Pharmakopsychology). 270. Lorazepam, flunitrazepam, fosazepam (comparison, sedative properties). 272. Prazepam (treatment of anxiety). 273. Prazepam (treatment of anxiety). 304. Clonazepam (treatment of epileptic seizures). 306. Diazepam (efficacy). 315. Chlordiazepoxide (+ alcohol, habituation). 330. Diazepam (sustained low doses, effect on aggression and mortality, male mice). 331. Chlordiazepoxide (male mice). 332. Nitrazepam, flurazepam (male mice). 340. Benzodiazepines (analgetic effects). 344. Halazepam, diazepam (motor coordinations). 345. Diazepam (muscle relaxant). 360. Diazepam (anticonvulsant action). 365. Oxazepam and chlordiazepoxide (hostility). 368. Clonazepam (antiepileptische Wirkung). 369. Diazepam (treatment of status epilepticus). 378. Diazepam (effect on conflicht behavior). 379. Chlordiazepoxide (+ chlorpromazine, effect on punishment discrimination). 384. Chlordiazepoxide (juvenile delinquent boys). 386. Lorazepam (pharmacology). 394. Chlordiazepoxide (pharmacological response following acute and chronic administration). 401. Chlordiazepoxide (+ amylobarbitone and placebo, treatment of tension and anxiety states). 422. Benzodiazepines (clinical practice). 423. Benzodiazepines (drug therapy). 441. Benzodiazepines (increased aggression and toxicity, grouped male mice). 444. Benzodiazepine (und andere, Pharmakologie und Toxikologie). 449. Benzodiazepines (+ barbiturates, synaptic pharmacology). 451. Diazepam (+ ethanol, mental and psychomotor effects). 463. Chlordiazepoxide (rat). 466. Chlordiazepoxide (pharmacology). 475. Chlordiazepoxide (taming action). 482. Chlordiazepoxide (calming zoo animals). 487. Nitrazepam, flurazepam, flunitrazepam (repeated dose comparison). 494. Diazepam (+acetophenazine, anxiety). 501. Diazepam (anaesthesia). 504. Chlordiazepoxide, diazepam (+ placebo). 526. Chlordiazepoxide, diazepam (+ amylobarbitone, comparison). 528. Diazepam (effect on food consumption in rats). 565. Chlordiazepoxide (patients with liver desease). 566. Diazepam, chlordiazepoxide (treatment of neurotic anxiety). 567. Benzodiazepines (general medical patients). 571. Benzodiazepines (effect of chronic administration on epileptic seizures, papio papio). 576. Prazepam (anxiety studies). 577. Diazepam, chlordiazepoxide (+ placebo). 588. Oxazepam (pharmacology). 621. Chlordiazepoxide (use for preparation for urography). 625. Diazepam (flight and defensive behavior, cat). 628. Benzodiazepines (role in nonpsychiatric medical practice). 629. Clobazam (effect on gastrointestinal disorders). 645. Chlorazepate (in epilepsy). 647. Chlordiazepoxide (early effects). 649. Diazepam (permeation through membranes). 686. Diazepam (antimetrazol activity). 689. Diazepam (species differences in anticonvulsant activity). 695. Oxazepam (increase of activity and tolerance during chronic administration). 704. Chlordiazepoxide (use in obese patients). 709. Diazepam (+ amylobarbitone, comparison). 710. Diazepam (+ ketamine, in the adult patient). 716. Chlorazepate (neurophysiological study). 774. Bromazepam, diazepam (versus placebo). 775. Diazepam (+ nabilone, comparison). 776. Diazepam (cardioversion). 783. Diazepam(and other drugs, effect on spinal relects of cat). 787. Nitrazepam, diazepam, flurazepam (matching behavior, macaca mulatta). 788. Diazepam, metabolites (behavioural activity). 789. Fosazepam (activity). 794. Clonazepam (epilepsy, children).

818. Flurazepam (electroencephalographic effects). 853. Chlordiazepoxide (+ secobarbital, effect on film-induced anxiety). 856. Chlordiazepoxide (psychiatric praxis). 874. Clobazam (efficacy and tolerance). 876. Chlordiazepoxide (pharmacology). 877. Chlordiazepoxide (pharmacology). 878. Benzodiazepines (pharmacology). 879. Diazepam (pharmacological and clinical studies). 880. Benzodiazepines (pharmacology). 881. Benzodiazepines (pharmacology). 882. Chlordiazepoxide (psychosedative properties). 883. Nitrazepam (Pharmakologie). 884. Diazepam (Pharmakologie). 885. Medazepam (Pharmakologie). 886. Flurazepam (Pharmacology). 887. Benzodiazepines (pharmacology). 888. Diazepam, Chlordiazepoxide, metabolites (pharmacology). 889. Medazepam, metabolites (pharmacology). 891. Chlordiazepoxide (mice). 892. Diazepam, clobazam (effect on central amine metabolism, rats). 901. Temazepam (anxiolytic properties). 905. Chlordiazepoxide (anxiety). 906. Diazepam (+ doxepine, in general practice and hospital clinic neurotic patients). 917. Chlorazepate, diazepam (clinical comparison). 931. Flurazepam (pharmacology). 932. Methylnitrazepam (pharmacology). 936. Chlordiazepoxide (properties). 937. Oxazepam (hostility). 940. Clobazam (anxiolytic activity). 941. Chlordiazepoxide (and MAO-inhibitors). 942. Benzodiazepines (+ morphine, mice). 943. Oxazepam (+ placebo, comparative study). 944. Benzodiazepines (anxiety states). 959. Chlordiazepoxide (and other drugs, effect on the limbic system). 960. Benzodiazepines (effect on central nervous system). 968. Lorazepam (clinical investigation). 1019. Diazepam (+ pyrithioxin, rat brain). 1022. Benzodiazepines (pharmacological aspects). 1023. Chlordiazepoxide, Diazepam, Desmethyldiazepam (conflict behavior, squirrel monkey). 1029. Prazepam, chlordiazepoxide (+ placebo, short term treatment of alcoholics). 1032. Diazepam (influence on the effect of neuromuscular blocking agents). 1039. Bromazepam (pharmacology). 1040. Bromazepam (pharmacology, central nervous system). 1041. Bromazepam (pharmacology, various administrations, rats). 1046. Prazepam (psychoneurotic outpatients). 1050. Benzodiazepine (Grundzüge einer Pharmakologie). 1081. Benzodiazepines (+ phenobarbital and diphenylhydantoin). 1104. Benzodiazepines (cats). 1113. Benzodiazepines (anticonvulsant properties). 1123. Flunitrazepam (neuromuscular blockade). 1135. Chlordiazepoxide (anxiety reactions). 1136. Chlordiazepoxide (anxiety states). 1164. Diazepam (man, cerebral blood flow and oxygen consumption). 1194. Clonazepam (dopamine related stereotyped behavior). 1200. Chlordiazepoxide (+ propanolol, anxiety states). 1212. Benzodiazepines (behavior in the pigeon). 1222. Benzodiazepines (laboratory and clinical correlations). 1232. Clonazepam (effect on epileptic seizures). 1234. Lorazepam, Diazepam (ventilatory patterns). 1235. Diazepam (treatment of spasmodic torticollis). 1236. Flunitrazepam (Pharmakologie und Klinik). 1237. Lorazepam (pharmacology). 1241. Diazepam (effect on evoked potential recorded from basal medial amygdaloid nucleus, lateral hypothalamus and midbrain reticular formation). 1242. Lorazepam (Erfahrungen als Tranquilizer). 1243. Diazepam (+ dixirazine, + opropramol, + placebo, comparison in anxiety states). 1245. Diazepam (influence of the route of administration on clinical action). 1246. Diazepam (i.v., effect on arterial oxygen-saturation during esophagogastroduodenoscopy). 1249. Hydrosoluble benzodiazepines (CNS-pharmacological properties). 1250. Clonazepam (absence seizures, treatment). 1251. 1-Phenyl-1,2,3,4-tetrahydro-5H-1,4-benzodiazepin-5-one (pharmacological activity). 1252. Diazepam (i.v., in dentistry). 1254. Clonazepam (als Antikonvulsivum). 1259. Diazepam (rat, chronic oral administration, plasma corticosterone responses). 1260. Clonazepam (treatment of epilepsy). 1261. Diazepam (acute tolerance in cats). 1262. Diazepam (effect on turnover of cerebral dopamine). 1263. Clobazam (pharmacological properties). 1267. Chlorazepate (Behandlung psychovegetativer Allgemeinstörungen). 1269. Clonazepam (EEG und klinische Bewertung). 1272. Clonazepam (+ aluminum exposure, effect on dialysis encephalopathy). 1273. Clobazam (effect on human coordination). 1275. Diazepam (+ doxepin, anxiety states, comparative trial). 1277. Clonazepam (effect in epilepsy). 1279. Clonazepam (anticonvulsant action). 1280. Clobazam (clinical survey). 1282. Lorazepam (premedicant, effect on recall). 1283. Lorazepam (parenteral, pilot clinical trial). 1285. Diazepam (mice, hypergravity, anticonvulsive effect). 1286. Chlorazepate (treatment of intractable epilepsy). 1300. Diazepam (i.v., patients with chronic liver disease). 1313. Clonazepam (therapy). 1314. Benzodiazepines (treatment of epilepsy). 1315. Clonazepam (effect on inhibited and non-inhibited behavior). 1316. Flunitrazepam (effect on circulation, coronary blood-pressure and margin of safety). 1317. Diazepam (high-dose, liver function test, therapy of tetanus). 1322. Benzodiazepines (étude, sommeil, comportement, humeur). 1327. Camazepam (trial versus chlordiazepoxide). 1329. Clonazepam (treatment of minor motor seizures). 1330. Benzodiazepines (drug response in different anxiety states). 1335. Benzodiazepines (review, general anesthesia and sedation). 1337. Clonazepam (treatment of petit mal). 1340. Diazepam (+ haloperidol, anxiety treatment, clinical trial). 1342. Clobazam (anticonvulsant action in reflex epilepsy). 1345. Diazepam (+ propanolol, comparative effects on sympathetic responses). 1351. Camazepam (anxiolytische Wirkung, Doppelblindversuch). 1352. Chlorazepate (premedication). 1356. Lorazepam (psychopharmacological study). 1357. Lorazepam (pharmacology of parenterally administered lorazepam). 1360. Benzodiazepines (effect on feelings and anxiety). 1367. Diazepam (i.v., cardioversion of supraventricular arrhythmias). 1371. Diazepam (role in orthopedic practice). 1372. Diazepam (hemodynamic and respiratory effects). 1374. Diazepam (oral, anxiety patients, concentration-effect relationship). 1375. Nitrazepam (+ amylobarbitone, sleep inducing effects). 1376. Water soluble benzodiazepines (response of spinal neurons to acetylcholine and excitatory amino acid analogues). 1377. Diazepam (i.v., report). 1378. Oxazepam-hemisuccinate(stereostructure activity, effects on CNS). 1379. Camazepam (Doppelblindversuch, psychoneurotische Patienten). 1380. Oxazepam (children, elderly, treatment of anxiety). 1381. Chlordiazepoxide (antiaggressive effects). 1383. Camazepam (Verwendung in der Allgemeinmedizin). 1385. Clonazepam (perorale Langzeittherapie schwerer Epilepsieformen des Kindesalters). 1386. Lorazepam, Diazepam (parenteral, chronic lung disease, respiratory effects). 1394. Benzodiazepines (effect on aggression). 1397. Diazepam (i.v., dentistry). 1398. Diazepam (i.v., dentistry, recovery). 1399. Diazepam (+ pentazocine, effects, comparison). 1403. Clobazam (versus placebo, neurotic anxiety and tension). 1404. Clobazam (versus diazepam, anxiety neurosis). 1405. Diazepam (i.v., sedation). 1406. (+ placebo, anxious outpatients, prediction of response). 1408. Diazepam (premedication, general anaesthesia for bronchoscopy and laryngoscopy). 1410. Benzodiazepines (review of actions relative to anaesthetic practice). 1412. Lorazepam (studies given before anaesthesia). 1414. Chlorazepate (comparison study, divided daily dose, single night dose). 1415. Diazepam (+ morphine, + chlorpromazine, shock-intensity discrimination). 1418. Clonazepam (anticonvulsant effectiveness). 1419. Clonazepam (treatment of epilepsy, mentally retarded children). 1420. Benzodiazepines (anticonvulsant properties). 1427. Lorazepam (CNS- and cardiovascular effects). 1428. General. 1431. Benzodiazepines (subcellular actions). 1433. Benzodiazepines (influence on aggressive behavior). 1434. Triazolam, Diazepam (+ placebo, treatment of insomnia and anxiety). 1435. Ketazolam, Diazepam (+ placebo, anxiety treatment, comparison). 1438. Clonazepam (treatment of epileptic seizures). 1441. Diazepam (treatment of acute convulsions in children). 1446. Diazepam (adjunct in obstetric analgesia). 1448. Oxazepam (clinical activity). 1449. Diazepam (+ thiopentone, induction agents to general anaes-

thesia, clinical comparison). 1450. Benzodiazepines (effect on age and vaginal perforation and first estrus in mice). 1453. Lorazepam (lack of precall and relief of anxiety). 1454. Water soluble benzodiazepines, Ro 21-3981 (induction of anesthesia). 1455. Clobazam (use in otorhinolaryngology). 1460. Lorazepam (as premedication). 1461. Triazolam, Alprazolam, Diazepam (pharmacology of metabolites). 1464. Clonazepam (children with epilepsy, trial). 1467. Oxazepam (biochemical and pharmacological properties). 1470. Diazepam (+ phenytoin, rat, actions, epileptiform focus). 1475. Benzodiazepines (central inhibitory mechanisms). 1476. Clobazam (neuropharmacological profile). 1478. Clonazepam (pediatrics, clinical experience). 1486. Clonazepam (+ lidocain, + penicillin, anticonvulsive actions). 1487. Clonazepam (treatment of intention myoclonus). 1488. Oxazepam, Flurazepam (+ chloralhydrate, geriatric patients, comparison as hypnotic sedatives). 1491. Lorazepam (i.v., acute anxiety crisis, report, 60 cases). 1492. Diazepam (for eclampsia). 1494. Diazepam, Oxazepam (normal subjects, subjective effects and vigilance). 1496. Lorazepam (effect on anxiety). 1513. Benzodiazepines (pharmacotherapy of anxiety). 1516. Prazepam, Lorazepam (therapy). 1520. Flurazepam x HCl (application). 1521. Flurazepam x HCl (hypnotic application). 1528. Clonazepam (als Antikonvulsivum). 1529. Camazepam (Therapie der Angina pectoris). 1531. Diazepam, Nitrazepam (degree of sedation with various doses). 1533. Benzodiazepines (actions on CNS). 1534. + 1535. Benzodiazepines (effect on cortical and subcortical epileptogenic tissues, cat, monkey). 1538. Diazepam, Clobazam (treatment of anxiety, comparison). 1541. Benzodiazepines (central actions, general introduction). 1550. Diazepam (+ doxepin, anxiety treatment). 1551. Diazepam, Chlordiazepoxide (premedicant for standard operation, study). 1553. Flunitrazepam (+ local anesthesia, report, 1400 operations). 1556. Diazepam, Lorazepam (+ pentobarbitone, effect on recall). 1559. Medazepam. 1563. Lorazepam (premedication for bronchoscopy). 1564. Clonazepam (+ valproic acid, epileptic seizures). 1577. Chlorazepate (clinical evaluation). 1581. + 1582. Clonazepam (treatment of intractable seizures). 1583. Flunitrazepam (+ ketamine, + muscle relaxants, general anesthesia). 1588. Clonazepam (treatment of epilepsy). 1589. Diazepam (Geburtshilfe und Frauenheilkunde, Wirkung, Übersicht). 1590. Clobazam (anxiety states, studies). 1592. Diazepam (comparison with pentazocine and pethidine in pediatric premedication). 1594. Oxazepam (treatment of anxiety). 1598. Diazepam (+ ketamine, haemodynamic studies, open heart surgery). 1603. Diazepam (mice, anticonvulsant activity). 1604. Flurazepam x HCl (comparative study). 1606. Lorazepam (effect on the vasoconstriction of fear). 1607. Diazepam + Ro 21-3981 (dogs, effect on cardiovascular-system). 1608. Diazepam (effect of low doses on human-performance). 1609. Diazepam (use in tetanus). 1611. Diazepam (+ hydralazine, treatment of severe pre-eclampsia). 1612. Diazepam (Einfluß auf Wehenschmerz). 1616. Benzodiazepines (treatment of alcohol withdrawal, studies). 1617. Chlordiazepoxide (treatment of epilepsy). 1619. Diazepam (treatment of eclampsia, 16 cases). 1624. CS-370 (pharmacological studies). 1625. Nitrazepam (premedication for minor surgery). 1626. Nitrazepam (correlation of plasma levels with subjective sedatory effects). 1628. Diazepam (as inductive agent). 1631. Flunitrazepam (Pharmakologie). 1633. Diazepam (management of eclampsia). 1634. Diazepam (i.v. administration). 1635. Diazepam (effects of i.v. administration). 1636. Clobazam (new hypnotic). 1638. Diazepam (high doses, treatment of neonatal tetanus). 1639. Lorazepam (i.v., anxiety states). 1640. Clonazepam (klinische Erfahrungen). 1643. Chlordiazepoxide (management of neurotic and psychotic states). 1647. Lorazepam (evaluation of the cardiopulmonary safety). 1648. Diazepam, Flunitrazepam (effects on ketamine side-effects). 1661. Diazepam, Flunitrazepam (comparison as adjuncts to local anesthesia for bronchoscopy). 1662. Flunitrazepam (effect of age on amnesia and sedation). 1663. Diazepam (effect on cognition via pupillometry). 1664. Diazepam (changes in the electrical activity of the cerebral cortical neurons in the rabbit). 1665. Medazepam (preliminary observations in psychiatric disorders). 1668. Clonazepam (Epilepsie verschiedener Formen, Wirksamkeit). 1669. Flunitrazepam (effect on behavior and psyche). 1672. Oxazepam (clinical pharmacology). 1675. Diazepam (management of eclampsia). 1679. Benzodiazepines (management of eclampsia). 1681. Triazolam, Flurazepam (long-term hypnotic efficacy and safety). 1683. Lorazepam (Anwendung in Psychiatrie und Innerer Medizin). 1684. Benzodiazepines (+ meprobamate, + barbiturates, effect on central monoamine neurons). 1685. Benzodiazepines (high-doses, treatment of severe neurotic anxiety). 1687. Chlordiazepoxide and metabolites (relationship of plasma levels to clinical response). 1690. Nitrazepam (comparison with alimemazine as hypnotics). 1695. Lorazepam (premedicant for day-case surgery). 1697. Clonazepam (treatment of epilepsy). 1698. Diazepam (use in early pregnancy). 1706. Chlordiazepoxide (effect on cardiac, smooth and skeletal muscle). 1707. Diazepam, Lorazepam (oral premedicants for surgery). 1708. Chlorazepate, Diazepam (comparison of nightly and daily doses). 1716. Lorazepam (treatment of sexual disorders). 1722. Diazepam (enhanced relief of phobia). 1723. Clonazepam (childhood, infancy, treatment of epilepsy). 1725. Chlordiazepoxide (compared with amitriptyline and perphenazine). 1726. Oxazepam (treatment of vegetative disorders). 1727. Nitrazepam (hypnotic safety). 1733. Diazepam (oral and i.m. routes, comparison of sedative effects). 1735. Diazepam (+ benzoctamine, + placebo, anxiety states, comparison). 1739. Diazepam, Clobazam (comparison in treatment of anxiety neurosis). 1740. Chlordiazepoxide (therapy in hepatic insufficiency). 1741. Diazepam (+ pethidine, analgesia for cytoscopy). 1742. Lorazepam (Prüfung in nervenärztlicher Praxis). 1743. Camazepam (Wirkung). 1744. Camazepam (Wirkung). 1745. Clonazepam (treatment of epilepsy). 1750. Chlordiazepoxide (modulation effect on PGO-spikes, rat). 1751. Diazepam (man, effects on EEG). 1755. Diazepam (use in gastrointestinal endoscopy). 1762. Clonazepam (treatment of epileptic seizures). 1763. Diazepam (liver disease). 1767. Clonazepam (rat brain, influence on monoamine containing neurons). 1768. Flunitrazepam (effect on turnover of serotonin, mouse brain). 1769. Benzodiazepines (effect on central serotonergic neuron systems). 1771. Clonazepam (treatment of epilepsy). 1774. Benzodiazepines (rats, influence on blood-coagulation). 1780. (i.v., anticonvulsant action). 1781. Diazepam, Flunitrazepam (+ neuroleptanalgesia, gastrointestinal endoscopy, comparative study). 1784. Flurazepam (lobster, frog, effect on amino-acid-evoked response). 1785. Diazepam (effect on meperidine requirements during labor). 1786. Lorazepam (use in premedication). 1788. Flurazepam (rabbits, EEG effects), 1789. Lorazepam (treatment of anxiety). 1790. Diazepam (i.v., minor oral surgery). 1791. Diazepam (man, relation between CNS-effects and plasma level). 1794. Clobazam (single doses morning or night, treatment of anxiety). 1797. Lorazepam (anti recall effect). 1798. Flunitrazepam (influence on memory). 1800. Clobazam (psychomotor performance). 1801. Diazepam (treatment of severe convulsive status epilepticus). 1802. Diazepam (Unterschiedliche Reaktionen bei verschiedenen i.v. Applikationsgeschwindigkeiten). 1803. Diazepam (effect on threshold of ventilatory responses to CO_2). 1806. Lorazepam (pre-operative medication). 1807. Diazepam (use of various solvents, effect on cardiac rhythm). 1814. Clonazepam (pharmacological properties and efficacy in epilepsy, review). 1816. Lorazepam (treatment of anxiety, safety and efficacy). 1819. Flunitrazepam (cardiovascular performances, other induction agents, comparison). 1820. Camazepam (Behandlung von Angstzuständen).

1821. Lorazepam (multicenter evaluation). 1824. Lorazepam (+ pentobarbital, as hypnotic, comparison). 1825. Lorazepam (+ glutethimide, as night before hypnotic, comparison). 1826. Diazepam (i.v., treatment of prolonged seizures activity). 1829. Diazepam (+ Doxepin, vergleichende Untersuchung, parenteral). 1830. Chlorazepat (Änderung der subjektiven Befindlichkeit). 1831. Camazepam (Behandlung des klimakterischen Syndroms). 1832. Diazepam (+ chlorpromazine, + imipramine, influence on central action of ethanol). 1833. Diazepam (cardiopulmonary effects). 1837. Diazepam (relationship between dose, plasma level, age, and central nervous system depression). 1838. Diazepam (relaxierende Wirkung auf Uterusmuskulatur). 1839. Benzodiazepines (alterations in binding-sites in Huntingdon-disease). 1840. Clonazepam (Therapie im Kindesalter, Möglichkeiten und Grenzen). 1841. Lorazepam (clinical profile). 1842. Benzodiazepines (anxious outpatients). 1843. Lorazepam (in anxiety). 1848. Diazepam (+ pethidine, + promethazine, comparison). 1855. Diazepam (+ hydroxyzine, pediatric premedication, oral versus i.m. route). 1857. Clonazepam (anticonvulsant properties). 1862. Chlordiazepoxide (+ amphetamine, effect on animal and human behavior). 1865. Chlordiazepoxide (clinical use in pre-operative anxiety states). 1866. Diazepam (anaesthetic for operative vaginal delivery). 1867. Oxazepam (long-term efficacy). 1868. Flurazepam (clinical and psychometric evaluation). 1869. Chlorazepate (expertise pharmacologique et toxicologique). 1870. Flurazepam (thymoleptic action of two salts). 1871. Diazepam (i.v., use in accident department). 1872. Chlordiazepoxide (+ amphetamine, effect on avoidance behavior of reserpinized mice). 1875. Benzodiazepines (recent developments in pharmacology). 1877. Clonazepam (Therapie kindlicher Epilepsien). 1878. Clonazepam (effect on neuronal-activity of sensomotor brain cortex in rats). 1879. Benzodiazepines (effect on CNS). 1880. Flunitrazepam (effect on respiration). 1882. Chlorazepat (einmalige Abenddosis). 1883. Bromazepam (Pharmakologie). 1887. Pinazepam (psychopharmacological properties). 1889. Diazepam (treatment of tetanus neonatorum). 1890. Benzodiazepines (clinical pharmacology and therapeutics). 1895. Chlordiazepoxide (+ promazine, comparative clinical evaluation in treatment of alcohol-withdrawal syndrome). 1898. Chlordiazepoxide (single versus repeated dose). 1900. Diazepam (newborn infant, in preeclamptic toxaemia). 1901. (i.v., intensity and duration of human psychomotor impairment, diazepam). 1902. Benzodiazepines (versus phenobarbital, treatment of anxiety). 1903. Lorazepam (long term use, safety and therapeutic effects). 1907. Lorazepam, Diazepam (+ placebo, treatment of anxiety states, comparison). 1914. Chlorazepat (24-Stunden-Tranquilizer). 1919. + 1920. Benzodiazepines (high-dose treatment of severe neurotic anxiety). 1921. Benzodiazepines (+ placebo, antianxiety effects, clinical research). 1924. Diazepam (in pre-eclamptic toxemia). 1927. Diazepam (parenteral, preanesthic medication). 1928. Lorazepam (squirrel monkey, rat, psychopharmacology). 1929. Benzodiazepines (antianxiety action). 1930. 1,4-Benzodiazepines (chemistry and structure-activity-relationship).

1937. Diazepam (treatment of tetanus). 1938. Benzodiazepines (+ phenobarbital, antagonists of dissimilar chemical convulsants). 1939. Benzodiazepines (chronic psychotic patients, comparative studies). 1940. Flunitrazepam (i.v., anaesthesia). 1944. Diazepam (rat, effect on isolated heart-muscle). 1949. Triazolam, Flurazepam x HCl (+ placebo, hypnotic activity, comparison). 1953. Diazepam (cat, effect on the gamma motor system). 1956. N-Desmethyldiazepam (+ amylobarbitone-sodium, anxious patients, clinical efficacy). 1957. Diazepam, Nor-diazepam (+ amylobarbitone, anxiety, short-term treatment). 1958. Diazepam, Flunitrazepam (Koronarchirurgie, Wirkung auf Kreislauf).

1959. Flurazepam (hypnotic activity in solution and in capsules). 1961. Flurazepam (+ chloral hydrate, acute disturbed psychiatric patients, effectiveness).

1962. Flurazepam (clinical evaluation as hypnotic in psychiatric patients). 1964. Chlordiazepoxide (high-dose treatment in anxiety). 1965. Diazepam (infusion in treatment of tetanus). 1969. Diazepam (oral, treatment of tetanus neonatal). 1971. Diazepam (infants, severe recurrent convulsions, continuous infusion). 1972. Benzodiazepines (in unselected obstetrical series). 1976. Diazepam (use in obstetrics). 1979. Diazepines (general study). 1982. Triazolam, Diazepam (low doses, behavioral and EEG-effect, comparison). 1984. Flunitrazepam (anaesthetic induction). 1987. Benzodiazepines (rats, mice, activity on aggressive behavior). 1993. Diazepam (i.v. administration). 1994. Clonazepam (treatment of infantile spasmus). 1995. Benzodiazepines (induction of anaesthetic sleep). 2001. Diazepam (management of functional gastrointestinal disorders). 2014. Triazolam (hypnotic efficacy). 2015. Lorazepam, Flurazepam (hypnotic efficacy). 2016. Prazepam (treatment of anxiety, multicenter evaluation). 2017. Diazepam (mice, + pentobarbital, + fentanyl-droperidol, study of the efficacy against toxicity, comparison). 2024. Lorazepam (as premedicant for general anaesthesia). 2025. Lorazepam (oral premedication, comparison with diazepam and heptabarbitone). 2027. Chlordiazepoxide (therapy and EEG correlates). 2028. Diazepam (use in military sick call). 2033. Pyrrolobenzodiazepines (anxiolytic agents). 2034. Benzodiazepines (comparison of effects, staircase method).

2039. Diazepam (i.v., sedation following cardiac operations). 2040. Diazepam (coronary vasodilation). 2041. Diazepam (pharmacological basis of coronary and systemic vasodilator actions). 2042. Diazepam (effect on left ventricular contractility on coronary blood flow). 2043. Diazepam (effect on left ventricular function and systemic vascular resistance). 2048. Benzodiazepines (+ barbiturates, + cannabinols, rats, hypothalamic injection, effect on food intake). 2049. Benzodiazepines (effect on evoked potentials, rats). 2053. Lorazepam (i.v., + placebo, treatment of acute anxiety states). 2054. Lorazepam (i.v., anxiety states, comparison of two dosages). 2057. Diazepam (in cardiac surgery). 2063. Sedatives (drug therapy of alcoholism). 2069. Diazepam (+ phenobarbital, comparison, anxiety-related symptoms, acute myocardial infarction). 2070. Diazepam (parenterally adminstered, relief of emotional factor in labor). 2071. Medazepam (EEG-Untersuchungen). 2080. Benzodiazepines (quantitative polygraphic study on emotional tension). 2081. Long-term sedatives (treatment of alcoholism). 2082. Psychotropic drugs (role in medical practice). 2083. Diazepam (dog, coronary and systemic hemodynamic effects). 2084. Diazepam (injectable, pilot study). 2085. Sedatives, hypnotics, minor tranquilizers (healthy problems). 2099. Chlordiazepoxide (+ chlorpromazine, effect on cognitive functioning). 2101. Diazepam (in dentistry). 2102. Diazepam (+morphine, disruption of taste-aversion learning by pretreatment with morphine). 2103. Clonazepam (anticonvulsant activity, review). 2106. Flunitrazepam (pharmacology). 2107. Diazepam (obstetric action). 2108. Diazepam (in anesthesia). 2114. Diazepam (i.v., use in outpatients procedures). 2122. Diazepam (evaluation in psychiatric disorders). 2123. Chlordiazepoxide (food preference test). 2134. Lorazepam (treatment of severe anxiety). 2135. Flunitrazepam (use in anesthesiology). 2136. Diazepam (in pulmonary surgery). 2138. Chlordiazepoxide (in psychotherapy). 2141. Chlordiazepoxide (+ meprobamate, + phenobarbital, clinical comparison). 2143. Diazepam (+ pentazocine, effects for premedication, comparison). 2144. Diazepam (i.v., in dentistry). 2150. Diazepam (i.v., sedation). 2163. Chlordiazepoxide (+ placebo, + trebenzomine, treatment of anxiety). 2165. Diazepam (experience in tetanus). 2166. Chlordiazepoxide (psychodynamic action as antialcoholic agent). 2171. Diazepam, bromazepam (EEG.-effects). 2172. Diazepam (in obstetric analgesia). 2173. Diazepam (i.v., in cardiovascular laboratory).

2174. Flurazepam x HCl (effect on EEG-characteristics). 2184. Diazepam (i.v., basal sedation, instrumental vaginal delivery). 2192. Lorazepam (pharmacology). 2193. Diazepam (therapy of depressed patients). 2194. Triazolam (rats, effects on behavior). 2195. Benzodiazepines (effects on speech). 2200. Diazepam (Behandlung des Abortus imminens und der drohenden Frühgeburt). 2202. Diazepam, Chlordiazepoxide (muscle-relaxant activity). 2204. Clonazepam (effect on human diphenylhydantoin-levels in epileptic patients). 2205. Benzodiazepines (use in glaucoma). 2206. Benzodiazepines (use in myoclonic epilepsy). 2207. Lorazepam (psychomotor depression). 2208. Diazepam (+ amylobarbitone, effect of low doses on human performance). 2209. Diazepam (effect on pituitary functions in man). 2211. Diazepam (i.v., apprehensive child). 2212. Diazepam (i.v., physiological responses to sedation). 2213. Lorazepam (central activity). 2215. Diazepam (single dose kinetic, liver function, neurophysiological effects). 2219. Diazepam (+ valproate, mice, comparison, convulsions in pentobarbital dependent mice). 2220. Diazepam (induction agent). 2222. Benzodiazepines (electrophysiological analysis). 2224. Benzodiazepines (action on isolated guinea-pigs ileum). 2225. Chlordiazepoxide (+ dipiperon, + amobarbital, humans, dose-effect study). 2226. Diazepam (man, effect on myocardial blood-flow). 2227. Diazepam (+ methohexitone, + ethanol, induction agent study). 2229. Chlordiazepoxide (effect on EEG). 2230. Clonazepam (in epilepsy). 2233. Diazepam (+flupenthixol, + nortriptyline, neurotic depression comparison). 2236. Diazepam (clinical evaluation in cerebral palsy). 2241. Diazepam (+ doxepin, gastrointestinal diseases and anxiety). 2242. Diazepam (i.v., circulatory responses in man). 2243. Diazepam (management of psychiatric disorders). 2244. Diazepam (i.v., psychological and physiological effects). 2245. Diazepam (supraventricular arrhythmias). 2246. Chlordiazepoxide (i.v., effects on EEG). 2250. Benzodiazepines and others (treatment of chronic alcoholism). 2252. Diazepam (effect on cognitive and psychomotor performance, review). 2253. Diazepam (as induction agent, cardiopulmonary disease). 2254. Diazepam (+ thiopental, as induction agent, cardiopulmonary disease). 2256. Chlordiazepoxide (epilepsy, clinical experience). 2257. Diazepam (in der Allgemeinpraxis). 2259. Diazepam (use in gastrointestinal endoscopy). 2261. Diazepam (+ fentanyl, + droperidol, action on the contractile of the isolated human myometrium). 2265. Diazepam (rats, effect on liver function). 2266. Diazepam (+ Thiopental, Kreislaufverhältnisse während Narkoseeinleitung). 2272. Diazepam (treatment of spasticity). 2275. Chlordiazepoxide (+ fluphenazine, effect on critical flicker frequency). 2284. Benzodiazepines (treatment of aggressive patients). 2287. Diazepam (injectable, therapy of tetanus). 2290. Benzodiazepines (Relaxation und Geburtsverkürzung). 2291. Nitrazepam (+ amylobarbitone sodium, single doses, persistant behavioral and EEG changes). 2293. Oxazepam (oral, as premedicant in minor surgery). 2295. Diazepam (+ chlorazepate, comparative psychophysiological and mood effects). 2296. Diazepam (effect on emergence from ketamin anesthesia). 2297. Diazepam (i.v., induction agent, general anesthesia). 2298. Lorazepam (treatment of anxiety). 2305. Diazepam (Einfluß auf Kreislauf). 2314. Diazepam, bromazepam (+ placebo, effects on feeling and psychomotor performance, man). 2323. Diazepam (i.v., in minor surgery). 2324. Diazepam (pharmacology). 2325. Clobazam (effects on anxiety, comparison). 2326. Chlorazepate (influence on psychomotor reaction). 2329. Diazepam (in spasticity). 2330. (use in U.S.adults). 2331. Camazepam (in psychovegetative disorders and psychomatic disorders). 2333. Chlordiazepoxide (+chlordimeform, + 2-deoxy-D-glucose, effect on responses in mice and rats). 2334. Diazepam (as adjuvant in childhood tetanus). 2335. Benzodiazepines (cardiopulmonary effects, comparison). 2339. Clonazepam (preliminary results of clinical trial). 2340. Diazepam (effect on evoked cerebral cortex activity). 2341. Diazepam (locus of CNS action). 2345. Diazepam (use in general dental practice). 2350. Lorazepam (treatment of irritable bowel syndrome). 2352. Diazepam (+ methocarbamol, treatment of skeletal muscle spasm, comparison). 2356. Diazepam (+ dihydrallazine, management of eclampsia and severe pre-eclampsia). 2357. Diazepam (+ sodium thiopental, comparison in cardioversion). 2361. Chlordiazepoxide (pigeons, effect on delayed pair comparison tasks). 2362. Nitrazepam, flurazepam (effects on visuo-motor performance). 2363. Nitrazepam, flurazepam (effect on mood states). 2366. Benzodiazepines (effects on spontaneous EEG and arousal responses, cats). 2367. Nitrazepam (cats, effect on response to stimulation). 2368. Lorazepam (+ amylobarbitone, anxiety states, comparison). 2376. Diazepam (Behandlung des Abortus imminens). 2379. Clonazepam (treatment of epilepsy, adults, clinical experience). 2386. Diazepam, lorazepam (comparison in general practice). 2387. Diazepam (treatment of tetanus, case following tooth extraction). 2388. Prazepam (effects on EEG and pressor response to hypothalamic stimulation). 2389. Prazepam (behavioral effects). 2392. Psychotropic drugs (normal human subjects, critical flicker frequency, review). 2394. Diazepam (dialysis encephalopathy). 2395. Flunitrazepam (induction agent). 2397. rat, behavioral effects). 2405. Diazepam (injectable, conscious dogs, cardiovascular response). 2408. Diazepam (in vitro, effect on human cells). 2409. Diazepam (in vivo, effect on chromosomes of human leukocytes). 2414. Diazepam (+ thiopentone, induction agent for Caesarean section, comparison). 2418. Diazepam, flunitrazepam, (+ ketamin, + fentanyl, induction of anesthesia, coronary-artery disease, hemodynamic study). 2419. Diazepam (dog, myocardial hemodynamic and metabolic effects). 2420. Flunitrazepam (sedative and amnesic effects during regional anesthesia). 2421. Diazepam, flunitrazepam (influence of sedation on post-operative pulmonary performance). 2422. N-Desmethyldiazepam (use in insomnia). 2423. Diazepam (use in anesthesiology). 2425. Diazepam (clinical use in anxiety states). 2431. Diazepam (Herzkatheterisierung ohne Narkose beim Säugling). 2438. Flunitrazepam (as hypnotic). 2439. Flurazepam (clinical trial). 2441. Psychotropic drugs (in addiction). 2445. Benzodiazepines (anxiety reducing activity). 2447. Minor tranquilizer (effect on psychomotor performance). 2448. Diazepam (long-term effect on plasma-lipids, aortic-artherosclerosis and blood pressures of atherogenic-fed roosters). 2450. Prazepam (behavioral effects). 2452. Flurazepam x HCl (+ placebo, insomnia treatment, comparison). 2453. Chlordesmethyldiazepam (normal subjects, effects). 2454. Diazepam (+ pentazocine, effect on venomotor reflexes in man).

2458. Camazepam (general description). 2459. Clobazam general description). 2461. Clobazam (anti-anxiety action). 2462. Clobazam (neuro-pharmacological profile). 2463. Clobazam (effects on human psychomotor performance). 2465. Clobazam (anticonvulsant actions in animal-models of epilepsy). 2470. Camazepam (versus diazepam, endoscopy inspection). 2471. Camazepam (double-blind study). 2472. Camazepam (neuropharmacological study). 2473. Camazepam (versus diazepam, in preparation for endoscopy inspection). 2474. Camazepam (effect on cardiac contractility and coronary hemodynamics). 2475. Camazepam (versus placebo, geriatric patients, psychic complaints). 2495. Diazepam (relationship between dose and activity). 2500. Flunitrazepam (experiences in anesthesiology and intensive-therapy). 2501. Flunitrazepam (pharmacological basis, clinical application). 2503. Flunitrazepam (clinical observations in prolonged asministration). 2505. Chlordiazepoxide (water intake and time course of drinking after single or repeated injections). 2531. Triazolam (general description). 2538. Flunitrazepam (parenteral in anesthesiology). 2540. Clotiazepam (psychopharmacological studies). 2549. Clotiazepam (general description). 2557. Clobazam (versus diazepam, comparison, in menopausal patients). 2558. Clobazam (versus lorazepam, in gynecology, comparison). 2559. Benzodiazepines (use in psychiatric inpatients). 2560. Lorazepam (i.v. premedication in general anesthesia). 2562. Diazepam (effect on brain-STEM evoked response). 2565. Diazepam (versus alprazolam, comparison, treatment of anxiety). 2566. Diazepam, lorazepam (ventilatory patterns). 2568. Chlordesmethyldiazepam, lorazepam (double blind comparison, neurotic inpatients). 2581. Clobazam (treatment of anxiety neurosis). 2583. Diazepam (cats, effect on rage reaction). 2584. Diazepam, ketazolam (versus placebo, comparison, once a day versus t.i.d. dosing). 2588. Diazepam (pigs, effects on aggression). 2589. Benzodiazepines (mice, potentiation of gnawing). 2590. Diazepam (+ fentanyl, balanced anesthesia). 2591. Diazepam (treatment of neonatal tetanum). 2594. Benzodiazepines (antagonism of neuronal responses, cerebral cortex). 2595. Chlordiazepoxide (effects on food and shock avoidance). 2597. Diazepam (+ ketamine, effect on spinal analgesia). 2598. Diazepam (humans, physostigmine reversal). 2602. Benzodiazepines (anxiolytic versus sedative properties, structure-activity relationship). 2604. Nitrazepam, temazepam (comparison as hypnotics). 2605. Benzodiazepines (anticholinergic drug synergism, mice). 2606. Diazepam (+ GABA, effects on serotonin-H-3 release from hippocampal synaptosomes). 2608. Clobazam (clinical trials). 2609. Diazepam (or phenobarbital, rats, changes in the convulsion threshold). 2612. Flunitrazepam (+ ketamine, + multiple relaxants, total anesthesia). 2613. Chlordiazepoxide (and phenobarbital, differential stimulus attributes). 2618. Diazepam (high-dose in schizophrenia). 2619. Diazepam (+ atropine, physostigmine reversal). 2621. Benzodiazepines (clinical pharmacology and therapeutic use). 2622. Diazepam, flurazepam (inhibition of adenosine uptake by rat brain). 2624. Nitrazepam (+ dixyrazine, + amylobarbitone, hypnotic medication in geriatric patients). 2626. Diazepam (failing to protect brain-tissue in hypoxic stress). 2628. Flunitrazepam (clinical trial in general psychiatry). 2630. Clonazepam (treatment of spasmodic torticollis). 2631. Benzodiazepines (RM-values and structure-activity relationship). 2632. Benzodiazepines (behavioral studies of workers engaged in benzodiazepine production). 2633.Camazepam (treatment of psycho-vegetative syndroms). 2634. Diazepam (antagonism by physostigmine). 2635. Diazepam (reversal of diazepam-induced postanesthetic somnolence by physostigmine). 2641. Clobazam (clinical experiences). 2646. Diazepam (+ atropine, pharmacology). 2648. Nitrazepam, triazolam (crossover study, young insomniac inpatients). 2653. Phenazepam, metabolites (changes in postsynaptic excitation processes). 2654. Clonazepam (treatment of restless legs). 2655. Diazepam (+ clorotepin, therapy of neurosis). 2656. Flurazepam (medical evaluation of left-ventricular function in cardiopathic patients during short and longterm treatment). 2657. Clonazepam (+ valproate, seizure management in acute hepatic porphyria). 2658. Ketazolam (hypnotic effectiveness in anxious subjects). 2659. Flurazepam (+ pentobarbital, + caffeine, effect on arousal threshold). 2662. Benzodiazepines (application of the free-wilson model to the analysis of pharmacological activity tests). 2665. Diazepam, clobazam (single dose, treatment of anxiety). 2669. Diazepam (effect on neuromuscular function). 2670. Diazepam (clinical effect on neuromuscular function). 2679. Temazepam (+ chlormethiazole, improved hypnotic treatment). 2681. Flunitrazepam (children, i.v., anesthesia). 2682. Clobazam (anxiety, pharmacological properties). 2683. Midazolam maleate (EEG- and other studies). 2685. Diazepam (+ morphine, disruption of taste aversion learning). 2687. Triazolam(depressive action). 2688. Triazolam (brief continous administration, depressive and disinhibitory effects). 2689. Benzodiazepines (plasma ACTH and cortisol levels, rat). 2690. Flunitrazepam (in practice of psychiatry). 2693. Diazepam (+ haloperidol, comparison, treatment of anxiety). 2694. Triazolam (+ flurazepam, comparison, hypnotic effects). 2696. Benzodiazepines (inhibition of calcium-dependent protein-phosphorylation in synaptosome and synaptic vesicle preparations). 2699. Chlordiazepoxide (food preference test). 2701. Chlordiazepoxide (+ ethanol, prenatal and postnatal development of rats). 2702. Diazepam, clobazam (rat, pharmacological activity in relation to brain level). 2703. Clobazam, Desmethylclobazam (brain concentrations and antileptazol activity). 2704. Clobazam (species differences of metabolism and antileptazol effect). 2705. Benzodiazepines (anticonflict effects, potentiation by intraventricular muscimol). 2709. Clorazepate (preoperative narcosis). 2710. Diazepam (neuromuscular function). 2718. Clonazepam (advantageous effects, treatment delirium tremens). 2727. Clonazepam (antimyoclonic action, effect of serotonin). 2729. Diazepam (+ ketamine, anesthesia for minorgynecological surgery). 2730. Diazepam (+ adenosine, potentiation of effects on isolated cardiac and smooth muscle). 2731. Diazepam (potentiation of the coronary vasodilator actions of adenosine in anesthized dogs). 2735. Flunitrazepam (in hospital psychiatry). 2736. Diazepam (diluting injection). 2739. Clorazepate (premedication). 2740. Ketazolam (+ placebo, comparison). 2743. Flunitrazepam (in insomnia). 2745. Clonazepam (children, i.v., status epilepticus). 2746. Diazepam (+ mianserin, comparison, anxiety). 2747. Benzodiazepines (relationship of GABA to anxiolytic effects). 2748. Benzodiazepines (relationship of GABA to anticonflict activity). 2749. Diazepam (male rats, effects on serum testosterone and ventral prostate gland). 2751. Diazepam, chlordiazepoxide (effect on feeding performance in a food-preference test). 2752. + 2753. Chlordiazepoxide (+ amphetamine, + fenfluramine, rat, interactions, feeding parameters). 2754. Chlordiazepoxide (food choice). 2755. Chlordiazepoxide (rat, feeding parameters, effect of acute or chronic administration). 2756. Chlordiazepoxide (rat, food choice). 2757. Chlordiazepoxide (pigeon, food and water intake). 2758. Diazepam (+ pentazocine, outpatient conservative dentistry). 2761. Benzodiazepines (effects in the leech). 2764. Benzodiazepines (and neurotransmitters). 2767. Diazepam (+ phenobarbital, effect on the EEG in the newborn). 2769. Benzodiazepines (simple animal behavioral model for anxiolytic effect). 2770. Diazepam (man, effect on spinal mono-synaptic reflex). 2771. Diazepam (+ xylazin, + ketamine, horses, short duration anesthesia). 2784. Oxazepam (treatment in crisis-intervention). 2790. Diazepam, flurazepam (effects on conditioned fear). 2791. Benzodiazepines (mice, effects on anxiety). 2792. Benzodiazepines (maintenance treatment). 2793. Triazolam (as hypnotic). 2795. Nitrazepam, estazolam (comparison of changes in the modification of the vigilance). 2796. Diazepam (effect on EEG in cirrhotic patients). 2798. Benzodiazepines (feeding in puppies and cats, structure-activity relationship). 2799. Clorazepate (and glaucomas). 2810. Flunitrazepam (hemodynamic effects in the coronary patient). 2811. + 2812. Flunitrazepam (influence on body functions). 2814. Flunitrazepam, diazepam (i.v., in conservative dentistry). 2815. Diazepam (in post-myocardial infarct period). 2819. Lormetazepam (i.v., hypnotic effect). 2824. Clobazam (versus placebo, for anxiety and tension). 2825. Clobazam (versus diazepam, anxiety neurosis). 2826. Triazolam (clinical trial as hypnotic). 2827. Diazepam i.v., temazepam oral (comparison, sedation for upper gastrointestinal endoscopy). 2830. Flunitrazepam (pharmacology). 2835. Diazepam (rat striatum and hypothalamus, rapid changes in enkephalin levels). 2838. Diazepam, lorazepam (comparison of action). 2839. Midazolam maleate (preliminary results). 2840. Midazolam maleate (studies). 2841. Midazolam maleate (amnesic action). 2842. Flunitrazepam (as i.v. induction agent). 2843. Diazepam (+ morphine, + chlorpromazine, discrimination of electric shock). 2854. Diazepam (effects on succinylcholine-induced myalgia, potassium increase, creatine phosphokinase elevation and relaxation). 2856. Diazepam (i.v., anesthesia and liver function). 2862. Diazepam (hemodynamic study in neurosurgical intensive-care). 2863. Cloxazolam, lorazepam (comparison as tranquilizer). 2864. Ketazolam (versus placebo and clorazepate, comparison, anxiety-treatment). 2865. Clorazepate, diazepam (comparison, anxious outpatients), 2866. Alprazolam (versus placebo, + imipramine, comparison, primary depression). 2867. Ketazolam, diazepam (long-term efficacy and safety studies). 2868. + 2869. + 2870. Diazepam, prazepam, clorazepate (+ placebo, comparison, anxious outpatients). 2872. Benzodiazepines (as hypnotics). 2875. Ketazolam, diazepam (+ placebo, comparison, treatment of anxiety). 2876. Diazepam (rats, and postwithdrawal drinking of ethanol). 2880. Benzodiazepines (social-interaction as method for detecting anxiolytic activity). 2882. Benzodiazepines (test of anxiety). 2888. Diazepam (+ d-amphetamine. effect on punished behavior, rats). 2890. Midazolam (i.v., induction agent). 2900. Benzodiazepines (+ ethanol, comparison of the central effects). 2904. Diazepam (+ baclofen, rats, effect on the anemic cerebrate rigitidy). 2905. Benzodiazepines (rats, effect on gamma-motor system). 2911. Triazolam, alprazolam, diazepam (pharmacology of some metabolites). 2917. Benzodiazepines (impact on clinical practice). 2918. Midazolam (as alternative to thiopentone). 2932. Benzodiazepines (and limbic system, anxiety and vigilance). 2933. Diazepam (+ methohexital, + fentanyl, comparison of recovery tests).

2935. Benzodiazepines (electrophysiological actions). 2937. Diazepam (memory-effects of single and 3-weeks administration). 2949. Diazepam, oxazepam (subjective effects and vigilance). 2950. Chlordiazepoxide (+ placebo, + prochlórperazine, psychoneurotic outpatients, treatment anxiety). 2952. Diazepam (+ dixyrazine, + placebo, premedication in gastroscopy). 2955. Flunitrazepam (rectal, in pediatric premedication). 2956. Diazepam (high-pressure and pH-influences on ketamine anesthesia, rat). 2957. Diazepam (treatment of children with drug-induced extrapyrimidal symptoms). 2959. Diazepam (+ phenobarbital, treatment of isolated seizures). 2970. Alprazolam (treatment of moderate to severe anxiety). 2974. + 2975. Lorazepam (treatment of status epilepticus). 2978. Diazepam (+ dipidolor, + pipilphen, effects on vasomotor reflex and respiration). 2981. Midazolam (dosage with the aid of EEG). 2984. Diazepam (and experimental tumour growth).

2990. Benzodiazepines (tool to explore the biochemical and neurophysiological basis of anxiety). 2992. Diazepam (study of tetanus neonatorum and treatment). 2993. Diazepam (high-doses in schizophrenia). 2994. Benzodiazepines (+ GABA, anticonvulsant action). 2998. Clonazepam (therapy in reading epilepsy). 3001. Pirenzepin (mechanism of action, gastric secretion inhibition). 3002. + 3003. Diazepam (+ mianserin, comparison, depressed outpatients). 3005. Clobazam (pharmacological and therapeutic profile). 3006. Benzodiazepines (CNS-activity). 3007. Diazepam (as induction agent, caesarean section). 3011. Diazepam (hypnotic and residual effects).

3012. Diazepam (effect on human learning). 3013. Lorazepam (multivariate symptoms analysis). 3014. Triazolam, flunitrazepam (preoperative stage, comparison of effects).

3015. Diazepam (versus N-desmethyldiazepam, anxiety treatment and sedation). 3016. Benzodiazepines (+ narcotics, comparison of cognitive impairment). 3018. Diazepam (effect on EEG-changes following intraseptal administration of atropine). 3019. Clonazepam (effect on atropine spikes in the limbic system). 3020. Diazepam (+ droperidol, as i.v. premedicants). 3023. 6-Aryl-4H-S-triazolo(4,3-A)(1,4)benzodiazepines (influence of 1-substitution on pharmacological activity). 3024. Midazolam (effect on the general, coronary and cerebral circulation). 3026. Clobazam (repeated doses, effects on aspects of performance, arousal and behavior). 3033. Flunitrazepam (study in 41 cases of severe insomnia). 3034. Diazepam (effect on the climacteric syndrome of natural estrogens). 3036. Nitrazepam (+ clonidine, sedative and cardiovascular effects). 3037. Nitrazepam (+ clonidine, sedative and hemodynamic effects, single dose comparison). 3038. Diazepam (+ pentobarbital, clinical effects comparison, preoperative medication). 3043. Diazepam and others (acute effects on higher nervous activity in man). 3046. Lorazepam (comparative use in cardiac bypass surgery). 3051. Flunitrazepam (as hypno-inducer in psychiatry). 3053. + 3054. Clonazepam (anti-myoclonic action). 3057. + 3058. Diazepam (diurnal variation of polyphagic effect). 3062. Diazepam (suppression of jaw opening reflex in rats). 3063. Diazepam (action on the discharge pattern of phrenic motoneurones, rats). 3064. Benzodiazepines (present status in psychopharmacology). 3065. Benzodiazepines (animal models of anxiety). 3066. Benzodiazepines (present status). 3069. Diazepam (rat, changes of the protein-metabolism). 3070. Chlordiazepoxide (+ amitriptyline, comparison of doses). 3073. Clorazepate (for premedication). 3074. Chlordiazepoxide (effect on punished and unpunished behavior). 3077. Clobazam (long-term study). 3078. Diazepam (cardioselective beta-blockade, comparison). 3079. Diazepam (drug preference and mood). 3087. Diazepam, midazolam (dog, cardiovascular responses). 3091. Flunitrazepam (+ thiopentone, + etomidate, rat, effect on cerebral energy metabolism). 3096. CS-430 (pharmacological studies). 3099. Nitrazepam (long-term treatment in insomnia). 3102. Oxazepam (relationship between plasma level and effect). 3104. Flunitrazepam (versus placebo, premedication for minor surgery). 3109. Flunitrazepam (+ piritramide, + nitrous oxide, termination of anesthesia in open-heart surgery). 3119. Benzodiazepines (correlation between anticonvulsive activity and antianxiety action). 3120. Diazepam (children, rectal, anti-pyretic effect to acetaminophen). 3122. Diazepam (effect on self-rated depression, anxiety and well-being). 3126. Diazepam (+ droperidol, oestrus rat uterus). 3230. Ketazolam, diazepam (versus placebo, comparison, anxiolytic efficacy and safety). 3131. Diazepam (anesthesia and myocardial-contractility). 3134. Diazepam (+ desipramine, comparison, mixed-anxiety-depression symptomatology). 3135. Ketazolam, diazepam (versus placebo, comparison, treatment of anxiety). 3136. Diazepam (+ ketamine, anesthesia for laparoscopy). 3145. Triazolam (hypnotic effect). 3146. Diazepam (rectal, infants and children, anticonvulsant effects). 3149. Clobazam (review of clinical studies). 3151. Lorazepam (and scopolamine-morphine, supplement conduction anesthesia). 3152. Diazepam (+ etomidate, + fentanyl, induction agents for general anesthesia). 3155. Chlordiazepoxide (+ pentobarbital, differentiation). 3156. Chlordiazepoxide (+ pentobarbital, + alcohol, discriminative effects). 3163. Diazepam (+ ketamine, + pancuronium, lack of cardiovascular stimulation during endotracheal intubation in cardiac surgical patients). 3164. Diazepam (i.v., epilepsy, diagnostic and prognostic significance of EEG). 3167. KA-2547 (treatment of anxiety neurosis, outpatients). 3168. Benzodiazepines (present-status in psychiatry and medicine). 3169. Clorazepate (man, physiological and psychological effects). 3180. Lorazepam (+ morphine, i.v., surgical premedication). 3184. Clobazam (treatment of gastrointestinal disorders). 3185. Benzodiazepines (maintenance treatment). 3186. Benzodiazepines (rat, blockade of the selective high increase in dopamine turnover induced by stress in mesocorticaldopaminergic-neurons). 3187. Diazepam (reduction of the behavior suppressing effects of meperidine and normeperidine). 3189. Flunitrazepam (in orthopedic-surgery and traumatology). 3191. Benzodiazepines and other drugs (effects on somatosensory evoked cortical potentials). 3191. Flunitrazepam (parenterally, for anesthesiology). 3195. Chlordiazepoxide, desmethyldiazepam, oxazepam, temazepam (alone or in combination with alcohol, effects on learning and memory). 3196. Diazepam, flunitrazepam (+ triclofos, children, as premedicants in otolaryngological surgery). 3197. Diazepam, flunitrazepam (+ pethidine, i.m., children, premedicants in otolaryngological surgery). 3204. Diazepam (+ phenobarbital, treatment of isolated seizures). 3205. Lorazepam (value in gas-encephalography). 3206. Clonazepam (in reading epilepsy). 3207. Diazepam (i.v., determinants of the dose required for gastroscopy). 3208. Flunitrazepam (+ placebo, in psychiatric setting). 3209. Diazepam, desmethyldiazepam (in spasticity and rigidity). 3210. Diazepam (+ d-amphetamine, effect on food competition).

3222. Diazepam (+ clomopramine, + chlorpromazine, effects on the cerebral energy-state and glycolytic metabolism, rat). 3226. Lorazepam (i.v., prevention of nausea and vomiting associated with cancer-chemotherapy). 3229. Benzodiazepines (oral premedication in minor gynecological surgery). 3230.

Alprazolam, diazepam (+ placebo, anxiolytic efficacy). 3231. Benzodiazepines + other drugs (comparison of anxiolytic activity). 3234. Flunitrazepam (+ thiopentone, induction of general-anesthesia, comparison). 3235. Flunitrazepam, lorazepam (clinical effects). 3245. Flunitrazepam (+ ketamine, dog). 3247. Bromazepam (+ alpha-methyldopa, in arterial hypertension). 3252. Benzodiazepines (potentiation of muscimol-induced hyperactivity). 3253. Clonazepam (treatment of restless legs). 3254. Flunitrazepam (review of pharmacological properties). 3263. Diazepam (+ nitrous oxide, hemodynamic effects, coronary artery disease). 3265. Benzodiazepines (short-time use). 3266. Flunitrazepam (rat, effect on reproduction). 3267. Flunitrazepam (oral, i.m., comparison of subjective effects and plasma-concentrations). 3268. Benzodiazepines (oral, effects on memory). 3269. Diazepam (+ cholecystokinin, + amphetamine, feeding, rats). 3270. + 3271. Alprazolam, chlordiazepoxide (anxiolytic effect in chronic withdrawal from alcohol). 3276. 1,5-Benzodiazepines (baboon, anticonvulsant activity). 3278. Benzodiazepines (use). 3280. Chlordiazepoxide (+ alcohol, mice, suppressed aggression). 3281. Flunitrazepam (survey, poison control center). 3289. Diazepam (therapy in post-natal pediatric tetanus). 3300. Diazepam (rectal, oral, i.v., single, man, comparison, biopharmaceutic activity). 3301. Diazepam (rat, stress-protective effects). 3302. Chlordiazepoxide (rats, effects on fear). 3304. Flunitrazepam (clinical study, pulmonary respiration, cardiovascular circulation). 3305. Lorazepam (effect on human gastric-secretion). 3310. Triazolam, flurazepam (comparison, hypnotic activity). 3311. Flurazepam (changes in EEG). 3322. 1,5-Benzodiazepines (psychotropic activity). 3323. Diazepam (versus methyl dopa, treatment of EPH-gestosis). 3330. 1,4- and 1,5-Benzodiazepines (healthy man, effect on performance). 3331. Diazepam, oxazepam, temazepam (performance studies). 3333. Flunitrazepam, triazolam (man, activity). 3339. Diazepam (antistress effects). 3343. Desmethyldiazepam (from clorazepate, effects of age and Billroth gastrectomy on absorption). 3349. Clobazam (treatment of anxiety in female patients with functional sexual disorders, double-blind trial against placebo). 3350. Flunitrazepam (as induction agent). 3351. Diazepam (restoration of sress and immune-response suppression of immune-responses by restraint). 3359. Benzodiazepines (effects of high and low environmental temperature on tranquilizer activity). 3362. Nitrazepam, tofisopam (+ placebo, comparison as premedicants). 3365. + 3366. Diazepam (compatibility with i.v. fluid containers and administration sets). 3367. Clonazepam (+ clomipramine, in cataplexy). 3368. Diazepam, flunitrazepam (+ droperidol, influence on smooth muscles of small arteries). 3372. Chlordiazepoxide (+ isoproterenol, effect on drinking and conflict behavior, rat). 3373. Diazepam (effect on threshold of ventilatory response to CO_2). 3382. Diazepam (and human memory). 3389. Diazepam (potentiation of purinergic depression of central neurons). 3390. Benzodiazepines (inhibition of adenosine uptake into rat brain synaptosomes). 3394. Diazepam (effects on EEG). 3397. Bromazepam (treatment of somatized psychogenic disorders). 3402. Bromazepam (clinical use on a long period). 3405. Benzodiazepines (systematic review). 3406. Diazepam (treatment of children with drug-induced extrapyramidal symptoms). 3408. Diazepam (+ chlorpromazine, + imipramine, +pyrazole, influence on ethanol-induced changes in activity of some enzymes in isolated rat-liver). 3409. Diazepam (+ phenytoin, + phenobarbital, brain uptake). 3418. Diazepam (prevention of laryngeal spasm). 3422. Midazolam maleate (hemodynamic observations). 3423. Midazolam maleate (+ thiopentone, comparison as hypnotics). 3430. Diazepam, flunitrazepam (human, competitive effects). 3431. Diazepam, flunitrazepam (older children, oral premedication). 3432. Diazepam, ketazolam (anxiety). 3438. Diazepam (+ morphine, + neuroleptic agents, unit activity of limbic system neurons). 3440. Flunitrazepam (+ ketamine, continuous i.v. drip in cardiovascular-surgery). 3441. + 3442. Lorazepam (i.v., cerebral circulatory and metabolic responses). 3448. Benzodiazepines (tardive dyskinesia). 3452. Clonazepam (+ valproate, treatment of refractory epileptic seizures in 12 children). 3458. Clonazepam (long term study, children with intractable seizures). 3462. Diazepam (+ thiopental, induction of general anesthesia, comparison of cardiorespiratory effects). 3463. Lorazepam (premedicant in dental surgery). 3468. Diazepam (effect on the lower esophageal sphincter). 3469. Benzodiazepines (in chronic schizophrenia). 3473. Benzodiazepines (depressive action, comparison). 3475. Chlordiazepoxide (+ amitriptyline, + mianserin, changes in clinical symptomatology and psychometric assessments in depressed patients, comparison). 3477. Clobazam (effects on mood and psychomotor performance, anxious patients). 3479. Flunitrazepam (study in psychiatric treatment). 3481. Lorazepam (treatment of anxiety associated with cardiovascular disorders). 3482. Diazepam (hemodynamics during induction of anesthesia for coronary-artery bypass grafting). 3484. Chlordiazepoxide (+ scopolamine in combination, mice, effects on shuttle-box avoidance performance of mice). 3485. Chlordiazepoxide (+ amitriptyline, + imipramine, and their combinations, effects on avoidance behavior in mice). 3486. Chlordiazepoxide (facilitating effects on locomotor activity and avoidance behavior of reserpinized mice). 3487. Chlordiazepoxide (effect when given during avoidance training in two inbred strains of mice). 3488. Chlordiazepoxide (repeated administration in mice, effects on spontaneous locomotor activity). 3489. Benzodiazepines (influence on scopolamine-induced locomotor stimulation in mice). 3490. Chlordiazepoxide (enhancement of the anticholinergic-induced locomotor stimulation in mice). 3491. Chlordiazepoxide (alone and in combination with amphetamine, facilitation of avoidance-behavior, effect on performance). 3493. Midazolam (+ sodium thiopental, bioassay). 3495. Lorazepam (oral and parenteral, clinical experiences). 3496. Diazepam, lorazepam (+ placebo, i.m., comparison, psychiatric effects). 3501. Diazepam (rat, effect on development of hypertension). 3502. Diazepam, clobazam (outpatients, neurotic disturbances). 3505. Benzodiazepines (in status epilepticus and nodding spasms). 3513. Diazepam (+ atropine, + meperidine, pre-endoscopic medication). 3517. Diazepam (+ warfarin, fatty-acid modulation). 3518. Diazepam (+ warfarin, changes in fatty-acid modulate reciprocal variations). 3527. Diazepam (+ pentobarbital, mode of action on hypothalamo-pituitary function, adult male rats). 3529. Clonazepam (+ valproate sodium, comparison, in chronic epilepsy). 3533. Flurazepam (evaluation in surgical patients). 3536. Clotiazepam (therapeutic experiences). 3539. Diazepam (in gastrointestinal endoscopy). 3541. Clobazam (+ nomifensin, treatment of anxious depression). 3545. Diazepam, lorazepam (+ placebo, i.m., treatment of acute anxiety). 3548. Diazepam (treatment of tardive-dyskinesia). 3563. Lorazepam, clonazepam (i.v., treatment of status epilepticus, comparison). 3564. Diazepam (+ doperidol, respiratory function following premedication). 3575. Diazepam (effects on locomotor activity and avoidance behavior, rats). 3581. Chlordiazepoxide (effects on conditioned and unconditioned behavior in mice with septal lesions). 3582. Diazepam (+ promethazine, effect on breathlessness induced by exercise or raised CO_2 in healthy subjects). 3583. Benzodiazepines (behavioral neurochemistry). 3584. Diazepam (+ thiopentone, + ketamine, + propanidid, + alphaxalone, man, relative potencies). 3585. Clonazepam (in migraine prophylaxis). 3602. Diazepam (+ caffeine, mood effects). 3605. Diazepam, clobazam (+ phenobarbital, + valproate, anticonvulsant profiles). 3608. Diazepam (effects on unit-activity of amygdaloid neurons). 3609. Diazepam (pharmacological consideration of substitute-F). 3616. Diazepam, camazepam (man, reaction-time). 3618. Benzodiazepines (long-term treatment). 3619. Flunitrazepam (pretreatment for prevention of adverse cardiovascular effects following ketamine). 3624. Diazepam (lack of effect on the ST segment of the electrocardiogram during exercise stress testing in normal subjects). 3625. Clobazam (in pre- and postoperative anxiety states). 3630. Diazepam (+ phenobarbital, prophylactic treatment of febrile convulsions). 3631. Flunitrazepam (use in dentistry). 3632.

Diazepam (+ ketamine, infusion anesthesia). 3634. Diazepam (effects on the somatosensory evoked responses following tooth pulp stimulation, rat). 3637. Flunitrazepam (+ benzoctamine, as sedative drugs in patients with preoperative decreased lung-function during spinal-anesthesia). 3638. Flunitrazepam (influence on the blood-gases during subarachnoid block in geriatric patients). 3640. Clonazepam (treatment of dialysis encephalopathy). 3641. Oxazepam (hemisuccinate, stereospecific influence on cyclic AMP accumulation elicited by adenosine in cerebral cortical slices). 3643. Clobazam (effectiveness in cerebellar and postural tremor). 3647. Benzodiazepines (effects on punished responding). 3650. Diazepam (action on biliary secretion, rat). 3660. Benzodiazepines (treatment of epilepsy, review). 3661. Chlordiazepoxide (loss of anxiolytic action with long-term treatment). 3663. Chlordiazepoxide (stimulatory effects on locomotor activity in mice). 3666. Chlordiazepoxide (attenuation of the effects of punishment by ethanol). 3668. Diazepam, clonazepam (comparison). 3669. Bromazepam (+ clorotepin, study in child instability). 3671. Lorazepam (in status epilepticus). 3674. Clobazam, clorazepate (single daily dose treatment of anxiety). 3675. Clobazam (as premedicant). 3678. Chlordiazepoxide (direct effect on mammalian cardiac tissues and crayfish and squid giant axons). 3681. Clonazepam (+ valproate sodium, absence status and concurrent administration). 3682. Diazepam (effect on hypothalamically elicited drinking and eating). 3684. Diazepam (i.v., effect on human lower oesophageal sphincter pressure). 3685. Diazepam (effect on prolactin secretion in acute schizophrenic-patients). 3686. Diazepam (individual and group effects on driver's ability, confidence and willingness to act in a gap-judging task). 3689. Midazolam (dog, cardiovascular effects). 3690. Diazepam (outpatient utilization in a military hospital). 3692. Benzodiazepines (+ zopiclone, comparison). 3693. Benzodiazepines (mode of action, clinical view). 3694. Clobazam (clinical view). 3695. Benzodiazepines (mode of action, clinical view). 3704. Diazepam (+ local-anesthetic spray, versus general-anesthesia in gastroduodenoscopy). 3716. Diazepam (+ propanolol, elevated plasma-free drug concentrations during cardiac-catheterization). 3719. Diazepam (effects on striatal met-enkephalin levels following long-term pharmacological manipulations). 3720. Benzodiazepines (influences on the hippocampal rhythmical slow activity during wakefulness and paradoxical sleep in chronically prepared cats). 3724. Diazepam (+ morphine, analgesic action). 3729. + 3730. Diazepam (+ catecholamines, mediation of the anticonvulsant activity). 3731. Diazepam (in morphine-diazepam-oxygen anesthesia, cardiovascular effects of dimethyl tubocurarine in patients with aortic valvular disease).

3733. Benzodiazepines (clinical pharmacology and therapeutics). 3734. Diazepam (+ careulein, + cholecystokinin octapeptide, anticonvulsant effects, comparison). 3735. Chlordiazepoxide (+ propanolol, effects on cardiac-arhythmias during alcohol withdrawal). 3736. Benzodiazepines (+ barbiturates, comparison of the porphyrin-inducing activity in chick-embryo liver-cells). 3737. Diazepam (psychological performance of anxious patients). 3738. Diazepam (+ amylobarbitone, comparison of clinical and psychological effects in anxious patients). 3739. Diazepam (counteraction of circulatory side-effects of ketamine by pretreatment with diazepam).

Poisoning (Treatment, Reports)
Vergiftungen (Behandlung, Kasuistik)

6. Nitrazepam (poisoning). 20. Oxazepam (poisoning). 26. Psycholeptic Drugs (acute poisoning, 28 cases). 29. Chlordiazepoxide (+ phenelzine, + amytal, overdosage). 64. Diazepam (poisoning, use of naloxone). 75. Diazepam (cardiac arrest). 132. Diazepam (+ barbiturates, suicidal attempt). 167. Diazepam (tödliche Vergiftung bei Drogenabhängigem). 168. Nitrazepam (alpha and beta coma in drug intoxication). 183. Chlordiazepoxide (persistant EEG-changes) 255. Diazepam (use of physostigmine as antidote). 294. Chlordiazepoxide (Klinik der Vergiftungen). 302. Diazepam (+ barbiturate, patient initially considered dead). 318. Chlordiazepoxide (+ amitriptyline, death). 358. Oxazepam (overdosage). 371. Sedatives (poisonings). 374. Diazepam (+ Alkohol, Häufigkeit in Blutproben). 385. Chlordiazepoxide + amitriptyline (death). 392. Chlordiazepoxide (poisoning). 404. Diazepam (intra arterial, hazards). 414. Benzodiazepines (acute overdosages). 491. Chlordiazepoxide (+ other drugs, overdoses). 524. Lorazepam (poisoning). 525. Benzodiazepines (related deaths). 534. Diazepam (34 cases of poisoning). 596. Nitroderivatives of benzodiazepines, Clonazepam, Nitrazepam, Nimetazepam (acute poisoning). 603. Lorazepam (abuse). 627. Benzodiazepines (acute intoxications). 631. Diazepam (and other drugs, overdose cases). 633. Diazepam (acute poisoning). 646. Chlordiazepoxide (and other drugs, use of extracorporeal hemisorption). 648. Nitrazepam (fatal poisoning). 721. Chlordiazepoxide (acute poisoning, children). 735. Allgemeine Behandlung. 737. Chlordiazepoxide (poisoning). 796. Drugs (abnormal distribution in fatal poisonings). 820. Nitrazepam (poisoning cases). 873. Chlordiazepoxide (+ alcohol, fatal overdose). 899. Diazepam (death following withdrawal). 958. Diazepam (poisoning). 1024. Oxazepam (poisoning, two-year-old child). 1042. Diazepam (poisoning, child). 1048. Diazepam (+ alcohol, death). 1118. Chlordiazepoxide (accidental poisonings in children, clinical aspects, emergency measures). 1121. Diazepam (two-year-old child, high dose poisoning and survival). 1125. Nitrazepam (overdosage). 1138. Nitrazepam (+ alcohol, suicide). 1181. Diazepam (acute intoxication, use of physostigmine). 1198. Clonazepam (overdose, cyclic coma). 1208. Diazepam, Chlordiazepoxide (tabulation of therapeutic, toxic and lethal concentrations of drugs and chemicals in blood). 1219. Oxazepam (grave poisoning). 1223. Oxazepam (non-keto-acidotic diabetic coma).

1341. Nitrazepam (intoxication). 1343. Benzodiazepines (+ meprobamate, intoxications). 1344. Diazepam (+ pyridoxine as antidots to isoniazid intoxications in rats and dogs). 1350. Chlordiazepoxide (two unsuccesful suicidal attempts). 1366. Chlordiazepoxide (toxicity, hemodialysis). 1465. Oxazepam (overdosage). 1480. Chlordiazepoxide (massive overdose). 1483. Chlordiazepoxide (poisoning). 1485. Benzodiazepines (abuse in alcoholics). 1527. Diazepam (rapid recovery from massive overdose). 1565. Diazepam (overdose). 1601. Chlordiazepoxide (large overdose). 1654. Diazepam (100 cases of acute intoxications, analysis). 1689. Diazepam (acute and chronic overdose). 1765. Diazepam (acute intoxications, experimental model for treatment). 1766. Diazepam (intoxication, physostigmine as antidote). 1808. Chlordiazepoxide (overdosage). 1828. Benzodiazepines and other drugs (changing patterns of drugs used for selfpoisoning). 1844. Nitrazepam (overdosage, bullous lesions). 1906. Chlordiazepoxide (poisoning, case report). 1915. Chlordiazepoxide (oral, suicidal attempt). 1923. Diazepam (intoxication, child). 1968. Diazepam (intoxication at birth, exchange transfusion). 1970. Chlordiazepoxide (large overdose). 2038. Oxazepam (pseudohyperosmolar non-ketoacitotic coma due to intoxication).

2497. Flurazepam (monointoxication). 2509. Nitrazepam (2 cases of lethal poisoning). 2518. Diazepam (detoxification). 2523. Benzodiazepines (+ barbiturates, intoxication cases, comparison). 2619. Diazepam (atropine in physostigmine reversal). 2620. Diazepam (naloxone reversal of diazepam effects). 2634. Diazepam (antagonism by physostigmine). 2635. Diazepam (postanesthic somnolence, reversal by physostigmine). 2639. Chlordiazepoxide (respiratory depression). 2667. Benzodiazepines (acute overdosage). 2692. Diazepam (frequency of use in methadone maintenance program). 2700. Benzodiazepines (emergencies in Toronto). 2719. Benzodiazepines (+ meprobamate, poisoning). 2726. Diazepam (naloxone does not antagonize diazepam induced sedation). 2774. Diazepam (atropine in physostigmine reversal of diazepam). 2806. Chlordiazepoxide (in acute alcoholism). 2837. Estazolam (intoxication). 2884. Diazepam and others (deaths, survey in USA and Canada). 2921. Diazepam (physostigmine reversal). 2922. Diazepam (atropine in physostigmine reversal). 2923. Diazepam (physostigmine-atropine solution fails to reverse diazepam sedation). 2936. Diazepam (physostigmine antagonism). 2944. Nitrosochlordiazepoxide (mice, lack of carcinogenic effect). 2953. Diazepam (treatment of alcohol withdrawal). 2954. Diazepam (large doses, treatment of delirium tremens). 3035. Lorazepam (oral, i.m., in acute alcohol withdrawal and incipient delirium tremens). 3049. Benzodiazepines (naloxone as antidote in poisoning). 3068. Benzodiazepines (hazards of poisoning). 3219. Diazepam (treatment of neonatal methadone abstinence). 3232. Benzodiazepines (+ alcohol, treatment of intoxications with naloxone). 3279. Clobazam (clinical study in alcohol detoxification). 3281. Flunitrazepam (survey in a poison control center). 3282. Flunitrazepam (acute overdosage). 3284. Diazepam (detoxification, single case). 3307. Diazepam (naloxone as antidote in acute intoxication). 3427. Prazepam (acute poisoning). 3467. Diazepam (physostigmine reversal). 3570. Lorazepam (i.v., use in alcohol withdrawal). 3677. Diazepam (poisoning in rodents, physostigmine and naloxone as antagonists). 3688. Chlordiazepoxide (in acute alcoholism). 3715. Benzodiazepines (massive requirements during acute alcohol withdrawal). 3778. Benzodiazepines and other drugs (treatment of poisoning).

Polarography / Polarographie

51. Diazepam, Nitrazepam, metabolites (polarographic behavior, differentiation of mixtures). 182. Chlordiazepoxide, Diazepam (in toxicological analysis). 193. 1,4-benzodiazepines (polarographic study on the acid-base-equilibria in aqueous solutions). 267. Nitrazepam, Diazepam (in man). 305. Oxazepam (determination). 314. Diazepam (in Leichenblut, ohne Extraktion). 395. Oxazepam, Lorazepam (quality control). 458. Nitrazepam (serum). 520. Diazepam (in pharmaceuticals). 596. Nitro-benzodiazepines, Clonazepam, Nitrazepam, Nimetazepam (acute poisoning). 597. Nimetazepam (in serum and whole blood). 653. Clonazepam, Flunitrazepam (pharmaceuticals). 654. Diazepam, Chlordiazepoxide (automated analysis, in tablets). 658. Chlordiazepoxide (other analytical data). 659. Diazepam (other analytical data). 802. Chlordiazepoxid (polarographisches Verhalten). 803. Flurazepam (in Arzneiformen). 805. Chlordiazepoxid (in Arzneiformen). 806. Medazepam (in Arzneiformen, Gleichspannungspolarographie). 807. Temazepam. 809. Prazepam (Gehaltsbestimmung). 810. Dikalium-chlorazepat (Gehaltsbestimmung). 811. Lorazepam (Bestimmung). 812. Chlordiazepoxid (Mechanismus der Reduktion). 813. Diazepam (Gehaltsbestimmung). 814. Nitrazepam (Auswertung von DC). 815. Nitrazepam (Auswertung von DC). 816. Nitrazepam. 817. Oxazepam (Reduktion an Hg-Tropfelektrode). 875. Chlorazepate (other analytical data). 922. Flurazepam (other analytical data). 1021. Benzodiazepines. 1034. Oxazepam (other analytical data). 1177. Clonazepam (in tablets, DC-polarography).

1321. 1,5-Benzodiazepines (study). 1324. 1,4-Benzodiazepines (+ spectrofluorometry). 1859. Chlordiazepoxide (effect of amitriptyline on polarography). 1918. 1,4-Benzodiazepines (polarographic identification). 2003. Cyclohexene-substituted Benzodiazepines.

2321. Benzodiazepine (Ringverengung während Polarographie). 2520. Bromazepam (study of the acid-base and complexing behavior).

Polarography (differential pulse polarography)
Polarographie (Differential-Puls-Polarographie)

1. Chlorazepate. 147. Chlordiazepoxide, Nor-Chlordiazepoxide, Demoxepam, Flurazepam, N-1-desalkyl-flurazepam, N-1-Hydroxyethyl-flurazepam, Diazepam, N-desmethyldiazepam, Temazepam, Oxazepam. 148. 1,4-Benzodiazepines. 149. 1,4-Benzodiazepines. 150. Drugs including benzodiazepines. 151. 1,4-Benzodiazepines (blood-level determination). 194. Flurazepam (in plasma). 229. 1,4-Benzodiazepines. 232. Lorazepam (urinary excretion). 233. Bromazepam and metabolites (urine). 241. Flurazepam and major metabolites (urine). 445. Chlordiazepoxide and metabolites (plasma). 521. Diazepam (serum). 870. Water soluble imidazobenzodiazepines(in urine).

2203. Chlorazepate (in plasma). 3004. Nitrazepam (HPLC-detection by DPP-detector).

Cathode-Ray-Polarography / Kathodenstrahl-Polarographie

81. Diazepam (in human plasma). 804. Medazepam and main metabolites. 1020. Bromazepam (im Blut).

Protein-Binding / Proteinbindung

145. General (independent binding of ligands to human serum albumin). 195. Chlorazepate (+ l-tryptophan, competitive binding action). 417. Diazepam (sex differences in protein binding in patients with renal insufficiency). 443. Diazepam (human serum albumin). 544. Diazepam, N-desmethyldiazepam (protein binding in patients with poor renal functions). 580. Diazepam (in man and different species). 583. Diazepam (man, dog, rabbit, guinea pig, rat). 584. Diazepam (food intake and plasma binding). 604. Diazepam (effect of food intake). 650. 1,4- Benzodiazepines (role of substituents on the hydrophobic binding by human plasma proteins). 749. Benzodiazepines (interaction with human serum albumin). 750. Benzodiazepines (interaction with human serum albumin). 751. Benzodiazepines (characterization of the binding to human serum albumin). 752. Benzodiazepines (human and bovine serum). 753. Benzodiazepines (influence of pH on the benzodiazepine- serum-albumin-complex, human). 754. Oxazepam (bovine serum albumin). 755. Benzodiazepines (competition with l-tryptophan). 756. Benzodiazepines (competitors for the binding of l-tryptophan to human serum albumin). 757. Oxazepam (human serum albumin). 758. Benzodiazepines (gel-filtration studies). 759. Benzodiazepines (circular dichroism studies). 1055. Diazepam (circular dichroism studies). 1057. Benzodiazepines (circular dichroism studies). 1058. General (affinity chromatography and circular dichroism measurements). 1128. Chlordiazepoxide (Bindung und Verteilung, Erythrozyten, Plasma). 1143. Diazepam (influence of a fatty acid on binding to human serum albumin). 1150. Diazepam (effect on hepatic microsomal enzymes). 1153. Chlordiazepoxide, Diazepam, Oxazepam (protein binding and lipophilic nature). 1347. Diazepam (reduced binding following chronic benzodiazepine treatment). 1354. Diazepam (after single dose of sodium oleate). 1439. Benzodiazepines (tryptophan modified human serum albumin). 1442. Clonazepam (+ valproate). 1641. Prazepam, Desalkylprazepam, Diazepam (human serum albumin). 1650. Diazepam (+ salicylic acid, + warfarin, effect of liver cirrhosis on the albumin binding-sites). 1653. Drugs (binding to serum albumin). 1667. General (Plasmaprotein-Bindung). 1700. ^{3}H-Diazepam (effects of cations and anions on binding to rat brain). 1701. ^{3}H-Diazepam (binding to rat-brain homogenates). 1717. ^{3}H-Diazepam (competitive inhibitor in bovine brain). 1817. Diazepam (plasma protein binding). 1912. ^{3}H-Diazepam (endogenous inhibitors of binding in CNS). 1913. Benzodiazepines

(reduction in receptors associated with purkinje-cell degeneration in nervous mutant mice). 1925. ^{3}H-Flunitrazepam (binding in human brain). 1954. Benzodiazepines (binding site activity, GABAergic modulation). 2139. Benzodiazepines (effect of heparin on plasma-binding). 2189. Benzodiazepines and others (protein-binding). 2294. Diazepam (pyrinergic inhibition of binding to rat-brain in vitro). 2308. Benzodiazepine (Bedeutung der Plasmaproteinbindung). 2371. ^{14}C-lorazepam (human plasma proteins). 2553. Lorazepam and conjugates. 2555. Diazepam (inter- and intrasubject variations). 2572. Diazepam (+ desmethyldiazepam, comparative protein-binding). 2607. Diazepam, metabolites (effects on binding of l-tryptophan). 2738. Benzodiazepines (human serum albumin, microcalorimetric study). 2742. Benzodiazepines (porcine brain, competitive inhibition). 2787. Diazepam (+ lidocaine, age-related changes). 2805. Chlordiazepoxide (+ heparin, effect on plasma binding). 2873. + 2874. Benzodiazepines (+ others, human serum albumin binding sites). 2913. Benzodiazepines (functional importance of binding in brain). 2914. Diazepam (alteration of binding in developing rat cerebral cortex). 2941. Diazepam (+ ethanol, interaction of effects of binding to bovine serum albumin). 2980. Diazepam (+ lidocaine, in renal disease). 3083. Benzodiazepines (plasma binding in humans). 3148. Diazepam (+ digitoxin in uremic and normal serum). 3228. Oxazepam-esters (correlation of hydrophobicity with serum binding, brain penetration and excretion). 3244. Diazepam (+ phenytoin, binding to plasma albumin and lipoproteins by gel-filtration and ultracentrifugation). 3246. Benzodiazepines (binding-proteins studies by affinity chromatography). 3317. Diazepam (unaltered plasma binding using indwelling heparinized cannulae for sampling). 3318. Diazepam (diurnal variations in plasma concentrations associated with reciprocal changes in free fraction). 3319. Diazepam (fatty-acid modulation of meal-induced variations in diazepam free fraction). 3357. Benzodiazepines (binding to bovine retina). 3383. Diazepam (plasma binding in patients with alcoholic cirrhosis). 3450. Diazepam (decreased binding as a specific response to chronic benzodiazepine treatment). 3460. Diazepam (determinants of plasma-protein binding). 3494. Flurazepam (NMR study of interaction with human serum albumin). 3543. Oxazepam-acetate (stereoselective binding to human-serum albumin). 3622. Chlordiazepoxide, diazepam, nitrazepam (+ phenprocoumon, binding to human and bovine serum albumin). 3714. Diazepam (intravascular factors affecting diazepam binding to human serum albumin). 3740. Diazepam, desmethyldiazepam (comparative protein binding).

Radioactive-Labelled Compounds
Radioaktiv markierte Substanzen

59. ^{14}C-Triflubazam (mice and dogs, blood level, excretion, distribution, metabolism). 124. Diazepam (Herkunftsbestimmung mittels ^{13}C und ^{3}H). 130. Pinazepam (^{3}H, rat, pharmacodynamics), 136. ^{3}H-Diazepam (specific receptors in rat brain, binding). 172. ^{14}C-Chlordiazepoxide (mice, brain distribution). 432. ^{14}C-Lorazepam (clinical pharmacokinetics, absorption and disposition). 483. ^{14}C-Nitrazepam (young and old rats, tissue distribution). 509. ^{14}C-Diazepam (monkey brain, fate). 572. ^{14}C-Chlordiazepoxide (dog, excretion). 600. ^{14}C-Chlordiazepoxide (man, dog, rat, metabolic fate). 694. N-Desmethyldiazepam (deuterated, metabolism). 714. ^{14}C-Diazepam (rabbits, distribution). 717. ^{14}C-Prazepam (synthesis). 732. ^{3}H-Diazepam (rat, binding to benzodiazepine receptors). 855. ^{14}C-Chlordiazepoxide (mice, distribution and metabolism). 994. ^{14}C-Medazepam (dog, rat, man, metabolism). 1010. ^{3}H-Diazepam (synthesis). 1289. ^{3}H-Diazepam, ^{3}H-Flunitrazepam (rat brain, specific binding). 1304. ^{3}H-Diazepam (binding receptor). 1338. ^{3}H-Flunitrazepam(receptors). 1373. ^{3}H-Flunitrazepam (rat brain, receptors). 1558. ^{3}H-Diazepam (receptor). 1632. ^{3}H-Diazepam (rat brain membranes). 1700. ^{3}H-Diazepam (rat brain, effect on anions). 1701. ^{3}H-Diazepam (rat-brain homogenates, binding). 1717. ^{3}H-Diazepam (bovine brain). 1759. ^{3}H-Diazepam (rat brain, receptor binding). 1912. ^{3}H-Diazepam (binding in CNS). 1925. ^{3}H-Flunitrazepam (binding in human brain).

2064. ^{3}H-Diazepam (enhancement of binding). 2142. ^{3}H-Diazepam (increased spezific binding in rat-brain following chronic administration). 2234. 7-Chloro-2,3-dihydro-1-methyl-5-phenyl-1H-1,4-benzodiazepine-5-^{14}C-hydrochloride (synthesis). 2353. ^{3}H-Diazepam (decreased binding as a specific response to chronic benzodiazepine treatment). 2371. ^{14}C-Lorazepam (binding, human plasma proteins). 2398. ^{3}H-Flunitrazepam (temperature dependence of binding). 2433. ^{3}H-Flunitrazepam (effects of GABA on binding in rat brain). 2443. ^{3}H-Diazepam (rat-brain).

2652. ^{14}C-Phenazepam (intrahepatic circulation). 2664. ^{3}H-Flunitrazepam (specific nuclear binding). 2680. ^{35}Cl-Diazepam (nuclear quadrupole resonance-spectra). 2695. ^{3}H-Diazepam (binding to benzodiazepine-GABA receptor). 2723. ^{3}H-Diazepam (binding in rat cortex). 2789. ^{3}H-Diazepam (inhibition of binding by an endogenous fraction from rat brain synaptosomes). 2833. ^{3}H-Flunitrazepam (binding to differentiating rat cerebral cells in culture). 2846. ^{14}C-Triazolam (disposition in man). 2945. ^{14}C-Lormetazepam (absorption, distribution and excretion in dogs, rabbits, rats and rhesus monkeys). 3048. ^{14}C-Lormetazepam (kinetics in humans). 3162. ^{3}H-Flunitrazepam (autoradiographic evidence for binding to melanin granules in cat eye). 3250. ^{3}H-Diazepam (modulation of binding in different brain-areas). 3258. ^{14}C-Lormetazepam (biotransformation in dogs, rats and rhesus monkeys). 3259. ^{14}C-Diazepam, ^{14}C-Flunitrazepam (high specific activity of C-11 labeling). 3260. C-11-labeled benzodiazepines (labeling procedure and invivo pharmacodynamics). 3340. ^{3}H-Diazepam (displacement by a peptide from brain receptors). 3414. ^{3}H-Flunitrazepam (characteristics of binding to bovine retinae). 3416. ^{3}H-Flunitrazepam (binding to bovine retinae). 3417. ^{3}H-Flunitrazepam (effect of GABA on binding in mouse-brains). 3428. ^{3}H-Diazepam (inhibition of binding to benzodiazepine receptors). 3450. ^{3}H-Diazepam (decreased binding as response to chronic benzodiazepine treatment). 3549. ^{3}H-Diazepam (enhancement of binding). 3552. ^{3}H-Diazepam (potentiation of GABA-enhanced binding to benzodiazepine receptors). 3553. ^{3}H-Diazepam (levels following i.v. administration). 3565. ^{3}H-Flunitrazepam (enhanced cortical binding). 3600. ^{3}H-Flunitrazepam (effect of temperature and chloride-ions on the stimulation of binding). 3617. ^{3}H-Diazepam (properties of binding to rat peritoneal mast cells). 3698. ^{3}H-Diazepam (enhancement of binding to rat brain membranes in vitro).

Radioimmunoassay and other Immunoassays /
Radioimmunoassays und andere Immunoassays

190. Diazepam (Radioimmunoassay = RIA). 229. 1,4-Benzodiazepines (RIA). 247. General (RIA). 260. Clonazepam (in plasma, ^{125}J-RIA). 261. Chlordiazepoxide (in plasma, RIA). 262. Clonazepam (RIA). 373. Diazepam (blood and serum (RIA). 845. Diazepam (blood, RIA). 1070. General (RIA). 1071. General (RIA). 1073. Clonazepam (+ diphenylhydantoin, + phenobarbital, blood, serum, plasma, RIA). 1291. Diazepam (plasma, RIA). 1396. Diazepam (micro samples, blood, plasma, saliva, RIA). 1540. Benzodiazepines (EMIT). 1911. Benzodiazepines (plasma, radioreceptor assay).

2110. Benzodiazepines and others (review, RIA). 2145. Chlordiazepoxide (RIA). 2147. Clonazepam (RIA). 2179. Diazepam (blood, serum, RIA). 2191. Flurazepam (plasma, RIA). 2268. Benzodiazepines and others (RIA). 2464. Clobazam (serum, radioreceptor assay). 2476. 1,4-Benzodiazepines (via oxazepamhemisuccinat, screening, RIA). 2481. Benzodiazepines (radioreceptor assay). 2488. Diazepam, + metabolites (radioreceptor assay). 2489. Diazepam, chlordiazepoxide, oxazepam (radioreceptor assay). 2527. Benzodiazepines (+ barbiturates, serum, homogeneous enzyme-immunoassay). 2691. Diazepam (EMIT and TLC). 2816. Desmethyldiazepam (specific RIA). 2817. Chlordiazepoxide (RIA). 2818. Nitrazepam (plasma, RIA). 2844. 1,4-Benzodiazepines (haptens useful in immunoassay development). 2903. Benzodiazepines (radioreceptor assay). 2947. Flunitrazepam (plasma, RIA). 2948. Flurazepam (plasma, RIA). 3048. ^{14}C-Lormetazepam (plasma, urine, RIA). 3147. Triazolam (RIA). 3211. Chlordiazepoxide (RIA). 3439. Benzodiazepines (RIA with broad specifity). 3470. Diazepam (RIA in forensic samples). 3471. Clonazepam (RIA). 3672. Diazepam, desmethyldiazepam (serum, urine, enzyme-immunoassay). 3745. Flunitrazepam (RIA).

Screening / Suchanalyse

43. urinary screening. 122. rapid screening. 146. rapid TLC-screening. 325. Diazepam, Flurazepam, Oxazepam, Chlordiazepoxide, Desmethyl-Diazepam (rapid GLC-screening in blood and tissues). 337. Alcaloids, narcotics.

364. Antiepileptic drugs (GLC-screening). 479. Nitrazepam, Chlordiazepoxide, Diazepam, Oxazepam (scheme for identification). 537. Diazepam, Oxazepam (screening). 538. Chlordiazepoxide, Diazepam (TLC-screening). 602. Benzodiazepines (+ methaqualone). 728. Diazepam, N-desmethyldiazepam, Flurazepam, N-desalkylflurazepam, N-1-hydroxyetthyl-flurazepam, Chlordiazepoxide, N-desmethyl-chlordiazepoxide, Oxazepam, Demoxepam, Lorazepam, Nitrazepam, Flunitrazepam, others (oxidative screening procedure).

760. Narcotics, barbiturates, amphetamines, tranquillizers, psychotomimetics (urine). 761. Diazepam, Chlordiazepoxide (+ phenothiazines, human urine). 762. Diazepam, Chlordiazepoxide (+ phenothiazines, XAD-2, urine). 896. Diazepam (rapid screening). 938. Diazepam (rapid screening, serum).

975. Diazepam, Chlordiazepoxide, Nitrazepam, Oxazepam, Medazepam, Prazepam, Chlorazepate, Clonazepam (urine, sreening, other substances). 981. Clobazam (urine).

1146. Diazepam, Chlordiazepoxide (GC / MS - screening).

1149. Benzodiazepines (fluorometric screening, blood, urine).

1618. Diazepam, Chlordiazepoxide (and major drugs of abuse).

2476. 1,4-Benzodiazepines (via oxazepamhemisuccinate, RIA-screening). 2477. 1,4-Benzodiazepines (broad screening). 2524. 1,4-Benzodiazepines. 2526. 1,4-Benzodiazepines. 2691. Diazepam (mass-screening and confirmation).

3382. Diazepam, chlordiazepoxide, flurazepam (screening by GLC/ECD and HPLC). 3509. Lormetazepam (via benzophenone-derivative). 3510. Triazolam (HPLC). 3665. Benzodiazepines (HPLC-screening). 3754. 1,4- and 1,5-benzodiazepines

3757. Benzodiazepines via benzophenones (TLC). 3759. Lormetazepam (urine). 3761. Benzodiazepines via benzophenones (TLC). 3774. Benzodiazepines and many other drugs (GLC-screening via retention indices).

Side-, adverse-, residual- and withdrawal-effects
Nebenwirkungen, Entzugserscheinungen,

27. Chlordiazepoxide (withdrawal, neonate). 47. Clonazepam (psychiatric side effects). 48. Diazepam (+ picrotoxin, effect on visual system). 50. Diazepam (ventricular arrhythmia). 63. Diazepam (dangers of treatment of status epilepticus). 72. Chlordiazepoxide (side effect). 127. Flurazepam (residual effects). 141. Diazepam (i.v., respiratory arrest). 169. Chlordiazepoxide, Oxazepam (+ Chlorpromazine and d-Amphetamine, effect on sexual responses, hamsters). 188. Diazepam (amnesic effect). 210. Flurazepam (adverse reaction). 214. Diazepam, Chlordiazepoxid (Sucht und Mißbrauch). 216. Benzodiazepines (severe reactions). 217. Diazepam (increased resistance to satiation, pigs). 221. Diazepam (complication to administration). 226. Diazepam (i.v., apnea). 248. Diazepam (and alcohol withdrawal). 258. Diazepam (i.v., apnea). 265. Diazepam (unexpected apnea). 274. Diazepam (psychosis). 286. Clonazepam (side effects). 308. Diazepam (+ glutethimide, hypothermia, cardiac arrest). 317. Diazepamm chlordiazepoxide (Geschmacksstörungen ?). 321. Diazepam (+pentazocine, amnesia) 382. Diazepam (and others, allergy). 389. Diazepam (floppy infant syndrome, maternal intake). 404. Diazepam (intra-arterial, hazards). 408. Diazepam, Lorazepam (i.v., thrombophlebitis). 409. Diazepam (i.v., thrombophlebitis). 433. Diazepam (amnesic action). 450. Benzodiazepines (leukopenia). 457. Diazepam (i.v., apnea). 461. Oxazepam (dependence). 462. Clonazepam (psychological symptoms). 464. Diazepam (floppy infant syndrome). 467. Oxazepam (dependence). 472. Diazepam, lorazepam, flunitrazepam (i.v., sequelea). 473. Benzodiazepines (i.v., sequelae). 477. Diazepam (and N-desmethyldiazepam, cumulation in cerebrospinal fluid after long term treatment in man). 492. Benzodiazepines (withdrawal). 493. Chlordiazepoxide (withdrawal reaction). 500. Diazepam (respiratory depression). 512. Nitrazepam (hypothermia). 515. Diazepam (hypothermia). 527. Diazepam, chlordiazepoxide (clinical depression of the central nervous system, age, smoking). 529. Flurazepam (hemodialysis). 532. Diazepam, chlordiazepoxide (effects on the metabolism of other drugs). 533. Diazepam (cerebellar involvement). 536. Psychopharmaka (Störwirkungen). 589. Diazepam (glaucoma, myasthenia gravis). 593. Diazepam (Einfluß auf Schock). 606. Flunitrazepam (amnesic action). 608. Chlordiazepoxide (intrahèpatic cholestasis). 612. Benzodiazepines (misuse, alcoholics). 623. Diazepam (thrombophlebitis). 624. Diazepam (thrombophlebitis after i.v.). 633. Chlordiazepoxide (withdrawal). 634. Diazepam (new particular syndrome by large doses). 635. Diazepam (thrombophlebitis after i.v.). 644. Diazepam (unusual reaction, i.v.). 656. Diazepam (allergic conjunctivitis). 696. Chlordiazepoxide (lipomobilizing effect). 697. Flurazepam (long term use in geriatrics). 700. Oxazepam (early pregnancy). 713. Psychotropic drugs (unusual abdominal complications, elderly patients). 726. Nitrazepam (dependence). 763. Chlordiazepoxide (covert effect). 777. Diazepam + lithium carbonate (hypothermia). 782. Diazepam (ventricular arrhythmias). 799. Tranquilizers (child abuse). 829. Diazepam (thrombosis). 830. Diazepam (allergy). 831. Lorazepam (histopathology of veins after i.v.). 838. Diazepam (dangers). 841. Benzodiazepines (abuse). 861. Benzodiazepines (withdrawal psychosis). 866. Diazepam (child, i.v.). 896. Diazepam (abuse). 903. Chlordiazepoxide (pulmonary edema). 904. Chlordiazepoxide (clyde mood scale changes in anxious patients). 912. Diazepam (withdrawal reaction). 913. Diazepam (withdrawal reaction). 924. Benzodiazepine (aktuelle Formen der Drogenabhängigkeit, neben Haschisch und LSD). 933. Chlordiazepoxide, + barbiturate and alcohol (chronic heart desease, fatty liver).

990. Chlordiazepoxide (adverse effects). 1035. Diazepam (cardiac arrest). 1036. Diazepam (cardiac arrest). 1044. Diazepam (reactions to i.v.). 1045. Diazepam (irritant properties). 1054. Clonazepam, 7-amino-metabolite (man, side effects). 1059. Chlordiazepoxide (dependence). 1067. Oxazepam (safety). 1069. Benzodiazepines (amnesic effects, rats). 1072. Diazepam, Nitrazepam (floppy infant syndrome). 1075. Chlordiazepoxide (respiratory insuffiency, delirium tremens). 1077. Diazepam + barbiturate (intrahepatic cholostasis, tetanus). 1078. Bromazepam (Einfluß auf basale Magensäureproduktion). 1112. Chlordiazepoxide (critique of overemphasis on side effects). 1122. Chlordiazepoxide,

N-desmethyl-diazepam (residual effects). 1126. Diazepam. chlordiazepoxide, nitrazepam (rat, effect on catecholamine metabolism). 1127. Diazepam (pulmonary complications). 1161. Diazepam (i.v., rare complications). 1163. Clonazepam (thrombocytopenia). 1178. Chlordiazepoxide (hallucinations). 1180. Flurazepam, fosazepam, flunitrazepam (psychogeriatric patients). 1186. Diazepam (withdrawal fits). 1202. Diazepam (i.v., chromosomal aberation, negative study). 1206. Chlordiazepoxide (effect on cholinesterase activity, blood). 1209. Chlordiazepoxide (+ thioridazine, subicterus following). 1210. Chlordiazepoxide (hiccups following oral ingestion). 1229. Diazepam (adverse behavioral effect). 1230. Diazepam (ventricular arrhythmias). 1231. Diazepam (+ meperidine, arterial blood gases, healthy volunteers). 1246. Diazepam (i.v., effect on arterial oxygen-saturation). 1247. Diazepam (amnesia and other effects after anesthesia). 1248. Chlorazepate (chronobiologic changes). 1253. Diazepam (delayed recovery). 1258. Nitrazepam (overdosage, cerebellar syndrome). 1262. Diazepam (effect on turnover of cerebral dopamine). 1276. Benzodiazepines (effects on transport of sugars and ions in rat skeletal-muscle in vitro). 1281. Benzodiazepines (especially oxazepam, abuse potential). 1282. Lorazepam (after injection, effect on recall). 1284. Chlordiazepoxide (attenuation of tetrabenazine "reversal"). 1287. Clonazepam (+ carbamazepine, metabolic drug interactions). 1288. Nitrazepam, Flurazepam x HCl (+ pentobarbitone-sodium, comparison of the residual effects on human performance). 1290. Diazepam, Chlordiazepoxide, (clinical depression of CNS in relation to cigarette smoking and age). 1301. Diazepam (effect on development of stretch reflex tension). 1303. Benzodiazepines (interactions with oral anticoagulants). 1305. Diazepam (dog, increase of cardiac toxicity of quabain after treatment with diazepam). 1309. Diazepam, Lorazepam (i.v., amnesic effects). 1311. Diazepam (induction agent, clinical studies). 1312. Chlordiazepoxide (withdrawal, neuroendocrine correlates). 1316. Flunitrazepam (effect on circulation, coronary blood pressure and margin of safety). 1331. Nitrazepam (increased sensitivity, old age). 1332. Diazepam (effect on the ventilatory response to carbon-dioxide and on steady-state gas exchange). 1348. Diazepam-metabolites (man, immediate and residual effects). 1353. Diazepam (+ meperidine, respiratory response to carbon dioxide). 1362. Diazepam (effect on experimental artherosclerosis). 1372. Diazepam (hemodynamic and respiratory effects). 1395. Diazepam (inhibition of elevated cyclic GMP-levels in hippocampus following tetanic stimulation of medial septal region). 1400. Flunitrazepam (histamine liberation). 1401. Flunitrazepam, Lormetazepam (influence on blood gas). 1409. Diazepam, Flunitrazepam, Lorazepam (man, amnesic action). 1411. Lorazepam (amnesic properties). 1413. Diazepam (+ hyoscine, + pethidine, adults, amnesic effects). 1417. General (risks at work). 1427. Lorazepam (man, CNS and cardiovascular effects). 1436. Diazepam (+ nitrous oxide, acute vasodilation following induction of anesthesia, i.v.). 1437. Flurazepam (cholestatic jaundice). 1451. + 1452. Benzodiazepines (abuse). 1471. Lorazepam (+ pentobarbital, + pentazocine, respiratory effects). 1477. Benzodiazepines (rat brain, effects on carbohydrate metabolism). 1493. Diazepam (addiction). 1499. Diazepam, Lorazepam (i.v., pain and clinical thrombophlebitis). 1508. Diazepam (i.v., adverse reactions). 1515. Benzodiazepines (dependence, tolerance and addiction). 1530. Diazepam (+ methohexitone, + sodium-4-hydroxy-butyrate, critical flicker frequency after small doses). 1547. Benzodiazepines (abuse). 1548. Nitrazepam, Flunitrazepam (+ placebo, long term study). 1554. Flunitrazepam, Lorazepam (amnesia). 1557. Diazepam (changes in hemodynamics). 1560. Diazepam (induktive Wirkung). 1561. Benzodiazepines (induktive Wirkung). 1566. Temazepam (+ alcohol, psychomotor performance). 1567. 1,5-Benzodiazepines (effects on sleep and psychomotor performance). 1576. Diazepam (Mißbrauch). 1589. Diazepam (Nebenwirkungen in der Geburtshilfe und Frauenheilkunde). 1673. Diazepam (increase of acetylcholine levels, mouse and rat brain). 1686. Diazepam (+ chlorpromazine, man, effect on memory-functions). 1688. Benzodiazepines (effect on uptake and efflux of serotonin in human blood-platelets in vitro). 1713. Diazepam (addiction). 1720. Benzodiazepines (+ barbiturates, residual effects). 1721. Benzodiazepines (interactions with other drugs). 1734. Benzodiazepines (oral, amnesic effects). 1783. Diazepam (+ pentazocine, + xylocain, effect on serum CPK-, GOT- and LDH-levels). 1795. Benzodiazepines (use, overuse, misuse and abuse). 1803. Diazepam (effect on threshold of ventilatory response to CO_2). 1811. Diazepam (Mißbrauch und Sucht). 1818. Sedatives (and drinking). 1833. Diazepam (cardiopulmonary effects). 1834. Bromazepam (effect on locomotor performance and brain mono-amine metabolism.). 1835. Benzodiazepines (synaptosomal uptake of norepinephrine and 5-hydroxytryptamine and synthesis of catecholamines during treatment). 1844. Nitrazepam (overdosage, bullous lesions). 1847. Chlordiazepoxide (reversal of an amphetamine-established aversion- dipsogenic effects). 1852. Diazepam,(irritant properties, answer). 1856. Diazepam (influence on carcadian-rhythm of glycine in rodent brain). 1860. Nitrazepam (depression of central respiratory drive). 1891. Diazepam (decline in plasma levels during fixed-dose therapy of alcohol withdrawal). 1891. Diazepam (induction effect on its own metabolism). 1894. Diazepam, Medazepam, Lorazepam (residual effects after single oral administration). 1897. Psychotropic drugs (interactions). 1910. Flunitrazepam (volumetric and gasometric values during induction of general anesthesia). 1956. N-Desmethyldiazepam (+ amylobarbitone-sodium, residual effects). 1997. Diazepam (+ succinylcholine, muscle pain). 2031. Diazepam (side-effects of maternal diazepam on newborn-infant). 2032. Diazepam (chronic administration, modification of ovine fetal respiratory-like activity). 2038. Oxazepam (intoxication, pseudohyperosmolar non-ketoacitotic coma). 2040. Diazepam (coronary vasodilation). 2041. Diazepam (pharmacological basis of coronary and systemic vasodilator actions). 2042. Diazepam (effect on left ventricular contractibility on coronary blood flow). 2043. Diazepam (effect on left ventricular function and systemic vascular resistance). 2055. Chlordiazepoxide (+ chlorpromazine, comparison of withdrawal symptomes). 2066. Diazepam (+ solubilizer, action on respiration). 2068. Diazepam (effect on unstimulated and stimulated gastric secretion). 2078. Diazepam (cardiovascular effects). 2079. Diazepam (effect on human gastric secretion). 2088. Hypnotics (residual effects). 2089. Flurazepam (residual effects). 2090. Flunitrazepam (residual effects). 2092. Chlorazepate (residual effects). 2112. Diazepam (cat, cardiovascular action). 2119. Tranquilizer (cytogenetic effects in vivo and in vitro). 2127. Anxiolytic Sedatives (length of treatment and response to sudden withdrawal). 2128. Diazepam (+ amitriptyline, acute hepatic necrosis). 2129. Diazepam (i.v., hemodynamic and respiratory effects). 2130. Diazepam (acute cardiovascular effects in patients with mitral valve disease). 2133. Diazepam (withdrawal syndrome). 2137. Diazepam (and lidocaine-induced cardiovascular changes). 2151. Prazepam (floppy-infant syndrome ?). 2161. Tranquilizer (addiction to). 2168. Diazepam, Chlordiazepoxide (hemodynamic and electrocardiographic effects following acute administration). 2181. Diazepam, flunitrazepam, lorazepam (relative amnesic action). 2185. Diazepam (effect on processes in memory). 2186. Diazepam (+ scopolamine, + physostigmine, effect on memory). 2187. Diazepam (+ fentanyl, effect on psychomotor and EEG-functions, rate of recovery). 2188. Diazepam (man, memory effects). 2214. Flunitrazepam (anterograde amnesia, reduction of blood-pressure, 3000 operations).

2238. Benzodiazepines (low dose treatment associated with oral-buccal dyskinesia symptoms). 2262. Diazepam (i.m., increased creatine-kinase concentrations). 2301. Flurazepam, triazolam (alone and together with alcohol, residual EEG-effects the morning after). 2306. Diazepam (effect on uteroplacental hemodynamics and metabolism). 2344. Diazepam (cardiorespiratory effects during endoscopy). 2403. Diazepam, chlordiazepoxide (absence of effects on the chromosomes of diploid human fibroblast cells). 2404. Diazepam (human lymphocytes treated with diazepam in vitro, chromosome studies). 2406. Diazepam (i.v., dogs, hemodynamic alterations). 2407. Diazepam, chlordiazepoxide (+ chlorpromazine, + chlorprothixene, effect on bile flow and intrabiliary pressure, cholecystectomized dog). 2417. N-Desmethyldiazepam (man, residual effects). 2420. Flunitrazepam (amnesic effects during regional anesthesia). 2430. Diazepam (Sucht und Mißbrauch). 2434. Diazepam (phlebitis). 2446. Psychotropic drugs (use and abuse). 2448. Diazepam (long term effects in roosters). 2449. Diazepam (misuse and abuse).

2554. Diazepam (effectiveness on ethanol and barbiturate withdrawal). 2561. Diazepam (addiction in Kenya). 2601. Benzodiazepines (dependance and withdrawal). 2603. Diazepam (withdrawal, neonate, presumptive intrauterine exposure). 2620. Diazepam (naloxone reversal of diazepam effects). 2623. Benzodiazepines (+ alcohol, withdrawal syndromes). 2625. Diazepam (reversal by physostigmine). 2635. Diazepam (postanesthetic somnolence, reversal by physostigmine). 2643. Benzodiazepines (physical dependance, 6 cases). 2678. Diazepam (i.v., apnea with maintenance of consciousness). 2711. Benzodiazepines (long-term use and abuse). 2721. Benzodiazepines (hangover-effects). 2722. Benzodiazepines + others (hangover). 2726. Diazepam (naloxone does not antagonize sedation). 2732. Diazepam (i.v., patterns of memory loss). 2733. Diazepam (amnesia). 2736. Diazepam (diluting injection). 2762. Clorazepate (failure to cause malformations or fetal wastage, rat). 2774. Diazepam (atropine in physostigmine reversal of diazepam). 2776. Diazepam (+ ethanol, humans, addition or potentiation). 2778. Benzodiazepines (+ alcohol, withdrawal effect). 2782. Benzodiazepines (in vitro effect on cholinesterase activity of human-fetal brain). 2783. Diazepam, desmethyldiazepam, nitrazepam (in vitro effects on atpase activity of human-fetal brain). 2797. Lorazepam (withdrawal seizures). 2811.+ 2812. Flunitrazepam (influence on body function). 2813. Diazepam (hemodilution against thrombophlebitis). 2821. Diazepam (man, enhancement of ketamine plasma-levels by diazepam). 2822. Diazepam (i.v., local complication). 2823. Diazepam (i.v., systemic complication). 2828. Benzodiazepines + others (i.v., thrombophlebitis). 2841. Midazolam (amnesic action). 2848. Benzodiazepines (advantages and disadvantages in prescription). 2850. Lorazepam (withdrawal seizures). 2851. Flurazepam (hostility reaction). 2852. Triazolam (hallucination). 2860. Benzodiazepines (withdrawal). 2871. Diazepam (preventation of some adverse-effects of succinylcholine). 2878. Diazepam (role in skin hyper-pigmentation). 2881. Lorazepam (impaired performance and sedation). 2885.+2886. Chlordiazepoxide (influence on gustatory contrast). 2887. Diazepam (+ alphaprodine, i.v., respiratory depression). 2891. Diazepam, midazolam (respiratory depression). 2892. Chlordiazepoxide (disruption of discrimination). 2898. Diazepam (effect of diazepam anesthesia on the radiosensitivity of the skin of the mouse foot). 2908. Benzodiazepines (caution in the elderly). 2909. Flurazepam (safety). 2983. Diazepam (alteration of cortical evoked-potentials). 3011. Temazepam (hypnotic and residual effects). 3039. Lorazepam (withdrawal seizures). 3050. Diazepam (complement-mediated reactions). 3052. Benzodiazepines (alterations in plasma-lipid and lipoprotein levels associated with benzodiazepines). 3056. Benzodiazepines (withdrawal reaction). 3067. Diazepam (absence of effects on tumors). 3068. Benzodiazepines (hazards of poisoning). 3075. Clonazepam (altered serotonergic activity in mouse brain). 3076. Benzodiazepines (withdrawal reactions). 3087. Diazepam, midazolam (dog, cardiovascular responses). 3088. Nitrazepam (+ hyoscine, effect on retention, human memory). 3089.+3090. Diazepam (effect of naloxone on respiratory changes). 3094. Benzodiazepines (rebound insomnia following withdrawal). 3097. Benzodiazepines (cholinesterase interactions). 3106. Benzodiazepines (withdrawal symptoms). 3108. Clorazepate (rage reaction). 3110. Diazepam (inhibition of prostaglandin synthesis in macrophages). 3111. Diazepam (effects on tumor growth and plasma prostaglandin, rats). 3123. Diazepam (prenatal exposure alters behavioral development in rats). 3124. Benzodiazepines (addiction potential). 3127. Benzodiazepines (withdrawal syndromes). 3146. Diazepam (infants, rectal, children, side-effects). 3150. Diazepam, flunitrazepam (+ thiopentone, + etomidate, i.v., venous complications). 3151. Lorazepam (+ scopolamine-morphine, amnesic effects). 3170. Benzodiazepines (rebound insomnia). 3171.+3172. Triazolam (trials and tribulations). 3181.+3182. Triazolam (Halcion-Story). 3188. Benzodiazepines (strong withdrawal syndrome, 6 cases). 3198. Diazepam (pharmacodynamics and pharmacokinetics in an abuser). 3200. Oxazepam, lorazepam, temazepam (side effects in psychogeriatric inpatients). 3217. Triazolam (behavioral reaction). 3219. Diazepam (treatment of neonatal methadone abstinence). 3221. Diazepam (thrombophlebitis after i.v. administration). 3223. Benzodiazepines (gynecomastia during abuse). 3241. Benzodiazepines (use and abuse). 3255. Diazepam (prevention of induced thrombophlebitis with chromophor). 3268. Benzodiazepines (oral, effect on memory). 3274. Benzodiazepines + others (insomnia). 3283. Diazepam, flunitrazepam (+ isotonic saline, i.v., local reactions). 3286. Diazepam (withdrawal). 3287. Diazepam (thrombophlebitis and prevention). 3290. Diazepam (+ ethanol, rhesus monkey, development of physical dependance). 3296. Diazepam (abuse and gynaecomastia). 3309. Diazepam (i.v., clinical study on local reactions). 3344. Triazolam (trials and tribulations). 3346. Nitrazepam, flurazepam, triazolam (residual effects). 3356. Benzodiazepines (adverse reactions). 3361. Benzodiazepines (cause small loss of body-weight). 3361. Clorazepate (jaundice induction). 3365. Diazepam (compatibility with i.v. fluid containers and administration sets). 3366. Diazepam (incompatibility in plastic intravenous bags). 3369. Clorazepate (delayed maze-learning after prenatal exposure, rats). 3370. Clorazepate (congenital malformations). 3371. Benzodiazepines (mice, blockade of passive-avoidance tasks). 3386. Benzodiazepines (use and abuse). 3398. Triazolam (anterograde amnesia, 3 cases). 3413. Diazepam (accidental intraarterial injection). 3448. Benzodiazepines (tardive dyskinesia). 3449. Flurazepam (central excitatory actions). 3466. Benzodiazepines (adverse reactions). 3508. Diazepam (i.v., local reactions). 3528. Diazepam (teratogenic effect, hamster). 3540. Benzodiazepines (anterograde amnesia). 3587. Lorazepam (withdrawal, case report). 3588. Diazepam (respiratory depression). 3601. Lorazepam (withdrawal). 3604. Nitrazepam (residual effects). 3627. Diazepam (i.v., prevention of pain and phlebitis). 3635. Diazepam (i.v. administration, provocation of tonic seizures). 3642. Triazolam (psychological disturbances). 3648. Lorazepam (withdrawal). 3654. Triazolam (innocent hypnotic ?). 3655. Triazolam (reactions). 3664. Diazepam (effects on human chromosomes). 3667. Phenazepam (role of GABA-ergic and dopaminergic mechanisms in the withdrawal syndrome). 3670. Diazepam (inhibition of myosin synthesis). 3696. Clonazepam (incontinence). 3708. Diazepam (withdrawal reaction from long-term low-dosage administration). 3709. + 3710.+3711. Benzodiazepines (effect on psychomotor performance). 3750. Benzodiazepines (paradoxical reactions).

Sleep-Effects / Schlafwirkungen

9. Fosazepam. 111. Flunitrazepam. 184. Diazepam, Fosazepam. 186. Clobazam, Triflubazam. 345. Diazepam. 487. Nitrazepam, Flurazepam, Flunitrazepam (repeated doses). 784. Diazepam, temazepam (man). 785. Diazepam, temazepam (sleep during the day). 786. Clobazam, Triflubazam (man). 914. Fosazepam, Nitrazepam (+ placebo, normal subjects).

1255. Lorazepam (versus glutethimide, sleep-induction, geriatric patients). 1299. Benzodiazepines (effect on growth-hormone and prolaction, secretion during nocturnal sleep). 1310. Lorazepam (+ pentobarbital, night-time sedation). 1334. Benzodiazepines (halothane-induced sleeping time, mouse). 1375. Nitrazepam (+ amylobarbitone, sleep-inducing effect). 1384. Flurazepam (sleep laboratory and clinical studies). 1434. Triazolam, Diazepam (+ placebo, treatment of insomnia). 1440. Flurazepam (effects on sleepEEG, visual computer and cycle analysis). 1567. 1,5-Benzodiazepines (effect on sleep and psychomotor performance morning following night-time sedation). 1610. Flunitrazepam (Vigilanzverlauf und Schlafqualitäten). 1620. Flurazepam (sleep laboratory studies). 1621. Triazolam (sleep laboratory evaluation). 1622. Flurazepam, Diazepam, Chlordiazepoxide, Flunitrazepam (sleep laboratory studies). 1680. Oxazepam (normal human volunteers, effect on sleep). 1752. Flunitrazepam (sleep cycle in normal subjects). 1753. Flunitrazepam (sleep cycle in insomniae patients). 1777. Diazepam and metabolites (effectiveness for sleep during day). 1778. Oxazepam (hypnotic activity). 1787. Nitrazepam, Flurazepam (comparison, effect on sleep). 1792. Benzodiazepines (effect on human sleep). 1904. Benzodiazepines (psychomotor-function, memory and subjective feelings after sleep induced by benzodiazepines).

2176. Nitrazepam, flunitrazepam, bromazepam (effect on sleep of normal subjects). 2216. Temazepam (effect on some psychological parameters of sleep and behavior). 2217. Temazepam (sub-chronic study, morning following night-time medication). 2218. Flunitrazepam (+ dichloralphenazone, + amylobarbitone, repeated-dose comparison, early-morning behavior). 2232. Flurazepam (effect on sleep in laboratory). 2318. Diazepam, fosazepam (effect on sleep in man). 2320. Benzodiazepines (+ alcohol, rat, effect on sleeping-time).

2498. Benzodiazepines (and sleep). 2499. Sleep Research. 2537. Flunitrazepam (treatment of severe insomnia). 2541. Thienodiazepines and benzodiazepines (humans, effect on sleep). 2542. Benzodiazepines and others (survey, sleeping agents). 2564. Benzodiazepines (effectiveness of bedtime dosing, clorazepate and halazepam comparison). 2663. Nitrazepam (+ pentobarbital,cat). 2728. Flurazepam (repeated use, mood and performance of poor sleepers). 2743. Flunitrazepam (in insomnia). 2773. Flurazepam (influence on human circadian rhythm of spontaneous motility). 2820. Midazolam (dependance of depth of sleep on length of injection and dosage). 2831. Flunitrazepam (insomnia of the aged). 2859. Flurazepam (insomnia in the elderly, treatment). 2943. Flurazepam (insomnia treatment). 2946. Flunitrazepam (treatment of insomnia in recently disintoxicated alcoholics). 2972. Diazepam (cats, effects on sleep). 3027. Triazolam, nitrazepam (effects on sleep quality, morning vigilance and psychomotor performance). 3029. Clobazam, clorazepate (+ placebo, effect on subjective ratings of sleep and early morning behavior). 3033. Flunitrazepam (41 cases of severe insomnia treatment). 3080. Ketazolam (effect on ocular motility during REM-sleep). 3081. Flurazepam (auditory arousal threshold). 3082. Flurazepam (effect on brain electrical activity during sleep). 3094. Benzodiazepines (rebound insomnia). 3095. Quazepam (sleep laboratory evaluation). 3099. Nitrazepam (long-term treatment in insomnia). 3183. Flunitrazepam (treatment of insomnia). 3199. Flurazepam (+ amobarbital, + secobarbital, in insomniac patients). 3200. Oxazepam, lorazepam, temazepam (efficacy in psychogeriatric inpatients). 3220. Diazepam, flurazepam (treatment of insomnia in general practice). 3298. Diazepam (+ gamma-hydroxybutyrate, rat, effect on sleep parameters). 3299. Diazepam (+ GABA, sleep-wakefulness cycle). 3316. Flurazepam, clorazepate (+ l-dopa, + thyrotropin-releasing hormone, effect on REM-sleep). 3329. Temazepam (effects on sleep and performance). 3332. Diazepam, temazepam (sleep of middle age). 3334. Benzodiazepines (effect on daytime sleep). 3358. Clonazepam (treatment of insomnia). 3385. Triazolam (chronic use, effects on sleep patterns of insomniacs). 3393. Triazolam (+ chloral hydrate, efficacy in geriatric insomniacs). 3433. Flunitrazepam (slow cerebral potentials in patients with sleep disturbances). 3455. Flurazepam, lorazepam, triazolam (effects on sleep and memory). 3456. Benzodiazepines (differential effects on nocturnal sleep and daytime performance). 3457. Flurazepam, temazepam (+ quinalbarbitone, effect on sleep). 3476. Oxazolam (nocturnal traffic noise and sleep). 3498. Flunitrazepam (long-term sleep evaluation). 3507. Flunitrazepam (action on sleep disturbances). 3524. Nitrazepam (treatment of insomnia). 3534. Triazolam (+ placebo, multiclinic comparison, hypnotic efficacy, insomniac outpatients). 3544. Flunitrazepam (treatment of insomnia, clinical psychiatry). 3546. Triazolam, flurazepam (crossover comparison, hospitalized psychiatric-patients with insomnia). 3590. Diazepam, + hydroxylated metabolites (man, studies on sleep). 3594. Lorazepam, diazepam (as night sedation and premedication, comparison). 2639. Diazepam (effect on sleep). 3676. Triazolam (in insomnia). 3707. Flurazepam (+ viloxazine, man, effect on sleep-EEG).

Synthesis / Synthesen

19. 5-Phenyl-1,4-benzodiazepine-2-thiones (synthesis and transformations). 21. Diazepam (Nachweis und Bestimmung von Synthese-Zwischenprodukten). 60. Diazepam, Chlordiazepoxide, Nitrazepam, Oxazepam (detection of impurities). 65. 5-Aryl-1,3-dihydro-2H-1,4-benzodiazepine-2-one-4-oxides (rearrangement). 66. 5-Phenyl-1,4-benzodiazepines (additional rearrangement). 67. 3-Substituted 1,4-benzodiazepine-2-ones. 68. 1,3-Dihydro-2H-1,4-benzodiazepine-2-ones and their N-Oxides. 103. Nitrazepam-Metaboliten (Synthesen). 113. 1,4-Benzodiazepines (new ring closure). 282. 3-Hydroxy-benzodiazepines (synthesis and analytical data). 289. Benzodiazepines (Synthesen). 333. Chlordiazepoxide (impurities in formulations). 338. 2-Phenyl-5H-imidazo (2,1-α)(2,4) benzodiazepines (synthesis). 339. 1,3-Dihydro-5-pyridyl-2H-1,4-benzodiazepines (synthesis). 470. Peptido-aminobenzophenones. 480. 1,4-Benzodiazepines (new synthetic approach). 511. Aminoacetamidobenzophenones (enzymic desalkylation and cyclization to the corresponding benzodiazepine in vitro). 516. Benzodiazepin-2-ones (diborane reduction). 519. Chlordiazepoxide (reduction at mercury electrodes). 561. Nitrazepam (polymorphic acetylation). 562. Diazepam, Chlordiazepoxide, Medazepam, Nitrazepam, Oxazepam (Mikrosublimation). 574. 7-Chlor-2N-nitrosomethylamino-5-phenyl-3H-1,4-benzodiazepin-4-oxid (Entstehung). 575. Chlordiazepoxide (Nitrosierbarkeit). 707. Diazepam, Nitrazepam (Hydrolyse, Ringverengung zu Chinolonderivaten). 712. 7-Chloro-2-hydrazino-5-phenyl-3H-1,4-benzodiazepines (synthesis and structure). 719. 2,3-Dihydro-1H-1,4-benzodiazepine-4-oxides (synthesis and reactions). 730. Chlordiazepoxide, Diazepam-N-oxide (reactions with dimethyl-acetylenedicarboxylate, rearrangement of quinoxaline derivatives, X-ray analysis of a resultant tetracyclic compound). 764. Benzodiazepines (hydroxylation in vitro). 797. 3-Oxy-substituted-1,4-benzodiazepines (water soluble derivatives). 860. Substituted benzophenones (nitration). 946. Trifluoromethyl-substituierte 1,4-Benzodiazepine (Synthese).

980. Flunitrazepam, Metaboliten (Synthesen auf DC). 1010. ^{3}H-labelled Diazepam (synthesis). 1083. 2-Carbobenzoxyglycilamidobenzophenones (conversion to 1,4-benzodiazepin-ones). 1084. 1,4-Benzodiazepin-2-one-4-oxides (enlargement of quinazoline-3-oxides with alkali). 1085. 1,4-Benzodiazepines (chemistry, structure-activity relationship). 1086. Aminoalkyl-substituted 1,4-benzodiazepin-2-ones (Flurazepam-Synthesis). 1087. 7-Nitro- and 7-trifluoromethyl-2,3-dihydro-5-phenyl-1H-1,4-benzodiazepines (transformations). 1088. Nitro-substituted 5-phenyl-1,4-benzodiazepin-derivatives. 1089. Halo-, methyl-, and methoxy substituted 1,3-dihydro-5-phenyl-2H-1,4-benzodiazepin-2-ones. 1090. 3,1,4-Benzoxadiazepines. 1091. 7-Chloro-2-methylamino-5-phenyl-3H-1,4-benzodiazepin-4-oxide (photoisomerization). 1092. 1,4-Benzodiazepines (structure-activating-relationship). 1093. 1,4-Benzodiazepines. 1094. 6-Chloro-2-chloromethyl-4-phenylquinazoline-3-oxide (conversion to 2Amino-derivatives of 7Chloro-5-phenyl-3H-1,4-benzodiazepin-4-oxide). 1095. 7-Chloro-2-methylamino-5-phenyl-3H-1,4-benzodiazepin-4-oxide (transformations). 1096. 7Chloro-2,3-dihydro- (and 2,3,4,5-tetrahydro)-5-phenyl-1H-1,4-benzodiazepines (synthesis and transformations). 1097. Substituted 2-Amino-5-phenyl-3H-1,4-benzodiazepine-N-oxides (synthesis).

1108. 1-Diethylaminoethyl-substituted 1,4-benzodiazepin-2-ones (new synthesis). 1213. 1,4-Benzodiazepinderivate (neues Verfahren zur Herstellung aus 2-Aminomethyl-indolderivaten).

1249. Hydrosoluble benzodiazepines (chemistry). 1251. 1-Phenyl-1,2,3,4-tetrahydro-5H-1,4-benzodiazepin-5-one (synthesis and pharmacological activity). 1346. 3-substituted-1,2-benzodiazepines (synthesis). 1421. Benzopyrano(4,3-B)-1,5-benzodiazepines (synthesis). 1422. Octahydro [1] -thiopyrano [4,3-b] - [1,5] - benzodiazepines (synthesis). 1423. Dihydrobenzothiopyrano [4,3-b] [1,5] benzodiazepin-7-ones and benzodiazepinium salts (synthesis). 1425. 2-Amino-4-aryl-3H-1,5-benzodiazepine analogs of clozapine (synthesis and biological evaluation). 1445. 1-Oxo-2-methyl-5-phenyl-2,5-dihydro-(1H)-2,3-benzodiazepine (synthesis). 1458. 3A,4,5,6-tetrahydro-3H-imidazo-(1,5A)-1,4-benzodiazepines (synthesis and rearrangements). 1459. Imidazothienodiazepines and Imidazopyrazolo-diazepines (synthesis). 1545. 6-Phenyl-4H-pyrrolo-(1,2-A)(1,4)-benzodiazepines (synthesis and biological action).

1568. Peptidoaminobenzophenones (open ring derivatives of 1,4-benzodiazepines). 1593. Substituted Acetamidobenzophenones (desalkylation and cyclization, in vitro and in vivo). 1637. 3-Substituted 1,4-Benzodiazepine-2-ones (synthesis). 1731. Nordiazepam, Clonazepam (Stabilität in Ampullen, Ringverengung). 1737. Benzodiazepin-2-on-Derivate (synthesis). 1738. Bridged 1,5-Benzodiazepines (by condensation of ortho-phenylenediamines with 4,6-dimethylbicyclo-3,3,1-nona-3,6-diene-2,8-dione). 1782. 7-Acido-5-phenyl-1,4-benzodiazepines (azido group as novel pharmacophoric substituent, synthesis). 1827. Group-IIb-metal-1,4-benzodiazepine complexes (synthesis and spectroscopic studies). 1845. H-3-1,5-Benzodiazepines (from ethynyl ketones and orthophenylendiamines). 1854. 2,4-Bisdialkylamino-3H-1,5-benzodiazepine (synthesis). 1932. O-Amino-benzophenones (synthesis). 1936. Tricyclic 1,4-Benzodiazepine (formation from benzoyl-DL-kynurenylglycine). 1952. 3-Methyloxazolo(3,2-D)-1,4-benzodiazepines (synthesis and configurational studies of their ketimine intermediates).

1979. 3H-1,2-Benzodiazepines (studies). 1980. 3-Substituted-1H-1,2-Benzodiazepines (synthesis). 1981. 1H-1,2-benzodiazepines (photosensitized oxygenation). 2006. Triazolo (5,1-A)-2,4-benzodiazepines (synthesis). 2012. 3-Substituted Imidazo-1,5-alpha-1,4-benzodiazepines (synthesis). 2013. 1-Phenylimidazo-and 3-Phenylimidazo (1,5-alpha)-1,4-benzodiazepines (synthesis).

2116. 5,6-dihydro-4-H-pyrrolo-(1,2-A)-4-benzodiazepines (synthesis). 2169. N-Oxides (photochemistry). 2223. 1,3-Dihydro-2,1,4-benzothiadiazepine (synthesis). 2234. 7-Chloro-2,3-dihydro-1-methyl-5-phenyl-1H-1,4-benzodiazepine-5-^{14}C-hydrochloride (synthesis). 2263. 2-(N-Beta-bromoethyl)-amino-5-substituted benzophenones (kinetics of cyclization into 1,4-benzodiazepines). 2269. 2-(Aminomethyl)-phthylimide (new reagent for the synthesis of 2,4-benzodiazepines). 2354. 7-Nitro-5-phenyl-2,3-dihydro-1H-1,4-benzodiazepin-2-on (photochemische Reduktion).

2910. Derivates from 2-(dialkylamino)-methyl-4H-triazol-4-yl-benzophenones and related heterocyclic benzophenones (synthesis and pharmacology). 2911. Triazolam, alprazolam, diazepam (3-hydroxy-metabolites prepared by a simple, one-step oxidation). 2912. Derivates from o-amino-o-phenyl-o-tolyl-4H-triazoles and -imidazoles. 2919. 3-unsubstituted and 3-alkylsubstituted H-1-1,2-benzodiazepines (synthesis). 2920. 1H-1,2-benzodiazepine-3-carboxylic acids (synthesis and thermochemical behavior). 2927. Diazepam (new synthesis). 3006. Benzodiazepines with a nitrogen atom-containing 5-membered ring fused to the 1,2-position of the diazepine ring (synthesis and CNS activity). 3030. Open-ring derivatives of 1,4-benzodiazepines. 3500. 3H-1,4-benzodiazepines with semicyclic hydroxamide structure (oxidoreductive 1,3-rearrangement to 2-alkylamino-3-acyloxy-3H-1,4-benzodiazepines). 3596. 1,4-Benzodiazepines (new simple synthesis). 3607. 2-Monoalkylamino and 2-dialkylamino-4-phenyl-3H-1,5-benzodiazepines (new synthesis). 3621. 2-^{14}C-labeled 3H-1,4-benzodiazepines (synthesis). 3644. 1H-1,3-benzodiazepines from isoquinoline-N-imides (photochemical synthesis). 3645. 5H-1,2-benzodiazepines (synthesis of the first examples). 3649. 1,5-Benzodiazepines (synthesis). 3771. Ketazolam (synthesis and proof of structure).

Theory of Action / Wirkungstheorie

10. Benzodiazepine receptors. 109. Diazepam (mechanism in cerebellar cortex). 123. Diazepam (GABA mechanisms). 131. Diazepam (receptor characterization). 135. Benzodiazepines (receptors in human cortical areas). 136. Diazepam (specific receptors in rat brain). 137. Benzodiazepines (brain specific receptors in rat and man). 213. Benzodiazepines (explaining, another approach). 643. Benzodiazepines (importance of glycine and GABA). 660. Benzodiazepines (mechanism). 729. Benzodiazepines (release of GABA). 731. Benzodiazepines (receptor). 732. Diazepam (receptors in rat cerebral cortex). 791. Benzodiazepines (brain specific receptors). 844. Diazepam (+ pentobarbital, GABA accumulation). 869. Diazepam (locus of central depressant action). 1074. Benzodiazepines (receptors in brain). 1140. Benzodiazepine analogues (locus of action). 1142. Benzodiazepines (+ pentobarbital, hippocampal neurons). 1187. Diazepam (model of its membrane action). 1190. Benzodiazepines (enhancement of GABA transmission). 1220. Benzodiazepines (GABA-ergic mechanism). 1257. Diazepam (+ GABA, regulation of high-affinity binding). 1274. Benzodiazepines (GABA-hypothesis). 1278. Diazepam (action on braincatecholamine metabolism). 1289. ^{3}H-Diazepam. ^{3}H-Flunitrazepam (specific binding, rat brain subfractions). 1294. Benzodiazepines (rat-brain, ontogenetic development of receptors). 1295. Benzodiazepines (receptors in brain). 1296. Benzodiazepines (lack of brain-specific receptors in mouse primary astroglial structures). 1297. Benzodiazepines (brain-specific receptors). 1298. Benzodiazepines (pharmacological characterization of brain receptors). 1304. ^{3}H-Diazepam (influence of GABA receptor agonists and antagonists on binding to receptor). 1338. ^{3}H-Flunitrazepam (receptors). 1355. Benzodiazepines (binding to specific rat-brain fractions).

1363. Diazepam (GABA-receptors, molecular mechanisms). 1364. Benzodiazepines (receptor, chloride anion channel). 1373. ^{3}H-Flunitrazepam (rat-brain receptors, membranes). 1462. Benzodiazepines (GABA theory). 1463. Benzodiazepines (GABA-ergic drugs, effect). 1536. Benzodiazepines (rat-brain, GABA-receptors). 1558. ^{3}H-Diazepam (localization of receptor). 1597. Benzodiazepines (GABA-receptors). 1632. ^{3}H-Diazepam (rat brain membranes). 1694. Benzodiazepines (mice, receptors, cerebellar purkinje-cells). 1724. Benzodiazepines (facilitation of binding by sodium-chloride and GABA). 1746. Benzodiazepines (receptors in normal and pathological human-brain).

1747. Benzodiazepines (rat-brain, receptor-binding after chronic administration of diazepam and phenobarbital).

1748. Benzodiazepines (human-brain, site of action, ^{3}H-Diazepam). 1759. ^{3}H-Diazepam (rat-brain, binding-receptor, synaptosomal membranes). 1760. Benzodiazepines (rat-brain, receptor binding in spinal-cord-membranes).

1799. Benzodiazepines (biogenic-amines as possible mediators). 1805. Benzodiazepines (rapid changes in brain-receptors). 1812. Clonazepam (Nachweis des kortikalen Angriffspunktes). 1954. Benzodiazepines (GABAergic modulation of binding site sensitivity). 1978. Benzodiazepines (+ pentobarbitone, effect on GABAergic recurrent inhibition of hippocampal neurons). 2007. Flurazepam (GABAergic activity). 2008. Oxazepam (stereospecific receptor binding by enantiomers). 2022. Benzodiazepines (labeling of receptors in vivo). 2023. ^{3}H-Diazepam (demonstration of binding to receptors in vivo).

2050. Benzodiazepines (effect of inosine and hypoxanthine as endogenous ligands for the brain-binding sites).

2056. Benzodiazepines (clonal-cell-lines, interaction with GABA). 2064. ^{3}H-Diazepam (enhancement of binding). 2097. Diazepam, lorazepam (rat, continous treatment, no changes in rat-receptor after withdrawal). 2117. Diazepam (GABA-receptor mediated binding). 2125. Benzodiazepines (mechanisms of action, monography).

2142. ^{3}H-Diazepam (increased specific binding in rat-brain after chronic administration). 2239. Benzodiazepines (stimulation of receptor-binding by GABA).

2285. Benzodiazepines (relationship between receptors and experimental anxiety in rats). 2289. ^{3}H-Diazepam (correlation between prevention of pentylene-tetrazole induced lethality and inhibition of ^{3}H-Diazepam-binding).

2312. Diazepam (site of action of anticonvulsant effect, rabbit). 2341. Diazepam (locus of CNS-action). 2343. 1,4-Benzodiazepines (structure-activity relations).

2351. Benzodiazepines (rats, differences in receptor-binding). 2353. ^{3}H-Diazepam (decreased binding as a specific response to chronic treatment). 2369. Benzodiazepines (role of the periaqueductal gray substance in anxiety action). 2398. ^{3}H-Flunitrazepam (temperature dependence of binding). 2399. Benzodiazepines (alterations of receptors in cerebellar of mutant mice). 2433. ^{3}H-Flunitrazepam (effect of GABA on binding in rat-brain). 2443. ^{3}H-Diazepam (enhancement of the binding to rat-brain membranes, invitro). 2445. Benzodiazepines (anxiety reducing activity by reduction of serotonin turnover in the brain). 2451. Benzodiazepines (autoradiography of receptors).

2519. Benzodiazepines (receptor, review). 2585. Benzodiazepines (possible ligands of receptor). 2586. Benzodiazepines (inhibition of GABA and benzodiazepine receptor-binding by penicillins). 2587. Benzodiazepines (receptor interactions may be involved in the neurotoxicity of various penicillin derivatives). 2592. Benzodiazepines (solubilization of the receptor from rat brain). 2610. GABA-receptors in clonal cell lines). 2615. Benzodiazepines (photoaffinity labeling and localization of receptor). 2636. Benzodiazepines (differential effects of kainic acid on receptors). 2637. Benzodiazepine receptor (differentiation from GABA receptor in the rat cerebellum by kainic acid). 2638. Benzodiazepine receptors (changes following GABA-ergic denervation of substantia nigra). 2640. Benzodiazepines + other drugs (theory of action). 2644. Benzodiazepine binding to rodent brain receptors (in vitro and in vivo inhibition by zopiclone). 2649. Benzodiazepines (use of an in vitro hippocampal slice preparation in studies of the action). 2660. Benzodiazepine receptor (with brain-like specifity, identification in bovine retina). 2664. ^{3}H-Flunitrazepam (specific binding, benzodiazepine receptor). 2666. Benzodiazepines (mechanism of action). 2671. Benzodiazepine receptor (review). 2672. Benzodiazepine receptor (searching for endogenous ligands). 2673. Benzodiazepine receptor (strychnine as a potent inhibitor). 2674. Benzodiazepine receptor (neuronal localization in cerebellum). 2675. Benzodiazepine receptor (special agonists). 2676. Benzodiazepine receptors (two or more confirmations of depending on GABA receptors and other variables). 2677. Benzodiazepine receptors (in brain, affection by different experimental stresses). 2695. ^{3}H-Diazepam (enhancement by ethanol of the binding at the benzodiazepine-GABA-receptor-ionophore complex). 2706. Benzodiazepine receptor (coupling to chloride anion channel). 2707. Benzodiazepine receptor (rat, postnatal development, cerebral cortex and cerebellum).

2717. Benzodiazepine receptor (neurotransmitter receptor localization). 2723. ^{3}H-Diazepam (rat cortex, GABA-receptor mediated modulation). 2724. Benzodiazepines (differential effects of triton X-100 on binding in a frozen-thawed synaptosomal fraction of rat brain). 2725. Benzodiazepine receptor (digitonin-solubilized systems). 2744. Flunitrazepam (live baboon, visualization of displacement in the brain). 2761. Benzodiazepine receptor (leech, GABA levels). 2763. Benzodiazepine receptor (role of GABA). 2765. Benzodiazepines (molecular mechanism in receptor action).

2766. Benzodiazepines (facilitation of GABA-ergic transmission). 2781. Benzodiazepine receptor (purinergic ?).

2788. Benzodiazepine receptor (identification of an endogenous peptide-ligand). 2789. ^{3}H-Diazepam (inhibition of binding by an endogenous fraction from rat brain synaptosomes). 2801. Diazepam (effects on GABA-evoked depolarization in rat dorsal root ganglia in vivo). 2807. Benzodiazepine receptor (localization in human and rat-brain by light and electron-microscopic autoradiography following photoaffinity-labeling). 2832. Benzodiazepine receptor (modulation of binding sites in calf cortex by an endogenous factor and GABAergic ligands). 2833. ^{3}H-Flunitrazepam (binding to differentiating rat cerebral cells in culture). 2834. Benzodiazepine receptor (in vivo occupation). 2836. Benzodiazepines (modulation of striatal enkephalin levels via a GABAergic mechanism). 2877. Benzodiazepine receptor (absence of brain specific benzodiazepine receptors in cyclostomes and elasmobranchs). 2897. Benzodiazepine receptors (loss from brains of mice after 6 months of ethanol-consumption). 2902. Benzodiazepine receptors (interactions with peptido-aminobenzophenones).

2916. Benzodiazepines (+ GABA, interaction). 2928. Benzodiazepine receptor (solubilization of histamine H-1).

2929. Benzodiazepine receptor (GABAergic regulation).

2930. Benzodiazepine receptor (properties of soluble gamma-aminobutyric acid). 2931. Benzodiazepine receptor (recognition sites). 2951. Benzodiazepine receptor (contribution of lipids and calcium). 2987. Benzodiazepine receptor (interaction with GABA-receptors). 2988. Benzodiazepines (modulation of GABA-coupled Cl-ionophore in neuroblastoma NB2A cells). 2989. 1,4-Benzodiazepines (pharmacological and biochemical correlates with GABA). 2991. Benzodiazepine receptor (and GABA receptors, molecular mechanisms regulation of interactions in the CNS). 3017. Diazepam (and GABA receptors, relationship in cerebellar purkinje-cells). 3022. Diazepam receptors (on mouse astrocytes in primary cultures, displacement by pharmacologically active concentrations of benzodiazepines or barbiturates). 3040. Benzodiazepines (binding sites present in retina). 3044. Benzodiazepine receptor (characterization in primary cultures of fetal mouse brain and spinal cord neurons). 3072. Benzodiazepines (+ valproic acid, proposed mechanisms of anticonvulsant action). 3084. Benzodiazepine receptors (photoaffinity labeling in bovine cerebral cortex). 3085. Benzodiazepine receptor (photoaffinity-labeling, solubilization and partial-purification from mammalian brain). 3092. Diazepam (effect on rat cerebellar GABAergic mechanisms). 3093. Diazepam (probable site of action in rat cerebellar GABA system). 3112. Benzodiazepines (molecular basis of actions). 3113. Flunitrazepam (modulation by picrotoxin and IPTBO of flunitrazepam-H-3 binding to the GABA-benzodiazepine receptor complex of rat cerebellum). 3114. Benzodiazepine receptor (thip and isoguvacine as partial agonists). 3115. Benzodiazepine receptor (pharmacological characterization of GABA-stimulated receptor-binding). 3116. Benzodiazepine receptor (is stimulation mediated by a novel GABA receptor ?). 3117. Benzodiazepine receptor (characterization of GABA-stimulated binding). 3118. Benzodiazepine receptor (unchanged after chronic ethanol administration). 3137. Benzodiazepine receptor (resolution of two biochemically and pharmacologically distinct receptors). 3157. Benzodiazepine receptor (pharmacological studies of the interactions with GABA receptors). 3158. (see 3157). 3161. Benzodiazepine receptors (radio-histochemical studies). 3162. ^{3}H-flunitrazepam (autoradiographic evidence for binding in the cat eye to melanin granules). 3177. Benzodiazepine receptor (study with valproic acid, evidence that GABA mechanisms mediate the anxiolytic action). 3179. Benzodiazepine receptor (putative, a protein solubilised from brain). 3201. Benzodiazepine receptor (synthetic non-benzodiazepine ligand). 3202. Benzodiazepine receptor (cellural and behavioral characteristics). 3203. Benzodiazepine receptor (the role of GABA in mediating the anticonvulsant properties). 3213. Benzodiazepine receptor (enhancement of GABA-mediated postsynaptic inhibition in cultured mammalian spinal-cord neurons). 3214. Benzodiazepine receptor (inosine as endogenous ligand on cultured spinal neurons). 3224. Benzodiazepine receptor (phylogenetic characteristics of muscimol-activated binding). 3233. Benzodiazepine receptor (ontogenetic changes in GABA modulation of brain binding). 3236. Benzodiazepine receptor (demonstration of 2 new endogenous benzodiazepine-like compounds from brain). 3237. Benzodiazepine receptor (putative endogenous ligands). 3242. Benzodiazepine receptor (facilitation of specific binding in rat brain membrane fragments by a number of anions). 3243. Diazepam (facilitation of the potassium-stimulated release of (3H)-dopamine from rat striatal-tissue). 3249. Benzodiazepine receptors (and GABA, in the offspring of cams receiving diazepam, ontogenetic studies). 3250. ^{3}H-Diazepam (and ^{3}H-GABA, modulation of binding in different brain-areas). 3251. Benzodiazepine receptor (endogenous regulators of recognition sites). 3257. Benzodiazepine receptor (GABA agonist THIP does not interfere with the benzodiazepine binding site on rats cortical membranes). 3272. Benzodiazepine receptor (repeated seizures induce long-term increase hippocampal benzodiazepine receptors). 3273.(see 3272.). 3277. Benzodiazepine receptor (changes during aging). 3285. Benzodiazepine receptor (decreased density in rat-brain following chronic phenytoin administration). 3288. Benzodiazepines (modification of the agonist responses at a presynaptic GABA receptor). 3292. Benzodiazepine receptor (protein identified and visualized in brain tissue by a photoaffinity label). 3293. Benzodiazepine receptor (rat brain, localization in regions of synaptic contacts). 3294. Benzodiazepine receptor (localization by photoaffinity labeling and isolation of a possible endogenous ligand). 3295. Benzodiazepine receptor (nicotinamide as a brain constituent with benzodiazepine-like actions). 3297. Benzodiazepine receptor (interactions with GABA in the cerebellar cortex). 3299. Diazepam (+ GABA, agonists and antagonists). 3324. Benzodiazepine receptor (electro-physiological evidence that GABA potentiation invivo correlates with benzodiazepine receptor affinity). 3325. Flurazepam (effects of microiontophoretically applied flurazepam on response of cerebral cortical neurones to putative neurotransmitters). 3335. Benzodiazepines (differential interactions with ethyl beta-carboline-3-carboxylate). 3336. ^{3}H-Diazepam (properties of displacing activity). 3337. Benzodiazepine receptors (specifically binding of propyl-H-3-beta-carboline-3-carboxylate to brain benzodiazepine receptors). 3340. Benzodiazepine receptor (isolation of a peptide which displaces diazepam-3-H from brain benzodiazepine receptors). 3341. Benzodiazepine receptor (inhibition of a GABA-stimulated benzodiazepine binding by a convulsant benzodiazepine). 3348. Benzodiazepine receptor (interaction between GABA-diazepam and benzodiazepine binding-sites in the frog spinal-cord). 3363. Benzodiazepine receptor (ontogeny, effects of triton X-100, bromide and muscimol). 3377. Benzodiazepine receptors (putative endogenous benzodiazepine-like compounds). 3378. (s. 3377.). 3379. Benzodiazepine-receptor (irreversible activation of the GABA-benzodiazepine-chloride-ionophore complex). 3380. Benzodiazepine receptor (correlation between receptor occupation and anticonvulsant effects of diazepam). 3381. Benzodiazepine receptor (demonstration of brain-specific receptors in rat retina). 3391. Diazepam (effects on adenosine and acetylcholine-release from rat-cerebral-cortex, purinergic mechanism). 3395. Benzodiazepine receptor (regional distribution of Na^+-independent GABA and benzodiazepine binding sites in rat CNS). 3396. Benzodiazepin receptor (diazepam binding in brain after sleep and wakefulness). 3399. Diazepam (effect on GABAergic cuneate neurons). 3410. Diazepam (modification of l-triiodothyronine-stimulated changes in behavior and the metabolism of brain norepinephrine, dopamine and 5-hydroxytryptamine, possible mechanisms of action). 3411. Diazepam (evidence for involvement of dopamine in the action). 3414. ^{3}H-Flunitrazepam (binding to bovine retinae). 3415. Benzodiazepine receptor (development and modulation by GABA). 3416. ^{3}H-Flunitrazepam (binding to bovine retina and effect og GABA). 3417. ^{3}H-Flunitrazepam (effect of GABA on the binding in mouse brains during development). 3420. Benzodiazepine receptor (effect of GABA on characteristics in human brain and alteration in Huntington's disease). 3421. Benzodiazepine receptor (alterations of Huntington's diseased human brain). 3428. Benzodiazepine receptor (irazepine and noncompetitive irreversible inhibition of ^{3}H-diazepam). 3429. Benzodiazepine receptor (synthesis and biological characterization of specific irreversible inhibitors). 3435. Benzodiazepine receptors (in emotional and non-emotional mice). 3436. Benzodiazepine receptor (in harmaline-induced tremor). 3437. Benzodiazepine receptor (the pharmacology of emotion). 3447. Benzodiazepine receptor (1-methyl-beta-carboline, harmane, as a potent endogenous inhibitor of binding). 3450. ^{3}H-Diazepam (decreased binding as a specific response to chronic benzodiazepine treatment). 3451. Benzodiazepine receptor (binding after in vivo elevation of GABA). 3497. Benzodiazepines (mechanism of action). 3503. Benzodiazepine receptor (modification of GABA-mediated depolarization of the cat ganglion by pentobarbital and two benzodiazepines). 3504. Benzodiazepine receptor (reduction of gamma-aminobutyric and GABA-mediated transmission by a convulsant benzodiazepine). 3506. Benzodiazepine actions (symposium report). 3521. Benzodiazepine actions (relationship of GABA to antianxiety effects). 3522. Benzodiazepine actions (mechanisms, behavioral aspects). 3530. Benzodiazepine receptor (possible involvement of GABA mechanisms in the anxiolytic action). 3531. Benzodiazepine receptor (solubilization and properties from calf cortex). 3532. Benzodiazepine receptor (supersensitivity to GABA's effect develops after striatonigral lesions). 3537. + 3538. Benzodiazepine receptor (molecular heterogeneity). 3542. Benzodiazepine receptor (a site for the potentiation of GABA-mediated responses by benzodiazepines). 3548. Benzodiazepine receptor (indirect evidence for the involvement of limbic, possible GABAergic mechanisms). 3549. Benzodiazepine receptor (enhancement of ^{3}H-diazepam-binding by EMD 28422, a novel purine). 3550. Benzodiazepine receptor (increased number elicited invitro by a novel purine, EMD 28422). 3551. Benzodiazepine receptor (physiological studies and putative endogenous ligands). 3552. Benzodiazepine receptor (potentiation by pentobarbital of GABA-enhanced ^{3}H-diazepam binding). 3554. Benzodiazepine receptor (purines as endogenous ligands). 3555. Benzodiazepine receptor (brain specific receptors localized in the inner plexiform layer of rat retina). 3556. Benzodiazepine receptor (inosine as endogenous ligand antagonizes pentylenetetrazole-evoked seizures). 3557. Benzodiazepine receptor (reduction associated with Purkinje cell degeneration in "nervous" mutant mice). 3558. Diazepam (+ muscimol, effects on GABA-mediated neurotransmission). 3565. ^{3}H-Flunitrazepam (enhanced cortical binding following stressful manipulations in rats). 3566. Benzodiazepine receptor (inhibition of cerebral binding by cimetidine and other antihistamines). 3567. Benzodiazepine receptor (antagonism of binding in brain by antilirium, benzyl alcohol and physostigmine). 3568. Benzodiazepine receptor (antagonism of binding in rat and human brain by antilirium). 3569. Benzodiazepine receptor (mammalian brain). 3571. Benzodiazepine receptor (reduction of binding sites in the caudate nucleus of the rat after kainic acid injections). 3572. Benzodiazepine receptor (acute administration of diazepam produces rapid increases in brain density). 3573. Benzodiazepine receptors (effects of tissue preincubation at 37°C). 3574. Benzodiazepine receptor (alterations in mutant mouse cerebellum). 3576. Benzodiazepine receptor (new evidence for multiple receptors). 3577. Benzodiazepine receptor (recognition sites coupling to GABA receptors and ionophores). 3578. Benzodiazepine receptor (increased thermolability in cerebral-cortex of a baboon with spontaneous seizures). 3591. Benzodiazepine receptor (binding to the high and low affinity GABA binding-sites). 3593. Benzodiazepine receptor (ligands independently stimulate phospholipid methylation). 3598. Benzodiazepine receptor (stimulation of binding by SQ 20009, chloride dependance and picrotoxin-sensitivity). 3599. Benzodiazepine receptor (interaction of SQ 20009 and GABA-like drugs as modulators to binding). 3600. ^{3}H-Flunitrazepam (effect of temperature and chloride-ions on the stimulation of its binding by the muscimol analogs THIP and piperidine-4-sulfonic acid). 3606. Benzodiazepine receptor (characterization of binding sites in cultured cells of neural origin). 3612. Benzodiazepine receptor (modulation of binding site sensitivity). 3613. Benzodiazepine receptor (studies). 3614. Benzodiazepine receptor (pharmacology). 3615. Diazepam (identification of binding in intact animals). 3636. Benzodiazepines (mechanism of action). 3646. Diazepam receptor (competition for binding by diphenylhydantoin and its enhancement by GABA). 3651. Diazepam receptor (role of GABAergic brain systems in the activating effect). 3652. Benzodiazepine actions (new trends on biochemical-mechanisms). 3697. Benzodiazepine receptor (heterogeneity in the CNS demonstrated with kenazepine, an alkylating benzodiazepine). 3698. ^{3}H-Diazepam (enhancement of binding to rat-brain membranes in vitro by SQ 20009, GABA and muscimol). 3699. Diazepam (enhancement of in vitro binding by avermectin B1A). 3703. Benzodiazepine receptor (retinal receptors are destroyed by kainic acid lesions). 3713. Benzodiazepine receptors (GABA activation in native and triton-treated membranes). 3718. ^{3}H-Diazepam (inhibition of binding to rat brain cortical synaptosomal membranes by adenosine uptake blockers). 3723. Benzodiazepine receptor (alterations in the human brain by Huntington's disease). 3726. Benzodiazepine receptor (autoradiographic localisation in the brain of humans and animals). 3727. Benzodiazepine receptor (radiohistochemical localization in rat brain). 3728. Diazepam (influence in the thalamic neurons). 3732. Benzodiazepine receptor (cerebral receptors and concept of endogenous ligand). 3776. The Benzodiazepine Receptor (importance on pharmacology, psychiatry and neurology, in German).

Thin-Layer-Chromatography / Dünnschichtchromatographie

33. Chlordiazepoxid (neben anderen). 34. Benzophenone. 36. Chlordiazepoxid (doping, Pferde). 37. Chlordiazepoxid (über Benzophenon). 38. Chlordiazepoxid (Schnellmethode). 57. Chlordiazepoxide, Diazepam (many other drugs). 60. Benzodiazepines (detection of impurities). 88. Arzneistoffgemische incl. Benzodiazepine. 93. Chlordiazepoxid, Medazepam (unverändert und über Benzophenone). 94. Chlordiazepoxid, Oxazepam, Nitrazepam, Diazepam (über Benzophenone). 96. Diazepam, Nitrazepam, Oxazepam, Chlordiazepoxid, Medazepam (zahlreiche andere analytische Daten und Angaben zur Biotransformation). 144. Benzodiazepines (and methaqualone, phenothiazines, opiates, screening). 146. Diazepam, Chlordiazepoxide (rapid screening, also other drugs). 196. Chlordiazepoxide (also phenothiazines, tranquilizers ans antihistaminics). 198. Chlordiazepoxide (also other drugs, screening). 220. Chlordiazepoxide (other drugs, screening). 277. Chlordiazepoxid (quant DC). 278. Diazepam, Chlordiazepoxid, Nitrazepam, Oxazepam, Medazepam (quant DC). 279. Chlordiazepoxide, Diazepam, Oxazepam, Nitrazepam, Medazepam, Chlorazepat, Clonazepam, Flurazepam, Bromazepam, Flunitrazepam, Medazepam, Prazepam (DC, photolytical N-desalkylation, benzophenones). 280. Clonazepam, Nitrazepam, Metaboliten (kontinuierliche Entwicklung). 281. Benzophenone (andere Pharmaka bzw. prim.aromat. Amine, screening). 282. 3-Hydroxybenzodiazepine. 283. Flunitrazepam, Metaboliten. 288. Screening. 292. Chlordiazepoxid (Remissionsmessung). 363. Oxazepam, Chlordiazepoxide, Diazepam, Nitrazepam (Blut, screening). 377. Chlordiazepoxid, Diazepam, Oxazepam, Medazepam, Chlorazepat, Prazepam (urin, Schnellnachweis, Methaqualon). 406. Flurazepam (neben zahlreichen anderen, Benzophenone), 446. Prim.Amine. 447. prim. aromat. Amine und Nitroverbind. 448. Bromazepam (plasma, quant.). 452. Benzodiazepine und Benzophenone (great review). 453. see 452. 481. Diazepam, Chlordiazepoxide (other drugs). 484. Diazepam, Nitrazepam, Chlordiazepoxide, Oxazepam, Medazepam (biological samples). 540. Chlordiazepoxide, Diazepam, (kleine Blutmengen). 541. Oxazepam (plasma quant.). 616. Benzodiazepine (urine). 617. Benzodiazepine (Notfallanalyse, Fluorometrie). 626. Diazepam. 630. Diazepam, Nitrazepam, Oxazepam, Chlordiazepoxid (Fluorometrie). 658. Chlordiazepoxide(other data). 659. Diazepam (other data). 667. Prazepam (other benzodiazepines). 676. Flurazepam, Metabolites (urine). 702. Chlordiazepoxide (other drugs). 718. Diazepam, desmethyldiazepam (serum). 720. Benzodiazepine und Benzophenone (Übersicht). 761. Diazepam, Chlordiazepoxide (fluorometry). 778. Nitrazepam (Nitrierungsumsetzungsprodukte). 795. Chlordiazepoxide (other drugs). 857. Benzodiazepine und Benzophenone (Blut, Mageninhalt Urin). 864. Chlordiazepoxid (Ausscheidungsstudien) 865. Nitrazepam (Ausscheidungsstudien). 875. Chlorazepate (other data). 919. Diazepam, Nitrazepam, Chlordiazepoxide, Oxazepam (Anwendung homogener azeotroper Fließmittelgemische). 922. Flurazepam (other data). 930. Diazepam, Nitrazepam (also isolation). 952. Benzodiazepines (urine, XAD-2). 954. Nitrazepam (and related compounds). 969. Benzodiazepine, Benzophenone (und Bromcarbamide, Fehlinterpretationen). 970. Diazepam, Chlordiazepoxid, Nitrazepam, Medazepam, Chlorazepate (TRT-Technik). 970. Diazepam, Chlordiazepoxid, Nitrazepam, Medazepam, Chlorazepate (2 dim.DC). 971. Oxazepam, Lorazepam (TRT-Technik, Benzophenone). 972. Lorazepam (Schnellnachweis, Benzophenone). 973. Nitrazepam, Diazepam, Chlorazepate (TRT-Technik). 974. Nitrazepam,

Metaboliten (TRT-Technik). 976. Benzodiazepine (Durchfluß-technik). 978. Benzodiazepine, Benzophenone (TRT-Technik u.a.) 982. Clobazam, Desmethylclobazam (andere). 983. Diazepam, Chlordiazepoxid, Nitrazepam, Oxazepam, Chlorazepate, Medazepam Prazepam, Clonazepam, Bromazepam, Flurazepam, Flunitrazepam, Clobazam, Fosazepam, Lorazepam (und 17 Metaboliten). 984. 19 Benzophenone. 985. Camazepam (und Metaboliten). 986. Clonazepam, Nitrazepam, Metaboliten (kontinuierliche Entwicklung). 987. Benzodiazepine (TRT-Technik). 1009. Benzodiazepines and others. 1034. Oxazepam (other data). 1066. Diazepam, Nor-Diazepam, Oxazepam, Temazepam. 1079. Benzodiazepine (und viele andere). 1098. Benzodiazepine-mixtures. 1101. Clobazam (biologisches Material). 1106. Chlordiazepoxide, Diazepam, metabolites (blood, plasma, spectrodensitometry). 1129. Benzodiazepines (biological material). 1131. Benzodiazepines (2 dim.TLC, biological fluids). 1133. Chlordiazepoxide. 1141. Chlordiazepoxide. 1160. Diazepam, N-desmethyldiazepam (serum, human). 1177. Clonazepam (in tablets, DC-polarography). 1188. Diazepam, metabolites (serum), clonazepam (serum). 1189. Diazepam, metabolites (serum). 1196. Oxazepam (biolog.Flüssigkeiten), 1197. Diazepam, Chlordiazepoxid, Oxazepam, Nitrazepam (und Thymoleptika). 1224. Tricyclic psychotropic drugs. 1225. Tricyclic psychotropic drugs. 1228. Chlordiazepoxide, metabolites (serum)(fluorescence densitometry, quant.).

1358. 1,4-Benzodiazepines (identification). 1618. Diazepam, Chlordiazepoxide (combination with major drugs of abuse). 1933. Benzodiazepines, Benzophenones (use of a color-reagent for detection). 1941. Chlordiazepoxide and metabolites (quantitation). 1946. Chlordiazepoxide and metabolites (fluorescence, quantitative densitometry). 1947. Diazepam and other 1,4-Benzodiazepines (fluorescence-TLC).

2199. 7-Nitrobenzodiazepines (human plasma, as 7-amino-metabolites).

2477. Benzodiazepines (TLC- and many other analytical data). 2528. 19 Benzodiazepines. 2548. Benzodiazepines and others (derivatization on TLC-plates). 2691. Diazepam (combination with EMIT). 2976. Diazepam (densitometric determination in formulations). 2996. Clobazam (serum). 3352. Benzodiazepines (reversed-phase mode). 3445. Benzophenones (TLC). 3509. Lormetazepam. 3510. Triazolam.

Toxicity / Toxicology

Toxizität / Toxikologie

4. Diazepam (cardiotoxicity in cultured heart cells). 116. Clonazepam (Pharmakologie und Toxikologie). 155. Chlorazepate (toxicology, teratological studies). 209. Chlordiazepoxide (toxicity, haemodialysis). 216. Benzodiazepines (severe reactions). 222. Chlordiazepoxide (overdosage). 265. Diazepam (apnea). 415. Flurazepam (high dose in elderly). 421. Chlordiazepoxide, Diazepam (relation to serum albumin concentration). 427. Nitrazepam (safety). 441. Benzodiazepines (toxicity). 564. Nitrazepam (toxicity). 627. Benzodiazepines (acute intoxications). 825. Lorazepam (toxicity). 826. Benzodiazepines (toxicity). 897. Chlordiazepoxide (clinical toxicology, experimental toxicology). 1037. Bromazepam, (rats, acute and subacute toxicity). 1038. Bromazepam (rats, chronic toxicity). 1162. Diazepam (+ chlorpromazine, chlormethiazole, pentobarbital, mice, combined toxicity with ethanol). 1208. Chlordiazepoxide, Diazepam (+ other drugs, tabulation of therapeutic, toxic and lethal concentrations of drugs and chemicals in blood). 1221. Chlordiazepoxide (experimental and clinical toxicology).

1258. Nitrazepam (cerebellar syndrome, overdosage).

1263. Clobazam (toxicological properties). 1264. Drugs (toxic concentrations in human biofluids). 1265. Drugs (toxic concentrations in serum, blood and plasma). 1305. Diazepam (increase of cardiac toxicity of quabain in dogs after repetitive treatment with). 1366. Chlordiazepoxide (hemodialysis). 1503. Nitrazepam (in elderly). 1869. Chlorazepate (expertise toxicologique). 1999. Benzodiazepines (toxicological research, blood and urine). 2428. Psychotropic drugs (influence of ethanol on toxicity). 2467. Clobazam (toxicology). 2579. Benzodiazepines and others (self-poisoning).

Traffic-Medicine Verkehrsmedizin

117. Diazepam (+ alcohol, causative agents in road traffic accidents). 121. Oxazepam, Chlordiazepoxide, Diazepam, Nitrazepam (Nachweis im Zusammenhang mit Verkehrsstraftaten). 170. Diazepam (blood alcohol levels and psychotropic drugs). 366. Drugs (+ alcohol, incidence in fatally injured motor vehicle drivers). 367. Drugs (detection in cases "Driving under the influence of"). 440. Große Übersicht. 488. Clobazam (and car driving ability). 568. Pharmaka, Drogenabhängigkeit und Verkehr. 569. + 570. (see 568.) 590. Diazepam (and traffic security). 605. Diazepam (after i.v. administration, relation to driving). 606. Flunitrazepam (after i.v. administration, relation to driving). 618. Nitrazepam (effect on manual skill, grip strength and reaction time). 632. Diazepam (+ alcohol, psychomotor performance). 637. Diazepam (+ codein + alcohol, driving). 640. Diazepam (+ alcohol, driving). 642. Chlordiazepoxide (+ flupenthixole + alcohol, driving). 669. Arzneimittel u. Alkohol (verkehrsmedizinisches Problem). 670. Arzneimittel (Beweissicherung , Verkehrsstraftaten, Harnproben). 673. Arzneimittel, Alkohol, Verkehr, Angaben von Alkoholtätern). 705. Diazepam (+ alcohol, + thrithiozine, effect on psychomotor skills related to driving). 724. Diazepam (+ haloperidol, driving safety). 732. Medikamente und Verkehr. 747. Prazepam (Leistungsminderung, Kraftfahrt). 977. Benzodiazepine, andere Medikamente, Alkohol, Verkehrstüchtigkeit, Literaturübersicht. 1076. Oxazepam (+Alkohol, Verkehrstüchtigkeit).

1473. Diazepam (verkehrsmedizinische Bedeutung, Einfluß auf Leistungsfähigkeit). 1655. Diazepam, Flunitrazepam, (+ droperidol, i.v., skills related to driving). 1657. Diazepam (+ meperidine, i.m., psychomotor skills related to driving). 1658. Diazepam (i.v., skills related to driving). 1691. Diazepam, Chlordiazepoxide (+ thioridazine, + haloperidol, + flupenthixole, + alcohol, effects on psychomotor skills related to driving).

1692. Diazepam (+ alcohol, combined effects related to driving). 1693. Diazepam (+ lithium, + alcohol, effects on psychomotor skills related to driving). 1729. Diazepam (+ alcohol, + GABA, actions and interactions on psychomotor skills). 1796. Chlordiazepoxide, Diazepam, (+ alcohol, effect on psychomotor skills related to driving). 1800. Clobazam (psychomotor performance).

1864. Bromazepam (effect on psychomotor skills). 1894. Diazepam, Medazepam, Lorazepam (skills related to driving after single oral administration). 1901. Diazepam (i.v., intensity and duration of human psychomotor impairment).

2051. Chlordiazepoxide (effect on visual field, extramuscular balance, colour matching ability and hand-eye-coordination in man). 2065. Lorazepam (effects on visuo-motor coordination and visual function in man). 2072. Oxazepam (effect on ocular re-adaption time). 2073. Diazepam (man, psycho-physical effects). 2075. Diazepam (time course of action). 2076. Diazepam (+ chlorpromazine, + barbiturates, time course of action of single dose, auditory flutter fusion, visual flicker fusion, man). 2077. Tranquilizer (effect on low-speed driving performance test). 2091. Benzodiazepine (+ Fahrtüchtigkeit). 2093. Diazepam (experimentalpsychologische Untersuchung). 2104. Benzodiazepine u. andere (Einfluß auf verkehrsmedizinische Leistungsbereitschaft). 2105. Chlordiazepoxide (Straßenverkehr, Beeinflussung der Alkoholwirkung). 2180. Benzodiazepines (effect on saccadic eye movements in man). 2248. Benzodiazepines and others (drug use and driving risk). 2249. Benzodiazepine und andere (Fahrversuche zur Beeinträchtigung der Verkehrstüchtigkeit). 2267. Medazepam (+ alcohol, effect on cognitive and motor skills related to driving). 2270. Diazepam (+ alcohol, effect on psychomotor performance). 2277. + 2278.+ 2279. Hypnotics (+ alcohol, effect on psychomotor performance and skills related to driving). 2282. + 2283. Benzodiazepines and others (drug interaction on driving skills). 2307. Medazepam (driving ability of anxious patients). 2346. Psychotropic drugs (and motorist). 2358. Bromazepam (+ thioridazine, combined effects with alcohol on psychomotor skills, subacute treatment). 2359. Hypnotics (alone and with alcohol, effect on psychomotor skills related to driving). 2360. Diazepam (+ thioridazine, modification of the psychomotor skills related to driving). 2362. Nitrazepam, flurazepam (effects on visuo-motor performance). 2378. Diazepam (+ Alkohol, visuelle Wahrnehmung). 2384. Bromazepam (or chlorpromazine, thioridazine, sulpiride, actions and interactions with alcohol on psychomotor skills related to driving). 2390. Psychoactive drugs (and traffic accidents). 2402. Chlorazepat (Auswirkungen auf das Reaktionsverhalten).

2460. Clobazam (and car-driving). 2463. Clobazam (effect on human psychomotor performance). 2521. Diazepam (+ ethanol, effect on psychomotor skills). 2551. Benzodiazepines and others (changes in relevance). 2552. Benzodiazepines and others (investigation of blood-samples). 2596. Diazepam (+ alcohol, effect on closed-course driving performance). 2776. Diazepam (+ ethanol, humans, addition or potentiation). 2895. Diazepam (changes in visual flicker fusion frequency). 2985. 1,4- and 1,5-Benzodiazepines (effects on aspects of car driving behavior). 3025. Benzodiazepines (and traffic accidents). 3028. Clobazam, lorazepam (effects on aspects of psychomotor performance and car handling ability). 3029. Clobazam, clorazepate (+ placebo, effects of repeated nocturnal doses on psychomotor performance). 3178. Diazepam (and traffic accidents). 3194. Nitrazepam, temazepam (acute effects on psychomotor skills and memory). 3523. Tofisopam (multiple-dose effects on psychomotor skills and memory, comparison with diazepam and interactions with ethanol). 3686. Diazepam (individual and group effects of 10-mg diazepam on drivers's ability, confidence and willingness to act in a gap-judging task). 3709. Benzodiazepines (effects on psychomotor performance). 3710. Benzodiazepines (psychomotor changes during initial day of medication). 3711. (see 3710.).

UV-Spectroscopy (also visible), Colorimetry
UV-Spektroskopie (auch im Sichtbaren), Kolorimetrie

96. Diazepam, Oxazepam, Nitrazepam, Chlordiazepoxide, Medazepam (UV-Spektren). 244. Flurazepam, major metabolites (spectrophotometry). 250. Benzodiazepine (und zahlreiche andere Pharmaka, neben IR-Spektren). 280. Nitrazepam, Clonazepam, Metaboliten (UV-Spektren und IR-Spektren).

282. Flunitrazepam, Metaboliten (UV- und IR-Spektren). 347. Nitrazepam (spectrophotometric determination). 356. Diazepam (spectrophotometric determination with Reinecke-salt-like compounds). 357. Chlordiazepoxide (mit Chromiaten). 438. Diazepam, Oxazepam, Nitrazepam (spectrophotometrisch, quantitativ). 523. Chlordiazepoxide (in plasma, UV). 658. Chlordiazepoxide (UV-Data and others). 659. Diazepam (UV-Data and others). 823. Chlordiazepoxide (spectrophotometric determination). 824. Chlordiazepoxide (colorimetric assay, rapid). 846. Medazepam (spectrophotometric determination of p_{ka}). 847. Diazepam (UV). 875. Chlorazepate (UV-Data and others). 907. Chlordiazepoxide (UV- and VIS-assay). 908. Nitrazepam (+ Hauptmetaboliten, Mensch, Ratte). 922. Flurazepam (UV-Data and others). 953. Nitrazepam (colorimetric determination). 982. Clobazam (UV- and IR-Spectra, MS). 985. Camazepam (UV-, IR- und Massen-Spektren). 1031. Diazepam, Oxazepam, Chlordiazepoxide (index of electronic spectra, other drugs). 1034. Oxazepam (UV-Data and others). 1192. Nitrazepam (colorimetric and spectrometric estimations in pharmaceuticals and urine samples). 1203. Flurazepam (UV, quantitative).

2003. Cyclohexene-substituted Benzodiazepines (spectrophotometric investigation).

2058. 1,4-Benzodiazepines (examination of acid-base equilibria). 2255. Clonazepam (+ metabolites, in serum). 2364. Nitrazepam (colorimetric method).

2477. Benzodiazepines (UV-data, many other analytical data). 2487. Benzodiazepines (many other analytical data). 2506. Chlordiazepoxide (photochemical decomposition). 2520. Bromazepam (spectral study of the acid-base and complexing behavior). 2906. Bromazepam (spectrophotometric determination). 2976. Diazepam (densitometric determination in preparations). 3509. Lormetazepam (many other analytical data). 3510. Triazolam (many other analytical data). 3753. Benzodiazepines (determination by derivative spectroscopy).

Other Themes / Andere Themen

18. Diazepam (pH controlled liquid extraction). 85. Oxazepam (distribution in pregnant guinea-pigs and rats). 100. Diazepam, Nitrazepam, Chlordiazepoxide, Oxazepam (Titration). 120. Nitrazepam (distribution in white rats organs). 155. Chlorazepate (teratological studies). 160. Allgemein (teratogenic effects). 172. Chlordiazepoxide (distribution in mice). 176. Prazepam (stability assay). 197. Chlorazepate (microcalorimetric method). 206. Chlordiazepoxide, diazepam, medazepam, nitrazepam (effect of solvents on the potency). 245. 1,4-Benzodiazepines (luminescence). 313. 1,4-Benzodiazepines (thermomicroextraction). 342. Bromazepam (quant. analysis by ring-oven method). 372. Benzodiazepines (isolation using XAD-2). 380. Nitrazepam (effect of temperature and humidity on stability). 383. Oxazepam (saliva concentrations after single oral dose). 388. Diazepam (influence of age and previous use on dosage required for endoscopy). 400. Diazepam and Nitrazepam metabolites (separation by column chromatography). 407. Benzodiazepine (p_k- und V_k-Messungen). 413. Chlordiazepoxide (gravimetrische und volumetrische Bestimmung). 435. Benzodiazepines (antibacterial properties). 483. Nitrazepam (tissue distribution in young and old rats). 496. Diazepam (stability in plasma samples when stored under varying conditions). 531. Organically bound fluorine (determination). 539. Diazepam (its role in a prison setting). 545. Nitrazepam (cerebrospinal concentrations). 553. Diazepam, metabolites (cerebrospinal concentrations). 554. Diazepam (concentrations in the adipose tissues of children). 579. Diazepam (factors influencing distribution and elimination). 663. Benzodiazepines (EMIT-assay in urine). 668. Chlordiazepoxide (brain levels in rat). 679. Benzodiazepine (enthalpiemetrische Messungen). 681. Diazepam (levels in adipose tissues of rats, mice and man). 690. Lorazepam, Oxazepam (brain concentrations and anticonvulsant activity). 693. Diazepam (brain levels in mice). 859. Benzodiazepines (microcrystalloscopic reactions). 1114. Benzodiazepines (problems, autopsy material). 1130. Benzodiazepines (paper electrophoretic detection and separation).

1308. Benzodiazepines (use in prison populations).

1320. Diazepam (cremophor EL as a diluent). 1326. 1,4-Benzodiazepines (patterns of use in Australia). 1361. 1,4-Benzodiazepines (photochemical decomposition). 1482. Oxazepam (crystal and molecular structure). 1613. Diazepam (precipitation from i.v. preparations). 1756. Diazepam (compatibility and stability of injections following dilution with intravenous fluids). 1775. Diazepam (potential source of error in official assays). 1861. Triazolobenzodiazepines. 1884. Benzodiazepines (students attitudes concerning therapeutic image).

1908. General (Nachweis in der Kniegelenkssynovialflüssigkeit). 1930. 1,4-Benzodiazepines (chemistry and structure-activity relationship). 1931. Benzodiazepines (story). 1967. 1,4-Benzodiazepines (identification by micro-crystal-tests). 2002. Brnzodiazepines (activity of enzymes of benzodiazepine alkaloid biosynthesis during development of penicillium-cyclopium).

2062. Diazepam (dilution in intravenous fluids). 2075. Diazepam (time course of action). 2076. Diazepam (time course of action, single doses, + chlorpromazine, + barbiturates, auditory flutter fusions, visual flicker fusion theshold, man). 2132. Diazepam (in emulsions for i.v. usage). 2152. Diazepam (in mixtures before anaesthesia). 2235. Patterns and problems of drug consumption in a developing country). 2239. 7-Chloro-5-(2,4-dichlorophenyl)-4,5-dihydro-1,4-dimethyl-3H-1,4-benzodiazepin-2-one (crystal and molecular structure).

2292. Popular attitudes and beliefs about tranquilizers .

2310. The desorption of medical substances from adsorbents in oral pharmaceutical suspensions. 2372. Diazepam (frequency of positive samples in postmortem examinations).

2373. Benzodiazepines (+ cyclophosphamide, chromosome studies, chinese hamsters). 2410. Chlordiazepoxide (discovery history). 2411. Benzodiazepines (story).

2506. Chlordiazepoxide (photochemical decomposition).

2517. Diazepam (absorption to plastic tubing). 2611. Benzodiazepines (acid-base equilibria in nonaqueous media).

2632. Benzodiazepines (behavioral studies of workers engaged in production of benzodiazepines). 2645. Oxazepam-enantiomers (chromatographic resolution of racemates).

2692. Diazepam (frequency of use in individuals on probation and in methadone maintenance programs). 2716. Medazepam hydrochloride (crystal studies). 2737. Diazepam (availability from plastic containers). 2759. Nitrazepam (photochemical decomposition). 2760. 1,4-Benzodiazepines (structure and photobiological activity). 2808. Benzodiazepines (friends, but also strangers). 2809. Benzodiazepines (which benzodiazepine, why and how ?). 2829. Triazolam (the Halcion story). 2857. 1,5-Benzodiazepines (as acid-base indicators). 2883. Pinazepam (physicochemical profile). 2907. Diazepam, nitrazepam, oxazepam (complex compounds with lead picrate). 2982. 7-Fluoro-1,4-benzodiazepines (acid-base equilibria). 2997. Triazolam (Halcion - the unmasking of a myth). 3021. Chlordiazepoxide (crystal-structure and protonation sites). 3107. 7-Bromo-5-(o-chlorophenyl)-1,3-dihydro-2H-1,4-benzodiazepine-2-one (crystal and molecular-structure). 3160. Clobazam (chemical aspects of the 1,4- and 1,5-benzodiazepines). 3173. N-Alkylaminobenzophenones (conversion to benzodiazepines in vivo). 3171. Triazolam (trials and tribulations). 3172. (see 3171.). 3181. Triazolam (Halcion story). 3182. (see 3181.). 3212. Benzodiazepines (correlation between the protein-binding, biological activity and the energy of the highest occupied molecular-orbital)). 3238. Benzodiazepines (thermogravimetric study with complex chromium(III)-compounds). 3291. Oxazepam (effects of visible and ultraviolet-radiation on chloroform solutions of oxazepam). 3303. Diazepam (solution and solid-state structural study of the copper(II)-complex of diazepam). 3313. Benzodiazepines (permeation through synthetic membranes).

3326. 2-Methylamino-5-chlorobenzophenone (pKa-value).

3344. Triazolam (trials and tribulations). 3403. 1,4-Benzodiazepines (palladium(II) and platinum(II)-complexes with 1,4-benzodiazepines as ligands).

3404. Diazepam (complexing behavior towards some bivalent 1st-row transition-metals). 3453. Diazepam (solubilization in bile-salts and in sodium-cholate-lecithin-water phases). 3454. Benzodiazepines (patterns of usage in a family medicine center). 3474. Diazepam (solubility and stability in sodium-salicylate solution). 3478. Benzodiazepines (Swedish doctors attitudes to benzodiazepines used as minor tranquilizers). 3499. 1,4-Benzodiazepine-4-oxides (the so-called Polonovski-reaction). 3597. Chiral 1,4-Benzodiazepines (kinetics of degenerate nucleophilic exchange of 3-C-hydroxy group). 3680. Chlordiazepoxide (variations among 10 chlordiazepoxide HCl 10-mg capsule products). 3687. Benzodiazepines (data compilation).

References

Literaturverzeichnis

Alphabetical List 1

1. Abruzzo,C.W., Brooks,M.A., Cotler,S., Kaplan,S.A.
Differential pulse polarographic assay procedure and in vitro biopharmaceutical properties of dipotassium chlorazepate.
J.Pharmacok.Biopharm. 4, 29 (1976)

2. Abruzzo,C.W., Macasieb,T., Weinfeld,R., Rider,J.A., Kaplan,S.A.
Changes in the oral absorption characteristics in man of dipotassium chlorazepate at normal and elevated gastric pH.
J.Pharmacok.Biopharm. 5, 377-90 (1977)

3. Ackermann,E., Richter,K., Sage,S.
Diazepam metabolism in human cortex kidney microsomes.
Biochem.Pharmacol. 25, 1557-60 (1967)

4. Acosta,D., Chappell,R.
Cardiotoxicity of diazepam in cultured heart cells.
Toxicology 8, 311-7 (1977)

5. Adoni,A., Kapitulnik,J., Kaufmann,N.A., Ron,M., Blondheim,S.H.
Effect of maternal administration of diazepam on the bilirubin-binding capacity of cord blood serum.
Amer.J.Obstet.Gynecol. 115, 577-9 (1973)

6. Agaltsova,T.B.
Forensic-chemical proof of eunoctin poisoning.
Sud.Med.Ekspert. 19, 23-7 (1976)

7. Agurell,S., Berlin,A., Ferngren,H., Hellstroem,B.
Plasma levels of diazepam after parenteral and rectal administration in children.
Epilepsia 16, 277-83 (1975)

8. Agurell,S., Berlin,A., Kallberg,N., Boreus,L.O.
Gaschromatographische Bestimmung antiepileptischer Heilmittel in kleinen Blutplasmaproben.
Dtsch.Apoth.-Ztg. 111, 1705 (1971)

9. Allen,S., Oswald,I.
Anxiety and sleep after fosazepam.
Brit.J.Clin.Pharmacol. 3, 165-8 (1976)

10. Ally,A.I., Manku,M.S., Horrobin,D.F., Karmali,R.A., Morgan,R.O., Karmazyn,M.
Thromboxane,A_2, as a possible natural ligand for benzodiazepine receptors.
Neurosci.Lett. 7, 31-5 (1978)

11. Alton,K.B., Grimes,R.M., Shaw,C., Patrick,J.E., McGuire,J.L.
Biotransformation of a 1,5-benzodiazepine, triflubazam, by man.
Drug Metab.Disposition 3, 352-60 (1975)

12. Alton,K.B., Patrick,J.E., Shaw,C., McGuire,J.L.
Comparative biotransformation of triflubazam in rats, dogs and monkeys.
Drug Metab.Disposition 3, 445-52 (1975)

13. Alvan,G., Siwers,B., Vessman,J.
Pharmacokinetics of oxazepam in healthy volunteers.
Acta Pharmacol.Toxicol. (KBH) 40, 40-51 (1977)

14. Ambrus,G., Albrecht,K., Horvath,G.
Microbiological degradation of diazepam.
Acta microbiol.Acad.Sci.Hung. 22, 145-52 (1975)

15. Andrê,M., Sibout,M., Petry,J.M., Vert,P.
Respiratory and neurologic depression in the premature newborn infant of a mother treated with diazepam.
J.Gynecol.Obstet.Biol.Reprod. (Paris) 2, 357-66 (1973)

16. Andreasen,P.B., Hendel,J., Greisen,G., Hvidberg,E.F.
Pharmacokinetics of diazepam in disordered liver function.
Eur.J.Clin.Pharmacol. 10, 115-20 (1976)

17. Andreoli,V., Maffei,F., Montanaro,N., Morandini,G.
Klinischer Vergleich von zwei 2'-Chlorbenzodiazepinen, Chlordesmethyldiazepam und Lorazepam, in einem Doppelblind Kreuzversuch bei Angstneurose.
Arzneim.-Forsch. (Drug Res.) 27, 436-40 (1977)

18. Andrew,K., Gupta,R.N., Keane,P.M.
Distribution of diazepam in pH-controlled liquid extraction.
Clin.Chem. 18, 1039-40 (1972)

19. Archer,G.A., Sternbach,L.H.
Quinazolines and 1,4-benzodiazepines. XVI. Synthesis and transformations of 5-phenyl-1,4-benzodiazepine-2-thiones.
J.Org.Chem. 29, 231-3 (1964)

20. Argren,T.
Oxazepam poisoning.
Tidsskr.Nor.Laegeforen 88, 280-1 (1968)

21. Arizan,S., Simionovici,R., Voinov,V.
Nachweis und Bestimmung von Zwischenprodukten bei der Synthese von Diazepam.
Pharmazie 24, 746-8 (1969)

22. Arnold,E.
A simple method for determining diazepam and its major metabolites in biological fluids: Application in bioavailability studies.
Acta Pharmacol.Toxicol. 36,335-52(1975)

23. Arrigoni,E., Manzo,L., Sarti,P.
Study of the metabolizing activities of organs "isolated in situ". II. Processes of glucurone-conjugation of oxazepam in the liver.
Boll.Soc.Ital.Biol.Sper. 43, 859-60 (1967)

24. Arrigoni,E., Manzo,L., Sarti,P.
Study on the metabolizing activities of organs isolated in situ. IV: Process of glucurone-conjugation of oxazepam in the brain.
Boll.Soc.Ital.Biol.Sper. 43, 1463-5 (1967)

25. Arrigoni-Martelli,E., Toth,E.
Effect of chlordiazepoxide on glucose metabolism in rats. In: European Society for the study of drug toxicity; Proceedings of the meeting held in Paris, Series No. 145, p. 73.
Excerpta Medica Foundation, Amsterdam, 1969

26. Assensio Biscogli,A., de Zorzi,C., Balducci,L., Midulla,M.
Acute accidental poisonings by psycholeptic drugs in children. Study of 28 cases.
Minerva Pediatr. 27, 1041-5 (1975)

27. Athinarayanan,P., Pierog,S.H., Nigam,S.K., Glass,L.
Chlordiazepoxide withdrawal in the neonate.
Amer.J.Obstet.Gynecol. 124, 212-3 (1976)

28. Auer,M., Dadisch,G.-L., Kolb,B., Machata,G., Pospisil,P., Vycudilik,W.
Gas-Chromatographische Bestimmung von basischen Arzneimitteln in Harn oder Blut und Anwendung zur Doping-Analyse.
Angewandte Chromatographie (1977), Heft 30, Bodenseewerk Perkin Elmer & Co. GmbH

29. Austin,T.R.
Mixed drug overdosage with phenelzine, amytal and chlordiazepoxide. A case report.
Anaesthesia 21, 249-52 (1966)

30. Auterhoff,H.
Lehrbuch der Pharmazeutischen Chemie.
7. Aufl., 1974, Wiss.Verlagsges. Stuttgart

31. Auterhoff,H., Kovar,K.-A.
Identifizierung von Arzneistoffen.
2. neubearbeitete und erweiterte Aufl. (1973). Wiss.Verlagsges. Stuttgart

32. Babbini,M., Montanaro,N., Strocchi,P., Gaiardi,M.
Enhancement of amphetamine-induced stereotyped behavior by benzodiazepines.
Eur.J.Pharmacol. 13, 330-40 (1971)

33. Bäumler,J.
Psychopharmaka und deren Nachweis bei Mißbrauch.
Chimia 17, 247-62 (1963)

34. Bäumler,J.
Zur Standardisierung der Dünnschichtchromatographie.
Toxichem 1, 5-8 (1976)

35. Bäumler,J., Brandenberger,H.
Einsatz der kombinierten Spektroskopie in der toxikologischen Analytik.
Z.Rechtsmed. 76, 159-86 (1975)

36. Bäumler,J., Brault,A.L., Im Obersteg,J.
Dopingnachweis im Speichel von Rennpferden.
Schweizer Archiv für Tierheilkunde 106, 346-54 (1964)

37. Bäumler,J., Rippstein,S.
Über den Nachweis von Librium und seiner Metaboliten.
Helv.Chim.Acta 44, 2208-10 (1961)

38. Bäumler,J., Rippstein,S.
Die Dünnschichtchromatographie als Schnellmethode zur Analyse von Arzneimitteln.
Pharm.Acta Helv. 36, 382-8 (1961)

39. Baggi,T.R., Mahajan,S.N., Rad,G.R.
Colorimetric determination of diazepam in pharmaceutical preparations.
J.Ass.Offic.Anal.Chem. 58, 875-8 (1975)

40. Bailey,L.C., Shroff,A.P.
GLC determination of 7-trifluormethyl-1-methyl-5-pentyl-1H-1,5-benzodiazepine-2,4-(3H,5H)-dione in plasma.
J.Pharm.Sci. 62, 1274 (1973)

41. Baird,E.S., Hailey,D.M.
Plasma levels of diazepam and its major metabolite following intramuscular administration.
Brit.J.Anesth. 45, 546-8 (1973)

42. Baird,E.S., Hailey,D.M., Malcolm,S.
A gas-chromatographic assay for medazepam and its major metabolites in plasma.
Clin.Chim.Acta 48,105-7 (1973)

43. Ballinger,B.R., Simpson,E., Stewart,M.J.
Urinary screening for drugs in a hospital for the mentally subnormal.
Acta Psychiat.Scand. 50, 619-24 (1974)

44. Banerjee,U., Yeoh,P.N.
Temporal dimensions on anticonvulsant action of some newer benzodiazepines against metrazol induced seizures in mice und rats.
Med.Biol. 55, 310-17 (1977)

45. Bant,W.
Diazepam withdrawal symptoms.
Brit.Med.J. 4, 285 (1975)

46. Banziger,R.F.
Anticonvulsant properties of chlordiazepoxide, diazepam, and certain other 1,4-benzodiazepines.
Arch.Int.Pharmacodyn.Ther. 154, 131-6 (1965)

47. Barfod,S., Wendelboe,J.
Severe psychiatric side effects of clonazepam treatment.
Ugeskr.Laeger 139, 2450 (1977)

48. Barnes,C.D., Moolenaar,G.M.
Effect of diazepam and picrotoxin on the visual system.
Neuropharmacology 10, 193-201 (1971)

49. Barrett,J.E., Dworkin,S.I., Zuccarelli,R.R.
Effects of d-amphetamine, chlordiazepoxide and promazine on responding of squirrel monkeys maintained unter fixed-interval schedules of food presentation and stimulus-shock termination.
Pharmacol.Biochem.Behav. 7, 529-37 (1977)

50. Barrett,J.S., Hey,E.B.,jr.
Ventricular arrhytmias associated with the use of diazepam for cardioversion.
J.Amer.Med.Ass. 214, 1323-4 (1976)

51. Barrett,J., Smyth,W.F., Hart,J.P.
The polarographic and spectral behaviour of some 1,4-benzodiazepine metabolites: Application to differentiation of mixtures.
J.Pharm.Pharmacol. 26, 9-17 (1974)

52. Bartosek,I., Kvetina,J., Guaitani,A., et al.
Comparative study of nitrazepam metabolism in perfused isolated liver of laboratory animals.
Eur.J.Pharmacol. 11, 378-82 (1970)

53. Bartosek,I., Mussini,E., Garattini,S.
Reduction of nitrazepam by rat liver.
Biochem.Pharmacol. 18, 2263-4 (1969)

54. Bartosek,I., Mussini,E., Saronio,C. et al.
Studies on nitrazepam reduction in vitro.
Eur.J.Pharmacol. 11, 249-53 (1970)

55. Baruzzi,A., Bordo,B., Bossi,L., Castelli,D., Gerna,M., Tognoni,G., Zagnoni,P.
Plasma levels of Di- n -propylacetate and clonazepam in epileptic patients.
Int.J.Clin.Pharmacol.Biopharm. 15, 403-8 (1977)

56. Baselt,R.C., Stewart,C.B., Franch,S.J.
Toxicological determination of benzodiazepines in biological fluids and tissues by flame-ionization gas chromatography.
J.Anal.Toxicol. 1, 10-3 (1977)

57. Bastos,M.L., Kananen,G.E., Young,R.M., Monforte,J.R., Sunshine,I.
Detection of basic organic drugs and their metabolites.
Clin.Chem. 16, 931-40 (1970)

58. Baute,L.
Clinical trial with lorazepam in pre-operative anxiety.
Acta Anaesthesiol.Belg. 28, 123-31 (1977)

59. Bechtel,W.D.
Proceedings: Blood Level, excretion, distribution and metabolism of ^{14}C-triflubazam, a new benzodiazepine, in mice and dogs.
Naunyn-Schmied.Arch.Pharmacol. 282, 6 (1974)

60. Beckstead,H.D., Smith,S.J.
Detection of impurities in medical 1,4-benzodiazepines and related compounds by thin-layer chromatography.
Arzneim.-Forsch. (Drug Res.) 18, 529-35 (1968)

61. Beharrell,G.P., Hailey,D.M., McLaurin,M.K.
Determination of nitrazepam in plasma by electron capture GLC.
J.Chromatogr. 70, 45-52 (1972)

62. Bekersky,I., Maggio,A.C., Mattaliano,v,J.R., Boxenbaum,H.G., Maynard,D.E., Cohn,P.D., Kaplan,S.A.
Influence of phenobarbital on the disposition of clonazepam and antipyrine in the dog.
J.Pharmacok.Biopharm. 5, 507-12 (1977)

63. Bell,D.S.
Dangers of treatment of status epilepticus with diazepam.
Brit.Med.J. 1, 159-61 (1969)

64. Bell,E.F.
The use of naloxone in the treatment of diazepam poisoning.
J.Pediat. 87, 803-4 (1975)

65. Bell,S.C., Childress,S.J.
A rearrangement of 5-aryl-1,3-dihydro-2H-1,4-benzodiazepine-2-one-4-oxides.
J.Org.Chem. 27, 1691-5 (1962)

66. Bell,S.C., Childress,S.J.
Additional rearrangements of 5-phenyl-1,4-benzodiazepines.
J.Org.Chem. 29, 506-7 (1964)

67. Bell,S.C., McCaully,R.J., Gochman,C., Childress,S.J., Gluckman,M.I.
3-Substituted 1,4-benzodiazepin-2-ones.
Arzneim.-Forsch. (Drug Res.) 11, 457-61 (1968)

68. Bell,S.C., Sulkowski,T.S., Gochman,C., Childress,S.J.
1,3-Dihydro-2H-1,4-benzodiazepine-2-ones and their 4-oxides.
J.Org.Chem. 27, 562-6 (1962)

69. Bellemonte,G.
Determination of diazepam and its metabolites in biological fluids.
Boll.Soc.Ital.Biol.Sper. 43, 460-4 (1967)

70. Belvedere,G., Frigerio,A., Malorni,A., Nardi,D.
Mass spectra of some 4-substituted phenyl-1,3-dihydro-2H-1,5-benzodiazepine-2-thiones.
Boll.Chim.Farm. 114, 151-60 (1975)

71. Ben-Neria,Y., Lass,Y.
Facilitation of synaptic transmission by diazepam in a perfused frog cerebellum.
Experientia 33, 1484 (1977)

72. Benor,D.
Side effect of chlordiazepoxide.
J.Clin.Pharmacol. 7, 180 (1967)

73. Benzi,G., Bertè,F., Crema,A.
Investigation of hepatic drug metabolism by isolated perfused liver in situ.
J.Pharm.Sci. 56, 893-5 (1967)

74. Benzi,G., Bertè,F., Crema,A., Frigo,G.M.
Cerebral drug metabolism investigated by isolated perfused brain in situ.
J.Pharm.Sci. 56, 1349-51 (1967)

75. Berger,R., Green,G., Melnick,A.
Cardiac arrest caused by oral diazepam intoxication.
Clin.Pediat. 14, 842-4 (1975)

76. Berlin,A., Dahlström,H.
Pharmacokinetics of the anticonvulsant drug clonazepam evaluated from single oral and intravenous doses and by repeated oral administration.
Eur.J.Clin.Pharmacol. 9, 155-9 (1975)

77. Berlin,A., Siwers,B., Agurell,S., Hiort,A., Sjöqvist,F.
Determination of bioavailability of diazepam in various formulations from steady state plasma concentration data.
Clin.Pharmacol.Ther. 13, 733-44 (1972)

78. Bernareggi,V., Bugada,G., Levi,G.
Absorption and pharmacological activities of a new diazepam preparation.
Arzneim.-Forsch. (Drug Res.) 20, 1230-2 (1970)

79. Berninger,H., Grünnagel,R., Mall,S., Möller,M.R.
Gaschromatographische Identifzierung unbekannter Substanzen aus Körperflüssigkeiten mittels der Retentionsindices.
Beitr.Gerichtl.Med. 33, 185-91 (1975)

80. Berninger,H., Möller,M.R.
Retentionsindices zur gaschromatographischen Identifzierung von Arzneimitteln.
Arch.Toxicol. 37, 295-305 (1977)

81. Berry,D.J.
The cathode-ray polarographic determination of diazepam, 7-chloro-1,3-dihydro-1-methyl-5-phenyl-2H-1,4-benzodiazepin-2-one, in human plasma.
Clin.Chim.Acta 32, 235-41(1971)

82. Berry,D.J., Grove,J.
Emergency toxicological screening for drugs commonly taken in overdose.
J.Chromatogr. 80, 205 (1973)

83. Bertagni,P., Bianchi,R., Marcucci,F., Mussini,E., Garattini,S.
The enterohepatic circulation of oxazepam-O-glucuronide in guinea-pigs.
J.Pharm.Pharmacol. 30, 185-7 (1978)

84. Bertagni,P., Marcucci,F., Mussini,E., Garattini,S.
Biliary excretion of conjugated hydroxyl benzodiazepines after administration of several benzodiazepines to rats, guinea pigs and mice.
J.Pharm.Sci. 61, 965-6 (1972)

85. Bertè,F., Benzi,G., Manzo,L. et al.
Investigation on tissue distribution and metabolism of oxazepam in pregnant guinea pig and rat.
Arch.Int.Pharmacodyn.Ther. 173, 377-81 (1968)

86. Bertè,F., Manzo,L., de Bernardi,M., Benzi,G.
Ability of the placenta to metabolize oxazepam and aminopyrine before and after drug stimulation.
Arch.Int.Pharmacodyn.Ther. 182, 182-5 (1969)

87. Bertè,F., Manzo,L., de Bernardi,M., Benzi,G.
Developmental patterns of drug metabolism in liver and in some non-hepatic tissues of fetal and newborn rabbits.
Farmaco(Pavia),Ediz.prat. 25, 177-85 (1970)

88. Bertram,J.
Die Identifzierung eines Arzneistoffgemisches durch Kombination von Dünnschichtchromatographie und chemischer Analytik.
Dtsch.Apoth.-Ztg. 114, 1395-8 (1974)

89. Besic,J.
Extraction of diazepam and metabolites from biological material and their gas chromatographic estimation.
Acta pharmac.jugosl. 26, 99 (1976)

90. Besic,J.
Plasma concentrations of diazepam and its metabolites in tetanus therapy.
Acta pharmac.jugosl. 26, 107 (1976)

91. Besner,J.-G., Caille,G., Plaa,G., Dugal,R.
Identification and quantitative determination of biliary metabolites of diazepam in rats.
Rev.Canad.Biol. 32, 241-50 (1973)

92. Besser,G.M., Steinberg,H.
L'interaction du chlordiazépoxide et du dexamphétamine chez l'homme.
Thérapie 17, 977-90 (1967)

93. Besserer,K., Henzler,S., Kohler,E., Mallach,H.J.
Mikrochemische Nachweismethoden von Chlordiazepoxid und Medazepam zur Prüfung der Pharmakokinetik.
Arzneim.-Forsch. (Drug Res.) 21, 2003-6 (1971)

94. Beyer,K.-H.
Zur Analytik von Benzodiazepinderivaten.
Dtsch.Apoth.-Ztg. 105, 1529 (1965)

95. Beyer,K.-H.
Zur Analytik von Benzodiazepinderivaten.
In: La medicine legale sociale, hrsg. von L.Roche, L.Cotte, J.J.Davod, A.Saury.
Masson, Paris 1966

96. Beyer,K.-H.
Zur Analytik der Tranquilizer/Zur Biotransformation der Tranquilizer.
Index der Psychopharmaka (Roche), 190-225 (1971)

97. Beyer,K.-H.
Die Biotransformation der Benzodiazepinderivate.
Dtsch.Apoth.-Ztg. 111, 1503-6 (1971)

98. Beyer,K.-H.
Biotransformation der Arzneimittel.
Wiss.Verlagsgesellschaft, Stuttgart, 1975

99. Beyer,K.-H., Sadée,W.
Über den Metabolismus von 5-Phenyl-1,4-benzodiazepinderivaten.
Pharmaz.Ztg. 112, 1394-5 (1967)

100. Beyer,K.-H., Sadée,W.
Titration von Benzodiazepinderivaten in wasserfreiem Medium.
Arch.Pharm. (Weinheim) 300, 667-73 (1967)

101. Beyer,K.-H., Sadée,W.
Spektrophotometrische Bestimmung von 5-Phenyl-1,4-benzodiazepinderivaten und Untersuchungen über den Metabolismus des Nitrazepams.
Arzneim.-Forsch. (Drug Res.) 19, 1929-31 (1969)

102. Beyer,K.-H., Sadée,W.
Analytische Daten von vier 5-Phenyl-1,4-benzodiazepinderivaten in Monographien.
Dtsch.Apoth.-Ztg. 109, 312-4 (1969)

103. Beyer,K.-H., Sadée,W.
Synthese und Analytik möglicher Nitrazepam-Metaboliten.
Arch.Pharm. (Weinheim) 302, 152-7 (1969)

104. Bianchi,G.N., Fennessy,M.R., Phillips,J., Everitt,B.S.
Plasma level of diazepam as a therapeutic predictor in anxiety states.
Psychopharmacology 35, 113-22 (1974)

105. Bickel,M.H.
The pharmacology and biochemistry of N-oxides.
Pharmacol.Rev. 21, 325-55 (1969)

106. Bickel,M.H.
Antidepressants and tranquillizers biochemical aspects.
Humangenetik 9, 202-4 (1970)

107. Bickel,M.H. et al.
Species and substrate differences of liver microsomal N-desalkylation and N-oxidation of N-oxides.
Xenobiotica 1, 533 (1971)

108. Bieger,R., Jonge,de,H., Loeliger,E.A.
Influence of nitrazepam on oral anticoagulation with phenprocoumon.
Clin-Pharmacol.Ther. 13, 361-5 (1972)

109. Biggio,G., Brodie,B.B., Costa,E., Guidotti,A.
Mechanisms by which diazepam, muscimol, and other drugs change the content of CGMP in cerebellar cortex.
Proc.Natl.Acad.Sci. USA 74, 3592-6 (1977)

110. Billets,S., Carruth,J., Einolf,N., Ward,R., Fenselau,C.
Rapid indentification of acute drug intoxications.
John Hopkins Med.J. 133, 148-55 (1973)

111. Bixler,E.D., Kales,A., Soldatos,C.R., Kales,J.D.
Flunitrazepam, an investigational hypnotic drug: Sleep laboratory evaluations.
J.Clin.Pharmacol. 17, 569-78 (1977)

112. Blair,H.M.
Fixed drug eruption from chlordiazepoxide.
Arch.Dermatol. 109, 914 (1974)

113. Blažević,N., Kaifez,F.
A new ring closure of 1,4-benzodiazepines.
J.Heterocycl.Chem. 7, 1173-4 (1970)

114. Bley,W., Nuhn,P., Benndorf,G.
NMR-spektroskopische Untersuchung von Arzneimitteln. 2.Mitt. Zur Konformation und Ringinversion von diazepam, nitrazepam und chlordiazepoxide.
Arch.Pharm. (Weinheim) 301, 444-51 (1968'

115. Bliding,A.
Effects of different rates of absorption of two benzodiazepines on sujective and objective parameters. Significance for clinical use and risk of abuse.
Eur.J.Clin.Pharmacol. 7, 201-11 (1974)

116. Blum,J.E., Haefely,W., Jalfre,M., Polc,P., Schärer,K.
Pharmakologie und Toxikologie des Antiepileptikums Clonazepam.
Arzneim.-Forsch. (Drug Res.) 23, 377-89 (1973)

117. Bo,O., Haffner,J.F.W., Langard,O., Trumpy,J.H., Bredesen,J.E., Lunde,P.K.M.
Ethanol and diazepam as causative agents in road traffic accidents.
pp. 439-48
Proc. 6Th Int.Conf. on Alcohol, Drugs and Driving Toronto 1974

118. Boer,de,A.G., Röst-Kaiser,J., Bracht,H., Breimer,D.D.
Assay of underivatized nitrazepam and clonazepam in plasma by capillary gas chromatography applied to pharmacokinetic and bioavailability studies in humans.
J.Chromatogr. 145, 105-15 (1978)

119. Boerner,U., Abbott,S., Eidson,J.C., Becker,C.E., Horio,H.T., Loeffler,K.
Direct mass spectrometric analysis of body fluids from acutely poisoned patients.
Clin.Chim.Acta 49, 445-54 (1973)

120. Bogatskii,A.V., Golovenko,N.I.A., Karaseva,T.L.
Distribution of nitrazepam and its metabolites in the subcellular fractions of several white rat organs.
Vopr.med.Khim. 92-6 (1977)

121. Bohn,G.
Über den Nachweis von Arzneimittelwirkstoffen in Blut und Urinproben im Zusammenhang mit Verkehrsstraftaten.
Mitteilungsblatt der GDCh-Fachgruppe Lebensmittelchemie und gerichtliche Chemie 24, 183-4 (1970)

122. Boissier,J.R., Simon,R., Aaron,C.
A new method for rapid screening of minor-tranquilizers in mice.
Eur.J.Pharmacol. 4, 145-51 (1969)

123. Bolme,P., Fuxe,K.
Possible involvement of GABA mechanisms in central cardiovascular and respiratory control-studies on interaction between diazepam, picrotoxin and clonidine.
Med.Biol. 55, 301-10 (1977)

124. Bommer,P., Moser,H., Stichler,W., Trimborn,P., Vetter,W.
Herkunftsbestimmung von Arzneimitteln durch Messung von natürlichen Isotopenverhältnissen: D/H und 13C/12C Verhältnisse einiger Proben von Diazepam.
Z.Naturforsch. 31, 111-4 (1976)

125. Bommer,P., Vane,F.M.
The application of various spectroscopies to the identification of drug metabolites.
In: Handbook of Experimental Pharmacology, Vol. 28, Part 2, edited by B.B.Brodie and J.R.Gillette, Springer-Verlag, Berlin-Heidelberg-New York, pp. 209-25 (1971)

126. Bond,A.J., Hailey,D.M., Lader,M.H.
Plasma concentrations of benzodiazepines.
Brit.J.Clin.Pharmacol. 4, 51-6 (1977)

127. Bond,A.J., Lader,M.H.
The residual effects of flurazepam.
Psychopharmacolog. 32, 223-35 (1973)

128. Booker,H.E., Celesia,G.G.
Serum concentrations of diazepam in subjects with epilepsy.
Arch.Neurol. 29, 191-4 (1973)

129. Borland,R.G., Nicholson,A.N.
Immediate effects on human performance of a 1,5-benzodiazepine (clobazam) compared with the 1,4-benzodiazepines, chlordiazepoxide-hydrochloride and diazepam.
Brit.J.Clin.Pharmacol. 2, 215-21 (1975)

130. Boselli,P.M., Scrollini,F.
Pharmacokinetics of ^{3}H-pinazepam in the rat brain.
Boll.Chim.Farm. 116, 363-9 (1977)

131. Bosmann,H.B., Case,K.R., Distefano,P.
Diazepam receptor characterization: Specific binding of a benzodiazepine to macromolecules in various areas of rat brain.
FEBS Lett. 82, 368-72 (1977)

132. Boucek,J., Skrabanek,P.
Suicidal attempt with valium in combination with barbiturates.
Act.Nerv.Super. (Praha) 10, 266-7 (1968)

133. Boxenbaum,H.G., Geitner,K.A., Jack,M.L., Dixon,W.R., Kaplan,S.A.
Pharmacokinetic and biopharmaceutic profile of chlordiazepoxide HCl in healthy subjects: Multiple dose oral administration.
J.Pharmacok.Biopharm. 5, 25-39 (1977)

134. Boxenbaum,H.G., Geitner,K.A., Jack,M.L., Dixon,W.R., Spiegel,H.E., Symington,J., Christian,R., Moore,J.D., Weissman,L., Kaplan,S.A.
Pharmacokinetics and biopharmaceutical profile of chlordiazepoxide HCl in healthy subjects: Single dose studies by the intraveneous, intramuscular and oral routes.
J.Pharmacok.Biopharm. 5, 3-23 (1977)

135. Braestrup,C., Albrechtsen,R., Squires,R.F.
High densities of benzodiazepine receptors in human cortical areas.
Nature 269, 702-4 (1977)

136. Braestrup,C., Squires,R.F.
Specific benzodiazepine receptors in rat brain characterized by high-affinity (^{3}H) diazepam binding.
Proc.Nat.Acad.Sci.US 74, 3805-9 (1977)

137. Braestrup,C., Squires,R.F., Nielsen,M.
Brain specific benzodiazepine receptors in rat and man.
Acta Pharm.Suec. 14, 9-10 (1977)

138. Brandt,R.
Passage of diazepam and desmethyldiazepam into breast milk.
Arzneim.-Forsch. (Drug Res.) 26, 454-7 (1976)

139. Bratton,A.C., Marshall,jr.,E.K.
A new coupling component for sulfanilamide determination.
J.Biol.Chem. 128, 537-50 (1939)

140. Braun,J., Caille,G., Martin,E.A.
Etude de la fluorescence de quelques derivês de la 1,4-benzodiazepine.
Can.J.Pharmacol.Sci. 3, 65-8 (1968)

141. Brauninger,G., Ravin,M.
Respiratory arrest following intravenous valium.
Ann.Ophthalmol. 6, 805-6 (1974)

142. Breckenridge,A., Orme,M.
Clinical implication of enzyme induction.
Ann.New York Acad.Sci. 179, 421-31 (1971)

143. Breimer,D.D., Bracht,H., de Boer,A.G.
Plasma level profile of nitrazepam (Mogadon) following oral administration.
Brit.J.Clin.Pharmacol. 4, 709-11 (1977)

144. Breiter,J., Helger,R., Interschick,E., Wüst,H.
Thin layer chromatographic screening for methaqualone, phenothiazines, opiates and benzodiazepines.
J.Clin.Chem.Clin.Biochem. 16, 127-35 (1978)

145. Brodersen,R., Sjoedin,T., Sjoeholm,I.
Independent binding of ligands to human serum albumin.
J.Biol.Chem. 252, 5067-72 (1977)

146. Broich,J.R., Hoffmann,D.B., Andryauskas,S., Galante,L., Umberger,C.J.
An improved method for rapid large-scale thin-layer chromatographic urine screening for drugs of abuse.
J.Chromatogr. 60, 95-101 (1971)

147. Brooks,M.A., D'Arconte,L.D., Hackman,M.R., de Silva,J.A.F.
Toxicological analysis of 1,4-benzodiazepines. I. Differential pulse polarography.
J.Anal.Toxicol. 1, 179-88 (1977)

148. Brooks,M.A., Bel Bruno,J.J., de Silva,J.A.F., Hackman,M.R.
A differential pulse polarographic examination of the 1,4-benzodiazepines.
Anal.Chim.Acta 74, 367-85 (1975)

149. Brooks,M.A., de Silva,J.A.F.
Determination of 1,4-benzodiazepines in biological fluids by differential pulse polarography.
Talanta 22, 849-60 (1975)

150. Brooks,M.A., de Silva,J.A.F., Hackman,M.R.
Differential pulse polarography determinations of drugs in biological fluids.
Amer.Lab. 5, 23-8 (1973)

151. Brooks,M.A., Hackman,M.R.
Trace level determination of 1,4-benzodiazepines in blood by differential polarography.
Anal.Chem. 47, 2059-62 (1975)

152. Brooks,M.A., Hackman,M.R., de Silva,J.A.F.
The toxicological analysis of 1,4-benzodiazepines. II. Electron-capture gas-liquid chromatography.
J.Anal.Toxicol.

153. Brooks,M.A., Hackman,M.R., Weinfeld,R.E., Macasieb,T.
Determination of chlorazepate and its major metabolites in blood and urine by ECD-GLC.
J.Chromatogr. 135, 123-31 (1977)

154. Brown,M.L., Sletten,I.W., Kleiman,K.M., Korol,B.
Effect of oxazepam on physiological responses to stress in normal subjects.
Curr.Ther.Res. 10, 543 (1968)

155. Brunaud,M., Navarro,J., Salle,J., Siou,G.
Pharmacological, toxicological, and teratological studies on Dipotassium-7-chlor-3-carboxy-1,3-dihydro-2,2-dihydroxy-5-phenyl-2H-1,4-benzodiazepin-chlorazepate (Dipotassium-chlorazepate, 4306 CB), a new tranquillizer.
Arzneim.-Forsch. (Drug Res.) 20, 123-5 (1970)

156. Buska,C., Cuparencu,B., Horak,J.
Influence of some benzodiazepines on serum lipids levels in hyperlipidaemic rabbits.
Agressiology 18, 265-9 (1977)

157. Butler,P.W.B., Besser,G.M., Steinberg,H.
Changes in plasma cortisol induced by dexamphetamine and chlordiazepoxide, given alone and in combination in man.
J.Endocrinol. 40, 391-2 (1968)

158. Butterfield,A.G., Matsui,F.F., Smith,S.J., Sears,R.W.
High-performance liquid chromatographic determination of chlordiazepoxide and major related impurities in pharmaceuticals.
J.Pharm.Sci. 66, 684-7 (1977)

159. Calanca,A.
Les médicaments psychotropes. (Effects et indications)
Revue Médicale de la Suisse Romande 94, 575-86 (1974)

160. Canfield,P.R.
Teratogenic effects of drugs during pregnancy.
J.Fam.Pract. 6, 26 (1978)

161. Cano,J.P., Baille,A.M., Viala,A.
Determination of bromazepam in plasma with an internal standard by GLC.
Arzneim.-Forsch. (Drug Res.) 25, 1012-6 (1975)

162. Cano,J.P., Catalin,J., Viala,A., Roger,J., Tassinari,C.A., Dravet,C., Gastraut,H.
Determination of clonazepam (RIVOTRIL) in plasma by GLC using an internal standard.
Eur.J.Toxicol.Environ.Hyg. 9, 213-25 (1976)

163. Cano,J.P., Guintrand,J., Aubert,C., Viala,A.
Determination of flunitrazepam, desmethylflunitrazepam and clonazepam in plasma by gas liquid chromatography with an internal standard.
Arzneim.-Forsch. (Drug Res.) 27, 338-42 (1977)

164. Cano,J.P., Soliva,M., Hartmann,D., Ziegler,W., Amrein,R.
Bioavailability from various galenic formulations of flunitrazepam.
Arzneim.-Forsch. (Drug Res.) 27, 2383-8 (1977)

165. Cano,J.P., Vignoli,L., Viala,A.
Determination du diazepam dans le sang et l'urine par GC.
Ann.pharm.franc. 25, 821-8 (1967)

166. Capron,J.P. et al.
Increased sulfobromophthalein clearance in a patient receiving phenobarbital and other anticonvulsant drugs.
Gastroenterology 69, 756 (1975)

167. Cardauns,H., Iffland,R.
Tödliche Diazepamvergiftung bei einem drogenabhängigen Jugendlichen.
Arch.Toxicol. 31, 147 (1973)

168. Carroll,W.M., Mastiglia,F.L.
Alpha and beta coma in drug intoxication.
Brit.Med.J. 2, 1518-9 (1977)

169. Carter,C.S., Daily,R.F., Leaf,R.
Effects of chlordiazepoxide, oxazepam, chlorpromazine, and d-amphetamine on sexual responses in male and female hamsters.
Psychopharmacology 55, 195 (1977)

170. Casier,H., Danechmand,L., Schaepdryver,de,A., Hermans,W., Piette,Y.
Blood alcohol levels and psychotropic drugs.
Arzneim.-Forsch. (Drug Res.) 16, 1505-7 (1966)

171. Cassano,G.B., Castrogiovanni,P., Gallevi,M.
Nitrazepam (RO 4-5360) in the treatment of anxiety states, double blind trial.
Pharmakopsychiatrie und Neuro-Pharmakopsychiatrie 3, 195-201 (1968)

172. Cassano,G.B., Gliozzi,E., Ghetti,B.
The relationship between dynamic features of the brain distribution of ^{14}C-chlordiazepoxide and motor behaviour changes in mice.
In: The Present Status of Psychotropic Drugs: Pharmacological and Clinical Aspects. Proc. 6th C.I.N.P., pp. 342-6. Congress, Tarragona, edited by A. Cerletti and F.J. Bovè. Excerpta Medica, Amsterdam. 1969

173. Castrogiovanni,P., Biagini,G.L., Canella,M., Gallevi,M., Cassano,G.B.
Confronto doppio cieco tra RO 5-4556 (Nobrium), chlordiazepossido e placebo in pazienti ansiosi.
Neopsichiatria 36, 1-14 (1968)

174. Cate,J.C., Jatlow,P.I.
Chlordiazepoxide overdose: Interpretation of serum drug concentrations.
Clin.Toxicol. 6, 533-61 (1973)

175. Celesia,G.G., Booker,H.E., Sato,S.
Brain and serum concentrations of diazepam in experimental epilepsy.
Epilepsia 15, 417-25 (1974)

176. Chafetz,L., Gaglia,C.A.,jr.
Stability assay for prazepam and related drugs.
J.Pharm.Sci. 56, 1681-2 (1967)

177. Chang,T.T.L. et al.
Identification of oxazepam and lorazepam glucuronides by chemical ionization mass spectroscopy.
Experientia 29, 653 (1973)

178. Chase,T.N., Katz,R.I., Kopin,I.J.
Effect of diazepam on fate of intracisternally injected serotonin ^{14}C.
Neuropharmacology 9, 103-8 (1970)

179. Childress,S.J., Gluckman,M.I.
1,4-benzodiazepines.
J.Pharm.Sci. 53, 577-90 (1964)

180. Christmas,A.J., Maxwell,D.R.
A comparison of the effects of some benzodiazepines and other drugs on aggressive and exploratory behaviour in mice and rats.
Neuropharmacology 9, 17-29 (1970)

181. Chun,A.H., Carrigan,P.J., Hoffman,D.J., Kershner,R.P., Stuart,J.D.
Effects of antacids on absorption of chlorazepate.
Clin.Pharmacol.Ther. 22, 329-35 (1977)

182. Cimbura,G., Gupta,R.C.
Polarographic determination of chlordiazepoxide and diazepam in toxicological analysis.
J.Forensic.Sci. 10, 282-93 (1965)

183. Clark,T.O., Arrowsmith,R.
Persistent EEG changes in chlordiazepoxide toxic state, a case report.
Can.Psychiatr.Assoc.J. 13, 279-80 (1968)

184. Clarke,C.H., Ferres,H.M., Nicholson,H.M., Stone,B.M.
Proceedings: Effects of diazepam and a soluble salt of diazepam (fosazepam) on sleep in man.
Brit.J.Pharmacol. 55, 262 (1975)

185. Clarke,C.H., Nicholson,A.N.
Activity of N-desmethyldiazepam (Nordiazepam) (Proceedings)
Brit.J.Clin.Pharmacol. 4, 647-8 (1977)

186. Clarke,C.H., Nicholson,A.N., Stone,B.M.
Effect of the 1,5-benzodiazepines, clobazam and triflubazam, on the sleep of man.
Brit.J.Pharmacol. 58, 439 (1976)

187. Clarke,E.G.C.
Isolation and Identification of Drugs,
The Pharmaceutical Press, London (1971)

188. Clarke,P.R., Eccersley,P.S., Frisby,J.P., Thornton,J.A.
The amnesic effect of diazepam (Valium).
Brit.J.Anaesth. 42, 690-7 (1970)

189. Clatworthy,A.J., Jones,L.V., Whitehouse,M.J.
The gas chromatography mass spectrometry of the major metabolites of flurazepam.
Biomed.Mass.Spectrom. 4, 248-54 (1977)

190. Cleeland,R., Christenson,J., Usategui-Gomez,M., Heveran,J., Davis,R., Grunberg,E.
Detection of drugs of abuse by radioimmunoassay: A summary of published data and some new information.
Clin.Chem. 22, 712-25 (1976)

191. Clifford,J.M.
Drug disposition and effect in sub-human primates used in pharmacology.
Comp.Biochem.Physiol. 57, 1-15 (1977)

192. Clifford,J.M., Smyth,W.F.
The determination of some 1,4-benzodiazepines and their metabolites in body fluids. A review.
The Analyst 99, 241-73 (1974)

193. Clifford,J.M., Smyth,W.F.
Polarographic study of the acid-base equilibria existing in aqueous solutions of the 1,4-benzodiazepines.
Z.Anal.Chem. 264, 149-53 (1973)

194. Clifford,J.M., Smyth,M.R., Smyth,W.F.
Assay of flurazepam in plasma by differential pulse polarography.
Z.Anal.Chem. 272, 198-201 (1974)

195. Coassolo,P., Briand,C., Bourdeaux,M., Sari,J.C.
Microcalorimetric method to determine competitive binding action of a psychotropic drug (dipotassium chlorazepate) on L-tryptophan human serum albumin complex.
Biochim.Biophys.Acta 538, 512-20 (1978)

196. Cochin,J., Daly,J.W.
The use of thin-layer chromatography for the analysis of drugs. Identification and isolation of phenothiazine tranquilizers and antihistaminics in body fluids and tissues.
J.Pharmacol.Exp.Ther. 139, 160 (1963)

197. Cohen,I.M., Harris,T.H.
Effects of chlordiazepoxide in psychiatric disorders.
Southern Med.J. 54, 1271 (1969)

198. Comer,J.P., Comer,I.
Applications of TLC in pharmaceutical analyses.
J.Pharm.Sci. 56, 413-36 (1967)

199. Comi,V., Fossati,A., Gervasi,G.B.
Specific metabolic pathway in vitro of pinazepam and diazepam by liver microsomal enzymes of different animal species.
Farmaco (Sci) 32, 278-85 (1977)

200. Consroe,P., Jones,B., Martin,P.
Lysergic acid diethylamide antagonism by chlorpromazine, haloperidol, diazepam, and pentobarbital in the rabbit.
Toxicil.Appl.Pharmacol. 42, 45-54 (1977)

201. Cooperman,M.L.
Plasma Diazepam Levels.
Lancet 1, 168 (1975)

202. Coutinho,C.B., Cheripko,J.A., Carbone,J.J.
Relationship between the duration of anticonvulsant activity of chlordiazepoxide and systemic levels of the parent compound and its major metabolites in mice.
Biochem.Pharmacol. 18, 303-16 (1969)

203. Coutinho,C.B., Cheripko,J.A., Carbone,J.J.
Correlation between the duration of the anticonvulsant activity of diazepam and its physiological disposition in mice.
Biochem.Pharmacol. 19, 363-79 (1970)

204. Coutinho,C.B., Cheripko,J.A., Carbone,J.J., Manning,J.E., Boff,E.
Behavioural changes in primates and diazepam metabolism.
Xenobiotica 3, 681-90 (1973)

205. Coutinho,C.B., King,M., Carbone,J.J., Manning,J.E., Boff,E., Crews,T.
Chlordiazepoxide metabolism as related to the reduction in the aggressive behaviour of cynomolgus primates.
Xenobiotica 1, 287-301 (1970)

206. Crankshaw,D.P., Raper,C.
The effect of solvents on the potency of chlordiazepoxide, diazepam, medazepam, and mitrazepam.
J.Pharm.Pharmacol. 23, 313-21 (1971)

207. Cravey,R.H., Jain,N.C.
The identification of non-barbiturate hypnotics from biological specimens.
J.Chromatogr.Sci. 12, 237-45 (1974)

208. Cree,J.E., Meyer,J., Hailey,D.M.
Diazepam in labour: Its metabolism and effect on clinical condition and thermogenesis of the newborn.
Brit.med.J. 4, 251-5 (1973)

209. Cruz,I.A., Cramer,N.C., Parrish,A.E.
Hemodialysis in chlordiazepoxide toxicity.
J.Amer.Med.Ass. 202, 438-40 (1967)

210. Cunningham,T.A.
Adverse reaction of flurazepam.
Can.med.Assoc.J. 112, 805 (1975)

211. Curry,S.H., Nicholson,A.N., Whelpton,R.
Plasma concentrations in the monkey (Macaca Mulatta) of six related benzodiazepines after intraperitoneal injection (Proceedings).
Brit.J.Pharmacol. 57, 427-8 (1976)

212. Curry,S.H., Whelpton,R., Nicholson,A.N.
Behavioural and pharmacokinetic studies in the monkey (MACACA MULATTA) with diazepam, nordiazepam and related 1,4-benzodiazepines.
Brit.J.Pharmacol. 61, 325-30 (1977)

213. Cutler,N.R., Shore,D.
Explaining benzodiazepines: Another approach.
Am.J.Psychiatry 134, 1155 (1977)

214. Czerwenka-Wenkstetten,H., Hofmann,G., Kryspin-Exner,K.
Tranquillizersucht und Missbrauch.
Wien.Med.Wochenschr. 115, 1012-6 (1965)

215. Dahl,S.G.
Accumulation and elimination of benzodiazepines.
Tidsskr.Nor.Laegeforen 95, 1142-5 (1975)

216. Daly,R.J., Kane,F.J.,jr.
Two severe reactions to benzodiazepine compounds.
Amer.J.Psychiatry 122, 577-8 (1965)

217. Dantzer,R.
Increased resistance to satiation in diazepam treated pigs.
Experientia 34, 81 (1978)

218. Dasberg,H.
Effects and plasma levels of N-desmethyldiazepam after oral administration in normal volunteers.
Psychopharmacologia 43, 191-8 (1975)

219. Dasberg,H., Kleijn,van der,E., Guelen,P.J., Pragg,van,H.M.
Plasma concentrations of diazepam and of its metabolite N-desmethyldiazepam in relation to anxiolytic effect.
Clin.Pharmacol.Ther. 15, 473-83 (1974)

220. Davidow,B., Petri,N.L., Quame,B.
A TLC screening procedure for detecting drug abuse.
Amer.J.Clin.Pathol. 50, 714-9 (1968)

221. Davies,G.
Complication of diazepam administration.
Can-Anaesth.Soc.J. 24, 418-9 (1977)

222. Davis,J.M., Bartlett,E., Termini,B.A.
Overdosage of psychotropic drugs: A Review. I. Major and minor tranquilizers.
Dis.Nerv.Syst. 29, 157-64 (1968)

223. De Bernardi,M., Manzo,L., Hokari,S., Berté,F.
Metabolic transformation of oxazepam and of aminopyrine in the rabbit placenta at various periods of pregnancy.
Boll.Soc.Ital.Biol.Sper. 44, 1937-41 (1968)

224. DeBoer,A.G., Roest-Kaiser,J., Bracht,H., Breimer,D.
Assay of underivatized nitrazepam and clonazepam in plasma by capillary gas chromatography applied to pharmacokinetic and bioavailability studies in humans.
J.Chromatogr. 145, 105-14 (1978)

225. Degkwitz,R.
Leitfaden der Psychopharmakologie.
Wiss.Verl.Ges., Stuttgart 1967

226. Del Vecchio,P.J.
Apnea after intravenous diazepam administration.
J.Amer.Med.Ass. 239, 614 (1978)

227. Demol,P., Singer,M., De Oliveira,J.P., Sarles,H.
Effect of diazepam on the exocrine pancreatic secretion in the alcoholized and nonalcoholized dog.
Z.Gastroenterol. 15, 572-6 (1977)

228. DeSilva,J.A.F.
Gas chromatography in drug research.
In: Gas Chromatography, 252-65, Grune and Stratton Inc., New York 1968

229. DeSilva,J.A.F.
Choice of sensitivity and specificity in the analysis of drugs in biological fluids: Use of electron capture GLC, spectrophotofluorometry, differential pulse polarography, and radioimmunoassay in the analysis of 1,4-benzodiazepines.
Quantitative Analystic Studies in Epilepsy, edited by Peter Kellaway and Ingemar Petersén. Raven Press, New York 1976, pp. 11-38

230. DeSilva,J.A.F.
Electron-capture-GLC in quantitation of 1,4-benzodiazepines.
In: Antiepileptic Drugs. Pippenger,C.E., Penry,J.K., Kutt,K., ED, Raven Press, New York 1978, pp. 111-139

231. DeSilva,J.A.F., Bekersky,I.
Determination of clonazepam and flunitrazepam in blood by Ecd-GLC.
J.Chromatogr. 99, 447-60 (1974)

232. DeSilva,J.A.F., Bekersky,I., Brooks,M.A.
ECD-GLC determination of blood levels of 7-chloro-1,3-dihydro-5-(2′-chlorophenyl)-2H-1,4-benzodiazepine-2-one (lorazepam) in humans and its urinary excretion as lorazepam determined by differential pulse polarography.
J.Pharm.Sci. 63, 1943-5 (1974)

233. DeSilva,J.A.F., Bekersky,I., Brooks,M.A., Weinfeld,R.E., Glover,W., Puglisi,C.V.
Determination of bromazepam in blood by electron-capture GLC and of its major urinary metabolites by differential pulse polarography.
J.Pharm.Sci. 63, 1440-5 (1974)

234. DeSilva,J.A.F., Bekersky,I., Puglisi,C.V.
The determination of lorazepam and its metabolite in blood and urine by electron-capture GLC.
J.Chromatogr.Sci. 11, 547-54 (1973)

235. DeSilva,J.A.F., Bekersky,I., Puglisi,C.V.
Spectrofluorodensitometric determination of flurazepam and its major metabolites in blood.
J.Pharm.Sci. 63, 1837-41 (1974)

236. DeSilva,J.A.F., Bekersky,I., Puglisi,C.V., Brooks,M.A., Weinfeld,R.E.
Determination of 1,4-benzodiazepines and diazepin-2-ones in blood by Ecd-GLC.
Anal.Chem. 48, 10-9 (1976)

237. DeSilva,J.A.F., Kaplan,J.
Determination of 7-bromo-1,3-dihydro-5(2-pyridyl)-2H-1,4-benzodiazepin-2-one (Ro 5-3350) in blood by gas-liquid-chromatography.
J.Pharm.Sci. 55, 1278-83 (1966)

238. DeSilva,J.A.F., Koechlin,B.A., Bader,G.
Blood level distribution patterns of diazepam and its major metabolite in man.
J.Pharm.Sci. 55, 692-702 (1966)

239. DeSilva,J.A.F., Munno,N., Strojny,N.
Determination of an indolyl-1,4-benzodiazepine in blood by spectrophotofluorometry.
Anal.Chem. 45, 665-71 (1973)

240. DeSilva,J.A.F., Puglisi,C.V.
Determination of medazepam (Nobrium), diazepam (Valium) and their major biotransformation products in blood and urine by electron capture gas-liquid chromatography.
Anal.Chem. 42, 1725-36 (1970)

241. DeSilva,J.A.F., Puglisi,C.V., Brooks,M.A., Hackman,M.R.
Determination of flurazepam (dalmane^{R}) and its major metabolites in blood by electron-capture GLC and in urine by differential pulse polarography.
J.Chromatogr. 99, 461-83 (1974)

242. DeSilva,J.A.F., Puglisi,C.V., Munno,N.
Determination of clonazepam and flunitrazepam in blood and urine by electron-capture GLC.
J.Pharm.Sci. 63, 520-6 (1974)

243. DeSilva,J.A.F., Schwartz,M.A., Stefanovic,V., Kaplan,J., D'Arconte,L.
Determination of diazepam (Valium) in blood by gas liquid chromatography.
Anal.Chem. 36, 2099-105 (1964)

244. DeSilva,J.A.F., Strojny,N.
Determination of flurazepam and its major biotransformation products in blood and urine by spectrofotofluorometry and spectrophotometry.
J.Pharm.Sci. 60, 1303-14 (1971)

245. DeSilva,J.A.F., Strojny,N., Stika,K.
Luminescence determination of pharmaceuticals of the tetrahydrocarbazole, carbazole and 1,4-benzodiazepine class.
Anal.Chem. 48, 144-55 (1976)

246. De Silverio,R.V., Rickels,K., Raab,E., Jameson,J.
Oxazepam and meprobamate in anxious neurotic outpatients.
J.Clin.Pharmacol. 9, 259-63 (1969)

247. Despaux,N., Duprey,F., Bohuon,Cl., Boudène,Cl.
Les radioimmunoessais. Leur application en toxicologie.
Pathol.Biol. 24, 419-29 (1976)

248. Deutsch,J.A., Walton,N.Y.
Diazepam maintenance of alcohol preference during alcohol withdrawal.
Science 198, 307-9 (1977)

249. Diab,A.M.
Colorimetric estimation of nitrazepam and metabolites in formulations and in blood and urine samples.
Pharmazie 30, 746 (1975)

250. Dibbern,H.-W.
UV- und IR-Spektren wichtiger pharmazeutischer Wirkstoffe.
Editio Cantor, Aulendorf (Germany) 1978

251. DiCarlo,F.J., Crew,M.C., Melgar,M.D., Haynes,L.J.
Prazepam metabolism by dogs.
J.Pharm.Sci. 58, 960-2 (1969)

252. DiCarlo,F.J., Viau,J.P.
Prazepam metabolism in dog urine.
J.Pharm.Sci. 59, 322-5 (1970)

253. DiCarlo,F.J., Viau,J.P., Epps,J.E., Haynes,L.J.
Biotransformation of prazepam in man.
Ann.N.Y.Acad.Sci. 179,487-92(1971)

254. DiCarlo,F.J., Viau,J.P., Epps,J.E., Haynes,L.J.
Prazepam metabolism by man.
Clin.Pharmacol.Ther. 11, 890-7 (1970)

255. DiLiberti,J., O'Brien,M.L., Turner,T.
The use of physostigmine as an antidote in accidental diazepam intoxication.
J.Pediat. 86, 106-7 (1975)

256. DiMascio,A., Barrett,J.E.
Comparative effects of oxazepam in "high" and "low" anxious student volunteers.
Psychosomatics 6, 298 (1965)

257. Ditt,J., Pauer,R.
Pharmakopsychologische Untersuchungen mit 7-chlor-2-methylamino-5-phenyl-3H-1,4-benzodiazepin-4-oxyd.
Arzneim.-Forsch. (Drug Res.) 15, 653-7 (1965)

258. Dixon,G.D.
Apnea after intraveneous diazepam.
J.Amer.Med.Ass. 239, 294 (1978)

259. Dixon,R., Brooks,M.A., Postma,E., Hackman,M.R., Spector,S., Moore,J.D., Schwartz,M.A.
N-desmethyldiazepam, a new metabolite of chlorodiazepoxide in man.
Clin.Pharmacol.Ther. 20, 450-7 (1976)

260. Dixon,R., Crews,T.
An ^{125}J-radioimmunoassay for the determination of the anticonvulsant agent clonazepam directly in plasma.
Res.Commun.Chem.Pathol.Pharm. 18, 477-86 (1977)

261. Dixon,W.R., Earley,J., Postma,E.
Radioimmunoassay of chlordiazepoxide in plasma.
J.Pharm.Sci. 64, 937-9 (1975)

262. Dixon,W.R., Young,R.L., Ning,R., Liebman,A.
Radioimmunoassay of the anticonvulsant agent clonazepam.
J.Pharm.Sci. 66, 235-7 (1977)

263. Dost,F.H.
Grundlagen der Pharmakokinetik.
Thieme, Stuttgart (1968)

264. Dost,F.H., Gladtke,E.
Ein Verfahren zur Ermittlung der Bilanz einverleibter Stoffe ohne Kenntnis der Ausscheidung.
Z.Klin.Chem.Klin.Biochem. 1, 14-8 (1963)

265. Doughty,A.
Unexpected danger of diazepam.
Brit.Med.J. 2, 239 (1970)

266. Dreifuss,F.E., Penry,J.K., Rose,S.W., Kupferberg, H.J., Dyken,P., Sato,S.
Serum clonazepam concentrations in children with absence seizures.
Neurology 25, 255-8 (1975)

267. Dugal,R., Caille,G., Cooper,S.F.
Urinary metabolites of diazepam in man: Chromatographie and polarographie methods.
Union Med.Can. 102, 2491-7 (1973)

268. Dundee,J.W. et al.
Plasma diazepam levels after single dose oral and intramuscular administration.
Anaesthesia 30, 164-9 (1975)

269. Dundee,J.W., Gamble,J.A., Assaf,R.A.
Plasma-diazepam levels following intramuscular injection by nurses and doctors.
Lancet 2, 1461 (1974)

270. Dundee,J.W., Johnston,H.M.L., Lilburn,J.K., Nair, S.G., Scott,M.G.
A placebo-controlled comparison of the sedative properties of three benzodiazepines, lorazepam, flunitrazepam and fosazepam.
Brit.J.Clin.Pharmacol. 4, 706-9 (1977)

271. Dundee,J.W., Lilburn,J.K., Toner,W., Howard,P.J.
Plasma lorazepam levels. A study following single dose administrations of 2 and 4 mg by different routes.
Anaesthesia 33, 15-20 (1978)

272. Dunlop,E., Weisberg,J.
Use of prazepam for treatment of patients with anxiety.
J.Psychopharmacol. 1, 75-8 (1966)

273. Dunlop,E., Weisberg,J.
Double-blind study of prazepam in the treatment of anxiety.
Psychosomatics 9, 235-8 (1968)

274. Dysken,M.W., Chan,C.H.
Diazepam withdrawal psychosis: A case report.
Amer.J.Psychiatry 134, 573 (1977)

275. Eatman,F.B., Colburn,W.A., Boxenbaum,H.G., Postmanter,H.N., Weinfeld,R.E., Ronfeld,R., Weisman,L., Moore,J.D., Gibaldi,M., Kaplan,S.A.
Pharmacokinetics of diazepam following multiple-dose oral administration to healthy human subjects.
J.Pharmacok.Biopharm. 5, 481-94 (1977)

276. Ebel,S.
Handbuch der Arzneimittelanalytik.
Verlag Chemie GmbH, Weinheim (1977)

277. Ebel,S., Kussmaul,H.
Quantitative Dünnschichtchromatographie.
Z.Anal.Chem. 269, 10-5 (1974)

278. Ebel,S., Kussmaul,H.
Quantitative Dünnschichtchromatographie: In situ Remissionsmessungen von Benzodiazepinen.
Arch.Pharm. 307, 230-1 (1974)

279. Ebel,S., Langer,B.-M., Schütz,H.
Verbesserter Nachweis für N-1-alkylierte 1,4-Benzodiazepine durch photolytische Abspaltung der N-Alkylgruppe.
Mikrochimica Acta (Wien) 1977 II, 261-77

280. Ebel,S., Schütz,H.
Untersuchungen zum Nachweis von Clonazepam (RIVOTRIL[R]) und seinen Hauptmetaboliten unter besonderer Berücksichtigung der dünnschichtchromatographischen Unterscheidung von Nitrazepam (MOGADAN[R]) und dessen wichtigsten Stoffwechselprodukten.
Arzneim.-Forsch. (Drug Res.) 27, 325-37 (1977)

281. Ebel,S., Schütz,H.
Dünnschichtchromatographischer Nachweis wichtiger Pharmaka über primäre aromatische Aminogruppen als Schlüsselfragment.
Dtsch.Apoth.-Ztg. 117, 1605-9 (1977)

282. Ebel,S., Schütz,H.
Analytik und Synthese wichtiger 3-Hydroxy-5-phenyl-1,4-benzodiazepin-2-on - Derivate.
Arzneim.-Forsch. 29, 1317-25 (1979)

283. Ebel,S., Schütz,H.
Zur Analytik von Flunitrazepam (Rohypnol), einem neuen Benzodiazepinderivat, unter besonderer Berücksichtigung der Metaboliten.
Z.Rechtsmedizin 81, 107-17 (1978)

284. Ebel,S., Schütz,H.
Biotransformation der Benzodiazepine.
Pharmazie in unserer Zeit 8, 87-93 (1979)

285. Eberts,jr.,F.S.
Disposition of triazolam, 8-chloro-6-(o-chlorophenyl)-1-methyl-4H-S-triazolo-(4,3-A)-benzodiazepine, in the dog.
Drug Metab.Disposition 5, 547-55 (1977)

286. Edwards,V.E.
Side effect of clonazepam therapy.
Proc.Aust.Assoc.Neurol. 11, 199-202 (1974)

287. Egg,H.
Über den Nachweis von Benzodiazepinen mit der Farbreaktion nach Sawicki und Johnson.
Arch.Pharm. 309, 433-8 (1976)

288. Egli,R.A.
DC-Identifizierung von Arzneisubstanzen.
Z.Anal.Chem. 259, 277-82 (1972)

289. Ehrhardt,G., Ruschig,H.
Arzneimittel, Band 1, S. 251-63
Verlag Chemie: Weinheim (Germany) 1972

290. Ehrsson,H., Knapp,D.
Rapid, efficient procedure for extraction of drugs for toxicological analysis.
Clin.Chem. 20, 1366-7 (1974)

291. Ehrsson,H., Tilly,A.
Electron capture gas chromatography of nitrazepam in human plasma as methyl derivatives.
Anal.Lett. 6, 197 (1973)

292. Eich,E., Geissler,H., Mutschler,E., Schunack,W.
Die direkte quantitative Messung von Dünnschicht-Chromatogrammen durch Remissions- und Fluoreszenzmessungen.
Arzneim.-Forsch. (Drug Res.) 19, 1895-7 (1969)

293. Eickstedt,K.-W.,von
Die Beeinflussung der Alkoholwirkung durch Valepotriate.
Arzneim.-Forsch. (Drug Res.) 19, 995-7 (1969)

294. Engelmann,L., Koehler,H.
Zur Klinik der Chlordiazepoxid-Intoxikationen.
Dtsch.Gesundheitsw. 26, 435-9 (1971)

295. Erkkola,R., Kanto,J., Sellman,R.
Perinatal metabolism of diazepam.
Brit.Med.J. 3, 472 (1974)

296. Erkkola,R., Kangas,L., Pekkarinen,A.
The transfer of diazepam across the placenta during labour.
Acta Obstet.Gynaecol.Scand. 52, 167-70 (1973)

297. Erkkola,R., Kanto,J.
Diazepam and breast-feeding.
Lancet 1, 1235-6 (1972)

298. Eschenhof,E.
Untersuchungen über das Schicksal des Antikonvulsivums Clonazepam im Organismus der Ratte, des Hundes und des Menschen.
Arzneim.-Forsch. (Drug Res.) 23, 390-400 (1973)

299. Etzler,K., Hoenle,R., Joswig,E.H., Köhler,C., Mallach,H.J.
Prüfung der statistischen Wechselwirkung zwischen Äthylalkohol und Carbamazepin, Methaqualon und Nitrazepam.
Arzneim.-Forsch. (Drug Res.) 19, 988-95 (1969)

300. Eustace,P.W., Hailey,D.M., Cox,A.G., Baird,E.S.
Biliary excretion of diazepam in man.
Brit.J.Anaesth. 47, 983-5 (1975)

301. Faber,D.B., Kok,R.M., Dijk,E.M.
Quantitative gas chromatographic analysis of flunitrazepam in human serum with electron-capture detection.
J.Chromatogr. 133, 319-26 (1977)

302. Fagrell,B.
A patient with severe barbiturate and diazepam intoxication who was initially considered dead by ambulance men and policemen.
Lakartidningen 71, 3241-2 (1974)

303. Fanelli,R., Marcucci,F., Mussini,E., Garattini,S.
The metabolism of diazepam by liver microsomal enzymes of rats und mice.
Eur.J.Pharmacol. 7, 307-13 (1969)

304. Fazio,C., Manfredi,M., Piccinelli,A.
Treatment of epileptic seizures with clonazepam.
Arch.Neurol. 32, 304-7 (1975)

305. Fazzari,F.R., Riggleman,O.H.
Polarographic determination of oxazepam.
J.Pharm.Sci. 58, 1530-1 (1969)

306. Feldman,P.E.
An analysis of the efficacy of diazepam.
J. Neuropsych. 3 (Suppl.) 62-7 (1962)

307. Feldmann,S.A., Crawley,B.E.
Diazepam and muscle relaxants.
Brit.Med.J. 1, 691 (1970)

308. Fell,R.H., Dendy,P.R.
Severe hypothermia and respiratory arrest in diazepam and glutethimide intoxication.
Anaesthesia 23, 636-40 (1968)

309. Fenner,H.
Untersuchungen zur Biotransformation von Arzneimitteln - ein Beitrag zur Arzneimittelsicherheit.
Dtsch.Apoth.-Ztg. 117, 1680-4 (1972)

310. Fennessy,M.R., Lee,J.R.
The effect of benzodiazepine on brain amines of the mouse.
Arch.Int.Pharmacodyn.Ther. 197, 37-44 (1972)

311. Fennessy,M.R., Sawnok,J.
The effect of benzodiazepines on the analgesic effect of morphine and sodium salicylate.
Arch.Int.Pharmacodyn.Ther. 204, 77-85 (1973)

312. Ferguson,J.L., Couri,D.
Electron capture gas chromatography determination of benzodiazepines and metabolites.
J.Anal.Toxicol. 1, 171-4 (1977)

313. Ficarra,P., Vigorita,M.G., Tommasini,A.
Some 1,4-benzodiazepine derivates, I. Thermomicroextraction of pharmaceutical preparations and analytical study.
Boll.chim.Farm. 115, 758-73 (1976)

314. Fidelus, J., Zietek,M., Mikolajek,A., Grochowska,Z.
Polarographische Bestimmung von Diazepam in Leichenblut ohne vorherige Extraktion.
Mikrochimica Acta 1972, 84-91

315. Finer,M.J.
Habituation to chlordiazepoxide in an alcoholic population.
J.Amer.Med.Ass. 213, 1342 (1970)

316. Fink,M., Irwin,P.
EEG and blood level relations of psychoactive drugs.
American Psychiatric Association 128th Ann.Mett., Anaheim/Cal. May 5-9, 1975, pp. 128

317. Finke,J.
Gibt es Geschmacksstörungen bei Benzodiazepin-Präparaten (Librium, Valium) ?
Med.Welt 26, 628 (1975)

318. Finkle,B.
Amitriptyline, chlordiazepoxide death.
Bull.Int.Ass.Forens.Toxicol. 11, 27 (1975)

319. Finkle,B.
Flurazepam and alcohol.
Bull.Int.Ass.Forens.Toxicol. 10, 6 (1974)

320. Finkle,B.S., Taylor,D.M., Bonelli,E.J.
A GC/MS reference data system for the identification of drugs of abuse.
J.Chromatogr.Sci. 10, 312-33 (1972)

321. Flinn,F.J., Wineland,P., Peterson,L.J.
Duration of amnesia during sedation with diazepam and pentazocine. Preliminary report.
J.Oral.Surg. 33, 23-6 (1975)

322. Florey,K.
Analytical Profiles of Drug Substances. Vol. 1
Academic Press, New York and London 1972

323. Florey,K.
Analytical Profiles of Drug Substances. Vol. 3
Academic Press, New York and London 1974

324. Florey,K.
Analytical Profiles of Drug Substances. Vol. 4
Academic Press, New York and London 1975

325. Foerster,E.H., Hatchett,D., Garriott,J.C.
A rapid comprehensive screening procedure for basic drugs in blood or tissues by gas chromatography.
J.Anal.Toxicol. 2, 50-5 (1978)

326. Foldes,E.G., Campbell,K.N., Wohlman,A.
Comparative blood level study of different brands of chlordiazepoxide hydrochloride and their coadministration with chymotrypsin.
Int.Z.Klin.Pharmakol.Ther.Toxikol. 3, 338-43 (1970)

327. Forgione,A., Martelli,P., Marcucci,F., Fanelli,R., Mussini,E., Jommi,G.C.
GLC and MS of various benzodiazepines.
J.Chromatogr. 59, 163-8 (1971)

328. Forth,W., Henschler,D., Rummel,W.
Allgemeine und spezielle Pharmakologie und Toxikologie.
2. überarbeitete und erweiterte Aufl.
B.I.-Wissenschaftsverlag: Mannheim/Wien/Zürich 1977

329. Foster,L.B., Frings,C.S.
Determination of diazepam (valium) concentrations in serum by GLC.
Clin.Chem. 16, 177-9 (1970)

330. Fox,K.A., Snyder,R.L.
Effect of sustained low doses of diazepam on aggression and mortality in grouped male mice.
J.Comparative and Physiological Psychology 69, 663-6 (1969)

331. Fox,K.A., Tockosh,J.R., Wilcox,A.H.
Increased aggression among grouped male mice fed chlordiazepoxide.
Eur.J.Pharmacol. 11, 119-21 (1970)

332. Fox,K.A., Webster,J.C., Guerriero,F.J.
Increased aggression among grouped male mice fed nitrazepam and flurazepam.
Pharmacologica Research Communications 4, 157-62 (1972)

333. French,W.N., Matsui,F.F., Smith,S.J.
Determination of major impurity in chlordiazepoxide formulations and drug substance.
J.Pharm.Sci. 64, 1545-7 (1975)

334. Frigerio,A., Baker,K.M., Belvedere,G.
GC-degradation of several drugs and their metabolites.
Anal.Chem. 45, 1846-51 (1973)

335. Frings,C.S.
Absence of interference of oxazepam with glucose determination.
J.Amer.Med.Ass. 217, 1244 (1971)

336. Frings,C.S., Cohen,P.S.
Rapid colorimetric method for the quantitative determination of librium in serum.
Amer.J.Clin.Pathol. 56, 216-9 (1971)

337. Frings,C.S., Queen,C.
Critical evaluation of Dole's method for screening alkaloids, narcotics, and other organic bases in urine.
Clin.Chem. 17, 664 (1971)

338. Fryer,R.I., Earley,J.V.
The synthesis of 2-phenyl-5H-imidazo(2,1-) (2,4) benzodiazepines.
J.Heterocycl.Chem. 14, 1435-9 (1977)

339. Fryer,R.I., Smith,R.A., Sternbach,L.H.
Quinazolines and 1,4-benzodiazepines: XVII. Synthesis of 1,3-dihydro-5-pyridyl-2H-1,4-benzodiazepine derivates.
J.Pharm.Sci. 53, 264-8 (1964)

340. Fujimura,H.
Anti-inflammatory and analgetic effects of benzodiazepine-derivates.
Folia Pharmacol.Jap. 69, 1-22 (1973)

341. Fukazawa,H., Iwase,H. et al.
Effects of chronic administration of bromazepam on its blood level profile and on the hepatic microsomal drug-metabolizing enzymes in the rat. Drug metabolism and disposition.
The Biological Pate of Chemicals 3, 235-44 (1975)

342. Fukumoto,M. et al.
Semi-quantitative analysis of bromazepam by ring-oven method.
Gifu Daigaku Igakubu Kiyo 20, 600-7 (1972)

343. Gänshirt,H.
In: E.Stahl, Dünnschichtchromatographie, S. 504, 2. Aufl. Berlin-Heidelberg-New York: Springer 1967

344. Gagnon,M.A., Langlois,Y., Boghen,D.R., Verdy,M.
Effects of halazepam and diazepam on the motor coordination of geriatric subjects.
Eur.J.Clin.Pharmacol. 11, 443-8 (1977)

345. Gaillard,J.M.
Comparison of two muscle relaxant drugs on human sleep: Diazepam and parachlorophenylGABA.
Acta Psychiatr.Belg. 77, 410-25 (1977)

346. Gallant,D.D., Bishop,M.P., Guerrero-Figuero,R., Selby,M., Phillips,R.
Doxepin versus diazepam. A controlled evaluation in 100 chronic alcoholic patients.
J.Clin.Pharmacol. 9, 57-65 (1969)

347. Gallo,N., Bianco,V.D., Doronzo,S., Laforgia,P.D.
A new spectrophotometric determination of nitrazepam.
Experientia 30, 439-40 (1974)

348. Gamble,J.A.S.
Factors influencing the absorption of diazepam.
Proc.Roy.Soc.Med. 68, 22 (1975)

349. Gamble,J.A.
Some factors influencing the absorption of diazepam.
Proc.Roy.Soc.Med. 68, 772 (1975)

350. Gamble,J.A., Assaf,R.A., Mackay,J.S., Kennedy,M.S., Howard,P.J.
Estimation of plasma diazepam, critique of a method using GLC and benzene extraction.
Anaesthesia 30, 159-63 (1975)

351. Gamble,J.A., Dundee,J.W., Assaf,R.A.
Plasma diazepam levels after single dose oral and intramuscular administration.
Anaesthesia 30, 164-9 (1975)

352. Gamble,J.A., Gaston,J.H., Nair,S.G., Dundee,J.W.
Some pharmacological factors influencing the absorption of diazepam following oral administration.
Brit.J.Anaesth. 48, 1181-5 (1976)

353. Gamble,J.A., Mackay,J.S., Dundee,J.W.
Plasma levels of diazepam.
Brit.J.Anaesth. 45, 1085 (1973)

354. Gamble,J.A., Mackay,J.S., Dundee,J.W.
Proceedings: Blood diazepam levels: preliminary results.
Brit.J.Anaesth. 45, 925-7 (1973)

355. Gamble,J.A., Moore,J., Lamki,H., Howard,P.J.
A study of plasma diazepam levels in mother and infant.
Brit.J.Obstet.Gynaecol. 84, 588-91 (1977)

356. Ganescu,I., Varhelyi,C., Brinzan,G., Boboc,L.
Thiocyanotochromium(III)somplexes in chemical analysis. 25. Oxydometric and spectrophotometric determination of diazepam with Reinecke salt-like compounds.
Pharmazie 31, 259 (1976)

357. Ganescu,I., Varhelyi,C., Brinzan,G., Boboc,L.
Thiocyanato-Chrom-III-Komplexe in der chemischen Analyse. 26. Mitt.: Oxydimetrische und spektrophotometrische Bestimmung des Chlordiazepoxids mit Tetrathiocyanato-diamin-chromiaten.
Pharmazie 32, 53 (1977)

358. Ganguli,L.K., Chatterjee,P., Mandal,J.N.
Oxazepam overdosage.
J.Indian Med.Assoc. 54, 424-5 (1970)

359. Garattini,S., Marcucci,F., Mussini,E.
Gas-chromatographic analysis of benzodiazepines.
In: Gas-Chromatography in Biology and Medicine, edited by R. Porter, pp. 161-72. Churchill, London 1969

360. Garattini,S., Marcucci,F., Mussini,E.
Studies on the anticonvulsant action of diazepam.
Brit.J.Pharmacol. 38, 455-7 (1970)

361. Garattini,S., Marcucci,F., Mussini,E.
Benzodiazepine metabolism in vitro.
Drug Metab.Rev. 1, 291-309 (1972)

362. Garattini,S., Mussini,E., Randall,L.O.
The Benzodiazepines, Raven Press, New York, 1973

363. Gardner-Thorpe,G., Parsonage,M.J., Toothill,C.
A comprehensive scheme for the evaluation of anticonvulsant concentrations in blood using TLC.
Clin.Chim.Acta 35, 39-47 (1971)

364. Gardner-Thorpe,G., Parsonage,M.J., Smethurst,P.F., Totthill,C.
A comprehensive gas-chromatographic scheme for the estimation of antiepileptic drugs.
Clin.Chim.Acta 36, 223-30 (1972)

365. Gardos,G., DiMascio,A., Salzman,C., Shader,R.I.
Differential actions of chlordiazepoxide and oxazepam on hostility.
Arch.General Psychiatr. 18, 757-60 (1968)

366. Garriott,J.C., DiMaio,V.J.M., Zumwalt,R.E., Petty,C.S.
Incidence of drugs and alcohol in fatally injured motor vehicle drivers.
J.Forens.Sci. 22, 383-9 (1977)

367. Garriot,J.C., Latman,N.
Drug detection in cases of "driving under the influence".
J.Forens.Sci. 21, 398-415 (1976)

368. Gastaut,H.
Propriétés anti épileptiques exceptionelles d'une benzodiazepine nouvelle, le Ro 5-4023 (Clonazepam).
Vie Med. 51, 5175-88 (1970)

369. Gastaut,H., Naquet,R., Poiré,R., Tassinari,C.A.
Treatment of status epilepticus with diazepam (VALIUM[R]).
Epilepsia (Amterdam) 6, 167-82 (1965)

370. Gastaut,H. et al.
Demonstration by a acreening-method of the exceptionel anticonvulsant properties of a new benzodiazepine.
Electroencephalog.Clin.Neurophysiol. 27, 105 (1969)

371. Gazzano,A.M., Poletto,T.A., Gorgerino,F., Sapienza,S.
Poisoning by sedatives.
Ann.Osp.Maria Vittoria Torino 17, 101-21 (1974)

372. Gelbke,H.P., Grell,T.H., Schmidt,Gg.
Isolation of drugs from blood by column chromatography on amberlite XAD-2
Arch.Toxicol. 39, 211-17 (1978)

373. Gelbke,H.P., Schlicht,H.J., Schmidt,Gg.
Radioimmunological screening and gas chromatographic identification of diazepam in blood and serum.
Arch.Toxicol. 38, 295-305 (1977)

374. Gelbke,H.P., Schlicht,H.J., Schmidt,Gg.
Häufigkeit positiver Diazepam-Befunde in Blutproben alkoholisierter Verkehrsteilnehmer.
Z.Rechtsmedizin 80, 319-28 (1978)

375. Geldmacher-von Mallinckrodt,M.
Forensische Toxikologie.
In: Gerichtliche Medizin, Bd. 2, S. 887 ff., hrsg. von B. Mueller, Springer-Verlag, Berlin Heidelberg New York, 1975

376. Geldmacher-von Mallinckrodt,M.
Einfache Untersuchungen auf Gifte im klinisch-chemischen Laboratorium.
Georg Thieme Verlag, Stuttgart, 1976

377. Geldmacher-von Mallinckrodt,M., Mang,U.
Schnellnachweis von Metaboliten des Methaqualon und der Chlordiazepoxid-Gruppe im Urin.
Z.Klin.Chem.Klin.Biochem. 8, 259-62 (1970)

378. Geller,I.
Relative potencies of benzodiazepines as measured by their effects on conflict behaviour.
Arch.Int.Pharmacodyn.Ther. 149, 243-7 (1964)

379. Geller,I., Kulak,J.T.,jr., Seifter,J.
The effect of chlordiazepoxide and chlorpromazine on a punishment discrimination.
Psychopharmacologia 3, 374-85 (1962)

380. Genton,D., Kesselring,U.W.
Effect of temperature and relative humidity on nitrazepam stability in solid state.
J.Pharm.Sci. 66, 676-80 (1977)

381. Gerna,M., Morselli,P.L.
A simple and sensitive GC-method for the determination of clonazepam in human plasma.
J.Chromatogr. 116, 445-50 (1976)

382. Ghosh,J.S.
Allergy to diazepam and other benzodiazepines.
Brit.Med.J. 1, 902-3 (1977)

383. Giles,H.G., Zilm,D.H., Frecker,R.C., MacLeod,S.M., Sellers,E.M.
Saliva and plasma concentrations of diazepam after a single oral dose.
Brit.J.Clin.Pharmacol. 4, 711-5 (1977)

384. Gleser,G.C., Gottschalk,L.A., Fox,R., Lippert,W.
Immediate changes in affect with chlordiazepoxide in juvenile delinquent boys.
Arch.General Psychiatry 13, 291-5 (1965)

385. Glogner,P., Heni,N., Herkel,L., Höfer,G.
Tödliche Limbatril -F- Intoxikation mit postmortaler gaschromatographischer Amitriptylin- und Nortriptylin-Gewebsspiegelbestimmung.
Dtsch.med.Wschr. 98, 2472-7 (1973)

386. Gluckmann,M.I.
Pharmacology of 7-chlor-5-(o-chlorphenyl)-1,3-dihydro-3-hydroxy-2H-1,4-benzodiazepin-2-on (Lorazepam).
Arzneim.-Forsch. (Drug Res.) 21, 1049-55 (1971)

387. Ghoneim,M.M., Mewaldt,S.P., Ambre,J.
Plasma levels of diazepam and mood ratings.
Anesth.Analg. (Cleve) 54, 173-7 (1975)

388. Giles,H.G., MacLeod,S.M., Wright,J.R., Sellers,E.M.
Influence of age and previous use on diazepam dosage required for endoscopy.
Can.Med.Ass.J. 118, 513-5 (1978)

389. Gillberg,C.
Floppy infant syndrom and maternal diazepam.
Lancet 2, 244 (1977)

390. Gillberg,C.
Diazepam intoxication during the neonatal period.
Lakartidningen 74, 2587-8 (1977)

391. Giudicelli,J.F., Berdeaux,A., Idrissi,N., Richer,Ch.
Clazepam: pharmacokinetics and effects on performance.
Brit.J.Clin.Pharmacol. 5, 65-71 (1978)

392. Gjerris,F.
Poisoning with chlordiazepoxide (Librium)
Dan.Med.Bull. 13, 170-2 (1966)

393. Glatt,M.M.
Benzodiazepines.
Brit.Med.J. 2, 444 (1967)

394. Goldberg,M.E., Manian,A.A., Efron,D.H.
A comparative study of certain pharmacological response following acute and chronic administration of chlordiazepoxide.
Life Sciences 6, 481-91 (1967)

395. Goldsmith,J.A., Jenkins,H.A., Grant,J., Smyth,W.F.
The polarographic behaviour of the 1,4-benzodiazepines oxazepam and lorazepam and a method for quality control.
Anal.Chim.Acta 66, 427-34 (1973)

396. Golovenko,N.I.A., Bogatskii,A.V., Orliuk,E.I., Kurushin,A.A., Karaseva,T.L.
Nitrazepam metabolism in the intestines of white rats.
Biull.Eksp.Biol.Med. 84, 53-6 (1977)

397. Golovenko,N.I.A., Bogatskii,A.V., Orlyuk,E.I., Kurushin,A.A., Karaseva,T.L.
Metabolism of nitrazepam in the intestine of albino rats.
Bull.Exp.Biol.Med. -Engl.Tr. 84, 981-5 (1977)

398. Golovenko,N.I.A., Zinkovsky,V.G.
Determination of 1,4-benzodiazepines in tranquilizers and their metabolites in biological media.
Khim.Farm.Zh.SSSR 12, 3-14 (1978)

399. Golovenko,N.I.A., Karaseva,T.L.
Biliary excretion of nitrazepam and its metabolites in rats.
Farmakol-Toksikol. 41, 17-9 (1978)

400. Golovenko,N.I.A., Zinkovski,V.G., Karaseva,T.L., Bogatskii,A.V.
Separation of diazepam and nitrazepam metabolites by column chromatography.
Farmatsiia 26, 39-41 (1977)

401. Gore,C.P., McComiskey,J.G.
A study of the comparative effectiveness of librium, amylobarbitone, and a placebo in the treatment of tension and anxiety states.
Proceedings of the Third World Congress of Psychiatry (Montreal), Vol. 2, pp. 979-82 (1961)

402. Gottschalk,L.A., Biener,R., Dinovo,E.C.
Effect of oral and intramuscular routes of administration on serum chlordiazepoxide levels and the prediction of these levels from predrug fasting serum glucose concentrations.
Res.Commun.Chem.Pathol.Pharmacol. 8, 697-702 (1974)

403. Goudie,J.H., Burnett,D.
A rapid method for the detection of methaqualone metabolites.
Clin.Chim.Acta 35, 133-5 (1971)

404. Gould,J.D., Lingam,S.
Hazards of intra-arterial diazepam.
Brit.Med.J. 2, 298-9 (1977)

405. Gräfe,G.
Zum Verhalten gebräuchlicher Psychopharmaka in der Arzneimittelanalyse.
Dtsch.Apoth.-Ztg. 112, 8-13 (1972)

406. Gräfe,G., Schmeling,W.
Zum chemischen Nachweis von Flurazepam (Dalmadorm).
Dtsch.Apoth.-Ztg. 116, 163-5 (1976)

407. Graf,E., El-Menshawy,M.
pK- und Vk-Messungen an Benzodiazepinen.
Pharmazie in unserer Zeit 6, 171-8 (1977)

408. Graham,C.W., Connor,J.T.
Pain and clinical thrombophlebitis following intravenous diazepam and lorazepam.
Anaesthesia 33, 187 (1978)

409. Graham,C.W., Pagano,R.R., Katz,R.L.
Thrombophlebitis after intravenous diazepam, - can it be prevented?
Anesth.Analg. (Cleve) 56, 409-13 (1977)

410. Grassi,E., Passetti,G.L., Trebbi,A.
Quantitative determination of pinazepam and its metabolites in blood and urine by high-performance liquid chromatography.
J.Chromatogr. 144, 132-5 (1977)

411. Greaves,M.S.
Quantitative determination of medazepam, diazepam, and nitrazepam in whole blood by flame-ionization gas-liquid-chromatography.
Clin.Chem. 20, 141-7 (1974)

412. Grecu,I., Barbu,S.
O noua metoda de determinare a chlordiazepoxidului.
Farmacia (Bucuresti) 16, 199-204 (1968)

413. Grecu,I., Barbu,S.
Gravimetric and volumetric determination of chlordiazepoxide.
Ann.Pharm.Fr. 26, 405-8 (1968)

414. Greenblatt,D.J., Allen,M.D., Noel,B.J., Shader,R.I.
Acute overdosage with benzodiazepine derivates.
Clin.Pharmacol.Ther. 21, 497-514 (1977)

415. Greenblatt,D.J., Allen,M.D., Shader,R.I.
Toxicity of high-dose flurazepam in the elderly.
Clin.Pharmacol.Ther. 21, 355-61 (1977)

416. Greenblatt,D.J., Comer,W.H., Elliott,H.W., Shader, R.I., Knowles,J.A., Ruelius,H.W.
Clinical pharmacokinetics of lorazepam. III. Intravenous injection. Preliminary results.
J.Clin.Pharmacol. 17, 490-4 (1977)

417. Greenblatt,D.J., Harmatz,J.S., Shader,R.I.
Sex differences in diazepam protein binding in patients with renal insuffiency.
Pharmacology 16, 26-30 (1977)

418. Greenblatt,D.J., Harmatz,J.S., Stanski,D.R., Shader,R.I., Franke,K., Koch-Weser,J.
Factors influencing blood concentrations of chlordiazepoxide: A use of multiple regression analysis.
Psychopharmacology 54, 277-82 (1977)

419. Greenblatt,D.J., Joyce,Th., Comer,W.H., Knowles,J.A., Shader,R.I., Kyriakopoulos,A.A., Maclaughlin,D.S., Ruelius,H.W.
Clinical pharmacokinetics of lorazepam. II. Intramuscular injection.
Clin.Pharmacol.Ther. 21, 222-30 (1977)

420. Greenblatt,D.J., Knowles,J.A., Comer,W.H., Shader,R.I., Harmatz,J.S., Ruelius,H.W.
Clinical pharmacokinetics of lorazepam. IV. Long-term administration.
J.Clin.Pharmacol. 17, 495-500 (1977)

421. Greenblatt,D.J., Koch-Weser,J.
Clinical toxicity of chlordiazepoxide and diazepam in relation to serum albumin concentration: A report from the Boston collaborative drug surveillance program.
Eur.J.Clin.Pharmacol. 7, 259-62 (1974)

422. Greenblatt,D.J., Shader,R.I.
In: Benzodiazepines in clinical practice.
Raven Press, New York, 1974, pp. 17-42

423. Greenblatt,D.J., Shader,R.I.
Drug Therapy. (Benzodiazepines)
N.Engl.J.Med. 291, 1011-5 (1974)

424. Greenblatt,D.J., Shader,R.I., Franke,K., MacLaughlin,D.S., Ransil,B.J., Koch-Weser,J.
Kinetics of intravenous chlordiazepoxide - sex differences in drug distribution.
Clin.Pharmacol.Ther. 22, 893-903 (1977)

425. Greenblatt,D.J., Shader,R.I., Harmatz,J.S., Franke,K., Koch-Weser,J.
Influence of magnesium and aluminium hydroxide mixture on chlordiazepoxide absorption.
Clin.Pharmacol.Ther. 19, 234-9 (1976)

426. Greenblatt,D.J., Shader,R.I., Koch-Weser,J.
Pharmacokinetic determinants of the response to single doses of chlordiazepoxide.
Am.J.Psychiatry 131, 1395-7 (1974)

427. Greenblatt,D.J., Shader,R.I., Koch-Weser,J.
Safety of nitrazepam.
Lancet 1, 315-23 (1974)

428. Greenblatt,D.J., Shader,R.I., Koch-Weser,J.
Slow absorption of intramuscular chlordiazepoxide.
N.Engl.J.Med. 291, 1116-8 (1974)

429. Greenblatt,D.J., Shader,R.I., Koch-Weser,J.
Pharmacokinetics in clinical medicine: Oxazepam versus other benzodiazepines.
Dis.Nerv.Syst. 36, 6-13 (1975)

430. Greenblatt,D.J., Shader,R.I., Koch-Weser,J.
Clinical pharmacokinetics of chlordiazepoxide.
In: Gottschalk,L.A., Merlis,S., ED. Pharmacokinetics of Psychoactive Drugs, New York, Spectrum Publications, 1976

431. Greenblatt,D.J., Shader,R.I., Koch-Weser,J., Franke,K.
Clinical pharmacokinetics of chlordiazepoxid.
Psychopharmacol.Bull.11, 34-5 (1975)

432. Greenblatt,D.J., Schillings,R.T., Kyriakopoulos,A.A., Shader,R.I., Sisenwine,S.F., Knowles,J.A., Ruelius,H.W.
Clinical pharmacokinetics of lorazepam. I. Absorption and disposition of oral ^{14}C-lorazepam.
Clin.Pharmacol.Ther. 20, 329-41 (1976)

433. Gregg,J.M., Ryan,D.E., Levin,K.H.
The amnesic actions of diazepam.
J.Oral.Surg. 32, 651-64 (1974)

434. Greizerstein,H.B., Wojtowicz,C.
Simultaneous determination of chlordiazepoxide and its N-demethyl metabolite in 50 ul blood samples by high pressure liquid chromatography.
Anal.Chem. 49, 2235-6 (1977)

435. Grieco,C., Silipo,C., Vittoria,A.
Structure-activity correlations for antibacterial 1,5-benzodiazepine derivates on gram-positive cells.
Farmaco (Sci) 32, 909-22 (1977)

436. Groot,de,G., Maes,R.A.A., Defoort,P., Thiery,M.
Placental transfer of lorazepam.
IRCS Med.Sci. 3, 594 (1975)

437. Groot,de,G., Maes,R.A.A., Lemmens,H.H.J.
Determination of lorazepam in plasma by electron capture GLC.
Arch.Toxicol. 35, 229-34 (1976)

438. Grom,O.L., Komar,V.S., Ladizhinskaia,N.S.
Spectrophotometric quantitative analysis of the prepared drugs diazepam, oxazepam and nitrazepam.
Farm.Z.H. 1976, 82-3

439. Gros,P., Raveux,R.
Etude de l'excretion du chlorazêpate dipotassique et de ses metabolites urinaires. Fractionnement, identification et dosage des metabolites urinaires.
Bull.Chim.Thêr. 4, 312-22 (1969)

440. Grüner,O.
Schädigung durch Alkohol oder alkoholähnliche Körper unter besonderer Berücksichtigung des Straßenverkehrs.
In: Gerichtliche Medizin, Bd. 2, S. 1023, 2. Aufl., hrsgb. von B.Mueller.
Berlin -Heidelberg-New York: Springer 1975

441. Guaitani,A., Marcucci,F., Garattini,S.
Increased aggression and toxicity in grouped male mice treated with tranquilizing benzodiazepines.
Psychopharmacologia 19, 241-5 (1971)

442. Guelan,P.J.M. et al.
Quantitative determination of the benzodiazepines by GLC.
Scan. 2, 4 (1973)

443. Guilbaud,P., Bourdeau,M., Sari,J.C., Briand,C.
Diazepam-human serum-albumin interaction study by a measure of fluorescence quenching.
Stud.Biophy. 69, 193-208 (1978)

444. Habermann,E., Löffler,H.
Spezielle Pharmakologie als Basis der Arzneitherapie.
Berlin-Heidelberg-New York: Springer 1975

445. Hackman,M.R., Brooks,M.A., Silva,de,J.A.F.
Determination of chlordiazepoxide hydrochloride (librium) and ist major metabolites in plasma by differential pulse polarography.
Anal.Chem. 46, 1075-82 (1974)

446. Haefelfinger,P.
Empfindlicher Nachweis von Substanzen mit primären Aminogruppen auf Dünnschichtplatten.
J.Chromatogr. 48, 184-90 (1970)

447. Haefelfinger,P.
Determination of nanogram amounts of primary aromatic amines and nitro compounds in blood and plasma.
J.Chromatogr. 111, 323-9 (1975)

448. Haefelfinger,P.
Determination of bromazepam in plasma by quantitative thin-layer chromatography.
Chromatographia 11, 10-3 (1977)

449. Haefely,W.E.
Synaptic pharmacology of barbiturates and benzodiazepines.
Agents Actions 7, 353-9 (1977)

450. Haerten,K., Poettgen,W.
Leukopenia following benzodiazepine derivates.
Med.Welt 26, 1712-4 (1975)

451. Haffner,J.F.W., Mørland,J., Setekleiv,J., Strømsaether,C.E., Danielsen,A., Frivik,P.T., Dybing,F.
Mental and psychomotor effects of diazepam and ethanol.
Acta Pharmacol.Toxicol. 32, 161-78 (1973)

452. Hailey,D.M.
Chromatography of 1,4-benzodiazepines.
Chromat.Rev. 18, 527 (1974)

453. Hailey,D.M.
Chromatography of the 1,4-benzodiazepines.
J.Chromatogr. 98, 527-68 (1974)

454. Hailey,D.M.
Gas chromatographic analysis of medazepam and its metabolites using an electrolytic conductivity detector.
J.Chromatogr. 100, 49-54 (1974)

455. Hailey,D.M., Cree,J.E., Meyer,J.
Perinatal metabolism of diazepam.
Brit.Med.J. 2, 670 (1974)

456. Hailey,D.M., Howard,A.G., Nickless,G.
Gas-chromatographic analysis of medazepam and its metabolites using an electrolytic conductivity detector.
J.Chromatogr. 100, 49 (1974)

457. Hall,S.C., Ovassapian,A.
Apnea after intravenous diazepam therapy.
J.Amer.Med.Ass. 238, 1052-5 (1977)

458. Halvorsen,S., Jacobsen,E.
Electroreduction and polarographic determination of nitrazepam in serum.
Anal.Chim.Acta 59, 127-36 (1972)

459. Han,W.W., Yakatan,G.J., Maness,D.D.
Kinetics and mechanisms of hydrolysis of 1,4-benzodiazepines I: Chlordiazepoxide and demoxepam.
J.Pharm.Sci. 65, 1198-204 (1976)

460. Han.W.W., Yakatan,G.J., Maness,D.D.
Kinetics and mechanisms of hydrolysis of 1,4-benzodiazepines II: Oxazepam and diazepam.
J.Pharm.Sci. 66, 573-7 (1977)

461. Hanna,S.M.
A case of oxazepam dependence.
Brit.J.Psychiatry 120, 443-5 (1972)

462. Hansson,O., Tonnby,B.
Serious psychological symptoms caused by clonazepam
Lakartidningen 13, 1209-10 (1976)

463. Haot,J., Djahanguiri,B., Richelle,M.
Action protectrice du chlordiazepoxide sur l'ulcère de contrainte chez le rat.
Arch.Int.Pharmacodyn.Ther. 148, 557-9 (1964)

464. Haram,K.
Floppy infant syndrome and maternal diazepam.
Lancet 2, 612-3 (1977)

465. Haram,K., Sagen,N., Brandt,R.D.
Transplacental passage of diazepam following intravenous injection immediately prior to operative vaginal delivery.
Int.J.Gynaecol.Obstet. 14, 545-9 (1976)

466. Harris,T.H.
Methamino diazepoxide (preliminary communications).
J.Amer.Med.Ass. 172, 1162-3 (1960)

467. Harry,T.V.
Oxazepam dependence.
Brit.J.Psychiatry 121, 235-6 (1972)

468. Hasegawa,M., Matsubara,I.
Metabolic fates of flurazepam. I. Gas chromatographic determination of flurazepam and its metabolites in human urine and blood using electron-capture-detector.
Chem.Pharm.Bull. (Tokyo) 23, 1826-33 (1975)

469. Hasegawa,M., Takai,H., Matsubara,I.
Metabolic fate of flurazepam. II: A new potent metabolite obtained by in vitro liver drug-metabolizing enzyme system.
J.Pharm.Sci. 64, 1732-3 (1975)

470. Hassall,C.H., Holmes,S.W., Johnson,W.H., Krohn,A., Smithen,C.E., Thomas,W.A.
Peptido-aminobenzophenones - Novel latentiated benzo-1,4-diazepines.
Experientia 33, 1492-3 (1977)

471. Hayes,S.L., Pablo,G., Radomski,G., Palmer,R.F.
Ethanol and oral diazepam absorption.
New Engl.J.Med. 296, 186-9 (1977)

472. Hegarty,J.E., Dundee,J.W.
Sequelae after the intraveneous injection of three benzodiazepines - diazepam, lorazepam, and flunitrazepam.
Brit.Med.J. 2, 1384-5 (1977)

473. Hegarty,J.E., Dundee,J.W.
Local sequelea following the i.v. injection of three benzodiazepines (proceedings).
Brit.J.Anaesth. 50, 78-9 (1978)

474. Heidbrink,V., Mallach,H.J., Moosmayer,A.
Zur gaschromatographischen Analytik der Benzodiazepine. 2. Mitteilung: Diazepam und seine Metabolite.
Arzneim.-Forsch. (Drug Res.) 25, 516-7 (1975)

475. Heise,G.A., Boff,E.
Taming action of chlordiazepoxide.
Fed.Proc. 20, 393 (1961)

476. Helstroem,B. et al.
Plasma levels of diazepam after parenteral and rectal administration in children.
Epilepsia 16, 27 (1975)

477. Hendel,J.
Cumulation in cerebrospinal fluid of the N-desmethyl metabolite after long-term treatment with diazepam in man.
Acta Pharmacol.Toxicol. 37, 17-22 (1975)

478. Hepner,G.W., Vesell,E.S., Lipton,A., Harvey,H.A., Wilkinson,G.R., Schenker,S.
Disposition of aminopyrine, antipyrine, diazepam, and indocyanine green in breath test and correlations in drug elimination.
J.Lab.Clin.Med. 90, 440-56 (1977)

479. Hermans,R.B., Kamp,P.E.
A scheme for the identification of sedatives and some psychotherapeutics in toxicological analysis.
Pharm.Weekbl. 102, 1123-41 (1967)

480. Hester,J.B., Duchamp,D.J., Chidester,C.G.
A synthetic approach to new 1,4-benzodiazepine derivates.
Tetrahedron Lett. 1609-12 (1971)

481. Hetland,L.B., Knowlton,D.A., Couri,D.
A method for the detection of drugs at therapeutic dosages in human urine using adsorption column chromatography and thin layer chromatography.
Clin.Chim.Acta 36, 473-8 (1972)

482. Heuschele,W.P.
Chlordiazepoxide for calming zoo animals.
J.Amer.Vet.Med.Assoc. 139, 996-8 (1961)

483. Hewick,D.S., Shaw,V.
Tissue distribution of radioactivity after injection of ^{14}C-nitrazepam in young and old rats.
J.Pharm.Pharmacol. 30, 318-9 (1978)

484. Heyndrickx,A., Leenheer,de,A.
Identification of 1,4-benzodiazepines in biological samples of man.
Farmaceutisch Tijdschrift voor Belgie 48, 1-9 (1971)

485. Hillestad,L., Hansen,T., Melsom,H., Drivenes,A.
Diazepam metabolism in normal man.
I. Serum concentrations and clinical effects after intraveneous, intramuscular, and oral administration.
Clin.Pharmacol.Ther. 16, 479-84 (1974)

486. Hillestad,L., Hansen,T., Melsom,H.
Diazepam metabolism in normal man.
II. Serum concentrations and clinical effect after oral administration and cumulation.
Clin.Pharmacol.Ther. 16, 485-9 (1974)

487. Hindmarch,I.
A repeated dose comparison of three benzodiazepine derivates (nitrazepam, flurazepam and flunitrazepam) on subjective appraisals of sleep and measures of psychomotor performance the morning following night-time medication.
Acta Psychiatr.Scand. 56, 373-81 (1977)

488. Hindmarch,I., Hanks,G.W., Hewett,A.J.
Clobazam, a 1,5-benzodiazepine, and car driving ability.
Brit.J.Clin.Pharmacol. 4, 573-8 (1977)

489. Hoffman,D.J., Chun,A.H.
GLC-determination of plasma drug levels after oral administration of chlorazepate potassium salts.
J.Pharm.Sci. 64, 1668-71 (1975)

490. Hokari,S., Manzo,L., De Barnardi,M., Bert,E.F.
Organotropism of oxazepam and of its glucuronoderivate in the guinea-pig at the maternal and fetal level.
Bo..Soc.Ital.Biol.Sper. 43, 861-4 (1967)

491. Hollister,L.E.
Overdose of psychotherapeutic drugs.
Clin.Pharmacol.Ther. 7, 142-6 (1966)

492. Hollister,L.E.
Withdrawal from benzodiazepine therapy.
J.Amer.Med.Ass. 237, 1432-4 (1977)

493. Hollister,L.E., Motzenbecker,F.P., Degan,R.O.
Withdrawal reactions from chlordiazepoxide (librium).
Psychopharmacologia 2, 63-8 (1961)

494. Hollister,L.E., Overall,J.E., Pokorny,A.D., Shelton,J.
Acetophenazine and diazepam in anxious depressions.
Arch.Gen.Psychiat. 24, 273-8 (1971)

495. Howard,A.G., Nickless,G., Hailey,D.M.
A rapid gas chromatographic method for the determination of diazepam and metabolites in body fluids.
J.Chromatogr. 90, 325-9 (1974)

496. Howard,P.J.
The stability of diazepam in plasma samples when stored under varying conditions.
J.Pharm.Pharmacol. 30, 136 (1978)

497. Howard,P.J. et al.
Estimation of plasma diazepam. Critique of a method using gas-liquid chromatography and benzene extraction.
Anaesthesia 30, 159-63 (1975)

498. Howard,P.J., Lilburn,J.K., Dundee,J.W., Tower,W., McIlroy,P.D.
Estimation of plasma lorazepam by gas-liquid chromatography and a benzene extraction.
Anaesthesia 32, 767-70 (1977)

499. Howard,P.J., Lilburn,J.K., Horellou,M.F., Mathe,D., Feiss,P., Dundee,J.W., Tower,W., McIlroy,P.D.A.
Estimation of plasma lorazepam by gas-liquid chromatography and benzene extraction.
Anaesthesia 33, 67-8 (1978)

500. Huch,R., Huch,A.
Respiratory depression after tranquillizers.
Lancet 2, 1267 (1974)

501. Hudson,M.W.
Drug combinations for anaesthesia.
Brit.Med.J. 4, 345 (1974)

502. Huettemann,R.E., Shroff,A.P.
High-pressure liquid chromatographic analysis of triflubazam und its metabolites in human and animal blood and urine.
J.Pharm.Sci. 64, 1339-42 (1975)

503. Hughes,F.W., Forney,R.B.
Combined effects of alcohol and other drugs.
Quart.J.Stud.Alcohol 25, 1085-6 (1964)

504. Hughes,F.W., Forney,R.B., Richards,A.B.
Comparative effect in human subjects of chlordiazepoxide, diazepam, and placebo on mental and physical performance.
Clin.Pharmacol.Ther. 6, 139-45 (1965)

505. Hulshoff,A., Perrin,J.H.
A comparison of the determination of partition coefficients of 1,4-benzodiazepines by high performance liquid chromatography and thin layer chromatography.
J.Chromatogr. 129, 249-63 (1976)

506. Hvidberg,E.F.
Plasma levels, antiepileptics and antidepressants.
Arzneim.-Forsch. (Drug Res.) 26, 1259 (1976)

507. Hvidberg,E.F., Sjoe,O.
Clinical pharmacokinetic experiences with clonazepam.
In: Schneider,H. et al., ED. Clinical Pharmacology of Anti-epileptic drugs. Berlin, Springer, 1975.

508. Idänpään-Heikkilä,J.E., Jouppila,P.I., Puolakka,J.O., Vorne,M.S.
Placental transfer and fetal metabolism of diazepam in early human pregnancy.
Amer.J.Obstet.Gynecol. 109, 1011-6 (1971)

509. Idänpään-Heikkilä,J.E., Taska,R.J., Allen,H.A., Schoolar,J.C.
Autoradiographic study of the fate of diazepam-^{14}C in the monkey brain.
Arch.Int.Pharmacodyn.Ther. 194, 68-77 (1971)

510. Iisalo,E., Kangas,L., Ruikka,I.
Pharmacokinetics of nitrazepam in young volunteers and aged patients (proceedings).
Brit.J.Clin.Pharmacol. 4, 646-64 (1977)

511. Illing,H.P., Yeomans,M.A., Rising,P.A., Johnson,P.
Enzymic desalkylation of a substituted aminoacetamidobenzophenone and cyclization to the correspondending benzodiazepine in vitro.
Xenobiotica 7, 439-54 (1977)

512. Impallomeni,M., Ezzat,R.
Hypothermia associated with nitrazepam administration.
Brit.Med.J. 1, 223-4 (1976)

513. Inaba,T., Tsutsumi,E., Mahon,W.A., Kalow,W.
Biliary excretion of diazepam in the rat.
Drug Metab.Dispos. 2, 429-32 (1974)

514. Ippen,H.
Index Pharmacorum, 2. unveränd.Aufl.
Stuttgart: Thieme 1974

515. Irvine,R.E.
Hypothermia due to diazepam.
Brit.Med.J. 2, 1007 (1966)

516. Ishizumi,K., Inaba,S., Yamamoto,H.
Benzodiazepines VIII. Diborane reduction of benzodiazepin-2-ones.
J.Org.Chem. 37, 4111-3 (1972)

517. Jabłońska,J.K., Knobloch,K., Majka,J., Wisniewska-Knypl,J.
Stimulatory effects of chlordiazepoxide, diazepam and oxazepam on the drug-metabolizing enzymes in microsomes.
Toxicology 5,103-11(1975)

518. Jackson,S.L.
Nitrazepam und diazepam.
Brit.Med.J. 2, 300-1 (1976)

519. Jacobsen,E., Jacobsen,T.V.
Electrochemical reduction of chlordiazepoxide at mercury electrodes.
Anal.Chim.Acta 55, 293-301 (1971)

520. Jacobsen,E., Jacobsen,T.V.
Polarographic determination of diazepam in pharmaceuticals.
Anal.Chim.Acta 60, 472-4 (1972)

521. Jacobsen,E., Jacobsen,T.V., Rojahn,T.
The determination of diazepam in serum by differential pulse polarography.
Anal.Chim.Acta 64, 473-6 (1973)

522. Jain,N.C., Kirk,P.L.
Systematic applications of gas-liquid chromatography in toxicology.
I. Extraction procedure and the alkaloids.
Microchem.J. 12, 229-72 (1967)

523. Jatlow,P.
Ultraviolet spectrophotometric measurement of chlordiazepoxid in plasma.
Clin.Chem. 18, 516-8 (1972)

524. Jeffery,D.I., Whitfield,M.F.
Lorazepam poisoning.
Brit.Med.J. 4, 719 (1974)

525. Jejurikar,S.G., Lowell,C.
Benzodiazepines related deaths.
Bull.Int.Ass.Foren.Toxicol. 12, (1) 14-6 (1976)

526. Jenner,F.A., Kerry,R.J.
Comparison of diazepam, chlordiazepoxide, and amylobarbitone (a multidose double-blind cross-over study).
Dis.Nerv.Syst. 28, 245-9 (1967)

527. Jick,H.
Clinical depression of the central nervous system due to diazepam and chlordiazepoxide in relation to cigarette smoking and age.
New England J.Med. 288, 277-80 (1973)

528. Johnson,D.N.
Effect of diazepam on food consumption in rats.
Psychopharmacology 56, 111-3 (1978)

529. Johnson,J., Padilla,B.G., Carter,J., Holt,J.H., Ozawa,T.
Adverse effects of flurazepam in a hemodialysis patient.
J.Am.Assoc.Nephrol.Nurs.Techn. 4, 93-5 (1977)

530. Jommi,G., Manito,P., Silanos,M.A.
Metabolism of diazepam in rabbits.
Arch.Biochem.Biophys. 108, 562-8 (1964)

531. Jones,C., Heveran,J.E., Senkowski,B.Z.
Determination of organically bound fluorine using sodium biphenyl reagent and a fluoride-specific ion electrode.
J.Pharm.Sci. 60, 1036-9 (1971)

532. Jori,A., Prestini,P.E., Pugliatti,C.
Effect of diazepam and chlordiazepoxide on the metabolism of other drugs.
J.Pharm.Pharmacol. 21, 387-90 (1969)

533. Julien,R.M.
Cerebellar involvement in the antiepileptic action of diazepam.
Neuropharmacology 11, 683-91 (1972)

534. Juul,P.
Diazepam (valium). II. Diazepam as a hypnotic. 34 cases of poisoning.
Ugeskr.Laeger 128, 112-5 (1966)

535. Juul,P.
Diazepam (valium). A method for its quantitative determination in serum.
Ugeskr. Laeger 128, 115-8 (1966)

536. Kähler,H.J.
Störwirkungen von Psychopharmaka und Analgetika.
Stuttgart: Wiss.Verlagsges. 1967

537. Kaistha,K.K.
Drug abuse screening programs: Detection procedures, development tests, street-sample analysis and field tests.
J.Pharm.Sci. 61, 655-78 (1972)

538. Kaistha,K.K., Jaffe,J.H.
TLC-techniques for identification of narcotics, barbiturates and CNS-stimulants in a drug abuse screening program.
J.Pharm.Sci. 61, 679-89 (1972)

539. Kalina,R.K.
Diazepam: Its role in a prison setting.
Dis.Nerv.Syst. 25, 101 (1964)

540. Kamm,G., Baier,R.
Nachweis von Chlordiazepoxid und Diazepam in kleinen Blutmengen.
Arzneim.-Forsch. (Drug Res.) 19, 213-5 (1969)

541. Kamm,G., Kelm,R.
Quantitativer Nachweis von Oxazepam im Plasma bei einmaliger und längerer Verabreichung.
Arzneim.-Forsch. (Drug Res.) 19, 1659-62 (1969)

542. Kangas,L.
Comparison of two gas-liquid chromatographic methods for the determination of nitrazepam in plasma.
J.Chromatogr. 136, 259-70 (1977)

543. Kangas,L., Kanto,J., Erkkola,R.
Transfer of nitrazepam across the human placenta.
Eur.J.Clin.Pharmacol. 12, 355-7 (1977)

544. Kangas,L., Kanto,J., Forsstroem,J., Isalo,E.
The protein binding of diazepam and N-demethyl-diazepam in patients with poor renal function.
Clin.Nephrol. 5, 114-8 (1976)

545. Kangas,L., Kanto,J., Siirtola,T., Pekkarinen,A.
Cerebrospinal-fluid concentrations of nitrazepam in man.
Acta Pharmacol.Toxicol. 41, 74-9 (1977)

546. Kangas,L., Kanto,J., Syvaelahti,E.
Plasma nitrazepam concentrations after acute intake and their correlation to sedation and serum growth hormone levels.
Acta Pharmacol.Toxicol. 41, 65-73 (1977)

547. Kangas,L., Pekkarinen,A., Sourander,C., Raijola,E.
A comparative gaschromatography study on absorption of diazepam tablets in man. A gaschromatographic study with ^{63}Ni-detector by determining diazepam concentrations in plasma.
Ann.Clin.Res. 6, 12-20 (1974)

548. Kanto,J.
Plasma concentrations of diazepam and its metabolites after peroral, intramuscular and rectal administration. Correlation between plasma concentration and sedatory effect of diazepam.
Int.J.Clin.Pharmacol.Biopharm. 12, 427-32 (1975)

549. Kanto,J., Erkkola,R.
The feto-maternal distribution of diazepam in early human pregnancy.
Ann.Chir.Gynaecol.Fenn. 63, 489-91 (1974)

550. Kanto.J., Erkkola,R., Sellman,R.
Accumulation of diazepam and N-demethyldiazepam in the fetal blood during the labour.
Ann.Clin.Res. 5, 375-9 (1973)

551. Kanto,J., Erkkola,R., Sellman,R.
Perinatal metabolism of diazepam.
Brit.Med.J. 1, 641-2 (1974)

552. Kanto,J., Iisalo,E., Lehtinen,V., Salminen,J.
The concentrations of diazepam and its metabolites in the plasma after an acute and chronic administration.
Psychopharmacologia 36, 123-31 (1974)

553. Kanto,J., Kangas,L., Siirtola,T.
Cerebrospinal-fluid concentrations of diazepam and its metabolites in man.
Acta Pharmacol.Toxicol. 36, 328-34 (1975)

554. Kanto,J.H., Pihlajamaki,K.K., Iisalo,E.U.
Concentrations of diazepam in adipose tissue of children.
Brit.J.Anaesth. 46, 168 (1974)

555. Kaplan,S.A., Alexander,K., Jack,M.L., Puglisi,C.V., de Silva,J.A.F., Lee,T.L., Weinfeld,R.E.
Pharmacokinetic profiles of clonazepam in dog and humans and of flunitrazepam in dog.
J.Pharm.Sci. 63, 527-32 (1974)

556. Kaplan,S.A., Jack,M.L., Alexander,K., Weinfeld,R.E.
Pharmacokinetic profile of diazepam in man following single intravenous and oral and chronic oral administrations.
J.Pharm.Sci. 62, 1789-96 (1973)

557. Kaplan,S.A., Jack,M.L., Weinfeld,R.E., Glover,W., Weissmann,L., Cutler,S.
Biopharmaceutical and clinical pharmacokinetic profile of bromazepam.
J.Pharmacok.Biopharm. 4, 1-16 (1976)

558. Kaplan,S.A., Lewis,M., Schwartz,M.A., Postma,E., Cutler,S., Abruzzo,C.W., Lee,T.L., Weinfeld,R.E.
Pharmacokinetik model for chlordiazepoxide HCl in the dog.
J.Pharm.Sci. 59, 1569-74 (1970)

559. Kaplan,S.A., de Silva,J.A.F.
Blood level profile in man following chronic administration of flurazepam hydrochloride.
J.Pharm.Sci. 62,1932-5 (1973)

560. Kaplan,S.A.F., de Silva,J.A.F., Jack,M.L., Alexander,K., Strojny,N., Weinfeld,R.W., Puglisi,C.V., Weissmann,L.
Blood level profile in man following chronic oral administration of flurazepam hydrochloride.
J.Pharm.Sci. 62, 1932-5 (1973)

561. Karim,A.K., Evans,D.A.
Polymorphic acetylation of nitrazepam.
J.Med.Genet. 13, 17-9 (1976)

562. Kassau,E.
Das Verhalten einiger Psychopharmaka bei der Mikrosublimation.
Dtsch.Apoth.-Ztg. 113, 1332-4 (1973)

563. Kaufman,A., Brickner,P.W.
Tranquilizer control.
J.Amer.Med.Ass. 224, 1190 (1973)

564. Kawai,J.
Toxicity of nitrazepam.
Psychiatr.Neurol.Jpn. 76, 667-75 (1974)

565. Kelly,D., Brown,C.C., Shafter,J.W.
A controlled physiological, clinical and psychological evaluation of chlordiazepoxide.
Brit.J.Psychiatry 115, 1387-92 (1969)

566. Kerry,R.J., Jenner,F.A., Pearson,I.B.
A double blind cross over comparison of Ro-3350, bromazepam, diazepam (valium) and chlordiazepoxide (librium) in the treatment of neurotic anxiety.
Psychosomatics 13, 122-4 (1972)

567. Kesson,C.M., Gray,J.M.B., Lawson,D.H.
Benzodiazepine drugs in general medical patients.
Brit.Med.J. 1, 680-2 (1976)

568. Kielholz,P., Pöldinger,W.
Pharmaka, Drogenabhängigkeit und Verkehr.
Schweiz.Med.Wschr. 97, 1-8 (1967)

569. Kielholz,P., Pöldinger,W.
Pharmaka, Drogenabhängigkeit und Verkehr.
Schweiz.Med.Wschr. 97, 49-54 (1967)

570. Kielholz,P., Goldborg,L., Im Obersteg,J., Poeldinger,W., Ramseyer,A., Schmid,P.
Straßenverkehr, Tranquilizer und Alkohol.
Deut.Med.Wochenschr. 92, 1525-31 (1967)

571. Killam,E.K., Matsuzaki, Killam,K.F.
Effects of chronic administration of benzodiazepines on epileptic seizures and brain electrical activity in Papio papio.
In: (362) pp. 443-60

572. Kimmel,H.B., Walkenstein,S.S.
Oxazepam excretion by chlordiazepoxide-^{14}C-dosed-dogs.
J.Pharm.Sci. 56, 538-9 (1967)

573. Kinawi,A., Baumgartl,I.
Studies on the interactions of phenprocoumon with chlordiazepoxide in rats.
J.Clin.Chem.Clin.Biochem. 15, 425-9 (1977)

574. Kinawi,A., Döring,D., Witte,I.
Reaktionskinetische Untersuchungen zur Entstehung von 7-Chlor-2N-nitrosomethylamino-5-phenyl-3H-1,4-benzodiazepin-4-oxid.
Arzneim.-Forsch. (Drug Res.) 27, 747 (1977)

575. Kinawi,A., Onken,A., Rozycka,B., Koenig,W.
Untersuchungen zur Nitrosierbarkeit von Chlordiazepoxid unter physiologischen Bedingungen.
Arzneim.-Forsch. (Drug Res.) 27, 363-7 (1977)

576. Kingstone,E., Villeneuve,A., Kossatz,I.
Prazepam in the treatment of anxiety and tension; a clinical study of a new benzodiazepine derivative.
Curr.Ther.Res. 8, 159-62 (1966)

577. Kingstone,E., Villeneuve,A., Kossatz,I.
Double-blind evaluation of diazepam, chlordiazepoxide and placebo in non-psychotic patients with anxiety and tension: Some methodological considerations.
Curr.Ther.Res. 11, 106-14 (1969)

578. Kleinrok,Z., Przegalinski,E., Czuczwar,S.
Participation of 5-hydroxytryptamine in anticonvulsive action of benzodiazepines.
Pol.J.Pharmacol.Pharm. 29, 385-91 (1977)

579. Klotz,U.
Wichtige Faktoren, die beim Menschen die Verteilung und Elimination von Valium beeinflussen.
Important factors determining human distribution and elimination of diazepam.
Fortschr.Med. 95, 1958-64 (1977)

580. Klotz,U., Antonin,K.H., Bieck,P.
Proceedings: Pharmacokinetics and protein bindung of diazepam in man and different species.
Naunyn-Schmied.-Arch.Pharmacol. 287, 90 (1975)

581. Klotz,U., Antonin,K.H., Bieck,P.R.
Hepatic elimination of diazepam and its active metabolites.
Arzneim.-Forsch. (Drug Res.) 26, 1265-6 (1976)

582. Klotz,U., Antonin,K.H., Bieck,P.R.
Comparison of the pharmacokinetics of diazepam after single and subchronic doses.
Eur.J.Clin.Pharmacol. 10, 121-6 (1976)

583. Klotz,U., Antonin,K.H., Bieck,P.R.
Pharmacokinetics and plasma binding of diazepam in man, dog, rabbit, guinea pig and rat.
J.Pharmacol.Exp.Ther. 199, 67-73 (1976)

584. Klotz,U., Antonin,H.K., Bieck,P.
Food intake and plasma binding of diazepam.
Brit.J.Clin.Pharmacol. 4, 85-6 (1977)

585. Klotz,U., Antonin,K.H., Bruegel,H., Bieck,P.R.
Disposition of diazepam and its major metabolite desmethyldiazepam in patients with liver disease.
Clin.Pharmacol.Ther. 21, 430-6 (1977)

586. Klotz,U., Avant,G.R., Hoyumpa,A., Schenker,S., Wilkinson,G.R.
Proceedings: Pharmacokinetics of diazepam in man.
Naunyn-Schmied.-Arch.Pharmacol. 282, 48 (1974)

587. Klotz,U., Avant,G.R., Hoyumpa,A., Schenker,S., Wilkinson,G.R.
The effects of age and liver disease on the disposition and elimination of diazepam in adult man.
J.Clin.Invest. 55, 347-59 (1975)

588. Klupp,H., Kähling,J.
The pharmacological action of 7-chloro-1,3-dihydro-3-hydroxy-5-phenyl-2H-1,4-benzodiazepine-2-one.
Arzneim.-Forsch. (Drug Res.) 15, 359-65 (1965)

589. Knaess,K.
Diazepam-glaucoma and myasthenia gravis.
Tidsskr.Nor.Laegeforen 91, 521-2 (1971)

590. Knaess,K.
Drugs and traffic security - once more.
Tidsskr.Nor.Laegeforen 91, 1899-901 (1971)

591. Knop,H.J. et al.
Detection of clonazepam in plasma by GLC.
Pharm.Weekbl. 110, 297 (1974)

592. Knop,H.J., van der Kleijn,E., Edmunds,L.C.
Pharmacokinetics of clonazepam in man and laboratory animals.
In: Schneider,H. et al. ED, Clinical Pharmacology of anti-epileptic drugs. Berlin, Springer, 1975

593. Knorpp,K.
Über den Einfluß von Diazepam (VALIUM[R]) auf den hämorrhagischen Schock bei Kaninchen.
Naunyn-Schmied.-Arch.Pharmacol. 267, 457-67 (1970)

594. Knowles,J.A., Comer,W.H., Ruelius,H.W.
Disposition of 7-chlor-5-(o-chlorphenyl)-1,3-dihydro-3-hydroxy-2H-1,4-benzodiazepin-2-on (lorazepam) in humans. Determination of the drug by electron capture gas chromatography.
Arzneim.-Forsch. (Drug Res.) 21, 1055-9 (1971)

595. Knowles,J.A., Ruelius,H.W.
Absorption and excretion of oxazepam in humans.
Arzneim.-Forsch. (Drug Res.) 22, 687-92 (1972)

596. Kobiela-Krzyżanowska,A.
Polarographic determination in whole blood of nitro-derivatives of benzodiazepine in acute poisoning.
Pharmazie 31, 649-50 (1976)

597. Kobiela-Krzyżanowska,A.
Polarographic-determinations of nimetazepam in serum and whole blood.
Pharmazie 32, 693-5 (1977)

598. Koechlin,B.A., D'Arconte,L.
Determination of chlordiazepoxide (librium) and of a metabolite of lactam character in plasma of humans, dogs and rats by a specific spectrofluorometric micro method.
Analyt.Biochem. 5, 195-207 (1963)

599. Koechlin,B.A., Schwartz,M.A.
The metabolic fate of chlordiazepoxide.
Fed.Proc. 20, 171 (1961)

600. Koechlin,B.A., Schwartz,M.A., Krol,G., Oberhansli,W.
The metabolic fate of ^{14}C-labelled chlordiazepoxide in man, in the dog and in the rat.
J.Pharm.Exp.Ther. 148, 399-411 (1965)

601. Kohler,E.
Über geeignete mikrochemische Nachweismethoden von Medazepam als Voraussetzung für pharmakokinetische Untersuchungen.
Inaug.Diss. Tübingen 1970

602. Kokoski,F.J., Hamner,S., Shiplet,M.
Detection of the use of methaqualone and benzodiazepines in urine screening programs.
Natl.Conf.Methadone Treat.Proc. 2, 1073-8 (1973)

603. Korsgaard,S.
Abuse of lorazepam (temesta).
Ugeskr.Laeger 138, 164-5 (1976)

604. Korttila,K., Kangas,L.
Unchanged protein binding and the increase of serum diazepam levels after food intake.
Acta Pharmacol.Toxicol. 40, 241-6 (1977)

605. Korttila,K., Linnoila,M.
Recovery and skills related to driving after intraveneous sedation: Dose-response relationship with diazepam.
Brit.J.Anaesth. 47, 457-63 (1975)

606. Korttila,K., Linnoila,M.
Amnesic action of and skills related to driving after intravenous flunitrazepam.
Acta Anaesthesiol.Scand. 20, 160-8 (1976)

607. Korttila,K., Sothman,A., Andersson,P.
Polyethylene glycol as a solvent for diazepam: Bioavailability and clinical effects after intramuscular administration, comparison of oral, intramuscular and rectal administration and precipitation from intravenous solutions.
Acta Pharmacol.Toxicol. 39, 104-17 (1976)

608. Kratzsch,K.H., Büttner,W., Reinhardt,G.
Intrahepatic cholestasis following chlordiazepoxide -- Contribution to the differential diagnosis of drug jaundice.
Z.Gesamte Inn.Med. 27, 408-11 (1972)

609. Krugers-Dagneaux,P.G.L.C.
Kwalitatieve aantoning van benzodiazepinepreparaten en / of metabolieten daarvan in urine.
Pharm.Weekbl. 108, 1025-37 (1973)

610. Krugers-Dagneaux,P.G.L.C., Klein-Elhorst,J.T.
Detection of a flurazepam metabolite in urine.
Pharm.Weekbl. 110, 1-9(1975)

611. Krugers-Dagneaux,P.G.L.C., Klein-Elhorst,J.T.
Detection of clonazepam and its metabolites in urine and plasma.
Pharm.Weekbl. 110, 419 (1975)

612. Kryspin-Exner,K.
Misuse of benzodiazepin derivates in alcoholics.
Brit.J.Addict. 61, 283-90 (1966)

613. Kvetina,J., Marcucci,F., Fanelli,R.
Metabolism of diazepam in isolated perfused liver of rat und mouse.
J.Pharm.Pharmacol. 20, 807-8 (1968)

614. Kyriakopoulos,A.A.
Bioavailability of lorazepam in humans.
In: Gottschalk,L.A., Merlis,S., ED. Pharmacokinetics of psychoactive drugs. New York, Spectrum Publications 1976

615. Lader,M.H., Wing,L.
Comparative bioassay of chlordiazepoxide and amylobarbitone sodium therapies in patients with anxiety states using physiological and clinical measures.
Psychiatry 28, 414-25 (1965)

616. Lafargue,P., Couture,J.C.
Recherche et identification dans les urines des derivées de la 1,4-benzodiazepines.
Ann.Biol.Clin. (Paris) 32, 443-6 (1974)

617. Lafargue,P., Meunier,J., Lemontey,Y.
Intérêt de la chromatographie sur couche mince d'adsorbant pou l'identification en toxicologie d'urgence des benzodiazépines-1,4 utilisées en therapeutique.
J.Chromatogr. 62, 423-9 (1971)

618. Lahtinen,U., Lahtinen,A., Pekkola,P.
The effect of nitrazepam on manual skill, grip strength, and reaction time with special reference to subjective evaluation of effects on sleep.
Acta Pharmacol.Toxicol. 42, 130-4 (1978)

619. Lai,A.A., Levy,R.H.
Pharmacokinetic profile of clonazepam in rhesus monkey.
J.Pharm.Sci. 67, 295-9 (1978)

620. Lal,S., Sourkes,T.L., Missala,K.
The effect of certain tranquilisers, chlorpromazine metabolites and diethyldithiocarbamate on tissue amphetamine levels in the rat.
Arch.Int.Pharmacodyn.Ther. 207, 122-30 (1974)

621. Lalli,A.F.
The use of chlordiazepoxide hydrochloride (librium) in preparation for urography.
J.Can.Assoc.Radiol. 25, 44-6 (1974)

622. Lampe,W.T.
Lactation following psychotropic agents.
Metabolism 16, 257-8 (1967)

623. Langdon,D.E.
Thrombophlebitis following diazepam.
J.Amer.Med.Ass. 225, 1389 (1973)

624. Langdon,D.E., Harlan,J.R., Bailey,R.L.
Thrombophlebitis with diazepam used intravenously.
J.Amer.Med.Ass. 223, 184-5 (1973)

625. Langfeldt,T., Ursin,H.
Diffential action of diazepam on flight and defensive behavior in the cat.
Psychopharmacologia 19, 61-6 (1971)

626. Langner,H.J.
Ein Nachweis von Ro 5-2807, einem neuen Psychopharmakon aus der Benzodiazepinreihe.
Z.Anal.Chem. 202, 28-34 (1964)

627. Larsson,S.O., Sundkvist,G.
Acute intoxication. A comparative investigation at a general city hospital for the years 1951, 1961 and 1971.
Acta Med.Scand. 195, 515-20 (1974)

628. Lasagna,L.
The role of benzodiazepines in nonpsychiatric medical practice.
Amer.J.Psychiat. 134, 656-8 (1977)

629. Laudano,O., Peralta,M., Lujan,L., Aparicio,N., Moizeszuwicz,J.
Effect of a new benzodiazepine derivate, clobazam, in anxious patients with gastro-intestinal disorders.
J.Clin.Pharmacol. 17, 441-6 (1977)

630. Lauffer,S., Schmid,E., Weist,F.
Dünnschichtchromatographische Trennung und spektrophoto-fluometrischer Nachweis psychotroper Pharmaka.
Arzneim.-Forsch. (Drug Res.) 19, 1965-71 (1969)

631. Law,N.C., Fales,H.M., Milne,G.W.A.
Identification of drugs taken in overdose cases.
Clin.Toxicol. 5, 17-21 (1972)

632. Lawton,M.P., Burton,C.
The effect of diazepam and alcohol on psychomotor performance.
J.Nerv.Ment.Dis. 136, 550-4 (1965)

633. Ledda,F.
Acute chlordiazepoxide poisoning in a drug addict, followed by withdrawal syndrome.
Clin.Ther. 44, 167-71 (1968)

634. Lingjaerde,O.
A new particular syndrome induced by large doses of diazepam ?
Tidsskr.Nor.Laegeforen 93, 606 (1973)

635. Lingjaerde,O.
Thrombophlebitis after intravenous injection of diazepam.
Tidsskr.Nor.Laegeforen 94, 455-6 (1974)

636. Linnoila,M., Dorrity,jr.,F.
Rapid gas chromatographic assay of serum diazepam, N-desmethyldiazepam, and desalkylflurazepam.
Acta Pharmacol.Toxicol. 41, 458-64 (1977)

637. Linnoila,M., Häkkinen,S.
Effects of diazepam and codeine, alone and in combination with alcohol, on simulated driving.
Clin.Pharmacol.Ther. 15, 368-73 (1974)

638. Linnoila,M., Korttila,K., Mattila,M.J.
Effect of food and repeated injections on serum diazepam levels.
Acta Pharmacol.Toxicol. 36, 181-6 (1975)

639. Linnoila,M., Markku,N., Floyd Dorrity,jr.,N.
Rapid gas chromatographic assay of serum diazepam, N-desmethyldiazepam and N-desalkylflurazepam.
Acta Pharmacol.Toxicol. 41, 458-64 (1977)

640. Linnoila,M., Mattila,J.
Drug interaction on psychomotor skills related to driving: Diazepam and alcohol.
Eur.J.Clin.Pharmacol. 5, 186-94 (1973)

641. Linnoila,M., Otterstroem,S., Anttila,M.
Chlordiazepoxide, diazepam and thioridazine serum concentrations after the simultaneous ingestion of alcohol or placebo drinks.
Ann.Clin.Res. 6, 4-6 (1974)

642. Linnoila,M., Saario,J., Olkoniemi,J., Liljequist,R., Himberg,J., Maeki,M.
Effect of two weeks' treatment with chlordiazepoxide and flupenthixole, alone or in combination with alcohol, on psychomotor skills related to driving.
Arzneim.-Forsch. (Drug Res.) 25, 1088-92 (1975)

643. Lippa,A.S., Regan,B.
Additional studies on importance of glycine and GABA in mediating actions of benzodiazepines.
Life Sci. 21, 1779-83 (1977)

644. Litchfield,N.B.
An unusual reaction to intravenous diazepam.
Dent.Anaesth.Sedat. 4, 9 (1975)

645. Livingston,S., Pauli,L.L.
Chlorazepate in epilepsy.
J.Amer.Med.Ass. 237, 1561 (1977)

646. Lopukhin,I.U.M., Isakov,I.U.F., Molodenkov,M.N., Burkov,I.V., Mosharov,O.P.
Use of method of extracorporeal hemosorption in treatment of experimental acute poisoning.
Eksp.Khir.Anasteziol. 3-6 (1975)

647. Lorr,M., McNair,D.M., Weinstein,G.J.
Early effects of chlordiazepoxide (librium) used with psychotherapy.
J.Psychatric Res. 1, 257-70 (1962)

648. Loveland,M.R.
Fatal nitrazepam poisoning.
Bull.Int.Ass.Forens.Toxicol. 10, (1) 16 (1974)

649. Lovering,E.G., Mainville,C.A., Rowe,M.L.
Drug permeation through membranes. V: Interaction of diazepam with common excipients.
J.Pharm.Sci. 65, 207-10 (1976)

650. Lucek,R.W., Coutinho,C.B.
The role of substituents in the hydrophobic binding of the 1,4-benzodiazepines by human plasma proteins.
Mol.Pharmacol. 12, 612-9 (1976)

651. Lucek,R.W., Coutinho,C.B., Cheripko,J.A., Ryan,J., Schwartz,M.A.
Further studies on medazepam metabolism in the rat.
Drug Metab.Dispos. 3, 297-302 (1975)

652. Luisi,G.
Detection and GLC-identification of benzodiazepine tranquilizing agents in biological material. (serum, urine, gastric content) in acute poisoning.
Boll.Soc.Ital.Biol.Sper. 49, 983-6 (1973)

653. Lumbantoruam,S.M.
Elektroanalytische Untersuchungen des Antiepileptikums Clonazepam und des Hypnotikums Flunitrazepam.
Dissertation Frankfurt/Main 1977

654. Lund,W., Opheim,L.-N.
Automated polarographic analysis. Part II: Determination of chlordiazepoxide and diazepam in tablets.
Anal.Chim.Acta 88, 275 (1977)

655. Lunde,I., Borchgrevink,C.F.
Use of diazepam in early pregnancy.
Lakartidningen 73, 1006 (1976)

656. Lutz,E.G.
Allergic conjunctivitis due to diazepam.
Amer.J.Psychiatry 132, 548 (1975)

657. MacBay,A.J., Algeri,E.J.
Ataraxics and nonbarbiturate sedatives.
Progr.Chem.Toxicol. 1, 157-90 (1963)

658. MacDonald,A., Michaelis,A.F., Senkowski,B.Z.
Chlordiazepoxide.
In: 322. (1972)

659. MacDonald,A., Michaelis,A.F., Senkowski,B.Z.
Diazepam.
In: 322. (1972)

660. MacDonald,R., Barker,J.L.
Benzodiazepines specifically modulate GABA-mediated postsynaptic inhibition in cultured mammalian neurones.
Nature 271, 563-4 (1978)

661. Macek,K., Rehák,V.
High-resolution liquid chromatography of some psychotropic drugs.
J.Chromatogr. 105, 182-5 (1975)

662. MacMahon,R.E.
Microsomal desalkylation of drugs.
J.Pharm.Sci. 55, 457-66 (1966)

663. Maden,B.H., McNeil,K.G., Huber,N.A., Khan,W.A., Singh,P., Schneider,R.S.
An EMIT-assay for benzodiazepines in urine.
Clin.Chem. 22, 1200 (1967)

664. Magbagbeola,J.A.
Interaction between chlordiazepoxide and propanidid.
Brit.J.Anaesth. 47, 161-2 (1975)

665. Mahon,W.A., Inaba,T., Stone,R.M.
Metabolism of flurazepam by the small intestine.
Clin.Pharmacol.Ther. 22, 228-33 (1977)

666. Mahon,W.A., Inaba,T., Umeda,T., Tsutsumi,E., Stone,R.
Biliary elimination of diazepam in man.
Clin.Pharmacol.Ther. 19, 443-50 (1976)

667. Maier,R.D., Wehr,K.H.
Zum Nachweis von Prazepam, einem neuen Tranquilizer aus der Reihe der Benzodiazepine.
Arch.Toxikol. 32, 341-5 (1974)

668. Maleque,A., Ahmad,K.
Brain levels of chlordiazepoxide in rats.
J.Physiol.Pharmacol. 21, 94-8 (1977)

669. Mallach,H.J.
Alkohol und Arzneimittel als verkehrsmedizinisches Problem.
Materia Medica Nordmark 20, 430-6 (1968)

670. Mallach,H.J., Ladusch,H.E.
Chemisch-toxikologische Harnuntersuchungen zur Beweissicherung bei Angaben über Arzneimitteleinnahmen durch alkoholbeeinflußte Pkw.Fahrer.
Blutalkohol 10, 42-9 (1973)

671. Mallach,H.J., Moosmayer,A., Gottwald,K., Staak,M.
Pharmakokinetische Untersuchungen über Resorption und Ausscheidung von Oxazepam in Kombination mit Alkohol.
Arzneim.-Forsch. (Drug Res.) 25, 1840-5 (1975)

672. Mallach,H.J., Moosmayer,A., Rupp,J.M.
Zur gaschromatographischen Analytik der Benzodiazepine. 1. Mitt.: Medazepam und seine Metabolite.
Arzneim.-Forsch. (Drug Res.) 23, 614-6 (1973)

673. Mallach,H.J., Seitz,J.
Angaben von Alkoholtätern über ihre Arzneimitteleinnahmen und deren Überprüfung.
Blutalkohol 12, 337-47 (1975)

674. Mandelli,M., Morselli,P.L., Nordio,S., Pardi,G., Principi,N., Sereni,F., Tognoni,G.
Placental transfer of diazepam and its disposition in the newborn.
Clin.Pharmacol.Ther. 17, 564-72 (1975)

675. Maness,D.D., Yakatan,G.J.
Fluorescence characteristics of benzodiazepines in strong acid.
J.Pharm.Sci. 64, 651-4 (1975)

676. Manno,B.R., Baker,J.R., Manno,J.E., Hughes,J.R.
Identification of flurazepam (Dalmane[R]) and a primary metabolite in urine by thin-layer chromatography.
J.Forens.Sci. 20, 38-44 (1975)

677. Manzo,L., deBernardi,M., Bertè,F.
Drug metabolism in the rabbit lung during pregnancy and in the perinatal period.
Farmaco 30, 491-7 (1975)

678. Manzo,L., Hokari,S., deBernardi,M., Bertè,F.
Effects of luminal and oxazepam on drug-metabolizing processes of the rabbit placenta in various periods of pregnancy.
Boll.Soc.Intal.Biol.Sper. 44, 1941-4 (1968)

679. Marcu,P., Grecu,I.
Enthalpimetrische Untersuchung einiger Benzodiazepinderivate.
Pharmazie 31, 167-8 (1976)

680. Marcucci,F., Bianchi,R., Airoldi,L., Salmona,M., Fanelli,R., Chiabrando,C., Frigerio,A., Mussini,E., Garattini,S.
Gas chromatographic - mass spectrometric determination of intact C_3-hydroxylated benzodiazepine glucuronides in urine.
J.Chromatogr. 107, 285-93 (1975)

681. Marcucci,F., Fanelli,R., Frova,M., Morselli,P.L.
Levels of diazepam in adipose tissues of rats, mice and man.
Eur.J.Pharmacol. 4, 464-6 (1968)

682. Marcucci,F., Fanelli,R., Mussini,E.
A method for gas chromatographic determination of benzodiazepines.
J.Chromatogr. 37, 318-20 (1968)

683. Marcucci,F., Fanelli,R., Mussini,E., Garattini,S.
The metabolism of diazepam by liver microsomal enzymes of rats and mice.
Eur.J.Pharmacol. 7, 307-13 (1969)

684. Marcucci,F., Fanelli,R., Mussini,E., Garattini,S.
Effect of phenobarbital on the in vitro metabolism of diazepam in several animal species.
Biochem.Pharmacol. 19, 1771-6 (1970)

685. Marcucci,F., Fanelli,R., Mussini,E., Garattini,S.
Further studies on species difference in diazepam metabolism.
Eur.J.Pharmacol. 9, 253-6 (1970)

686. Marcucci,F., Fanelli,R., Mussini,E., Garattini,S.
Further studies on the long lasting antimetrazol activity of diazepam in mice.
Eur.J.Pharmacol. 11, 115-6 (1970)

687. Marcucci,F., Guaitani,A., Fanelli,R., Mussini,E., Garattini,S.
Metabolism and anticonvulsant activity of diazepam in guinea pigs.
Eur.J.Pharmacol. 20, 1711-3 (1971)

688. Marcucci,F., Guaitani,A., Kvetina,J., Mussini,E., Garattini,S.
Species difference in diazepam metabolism and anticonvulsant effect.
Eur.J.Pharmacol. 4, 467-70 (1968)

689. Marcucci,F., Mussini,E.
A metabolic explanation for differences between species of the anticonvulsant activity of diazepam.
Brit.J.Pharmacol. 34, 667-8 (1968)

690. Marcucci,F., Mussini,E., Airoldi,E., Guaitani,A., Garattini,S.
Brain concentrations of lorazepam and oxazepam at equal degree of anticonvulsant activity.
J.Pharm.Pharmacol. 24, 63-4 (1972)

691. Marcucci,F., Mussini,E., Airoldi,L., Guaitani,A., Garattini,S.
Diazepam metabolism and anticonvulsant activity in newborn animals.
Biochem.Pharmacol. 22, 3051-9 (1973)

692. Marcucci,F., Mussini,E., Fanelli,R., Garattini,S.
Species differences in diazepam metabolism.
I. Metabolism of diazepam metabolites.
Biochem.Pharmacol. 19, 1847-51 (1970)

693. Marcucci,F., Mussini,E., Guaitani,A., Fanelli,R., Garattini,S.
Anticonvulsant activity and brain levels of diazepam and its metabolites in mice.
Eur.J.Pharmacol. 16, 311-4 (1971)

694. Marcucci,F., Mussini,E., Martelli,P., Guaitani,A., Garattini,S.
Metabolism and anticonvulsant activity of deuterated N-demethyldiazepam.
J.Pharm.Sci. 62, 1900-2 (1973)

695. Margules,D.L., Stein,L.
Increase of "antianxiety" activity and tolerance of behavioral depression during chronic administration of oxazepam.
Psychopharmacologia 13, 74-80 (1968)

696. Martelli,E.A., Corsico,N.
On the mechanism of lipomobilizing effect of chlordiazepoxide.
J.Pharm.Pharmacol. 21, 59 (1969)

697. Marttila,J.K., Hammel,R.J., Alexander,B., Zustiak,R.
Potential untoward effects of long-term use of flurazepam in geriatric patients.
J.Amer.Pharm.Ass. 17, 692-5 (1977)

698. Mascherpa,P.
Studies of fetal pharmacology. 3. Possibilities of using the technique of "organs isolated in situ" in the fetus and the newborn infant.
Boll.Soc. Ital.Biol.Sper. 44, 1552-3 (1968)

699. Mascherpa,P.
Studies on drug organotropism and drug metabolizing activity in the fetus and the newborn.
Boll.Chim.Farm. 107, 589-97 (1968)

700. Maslowsky,J.
Case of early oxazepam addiction treated at the outpatients clinic.
Psychiatr.Pol. 6, 223-4 (1972)

701. Massotti,M.
Effect of diazepam on dopamine and homovanillic acid levels in the corpus striatum of rats pretreated with -hydroxybutyric acid.
Neurochem.Res. 2, 689-95 (1977)

702. Masuda,T.
Medico-legal studies on isolation and identification of hypnotics by thin-layer chromatography.
1. Thin-layer chromatography of hypnotics and tranquilizers.
J.Kumamoto Med.Soc. 46, 105-18 (1972)

703. Masuda,Y.
Determination of nitrazepam in blood and urine by gas liquid chromatography.
Jap.J.Legal Med. 25, 445 (1971)

704. Matlin,E.
Use of chlordiazepoxide in obese patients.
Clin.Med. 70, 780-4 (1963)

705. Mattila,M.J., Palva,E., Seppala,T., Saario,I.
Effects of thrithiozine on psychomotor skills related to driving - comparison with diazepam and interactions with alcohol.
Curr.Ther.Res. 22, 875-6 (1977)

706. Maulding,H.V., Nazareno,J.P., Pearson,J.E., Michaelis,A.F.
Practical kinetics: III: Benzodiazepine hydrolysis.
J.Pharm.Sci. 64, 278-84 (1975)

707. Mayer,W., Erbe,S., Voigt,R.
Beiträge zur Analytik und Stabilität einiger pharmazeutisch interessanter Benzodiazepine.
1. Diazepam und Nitrazepam, Hydrolyseverlauf und Feststellung einer Ringverengung zu isomeren Chinolonderivaten.
Pharmazie 27, 32-42 (1972)

708. McAllister,C.B.
Use of internal standards in the estimation of diazepam in plasma.
J.Chromatogr. 151, 62-6 (1978)

709. McDonall,A., Owen,S., Robin,A.A.
A controlled comparison of diazepam and amylobarbitone in anxiety states.
Brit.J.Psychiatry 112, 629-31 (1966)

710. McLean,A.G.
Ketamine and diazepam in the adult patient.
Med.J.Aust. 2, 594 (1971)

711. McMartin,C.M., Street,H.V.
Gas-liquid chromatography of submicrogram amounts of drugs. I. Preparation, scope and limitation of columns.
J.Chromatogr. 22, 274-85 (1966)

712. Meguro,K., Kuwada,Y.
Synthesis and structures of 7-chloro-2-hydrazino-5-phenyl-3H-1,4-benzodiazepines and some isomeric 1,4,5-benzotriazocines.
Tetrahedron Lett. 4039-42 (1970)

713. Mehta,D., Mehta,S., Mathew,P.
Unusual abdominal complications of a suicidal overdose of analgesic and psychotropic drugs in an elderly patient.
J.Am.Geriatr.Soc. 26, 43-6 (1978)

714. Meissner,J., Preil,P.
Distribution of ^{14}C-diazepam (valium) in pregnant and lactating rabbits.
Nucl.Med. (Stuttg.) 14, 272-84 (1975)

715. Melander,A., Danielson,K., Vessman,J., Waehlin,E.
Bioavailability of oxazepam: Absence of influence of food intake.
Acta Pharmacol.Toxicol. 40, 584-8 (1977)

716. Mercier,J., Dessaigne,S., Manez,J.
Neurophysiological study of dipotassium chlorazepate (4306 CB).
Arzneim.-Forsch. (Drug Res.) 20, 125-7 (1970)

717. Merrill,E.J.
Synthesis of 7-chloro-1-cyclopropylmethyl-(methylene-^{14}C)-5-phenyl-1H-1,4-benzodiazepine-2(3H)-one and 7-chloro-1-(cyclopropylmethyl)-5-phenyl-1H-1,4-benzodiazepine-2(3H)-one-5-^{14}C.
J.Lab.Compounds (in the press)

718. Merwe,van der,P.J., Steyn,J.M.
Thin-layer chromatographic method for determination of diazepam and its major metabolite, N-desmethyldiazepam, in human serum.
J.Chromatogr. 148, 549-53 (1978)

719. Metlesics,W., Silverman,G., Sternbach,L.H.
Quinazolines and 1,4-benzodiazepines.
XII. Preparation and reactions of 2,3-dihydro-1H-1,4-benzodiazepine-4-oxides.
J.Org.Chem. 28, 2459-60 (1963)

720. Metter,D., Magerl,H., Tönnes,H.-W.
Nachweisbarkeit von acht gebräuchlichen Benzodiazepinen im Blut und im Harn.
Arch.Toxicol. (im Druck)

721. Mikhelson,V.A., Baryshkov,I.U.A., Lutskii,I.M., Silin,N.N., Maceret,N.A.
Acute elenium poisoning in children.
Pediatriia 53, 27-30 (1974)

722. Milkovich,L., van den Berg,B.J.
Effects of prenatal meprobamate and chlordiazepoxide hydrochloride on human embryonic and fetal development.
N.Engl.J.Med. 291, 1268-71 (1974)

723. Milne,G.W.A., Fales,H.M., Axenrod,Th.
Identification of dangerous drugs by isobutane chemical ionization mass spectrometry.
Anal.Chem. 13, 1815-20 (1971)

724. Milner,G., Landauer,A.A.
Haloperidol and diazepam, alone and together with alcohol, in relation to driving safety.
Blutalkohol 10, 247-54 (1973)

725. Min,B.H., Garland,W.A.
Determination of clonazepam and its 7-amino-metabolite in plasma and blood by gas chromatography-chemical ionization mass spectrometry.
J.Chromatogr. 139, 121-33 (1977)

726. Misra,P.C.
Nitrazepam (mogadon) dependence.
Brit.J.Psychiatry 126, 81-2 (1975)

727. Missen,A.W.
Procedures compared for extracting benzodiazepines from blood.
Clin.Chem. 22, 927-8 (1976)

728. Missen,A.W.
An oxidative screening procedure for nanogram amounts of benzodiazepines and other drugs in blood.
J.Anal.Toxicol. 1, 224-6 (1977)

729. Mitchell,P.R., Martin,I.L.
Effects of benzodiazepines on K-T-stimulated release of GABA.
Neuropharm 17, 317-20 (1978)

730. Miyadera,T., Kawano,Y., Hata,T., Tamura,C., Tachikawa,R.
Reactions of chlordiazepoxide and diazepam-N-oxide with dimethyl acetylenedicarboxylate with rearrangement of quinoxaline derivates and X-ray analysis of a resultant tetracyclic compound.
Chem.Pharm.Bull. Tokyo 25, 3247-70 (1977)

731. Moehler,H., Okada,T.
Benzodiazepine receptor: Demonstration in the central nervous system.
Science 198, 849-51 (1977)

732. Moehler,H., Okada,T.
Properties of ^{3}H-diazepam binding to benzodiazepine receptors in rat cerebral cortex.
Life Sci. 20, 2101-10 (1977)

733. Möller,M.R.
Habil.Schrift, Homburg/Saar 1977

734. Möller,M.R., Witzmann,K.H., Tausch,D.
Beitrag zum Nachweis der kombinierten Einnahme von Alkohol und Arzneimitteln.
Beiträge gerichtl.Med. 31, 259-66 (1973)

735. Moeschlin,S.
Klinik und Therapie der Vergiftungen.
5. Aufl., Stuttgart: Thieme 1972

736. Moffat,A.C.
Use of SE-30 as a stationary phase for the GLC of drugs.
J.Chromatogr. 113, 69-95 (1975)

737. Mohseni,H.
Fatal case of chlordiazepoxide (librium) poisoning.
Bull.Int.Ass.Forens.Toxicol. 11, (2) 17 (1975)

738. Møller Jensen,K.
Determination of nitrazepam in serum by gas-liquid chromatography.
Application in bioavailability studies.
J.Chromatogr. 111, 389-96 (1975)

739. Monaco,F., Durelli,L., Furlan,P.M.
Does a drug-induced stimulation of diazepam metabolism exist ?
Riv.Neurol. 45, 171-6 (1975)

740. Moore,B., Nickless,G., Hallett,C., Howard,A.G.
Analysis of nitrazepam and its metabolites by high-pressure liquid chromatography.
J.Chromatogr. 137, 215-7 (1977)

741. Moosmayer,A., Mallach,H.J., Staak,M.
Pharmakokinetische Untersuchungen nach oraler Applikation von Oxazepam in Kombination mit Alkohol.
Beitr.gerichtl.Med. 34, 85 (1976)

742. Mørland,J., Setekleiv,J., Haffner,J.F.W., Strømsaether,C.E., Danielse,A., Holst Wethe,G.
Combined effects of diazepam and ethanol on mental and psychomotor functions.
Acta Pharmacol.Toxicol. 34, 5-15 (1974)

743. Morris,R.W.
Drinking, smoking and drug interactions.
Pharmindex 14, 10 (1972)

744. Morselli,P.L., Mandelli,M., Tognoni,G., Principi,N., Pardi,G., Sereni,F.
Drug interactions in the human fetus and in the newborn infant. p. 259-70
In: Morselli,P.L. et al., ED Drug Interactions. New York, Raven Press, 1974

745. Morselli,P.L., Principi,N., Tognoni,G., Reali,E., Belvedere,G., Standen,S.M., Sereni,F.
Diazepam elimination in premature and full term infants and children.
J.Perinat.Med. 1, 133-41 (1973)

746. Morselli,P.L., Veneroni,E., Zaccala,M., Bizzi,A.
Further observations on the interaction between ethanol and psychotropic drugs.
Arzneim.-Forsch. (Drug Res.) 21, 20-3 (1971)

747. Moser,L.
Die Untersuchung kraftfahrwesentlicher Leistungsminderungen durch Arzneimittel.
Blutalkohol 11, 285 (1974)

748. Müller,R.K.
Die toxikologisch-chemische Analyse.
Verlag Theodor Steinkopff, Dresden / Verlag Chemie Weinheim, West Germany, 1976

749. Müller,W., Wollert,U.
The interaction of some benzodiazepine derivates with human serum albumin. Circular dichroism studies.
Naunyn-Schmied.-Arch.Pharmacol. 277, Suppl.R.49 (1973)

750. Müller,W., Wollert,U.
Interactions of benzodiazepines with human serum albumin.
Naunyn-Schmied.-Arch.Pharmacol. 278, 301-12 (1973)

751. Müller,W., Wollert,U.
Characterization of the binding of benzodiazepines to human serum albumin.
Naunyn-Schmied.-Arch.Pharmacol. 280, 229-37 (1973)

752. Müller,W., Wollert,U.
Large differences between human and bovine serum albumin reflected in the binding behaviour for benzodiazepine derivates, circular dichroism and gelfiltration studies.
Naunyn-Schmied.-Arch.Pharmacol. 282, 68 (1974)

753. Müller,W., Wollert,U.
Influence of pH on the benzodiazepine-human-serum albumin complex, circular dichroism studies.
Naunyn-Schmied.-Arch.Pharmacol. 283, 67-82 (1974)

754. Müller,W., Wollert,U.
Binding of d- and l-oxazepam hemisuccinate to bovine serum albumin.
Res.Commun.Chem.Pathol.Pharmacol. 9, 413-20 (1974)

755. Müller,W., Wollert,U.
Proceedings: Benzodiazepines, very specific competitors for the binding of l-tryptophan to human serum albumin.
Naunyn-Schmied.-Arch.Pharmacol. 287, 66 (1975)

756. Müller,W.E., Wollert,U.
Benzodiazepines: Specific competitors for the binding of L-tryptophan to human serum albumin.
Naunyn-Schmied.-Arch.Pharmacol. 288, 17-27 (1975)

757. Müller,W., Wollert,U.
High stereospecificity of the benzodiazepine binding site on human serum albumin, -studies with D- and L-oxazepam hemisuccinate.
Mol.Pharmacol. 11, 52-60 (1975)

758. Müller,W., Wollert,U.
Interaction of benzodiazepine derivates with bovine serum albumin. - I. Gel filtration studies.
Biochem.Pharmacol. 25, 141-5 (1976)

759. Müller,W., Wollert,U.
Interaction of benzodiazepine derivates with bovine serum albumin. - II. Circular dichroism studies.
Biochem.Pharmacol. 25, 147-52 (1976)

760. Mulé,S.J.
Identification of narcotics, barbiturates, amphetamines, tranquillizers and psychotomimetics in human urine.
J.Chromatogr. 39, 302-11 (1969)

761. Mulé,S.J.
Routine identification of drugs of abuse in human urine.
I. Application of fluorometry, TLC & GLC.
J.Chromatogr. 55, 255-66 (1971)

762. Mulé,S.J., Bastos,M.L., Jukofsky,D., Saffer,E.
Routine identification of drugs of abuse in human urine.
II. Development and application of the XAD-2 resin column method.
J.Chromatogr. 63, 289-301 (1971)

763. Murray,N.
Covert effect of chlordiazepoxide therapy.
J.Neuropsychiatry 3, 168 (1962)

764. Mussini,E., Marcucci,F., Airoldi,L., Facchinetti,T., Garattini,S.
Hydroxylation of three benzodiazepines in vitro.
J.Pharm.Sci. 66, 1482-3 (1977)

765. Mussini,E., Marcucci,F., Fanelli,R., Garattini,S.
Metabolism of diazepam in guinea pigs.
Chem.Biol.Interact. 5, 73-6 (1972)

766. Mussini,E., Marcucci,F., Fanelli,R., Garattini,S.
Metabolism of diazepam and its metabolites by guinea pig liver microsomes.
Biochem.Pharmacol. 20, 2529-31 (1971)

767. Mussini,E., Marcucci,F., Fanelli,R., Guaitani,A., Garattini,S.
Analytical and pharmacokinetic studies on the optic isomers of oxazepam succinate half-ester.
Biochem.Pharmacol. 21, 127-9 (1972)

768. Mutschler,E.
Arzneimittel-Wirkungen.
Ein Lehrbuch der Pharmakologie für Pharmazeuten, Chemiker und Biologen. 3. Aufl.
Wiss.Verlagsgesellschaft mbH, Stuttgart, 1975

769. Myrsten,A.-L., Goldberg,L., Neri,A.
Interaction between alcohol and tranquilizing drugs.
Report from the Psychological Laboratories, The University of Stockholm, 1971, 1-24

770. Naess,K.
Pharmacokinetics of benzodiazepines. Practical comments.
Tidsskr.Nor.Laegeforen 95, 1170-1 (1975)

771. Naestoft,J., Larsen,N.E.
Quantitative determination of clonazepam and its metabolites in human plasma by gas chromatography.
J.Chromatogr. 93, 113-22 (1974)

772. Naestoft,J., Lund,M., Larsen,N.E., Hvidberg,E.
Assay and pharmacokinetics of clonazepam in humans.
Acta Neurol.Scand. 49, 103-8 (1973)

773. Nakamura,M., Fukushima,H.
Effect of 5,6-dihydroxytryptamine on the head twitches induced by 5-HTP, 5-HT, mescaline and fludiazepam in mice.
J.Pharm.Pharmacol. 30, 56-8 (1978)

774. Nakano,S. et al.
Human pharmacological study. Bromazepam, diazepam, placebo.
J.Jap.Psychosomatic Soc. 13, 111-8 (1973)

775. Nakano,S., Gillespie,H.K., Hollister,L.E.
Model for evaluation of antianxiety drugs with use of experimetally induced stress. Comparison of nabilone and diazepam.
Clin.Pharmacol.Ther. 23, 54-63 (1978)

776. Naney,A.P., Chaffee,W.G.
Diazepam for cardioversion.
J.Amer.Med.Ass. 215, 487 (1971)

777. Naylor,G.J., McHarg,A.
Profound hypothermia on combined lithium carbonate and diazepam treatment.
Brit.Med.J. 2, 22 (1977)

778. Negritescu,S., Mihalas,E., Sterescu,M., Joan,C.
Dünnschichtchromatographische Trennung der bei der Nitrierung im Rahmen der Nitrazepamsynthese entstehenden Umsetzungsprodukte.
Pharmazie 31, 823 (1976)

779. Negwer,M.
Organisch-chemische Arzneimittel und ihre Synonyma, 3 Bände,
5. neubearbeitete und stark erweiterte Aufl. 1978. Akademie-Verlag, Berlin

780. Netter,K.J.
Grundlagen des Arzneimittelstoffwechsels.
Arzneim.-Forsch. (Drug Res.) 25, 1110 (1975)

781. Neves,M.H., Brites,V.L., Andrade,A.T., Guerra,M.O.
Effect of diazepam diluent on fertility and gestation in female rats.
Rev.Ginecol.Obstet. (Rio de J.) 134, 161-5 (1977)

782. Nevins,M.A.
Ventricular arrhythmias and diazepam.
J.Amer.Med.Ass. 215, 643 (1971)

783. Ngai,S.H., Tseng,D.T.C., Wang,S.C.
Effects of diazepam and other central nervous system depressants on spinal reflects of cat.
J.Pharmacol.Exp.Ter. 153, 344-51 (1966)

784. Nicholson,A.N., Stone,B.M.
Effects of a metabolite of diazepam, 3-hydroxydiazepam (temazepam), on sleep in man.
Brit.J.Clin.Pharmacol. 3, 543 (1976)

785. Nicholson,A.N., Stone,B.M.
Effectiveness of diazepam and its metabolite 3-hydroxydiazepam (temazepam) for sleep during the day (proceedings).
J.Physiol. (London) 270, 29-30 (1977)

786. Nicholson,A.N., Stone,B.M., Clarke,C.H.
Effect of the 1,5-benzodiazepines, clobazam and triflubazam, on sleep in man.
Brit.J.Clin.Pharmacol. 4, 567-72 (1977)

787. Nicholson,A.N., Wright,C.M.
Inhibitory and disinhibitory effects of nitrazepam, diazepam and flurazepam hydrochloride on delayed matching behaviour in monkeys (macaca mulatta).
Neuropharmacology 13, 919-26 (1974)

788. Nicholson,A.N., Wright,C.M.
Behavioural activity in the monkey (macaca mulatta) of the metabolites of diazepam in man.
Brit.J.Pharmacol. 57, 428 (1976)

789. Nicholson,A.N., Wright,C.M.
Activity of fosazepam, a soluble analogue of diazepam.
Brit.J.Clin.Pharmacol. 4, 494-6 (1977)

790. Nielsen,B.L., Clausen,J.
Diazepamum (valium). 3. En methode til kvantitativ bestemmelse i serum.
Ugeskr.Laeger 128, 119 (1966)

791. Nielsen,M., Braestrup,C., Squires,R.F.
Evidence for a late evolutionary appearance of brain specific benzodiazepine receptors: An investigation of 18 vertebrate and 5 invertebrate species.
Brain Res. 141, 342-6 (1978)

792. Nishikawa,T., Mineura,K., Takahira,H.
Studies on the fate of flurazepam. Absorption, excretion and distribution of flurazepam in the rat.
Yakugaku Zasshi 93, 226-31 (1973)

793. Nishikawa,T., Mineura,K., Takahira,H.
Studies on the fate of flurazepam. 2. The metabolism of flurazepam in the rat.
Yakugaku Zasshi 93, 232-8 (1973)

794. Nogen,A.G.
The utility of clonazepam in epilepsy of various types. Observations with 22 childhood cases.
Clin.Pediat. 17, 71-85 (1978)

795. Noirfalise,A.
Dünnschichtchromatographie von Psychopharmaka.
J.Chromatogr. 20, 61-77 (1965)

796. Norheim,G.
Abnormal drug distribution in fatal intoxications.
Forens.Sci. 3, 271-4 (1974)

797. Nudelman,A., McCaully,R.J., Bell,S.C.
Water soluble derivates of 3-oxy-substituted 1,4-benzodiazepines.
J.Pharm.Sci. 64, 1880-5 (1974)

798. Nuhn,P., Bley,W.
NMR-spektroskopische Untersuchung von Arzneimitteln. Zur Konfiguration von Diazepam, Nitrazepam und Chlordiazepoxid.
Pharmazie 22, 532-3 (1967)

799. Oates,R.K.
Tranquilizers and child abuse.
Med.J.Aust. 1, 40-1 (1977)

800. O'Connell,B., McCarthy,G., Robinson,A.E.
Diazepam in the newborn.
Brit.Med.J. 4, 610 (1973)

801. Odar-Cederloef,I., Vessman,J., Alvan,G., Sjoeqvist,F.
Oxazepam disposition in uremic patients.
Acta Pharmacol.Toxicol. 40, 52-62 (1977)

802. Oelschläger,H.
Über das polarographische Verhalten des Chlordiazepoxids (Librium).
Arch.Pharm. 296, 396-403 (1963)

803. Oelschläger,H., Druckrey,F., Sengün,F.I.
Polarographische Bestimmung des Euhypnicums Flurazepam in seinen Arzneiformen.
Pharm.Acta Helv. 51, 353-61 (1976)

804. Oelschläger,H., Geppert,V.
Drug analysis by polarographic methods, XIX: Determination of medazepam and its main metabolites by cathode ray polarography.
Arch.Pharm. 309, 1000-6 (1976)

805. Oelschläger,H., Kurek,E., Sengün,F.I., Volke,J.
Polarographische Gehaltsbestimmung des Chlordiazepoxids (LIBRIUM®) in seinen Arzneiformen.
Z.Anal.Chem. 282, 123-8 (1976)

806. Oelschläger,H., Oehr,H.-P.
Gehaltsbestimmung von Medazepam in galenischen Zubereitungen mit Hilfe der Gleichspannungspolarographie.
Pharm.Acta Helv. 45, 708 (1970)

807. Oelschläger,H., Oehr,H.P.
Polarographische Bestimmung des Temazepams.
Pharm.Acta Helv. 49, 179-86 (1974)

808. Oelschläger,H., Oehr,H.-P., Lim,G.T.
Polarographisch reines Dimethylformamid.
Pharm.Acta Helv. 48, 662-7 (1973)

809. Oelschläger,H., Sengün,F.I.
Elektrochemische Eigenschaften und polarographische Gehaltsbestimmung des Prazepams.
Arch.Pharm. 306, 737-46 (1973)

810. Oelschläger,H., Sengün,F.I.
Gehaltsbestimmung von Dikaliumchlorazepat.
Arch.Pharm. 307, 401-9 (1974)

811. Oelschläger,H., Sengün,F.I.
Polarographische Bestimmung von Lorazepam.
Pharmazie 29, 770-3 (1975)

812. Oelschläger,H., Volke,J., Hoffmann,H., Kurek,E.
Mechanismus der Polarographischen Reduktion des Chlordiazepoxids.
Arch.Pharm. 300, 250-7 (1967)

813. Oelschläger,H., Volke,J., Kurek,E.
Polarographische Gehaltsbestimmung des Diazepams (Valium® "Roche").
Arch.Pharm. 297, 431-42 (1964)

814. Oelschläger,H., Volke,J., Lim,G.T.
Polarographische Auswertung von Dünnschicht-Chromatogrammen.
Arch.Pharm. 298, 213-9 (1965)

815. Oelschläger,H., Volke,J., Lim,G.T.
Polarographische Auswertung von Magnesiumsilikat-Dünnschichtchromatogrammen.
Arzneim.-Forsch. (Drug Res.) 17, 637 (1967)

816. Oelschläger,H., Volke,J., Lim,G.T., Frank,U.
Zur Analytik des Euhypnicums 1,3-Dihydro-7-nitro-5-phenyl-2H-1,4-benzodiazepin-2-on.
Arzneim.-Forsch. (Drug Res.) 16, 82 (1966)

817. Oelschläger,H., Volke,J., Lim,G.T., Spang,R.
Reduktion des Oxazepams an der Hg-Tropfelektrode.
Arch.Pharm. 302, 946-51 (1969)

818. Ohmori,K., Watanabe,S., Ueki,S.
Electroencephalographic effects of flurazepam in rabbits.
Folia Pharmacol.JPN 73, 939-55 (1977)

819. Olive,G., Dreux,C.
Bases pharmacologiques de l'utilisation des benzodiazepines en médecine perinatale.
Arch.Fr.Pediatr. 34, 74-89 (1977)

820. Oliver,J.S., Smith,H.
Determination of nitrazepam in poisoning cases.
Forens.Sci. 4, 183-6 (1974)

821. Orme,M., Breckenridge,A., Brooks,R.V.
Interactions of benzodiazepines with warfarin.
Brit.Med.J. 3, 611-4 (1972)

822. Osselton,M.D., Hammond,M.D., Twitchett,P.J.
The extraction and analysis of benzodiazepines in tissues by enzymic digestion and high-performance liquid chromatography.
J.Pharm. (Lond.) 29, 460-2 (1977)

823. Ossmann,A.R.E.N., Hassany,A.H.E.
Spectrophotometric determination of chlordiazepoxide.
Pharmazie 30, 257 (1975)

824. Ossman,A.R., Hassany,A.H.
Rapid sensitive colorimetric assay for determination of chlordiazepoxide.
Pharmazie 31, 744-5 (1976)

825. Owen,G., Hatfield,G.K., Pollock,J.J., Steinberg, A.J., Tucker,W.E., Agersborg,jr.,H.P.K.
Toxicity studies of lorazepam, a new benzodiazepine in animals.
Arzneim.-Forsch. (Drug Res.) 21, 1065 (1971)

826. Owen,G., Smith,T.H.F., Agersborg,H.P.K.
Toxicity of some benzodiazepine compounds with CNS activity.
Toxicol.Appl.Pharmacol. 16, 556-70 (1970)

827. Owen,J.R., Iranis,S.F., Blair,A.W.
Effect of diazepam administered to mothers during labour on temperature regulation of neonate.
Arch.Dis.Child. 47, 107-10 (1972)

828. Pacifici,G.M., Placidi,G.F.
Rapid and sensitive electron-capture gas chromatographic method for the determination of pinazepam and its metabolites in human plasma, urine and milk.
J.Chromatogr. 135, 133-9 (1977)

829. Padfield,A.
Thrombosis following diazepam.
Brit.J.Anaesth. 46, 413 (1974)

830. Padfield,A., Watkins,J.
Allergy to diazepam.
Brit.Med.J. 1, 575-6 (1977)

831. Pagano,R.R., Graham,C.W., Galligan,M., Conner,J.T., Katz,R.L.
Histopathology of veins after intravenous lorazepam and Ro 21-3981.
Can.Anaesth.Soc.J. 25, 50-2 (1978)

832. Pantoja,O., Vianna,A.D.S.
Acetyl-salicylic acid plus diazepam - New analgesic formulation.
Rev.Bra.Med. 35, 88-90 (1978)

833. Pape,B.E.
Analytical toxicology: Applications of element-selective electrolytic conductivity detection for gas chromatography.
Clin.Chem. 22, 739-48 (1976)

834. Pape,B.E., Ribick,M.A.
Analysis of medazepam, diazepam, and metabolites in plasma by gas-liquid chromatography with electrolytic conductivity detection.
J.Chromatogr. 136, 127-39 (1977)

835. Parke,D.V.
The Biochemistry of Foreign Compounds.
Pergamon Press, Oxford (1968)

836. Parry,G.J.
Concentration of clonazepam in serum and cerebrospinal fluid of the sheep.
Pharmacology 15, 318-23 (1977)

837. Parry,G.J.G., Ferry,D.G.
Rapid gas chromatographic method for the determination of clonazepam in serum and cerebrospinal fluid.
J.Chromatogr. 128, 166 (1976)

838. Patch,V.D.
The dangers of diazepam, a street drug.
N.Engl.J.Med. 290, 807 (1974)

839. Patrick,M.J., Tilstone,W.J., Reavey,P.
Diazepam and breast-feeding.
Lancet 1, 542-3 (1972)

840. Paul,C.J., Whitehouse,L.W.
Metabolic bases for the supra additive effect of the ethanol-diazepam combination in mice.
Brit.J.Pharmacol. 60, 83-90 (1977)

841. Peet,M., Moonie,L.
Abuse of benzodiazepines.
Brit.Med.J. 1, 714 (1977)

842. Pelzer,H., Maass,D.
Pharmakokinetik und Metabolismus von 7-Chlor-1,3-dihydro-3-hydroxy-5-phenyl-2H-1,4-benzodiazepin-2-on und dessen Hemisuccinat beim Menschen.
Arzneim.-Forsch. (Drug Res.) 19, 1652-6 (1969)

843. Pentz,R., Schütt,A.
A rapid gas-chromatographic method for the determination of drugs in clinical toxicology.
Arch.Toxicol. 39, 225-33 (1978)

844. Pericic,D., Walters,J.R., Chase,T.N.
Effect of diazepam and pentobarbital on aminooxyacetic acid-induced accumulation on GABA.
J.Neurochem. 29, 539-46 (1977)

845. Peskar,B., Spector,S.
Quantitative determination of diazepam in blood by radioimmunoassay.
J.Pharmacol.Exp.Ther. 186, 167-72 (1973)

846. le Petit,G.F.

Medazepam pka determined by spectrophotometric and solubility methods.

J.Pharm.Sci. 65, 1094-5 (1976)

847. le Petit,G.

UV-spectrophotometric determination of the benzodiazepine derivative diazepam.

Z.Anal.Chem. 283, 199-203 (1977)

848. Pfeifer,S.

Biotransformation von Arzneimitteln, Bd. 1

VEB Verlag Volk und Gesundheit, Berlin, 1975

849. Pfeifer,S.

Biotransformation von Arzneimitteln, Bd. 2

VEB Verlag Volk und Gesundheit, Berlin, 1977

850. Pfeifer,S.

Biotransformation von Arzneimitteln, Bd. 3

VEB Verlag Volk und Gesundheit, Berlin, 1978

851. Piazza,L., Delfino,U., Zuccaro,G.M., Graziani,M., Giribone,G.

Histological findings in animals exposed to acute and chronic intoxication with methyldiazepinone.

Minerva Anestesiol. 35, 400-5 (1969)

852. Pierce,W.O., Lamoreaux,T.C., Urry,F.M., Kopjak,L., Finkle,B.S.

A new rapid gas chromatography method for the detection of basic drugs in postmortem blood, using a nitrogen phosphorus detector.
Part I: Qualitative analysis.

J.Anal.Toxicol. 2, 26-31 (1978)

853. Pillard,R.C., Fisher,S.

Effects of chlordiazepoxide and secobarbital on film-induced anxiety.

Psychopharmacologia 12, 18-23 (1967)

854. Placidi,G.F. et al.

Regional distribution of diazepam and its metabolites in the brain of cat after chronic treatment.

Psychopharmacologia 48, 133 (1976)

855. Placidi,G.F., Cassano,G.B.

Distribution and metabolism of ^{14}C-labelled chlordiazepoxide in mice.

Int.J.Neuropharmacol. 7, 383-9 (1968)

856. Podobnikar,I.G.

Implementation of psychotherapy by librium in a pioneering rural-industrial psychiatric practice.

Psychosomatics 12, 205-9 (1971)

857. Pohl,K.D., Ropohl,D.

Qualitative und quantitative Nachweismöglichkeiten von Benzodiazepinen und ihren Metaboliten in Mageninhalt, Blut und Urin.

Z.Rechtsmed. (im Druck)

858. Post,D.

Gaschromatographischer Beitrag zur Analytik pyridinchromophorer und phenylchromophorer Basen.

Beitr.Gerichtl.Med. 34, 219-27 (1976)

859. Prach,P.M., Lapysh,M.M.

Microcrystalloscopic reactions of benzodiazepine derivates.

Farmatsiia 26, 74-6 (1977)

860. Prashad,M., Ray,S., Bhaduri,A.P.

Nitration of substituted benzophenones.

Ind.J.Chem.B. 16, 142-3 (1978)

861. Preskorn,S.H., Denner,L.J.

Benzodiazepines and withdrawal psychosis, report of three cases.

J.Amer.Med.Ass. 237, 36-8 (1977)

862. Preuß,Fr.R.

Gadamers Lehrbuch der chemischen Toxikologie und Anleitung zur Ausmittelung der Gifte. Band I. Grundlagen, Ausmittelung, Chemie und Biochemie der Gifte. 1. Hälfte.

Vandenhoeck & Ruprecht, Göttingen 1969

863. Preuß,Fr.R.

Gadamers Lehrbuch der chemischen Toxikologie und Anleitung zur Ausmittelung der Gifte. Band I. Grundlagen, Ausmittelung, Chemie und Biochemie der Gifte. 2. Hälfte.

Vandenhoeck & Ruprecht, Göttingen 1979

864. Pribilla,O.

Chlordiazepoxid - Studien zum Nachweis der Ausscheidung beim Menschen.

Arzneim.-Forsch. (Drug Res.) 14, 723-33 (1964)

865. Pribilla,O.

Zum chemischen Nachweis von 1,3-Dihydro-7-nitro-5-phenyl-2H-1,4-benzodiazepin-2-on.

Arzneim.-Forsch. (Drug Res.) 15, 1148-52 (1965)

866. Prior,P.F., MacLaine,G.M., Scott,D.F., Laurance,B.M.

Tonic status epilepticus precipitated by intravenous diazepam in a child with petit mal status.

Epilepsia 13, 467-72 (1972)

867. Proelss,H.F., Lohmann,H.J.

Profile of sedatives and tranquilizers in serum as measured by gas-liquid chromatography.

Clin.Chem. 17, 222-8 (1971)

868. Pryor,G.T., Larsen,F.F., Carr,J.D., Braude,M.C.

Interactions of ^{9}-tetrahydrocannabinol with phenobarbital, ethanol, and chlordiazepoxide in rats.

Pharmacol.Biochem. and Behav. 7, 331-45 (1977)

869. Przybyla,A.C., Wang,S.C.

Locus of central depressant action of diazepam.

J.Pharmacol.Exp.Ther. 163, 439 (1968)

870. Puglisi,C.V., Meyer,J.C., D'Arconte,L., Brooks,A., de Silva,J.A.

Determination of water soluble imidazo-1,4-benzodiazepines in blood by electron-capture gas-liquid-chromatography and in urine by differential pulse polarography.

J.Chromatogr. 145, 81-96 (1978)

871. Puglisi,C.V., de Silva,J.A.F.
Determination of 7-iodo-1,3-dihydro-1-methyl-5-(2'-fluorophenyl)-2H-1,4-benzodiazepin-2-one (Ro 7-9957) and its major biotransformations products in blood and urine by ECD-GLC.
J.Chromatogr. 118, 370-86 (1976)

872. Raaflaub,J., Speiser,Courvoisier,J.
Zur Pharmakokinetik von Bromazepam beim Menschen.
Arzneim.-Forsch. (Drug Res.) 24, 1841-4 (1974)

873. Rada,R.T., Kellner,R., Buchanan,J.G.
Chlordiazepoxide and alcohol: A fatal overdose.
J.Forens.Sci. 20, 544-7 (1975)

874. Radmayr,E., Koeppen,D.
Clobazam (frisium) in everyday practice, an open six-month's study of its efficacy and tolerance.
Münchner Med.Wschr. 119, 1623-6 (1977)

875. Raihle,J.A., Papendick,V.E.
Chlorazepate dipotassium.
In: 324., 91-112 (1975)

876. Randall,L.O.
Pharmacology of methaminodiazepoxide.
Dis.Nerv.Syst. 21, Suppl 7-10 (1960)

877. Randall.L.O.
Pharmacology of chlordiazepoxide (librium).
Dis.Nerv.Syst. 22, 7-15 (1961)

878. Randall,L.O.
Chemistry and pharmacology of the benzodiazepines.
Nordisk Psykiatrisk Tidsskrift 25, 9-11 (1971)

879. Randall,L.O., Heise,G.A., Schallek,W., Bagdon,R.E., Banziger,R.F., Boris,A., Moe,R.A., Abrams,W.B.
Pharmacological and clinical studies on valium,a new psychotherapeutic agent of the benzodiazepine class.
Curr.Ther.Res. 3, 405-25 (1961)

880. Randall,L.O., Kappell,B.
Pharmacological activity of some benzodiazepines and their metabolites.
In: 362., p. 27-51

881. Randall,L.O., Schallek,W.
Pharmacological activity of certain benzodiazepines.
In: Psychopharmacology: A review of grogress 1957 - 1967, edited by D.H. Efron, pp. 153-84, United States Public Health Service Publication Number 1836 (1968)

882. Randall,L.O., Schallek,W., Heise,G.A., Keith,E.F., Bagdon,R.E.
The psychosedative properties of methaminodiazepoxide.
J.Pharmacol.Exp.Ther. 129, 163-71 (1960)

883. Randall,L.O., Schallek,W., Scheckel,C., Bagdon,R.E., Rieder,R.E.
Zur Pharmakologie von Mogadon, einem Schlafmittel mit neuartigem Wirkungsmechanismus.
Schweiz.Med.Wschr. 95, 334-7 (1965)

884. Randall,L.O., Schallek,W., Scheckel,C., Banziger,R., Boris,A., Moe,R.A., Bagdon,R.E., Schwartz,M.A., Zbinden,C.
Zur Pharmakologie von Valium, einem neuen Psychopharmakon der Benzodiazepinreihe.
Schweiz.Med.Wschr. 93, 794-7 (1963)

885. Randall,L.O., Schallek,W., Scheckel,C., Banziger,R.U., Moe,R.A.
Zur Pharmakologie des neuen Psychopharmakons 7-Chlor-2,3-dihydro-1-methyl-5-phenyl-1H-1,4-benzodiazepin.
Arzneim.-Forsch. (Drug Res.) 18, 1542-5 (1968)

886. Randall,L.O., Schallek,W., Scheckel,C.L., Stefko, P.L., Banziger,R.F., Pool,W., Moe,R.A.
Pharmacological studies on flurazepam hydrochloride (Ro 5-6901), a new psychotropic agent of the benzodiazepine class.
Arch.Int.Pharmacodyn.Ther. 178, 216-41 (1969)

887. Randall,L.O., Schallek,W., Sternbach,L., Ning,R.Y.
Chemistry and pharmacology of the 1,4-benzodiazepines.
In: de Stevens,F., Gordon,M. (Ed.), Psychopharmacological agents, Vol. 3 / Medicinal Chemistry - Monographs, Vol. 4, Part 3, pp. 175-281, Acad.Press, New York / N.Y. 1974

888. Randall,L.O., Scheckel,C.L., Banziger,R.F.
Pharmacology of the metabolites of chlordiazepoxide and diazepam.
Curr.Ther.Res. 7, 590-606 (1965)

889. Randall,L.O., Scheckel,C.L., Pool,W.
Pharmacology of medazepam and metabolites.
Arch.Int.Pharmacodyn.Ther. 185, 135-48 (1970)

890. Randerath,K.
Dünnschicht-Chromatographie.
Verlag Chemie: Weinheim (Germany)

891. Rao,K.P., Rao,M.S.
Induction of dominant lethal mutations in mice with chlordiazepoxide hydrochloride.
Indian J.Med.Res. 66, 847-52 (1977)

892. Rastogi,R.B., Agarwal,R.A., Lapierre,Y.D., Singhal,R.L.
Effects of acute diazepam and clobazam on spontaneous locomotor activity and central amine metabolism in rats.
Eur.J.Pharmacol. 43, 91-8 (1977)

893. Raveux,R., Gros,P.
III. Etude de l'excretion du chlorazépate dipotassique et de ses metabolites urinaires.
Chim.Ther. 1969, 481-7 (1969)

894. Raveux,R., Gros,P., Navarro,J.
II. Etude de l'excretion du chlorazepate dipotassique et de ses metabolites urinaires.
Chim.Ther. 1969, 357-60 (1969)

895. Reeder,E., Stempel,A., Sternbach,L.H.
Benzodiazepines.
Chemical Abstracts 60, 13261 d (1964)

896. Rejgent,T.A., Wahl,K.C.
Diazepam abuse: Incidence, rapid screening, and confirming methods.
Clin.Chem. 22, 889-91 (1976)

897. Reggiani,A., Hürlimann,A., Theiss,E.
Some aspects of the experimental and clinical toxicology of chlordiazepoxide.
Proceedings of the European Society for the Study of Drug Toxicity 9, 79-97 (1968)

898. Rein,E.
Assay of drugs and other trace compounds in biological fluids.
North-Holland Publishing Company, Amsterdam-New York-Oxford, 1976

899. Relkin,R.
Death following withdrawal of diazepam.
N.Y.State J.Med. 66, 1770-1 (1966)

900. Rey,E., Turquais,J.M., Olive,G.
Micromethod for determination of diazepam by electron-capture gas-liquid chromatography.
Clin.Chem. 23, 1338-9 (1977)

901. Riccioni,R., Gallevi,M., Sacchetti,G., Castrogiovanni,P., Cassano,G.P.
Il temazepam: nuovo ansiolitico della serie 1,4-benzodiazepinica. Studio pilota nell'uomo.
Neopsichiatria 39, 1-22 (1968)

902. Rice,A.J., Wilson,W.R.
Rapid identification of drugs in body fluids of comatose patients.
Clin.Toxicol. 6, 59-73 (1973)

903. Richman,S., Harris,R.D.
Acute pulmonary edema associated with librium abuse, a case report.
Radiology 103, 57-8 (1972)

904. Rickels,K., Clyde,D.J.
Clyde mood scale changes in anxious outpatients produced by chlordiazepoxide therapy.
J.Nerv.Ment.Dis. 145, 154-7 (1967)

905. Rickels,K., Downing,R.W., Howard,K.
Predictors of chlordiazepoxide response in anxiety.
Clin.Pharmacol.Ther. 12, 263-73 (1971)

906. Rickels,K., Perloff,M., Stepansky,W., Dion,H.S., Case,W.G., Sapra,R.K.
Doxepin and diazepam in general practice and hospital clinic neurotic patients: A collaborative controlled study.
Psychopharmacologia 15, 265-79 (1969)

907. Riddick,J.H.
An ultraviolet and visible spectrophotometric assay method for chlordiazepoxide.
Clin.Biochem. 6, 189-99 (1973)

908. Rieder,J.
Methoden zur Bestimmung von Nitrazepam und seinen Hauptmetaboliten in biologischen Proben und Ergebnisse von Versuchen über die Pharmakokinetik der Substanz bei Mensch und Ratte.
Arzneim.-Forsch. (Drug Res.) 15, 1134-48 (1965)

909. Rieder,J.
A fluorimetric method for determining nitrazepam and the sum of its main metabolites in plasma and urine.
Arzneim.-Forsch. (Drug Res.) 23, 207-11 (1973)

910. Rieder,J.
Plasma levels and derived pharmacokinetic characteristics of unchanged nitrazepam in man.
Arzneim.-Forsch. (Drug Res.) 23, 212-8 (1973)

911. Rieder,J., Rentsch,G.
Metabolismus und Pharmakokinetik des neuen Psychopharmakons Medazepam beim Menschen.
Arzneim.-Forsch. (Drug Res.) 18, 1545-56 (1968)

912. Rifkin,A., Quitkin,F., Klein,D.F.
Withdrawal reaction to diazepam.
J.Amer.Med.Ass. 236, 2172-3 (1976)

913. Rifkin,A., Klein,D.F., Quitkin,F.
Withdrawal from diazepam.
J.Amer.Med.Ass. 238, 306 (1977)

914. Risberg,A.M., Henricsson,S., Ingvar,D.H.
Evaluation of the effect of fosazepam (a new benzodiazepine), nitrazepam and placebo on sleep patterns in normal subjects.
Eur.J.Clin.Pharmacol. 12, 105-9 (1977)

915. Rise,A.
Drugs and the fetus. Anxiolytic agents. Meprobamate and chlordiazepoxide.
Lakartidningen 73, 1004-6 (1976)

916. Rising,P.A., Illing,H.P., Johnson,P., Yeomans,M.A.
The metabolism of a substituted aminoacetamidobenzophenone and cyclization to the corresponding benzodiazepine in the rat in vivo.
Xenobiotica 7, 425-37 (1977)

917. Robin,A., Curry,S.H., Whelpton,R.
Clinical and biochemical comparison of chlorazepate and diazepam.
Psychol.Med. 4, 388-92 (1974)

918. Rodgers,D.H.
Separation and analysis of psychopharmacologic drugs by high efficiency liquid chromatography.
J.Chromatogr.Sci. 12, 742-6 (1975)

919. Röder,E., Mutschler,E., Rochelmeyer,H.
Über die Verwendung von homogenen azeotropen Gemischen in der DC.
II. Über die Trennung von Diazepinen.
Z.Anal.Chem. 244, 45-6 (1969)

920. Rosanelli,K.
Effect of prenatylly administered diazepam on the premature infant.
Geburtshilfe Frauenheilkd. 30, 713-24 (1970)

921. Rossum,van,J.M., Breimer,D.D., Ginneken,van,G.A.M., Kordelaar,van,J.M.G., Vree,T.B.
Gas-liquid chromatography in pharmacology and toxicologie.
Clin.Chim.Acta 34, 311-9 (1971)

922. Rudy,B.C., Senkowski,B.Z.
Flurazepam hydrochloride.
In: 323., 307-31 (1974)

923. Ruelius,H.W., Lee,J.M., Alburn,H.E.
Metabolism of diazepam in dogs: Transformation to oxazepam.
Arch.Biochem.Biophys. 111, 376-80 (1965)

924. Runge,M., Arnold,W., Schreiber,D.
Aktuelle Formen der Drogenabhängigkeit unter besonderer Berücksichtigung von Haschisch und LSD.
Med.Welt 22, 1301-8 (1971)

925. Rupp,W., Heptner,W., Uihlein,M., Bender,R., Taeuber,K.
Kinetic interaction of nomifensine with a 1,5-benzodiazepine (clobazam).
Brit.J.Clin.Pharmacol. 4, 143-6 (1977)

926. Rushton,R., Steinberg,H.
Combined effects of chlordiazepoxide and dexamphetamine on activity of rats in an unfamiliar environment.
Nature 211, 1312-3 (1966)

927. Rutherford,D.M.
Rapid micro-method for the measurement of diazepam and desmethyldiazepam in blood plasma by gas-liquid chromatography.
J.Chromatogr. 137, 439-48 (1977)

928. Saario,I. et al.
Interaction of drugs with alcohol on human.
J.Clin.Pharmacol. 15, 52-9(1975)

929. Sadée,W., Kleijn,van der,E.
Thermolysis of 1,4-benzodiazepines during GC and MS.
J.Pharm.Sci. 60, 135-7 (1971)

930. Saito,S.
Isolation and identification of hypnotics. 8. Isolation and identification of benzalin and cercine by TLC in vitro.
Jap.J.leg.Med. 25, 402-8 (1971)

931. Sakai,S., Inukai,T., Hara,Y., Kitagawa,S.
Benzodiazepine flurazepam / ID-480 /. Pharmacological studies of a new benzodiazepine compound, flurazepam / ID-480.
Pharmacometrics 5, 581-97 (1971)

932. Sakai,S., Kitagawa,S., Yamamoto,H.
Pharmacological studies on 1-methyl-7-nitro-5-phenyl-1,3-dihydro-2H-1,4-benzodiazepin-2-one / S-1530.
Arzneim.-Forsch. (Drug Res.) 22, 534-9 (1972)

933. Saldeen,T., Johansson,O.
The significance of chronic heart disease, fatty liver, and consumption of barbiturate and librium on the tolerance of ethyl alcohol, as judged in a postmortem series.
J.Forens.Sci. 12, 273-94 (1967)

934. Saletu,B., Gruenberger,J., Linzmayer,L.
Classification and determination of cerebral bioavailability of psychotropic drugs by quantitative "pharmaco-EEG and psychometric investigations (studies with AX-A 411-BS)".
Int.J.Clin.Pharmacol.Biopharm. 15, 449-59 (1977)

935. Salim,E.F., Deuble,J.L., Papariello,G.
Qualitative and quantitative tests for oxazepam.
J.Pharm.Sci. 57, 311-3 (1968)

936. Salzman,C., DiMascio,A., Shader,R.I., Harmatz,J.S.
Chlordiazepoxide, expection, and hostility.
Psychopharmacologia 14, 38-45 (1969)

937. Salzman,C., Kochansky,G.E., Shader,R.I., Harmatz,J.S., Ogletree,A.M.
Is oxazepam associated with hostility.
Dis.Nerv.Syst. 36, 30-2 (1975)

938. Samuels,R.W.
A rapid screening test for diazepam in serum.
J.Anal.Toxicol. 1, 208-10 (1977)

939. Sanchez,M.C., Comoñe,J., Gelpí,E.
Electron capture and multiple ion detection of benzodiazepine esters in pharmacokinetic studies.
J.Chromatogr. 126, 601-13 (1976)

940. Sandler,K., Brunswick,D., Digiacomo,J., Mendels,J.
A preliminary evaluation of the anxiolytic activity of clobazam.
Curr.Ther.Res. 21, 114-6 (1977)

941. Sansone,M.
Chlordiazepoxide and monoamine oxidase inhibitors on avoidance behaviour in mice.
Pharmacol.Res.Commun. 9, 729-35 (1977)

942. Sansone,M., Castellano,C., Vetulani,J.
Improvement of shuttle-box performance of mice by combination of benzodiazepines and morphine during training.
Arch.Int.Pharmacodyn.Ther. 230, 83-92 (1977)

943. Sarteschi,P., Cassano,G.B., Castrogiovanni,P., Gallevi,M.
Valutazione comparativa dell´oxazepam (Wy 3498) e del placebo su nevrotici e depressi endogeni.
Medicina Psicosomatica 13, 3-27 (1968)

944. Sarteschi,P., Cassano,G.P., Castrogiovanni,P., Placidi,G.F., Sacchetti,G.
Major and minor tranquilizers in the treatment of anxiety states.
Arzneim.-Forsch. (Drug Res.) 22, 93-7 (1972)

945. Sarteschi,P. et al.
Placental penetration and foetal uptake of neuropharmacological agents.
Pharmakopsychiatrie, Neuropsychopharmakologie 6, 50 (1973)

946. Saucy,G., Sternbach,L.H.
Chinazoline und 1,4-Benzodiazepine. VII. Trifluoromethyl-substituierte Verbindungen.
Helv.Chim.Acta 45, 2226-41 (1962)

947. Sawada,H.
An urinary metabolite of bromazepam.
Experientia 28, 393-4 (1972)

948. Sawada,H. et al.
Studies on metabolism of bromazepam. I. Isolation and identification of the metabolites of bromazepam in urine.
J.Pharm.Soc.Jap. 92, 1237-41 (1972)

949. Sawada,H. et al.
Studies on metabolism of bromazepam. IV. Hydroxylation of 2-(2-amino-5-bromobenzoyl)-pyridine by liver microsomal enzymes.
Yakugaku Zasshi 94, 991-7 (1974)

950. Sawada,H., Hara,A.
Studies on metabolism of bromazepam. V. Identification of new urinary metabolites and their excretion pattern in various animal species.
J.Pharm.Soc.Jpn. 95, 430-8 (1975)

951. Sawada,H., Hara,A.
Novel metabolite of nitrazepam in the rabbit urine.
Experientia 32, 987-8 (1976)

952. Sawada,H., Hara,A., Asano,S., Matsumoto,Y.
Isolation and identification of benzodiazepine drugs and their metabolites in urine by use of amberlite XAD-2 resin and thin-layer chromatography.
Clin.Chem. 22, 1596-1603 (1976)

953. Sawada,H., Shinohara,K.
Colorimetric determination of nitrazepam.
J.Hyg.Chem. 16, 318-21 (19707

954. Sawada,H., Shinohara,K.
Detection and identification of nitrazepam and related compounds by thin-layer chromatography.
Arch.Toxicol. 27, 71-8 (1970)

955. Sawada,H., Shinohara,K.
On the urinary excretion of nitrazepam and its metabolites.
Arch.Toxikol. 28, 214-21 (1971)

956. Scagliola,N., Julien,R., Dreux,C.
Micromethod of diazepam determination in the blood by GLC. Application in neonatal pharmacology.
Ann.Biol.Clin. (Paris) 34, 27-32 (1976)

957. Scanlon,J.W.
Effect of benzodiazepines in neonates.
N.Engl.J.Med. 292, 649-50 (1975)

958. Scarzella,M.
A case of diazepam poisoning.
Minerva Pediat. 20, 581-2 (1968)

959. Schallek,W., Kuehn,A., Jew,N.
Effects of chlordiazepoxide (librium) and other psychotropic agents on the limbic system of the brain.
Ann.N.Y. Acad.Sci. 96, 303-12 (1962)

960. Schallek,W., Zabransky,F., Kuehn,A.
Effect of benzodiazepines on central nervous system of cat.
Arch.Int.Pharmacodyn.Ther. 149, 343-61 (1970)

961. Schillings,R.T., Shrader,S.R., Ruelius,H.W.
Urinary metabolites of lorazepam in humans and four animal species.
Arzneim.-Forsch. (Drug Res.) 21, 1059-65 (1971)

962. Schillings,R.T., Sisenwine,S.F., Ruelius,H.W.
Disposition and metabolism of lorazepam in the male rat.
Drug Metab.Disposition 5, 425-35 (1977)

963. Schillings,R.T., Sisenwine,S.F., Schwartz,M.A., Ruelius,H.W.
Lorazepam: Glucuronide formation in the cat.
Drug Metab.Disposition 3, 85-8 (1975)

964. Schlicht,H.J., Gelbke,H.P.
A micromethod for the isolation of drugs from blood using amberlite XAD-2.
Z.Rechtsmedizin 81, 25-30 (1978)

965. Schmidt,Gg.
Postmortale Veränderungen von Arzneistoffen und Giften in Organen und Körperflüssigkeiten einschließlich Neubildung von Störsubstanzen.
In: Gadamers Lehrbuch der chemischen Toxikologie und Anleitung zur Ausmittelung der Gifte. Hrsgb. E.Graf und Fr.R.Preuß, Band I, 1, S. 189-237, Vandenhoeck & Ruprecht, Göttingen 1969

966. Schmidt,Gg.
Der forensische Beweiswert toxikologischer Untersuchungen.
Beitr.gerichtl.Med. 25, 122 (1969)

967. Schneider,J., Kamm,G.
Does oxazepam (adumbran) interfere with anticoagulant treatment. A controlled study.
Med.Klin. 73, 153-6 (1978)

968. Schrappe,O. et al.
Klinische Untersuchungen mit WY 4036 (Lorazepam), einem neuartigen Tranquilizer.
Arzneim.-Forsch. (Drug Res.) 21, 1079-82 (1971)

969. Schütz,C., Muskat,E., Schütz,H.

Fehlerquellen bei der Interpretation chemisch-toxikologischer Befunde unter besonderer Berücksichtigung des Bromoureid- und Benzodiazepinnachweises.

Beitr.gerichtl.Med. 33, 224-7 (1975)

970. Schütz,C., Post,D., Schewe,G., Schütz,H., Muskat,E.

Mikrochemischer Nachweis und Unterscheidung von fünf Tranquilizern aus der Klasse der 5-Phenyl-1,4-Benzodiazepine mit Hilfe der dünnschicht-chromatographischen TRT-Technik.

Z.Anal.Chem. 262, 282-6 (1972)

971. Schütz,C., Schütz,H.

Zur Unterscheidung der Benzodiazepine Lorazepam und Oxazepam mit Hilfe der dünnschichtchromatographischen Trennung-Reaktion-Trennung-Technik.

Z.Klin.Chem.Klin.Biochem. 10, 528-30 (1972)

972. Schütz,C., Schütz,H.

Der Schnellnachweis von Lorazepam (TAVOR[R]),einem neuen Tranquilizer aus der Reihe der Benzodiazepine.

Arch.Toxikol. 30, 183-6 (1973)

973. Schütz,C., Schütz,H., Ha,Y.D., Muskat,E.

Reaktionschromatographischer Nachweis von Diazepam (Valium), Nitrazepam (Mogadan) und Chlorazepate (Tranxilium).

Dtsch.Apoth.-Ztg. 113, 1967-9 (1973)

974. Schütz,H.

Möglichkeiten der Reaktionschromatographie, dargestellt am Beispiel des reaktionschromatographischen Nachweises von Nitrazepam (Mogadan) und seiner Hauptmetaboliten.

J.Chromatogr. 94, 159-67 (1974)

975. Schütz,H.

Ein Screening-Test für einige wichtige Pharmaka mit Hilfe der Reaktion nach Bratton-Marshall im Rahmen der Routineprüfung auf Benzodiazepine.

Schriftenreihe der Deutschen Verkehrswissenschaftlichen Gesellschaft,
In: Verkehrssicherheit durch Technik und Medizin.
Köln: 1976, S. 277-86

976. Schütz,H.

Anordnung zur kontinuierlichen Verlaufskontrolle dünnschichtchromatographischer Trennungen anhand der Fluoreszenzlöschung bei UV-Bestrahlung in der Entwicklungskammer.

Bundesrepublik Deutschland: Deutsches Patentamt München, Offenlegungsschrift 24 57 421 (1976)

977. Schütz,H.

Alkohol, Medikamente, Wechselwirkungen und Verkehrstüchtigkeit - eine Literaturübersicht.

Schriftenreihe der Deutschen Verkehrswissenschaftlichen Gesellschaft,
In: Verkehrssicherheit durch Technik und Medizin.
Köln: 1976, S. 287-94

978. Schütz,H.

Reaktionen auf der Dünnschichtplatte - eine Mikromethode für analytische und präparative Spezialprobleme.

Dissertation Marburg/Lahn 1977

979. Schütz,H.

In: Gadamers Lehrbuch der chemischen Toxikologie und Anleitung zur Ausmittelung der Gifte.
Bd. I, 2 (1. Hälfte), Hrsgb. Fr.R.Preuß,
Vandenhoeck & Ruprecht, Göttingen 1979

980. Schütz,H.

Mikropräparation wichtiger Flunitrazepam-Metaboliten durch Reaktionen auf der Dünnschichtplatte.

J.Chromatogr. 168, 429-34 (1979)

981. Ein screening-test auf Nor-Clobazam, einen Hauptmetaboliten des neuen 1,5-Benzodiazepins Clobazam (Frisium[R]).

Arch.Kriminol. 163, 91-4 (1979)

982. Schütz,H.

Analytische Daten des neuen 1,5-Benzodiazepins Clobazam (Frisium[R]) und seines Hauptmetaboliten Nor-Clobazam.

Arch.Toxicol. 41, 233-8 (1978)

983. Schütz,H.

Dünnschichtchromatographische Trennung und Detektion von 14 1,4- bzw. 1,5-Benzodiazepin-Handelspräparaten und 17 Hauptmetaboliten.

Z.Anal.Chem. 294, 135-9 (1979)

984. Schütz,H.

TLC-data of 19 main hydrolysis-derivates of 1,4- and 1,5-benzodiazepines and major metabolites.

J.Anal.Toxicol. 2, 147-8 (1978)

985. Schütz,H.

Zum Nachweis von Camazepam (Albego[R]), einem neuen Benzodiazepinderivat.

Ärztl.Lab. 25, 75-8 (1979)

986. Schütz,H., Meurer,G.

Untersuchungen zur kontinuierlichen DC-Entwicklung mit simultaner Kontrolle der Fluoreszenzlöschung.

Beitr.gerichtl.Med. 35, 337-41 (1977)

987. Schütz,H., Schütz,C.

Zur Anwendung der dünnschichtchromatographischen TRT-Technik in der forensischen Toxikologie.

Beitr.gerichtl.Med. 31, 330-2 (1973)

988. Schütz,H., Westenberger,V.

Gas-chromatographic data of 31 benzodiazepines and metabolites.

J.Chromatogr. 169, 409-11 (1979)

989. Schütz,H., Westenberger,V.

Gaschromatographische Daten von 19 Hydrolysederivaten aus 12 wichtigen Benzodiazepinen und 17 Hauptmetaboliten.

Z.Rechtsmedizin 82, 43-53 (1978)

990. Schulze,B.

Problem of drug-induced cerebral reactions: A case of myoclonic state under treatment with tricyclic antidepressive agents.

Nervenarzt 43, 332-6 (1972)

991. Schwartz,D.E., Vecchi,M., Ronco,A., Kaiser,K.
Blood levels after administration of diazepam in various forms.
Arzneim.-Forsch. (Drug Res.) 16, 1109-10 (1966)

992. Schwartz,M.A.
In: 362., pp. 53-73

993. Schwartz,M.A., Bommer,P., Vane,F.M.
Diazepam metabolites in the rat: Characterization by high-resolution mass spectrometry and nuclear magnetic resonance.
Arch.Biochem.Biophys. 121, 508-16 (1967)

994. Schwartz,M.A., Carbone,J.J.
Metabolism of ^{14}C-medazepam hydrochloride in dog, rat and man.
Biochem.Pharmacol. 19, 343-61 (1970)

995. Schwartz,M.A., Koechlin,B.A., Krol,G.
Metabolism of diazepam in rat, dog and man.
Fed.Proc.Fed.Amer.Soc.Exp.Biol. 22, 367 (1963)

996. Schwartz,M.A., Koechlin,B.A., Postma,E., Palmer,S., Krol,G.
Metabolism of diazepam in rat, dog and man.
J.Pharmacol.Exp.Ther. 149, 423-35 (1965)

997. Schwartz,M.A., Kolis,S.J.
Pathways of medazepam metabolism in the dog and rat.
J.Pharm.Exp.Ther. 180, 180-8 (1972)

998. Schwartz,M.A., Kolis,S.J.
Oxidation of an amino carbinol by an NAD^{+} - dependent microsomal dehydrogenase.
Drug Metab.Disposition 1, 322-31 (1973)

999. Schwartz,M.A., Postma,E.
Metabolic N-demethylation of chlordiazepoxide.
J.Pharm.Sci. 55, 1358-62 (1966)

1000. Schwartz,M.A., Postma,E.
Metabolism of diazepam in vitro.
Biochem.Pharmacol. 17, 2443-9 (1968)

1001. Schwartz,M.A., Postma,E.
Metabolism of flurazepam, a benzodiazepine in man and dog.
J.Pharm.Sci. 59, 1800-6 (1970)

1002. Schwartz,M.A., Postma,E.
Metabolites of demoxepam, a chlordiazepoxide metabolite in man.
J.Pharm.Sci. 61, 123-5 (1972)

1003. Schwartz,M.A., Postma,E., Gaut,Z.
Biological half-life of chlordiazepoxide and its metabolite, demoxepam, in man.
J.Pharm.Sci. 60, 1500-3 (1971)

1004. Schwartz,M.A., Postma,E., Kolis,S.J.
Metabolism of demoxepam, a chlordiazepoxide metabolite in a dog.
J.Pharm.Sci. 60, 438-44 (1971)

1005. Schwartz,M.A., Postma,E., Kolis,S.J., Leon,A.S.
Metabolites of bromazepam, a benzodiazepine, in the human, dog, rat and mouse.
J.Pharm.Sci. 62, 1776-9 (1974)

1006. Schwartz,M.A., Vane,V.M., Postma,E.
Chlordiazepoxide metabolites in the rat. Characterization by high resolution mass spectrometry.
Biochem.Pharmacol. 17, 965-74 (1968)

1007. Schwartz,M.A., Vane,V.M., Postma,E.
Metabolism of flurazepam, a benzodiazepine, in man and dog.
J.Pharm.Sci. 59, 1800-6(1970)

1008. Schwartz,M.A., Vane,F.M., Postma,E.
Urinary metabolites of flurazepam.
J.Med.Chem. 11, 770 (1968)

1009. Schweda,P.
Thin-layer chromatography of toxicologically significant substanzes on silica gel - coated glass plates and polyester sheets.
Anal.Chem. 39, 1019-23 (1967)

1010. Schwob,R., Wuersch,J.
Novel method for preparation of highly tritiated methyl-iodide, and its use for syntheses of methyl-H-3-labeled diazepam and methiodides of (+)-bicuculline and (-)-bicuculline.
J.Label.C.R. 14, 355-60 (1978)

1011. Scott,C.G., Bommer,P.
The liquid chromatography of some benzodiazepines.
J.Chromatogr.Sci. 8, 446-8 (1970)

1012. Seeds,A.E., Stolee,A., Eichhorst,B.C.
Permeability of human chorion laeve to diazepam and meperidine.
Obstet.Gynecol. 47, 28-30 (1976)

1013. Sellers,E.M., Zilm,D.H., Degani,N.C.
Comparative efficacy of propanolol and chlordiazepoxide in alcohol withdrawal.
J.Stud.Alcohol 38, 2096-109 (1977)

1014. Sellman,R., Hurme,M., Kanto,J.
Biliary excretion of diazepam and its metabolites in man after repeated oral doses.
Eur.J.Clin.Pharmacol. 12, 209-12 (1977)

1015. Sellman,R., Kanto,J., Pekkarinen,J.
Biliary excretion of diazepam and its metabolites in man.
Acta Pharmacol.Toxicol. 37, 242-9 (1975)

1016. Sellman,R., Kanto,J., Raijola,E., Pekkarinen,A.
Human and animal study on elimination from plasma and metabolism of diazepam after chronic alcohol intake.
Acta Pharmacol.Toxicol. 36, 33-8 (1975)

1017. Sellman,R., Pekkarinen,A., Kangas,L., Raijola,E.
Reduced concentrations of plasma diazepam in chronic alcoholic patients following an oral administration of diazepam.
Acta Pharmacol.Toxicol. 36, 25-32 (1975)

1018. Sellman,R., Kanto,J., Raijola,E., Pekkarinen,A.
Induction effect of diazepam on its own metabolism.
Acta Pharmacol.Toxicol. 37,345-51(1975)

1019. Semiginovský,B., Jakoubek,B., Pavlik,A., Sobotka,P.
Effects of early experimence, pyrithioxin and diazepam on U 14 C glucose utilization in rat brain during emotional stress.
Activ.Nerv.Super 19, 307-9 (1977)

1020. Sengün,F.I., Oelschläger,H.
Arzneimittelanalysen mittels Polarographie oder Oszillopolarographie.
18. Mitt.: Elektroanalytische Eigenschaften des Bromazepams und seine Bestimmung im Blut durch Kathodenstrahlpolarographie.
Arch.Pharm. 720-3 (1975)

1021. Senkowski,B.Z., Levin,M.S., Urbigkit,J.R., Wollish,E.G.
Polarography of some benzodiazepines.
Anal.Chem. 36, 1991-4 (1964)

1022. Sepinwall,J.
Some pharmacological aspects of benzodiazepines.
Folha Medica 67, 727-35 (1973)

1023. Sepinwall,J., Grodsky,F.S., Cook,L.
Conflict behavior in the squirrel monkey: Effects of chlordiazepoxide, diazepam and N-desmethyl-diazepam.
J.Pharmacol.Exp.Ther. 204, 88-103 (1978)

1024. Serra,F., Poggi,F.
Oxazepam poisoning in a two year old child.
Clin.Ter. 42, 357-60 (1967)

1025. Settel,E.
Combined d-amphetamine and chlordiazepoxide therapy in the emotionally disturbed obese patient.
Clin.Med. 70, 1077-88 (1963)

1026. Shader,R.I., Greenblatt,D.J.
Clinical implications of benzodiazepine pharmacokinetics.
Am.J.Psychiatry 134, 652-6 (1977)

1027. Shader,R.I., Greenblatt,D.J., Harmatz,J.S. Franke,K., Koch-Weser,J.
Absorption and disposition of chlordiazepoxide in young and elderly male volunteers.
J.Clin.Pharmacol. 17, 709-18 (1977)

1028. Shader,R.I., Greenblatt,D.J., Salzman,C., Kochansky,G.E., Harmatz,J.S.
Benzodiazepines: Safety and toxicity.
Dis.Nerv.Syst. 36, 23-6 (1975)

1029. Shaffer,J.W., Yeganeh,M.L., Foxwell,N., Kurland,A.A.
A comparison of the effects of prazepam, chlordiazepoxide, and placebo in the short-term treatment of convalescing alcoholics.
J.Clin.Pharmacol. 8, 392-9 (1968)

1030. Shapcott,D., Lemieux,B.
The measurement of rivotril in whole blood by gas-liquid chromatography.
Clin.Biochem. 8,283-7 (1975)

1031. Sharkey,M.F., Andres,C.N., Snow,S.W., Major,jr.,A., Kram,T., Warner,V., Alexander,T.G.
An index of electronic spectra.
J.Ass.Offic.Anal.Chem. 51, 1124-54 (1968)

1032. Sharma,K.K., Sharma,U.C.
Influence of diazepam on the effect of neuromuscular blocking agents.
J.Pharm.Pharmacol. 30, 64 (1978)

1033. Shaw,W.L.
Poisoning with mianserin (letter).
Brit.Med.J. 2, 459 (1977)

1034. Shearer,C.M., Pilla,C.R.
Oxazepam.
In: 323., 441-64 (1974)

1035. Sherman,P.M.
Cardiac arrest with diazepam.
J.Oral Surg. 32, 567 (1974)

1036. Sherman,P.M.
Further comments on cardiac arrest from diazepam.
J.Oral Surg. 33, 86 (1975)

1037. Shibuya,T.
Pharmacological studies of 7-bromo-1,3-dihydro-5-(2-pyridyl)-2H-1,4-benzodiazepin-2-one, Ro-3350, bromazepam. Report 1. Studies on the acute and subacute toxicity of bromazepam in rats.
J.Tokyo Med.Coll. 31, 213-32 (1973)

1038. Shibuya,T. et al.
Pharmacological studies of 7-bromo-1,3-dihydro-5-(2-pyridyl)-2H-1,4-benzodiazepin-2-one, Ro-3350, bromazepam. Report 2. Studies on the chronic toxicity of bromazepam in rats.
J.Tokyo Med.Coll. 31, 233-51 (1973)

1039. Shibuya,T. et al.
Pharmacological studies of 7-bromo-1,3-dihydro-5-(2-pyridyl)-2H-1,4-benzodiazepin-2-one, Ro-3350, bromazepam. Report 3. Studies on the general pharmacological action of bromazepam.
J.Tokyo Med.Coll. 31, 253-8 (1973)

1040. Shibuya,T. et al.
Pharmacological studies of 7-bromo-1,3-dihydro-5-(2-pyridyl)-2H-1,4-benzodiazepin-2-one, Ro-3350, bromazepam. Report 4. Studies on the central nervous system.
J.Tokyo Med.Coll. 31, 287-301 (1973)

1041. Shibuya,T., Matsuda,H.
Pharmacological studies of 7-bromo-1,3-dihydro-5-(2-pyridyl)-2H-1,4-benzodiazepin-2-one,Ro-3350, bromazepam. Report 5. Variation of body weight curve, especially recovery test by various administration methods in rats.
J.Tokyo Med.Coll. 31, 307-14 (1973)

1042. Shimkin,P.M., Shaivitz,S.A.
Diazepam poisoning in a child.
J.Amer.Med.Ass. 196,662-3 (1966)

1043. Shull,H.J., Wilkinson,G.R., Johnson,R., Schenker,S.
Normal disposition of oxazepam in acute viral hepatitis and cirrhosis.
Ann.Intern.Med. 84, 420-5 (1976)

1044. Siebke,H., Ellertsen,B.B., Lind,B.
Reactions to intraveneous injections of diazepam.
Brit.J.Anaesth. 48, 1187-9 (1976)

1045. Sillers,B.R.
Irritant properties of diazepam.
Brit.Dent.J. 124, 295 (1968)

1046. Silver,D., Ban,T.A., Kristof,F.E., Saxena,B.M., Bennett,J.
Prazepam in the treatment of psychoneurotic outpatients. A brief report.
Curr.Ther.Res. 11, 596-9 (1969)

1047. Silvermann,G., Braithwaite,R.A.
Benzodiazepines and tricyclic antidepressant plasma levels.
Brit.Med.J. 3, 18-20 (1973)

1048. Simon,R.K.
Ethanol, valium death.
Bull.Int.Ass.Forens.Toxicol. 12, 19-20 (1976)

1049. Sine,H.E., McKenna,M.J., Law,M.R., Murray,M.H.
Emergency drug analysis.
J.Chromatogr.Sci. 10, 297-302 (1972)

1050. Sinz,P.
Grundzüge einer Pharmakologie der Benzodiazepine.
Medicamentum 17, 11-5 (1976)

1051. Siris,J.H., Pippenger,C.E., Werner,W.L., Masland,R.L.
Anticonvulsant drug-serum levels in psychiatric patients with seizure disorders. Effects of certain psychotropic drugs.
N.Y. State J.Med. 74, 1554-6 (1974)

1052. Sisenwine,S.F., Tio,C.O., Ruelius,H.W.
The metabolic transformation of oxazepam in man, pig and rat.
Pharmacologist 12, 272 (1970)

1053. Sisenwine,S.F., Tio,C.O., Shrader,S.R., Ruelius,H.W.
The biotransformation of oxazepam in man, miniature swine and rat.
Arzneim.-Forsch. (Drug Res.) 22, 682-7 (1972)

1054. Sjö,O., Hvidberg,E.F., Naestoft,J., Lund,M.
Pharmacokinetics and side-effects of clonazepam and its 7-amino-metabolite in man.
Eur.J.Clin.Pharmacol. 8, 249-54 (1975)

1055. Sjoedin,T.
Circular dichroism studies on the inhibiting effect of oleic acid on the binding of diazepam to human serum albumin.
Biochem.Pharmacol. 26, 2157-61 (1977)

1056. Sjoedin,T., Hansson,R., Sjoeholm,I.
Isolation and identification of an trypsin-resistant fragment of human serum albumin with bilirubin- and drug-binding properties.
Biochim.Biophys.Acta 494, 61-75 (1977)

1057. Sjoedin,T., Roosdorp,N., Sjoeholm,I.
Studies on the binding of benzodiazepines to human serum albumin by circular dichroism measurements.
Biochem.Pharmacol. 25, 2131-40 (1976)

1058. Sjoeholm,I., Ljungstedt,I.
Studies on the tryptophan and drug-binding properties of human serum albumin fragments by affinity chromatography and circular dichroism measurements.
J.Biol.Chem. 248, 8434-41 (1973)

1059. Slater,J.
Suspected dependence on chlordiazepoxide hydrochloride (librium).
Can.Med.Assoc.J. 95, 416 (1966)

1060. Smart,L.C.
Detection of diazepam in forensic toxicology.
J.Can.Soc.Forens.Sci. 8, 27 (1975)

1061. Smith,A., Rawlins,M.D.
Benzodiazepines.
Brit.Med.J. 2, 447 (1977)

1062. Smith,L.R., Williams,R.T.
Implication of the conjugation of drugs and other endogenous compounds.
In: Glucuronic Acid Free and Combined, edited by G.J.Dutton, Academic Press, New York, pp. 457-91 (1966)

1063. Smith,T.C., Moyer,C.E.
Bioavailability of two preparations of chlordiazepoxide.
Curr.Ther.Res. 20, 204-10 (1976)

1064. Sohn,D., Simon,J.
Rapid identification of psychopharmacologic agents in cases of drug abuse.
Clin.Chem. 18, 405-10 (1972)

1065. Sokol,G.H., Greenblatt,D.J., Littman,P., Franke,K., Koch-Weser,J.
Chlordiazepoxide metabolism in mice following hepatic irradiations.
Pharmacology 13, 248-51 (1975)

1066. Soljic,Z., Grba,V., Besic,J.
Separation of some compounds from the 1,4-benzodiazepine group by TLC.
Chromatographia 10, 751-2 (1977)

1067. Solomon,K.
Safety of oxazepam.
N.Y.State J.Med. 78, 91-2 (1978)

1068. Solow,E.B., Kenfield,C.P.
A micromethod for the determination of clonazepam in serum by electron-capture gas-liquid chromatography.
J.Anal.Toxicol. 1, 155-7 (1977)

1069. Soubrie,P., Simon,P., Boissier,J.R.
An amnesic effect of benzodiazepines in rats ?
Experientia 32, 359-60 (1976)

1070. Spector,S.
Radioimmunoassay.
Ann.Rev.Pharmacol. 13, 359-70 (1973)

1071. Spector,S.
Radioimmunoassay of drugs.
Radioimmuniassay Related Procedures Medicine 2, 233-49 (1974)

1072. Speight,A.N.
Floppy-infant syndrome and maternal diazepam and/ or nitrazepam.
Lancet 2, 878 (1977)

1073. Spiegel,H.E., Symingto,J., Savulich,A.
Stability and reliability of radioimmunoassays for clonazepam, diphenylhydantoin and phenobarbital in blood, serum or plasma.
Res.Commun.Chem.Pathol.Pharm. 19, 271-80 (1978)

1074. Squires,R.F., Brastrup,C.
Benzodiazepine receptors in rat brain.
Nature 266, 732-4 (1977)

1075. Sroczynski,Z., Lunding,M.
Acute respiratory insufficiency following treatment with chlordiazepoxide in patients with delirium tremens.
Ugeskr.Laeger 136, 1444-6 (1974)

1076. Staak,M., Mallach,H.J., Moosmayer,A.
Untersuchungen über die Auswirkung von Oxazepam und Alkohol auf die Verkehrstüchtigkeit.
Beitr.gerichtl.Med. 34, 91-6 (1976)

1077. Stacher,G.
Intrahepatic cholostasis following combined diazepam-barbiturate therapy in patients with tetanus.
Wien.Klin.Wochenschr. 85, 401-6 (1973)

1078. Stacher,G.
Der Einfluß eines neuen Psychopharmakons der Benzodiazepinreihe (Bromazepam) auf die basale Magensäureproduktion.
Z.Gastroenterologie 12, 179-84 (1974)

1079. Stahl,E.
Dünnschichtchromatographie.
2. Aufl., Springer, Berlin-Heidelberg-New York, 1967

1080. Stanski,D.R., Greenblatt,D.J., Selwyn,A., Shader,R.I.
Plasma and cerebrospinal fluid concentrations of chlordiazepoxid and its metabolites in surgical patients.
Clin.Pharmacol.Ther. 20, 571-8 (1976)

1081. Stark,L.G., Killam,K.F., Killam,E.K.
The anticonvulsant effects of phenobarbital, diphenylhydantoin and two benzodiazepines in the baboon Papio Papio.
J.Pharm.Exp. 173, 125-32 (1970)

1082. Steidinger,J., Schmid,E.
Untersuchungen über den Stoffwechsel von 7-Chlor-1,3-dihydro-3-hydroxy-5-phenyl-2H-1,4-benzodiazepin-2-on.
Arzneim.-Forsch. (Drug Res.) 20, 1232-5 (1970)

1083. Stempel,A., Landgraf,F.W.
Quinazolines and 1,4-benzodiazepines.
IX. 2-Carbobenzoxyglycylamidobenzophenones and their conversion to 1,4-benzodiazepines.
J.Org.Chem. 27, 4675-6 (1962)

1084. Stempel,A., Reeder,E., Sternbach,L.H.
Quinazolines and 1,4-benzodiazepines.
XXVII. Mechanisms of ring enlargement of quinazoline-3-oxides with alkali to 1,4-benzodiazepin-2-one-4-oxides.
J.Org.Chem. 30, 4267-71 (1965)

1085. Sternbach,L.H.
1,4-Benzodiazepines. Chemistry and some aspects of the structure-activity relationship.
Angew.Chem. (Intern.Ed.) 10, 34-43 (1971)
Angew.Chem. 83, 70-9 (1971)

1086. Sternbach,L.H., Archer,G.A., Earley,J.V., Fryer,R.I., Reeder,E., Wasyliw,N., Randall,L.O., Banziger,R.
Quinazolines and 1,4-benzodiazepines.
XXV: Structure activity relationships of aminoalkyl-substituted 1,4-benzodiazepin-2-ones.
J.Med.Chem. 8, 815-21 (1965)

1087. Sternbach,L.H., Archer,G., Reeder,E.
Quinazolines and benzodiazepines.
XV: 7-nitro-and 7-trifluoromethyl-2,3-dihydro-5-phenyl-1H-1,4-benzodiazepines and their transformations.
J.Org.Chem. 28, 3013-6 (1963)

1088. Sternbach,L.H., Fryer,R.J., Keller,O., Metlesics,W., Sach,G., Steiger,N.
Quinazolines and 1,4-benzodiazepines.
X: Nitro-substituted 5-phenyl-1,4-benzodiazepin-derivates.
J.Med.Chem. 6, 261-5 (1963)

1089. Sternbach,L.H., Fryer,R.I., Metlesics,W., Reeder,E., Sach,G., Saucy,G., Stempel,A.
Quinazolines and 1,4-benzodiazepines.
VI: Halo-, methyl-, and methoxy substituted 1,3-dihydro-5-phenyl-2H-1,4-benzodiazepin-2-ones.
J.Org.Chem. 27, 3788-96 (1962)

1090. Sternbach,L.H., Kaiser,S., Reeder,E.
Quinazoline 3-oxide structure of compounds previously described in the literature as 3,1,4-benzodiazepines.
J.Am.Chem.Soc. 82, 475-80 (1960)

1091. Sternbach,L.H., Koechlin,B.A., Reeder,E.
Quinazolines and 1,4-benzodiazepines.
VIII: The photoisomerization of 7-chloro-2-methylamino-5-phenyl-3H-1,4-benzodiazepine-4-oxide.
J.Org.Chem. 27, 4671-2 (1962)

1092. Sternbach,L.H., Randall,L.O., Banziger,R., Lehr,H.
Structure-activating relationship in the 1,4-benzodiazepine series.
In: Drugs affecting the central nervous system, Vol. 2, edited by A.Burger.
Marcel Dekker Inc., New York, pp. 237-64 (1967)

1093. Sternbach,L.H., Randall,L.O., Gustafson,S.R.
1,4-Benzodiazepines (chlordiazepoxide and related compounds).
In: Psychopharmacological Agents, Vol. 1, edited by M.Gordon.
Academic Press, New York, pp. 137-224 (1964)

1094. Sternbach,L.H., Reeder,E.
Quinazolines and 1,4-benzodiazepines.
II: The rearrangement of 6-chloro-2-chloromethyl-4-phenylquinazoline 3-oxide into 2-amino derivatives of 7-chloro-5-phenyl-3H-1,4-benzodiazepine 4-oxide.
J.Org.Chem. 26, 1111-18 (1961)

1095. Sternbach,L.H., Reeder,E.
Quinazolines and 1,4-benzodiazepines.
IV: Transformations of 7-chloro-2-methylamino-5-phenyl-3H-1,4-benzodiazepine 4-oxide.
J.Org.Chem. 26, 4936-41 (1961)

1096. Sternbach,L.H., Reeder,E., Archer,C.A.
Quinazolines and 1,4-benzodiazepines.
XI: Synthesis and transformations of 7-chloro-2,3-dihydro (and 2,3,4,5-tetrahydro)-5-phenyl-1H-1,4-benzodiazepine.
J.Org.Chem. 28, 2456-9 (1963)

1097. Sternbach,L.H., Reeder,E., Keller,O., Metlesics,W.
Quinazolines and 1,4-benzodiazepines.
III: Substituted 2-amino-5-phenyl-3H-1,4-benzodiazepine 4-oxides.
J.Org.Chem. 26, 4488-97 (1961)

1098. Stevens,H.M., Jenkins,R.W.
The chromatographic separation of mixtures of benzodiazepine drugs.
J.Forens.Sci.Soc. 11, 183-6 (1971)

1099. Stewart,J.T., Williamson,J.L.
Fluorometric determination of chlordiazepoxide in dosage forms and biological fluids with fluorescamine.
Anal.Chem. 48, 1182-5 (1976)

1100. Steyn,J.M., Hundt,H.K.
Quantitative gas chromatographic determination of diazepam and its major metabolite in human serum.
J.Chromatogr. 107, 196-200 (1975)

1101. Sticht,G., Käferstein,H.
Nachweis von Clobazam (Frisium[R]) in biologischem Material.
Z.Rechtsmedizin 82, 105-12 (1978)

1102. Stirrat,G.M., Edington,P.T., Berry,D.J.
Transplacental passage of chlordiazepoxide.
Brit.Med.J. 2, 729 (1974)

1103. Stjernholm,M.R., Katz,F.H.
Effect of diphenylhydantoin, phenobarbital, and diazepam on the metabolism of methylprednisolone and its sodium succinate.
J.Clin.Endocr. 41, 887 (1975)

1104. Straw,R.N.
The effect of certain benzodiazepines of the threshold for pentylenetetrazol-induced seizures in cats.
Arch.Int.Pharmacodyn.Ther. 175, 465-9 (1968)

1105. Street,H.V.
Rapid methods of toxicological analysis.
In: A.Stolman (Ed.), Progress in Toxicology.
Academic Press, New York, 1965, 2: 239-81

1106. Strojny,N., Bratin,K., Brooks,M.A., DeSilva,J.A.F.
Determination of chlordiazepoxide, diazepam and their major metabolites in blood and plasma by spectrodensitometry.
J.Chromatogr. 143, 363-74 (1977)

1107. Strojny,N., Puglisi,C.V., DeSilva,J.A.F.
Determination of chlordiazepoxide and its metabolites in plasma by high-pressure liquid-chromatography.
Anal.Letters 11, 135-60 (1978)

1108. Sumitomi-Inaba,S., Ishizumi,K., Yamamoto,H.
Benzodiazepines. IV. A new synthesis of 1-diethylaminoethyl-substituted 1,4-benzo-diazepine-2-ones.
Chem.Pharm.Bull. 19, 263-72 (1971)

1109. Sunshine,I.
Handbook of Analytical Toxicology.
The Chemical Rubber Company, Cleveland (Ohio) 1969

1110. Sutherland,J.W., Williamson,D.E., Theivagt,J.G.
Pharmaceuticals and related drugs.
Anal.Chem. 43, 206-66 (1971)

1111. Svenson,S.E., Gordon,L.E.
Diazepam: A progress report.
Curr.Ther.Res. 7, 367-91 (1965)

1112. Svenson,S.E., Hamilton,R.G.
A critique of overemphasis on side effects with the psychotropic drugs: An analysis of 18,000 chlordiazepoxide-treated cases.
Curr.Ther.Res. 8, 455-64 (1966)

1113. Swinyard,E.A., Castellion,A.W.
Anticonvulsant properties of some benzodiazepines.
J.Pharmacol.Exp.Ther. 151, 369-75 (1966)

1114. Sybirska,H., Gajzińska,H.
Problems of identification of benzodiazepine-derivates in autopsical material.
Arch.Med.Sadowej 27, 107-14 (1977)

1115. Syvaelahti,E.K., Kanto,J.H.
Serum growth hormone, serum immunoreactive insulin and blood glucose response to oral and intravenous diazepam in man.
Int.J.Clin.Pharmacol.Biopharm. 12, 74-82 (1975)

1116. Szafranowa,H., Krysicka-Doczkal,H., Lewandowska,I., Wutkiewicz,M.
The influence of protein deficiency in rats on chlordiazepoxide and chlorpromazine kinetics.
Pol.J.Pharmacol.Pharm. 27, 1-8 (1975)

1117. Szcawinska,K., Cenajek,D.
Influence of cystamine on pharmacokinetics and pharmacodynamics of nitrazepam.
Arch.Immunol.Ther.Exp. (Warsz.) 25, 157-62 (1977)

1118. Tabolin,V.A., Vakhush,A.M., Almazova,I.G., Radilov,I.U.O., Lutskii,I.M.
Clinical aspects and emergency measures in accidental poisoning with elenium (librium) in children.
Vopr.Okhr.Materin.Det. 14, 79-81 (1969)

1119. Tanja,J.J., Clark,C.R., Griffies,D.E.
Serum levels of diazepam and N-desmethyldiazepam in hospitalized patients.
J.Anal.Toxicol. 1, 175-8 (1977)

1120. Tank,F.-W.
Anwendungsmöglichkeiten der Hochdruckflüssigkeitschromatographie in der pharmazeutischen Analytik.
Dissertation Marburg/Lahn 1976

1121. Tanner,T.B., Moorhead,S.H.
High dose poisoning with diazepam (valium) and survival in a two-year-old child.
J.Med.Ass.Can. 57, 534-6 (1968)

1122. Tansella,M., Zimmermann-Tansella,C., Lader,M.
The residual effects of N-desmethyldiazepam in patients.
Z.Ges.Inn.Med. 29, 81-90 (1974)

1123. Tassonyi,E.
Effects of flunitrazepam (rohypnol) on neuromuscular blockade, clinical study.
Ann.Anesthesiol.Fr. 18, 741-6 (1977)

1124. Tateishi,M., Shimizu,H.
A new metabolic pathway of bromazepam involving attachment of a methylthio group.
Xenobiotica 6, 431 (1976)

1125. Taylor,J.F., Fysh,R.R.
Nitrazepam overdosage.
Bull.Int.Ass.Forens.Toxicol. 11, 14-5 (1975)

1126. Taylor,K.M., Laverty,R.
The effect of chlordiazepoxide, diazepam, and nitrazepam on catecholamine metabolism in regions of the rat brain.
Eur.J.Pharmacol. 8, 296-301 (1969)

1127. Taylor,P.A., Cotton,P.B., Towey,R.M., Gent,A.E.
Pulmonary complications after oesophagogastroscopy using diazepam.
Brit.Med.J. 1, 666 (1972)

1128. Terhaag,B.
Über Bindung und Verteilung von Chlordiazepoxid (Radepur) und seiner Metaboliten im Erythrozyten-Plasma und Erythrozyten-Puffer-System.
Acta Biol.Med.Ger. 35, 1373-8 (1976)

1129. Tewari,S.N., Shukla,S.K.
Thin layer chromatographic technique for the separation and identification of 1,4-benzodiazepine drugs in biological material.
Pharmazie 31, 893-4 (1976)

1130. Tewari,S.N., Shukla,S.K.
Paper electrophoretic detection and separation of some psychotropic drugs of 1,4-benzodiazepine series in autopsy materials.
Pharmazie 32, 243 (1977)

1131. Tewari,S.N., Shukla,S.K.
Separation and identification of 1,4-benzodiazepine drugs present in the biological fluids by two dimensional TLC.
Pharmazie 32, 536 (1977)

1132. Thiessen,J.J., Sellers,E.M., Denbeigh,P., Dolman,L.
Plasma protein binding of diazepam and tolbutamide in chronic alcoholics.
J.Clin.Pharmacol. 16, 345-51 (1976)

1133. Thomas,J.J., Dryon,L.
Identification de médicaments psychotropes par chromatographie sur couche mince.
J.Pharm.Belg. 19, 481-504 (1964)

1134. Toaff,M.E., Hezroni,J., Toaff,R.
Effect of diazepam on uterine activity during labor.
Isr.J.Med.Sci. 13, 1007-12 (1977)

1135. Tobin,J.M., Bird,I.F., Boyle,D.E.
Preliminary evaluation of librium (Ro-0690) in the treatment of anxiety reactions.
Dis.Nerv.Syst. 21, 11 (1960)

1136. Tobin,J.M., Lewis,N.D.C.
New psychotherapeutic agent, chlordiazepoxide. Use in treatment of anxiety states and related symptoms.
J.Amer.Med.Ass. 174, 1242-9 (1960)

1137. Tompsett,S.L.
Nitrazepam in blood serum and urine and librium in urine.
J.Clin.Path. 21, 366-71 (1968)

1138. Torry,J.M.
A case of suicide with nitrazepam and alcohol.
Practitioner 217, 648-9 (1976)

1139. Trebbi,A., Gervasi,G.B., Comi,V.
Determination of pinazepam and its metabolites in serum, urine and brain by gas-liquid chromatography and mass spectrometry.
J.Chromatogr. 110, 309-19 (1975)

1140. Tseng,T.-C., Wang,S.C.
Locus of central depressant action of some benzodiazepine analogues.
Proc.Soc.Exp.Biol.Med. 137, 526-31 (1971)

1141. Truhaut,R., Boudène,C., Claude,J.-R.
Apercus sur les applications de la chromatographie en couche mince en analyse toxicologique.
Ann.Biol.Clin. 26, 93-111 (1968)

1142. Tsuchiya,T., Fukushim,H.
Effects of benzodiazepines and pentobarbital on gaba-ergic recurrent inhibition of hippocampal neurons.
Eur.J.Pharm. 48, 421-4 (1978)

1143. Tsutsumi,E., Inaba,T., Mahon,W.A.
The displacing effect of a fatty acid on the binding of diazepam to human serum albumin.
Biochem.Pharmacol. 24, 1361-2 (1975)

1144. Tulzer,W.
Die Bedeutung praenatal verabreichter Medikamente für Früh- und Neugeborene.
Wien.Klin.Wochenschr. 82, 304-7 (1970)

1145. Uihlein,M., Hajdú,P.
High performance liquid chromatography in research of pharmacokinetics and metabolism.
Arzneim.-Forsch. (Drug Res.) 27, 98-102 (1977)

1146. Ullucci,P.A., Cadoret,R., Stasiowski,P.D., Martin,H.F.
A comprehensive GC/MS drug screening procedure.
J.Anal.Toxicol. 2, 33-8 (1978)

1147. Unterhalt,B., Keil,B., Reinhold,K.
Untersuchung von Tranquillantien, insbesondere von Medazepam.
Dtsch.Apoth.-Ztg. 111, 1775-7 (1971)

1148. Vajda,F.J.E., Prineas,R.J., Lovell,R.R.H.
Interactions between phenytoin and the benzodiazepines.
Brit.Med.J. 1971, 346

1149. Valentour,J.C., Monforte,J.R., Lorenzo,B., Sunshine,I.
Fluorometric screening method for detecting benzodiazepines in blood and urine.
Clin.Chem. 21, 1976-9 (1975)

1150. Valerino,D.M. et al.
Effect of various centrally active drugs on hepatic microsomal enzymes: A comparative study.
Drug.Metab.Disposition 1, 669 (1973)

1151. Vallner,J.
Binding of drugs by albumin and plasma protein.
J.Pharm.Sci. 66, 447-65 (1977)

1152. Van der Kleijn,E.
Kinetics of distribution and metabolism of diazepam and chlordiazepoxide in mice.
Arch.Int.Pharmacodyn.Ther. 178, 193-215 (1969)

1153. Van der Kleijn,E.
Protein binding and lipophilic nature of ataractics of the meprobamate- and diazepine-group.
Arch.Int.Pharmacodyn.Ther. 179, 225-50 (1969)

1154. Van der Kleijn,E.
Kinetics of distribution and metabolism of diazepam in animals and humans.
Arch.Int.Pharmacodyn.Ther. 182, 433-6 (1969)

1155. Van der Kleijn,E.
Pharmacokinetics of distribution and metabolism of ataractic drugs and an evaluation of the site of antianxiety activity.
Ann.N.Y. Acad.Sci. 179, 115-25 (1971)

1156. Van der Kleijn,E., Beelen,G., Frederick,M.
Determination of tranquillizers by GLC in biological fluids.
Clin.Chim.Acta 34, 345-56 (1971)

1157. Van der Kleijn,E., Guelen,P.J.M., Beelen,T.C.M., Rijntjes,M.V.M., Zuidgeest,T.L.B.
Kinetics of general and regional brain distribution of closely related 7-chloro-1,4-benzodiazepines.
In: 362., pp. 145-159

1158. Van der Kleijn,E., Rossum,van,J.M., Muskens,A.T., Rijntjes,N.V.
Pharmacokinetics of diazepam in dogs, mice, and humans.
Acta Pharmacol.Toxicol. 29, 109-29 (1971)

1159. Van der Kleijn,E., Wijffels,C.C.
Whole-body and regional brain distribution of diazepam in newborn rhesus monkeys.
Arch.Int.Pharmacodyn.Ther. 192, 255-64 (1971)

1160. Van der Meren,P.J., Steyn,J.M.
Thin-layer chromatographic method for determination of diazepam and its major metabolite, N-desmethyldiazepam, in human serum.
J.Chromatogr. 148, 549-52 (1978)

1161. Van Melkebeek,A., Barsy,de,A.M.
A rare but severe complication arising from the intravenous use of diazepam.
Acta Neurol.Belg. 70, 286-94 (1970)

1162. Vapaatalo,H., Karppanen,H.
Combined toxicity of ethanol with chlorpromazine, diazepam, chlormethiazole or pentobarbital in mice.
Agents Actions 1, 43-5 (1969)

1163. Veall,R.M., Hogarth,H.C.
Thrombocytopenia during treatment with clonazepam.
Brit.Med.J. 4, 462 (1975)

1164. Vernhiet,J., Renou,A.M., Orgogozo,J.M., Constant,P., Caille,J.M.
Effects of a diazepam-fentanyl mixture on cerebral blood flow and oxygen consumption in man.
Brit.J.Anaesth. 50, 165-9 (1978)

1165. Vessmann,J., Freij,G., Strömberg,S.
Determination of oxazepam in serum and urine by electron capture gas chromatography.
Acta Pharm.Suecica 9,447-56(1972)

1166. Vessmann,J., Johansson,M., Magnusson,P., Stroemberg,S.
Determination of intact oxazepam by electron-capture gas chromatography after an extractive alkylation reaktion.
Anal.Chem. 49, 1545-9 (1977)

1167. Viala,A., Cano,J.P.
Diazepam (valium) blood levels after administration of the drugs in capsules.
Therapie 23, 775-8 (1968)

1168. Viala,A., Cano,J.P.
Blood levels of diazepam (valium) after administration of the drug in solution or syrup form.
Therapie 24, 1115-21 (1969)

1169. Viala,A., Cano,J.P., Dravet,C., Tassinari,C.A., Roger,J.
Blood levels of diazepam (valium) and N-desmethyldiazepam in the epileptic child, a preliminary report.
Psychiatr.Neurol.Neurochir. 74, 153-8 (1971)

1170. Viala,A., Cano,J.P., Reynier,J.P., Rispe,R.
Determination of N-desmethyldiazepam in plasma by gas chromatography with an internal standard.
J.Chromatogr. 147, 349-57 (1978)

1171. Viau,J.P., Epps,J.E., DiCarlo,J.
Prazepam metabolism after chronic administration to humans.
Xenobiotica 3, 581-7 (1973)

1172. Viau,J.P., Epps,J.E., DiCarlo,F.J.
Metabolism of prazepam in vitro.
Fed.Proc.Fed.Amer.Soc.Exp.Biol. 30, 225 (1971)

1173. Viau,J.-P., Epps,J.E., DiCarlo,F.J.
Prazepam metabolism in vitro.
Biochem.Pharmacol. 21, 563-9 (1972)

1174. Viau,J.-P., Epps,J.E., DiCarlo,F.J.
Prazepam metabolism in the rat.
J.Pharm.Sci. 62, 641-5 (1973)

1175. Vidic,E.
Nachweis und Beständigkeit von Arzneistoffen in Blutproben.
Arch.Toxikol. 27, 19-39 (1970)

1176. Vidic,E., Klug,E.
Papier- und dünnschichtchromatographische Systematik für basische Arzneistoffe.
Z.Rechtsmedizin 76, 283-91 (1975)

1177. Vinh,C.T., Braun,J., Plourde,J.R.
Determination of clonazepam in tablets by DC-polarography.
J.Pharm.Sci. 67, 731-3 (1978)

1178. Viscott,D.S.
Chlordiazepoxide and hallucinations. Report of cases.
Arch.Gen.Psychiatry 19, 370-6 (1968)

1179. Viukari,M., Linnoila,M.
Serum medazepam, diazepam, and N-desmethyldiazepam levels after single and multiple oral doses of medazepam.
Ann.Clin.Res. 9, 284-7 (1977)

1180. Viukari,M., Linnoila,M., Aalto,U.
Efficacy and side-effects of flurazepam, fosazepam and nitrazepam as sleeping aids in psychogeriatric patients.
Acta Psychiat.Scand. 57, 27-36 (1978)

1181. Vogel,H.L.
Intravenous use of physostimine in the management of acute diazepam intoxication.
J.Am.Osteopath.Assoc. 76, 349-51 (1977)

1182. Volkova,I.V.
Determination of chlordiazepoxide and its main metabolites in blood in chemical and toxicological studies.
Farmatsiia 26, 35-8 (1977)

1183. Vorne,M. et al.
Diazepam, ethanol and drug-metabolizing enzymes in rat liver.
Arch.Int.Pharmacodyn.Thér. 216, 280 (1975)

1184. Vorne,M., Idänpään-Heikkilä,J.
Inhibition of drug-metabolizing enzymes by diazepam in rat liver.
Experientia 31, 962 (1975)

1185. Vree,T.B., Lenselink,B., van der Kleijn,E., Nijhuis,G.M.
Determination of flunitrazepam in body fluids by means of high-performance liquid chromatography.
J.Chromatogr. 143, 530-4 (1977)

1186. Vyas,I., Carney,M.W.
Diazepam withdrawal fits.
Brit.Med.J. 4, 44 (1975)

1187. Vyskocil,F.
Diazepam blockade of repetitive action potentials in skeletal muscle fibres, a model of its membrane action.
Brain Res. 133, 315-28 (1977)

1188. Wad,N.T., Hanifl,E.J.
Simplified thin-layer chromatographic method for the simultaneous determination of clonazepam, diazepam, and their metabolites in serum.
J.Chromatogr. 143, 214-8 (1977)

1189. Wad,N., Rosenmund,H., Hanifl,E.
A simplified quantitative method for the simultaneous determination of diazepam and its metabolites in serum by thin-layer chromatography.
J.Chromatogr. 128, 231-4 (1976)

1190. Waddington,J.L., Longden,A.
Rotational behaviour and cGMP responses following manipulation of nigral mechanisms with chlordiazepoxide. Evidence for enhancement of GABA transmission by benzodiazepines.
Naunyn-Schmied. Arch.Pharmacol. 300, 233-9 (1977)

1191. Walkenstein,S.S., Wiser,R., Gudmundsen,C.H., Kimmel,H.B., Corradino,R.A.
Absorption, metabolism and excretion of oxazepam and its succinate half-ester.
J.Pharm.Sci. 1181-6 (1964)

1192. Wassel,G.M., Diab,A.M.
Colorimetric and spectrometric estimations of nitrazepam in pharmaceuticals and urine samples.
Pharmazie 28, 790-1 (1973)

1193. Weber,D.J.
High pressure liquid chromatography of benzodiazepines: Analysis of ketazolam.
J.Pharm.Sci. 61, 1797-1800 (1972)

1194. Weiner,W.J., Goetz,C., Nausleda,P.A., Klawans,H.L.
Clonazepam and dopamine-related stereotyped behavior.
Life Sci. 21, 901-6 (1977)

1195. Weinfeld,R.E., Posmanter,H.N., Khoo,K.C., Puglisi,C.V.
Rapid determination of diazepam and nordiazepam in plasma by electron capture gas-liquid chromatography. Application in clinical pharmacokinetic studies.
J.Chromatogr. 143, 581-95 (1977)

1196. Weist,F.R.
Zum Nachweis von 7-Chlor-1,3-dihydro-3-hydroxy-5-phenyl-2H-1,4-benzodiazepin-2-on in biologischen Flüssigkeiten.
Arzneim.-Forsch. (Drug Res.) 18, 87-9 (1968)

1197. Weist,F., Schmid,E.
Dünnschichtchromatographischer Schnellnachweis von Tranquilizern der Benzodiazepin-Reihe und von thymoleptischen Medikamenten.
Med.Welt 7, 369-72 (1969)

1198. Welch,T.R., Rumack,B.H., Hammond,K.
Clonazepam overdose resulting in cyclic coma.
Clin.Toxicol. 10, 433-6 (1977)

1199. Wellhöner,H.-H.
Allgemeine und systematische Pharmakologie und Toxikologie.
Springer, Berlin-Heidelberg-New York 1975

1200. Wheatley,D.
Comparative effects of propanolol and chlordiazepoxide in anxiety states.
Brit.J.Psychiatr. 115, 1411-2 (1969)

1201. Whelpton,R., Curry,S.H.
Gas-chromatographic separation of chlorpromazin, diazepam, and N-desmethyldiazepam.
J.Pharm.Pharmacol. 27, 970-1 (1975)

1202. White,B.J., Driscoll,E.J., Tijio,J.H., Smilack,Z.H.
Chromosomal aberration rates and intravenously given diazepam, a negative study.
J.Amer.Med.Ass. 230, 414-7 (1974)

1203. White,J.M.
A note on the quantitation of fluorazepam by ultraviolet absorption spectrometry.
Bull.Int.Ass.Forens.Toxicol. 10, 4 (1974)

1204. Whitehouse,L.W., Paul,C.J., Coldwell,B.B., Thomas,B.H.
Effect of ethanol on diazepam distribution in rat.
Res.Commun.Chem.Pathol.Pharmacol. 12, 221-42 (1975)

1205. Wiersema,S.
Unusually high diazepam level in a chronic user.
Bull.Int.Ass.Forens.Toxicol. 11, 13-4 (1975)

1206. Wiezorek,W.D., Liebmann,H., Stremmel,D.
Effects of benzodiazepine derivates on cholinesterase activity of rat blood.
Pharmazie 32, 530-2 (1977)

1207. Williams,R.T.
Detoxication Mechanisms.
John Wiley and Sons, Inc., New York 1959

1208. Winek,C.L.
Tabulation of therapeutic, toxic, and lethal concentrations of drugs and chemicals in blood.
Clin.Chem. 22, 832-6 (1976)

1209. Winkelmayer,R.
Subicterus following the administration of thioridazine and chlordiazepoxide.
Del.Med.J. 38, 334-6 (1966)

1210. Winstead,D.K.
Hiccups following ingestion of oral chlordiazepoxide.
Am.J.Psychiatry 133, 719 (1976)

1211. Wretlind,M., Pilbrant,A., Sundwall,A., Vessman,J.
Disposition of three benzodiazepines after single oral administration in man.
Acta Pharm.Toxicol. 40, 28-39 (1977)

1212. Wuttke,W., Kelleher,R.T.
Effects of some benzodiazepines on punished and unpunished behavior in the pigeon.
J.Pharm.Exp. 172, 397-405 (1970)

1213. Yamamoto,H., Inaba,S., Hirohashi,T., Ishizumi,K.
Notiz über ein neues Verfahren zur Herstellung von 1,4-Benzodiazepinderivaten aus 2-Aminomethyl-indol-derivaten.
Chem.Ber. 101, 4245-7 (1968)

1214. Yamamoto,K., Kuze,S., Murakami,S., Takeshita,M.
Simultaneous determination of pentazocine and diazepam in the blood by gas chromatography.
Jpn.J.Anestesiol. 25, 680-5 (1976)

1215. Yanagi,Y., Haga,F., Endo,M., Kitagawa,S.
Comparative metabolic study of nimetazepam and its desmethyl derivative (nitrazepam) in man.
Xenobiotica 5, 245-7 (1975)

1216. Yanagi,Y., Haga,F., Endo,M., Kitagawa,S.
Comparative metabolic study of nimetazepam and its desmethyl derivative (nitrazepam) in dogs.
Xenobiotica 6, 101-12 (1976)

1217. Yasumura,A., Murata,H., Hattori,K., Matsuda,K.
Studies of metabolism of oxazolam.
II: Isolation and identification of the metabolites of oxazolam in rats.
Chem.Pharm.Bull. 19, 1929 (1971)

1218. Young,R.L., Albano,R.F., Charnecki,A.M., Demcsak,G.
Effect of diazepam on regional levels of glucose and malate in the central nervous system.
Fed.Proc.Fed.Amer.Soc.Exp.Biol. 28, 444 (1969)

1219. Zaffiri,O., Francescato,F., Ruggerini,R., Bisiani,M.
Prolonged resuscitation in a case of grave poisoning with oxazepam.
Minerva Anestesiol. 33, 729-31 (1967)

1220. Zakusov,V.V., Ostrovskaya,R.U., Kozhechkin,S.N., Markovich,V.V., Molodavkin,G.M., Voronina,T.A.
Further evidence for GABA-ergic mechanisms in the action of benzodiazepines.
Arch.Int.Pharmacodyn.Ther. 229, 313-27 (1977)

1221. Zbinden,G., Bagdon,R.E., Keith,E.F., Phillips.R.D., Randall,L.O.
Experimental and clinical toxicology of chlordiazepoxid (librium).
Toxicol.Appl.Pharmacol. 3, 619-37 (1961)

1222. Zbinden,G., Randall,L.O.
Pharmacology of benzodiazepines: Laboratory and clinical correlations.
In: Advances of Pharmacology, Vol. 5, edited by S.Garattini and P.A.Shore.
Academic Press, New York, pp. 213-91 (1967)

1223. Zileli,M.S., Teletar,F., Deniz,S., Ilter,E., Adalar,N.
Oxazepam intoxication stimulating non-keto-acidotic diabetic coma.
J.Amer.Med.Ass. 215, 1986 (1971)

1224. Zingales,I.A.
Systematic identification of tricyclic psychotropic drugs.
J.Chromatogr. 31, 405-19 (1967)

1225. Zingales,I.
Systematic identification of psychotropic drugs by thin-layer chromatography.
J.Chromatogr. 34, 44-51 (1968)

1226. Zingales,I.A.
Determination of chlordiazepoxide plasma concentrations by electron capture GLC.
J.Chromatogr. 61, 237-52 (1971)

1227. Zingales,I.A.
Diazepam metabolism during chronic medication. Unbound fraction in plasma, erythrocytes and urine.
J.Chromatogr. 75, 55-78 (1973)

1228. Zingales,I.A.
Quantitative-determination of chlordiazepoxide and its metabolites in serum by fluorescence TLC-densitometry.
J.Pharm.Sci. 67, 639-41 (1978)

1229. Zisook,S., Devaul,R.A.
Adverse behavioral effects of benzodiazepines.
J.Fam.Pract. 5, 963-6 (1977)

1230. Zsigmond,E.K.
Causes of ventricular arrhythmias.
J.Amer.Med.Ass. 221, 712-3 (1972)

1231. Zsigmond,E.K., Flynn,K., Martinez,O.A.
Diazepam and meperidine on arterial blood gases in healthy volunteers.
J.Clin.Pharmacol. 14, 377-81 (1974)

Alphabetical List 2

1232. Aarli,J.A.
Effect of clonazepam (Ro 5-4023) on epileptic seizures.
Acta Neurol.Scand. 49, 11 (1973)

1233. Ackermann,E., Richter,K.
Diazepam metabolism in the human fetus.
In Morselli,P.L., Garattini,S. u. Sereni,F. ED:
Basic and therapeutic aspects of perinatal pharmacology.
Raven Press - New York 1975

1234. Adeoshun,I.O., Healy,T.E.J., Patrick,J.M.
Ventilatory patterns in surgical patients premedicated with lorazepam or diazepam.
Brit.J.Clin.Pharmacol. 6, 466-7 (1978)

1235. Ahmad,S., Meeran,M.K.
Treatment of spasmodic torticollis with diazepam.
Brit.Med.J. 1, 127 (1979)

1236. Ahnefeld,F.W., Bergmann,H., Burri,C., Dick,W., Halmágyi,M., Hossli,G., Rügheimer,E.
Rohypnol (Flunitrazepam). - Pharmakologische Grundlagen - klinische Anwendungen.
Springer Verlag, Berlin Heidelberg New York 1978

1237. Alps,B.J., Harry,T.V.A., Southgate,P.J.
The pharmacology of lorazepam, a broad-spectrum tranquillizer.
Curr.Med.Res.Opinion 1, 239 (1973)

1238. Alvan,G., Jönsson,M., Sundwall,A., Vessman,J.
Intravenous tolerance, first pass conjugation and enterohepatic recycling of oxazepam in dogs.
Acta Pharmacol.Toxicol. 40, 16-27 (1977)

1239. Alvan,G., Odar-Cederloef,I.
Pharmacokinetic profile of oxazepam.
Acta Psych.Scand. 1978, 47-55 (1978)

1240. Amrein,R.
Zur Pharmakokinetik und zum Metabolismus von Flunitrazepam.
The pharmacokinetics and metabolism of flunitrazepam.
Klin.Anaesthesiol.Intensivther. 17, 8-24 (1978)

1241. Anezaki,K., Ando,R., Shima,K., Sakurada,T., Kisara,K.
Effects of diazepam on evoked-potential recorded from basal medial amygdaloid nucleus, lateral hypothalamus and midbrain reticular formation.
Fol.Pharm.J. 74, 491-8 (1978)

1242. Appel,P., Berger,I., Harrer,G.
Erfahrungen mit Wy 4036, einem neuen Tranquilizer aus der Benzodiazepin-Reihe.
Arzneim.-Forsch. (Drug Res.) 21, 1083 (1971)

1243. Arfwidson,L., Arn,L., Beskow,J., Ottoson,J.O., Person,G.
A comparison between diazepam, dixirazine, opropramol and placebo in anxiety states.
Acta Psychiatr.Scand. 221, 19-32 (1971)

1244. Arndts,D., Rominger,K.L.
Isolierung von Metaboliten neuer Arzneimittel zur massenspektrometrischen Strukturaufklärung.
Arzneim.-Forsch. (Drug Res.) 28, 1951-60 (1978)

1245. Assaf,R.A.E., Dundee,J.W., Gamble,J.A.S.
The influence of the route of administration on the clinical action of diazepam.
Anaesthesia 30, 152-8 (1975)

1246. Atluri,R., Ravry,M.J.R.
Effect of intravenous diazepam on arterial oxygen-saturation levels during esophagogastroduodenoscopy.
Gastrointest.Endoscopy 24, 191 (1978)

1247. Authier,L., Chapados,R., Sindon,A., Gagnon,M.A.
Amnesia and other effects of diazepam in premedication and induction of anesthesia.
Can.Anaest.Soc.J. 25, 297-302 (1978)

1248. Aymard,N., Soulaira,A.
Chronobiologic changes in pharmacokinetics of dipotassic chlorazepate, a benzodiazepine.
Chronobiol. 5, 187-8 (1978)

1249. Babbini,M., DeMarchi,F., Montanaro,N., Strocchi,P., Torrielli,M.V.
Chemistry and CNS-pharmacological properties of two hydrosoluble benzodiazepine derivatives.
Arzneim.-Forsch. (Drug Res.) 19, 1931-6 (1969)

1250. Bachman,D.S.
Clonazepam in treatment of absence seizures with automatisms.
Arch.Neurol. 35, 773-4 (1978)

1251. Bagolini,C., De Witt,P., Pacifici,L., Ramacci,M.T.
Synthesis and pharmacological activity of some derivatives of 1-Phenyl-1,2,3,4-tetrahydro-5H-1,4-benzodiazepin-5-one.
J.Med.Chem. 21, 476-80 (1978)

1252. Baird,E.S., Flowerdew,G.D.
Intravenous diazepam in conservative dentistry.
Brit.Dent.J. 128, 11 (1970)

1253. Baird,E.S., Hailey,D.M.
Delayed recovery from a sedative: Correlation of the plasma levels of diazepam with clinical effects after oral and intravenous administration.
Brit.J.Anaest. 44, 803-7 (1972)

1254. Balassa,M., Deisenhammer,E.
Erste Untersuchungsergebnisse mit einem neuen Antikonvulsivum der Benzodiazepinreihe (Clonazepam).
Wien.Med.Wschr. 22, 27-31 (1972)

1255. Banen,D.M., Resnick,O.
Lorazepam versus glutethimide as a sleep-inducing agent for geriatric patients.
J.Amer.Geriatr.Soc. 21, 507-11 (1973)

1256. Bankmikk,O.K., Steiness,E., Arnold,E., Hansen,T., Sobye,M., Lunding,M.
Serum diazepam and serum creatine-kinase after intramuscular injection of diazepam in two different vehicles.
Act.Anae.Sc. 1978, 91-5 (1978)

1257. Baraldi,M., Schwartz,J., Guidotti,A., Costa,E.
Regulation of high affinity binding of diazepam and GABA TC membranes of neuroelastoma and glioma cells.
Pharmacology 20, 273 (1978)

1258. Bardhan,K.G.
Cerebellar syndrome after nitrazepam overdosage.
Lancet 1, 1319-20 (1969)

1259. Barlow,S.M., Knight,A.F., Sullivan,F.M.
Plasma corticosterone responses to stress following chronic oral-administration of diazepam in the rat.
J.Pharm.Pharmacol. 31, 23-6 (1979)

1260. Barnett,A.M.
Treatment of epilepsy with clonazepam.
S.Afr.Med.J. 47, 1683 (1973)

1261. Barnett,A., Fiore,J.W.
Acute tolerance to diazepam in cats.
In: 362. pp. 545-58

1262. Bartholini,G., Keller,H.H., Pieri,L., Pletscher,A.
The effect of diazepam on the turnover of cerebral dopamine.
In: 362. pp. 235-40

1263. Barzaghi,F., Fournex,R., Mantegazza,P.
Pharmacological and toxicological properties of clobazam (1-phenyl-5-methyl-8-chloro-1,2,4,5,-tetrahydro-2,4-diketo-3H-1,5-benzodiazepine), a new psychotherapeutic agent.
Arzneim.-Forsch. (Drug Res.) 23, 683-6 (1973)

1264. Baselt,R.C., Cravey,R.H.
A compendium of therapeutic and toxic concentrations of toxicologically significant drugs in human biofluids.
J.Anal.Toxicol. 1, 81-103 (1977)

1265. Baselt,R.C., Wright,J.A., Cravey,R.H.
Therapeutic und toxic concentrations of more than 100 toxicologically significant drugs in blood, plasma, or serum: a tabulation.
Clin.Chem. 21, 44-62 (1975)

1266. Belvedere,G., Tognoni,G., Frigerio,A., Morselli,P.L.
A specific, rapid and sensitive method for gas-chromatographic determination of methyl-oxazepam in small samples of blood.
Anal.Lett. 5, 531-3 (1972)

1267. Bentel,H.U., Schoenmeyer,J.
Die Behandlung psychovegetativer Allgemeinstörungen mit einer abendlichen Einmaldosis Dikaliumchlorazepat im Rahmen einer Multicenter-Studie.
Wien.klin.Wschr. 90, 1-12, Suppl. 92 (1978)

1268. Bepko,F., Lowe,E., Waxman,B.
Relief of the emotional factor in labor with parenterally administered diazepam.
Obstet.Gynecol. 26, 852-7 (1965)

1269. Bergamini,L., Mutani,R., Fariello,R. et al.
Elektroenzephalographische und klinische Bewertung des neuen Benzodiazepins Ro 5-4023.
EEG-EMG 1, 182-8 (1970)

1270. Berger,M.
Untersuchungen der Wirkungsqualität von Valium am Uterus.
In: Relaxation und Sedation des menschlichen Uterus. II. Symposium Bern 1963, S.Karger, Basel

1271. Berger,M.
Die Anwendung von Diazepam bei 3000 Gebärenden.
Arzneim.-Forsch. (Drug Res.) 16, 1110-3 (1966)

1272. Berkseth,R.O., Anderson,D.C., Mahowald,M.W., Shapiro,F.L.
Dialysis encephalopathy - effects of continued aluminum exposure and clonazepam on prognosis.
Kidney Int. 14, 670 (1978)

1273. Berry,P.A., Burtles,R., Grubb,D.J., Hoare,M.V.
An evaluation of the effects of clobazam on human co-ordination, mental activity and mood.
Brit.J.Clin.Pharmacol. 1, 346 (1974)

1274. Bertilsson,L.
Mechanism of action of benzodiazepines - GABA hypothesis.
Acta Psych.Scand. 1978, 19-26 (1978)

1275. Bianchi,G.N., Philips,J.
A comparative trial of doxepin and diazepam in anxiety states.
Psychopharmacologia 25, 86-95 (1972)

1276. Bihler,I., Sawh,P.C.
Effects of benzodiazepines on transport of sugars and ions in rat skeletal-muscle in vitro.
Molec.Pharm. 14, 879-83 (1978)

1277. Birket-Smith,E., Mikkelsen,R.
Preliminary observations on the effect of a new benzodiazepine (Ro 5-4023) in epilepsy.
Acta Neurol.Scand. 48, 22-7 (1972)

1278. Biswas,B., Carlsson,A.
Mode of action of diazepam on brain catecholamine metabolism.
Naunyn-Schmied.Arch.Toxicol. 303, 73-8 (1978)

1279. Bladin,P.F.
The use of clonazepam as an anticonvulsant - clinical evaluation.
Med.J.Aust. 1, 683-8 (1973)

1280. Blaha,L.
Clobazam - clinical survey.
Med.Welt 29, 1460-2 (1978)

1281. Bliding,A.
Abuse potential of benzodiazepines with special reference to oxazepam.
Acta Psych.Scand. 1978, 111-6 (1978)

1282. Blitt,C.D., Petty,W.C., Wright,W.A., Wright,B.
Clinical evaluation of injectable lorazepam as a premedicant. The effect on recall.
Anesth.Analg. 55, 522-5 (1976)

1283. Bobon,J., Bourdouxhe,S., Breulet,M., Parent,M., Bobon,D.P.
Pilot clinical trial of parenteral lorazepam (Temesta) in anxiety states.
Psychopharmacologia 33, 377-84 (1973)

1284. Boff.E., Heise,G.A.
Attenuation of tetrabenazine "reversal" by chlordiazepoxide hydrochloride.
Fed.Proc. 22, 510 (1963)

1285. Bogatsky,A.V., Golovenko,N.Y., Andronati,S.A., Kolomeichenko,G.Y., Meteshkin,Y.V.
Anticonvulsive effect, metabolism and pharmacokinetics of diazepam in mice, exposed to hypergravity.
Kosm.Biol.AV.M. 12, 75-8 (1978)

1286. Booker,H.E.
Clorazepate dipotassium in the treatment of intractable epilepsy.
J.Amer.Med.Assoc. 229, 552-5 (1974)

1287. Borchert,H.H., Szolomic. I., Pfeifer,S.
Metabolic drug interactions of carbamazepine and clonazepam.
Pharmazie 33, 816-20 (1978)

1288. Borland,R.G., Nicholson,A.N.
Comparison of the residual effects of two benzodiazepines (nitrazepam and flurazepam hydrochloride) and pentobarbitone sodium on human performance.
Brit.J.Clin.Pharmacol. 2, 9-17 (1975)

1289. Bosmann,H.B., Penney,D.P., Case,K.R., DiStefano,P., Averill,K.
Diazepam receptor: Specific binding of ^{3}H-diazepam and ^{3}H-flunitrazepam to rat brain subfractions.
FEBS Lett. 87, 199-202 (1978)

1290. Boston Collaborative Surveillance Program.
Clinical depression of the central nervous system due to diazepam and chlordiazepoxide in relation to cigarette smoking and age.
N.Engl.J.Med. 288, 277-80 (1973)

1291. Bourne,R.C., Robinson,J.D., Teale,J.D.
Simple radioimmunoassay for plasma diazepam and its application to single dose studies in man.
Brit.J.Pharm. 63, 371 (1978)

1292. Boxenbaum,H.G., Posmanter ,H.N., Macasieb,T., Geitner,K.A., Weinfeld,R.E., Moore,J.D., Darragh,A., Okelly,D.A., Weissman,L., Kaplan,S.A.
Pharmacokinetics of flunitrazepam following single-dose and multiple-dose oral administration to healthy human subjects.
J.Pharm.Biopharm. 6, 283-93 (1978)

1293. Bozza-Marrubini,M., Selenati,A.
Clinical use of diazepam in intensive therapy: Indications and results.
In: 362. pp. 565-70

1294. Braestrup,C., Nielsen,M.
Ontogenetic development of benzodiazepine receptors in rat-brain.
Brain Res. 147, 170-3 (1978)

1295. Braestrup,C., Nielsen,M., Squires,R.F., Laurberg,S.
Benzodiazepine receptor in brain.
Acta Psych.Scand. 1978, 27-32 (1978)

1296. Braestrup,C., Nissen,C., Squires,R.F., Schousbo,A.
Lack of brain specific benzodiazepine receptors on mouse primary astroglial cultures.
Neurosci.Lett. 9, 45-9 (1978)

1297. Braestrup,C., Squires,R.F.
Brain specific benzodiazepine receptors.
Brit.J.Psychiatry 133, 249-60 (1978)

1298. Braestrup,C., Squires,R.F.
Pharmacological characterization of benzodiazepine receptors in the brain.
Eur.J.Pharmacol. 48, 263-70 (1978)

1299. Brambill. ,F., Ponzano,M., Maffei,C., Scarone,S., Resele,L.F., Musetti,L.
Growth-hormone and prolactin secretion during nocturnal sleep - effect of benzodiazepine therapy.
Chronobiol. 4, 102 (1977)

1300. Branch,R.A., Morgan,M.H., Read,A.E.
Intravenous administration of diazepam in patients with chronic liver desease.
Gut 17, 975-83 (1976)

1301. Brausch,U., Henatsch,H.-D., Student,C., Takano,K.
Effect of diazepam on development of stretch reflex tension.
In: 362. pp. 531-44

1302. Breckenridge,A.
Discussion Summary
In: 362. pp. 175-6

1303. Breckenridge,A., Orme,M.
Interaction of benzodiazepines with oral anticoagulants.
In: 362. pp. 647-54

1304. Briley,M.S., Langer,S.Z.
Influence of GABA receptor agonists and antagonists on binding of ^{3}H-diazepam to benzodiazepine receptor.
Eur.J.Pharmacol. 52, 129-32 (1978)

1305. Brisette,Y., Gascon,A.L.
Increase in cardiac toxicity of quabain in dogs after repetitive treatment with diazepam.
Tox.Appl.Ph. 44, 127-35 (1978)

1306. Brodie,R.R., Chasseaud,L.F., Taylor,T.
High-performance liquid chromatographic determination of benzodiazepines in human plasma.
J.Chromatogr. 150, 361-6 (1978)

1307. Brown,A.A.
Sedatives, hypnotics and anxiolytics.
Ont.Dent. 54, 15-6 (1977)

1308. Brown,C.R.
Use of benzodiazepines in prison populations.
J.Clin.Psychology 39, 219-22 (1978)

1309. Brown,J., Lewis,V., Brown,M.W., Horn,G., Bowes,J.B.
Amnesic effects of intravenous diazepam and lorazepam.
Experientia 34, 501-2 (1978)

1310. Brown,P.J., Forrest,W.H., Brown,C.R.
Lorazepam compared with pentobarbital for nighttime-sedation.
J.Clin.Pharmacol. 15, 752-9 (1975)

1311. Brown,S.S., Dundee,J.W.
Clinical studies of induction agents: XXV: Diazepam.
Brit.J.Anaesth. 40, 108-12 (1968)

1312. Brown,W.A., Laughren,T.P., Williams,B.W.
Neuroendocrine correlates of clinical response during withdrawal from chlordiazepoxide.
Comm.Psycho. 2, 251-4 (1978)

1313. Browne,T.R.
Drug-Therapy - Clonazepam.
New Engl.J.Med. 299, 812-6 (1978)

1314. Browne,T.R., Penzy,J.K.
Benzodiazepines in the treatment of epilepsy.
Epilepsia 14, 277 (1973)

1315. Brucato,A., Coppola,A., Antona,A., Gianguzza,S.
Effect of clonazepam on a model of inhibited and non-inhibited behavior.
Boll.Soc.Ital.Biol.Sper. 53, 2031-5 (1977)

1316. Brueckner,J.B., Hess,W., Johannsen,H.J., Kielmann,D., Oser,G., Schweichel,E.
Kreislaufbeeinflussung, Koronardurchblutung und Sicherheitsbreite von Rohypnol (Flunitrazepam).
The effect on circulation, coronary blood pressure and margin of safety of rohypnol (flunitrazepam).
Klin.Anaesthesiol.Intensivther. 17, 82-92 (1978)

1317. Buchanan,N., Cane,R.D.
Liver-function tests and prolonged use of high-dose diazepam, with special reference to tetanus.
S.Afr.Med.J. 54, 768 (1978)

1318. Bugge,A.
Quantitative high-performance liquid chromatography of diazepam and N-desmethyl-diazepam in blood.
J.Chromatogr. 128, 111-6 (1976)

1319. Burn,J.M.
Effect of maternal diazepam on the newborn.
Brit.Med.J. 1, 1216-7 (1978)

1320. Burton,G.W., Lenz,R.J., Thomas,T.S., Midda,M.
Cremophor EL as a diluent for diazepam.
Brit.Med.J. 3, 258 (1974)

1321. Butkiewicz,K.
Polarographic study of some derivatives of 3H-1,5-benzodiazepine-H-3.
J.Electr.Chem. 90, 271-81 (1978)

1322. Caille,E.J., Bassano,J.-L.
Etude de quatre benzodiazépines au niveau de l'électrogenèse cérébrale, du sommeil, du comportement et de l'humeur.
J.Pharmacol.Clin. 4, 241-55 (1974)

1323. Caille,G., Braun,J., Gravel,D., Plourde,R.
Dosage spectrofluorométrique de l'oxazepam et structure du dérive fluorescentforme.
Can.J.Pharm.Sci. 8, 42-5 (1973)

1324. Caille,G., Braun,J., Mockle,J.A.
Analyse spectrofluorométrique et polarographique des formes pharmaceutiques renfermant des dérivés de la 1,4-Benzodiazépine.
Can.J.Pharm.Sci. 5, 78-80(1970)

1325. Cano,J.P., Vignoli,L., Viala,A.
Détermination du diazépam dans le sang et l'urine par chromatographie en phase gazeuse.
I. matériel et méthode.
Ann.Pharm.Franc. 25, 697-703 (1967)

1326. Carmody,J., Boyle,R., Butler,P., Douglas,P., Dwyer,D.
Patterns of the use of benzodiazepines in Australia.
Med.J.Aust. 64, 666-8 (1977)

1327. Carrara,S., Mauri,M., Guazell. ,M., Maggini,C., Castrogi,P.
Controlled double-blind trial of camazepam, a new benzodiazepine derivative, versus chlordiazepoxide.
Eur.J.Clin.Pharm. 13, 335-7 (1978)

1328. Carrigan,P.J., Chao,G.C., Barker,W.M., Hoffman,D.J., Chun,A.H.C.
Steady-state bioavailability of two chlorazepate dipotassium dosage forms.
J.Clin.Pharm. 17, 18-28 (1977)

1329. Carson,M.J. et al.
Treatment of minor motor seizures with clonazepam.
Dev.Med.Child Neurol. 17, 306 (1975)

1330. Cassano,G.B., Castrogiovanni,P., Conti,L.
Drug response in different anxiety states under benzodiazepine treatment. Some multivariate analyses for the evaluation of "rating scale for depression" scores.
In: 362. pp. 379-90

1331. Castleden,C.M., George,C.F., Marcer,D., Hallett,C.
Increased sensitivity to nitrazepam in old age.
Brit.Med.J. 1, 10-2 (1977)

1332. Catchlove,R.F.H., Kafer,E.R.
The effects of diazepam on the ventilatory response to carbon dioxide and on steady-state gas exchange.
Anesthesiology 34, 9-13 (1971)

1333. Cavanagh,D., Condo,C.S.
Diazepam - a pilot study of drug concentrations on maternal blood, amniotic fluid and cord blood.
Curr.Ther.Res. 6, 122 (1964)

1334. Chambers,D.M., Jefferson,G.C., Ruddick,C.A.
Halothane-induced sleeping time in mouse - its modification by benzodiazepines.
Eur.J.Pharm. 50, 103-12 (1978)

1335. Chambiras,P.G.
General anaesthesia and sedation: A Review.
Aust.dent.J. 15, 44 (1970)

1336. Chan,A.W.K., Greizerstein,H.E., Strauss,W.
Interaction of chlordiazepoxide with ethanol.
Pharmacology 20, 159 (1978)

1337. Chandra,B.
Clonazepam in the treatment of petit mal.
Asian J.Med. 9, 433 (1973)

1338. Chang,R.S., Snyder,S.H.
Benzodiazepine receptors: Labeling in intact animals with ^{3}H-flunitrazepam.
Eur.J.Pharmacol. 48, 213-8 (1978)

1339. Chang,T., Peterson,F., Johnson,E., Croskey,L., Goulet,J.R., Smith,T.C., Glazko,A.J.
Metabolic disposition of prazepam in man.
Pharmacology 20, 215 (1978)

1340. Channaba,S.M., Jayram,S.S., Kodandar,P.
Clinical study of haloperidol and diazepam in anxiety states - double blind trial.
Curr.Ther.Res. 24, 381-7 (1978)

1341. Chapallaz,S.
Intoxications aigues par le nitrazepam (Mogadon^{R}).
Schweiz.Apotheker-Ztg. 111, 95-9 (1973)

1342. Chapman,A.G., Horton,R.W., Meldrum,B.S.
Anticonvulsant action of a 1,5-benzodiazepine, clobazam, in reflex epilepsy.
Epilepsia 19, 293-9 (1978)

1343. Charbonne,P., Bazin,C.
Intoxication by benzodiazepines and meprobamate.
Rev.Prat. 28, 4533 (1978)

1344. Chin,L., Sievers,M.L., Laird,H.E., Herrier,R.N., Picchion. ,A.L.
Evaluation of diazepam and pyridoxine as antidotes to isoniazid intoxication in rats and dogs.
Tox.Appl.Pharm. 45, 713-22 (1978)

1345. Chinn,C., Earnes,C.D.
Comparative effects of propanolol and diazepam on hypothalamically-evoked sympathetic responses.
Pharmacology 20, 207 (1978)

1346. Chiodini,L., Garanti,L., Zecchi,G.
Synthesis of 3-substituted 1-H-1,2-benzodiazepines.
Synthesis 1978, 603-5 (1978)

1347. Chiu,T.H., Rosenberg,H.C.
Reduced diazepam binding following chronic benzodiazepine treatment.
Life Sci. 23, 1153-7 (1978)

1348. Clarke,C.H., Nicholson,A.N.
Immediate and residual effects in man of metabolites of diazepam.
Brit.J.Clin.Pharmacol. 6, 325-31 (1978)

1349. Clarke,E.G.C.
Isolation and Identification of Drugs. Vol. 2
The Pharmaceutical Press, London (1975)

1350. Clarke,T.P., Simpson,T.R., Wise,S.P.
Two unsuccesful suicidal attempts with a new drug: Metaminodiazepoxide (Librium).
Texas State J.Med. 57, 24-6 (1961)

1351. Cloquette,R.
Doppelblindversuch mit B 5833 (Camazepam) als anxiolytische Substanz.
Acta Psych.Belgica 74, 317-26 (1974)

1352. Cohen,A.R., Levin,A., Houltin,P.J.C., Wolhuter,A.
Use of chlorazepate for premedication on night before surgery.
Brit.J.Anaest. 50, 821-3 (1978)

1353. Cohen,R.B., Finn,H., Steen,S.M.
Effect of diazepam and meperidine, alone and in combination on respiratory response to carbon dioxide.
Anesth.Analg. 48, 353-5 (1969)

1354. Colburn,W.A., Gibaldi,M.
Plasma-protein binding of diazepam after single dose of sodium oleate.
J.Pharm.Sci. 67, 891-2 (1978)

1355. Colello,G.D., Case,K., Bosmann,H.B.
Benzodiazepine binding to specific rat-brain fractions - assay parameters.
Pharmacology 20, 273 (1978)

1356. Collard,J.
Initial psychopharmacological study of lorazepam (Wy 4036).
Arzneim.-Forsch. (Drug Res.) 21, 1091 (1971)

1357. Comer,W.H., Elliott,H.W., Nomof,N., Navarro,G., Kokka,N., Ruelius,H.W., Knowles,J.A.
Pharmacology of parenterally administered lorazepam in man.
J.Int.Med.Res. 1, 216-25 (1973)

1358. Constant,T., Enache,S., Vasiliev,R.
Identification by chromatography on thin-layer of 1,4-benzodiazepinic medical drugs.
Rev.Chim. 29, 166-8 (1978)

1359. Cook,L., Davidson,A.B.
Effects of behaviorally active drugs in a conflict-punishment procedure in rats.
In: 362. pp. 327-46

1360. Cooper,S.J.
Benzodiazepines - relations between their effects on feeding and on anxiety.
Irish J.Med. 147, 14-8 (1978)

1361. Cornelissen ,P.J., Vanhenegouwen,G.M., Gerritsma ,K.W.
Photo-chemical decomposition of 1,4-benzodiazepines - diazepam.
Int.J.Pharm. 1, 173-81 (1978)

1362. Cornhill,J.F., Levesque,M.J., Nerem,R.M., Patel,D.J.
Effect of diazepam on development of experimental artherosclerosis.
Circulation 58, 128 (1978)

1363. Costa,E., Guidotti,A., Toffano,G.
Molecular mechanisms mediating action of diazepam on GABA receptors.
Brit.J.Psychiatry 133, 239-48 (1978)

1364. Costa,T., Rodbard,D., Pert,C.B.
Is the benzodiazepine receptor coupled to a chloride anion channel?
Nature 277, 315-7 (1979)

1365. Craig,J.C., Purushothaman,K.K.
An improved preparation of tertiary amine N-Oxides.
J.Org.Chem. 35, 1721-2 (1970)

1366. Cruz,I.A., Cramet,N.C., Parrish,A.E.
Hemodialysis in chlordiazepoxide toxicity.
J.Amer.Med.Assoc. 202, 438 (1967)

1367. Cullhed,I., Delius,W., Holmdahl,M.H.
Intravenous diazepam in cardioversion of supraventricular arrhythmias.
Med.Welt 29, 1049-52 (1978)

1368. Curry,A.
Poison detection in human organs.
Charles C.Thomas, Springfield Ill., 1969

1369. Curry,S.H.
Drug disposition and pharmacokinetics.
pp. 88-90. Oxford: Blackwell Scientific Publications 1974

1370. Curry,S.H.
Concentration-effect relationship with major and minor tranquilizers.
Clin.Pharmacol.Ther. 16, 192-7 (1974)

1371. Dabral,P.K., Tripathi,R.P., Varma,A.N.
Role of diazepam in orthopedic practice.
Clinician 42, 86-90 (1978)

1372. Dalen,J.E., Evans,G.L., Banas,J.S., Brooks,H.L., Paraskos,J.A., Dexter,L.
The hemodynamic and respiratory effects of diazepam (Valium).
Anesthesiology 30, 259 (1969)

1373. Damm,H.W., Müller,W.E., Schlafer,U., Wollert,U.
^{3}H-Flunitrazepam - its advantages as a liquid for identification of benzodiazepine receptors in rat-brain membranes.
Res.Comm.Chem.Path.Pharmacol. 22, 597-600 (1978)

1374. Dasberg,H.H.
Oral diazepam in hospitalized anxiety patients (with observation on concentration-effect relationship).
Pharmacopsych. 8, 162-9 (1975)

1375. Davies,C., Levine,M.
A controlled comparison of nitrazepam (Mogadon) with sodium amylobarbitone as a sleep-inducing agent.
Brit.J.Physiol. 113, 1005-8 (1967)

1376. Davies,J., Polc,P.
Effect of a water soluble benzodiazepine on the response of spinal neurones to acetylcholine and excitatory amino acid analogues.
Neuropharmacology 17, 217-20 (1978)

1377. Davis,R.C.
Intravenous diazepam administration.
J.Amer.Med.Assoc. 225, 750 (1973)

1378. DeAngelis,L., Predominato,M., Vertua,R.
Stereostructure-activity relationship for oxazepam hemisuccinate. Effects on central nervous system.
Arzneim.-Forsch. (Drug Res.) 22, 1328-33 (1972)

1379. Deberdt,R.
Camazepam gegen ein Standardvergleichspräparat: Ein Doppelblindversuch bei psychoneurotischen Patienten.
Curr.Ther.Res. 17, 32-9 (1975)

1380. Deberdt,R.
Oxazepam in the treatment of anxiety in children and the elderly.
Acta Psych.Scand. 1978, 104-10 (1978)

1381. Delgado,J.M.R.
Antiaggressive effects of chlordiazepoxide.
In: 362. pp. 419-32

1382. Delia,T.J., Olsen,M.J., Brown,G.B.
Cytosine 3-N-Oxide and its rearrangement on acetylation.
J.Org.Chem. 30, 2766-8 (1965)

1383. De Longhi,B., Pavan,P.A.
Beiträge zur Verwendung von Camazepam in der Allgemeinmedizin.
Gazzetta Medica Italiana 135, 477-82 (1976)

1384. Dement,W.C., Zarcone,V.P., Hoddes,E., Smythe,H., Carskadon,M.
Sleep laboratory and clinical studies with flurazepam.
In: 362. pp. 599-612

1385. Demermuth,G., Kovacs,E.
Die Wirkung von Clonazepam in der peroralen Langzeittherapie schwerer Epilepsieformen des Kindesalters.
Schweiz.Med.Wochenschr. 104, 608 (1974)

1386. Denaut,M., Yernault,J.C., DeCoster,A.
Double-blind comparison of the respiratory effects of parenteral lorazepam and diazepam in patients with chronic obstructive lung disease.
Curr.Med.Res.Opin. 2, 611 (1975)

1387. DeSilva,J.A.F., D'Arconte,L., Kaplan,J.
The determination of blood levels and the placental transfer of diazepam in humans.
Curr.Ther.Res. 6, 115-21 (1964)

1388. DeSilva,J.A.F., Strojny,N.
Spectrofluorometric determination of pharmaceuticals containing aromatic or aliphatic primary amino groups as their fluorescamine (Fluram) derivatives.
Anal.Chem. 47, 714-8 (1975)

1389. Desmond,P.V., Roberts,R.K., Wilkinson,G.R., Schenker,S.
Effect of sex and oral-contraceptive steroids on disposition of chlordiazepoxide.
Clin.Res. 26, 701 (1978)

1390. Desmond,P.V., Roberts,R.K., Wilkinson,G.R., Schenker,S.
No effect of smoking on metabolism of chlordiazepoxide.
N.Engl.J.Med. 300, 199-200 (1979)

1391. Dhar,A.K., Kutt,H.
Monitoring diazepam and desmethyldiazepam concentrations in plasma by gas-liquid-chromatography, with use of a nitrogen-sensitive detector.
Clin.Chem. 25, 137-40 (1979)

1392. Diamond,M.J.
Serum concentrations of lorazepam.
Brit.J.Anaesth. 50, 730 (1978)

1393. DiGregorio,G.J., Piraino,A.J., Ruch,E.
Diazepam concentrations in parotid saliva, mixed saliva, and plasma.
Clin.Pharm. 24, 720-5 (1978)

1394. DiMascio,A.
The effects of benzodiazepines on aggression: Reduced or increased?
In: 362. pp. 433-40

1395. Divakara. ,P., Taber,K., Stanley,J.C., Marchand,J., Defrance,J., Clementc. ,Y.
Diazepam inhibition of elevated cyclic-GMP levels in hippocampus following tetanic stimulation of medial septal region.
Pharmacology 20, 231 (1978)

1396. Dixon,R., Crews,T.
Diazepam: Determination in Micro samples of blood, plasma, and saliva by radioimmunoassay.
J.Anal.Toxicol. 2, 210-3 (1978)

1397. Dixon,R.A., Day,C.D., Eccersley,P.S., Thornton,J.A.
Intravenous diazepam in dentistry: Monitoring results from a controlled clinical trial.
Brit.J.Anaesth. 45,202-6 (1973)

1398. Dixon,R.A., Thornton,J.A.
Tests of recovery from anaesthesia and sedation: Intravenous diazepam in dentistry.
Brit.J.Anaesth. 45,207-15(1973)

1399. Dixon,R.H., Tilton,B.E., Griggs,B.D.
A comparison of the sedative and cardiorespiratory effects of diazepam and pentazocine for premedication.
Anesth.Analg. 49, 546-50 (1970)

1400. Doenicke,A., Lorenz,W.
Histaminliberierung durch Flunitrazepam.
Histamine liberation by flunitrazepam.
Klin.Anaesthesiol.Intensivther. 17, 62-6 (1978)

1401. Doenicke,A., Suttmann,H., Sohler,W.
Der Einfluß von Flunitrazepam und Lormetazepam auf die Blutgase.
The effect of flunitrazepam und lormetazepam on blood gas.
Klin.Anaesthesiol.Intensivther. 17, 93-8 (1978)

1402. Dole,V.P., Kim,V.K., Eglitis,I.
Detection of narcotic drugs, tranquilizers, amphetamines and barbiturates in urine.
J.Amer.Med.Ass. 198, 349 (1966)

1403. Donlon,P.T., Green,W., Johnson,M.
Clobazam versus placebo for neurotic anxiety and tension.
Curr.Ther.Res. 22, 894-9 (1977)

1404. Doongaji,D.R., Sheth,A., Apte,J.S., Akdawala,P.D., Khare,C.B., Thatte,S.S.
Clobazam versus diazepam - double-blind study in anxiety neurosis.
J.Clin.Pharm. 18, 358-64 (1978)

1405. Driscoll,E.J., Smilack,Z.H., Lightbody,P.M., Fiorucci,R.D.
Sedation with intravenous diazepam.
J.Oral.Surg. 38, 580 (1972)

1406. Downing,R.W., Rickels,K.
Prediction of response to chlordiazepoxide and placebo in anxious outpatients.
Pharmakopsychiatry 11, 207-19 (1978)

1407. Dulac,O., Alcardi,J., Rey,E.
Blood-levels of diazepam after single rectal administration in infants and children.
J.Pediat. 93, 1039-41 (1978)

1408. Duncan,A.W., Barr,E.M.
Diazepam premedication and awareness during the general anaesthesia for bronchoscopy and laryngoscopy.
Brit.J.Anaesth. 45, 1150-2 (1973)

1409. Dundee,J.W., George,K.A.
The amnesic action of diazepam, flunitrazepam and lorazepam in man.
Acta.Anaesthesiol.Belg. 27, 3 (1976)

1410. Dundee,J.W., Haslett,W.H.K.
The benzodiazepines. - A review of their actions and uses relative to anaesthetic practice.
Brit.J.Anaesth. 42, 217-34 (1970)

1411. Dundee,J.W., Johnstone,H.M.L., Gray,R.C.
Lorazepam as a sedative-amnesic in an intensive care unit.
Curr.Med.Res.Opinion 4, 290 (1976)

1412. Dundee,J.W., Lilburn,J.K., Nair,S.G., George,K.A.
Studies of drugs given before anaesthesia. XXVI: Lorazepam.
Brit.J.Anaesth. 49, 1047 (1977)

1413. Dundee,J.W., Pandit,S.K.
Anterograde amnesic effects of pethidine, hyoscine and diazepam in adults.
Brit.J.Pharmacol. 44, 140-4 (1972)

1414. Dureman,I., Malmgren,H., Norrman,B.
Comparison studies of chlorazepate administered as a divided daily dose and as a single dose at night.
Psychopharmacology 57, 123-6 (1978)

1415. Dykstra,L.A.
Effects of morphine, diazepam and chlorpromazine on shock-intensity discrimination.
Pharmacology 20, 270 (1978)

1416. Edelbroek ,P.M., DeWolff,F.A.
Improved micromethod for determination of underivatized clonazepam in serum by gas-chromatography.
Clin.Chem. 24, 1774-7 (1978)

1417. Edwards,F.
Risks at work from medication.
J.R.Coll.Physicians Lond. 12, 219-29 (1978)

1418. Edwards,V.E., Eadie,M.J.
Clonazepam: A clinical study of its effectiveness as an anticonvulsant.
Proc.Aust.Assoc.Neurol. 10, 61 (1973)

1419. Eeg-Orlofsson,O.
Experiences with Rivotril[R] in treatment of epilepsy - particularly minor motor epilepsy- in mentally retarded children.
Acta Neurol.Scand. 40, 29 (1973)

1420. Eidelberg,E., Neer,H.M., Miller,M.K.
Anticonvulsant properties of some benzodiazepine derivates.
Neurology (Minneap.) 15, 223-30 (1965)

1421. Eiden,F., Heja,G.
Benzopyrano(4,3-B)-1,5-benzodiazepines.
Arch.Pharm. (Weinheim) 310, 964-72 (1977)

1422. Eiden,F., Schmiz,E.
Pyrone u. Pyridone. - 75. Octahydro [1]-thiopyrano [4,3-b] -[1,5] - benzodiazepines.
Arch.Pharm. 311, 799-804 (1978)

1423. Eiden,F., Schmiz,E.
Dihydrobenzothiopyrano[4,3-b] [1,5]benzodiazepine-7-ones and benzodiazepinium salts.
Arch.Pharm. 311, 867-73 (1978)

1424. Eliot,B.W., Hill,J.G., Cole,A.P. et al.
Continuous pethidine-diazepam infusion during labour and its effects on the newborn.
Brit.J.Obstet.Gynaecol. 82, 126-31 (1975)

1425. Ellefson,C.R., Woo,C.M., Miller,A., Kehr,J.R.
Synthesis and biological evaluation of some 2-amino-4-aryl-3H-1,5-benzodiazepine analogs of clozapine.
J.Med.Chem. 21, 952-7 (1978)

1426. Elliott,H.W.
Metabolism of lorazepam.
Brit.J.Anaesth. 48, 1017-23 (1976)

1427. Elliott,H.W., Nomof,N., Navarro,G., Ruelius,H.W., Knowles,J.A., Comer,W.H.
Central nervous system and cardiovascular effects of lorazepam in man.
Clin.Pharmacol.Ther. 12, 468-81 (1971)

1428. Emmitt,R.B.
Tranquilizers and other psychotherapeutic medicines.
Health Care 9, 1-67 (1974)

1429. Erkkola,R., Kanto,J., Sellman,R.
Diazepam concentrations in mother and foetus in early pregnancy.
Excerpta Medica International Congress Series 1973a, No. 279, pp. 321

1430. Erkkola,R., Kanto,J., Sellman,R.
Diazepam in early human pregnancy.
Acta Obstet.Gynec.Scand. 53, 135-8 (1974)

1431. Essman,W.B.
Subcellular actions of benzodiazepines.
In: 362. pp. 177-90

1432. Essman,W.B.
Discussion Summary.
In: 362. p. 281

1433. Essman,W.B.
Benzodiazepines and aggressive behavior.
Mod.Probl.Pharmacopsychiatry 13, 13-28 (1978)

1434. Fabre,L.F., McLendon,D.M.
Comparison of triazolam, diazepam and placebo in treatment of insomnia and anxiety in out-patients with anxiety neurosis.
Clin.Res. 26, 590 (1978)

1435. Fabre,L.F., McLendon,D.M., Gainey,A.
Double-blind comparison of ketazolam administered once a day with diazepam and placebo in anxious out-patients.
Curr.Ther.Res. 24, 875-83 (1978)

1436. Falk,jr.R.B., Denlinger,J.K., Nahrwold,M.L., Todd,R.A.
Acute vasodilation following induction of anesthesia with intravenous diazepam and nitrous oxide.
Anesthesiology 49, 149-50 (1978)

1437. Fang,M.H., Ginsberg,A.L., Dobbins,W.O.
Cholestatic jaundice associated with flurazepam hydrochloride.
Ann.Intern.Med. 89, 363-4 (1978)

1438. Fazio,C. et al.
Treatment of epileptic seizures with clonazepam.
Arch.Neurol. 32, 304 (1975)

1439. Fehske,K.J., Müller,W.E., Wollert,U.
Modification of lone tryptophan residue in human-serum albumin by 2-hydroxy-5-nitrobenzyl bromide-characterization of modified protein and binding of 1-tryptophan and benzodiazepines to tryptophan-modified albumin.
Hoppe-Seyler's Zeitschrift für physiologische Chemie 359, 709-17 (1978)

1440. Feinberg,I., Fein,G., Walker,J.M., Price,L.J., Floyd,T.C., March,J.D.
Flurazepam effects on sleep EEG - visual computer, and cycle analysis.
Arch.General Psychiatry 36, 95-102 (1979)

1441. Ferngren,H.
Diazepam treatment for acute convulsions in children.
Epilepsia 15, 27 (1974)

1442. Ferry,D.G., McQueen,E.G.
Protein-binding of clonazepam and valproate.
Clin.Exp.Ph. 5, 258 (1978)

1443. Ficarra,P., Vigorita,M.G., Tommasini,A.
Various 1,4-benzodiazepine derivatives.
II. Thermomicroextraction from pharmaceutical preparations and analytical study.
Boll.Chim.Farm. 116, 720-30 (1977)

1444. Finkle,B.S., Cherry,E.J., Taylor,D.M.
A GLC based system for the detection of poisons, drugs and human metabolites encountered in forensic toxicology.
J.Chromatogr.Sci. 9, 393 (1971)

1445. Flammang,M.
Benzodiazepine-2,3-system- synthesis of 1-oxo-2-methyl-5-phenyl-2,5-dihydro- (1H) 2,3-benzodiazepine.
Cr.Ac.Sci.C. 286, 671-3 (1978)

1446. Flowers,C.E., Rudolph,A.J., Desmond,M.M.
Diazepam (Valium) as an adjunct in obstetric analgesia.
Abstet.Gynecol. 34, 68-81 (1969)

1447. Fontani,F., Targa,G., Nardi,D.
Physicochemical profile of tibezonium iodide.
Boll.Chim.Farm. 116, 705-13 (1977)

1448. Fouks,L., Pinalie,B., Porchero ,J.E., Cardon,A.
Clinical activity of oxazepam.
Act.Psych.Scand. 1978, 99-103 (1978)

1449. Fox,G.S., Wynards,J.E., Bhambhami,M.
A clinical comparison of diazepam and thiopentone as induction agents to general anaesthesia.
Can.Anaesth.Soc.J. 15, 281 (1968)

1450. Fox,K.A., Guerriero,F.J.
Effect of benzodiazepines on age of vaginal perforation and first estrus in mice.
Res.Commun.Chem.Pathol.Pharmacol. 21, 181-4 (1978)

1451. Fox,R.
Abuse of benzodiazepines (letter).
Lancet 2, 681-2 (1978)

1452. Fox,R.
Abuse of benzodiazepines - reply.
Lancet 2, 1045 (1978)

1453. Fragen,R.J., Caldwell,N.
Lorazepam premedication: Lack of precall and relief of anxiety.
Anesth.Analg. (Cleve.) 55, 792-6 (1976)

1454. Fragen,R.J., Gahl,F., Caldwell,N.
Water-soluble benzodiazepine, Ro 21-3981, for induction of anesthesia.
Anesthesiol. 49, 41-3 (1978)

1455. Freche,C.
Study on an anxiolytic, clobazam, in otorhinolaryngology inpsychosomatic pharyngeal manifestations.
Sem.Hop.Ther. 51, 261-3 (1975)

1456. Friedman,E.A., Niswander,K.R., Sachtleben,M.R.
Effect of diazepam on labor.
Obstet.Gynecol. 34, 82-6 (1969)

1457. Frigerio,A., Chisalberti,E.L.
Mass Spectrometry in Drug-Metabolism.
Plenum Press, New York - London 1977

1458. Fryer,R.I., Blount,J., Reeder,E., Trybulsky,E.J., Walser,A.
Quinazolines and 1,4-benzodiazepines. 88. Synthesis and rearrangement of 3A,4,5,6,-tetrahydro-3H-imidazo (1,5A)-1,4-benzodiazepines.
J.Org.Chem. 43, 4480-4 (1978)

1459. Fryer,R.I., Early,J.V., Walser,A.
Quinazolines and 1,4-benzodiazepines. 86. Synthesis of imidazothienodiazepines and imidazopyrazolo-diazepines.
J.Heterocycl.Chem. 15, 619-24 (1978)

1460. Gale,S., Galloon,S.
Lorazepam as a premedication.
Can.Anaesth.Soc.J. 23, 22-9 (1976)

1461. Gall,M., Kamdar,B.V., Collins,R.J.
Pharmacology of some metabolites of triazolam, alprazolam, and diazepam prepared by a simple, one-step oxidation of benzodiazepines.
J.Med.Chem. 21, 1290-4 (1978)

1462. Gallager,D.W.
Benzodiazepines- potentiation of a GABA inhibitory response in dorsal raphe nucleus.
Eur.J.Pharm. 49, 133-43 (1978)

1463. Gallager,D.W., Thomas,J.W., Tallman,J.F.
Effect of GABA ergic drugs on benzodiazepine binding-site sensitivity in rat cerebral-cortex.
Biochem.Pharmacol. 27, 2745-9 (1978)

1464. Gamstorp,I., Kubista,J.
A trial with clonazepam (Ro 5-4023) in children with epilepsy.
Epilepsia 14, 103 (1973)

1465. Ganguli,L.K., Sen,D., Chatterjee,P., Mandal,J.N.
Oxazepam overdosage.
J.Indian Med.Assoc. 54, 424-5 (1970)

1466. Garattini,S.
Metabolism of diazepam in animals and man.
In: The present status of psychotropic drugs. Editê par A.Cerletti et F.J.Bovê, pp. 84-93, Excerpta Medica Foundation, 1969

1467. Garattini,S.
Biochemical and pharmacological properties of oxazepam.
Acta Psych.Scand. 1978, 9-18 (1978)

1468. Garattini,S., Marcucci,F., Morselli,P.L., Mussini,E.
The significance of measuring blood levels of benzodiazepines.
In: D.S.Davies and B.N.C.Prichard (Eds.). Biological effects of drugs in relation to their plasma concentrations.
MacMillan Publishers, London, 1973, 211-25

1469. Garattini,S., Mussini,E., Marcucci,F., Guaitani,A.
Metabolic studies on benzodiazepines in various animal species.
In: 362. pp. 75-98

1470. Gartside,I.B.
The actions of diazepam and phenytoin on a low dose penicillin epileptiform focus in the anaesthetised rat.
Brit.J.Pharmacol. 62, 289-92 (1978)

1471. Gasser,Y.C., Kaufman,R.D., Bellville,J.W.
Respiratory effects of lorazepam, pentobarbital and pentazocine.
Clin.Pharmacol.Ther. 18, 170-4 (1975)

1472. Gastaut,H., Courjon. J., Poire,R. et al.
Treatment of status epilepticus with a new benzodiazepine more active than diazepam.
Epilepsia 12, 197-214 (1971)

1473. Gelbke,H.-P.
Untersuchungen zur verkehrsmedizinischen Bedeutung von Diazepam: Analytik, quantitative Bedeutung im Verkehrsgeschehen und Einfluß auf die Leistungsfähigkeit.
Habil.Schrift Heidelberg 1978

1474. Gelbke,H.P., Schlicht,H.J.
Formation of thermally stable derivatives of chlordiazepoxide and its desmethyl metabolite for GLC.
J.Pharm.Sci. 67, 1176-7 (1978)

1475. Geller,H.M., Taylor,D.A., Hoffer,B.J.
Benzodiazepines and central inhibitory mechanisms.
Naunyn-Schmied.-Arch.Pharmacol. 304, 81-8 (1978)

1476. Gerhards,H.J.
Neuropharmacological profile of clobazam, a new 1,5-benzodiazepine.
Psychopharmacology 58, 27-33 (1978)

1477. Gey,K.
Effect of benzodiazepines on carbohydrate metabolism in rat brain.
In: 362. pp. 243-56

1478. Giardini,M., Guareschi-Cazzullo,A.
Clinical experience with clonazepam (Ro 5-4023) in pediatrics.
Electroenceph.Clin.Neurophysiol. 35, 406 (1973)

1479. Gibaldi,M., Perrier,D.
Pharmacokinetics.
Marcel Dekker, New York, 1975

1480. Gilbert,J.E.
Ingestion of a massive dose of librium.
South Dakota J.Med.Pharm. 14, 307-9 (1961)

1481. Giles,H.G., Fan,T., Naranjo,C.A., Sellers,E.M.
Simple electron-capture gas-chromatographic analysis of oxazepam in plasma by determination of its thermal-degradation product.
Can.J.Pharm.Sci. 13, 64-5 (1978)

1482. Gilli,G., Bertolas,V., Sacerdotti,M., Borea,P.A.
Crystal and molecular-structure of 7-chloro-1,3-dihydro-3-hydroxy-5-phenyl-2H-1,4-benzodiazepin-2-one (oxazepam).
Acta Cryst. B 34, 2826-9 (1978)

1483. Gjerris,F.
Poisoning with chlordiazepoxide (Librium).
Dan.Med.Bull. 13, 170 (1966)

1484. Gladtke,E., von Hattingberg,H.M.
Pharmakokinetik - eine Einführung.
Springer-Verlag: Berlin-Heidelberg-New York 1973

1485. Glatt,M.M.
Benzodiazepine abuse in alcoholics.
Lancet 2, 1205 (1978)

1486. Gogolák,G., Stumpf,Ch., Tschakaloff,Ch.
Anticonvulsive Wirkung von Clonazepam und Ro 8-4192 gegenüber Penicillin und Lidocain.
Arzneim.-Forsch. (Drug Res.) 23, 545-9 (1973)

1487. Goldberg,M., Dorman,J.
Intention myoclonus: Successful treatment with clonazepam.
Neurology 26, 24 (1976)

1488. Goldstein,S.E., Birnbom,F., Lancee,W.J., Darke,A.C.
Comparison of oxazepam, flurazepam and chloral hydrate as hypnotic sedatives in geriatric-patients.
J.Amer.Ger.Soc. 26, 366-71 (1978)

1489. Golovenko,N.I.A., Bogatskii,A.V., Karaseva,T.L.
Dependence of nitrazepam metabolism on the method of its administration and species of experimental animals.
Ukr.Biohk.ZH. 50, 302-6 (1978)

1490. Golovenko,N.I.A., Meteshkii,J.V.
Hydroxylation of 1,4-benzodiazepines and parent compounds in endoplasmic-reticulum of albino-rat liver.
Dop.Ukr.B. 1978, 921-3 (1978)

1491. Gomez-Lozano,P.
Intravenous lorazepam in the acute anxiety crisis: a preliminary report on 60 cases.
Curr.Therap.Res. 19, 469 (1976)

1492. Gorbach,A.C.
Diazepam for eclampsia.
Amer.J.Abstet.Gynecol. 102, 611 (1968)

1493. Gordon,E.B.
Addiction to diazepam (Valium)
Brit.Med.J. 1, 112 (1967)

1494. Gotestam,K.G., Andersson,B.E.
Subjective effects and vigilance after diazepam and oxazepam in normal subjects.
Acta Psych.Scand. 1978, 117-21 (1978)

1495. Gottschalk,L.A., Cohn,J.B.
The relationship of diazepam and ketazolam blood levels to anxiety and hostility in chronic alcoholics.
Psychopharmacol. Bull. 14, 39-43 (1978)

1496. Gottschalk,L.A., Elliott,H.W., Bates,D.A., Cable,C.G.
Content analysis of speech samples to determine effect of lorazepam on anxiety.
Clin.Pharmacol.Ther. 13, 323-8 (1972)

1497. Gottschalk,L.A., Kaplan,S.A.
Chlordiazepoxide plasma-levels and clinical responses.
Compr.Psychiatry 13, 519-27 (1972)

1498. Gottschalk,L.A., Noble,E.P., Stolzoff,G.E., Bates,D.E., Cable,C.G., Uliana,R.L., Birch,H., Fleming,E.W.
Relationship of chlordiazepoxide blood levels to psychological and biochemical responses.
In: 362. pp. 257-80

1499. Graham,C.W., Pagano,R.R., Conner,J.T.
Pain and clinical thrombophlebitis following intravenous diazepam and lorazepam.
Anaesthesia 33, 188-91 (1978)

1500. Greenblatt,D.J.
Kinetics of lorazepam in humans - effect of dose and route of administration.
Clin.Res. 26, 609 (1978)

1501. Greenblatt,D.J.
Determination of desmethyldiazepam in plasma by electron-capture GLC: Application to pharmacokinetic studies of chlorazepate.
J.Pharm.Sci. 67, 427-9 (1978)

1502. Greenblatt,D.J.
Simultaneous gas-chromatographic analysis for diazepam and its major metabolite, desmethyldiazepam, with use of double internal standardization.
Clin.Chem. 24, 1838-41 (1978)

1503. Greenblatt,D.J., Allen,M.D.
Toxicity of nitrazepam in elderly - report from Boston collaborative drug surveillance program.
Brit.J.Clin.Pharmacol. 5, 407-13 (1978)

1504. Greenblatt,D.J., Allen,M.D., MacLaughlin,D.S., Harmatz,J.S., Shader,R.I.
Diazepam absorption - effect of antacids and food.
Clin.Pharm. 5, 600-9 (1978)

1505. Greenblatt,D.J., Comer,W.H., Elliott,H.W. et al.
Clinical pharmacokinetics of lorazepam.
III. Intravenous injection.
J.Clin.Pharm. 17, 490-4 (1977)

1506. Greenblatt,D.J., Franke,K., Shader,R.I.
Analysis of lorazepam and its glucuronide-metabolite by electron-capture gas-liquid chromatography-use in pharmacokinetic studies of lorazepam.
J.Chromatogr. 146, 311-20 (1978)

1507. Greenblatt,D.J., Harmatz,J.S., Shader,R.I.
Factors influencing diazepam pharmacokinetics: Age, sex, and liver disease.
Int.J.Clin.Pharmacol.Biopharm. 16, 177-9 (1978)

1508. Greenblatt,D.J., Koch-Weser,J.
Adverse reactions to intravenous diazepam: A report from the Boston collaborative drug surveillance program.
Am.J.Med.Sci. 266, 261-6 (1973)

1509. Greenblatt,D.J., Koch-Weser,J.
Clinical pharmacokinetics.
New Engl.J.Med. 293, 702-5 (1975)

1510. Greenblatt,D.J., Schillings,R.T., Kyriakopoulos, A.A., Shader,R.I., Sisenwine,S.F., Knowles,J.A., Ruelius,H.W.
Clinical pharmacokinetics of lorazepam. I. Absorption and disposition of oral ^{14}C-lorazepam.
Clin.Pharmacol.Ther. 20,329-41(1976)

1511. Greenblatt,D.J., Shader,R.I.
Benzodiazepines.
New Engl.J.Med. 291, 1011-4 (1974)

1512. Greenblatt,D.J., Shader,R.I.
Benzodiazepines.
New Engl.J.Med. 291, 1239-42 (1974)

1513. Greenblatt,D.J., Shader,R.I.
Pharmacotherapy of anxiety with benzodiazepines and ß-adrenergic blockers.
In: Lipton,M.A., DiMascio,A., Killam,K.F. editors: Psychopharmacology: A generation of progress. New York 1978, Raven Press, pp. 1381-9

1514. Greenblatt,D.J., Shader,R.I.
Pharmacokinetic understanding of antianxiety drug therapy.
South.Med.J. 71, 2-9 (1978)

1515. Greenblatt,D.J., Shader,R.I.
Dependence, tolerance, and addiction to benzodiazepines - clinical and pharmacokinetic considerations.
Drug Metab.Rev. 8, 13-28 (1978)

1516. Greenblatt,D.J., Shader,R.I.
Drug-therapy - Prazepam and lorazepam, 2 new benzodiazepines.
N.Engl.J.Med. 299, 1342-4 (1978)

1517. Greenblatt,D.J., Shader,R.I., Franke,K., Harmatz,J.S.
Pharmacokinetics of chlordiazepoxide and metabolites following single and multiple oral doses.
Int.J.Clin.Pharmacol.Biopharm. 16, 486-93 (1978)

1518. Greenblatt,D.J., Shader,R.I., Franke,K., MacLaughlin, D.S., Harmatz,J.S., Allen,M.D., Werner,A., Woo,E.
Pharmacokinetics and bioavailability of intravenous, intramuscular, and oral lorazepam in humans.
J.Pharm.Sci. 68, 57-63 (1979)

1519. Greenblatt,D.J., Shader,R.I., Harmatz,J.S., Franke,K., Koch-Weser,J.
Absorption rate, blood concentrations, and early response to oral chlordiazepoxide.
Amer.J.Psychiatry 134, 559-62 (1977)

1520. Greenblatt,D.J., Shader,R.I., Koch-Weser,J.
Flurazepam hydrochloride.
Clin.Pharmacol.Ther. 17, 1-14 (1975)

1521. Greenblatt,D.J., Shader,R.I., Koch-Weser,J.
Flurazepam hydrochloride, a benzodiazepine hypnotic.
Ann.Intern.Med. 83, 237-41 (1975)

1522. Greenblatt,D.J., Shader,R.I., Koch-Weser,J.
Serum creatine phosphokinase concentrations after intramuscular chlordiazepoxide and its solvent.
J.Clin.Pharmacol. 16, 118-21 (1976)

1523. Greenblatt,D.J., Shader,R.I., Koch-Weser,J., Franke,K.
Clinical pharmacokinetics of chlordiazepoxide.
In: Gottschalk,L.A., and Merlis,S., editors: Pharmacokinetics of psychoactive drugs: Blood levels and clinical response, Flushing, N.Y., 1976, Spectrum Publications, pp. 127-39

1524. Greenblatt,D.J., Shader,R.I., MacLeod,S.M., Sellers,E.M.
Clinical pharmacokinetics of chlordiazepoxide.
Clin.Pharm. 3, 381-94 (1978)

1525. Greenblatt,D.J., Shader,R.I., MacLeod,S.M., Sellers,E.M., Franke,K., Giles,H.G.
Absorption of oral and intramuscular chlordiazepoxide.
Eur.J.Clin.Pharmacol. 13, 267-74 (1978)

1526. Greenblatt,D.J., Shader,R.I., Weinberger,D.R., Allen,M.D., MacLaughlin,D.S.
Effect of a cocktail on diazepam absorption.
Psychopharmacology 57, 199-203 (1978)

1527. Greenblatt,D.J., Woo,E., Allen,M.D., Orsulak,P.J., Shader,R.I.
Rapid recovery from massive diazepam overdose.
J.Amer.Med.Ass. 240, 1872-4 (1978)

1528. Groh,C., Rosenmayr,F.W.
Clonazepam (Ro 5-4023), ein neues Antikonvulsium.
Wien.Klin.Wschr. 19, 334-7 (1971)

1529. Grosso,F.
Camazepam in der Therapie der Angina pectoris.
La Clinica Therapeutica 71, 49-55 (1974)

1530. Grove-White,I.G., Kelman,G.R.
Critical flicker frequency after small doses of methohexitone, diazepam and sodium 4-hydroxy-butyrate.
Brit.J.Anaesth. 43,110-2 (1971)

1531. Grundstroem,R., Holmberg,G., Hansen,T.
Degree of sedation obtained with various doses of diazepam and nitrazepam.
Acta Pharmacol.Toxicol. 43, 13-8 (1978)

1532. Guelen,P.J.M., van der Kleyin,E.
Determination of benzodiazepines by GLC. Proceedings of the workshop on the determination of anti-epileptic drugs. Amsterdam, 1973. Excerpta Medica Foundation

1533. Guerrero-Figueroa,R., Gallant,D.M., Guerrero-Figueroa,C., Gallant,J.
Electrophysiological analysis of the action of four benzodiazepine derivatives on the central nervous system.
In: 362. pp. 489-512

1534. Guerrero-Figueroa,R., Rye,M.M., Heath,R.G.
Effects of two benzodiazepine derivatives on cortical and subcortical epileptogenic tissues in the cat and monkey.
Curr.Ther.Res. 11, 27-39 (1969)

1535. Guerrero-Figueroa,R., Rye,M.M., Heath,R.G.
Effect of two benzodiazepine derivatives on cortical and subcortical epileptogenic tissues in the cat and monkey.
II. Cortical and centroencephalic structures.
Curr.Ther.Res. 11, 40-50 (1969)

1536. Guidotti,A., Toffano,G., Costa,E.
Endogenous protein modulates affinity of GABA and benzodiazepine receptors in rat-brain.
Nature 275, 553-5 (1978)

1537. Guthy,H.
Zur medikamentösen Behandlung der Angst bei Alkoholismus im Entzugsstadium.
Münch.med.Wschr. 117, 1387-90 (1975)

1538. Guz,I.
Controlled comparison of clobazam and diazepam in treatment of anxiety in neurotic patients.
Rev.Bra.Med. 35, 431-5 (1978)

1539. Haataja,M., Nieminen,L., Kangas,L., Möttönen,M., Bjöndahl,K.
Effect of spironolactone on pentobarbital anaesthesia, diazepam metabolism and toxicity of spironolactone and frusemide.
Ann.Med.Exp.Biol.Fenn. 50, 57 (1972)

1540. Haden,B.H., McNeil,K.G., Huber,N.A., Khan,W.A., Singh,P., Schneider,R.S.
An EMIT assay for benzodiazepines in urine.
Clin.Chem. 22, 1200 (1978)

1541. Haefely,W.E.
Central actions of benzodiazepines - general introduction.
Brit.J.Psychiatry 133, 231-8 (1978)

1542. Hajdú,P., Uihlein,M., Damm,D.
Clobazam: Physikalisch-chemische und analytische Untersuchungen.
J.Chromatogr. (in the press)

1543. Hall,R.C., Kirkpatrick,B.
The Benzodiazepines.
Am.Fam.Physician 17, 131-4 (1978)

1544. Hansen,C.R., Boyd,R.L.
Preparation and some reactions of 3-oxazoline-N-oxides.
J.Heterocycl.Chem. 7, 911-5 (1970)

1545. Hara,T., Kayama,Y., Mori,T., Itoh,K., Fujimori,H., Sunami,T., Hashimoto,Y., Ishimoto,S.
Diazepines: 5. Synthesis and biological action of 6-phenyl-4H-pyrrolo (1,2-A) (1,4) benzodiazepines.
J.Med.Chem. 21, 263-8 (1978)

1546. Haram,K., Bakke,O.M., Johannesson,K.H., Lund,T.
Transplacental passage of diazepam during labor - influence of uterine contractions.
Clin.Pharm. 5, 590-9 (1978)

1547. Harry,T.V.A.
Abuse of benzodiazepines.
Lancet 2, 1045 (1978)

1548. Hartelius,H., Larsson,A.K., Lepp,M., Malm,U., Arvidsson,A., Dahlstroem,H.
Controlled long-term study of flunitrazepam, nitrazepam and placebo, with special regard to withdrawal effects.
Acta Psych.Scand. 58, 1-15 (1978)

1549. Harzer,K., Barchet,R.
Analyse von Benzodiazepinen und deren Hydrolysenprodukte, den Benzophenonen, durch Hochdruckflüssigkeitschromatographie in umgekehrter Phase und ihre Anwendung auf biologisches Material.
J.Chromatogr. 132, 83-90 (1977)

1550. Haskell,D.S., Gambill,J.D., Gardos,G., McNair,D.M., Fisher,S.
Doxepin or diazepam for anxious and anxious-depressed putpatients.
J.Clin.Psy. 39, 135-9 (1978)

1551. Haslett,W.H.
A controlled study of diazepam and chlordiazepoxide as premedicant for a standard operation.
In: P.F. Knight, C.G. Burgess (Ed.): Diazepam in anaesthesia.
J. Wright and Sons Ltd., Bristol 1968

1552. Hattingberg,von,H.M.
Mathematische Verfahren zur Auswertung von pharmakokinetischen Untersuchungen.
Arzneim.-Forsch. (Drug Res.) 23, 1646-9 (1973)

1553. Heermann,J.
Flunitrazepam combined with local-anesthesia in 1400 operations.
Clin.Otolaryng. 3, 509-10 (1978)

1554. Heipertz,W., Vontin,H., Schorer,R., Junger,H.
Die Amnesie nach den Benzodiazepinen Flunitrazepam und Lorazepam.
Amnesia after the benzodiazepines flunitrazepam und lorazepam.
Klin.Anaesthesiol.Intensivther. 17, 163-8 (1978)

1555. Heise,G.A., McConnell,H.
Differences between chlordiazepoxide-type and chlorpromazine-type action in "trace" avoidance.
Proc. 3rd World Congr. Psychiat., Montreal, Canada 2, 917 (1961)

1556. Heisterkamp,D.V., Cohen.J.P.
The effect of intravenous premedication with lorazepam (Ativan), pentobarbitone or diazepam on recall.
Brit.J.Anaesth. 47, 79-81 (1975)

1557. Hempelmann,G., Seitz,W., Piepenbrink,S.
Diazepam (Valium) - changes in hemodynamics. Myocardial oxygen-consumption and vascular tone.
Anaesthesis 27, 357-63 (1978)

1558. Henn,F.A., Henke,D.J.
Cellular, localization of diazepam-H-3 receptors.
Neuropharm. 11, 985-8 (1978)

1559. Herlofsen,H.B.
Brief report on a new benzodiazepin preparation RO 5-4556/B-5.
Acta Psychiat.Scand. 203, 243-6 (1967)

1560. Heubel,F., Frank,R.
Zur induktiven Wirkung von Diazepam.
Arzneim.-Forsch. (Drug Res.) 20, 1706-8 (1970)

1561. Heubel,F., Patutschnick,H.
Vergleichende Untersuchungen über die induktive Wirkung verschiedener Benzodiazepine an Hand der durch Pentobarbital bedingten Schlafzeit der Ratte.
Arzneim.-Forsch. (Drug Res.) 22, 1196-9 (1972)

1562. Hewick,D.S., Shaw,V.
The importance of the intestinal microflora in nitrazepam metabolism in the rat.
Brit.J.Pharmacol. 62, 427 (1978)

1563. Hewitt,J.M., Barr,A.M.
Premedication with lorazepam for bronchoscopy under general-anesthesia.
Brit.J.Anaest. 11, 1149-54 (1978)

1564. Hildebrand,W.K.
Concomitant use of clonazepam and valproic acid in treatment of epileptic seizures.
Am.J.Hosp.P. 36, 22 (1979)

1565. Hillyer,D.M.
An overdose of valium.
Med.J.Aust. 1, 565 (1965)

1566. Hindmarch,I.
The effect of repeated doses of temazepam taken in conjunction with alcohol on aspects of psychomotor performance the morning following night time medication.
Arzneim.-Forsch. (Drug Res.) 28, 2357-60 (1978)

1567. Hindmarch,I., Parrott,A.C.
Effect of a sub-chronic administration of 3 dose levels of a 1,5-benzodiazepine derivative, clobazam, on subjective assessments of sleep and aspects of psychomotor performance morning following night time medication.
Arzneim.-Forsch. (Drug Res.) 28, 2169-72 (1978)

1568. Hirai,K., Ishiba,T., Sugimoto,M., Sasakura,K., Fujishit,T., Tsukinok,Y., Hirose,K.
Benzophenone related compounds. 1. Peptido-aminobenzophenones. Novel open-ring derivatives of 1,4-Benzodiazepines.
Chem.Pharm. 26, 1947-50 (1978)

1569. Hoffmann-La Roche (Firmenschrift)
Sicherheitsanalyse eines Medikaments, eine kritische, klinische Auswertung.
Valium Roche, Hämodynamik
Hoffmann-La Roche AG - Grenzach

1570. Hoffmann-La Roche (Firmenschrift)
Sicherheitsanalyse eines Medikaments, Valium Roche, Pharmakokinetik.
Hoffmann-La Roche AG - Grenzach

1571. Hoffmann-La Roche (Firmenschrift)
Sicherheitsanalyse eines Medikaments, eine kritische, klinische Auswertung.
Valium Roche, Frühschwangerschaft und Stillperiode
Hoffmann-La Roche AG - Grenzach

1572. Hoffmann-La Roche (Firmenschrift)
Sicherheitsanalyse eines Medikaments, eine kritische, klinische Auswertung.
Valium Roche, Leberverträglichkeit
Hoffmann-La Roche AG - Grenzach

1573. Hoogland,D.R., Miya,T.S., Bousquet,W.F.
Metabolism tolerance studies with chlordiazepoxide -2-C^{14} in the rat.
Toxicol.appl.Pharmacol. 9, 116-23 (1966)

1574. Hollister,L.E.
Antianxiety drugs in clinical practice.
In: 362. pp. 367-78

1575. Hollister,L.E.
Discussion Summary.
In: 362. pp. 441-2

1576. Holmberg,G.
Missbrukas diazepam?
Läkartidningen 66, 77 (1967)

1577. Holmberg,G., Livstedt,B.
Clinical evaluation of a new benzodiazepine derivative, chlorazepate.
Arzneim.-Forsch. (Drug Res.) 22, 916-9 (1972)

1578. Holmberg,G., William-Olsson,U.
The effect of benzquinamide, in comparison with chlordiazepoxide and placebo, on performance in some psychological tests.
Psychopharmacologia 4, 402-17 (1963)

1579. Holmes,J.H., Kanfer,I., Zwarensteyn,H.
Effect of benzodiazepine-derivatives on human-blood cholinesterase in vitro.
Res.Comm.Chem.Pathol. 21, 367-70 (1978)

1580. Holmes,J.H., Kanfer,I., Zwarensteyn,H.
Effect of benzodiazepine derivatives on purified blood cholinesterases in vitro.
Res.Comm.C.P. 22, 431-2 (1978)

1581. Hooshmand,H.
Intractable seizures: Treatment with a new benzodiazepine anticonvulsant.
Arch.Neurol. 27, 205-8 (1972)

1582. Hooshmand,H.
A new benzodiazepine anticonvulsant in intractible seizures.
Curr.Psychiatr.Ther. 13, 67 (1973)

1583. Houlton,P.J.C., Downing,J.W.
General-anesthesia with intravenous flunitrazepam, continous ketamine infusion and muscle-relaxant. Preliminary report.
S.Afr.Med.J. 54, 1048-9 (1978)

1584. Howard,P.J., Toner,W.
Plasma lorazepam estimation in neonates.
Anaesthesia 33, 276-7 (1978)

1585. Howd,R.A., Pryor,G.T.
Alterations in disposition and effects of pentobarbital and diazepam after chronic morphine in rats.
Pharmacology 20, 268 (1978)

1586. Hoyumpa,jr.,A.M.
Disposition and elimination of minor tranquilizers in the ages and in patients with liver disease.
South.Med.J. 71, 23-8 (1978)

1587. Hoyumpa,A., Desmond,P., Roberts,R., Nichols,S., Johnson,R., Schenker,S.
Effect of ethanol on benzodiazepine disposition in dogs.
Clin.Res. 26, 793 (1978)

1588. Huang,C.Y., McLeod,J.G., Sampson,D., Hensley,W.J.
Clonazepam in the treatment of epilepsy.
Proc.Aust.Assoc.Neurol. 10, 67 (1973)

1589. Hüter,J.
Über Wirksamkeit, Nebenwirkungen, Indikationen und Kontraindikationen von Diazepam (Valium[R]) in der Geburtshilfe und Frauenheilkunde.
Klin.Wschr. 46, 685-7 (1968)

1590. Hunt,B.J., George,A.J., Ridges,A.P.
Preliminary studies in humans on clobazam (HR376) - a new antianxiety agent.
Brit.J.Clin.Pharm. 1, 174-5 (1974)

1591. Idänpään-Heikkilä,J.E., Taska,R.J., Allen,H.A., Schoolar,J.G.
Placental transfer of diazepam-^{14}C in mice, hamsters and monkeys.
J.Pharmacol.Exp.Ther. 176, 752 (1971)

1592. Iisalo,E.U.M., Iisalo,E.
Comparison of high-dose pentazocine with pethidine and diazepam in pediatric premedication.
Ann.Chir.Gyn. 67, 123-8 (1978)

1593. Illing,H.P.A., Johnson,P., Rising,P.A., Yeomans,M.A.
Desalkylation and cyclization of a substituted acetamidobenzophenone to form corresponding benzodiazepine in vivo and in vitro.
Xenobiotica 7, 99 (1977)

1594. Imlah,N.W.
Episodic nature of anxiety and its treatment with oxazepam.
Acta Psych.Scand. 1978, 94-8 (1978)

1595. Ishihama,H., Kabuto,S., Kimata,H., Tamaki,T., Yonemitsu,M.
Studies on metabolism of prazepam.
1. Metabolic fate of prazepam in rats.
Yakugaku Za. 98, 720-36 (1978)

1596. Ishihama,H., Kimata,H., Yonemitsu,M., Matsumoto,S., Ota,T., Koga,T., Otani,G.
Studies on metabolism of prazepam. 3. Metabolic-fate of cyclopropylmethyl group of prazepam in rats.
Yakugaku Za. 98, 937-43 (1978)

1597. Iversen,L.L.
GABA and benzodiazepine receptors.
Nature 275, 477 (1978)

1598. Jackson,A.P., Dhadphale,P.R., Callaghan,M.L., Alseri,S.
Haemodynamic studies during induction of anaesthesia for open-heart surgery using diazepam and ketamine.
Brit.J.Anaesth. 50, 375-8 (1978)

1599. Jäättelä,A., Mannistö,P., Paatero,H., Tuomist,J.
The effects of diazepam or diphenhydramine on healthy subjects.
Psychopharmacologia 21, 202-11 (1971)

1600. Jalfre,M., Monachon,M.A., Haefely,W.
Effects on the amygdalohippocampal evoked potential in the cat of four benzodiazepines and some other psychotropic drugs.
Naunyn-Schmied.-Arch.-Pharmacol. 270, 180-91 (1971)

1601. Jenner,F.A., Parkin,D.
A large overdose of chlordiazepoxide.
Lancet 2, 322-3 (1961)

1602. Jensen,K.M.
Determination of nitrazepam in serum by gas-liquid-chromatography.
J.Chromatogr. 111, 389-96 (1975)

1603. Jeppson,R., Ljungberg,S.L.
Anticonvulsant activity in mice of diazepam in an emulsion formulation for intravenous administration.
Acta pharmacol.et toxicol. 36, 312-20 (1975)

1604. Jick,H.
Comparative studies with a hypnotic (Ro 5-6901) under current investigation.
Curr.Ther.Res. 9, 355-7 (1967)

1605. Jick,H.
Drugs - remarkably nontoxic.
N.Engl.J.Med. 291, 824-8 (1974)

1606. Johnstone,M.
The effect of lorazepam on the vasoconstriction of fear.
Anaesthesia 31, 868 (1976)

1607. Jones,D.J., Stehling,L.C., Zauder,H.L.
Comparison of effects of Ro 21-3981 and Diazepam on cardiovascular-system in dogs.
Pharmacology 20, 254 (1978)

1608. Jones,D.M., Lewis,M.J., Springgs,T.L.B.
Effects of low-doses of diazepam on human-performance in group administered tasks.
Brit.J.Clin.Pharmacol. 6, 333-7 (1978)

1609. Joseph,A., Pulimood,B.M.
Use of diazepam in tetanus - comparative study.
Ind.J.Med.Res. 68, 489-91 (1978)

1610. Jovanovic,H.J.
Vigilanzverlauf und Schlafqualitäten unter Einwirkung von Flunitrazepam.
Vigilance pattern and sleep quality under the effect of flunitrazepam.
Klin.Anaesthesiol.Intensivther. 17, 25-53 (1978)

1611. Joyce,D.N., Kenyon,V.G.
The use of diazepam and hydralazine in the treatment of severe pre-eclampsia.
J.Obstet.Gynaecol.Br.Commonw. 79, 250-4 (1972)

1612. Jung,H., Niebel,B.
Der Wehenschmerz unter dem Einfluß von Valium-Roche und die Objektivierbarkeit durch das Algotokogramm.
Geburtsh.u.Frauenheilk. 26, 937 (1966)

1613. Jusko,W.J., Gretch,M., Gasset,R.
Precipitation of diazepam from intravenous preparations.
J.Amer.Med.Ass. 225, 176 (1973)

1614. Kabra,P.M., Stevens,G.L., Marton,L.J.
High-pressure liquid chromatographic analysis of diazepam, oxazepam and N-desmethyldiazepam in human blood.
J.Chromatogr. 150, 355-60 (1978)

1615. Kabuto,S., Tamaki,T., Koide,T., Ishihama,H.
Studies on metabolism of prazepam. 4. Metabolic fate of prazepam in monkeys.
Yakugaku Za. 98, 944-9 (1978)

1616. Kaim,S.C.
Benzodiazepines in the treatment of alcohol withdrawal states.
In: 362. pp. 571-576

1617. Kaim,S.C., Rosenstein,I.N.
Experience with chlordiazepoxide in the management of epilepsy.
J.Neuropsychiatry 3, 12-7 (1961)

1618. Kaistha,K.K., Tadrus,R.
Thin-layer detection of diazepam and-or chlordiazepoxide alone or in combination with major drugs of abuse in drug-abuse urine screening programs.
J.Chromatogr. 154, 211-8 (1978)

1619. Kaivathekar,P., Anusuya,S.R., Sriniwas,P. et al.
Diazepam (calmpose) in eclampsia: a preliminary report of 16 cases.
Curr.Ther.Res. 15, 845-55 (1973)

1620. Kales,A., Bixler,E.O., Scharf,M., Kales,J.D.
Sleep laboratory studies of flurazepam: A model for evaluating hypnotic drugs.
Clin.Pharmacol.Ther. 19, 576-83 (1976)

1621. Kales,A., Kales,J.D., Bixler,E.O., Russek,E., Scharf,M.B.
Hypnotic efficacy of triazolam: Sleep laboratory evaluation of intermediate-term effectiveness.
J.Clin.Pharmacol. 16, 399 (1976)

1622. Kales,A., Scharf,M.B.
Sleep laboratory and clinical studies of the effects of benzodiazepines on sleep: Flurazepam, diazepam, chlordiazepoxide, and RO 5-4200.
In: 362. pp. 577-98

1623. Kales,A., Scharf,M.B., Kales,J.D.
Rebound insomnia: A new clinical syndrome.
Science 201, 1039-41 (1978)

1624. Kamioka,T., Takagi,H., Kobayashi,S., Suzuki,Y.
Pharmacological studies on 10-Chloro-11b-(2-chlorophenyl)-2,3.5,6,7,11b-hexahydrobenzo-(6,7)-1,4-diazepino(5,4-b)-oxazol-6-one (CS-370), a new psychosedative agent.
Arzneim.-Forsch. (Drug Res.) 22, 884-91 (1972)

1625. Kangas,L., Kanto,J., Mansikka,M.
Nitrazepam premedication for minor surgery.
Upsal.J.Med. 1977, 102 (1977)

1626. Kangas,L., Kanto,J., Syvälahti,E.
Correlation of plasma levels with subjective sedatory effects of nitrazepam.
Acta physiol.Scand. 440, 122 (1976)

1627. Kanto,J.
Plasma levels of diazepam after oral and intramuscular administration.
Brit.J.Anaesth. 46, 817 (1974)

1628. Kanto,J., Iisalo,E.U.M.
Diazepam as an inductive agent in two kinds of combination anaesthesia.
Scand.J.Clin.Lab.Invest. 31, 14 (1973)

1629. Kanto,J., Pihlajamäki,K.
Interaction of diazepam and halothane in rats.
Ann.Chir.Gynaec.Fenn. 62, 247-50 (1973)

1630. Kanto,J.H., Sellman,R., Haataja,M., Hurme,P.
Plasma and urine concentrations of diazepam and its metabolites in children, adults and in diazepam intoxicated patients.
Int.J.Clin. 16, 258-64 (1978)

1631. Kapp,W.
Zur Pharmakologie von Flunitrazepam (Rohypnol).
The pharmacology of flunitrazepam (Rohypnol).
Klin.Anaesthesiol.Intensivther. 17, 1-7 (1978)

1632. Karobath,M., Sperk,G., Schoenbeck,G.
Evidence for an endogenous factor interfering with diazepam-H-3-bindings to rat-brain membranes.
Eur.J.Pharm. 49, 323-6 (1978)

1633. Kasturilal,K., Shetti,R.N.
Role of diazepam in the management of eclampsia.
Curr.Ther.Res. 18, 627-35 (1976)

1634. Keller,M.F.
Intravenous diazepam administration.
J.Amer.Med.Assoc. 225, 750 (1973)

1635. Kelly,D., Pick,R., Chen,C.-N.
A psychological and physiological evaluation of the effects of intravenous diazepam.
Brit.J.Psychiat. 122, 419-26 (1973)

1636. Kesson,C.M., Gray,J.M.B., Lawson,D.H.
Clobazam - new hypnotic.
Brit.J.Clin.Pharmacol. 6, 243-6 (1978)

1637. Khan,W.A., Singh,P.
Synthesis of 3-substituted 1,4-benzodiazepine-2-ones.
Org.Prep.Pr. 10, 105-11 (1978)

1638. Khoo,B.H., Lee,E.L., Lam,K.L.
Neonatal tetanus treated with high dosage diazepam.
Arch.Dis.Childr. 53, 737-9 (1978)

1639. Khorana,A.B.
Intravenous lorazepam in acute anxiety states.
Curr.Med.Res.Opin. 3, 453 (1975)

1640. Kick,H., Dreyer,R.
Klinische Erfahrungen mit Ro 5-4023.
Zentralbl.Ges.Neurol.Psychiatr. 201, 106 (1971)

1641. Kimata,H., Ishihama,H.
Binding of prazepam, desalkylprazepam and diazepam to human serum albumin.
Yakugaku Za. 98, 715-9 (1978)

1642. Kinawi,A., Teller,C.
Studies on interaction of phenprocoumon with diazepam and with nitrazepam.
J.Clin.Chem. 16, 313-4 (1978)

1643. Kinross-Wright,J., Cohen,I.M., Knight,J.A.
The management of neurotic and psychotic states with Ro 5-0690 (Librium).
Dis.Nerv.Syst. 21, 23-6 (1960)

1644. Kitagawa,H., Kurahashi,K., Fujiwara,M., Kohei,H.
Anti-ulcerogenic effect of a pyrido-benzodiazepine derivative (L-S 519) on experimental ulcers.
Arzneim.-Forsch. (Drug Res.) 28, 2122-7 (1978)

1645. Klotz,U.
Clinical pharmacokinetics of diazepam and its biologically-active metabolites.
Klin.Wschr. 56, 895-904 (1978)

1646. Klotz,U., Antonin,K., Bieck,P.
Elimination of diazepam after single and subchronic dosage.
Clin.Pharmacol.Ther. 17, 237-8 (1975)

1647. Knapp,R.B., Fierro,L.
Evaluation of the cardiopulmonary safety and effects of lorazepam as a premedicant.
Anesth.Analg. 53, 122-4 (1974)

1648. Knoche,E., Traub,E., Dick,W.
Effects of diazepam and flunitrazepam on undesired post-operative side-effects of ketamine anesthesia.
Anaesthesis 27, 302-8 (1978)

1649. Knudsen,F.U.
Plasma-diazepam in infants after rectal administration in solution and by suppository.
Acta paediat.Scand. 66, 563-7 (1977)

1650. Kober,A., Jenner,A., Sjöholm,I., Borga,D., Odarcederloef,I.
Differentiated effects of liver-cirrhosis on the albumin binding-sites for diazepam, salicylic-acid and warfarin.
Biochem.Pharmacol. 27, 2729-35 (1978)

1651. Koch-Weser,J.
Drug therapy: serum drug concentrations as therapeutic guides.
N.Engl.J.Med. 287, 227-31 (1972)

1652. Koch-Weser,J.
Bioavailability of drugs.
N.Engl.J.Med. 291, 233-7 (1974)

1653. Koch-Weser,J., Sellers,E.M.
Binding of drugs to serum albumin.
N.Engl.J.Med. 294, 311-6 (1976)

1654. Kop,P., Cosic,V., Simic,B., Andelski,A., Brdjovic,P.
Analysis of the clinical experience in 100 cases of acute intoxication with Apaurin (Diazepam).
Bull.Méd.Lég.Toxicol. 15, 243-51 (1972)

1655. Korttila,K., Linnoila,M.
Skills related to driving after intravenous diazepam, flunitrazepam or droperidol.
Brit.J.Anaesth. 46, 961-9 (1974)

1656. Korttila,K., Linnoila,M.
Absorption and sedative effects of diazepam after oral administration and intramuscular administration into vastus lateralis muscle and deltoid muscle.
Brit.J.Anaesth. 47, 857-62 (1975)

1657. Korttila,K., Linnoila,M.

Psychomotor skills related to driving after intramuscular administration of diazepam and meperidine.

Anaesthesiology 42, 685-91 (1975)

1658. Korttila,K., Linnoila,M.

Skills related to driving after intravenous sedation: Dose-response relationship with diazepam.

Brit.J.Anaesth. 47, 457-63 (1975)

1659. Korttila,K., Mattila,M.J., Linnoila,M.

Saturation of tissues with N-desmethyldiazepam as a cause for elevated serum levels of this metabolite after repeated administration of diazepam.

Acta Pharmacol.et Toxicol. 36, 190-2 (1975)

1660. Korttila,K., Mattila,M.J., Linnoila,M.

Prolonged recovery after diazepam sedation: The influence of food, charcoal ingestion and injection rate on the effects of intravenous diazepam.

Brit.J.Anaesth. 48, 333-40 (1976)

1661. Korttila,K., Saarniva ,L., Himberg,J.J., Hytonen,M.

Comparison of diazepam and flunitrazepam as adjuncts to local-anesthesia for bronchoscopy.

Upsal.J.Med. 1977, 100 (1977)

1662. Korttila,K., Saarniva ,L., Tarkkanen,J., Himberg,J.J., Hytonen,M.

Effect of age on amnesia and sedation induced by flunitrazepam during local-anesthesia for bronchoscopy.

Brit.J.Anaesth. 50, 1211-8 (1978)

1663. Kotzan,J.A.

Effect of diazepam on cognition via pupillometry.

J.Pharm.Sci. 67, 956-8 (1978)

1664. Kozhechkin,S.N.

Changes in the electrical activity of the cerebral cortical neurons in the rabbit under the effect of diazepam.

Biull.Eksp.Biol.Med. 85, 41-5 (1978)

1665. Krakowski,A.J.

Preliminary observations on the use of Ro-4556 in psychiatric disorders characterized by anxiety-tension.

Psychosomatics 7, 150-1 (1966)

1666. Kraus,J.W., Desmond,P.V., Marshall,J.P., Johnson,R.F., Schenker,S., Wilkinson,G.R.

Effect of aging and liver-disease on disposition of lorazepam.

Clin.Pharm. 24, 411-9 (1978)

1667. Krieglstein,J.

Zur Plasmaproteinbindung von Arzneimitteln.

Klin.Wschr. 47, 1125-30 (1969)

1668. Kruse,R., Blakenhorn,V.

Zusammenfassender Erfahrungsbericht über die klinische Anwendung und Wirksamkeit von Ro 5-4023 (clonazepam) auf verschiedene Formen epileptischer Anfälle.

Acta Neurol.Scand. 49, 60 (1973)

1669. Kugler,J., Doenicke,A., Suttmann,H., Laub,M., Späth,M., Woeller,L.

Einfluß von Flunitrazepam auf Verhalten und Psyche. The effect of flunitrazepam on behavior and psyche.

Klin.Anaesthesiol.Intensivther. 17, 54-61 (1978)

1670. Kyriakopoulos,A.A., Greenblatt,D.J., Shader,R.I.

Clinical pharmacokinetics of lorazepam. Review.

J.Clin.Psych. 39, 16-23 (1978)

1671. Lader,M.H.

Plasma concentrations of tricyclic antidepressive drugs.

Brit.J.Clin.Pharmacol. 1, 281-3 (1974)

1672. Lader,M.H.

Clinical pharmacology of oxazepam.

Acta Psych.Scand. 1978, 89-93 (1978)

1673. Ladinsky,H., Consolo,S., Peri,G., Garattini,S.

Increase in mouse and rat brain acetylcholine levels by diazepam.

In: 362. pp. 241-2

1674. Lal,A.A., Levy,R.H., Cutler,R.E.

Time-course of interaction between carbamazepine and clonazepam in normal man.

Clin.Pharm. 24, 316-23 (1978)

1675. Lal,K., Sharma,T.C.

Experiences with diazepam in management of eclampsia.

Medikon 9, 14-7 (1978)

1676. Langslet,A., Meberg,A., Bredesen,J.E., Lunde,P.K.M.

Plasma concentrations of diazepam and N-desmethyl-diazepam in newborn-infants after intravenous, intramuscular, rectal and oral-administration.

Acta Paed.Sci. 67, 699-704 (1978)

1677. Lanzoni,J., Airoldi,L., Marcucci,F., Mussini,E.

Gas-chromatographic determination of chlor-desmethyldiazepam and lorazepam in rats and mice.

J.Chromatogr. 168, 260-5 (1979)

1678. Law,N.C.

A modern approach for drug identification.

Amer.J.Med.Technol. 39, 237 (1973)

1679. Lean,T.H., Ratman,S.S., Sivasamboo,R.

Use of benzodiazepines in the management of eclampsia.

J.Obstet.Gynaecol.Brit.Commonw. 75, 856-62 (1968)

1680. Lehmann,W.

Effect of oxazepam on sleep in normal human volunteers.

Acta Psych.Scand. 1978, 33-39 (1978)

1681. Leibowitz,M., Sunshine,A.
Long-term hypnotic efficacy and safety of triazolam and flurazepam.
J.Clin.Pharmacol. 18, 302-9 (1978)

1682. Leinzinger,E., Lechner,G., Zwinz,G.
Geburtsverlauf bei Anwendung eines Benzodiazepin-Derivates.
Fortschr.Geburtsh.Gynäk. 19, 303 (1964)

1683. Leube,H., Höffkes,H.
Erfahrungen mit dem neuen Tranquilizer Wy 4036 (Lorazepam) auf dem psychiatrisch-neurologischen Fachgebiet und im Rahmen der inneren Medizin.
Arzneim.-Forsch. (Drug Res.) 21, 1098 (1971)

1684. Lidbrink,P., Corrodi,H., Fuxe,K., Olson,L.
The effect of benzodiazepines, meprobamate, and barbiturates on central monoamine neurons.
In: 362. pp. 203-24

1685. Liepman,M.
High-dose benzodiazepines in the treatment of severe neurotic anxiety.
J.Clin.Psych. 40, 54 (1979)

1686. Liljequist,R., Linnoila,M., Mattila,M.J.
Effect of diazepam and chlorpromazine on memory functions in man.
Eur.J.Clin.Pharmacol. 13, 339-43 (1978)

1687. Lin,K.M., Friedel,R.O.
Relationship of plasma-levels of chlordiazepoxide and metabolites to clinical response.
Amer.J.Psychiatry 136, 18-23 (1979)

1688. Lingjaerde,jr.,O.
Effect of benzodiazepines on uptake and efflux of serotonin in human blood platelets in vitro.
In: 362. pp. 225-34

1689. Lingjaerde,O.
Acute og kronik overdosering av diazepam (Valium).
Nord.psykiat.T. 19, 73-8 (1965)

1690. Lingjaerde,O., Berglund,J., Bratland,S.Z., Christen, J.E., Eikrem,A., Hercz,I., Joakimse,R., Moe,F., Olsen,T.I., Stenvold,S.E.
Alimemazine as a hypnotic in general practice patients - controlled comparison with nitrazepam.
Curr.Ther.Res. 24, 388-96 (1978)

1691. Linnoila,M.
Effects of diazepam, chlordiazepoxide, thioridazine, haloperidol, flupenthixole and alcohol on psychomotor skills related to driving.
Ann.Med.Exp.Biol.Fenn. 51, 125 (1973)

1692. Linnoila,M., Mattila,M.J.
Combined effects of diazepam and alcohol on skills related to driving.
Scand.J.Clin.Lab.Invest. 29, Suppl. 172 24 (1972)

1693. Linnoila,M., Saario,I., Måki,M.
Effect of treatment with diazepam or lithium and alcohol on psychomotor skills related to driving.
Eur.J.Clin.Pharmacol. 7, 337-42 (1974)

1694. Lippa,A.S., Sano,M.C., Coupet,J., Klepner,C.A., Beer,B.
Evidence that benzodiazepine receptors reside on cerebellar purkinje-cells - studies with nervous mutant mice.
Life Sci. 23, 2213-7 (1978)

1695. Loach,A., Fisher,A.
Lorazepam as a premedicant for day-case surgery: An assessment.
Anaesthesia 30, 545-9 (1975)

1696. Longoni,A., Mandelli,V., Pessotti,I.
Study of antianxiety effects of drugs in the rat with a multiple punishment and reward schedule.
In: 362. pp. 347-54

1697. Lund,M., Trolle,E.
Clonazepam in the treatment of epilepsy.
Acta Neurol.Scand. 49, 82 (1973)

1698. Lunde,I., Borchgrevink,C.F.
Use of diazepam in early pregnancy.
Nor.Tannlaegeforen Tid. 86, 431-2 (1976)

1699. Machata,G.
Grenzen der Nachweismöglichkeiten von Substanzen in Körperflüssigkeiten und -geweben.
Z.Rechtsmedizin 70, 191-6 (1972)

1700. Mackerer,C.R., Kochman,R.L.
Effects of cations and anions on binding of ^{3}H-diazepam to rat-brain.
Proc.Soc.Exp.Med. 158, 393-7 (1978)

1701. Mackerer,C.R., Kochman,R.L., Bierschenk,B.A., Bremner,S.S.
Binding of ^{3}H-diazepam to rat-brain homogenates.
J.Pharm.Exp. 206, 405-13 (1978)

1702. MacLeod,S.M., Giles,H.G., Bengert,B., Liu,F.F., Sellers,E.M.
Age-related and gender-related differences in diazepam pharmacokinetics.
J.Clin.Pharm. 19, 15-9 (1979)

1703. MacLeod,S.M., Giles,H.G., Patzalek,G., Thiessen,J.J., Sellers,E.M.
Diazepam actions and plasma concentrations following ethanol ingestion.
J.Clin.Pharmacol. 11, 345-9 (1977)

1704. MacLeod,S.M., Greenblatt,D.J., Sellers,E.M.
Determination of intravenous chlordiazepoxide pharmacokinetics: Plasma versus blood.
Clin.Res. 25, 273 (1977)

1705. MacLeod,S.M., Sellers,E.M., Giles,H.G., Billings,B.J., Martin,P.R., Greenblatt,D.J., Marshman,J.A.
Interaction of disulfiram with benzodiazepines.
Clin.Pharm. 5, 583-9 (1978)

1706. Madan,B.R., Sharma,J.D., Uyas,D.E.
Actions of methaminodiazepoxide on cardiac, smooth and skeletal muscles.
Arch.Int.Pharmacodyn. 143, 127-37 (1963)

1707. Magbagbeola,J.A.O.
A comparison of lorazepam and diazepam as oral premedicants for surgery under regional anaesthesia.
Brit.J.Anaesth. 46, 449-51 (1974)

1708. Magnus,R.V., Dean,B.C., Curry,S.H.
Clorazepate: Double blind crossover comparison of a single nightly dose with diazepam thrice daily in anxiety.
Dis.Nerv.Syst. 38, 918-21 (1978)

1709. Magnussen,M.P., Frey,H.H.
Einfluß von Alkohol auf die Resorption zentral depressiver Pharmaka aus dem Magen.
Naunyn-Schmied.-Arch.Pharmacol. 257, 39-40 (1967)

1710. Mahon,W.A., Inaba,T., Tsutsimi,E., Umeda,T.
The metabolism of diazepam in man.
Clin.Res. 22, 726 (1974)

1711. Maksay,G., Tegyey,Z., Otvos,L.
Kinetic investigations of liver microsomal esterases with oxazepam esters.
Hoppe-Seyler's Zeitschrf.Physiol.Chem. 359, 879-86 (1978)

1712. Maksay,G., Tegyey,Z., Otvos,L.
Stereospecifity of esterases hydrolysing oxazepam acetate.
J.Pharm.Sci. 67, 1208-10 (1978)

1713. Maletzky,B.M., Klotter,J.
Addiction to diazepam.
Int.J.Addict. 11, 95 (1976)

1714. Malmgren,G., Arnold,E., Schubert,B., Hansen,T.
Klinisk-analytisk undersökning.
Farm.Rev. 22, 702-6 (1972)

1715. Mandelli,M., Tognoni,G., Garattini,S.
Clinical pharmacokinetics of diazepam.
Clin.Pharmacokinetics 3, 72-91 (1978)

1716. Maneksha,S., Harry,T.V.A.
Lorazepam in sexual disorders.
Brit.J.Clin.Pract. 29, 175-6 (1975)

1717. Marangos,P.J., Paul,S.M., Greenlaw,P., Goodwin, F.K., Skolnick,P.
Demonstration of an endogenous, competitive inhibitor of H-3-diazepam binding in bovine brain.
Life Sci. 22, 1893-1900 (1978)

1718. Marcucci,F., Fanelli,R., Mussini,E., Garattini,S.
Species differences in diazepam metabolism: I. Metabolism of diazepam metabolites.
Biochem.Pharmacol. 19, 1847-51 (1970)

1719. Marcucci,F., Mussini,E., Cotellessa ,L., Ghirardi,P., Parenti,M., Riva,R., Salva,P.
Distribution of camazepam in rats and mice.
J.Pharm.Sci. 67, 1470-1 (1978)

1720. Mariani,L.
Performance capacity and hypnotics: Residual effect of benzodiazepine and barbiturates.
Clin.Ther. 83, 347-52 (1977)

1721. Marino,A.
Behavioral and psychosomatic effects of benzodiazepines: Interactions with other drugs.
In: 362. pp. 631-40

1722. Marks,I.M., Visvanathan,R., Lipsedge,M.S., Gardner,R.
Enhanced relief of phobia by flooding during waning diazepam effect.
Brit.J.Psychiat. 121, 493-505 (1972)

1723. Martin,A., Hirt,H.R.
Clinical experience with clonazepam (Rivotril) in the treatment of epilepsies in infancy and childhood.
Neuropaediatrie 4, 245 (1973)

1724. Martin,I.L., Candy,J.M.
Facilitation of benzodiazepine binding by sodium-chloride and GABA.
Neuropharm. 11, 993-8 (1978)

1725. Martins,J.K.
Combined amitriptyline -perphenazine (Etrafon) compared with chlordiazepoxide hydrochloride, a double-blind crossover study.
Curr.Therap.Res. 8, 17 (1966)

1726. Mathej,H.G.
Il trattamento della sindrome vegetativa funzionale con oxazepam.
Arzneim.-Forsch. (Drug Res.) 15, 374-6 (1965)

1727. Matthew,H., Proudfoot,A.T., Aitkin,R.C.B., Raeburn,J.A., Wright,N.
Nitrazepam - a safe hypnotic.
Brit.med.J. 3, 23-5 (1969)

1728. Matsumoto,S., Kimata,H., Ishihama,H., Yakugaku,Z.A.
Studies on metabolism of prazepam. 2. Metabolism of prazepam, diazepam and desalkylprazepam by rat-liver microsomes.
Yakugaku Za. 98, 737-43 (1978)

1729. Mattila,M.J., Palva,E., Seppala,T., Ostrovski,R.U.
Actions and interactions with alcohol of drugs on psychomotor-skills- comparison of diazepam and gamma-hydroxybutyric acid.
Arch.Int.Pharmacodyn.Ther. 234, 236-46 (1978)

1730. Mattson, R.H.
The Benzodiazepines.
In: Woddbury, D.M. et al. (eds):
Antiepileptic Drugs, New York, Raven Press 1972, pp. 497-516

1731. Mayer, W., Erbe, S., Wolf, G., Voigt, R.
Beiträge zur Analytik und Stabilität einiger pharmazeutisch interessanter 1,4-Benzodiazepine.
2. Mitteilung: Ringverengung bei Nordiazepam und Clonazepam. pH-Abhängigkeit der hydrolytischen Spaltung des Diazepams Faustan[R] und Anwendung kinetischer Methoden zur Ermittlung des Stabilitätsverhaltens von Diazepam in Ampullenlösungen.
Pharmazie 29, 700-7 (1974)

1732. McCarthy, G.T., O'Connell, B., Robinson, A.E.
Blood levels of diazepam in infants of two mothers given large doses of diazepam during labour.
J.Obstet.Gynaecol.Brit.Commonw. 80, 349-52 (1973)

1733. McCaughey, W., Dundee, J.W.
Comparison of sedative effects of diazepam given by the oral and intramuscular routes.
Brit.J.Anaesth. 44, 901-2 (1972)

1734. McKay, A.C., Dundee, J.W., George, K.A.
Amnesic effects of orally-administered benzodiazepines.
Brit.J.Anaesth. 50, 1080-1 (1978)

1735. McLeod, W.R.
A comparison of diazepam, benzoctamine and placebo in anxiety states.
Curr.Ther.Res. 14, 239-45 (1972)

1736. Meberg, A., Langslet, A., Bredesen, J.E., Lunde, P.K.M.
Plasma concentrations of diazepam and N-desmethyldiazepam in children after a single rectal or intramuscular dose of diazepam.
Eur.J.Clin.Pharmacol. 14, 273-6 (1978)

1737. Meguro, K., Masuda, T., Kuwada, Y., Tawada, H.
Verfahren zur Herstellung von Benzodiazepin-2-on-Derivaten und neue Benzodiazepin-2-on-Derivate.
Ger.Offen. 1944404 (to Takeda chemical Industries Ltd. assued March 12, 1970)

1738. Mellor, J.M., Stibbard, J.H., Rawlins, M.F.
Synthesis of bridged 1,5-benzodiazepines by condensation of ortho-phenylene-diamines with 4,6-dimethylbicyclo-3,3,1-nona-3,6-diene-2,8-dione.
J.Chem.Soc. 1978, 557-8 (1978)

1739. Mendels, J., Secunda, S., Schless, A., Sandler, K., Singer, J.
Double-blind comparison of clobazam and diazepam in treatment of anxiety neurosis.
J.Clin.Pharm. 18, 353-7 (1978)

1740. Mendenhall, C.L., Robinson, J.D., Morgan, D.D.
Chlordiazepoxide, Librium[R], therapy in hepatic insufficiency.
Gastroeterology 69, 845 (1975)

1741. Metz, P., Halveg, J.O.
Pethidine-diazepam analgesia for cytoscopy.
Anaesthesia 29, 92 (1974)

1742. Meusert, W.
Prüfung von Lorazepam (Wy 4036) in der nervenärztlichen Praxis.
Arzneim.-Forsch. (Drug Res.) 21, 1087 (1971)

1743. Meusert, W.
Vorläufige Mitteilung über die Wirkung von SB 5833 (Camazepam) - einem neuen Derivat aus der Benzodiazepinreihe.
Therapiewoche 25, 3436-9 (1975)

1744. Meusert, W.
Doppelblindversuch mit einem neuen Derivat aus der Benzodiazepinreihe (Camazepam).
Med.Mschr. 30, 413-5 (1976)

1745. Mikkelsen, B., Birkett-Smith, F.
A clinical study of the benzodiazepine Ro 5-4023 (clonazepam) in the treatment of epilepsy.
Acta Neurol.Scand. 49, 91 (1973)

1746. Moehler, H., Okada, T.
Benzodiazepine receptors in normal and pathological human-brain.
Brit.J.Psychiatry 133, 261-8 (1978)

1747. Moehler, H., Okada, T., Enna, S.J.
Benzodiazepine and neurotransmitter receptor-binding in rat-brain after chronic administration of diazepam or phenobarbital.
Brain Res. 156, 391-5 (1978)

1748. Moehler, H., Okada, T., Heitz, P., Ulrich, J.
Biochemical identification of the site of action of benzodiazepines in human brain by ^{3}H-diazepam binding.
Life Sci. 22, 985-95 (1978)

1749. Molander, L., Duvhök, C.
Acute effects of oxazepam, diazepam and methylperone, alone and in combination with alcohol on sedation, coordination and mood.
Acta Pharmacol.Toxicol. 38, 145-60 (1976)

1750. Monachon, M.-A., Jalfre, M., Haefely, W.
A modulation effect of chlordiazepoxide on drug-induced PGO spikes in the cat.
In: 362. pp. 513-30

1751. Montagu, J.D.
Effects of diazepam on the EEG in man.
Eur.J.Pharmacol. 17, 167-70 (1972)

1752. Monti, J., Altier, H.
Flunitrazepam (Ro 5-4200) and sleep cycle in normal subjects.
Psychopharmacologia 32, 343 (1973)

1753. Monti,J., Trenchi,H.M., Morales,F., Monti,L.
Flunitrazepam (Ro 5-4200) and sleep cycle in insomniae patients.
Psychopharmacologia 35, 371 (1974)

1754. Moore,R.G., McBride,W.G.
Disposition kinetics of diazepam in pregnant-women at parturition.
Eur.J.Clin.Pharm. 13, 275-84 (1978)

1755. Morris,E.
Use of diazepam in gastrointestinal endoscopy.
S.Afr.Med.J. 54, 1118 (1978)

1756. Morris,M.E.
Compatibility and stability of diazepam injection following dilution with intravenous fluids.
Amer.J.Hosp.Pharm. 35, 669-72 (1978)

1757. Morselli,P.L., Cassano,G.B., Placidi,G.F., Muscettola,G.B., Rizzo,M.
Kinetics of the distribution of ^{14}C-diazepam and its metabolites in various areas of cat brain.
In: 362. pp. 129-44

1758. Moser,L., Huther,K.J., Koch-Weser,J., Lundt,P.V.
Effects of terfenadine and diphenhydramine alone or in combination with diazepam or alcohol on psychomotor performance and subjective feelings.
Eur.J.Clin.Pharmacol. 14, 417-23 (1978)

1759. Müller,W.E., Schlafer,U., Wollert,U.
Benzodiazepine receptor-binding - Interactions of some none-benzodiazepine drugs with specific ^{3}H-diazepam binding to rat-brain synaptosomal membranes.
Naunyn-Schmied.-Arch.Pharmacol. 305, 23-6 (1978)

1760. Müller,W.E., Schlafer,U., Wollert,U.
Benzodiazepine receptor-binding in rat spinal-cord membranes.
Neurosci.L. 9, 239-43 (1978)

1761. Mulley,B.A., Potter,B.I., Rye,R.M., Takeshit. ,K.
Interactions between diazepam and paracetamol.
J.Clin.Pharmacol. 3, 25-35 (1978)

1762. Munthe-Kaas,A., Strandjord,R.
Clonazepam in the treatment of epileptic seizures.
Acta Neurol.Scand. 49, 97 (1973)

1763. Murray-Lyon,I.M., Young,J., Parkes,J.D., Knill-Jones,R.P., Williams,R.
Clinical and electroencephalographic assessment of diazepam in liver disease.
Brit.Med.J. 4, 265-6 (1972)

1764. Naess,K.
Diazepam and alcohol.
Tidsskr.Nor.Laegeforen 98, 1019 (1978)

1765. Nagy,J.
Experimental-model for treatment of acute diazepam intoxication.
EEG Cl.Neur. 44, 538 (1978)

1766. Nagy,J., Decsi,L.
Physostigmine, a highly potent antidote for acute experimental diazepam intoxication.
Neuropharm. 17, 469-75 (1978)

1767. Nakamura,K., Shimokawa,Y., Oikawa,Y., Nakamura,K.
Influence of clonazepam, an anticonvulsant benzodiazepine drug, on the rat brain monoamine containing neurons especially on dopaminergic neurons.
Nippon Yakurigaku Zasshi 74, 251-65 (1978)

1768. Nakamura,M., Fukushima,H.
Effect of fludiazepam on turnover of serotonin in mouse brain.
Jap.J.Pharmacol. 27, 905-8 (1977)

1769. Nakamura,M., Fukushima,H.
Effect of benzodiazepines on central serotonergic neuron systems.
Psychopharmakology (Berl.) 53, 121-6 (1977)

1770. Nakano,S., Ogawa,N., Kawazu,Y., Osato,E.
Effects of antianxiety drug and personality on stress-inducing psychomotor performance test.
J.Clin.Pharmacol. 18, 125-30 (1978)

1771. Nanda,R.N., Johnson,R.H., Keogh,H.J. et al.
Treatment of epilepsy with clonazepam and its effect on other anticonvulsants.
J.Neurol.Neurosurg.Psychiatry 40, 538 (1977)

1772. Naranjo,C.A., Sellers,E.M., Giles,H.G., Abel,J.G.
Diurnal-variations of plasma total diazepam and desmethyldiazepam concentrations and drug free fraction.
Clin.Res. 26, 836 (1978)

1773. Nau,H., Liddiard,C., Jesdinsky,D., Wittfoht,W., Brendel,K.
Quantitative-analysis of prazepam and its metabolites by electron-capture gas-chromatography and selected ion monitoring. Application to diaplacental passage and fetal hepatic-metabolism in early human pregnancy.
J.Chromatogr. 146, 227-39 (1978)

1774. Neumann,E., Horak,J., Cuparenco,B., Cucuianu,M., Seusan,E.
Influence of some benzodiazepine derivatives on blood-coagulation in rats.
Agressolog. 19, 201-9 (1978)

1775. Newton,D.W.
Potential source of error in official diazepam assays.
J.Pharm.Sci. 67, 550-1 (1978)

1776. Niada,R., Omini,C., Prino,G., Folco,G.C., Milani,S., Berti,F.
Synergistic interaction between diazepam and octatropine-methylbromide at the gastrointestinal level.
Pharmacol.Res. 10, 951-60 (1978)

1777. Nicholson,A.N., Stone,B.M.
Effectiveness of diazepam and its metabolites 3-Hydroxydiazepam (Temazepam) and 3-hydroxy-N-desmethyldiazepam (Oxazepam) for sleep during day.
Chronobiol. 5, 191 (1978)

1778. Nicholson,A.N., Stone,B.M.
Hypnotic activity of 3-Hydroxy-, N-desmethyldiazepam (Oxazepam).
Brit.J.Clin.Pharmacol. 5, 469-72 (1978)

1779. Nicholson,J.D.
Derivative formation in the quantitative gas-chromatographic analysis of pharmaceuticals.
Analyst 103, 1-28 (1978)

1780. Niedermeyer,E.
Intravenous diazepam and its anticonvulsant action.
Johns Hopkins Med.J. 127, 79-96 (1970)

1781. Nimmo,W.S., Forrest,J.A.H., Haeding,R.C., Finlaysc.,N.D., Prescott,L.F.
Premedication for upper gastrointestinal endoscopy - comparative-study of flunitrazepam, diazepam and neuroleptanalgesia.
Endoscopy 10, 183-6 (1978)

1782. Ning,R.Y., Sternbach,L.H., Pool,W., Randall,L.O.
Quinazolines and 1,4-Benzodiazepines. 58. The azido group, a novel pharmacophoric substituent. 7-Acido-5-phenyl-1,4-benzodiazepines.
J.Med.Chem. 16, 879-82 (1973)

1783. Nissel,H.
Die Wirkung von Diazepam, Pentazocin und Xylocain auf die Serum-CPK-, GOT- und LDH-Spiegel.
Wien.klin.Wschr. 86, 472-4 (1974)

1784. Nistri,A., Constanti,A.
Effects of flurazepam on amino acid-evoked response recorded from the lobster muscle and the frog spinal cord.
Neuropharmacology 17, 127-35 (1978)

1785. Niswander,K.R.
Effect of diazepam on meperidine requirements of patients during labor.
Obstet.Gynecol. 34, 62-7 (1969)

1786. Norris,W., Wallace,P.G.M.
Wy 4036 (Lorazepam): A study of its use in premedication.
Brit.J.Anaesth. 43, 785-9 (1971)

1787. Ogura,C., Majima,K., Nakasawa,K., Nakamura,I., Umezawa,Y., Ueda,H.
Comparative-study of effects of flurazepam and nitrazepam on sleep by 24-hour polygraphy.
Eur.J.Clin.Pharmacol. 13, 413-8 (1978)

1788. Ohmori,K.
Electroencephalographic effects of flurazepam in rabbits.
Nippon Yakurigaku Zasshi 73, 939-54 (1977)

1789. Olgiati,S.G.
Clinical assessment of lorazepam in anxiety: A double-blind study.
Curr.Ther.Res. 17, 13-22 (1975)

1790. O'Neil,R., Verril,P.J., Aelling,W.H., Laurence,D.R.
Intravenous diazepam in minor oral surgery.
Brit.Dent.J. 127, 15-8 (1970)

1791. Orr,J., Dussault,P., Chappel,C., Goldberg,L., Reggiani,G.
Relation between drug-induced central nervous system effects and plasma levels of diazepam in man.
In: Alcohol, drugs and driving. Eds. M.J.Mattila & M.Linnoila. Karger, Basel, 1976

1792. Oswald,I., Lewis,S.A., Tagney,J., Firth,H., Haider,I.
Benzodiazepines and human sleep.
In: 362. pp. 613-26

1793. Otvoes,L., Tegyey,Z., Vereczkey,L., Ledniczky,M., Tamas,J., Palosi,E., Szporny,L.
Metabolism of levorotary 4,5-dihydrodiazepam in the rat.
Drug Metab.Dispos. 6, 213-7 (1978)

1794. Padilla,J., Camacho,R.
Clinical evaluation of clobazam in patients with anxiety - single dose morning or night.
Inv.Med.Int. 5, 323-8 (1978)

1795. Palmer,G.C.
Use, Overuse, Misuse, and abuse of benzodiazepines.
Alab.J.Med.Sci. 15, 383-99 (1978)

1796. Palva,E.S., Linnoila,M.
Effect of active metabolites of chlordiazepoxide and diazepam, alone or in combination with alcohol, on psychomotor-skills related to driving.
Eur.J.Clin.Pharm. 13, 345-50 (1978)

1797. Pandit,S.K., Heisterkamp,D.V., Cohen,P.J.
Further studies of the anti-recall effect of lorazepam: A dose-time-effect relationship.
Anesthesiology 45, 495-500 (1976)

1798. Paquet,C., Gaillard,J.M., Tissot,R.
Flunitrazepam and memory.
Acta Psychiatr.Belg. 78, 374-82 (1978)

1799. Parmar,S.S., Yutrzenkow,G.J., Davis,J.S., Brumleve,S.J.
Involvement of biogenic-amines as possible mediators in anticonvulsant activity of benzodiazepines.
Pharmacology 20, 240 (1978)

1800. Parrott,A.C., Hindmarch,I.
Clobazam- 1,5-benzodiazepine derivative-effects upon human psychomotor performance under different levels of task reinforcement.
Arch.Int.Pharm. 232, 261-8 (1978)

1801. Parsonage,M.J., Norris,J.W.
Use of diazepam in treatment of severe convulsive status epilepticus.
Brit.Med.J. 3, 85-8 (1967)

1802. Pateisky,K., Wessely,P.
Unterschiedliche Reaktion auf Diazepam bei verschiedener intravenöser Applikationsgeschwindigkeit (polygraphische Studie).
Schweiz.Rundschau Med. 64, 962-5 (1975)

1803. Patrick,J.M., Sempik,A.K.
Effect of diazepam on threshold of ventilatory response to CO_2.
Brit.J.Clin.Pharmacol. 6, 462-3 (1978)

1804. Paul,H.H., Sapper,H., Lohmann,W.
H-1-NMR investigations on the hydrogen-bond formation between the tranquilizers diazepam and nitrazepam and some nucleobases.
Z.Naturforsch. C 33, 870-5 (1978)

1805. Paul,S.M., Skolnick,P.
Rapid changes in brain benzodiazepine receptors after experimental seizures.
Science 202, 892-4 (1978)

1806. Paymaster,N.J.
Lorazepam (WY 4036) as a pre-operative medication.
Anaesthesia 28, 521-6 (1973)

1807. Pearl,D.S., Quest,J.A., Gillis,R.A.
Use of various solvents to study the effect of diazepam on cardiac rhythm.
Toxicol.Appl.Pharmacol. 44, 653-6 (1978)

1808. Pennington,G.W., Synge,V.M.
Chlordiazepoxide (Librium) overdosage.
J.Ir.Med.Assoc. 49, 187-8 (1961)

1809. Perchalski,R.J., Wilder,B.J.
Determination of benzodiazepine anticonvulsants in plasma by high-performance liquid chromatography.
Anal.Chem. 50, 554-7 (1978)

1810. Perry,P.J., Wilding,D.C., Fowler,R.C., Hepler,C.D., Caputo,J.F.
Absorption of oral and intramuscular chlordiazepoxide by alcoholics.
Clin.Pharmacol.Ther. 23, 535-41 (1978)

1811. Peters,U.H., Seidel,M.
Medikamentenmißbrauch und Sucht bei Diazepam.
Arzneim.-Forsch. (Drug Res.) 20, 876-7 (1970)

1812. Petsche,H.
Zum Nachweis des kortikalen Angriffspunktes des antikonvulsiven Benzodiazepinderivats Clonazepam (Ro 5-4023).
EEG-EMG 3, 145-53 (1972)

1813. Pilbrant,A., Glenne,P.-O., Sundwall,A., Vessman,J., Wretlind,M.
Comparative bioavailability of oral dosage forms of oxazepam. - Correlation with in vitro dissolution rates.
Acta Pharmacol.Toxicol. 40, 7-15 (1977)

1814. Pinder,R.M., Brogden,R.N., Speight,T.M., Avery,G.S.
Clonazepam: A review of its pharmacological properties and therapeutic efficacy in epilepsy.
Drugs 12, 321 (1976)

1815. Pinelli,P.
Electromyographic evaluation of drug-induced muscle relaxation.
In: 362. pp. 559-64

1816. Pinosky,D.G.
Clinical-assessment of safety and efficacy of lorazepam - new benzodiazepine derivative. - in treatment of anxiety.
J.Clin.Psych. 39, 24-9 (1978)

1817. Piraino,A.J., DiGregorio,G.J.
Comparative availability of diazepam in human plasma, parotid saliva and mixed saliva and its relationship to plasma protein binding.
The Pharmacologist 19, 128 (1977)

1818. Plumb,J.
Sedatives and drinking.
Brit.Med.J. 2, 1135 (1976)

1819. Popescu,D.T., Nauta,J.
Cardiovascular performances of flunitrazepam compared with that of other induction-agents.
Upsal.J.Med. 1977, 95 (1977)

1820. Porta,V., Jann,G.
Klinischer Versuch mit Camazepam in der Behandlung von Angstzuständen.
Min.Psich.e Psicol. 15, 106 (1974)

1821. Porter,W.R., Lancee,W.J.
Multicenter evaluation of lorazepam, a new benzodiazepine.
Clin.Ther. 2, 31-40 (1978)

1822. Post,C., Lindgren,S., Bertler,A., Malmgren,H.
Pharmacokinetics of N-desmethyldiazepam in healthy volunteers after single daily doses of dipotassium chlorazepate.
Psychopharmacology 53, 105-9 (1977)

1823. Post,D.
Persönl. Mitteilung / Personal Comm.

1824. Powell,W.F., Comer,W.H.
Controlled comparison of lorazepam and pentobarbital as hypnotics for presurgical patients.
Anesth.Analg. 52, 267-71 (1973)

1825. Powell,W.F., Comer,W.H.
Double-blind controlled comparison of lorazepam and glutethimide as night-before-operation hypnotics.
Anesth.Analg. 52, 313-6 (1973)

1826. Prensky,A.L., Raff,M.C., Moore,M.J., Schwaab,R.S.
Intravenous diazepam in the treatment of prolonged seizures activity.
New Engl.J.Med. 276, 779-84 (1967)

1827. Preti,C., Tosi,G.
Syntheses and spectroscopic studies on group IIb-metal-1,4-benzodiazepine complexes.
Transit.Met. 3, 246-50 (1978)

1828. Proudfoot,A.T., Park.J.
Changing patterns of drugs used for selfpoisoning.
Brit.Med.J. 1, 90 (1978)

1829. Radmayr,E.
Vergleichende Untersuchung mit Doxepin und Diazepam parenteral.
Wien.Med.Wschr. 122, 336 (1972)

1830. Raff,G., Staak,M., Strohm,H.
Experimentelle Untersuchungen über die Änderung der subjektiven Befindlichkeit unter Dikalium-Chlorazepat.
Blutalkohol 15, 193-9 (1978)

1831. Ragni,N.
Camazepam beim klimakterischen Syndrom.
Il Progr. Medico 30, 479-83 (1974)

1832. Rajtar,G.
The influence of chlorpromazine, diazepam and imipramine on the central action of ethanol.
Arch.Immunol.Ther.Exp. (Warsz.) 25, 813-8 (1977)

1833. Rao,S., Shebarniuk,K., Prasad,S., Lee,K.J., Sproule,B.J.
Cardiopulmonary effects of diazepam.
Clin.Pharmacol.Ther. 14, 182 (1973)

1834. Rastogi,R.B., Lapierre,Y.D., Singhal,R.L.
Effect of a new benzodiazepine bromazepam on locomotor performance and brain mono-amine metabolism.
J.Neural.Tr. 42, 251-61 (1978)

1835. Rastogi,R.B., Lapierre,Y.D., Singhal,R.L.
Synaptosomal uptake of norepinephrine and 5-hydroxytryptamine and synthesis of catecholamines during benzodiazepine treatment.
Can.J.Physiol. 56, 777-84 (1978)

1836. Reggiani,G.
Discussion summary.
In: 362. pp. 627-30

1837. Reidenberg,M.M., Levy,M., Warner,H., Coutinho,C.B., Schwartz,M.A., Yu,G., Cheripko,J.
Relationship between diazepam dose, plasma level, age, and central nervous system depression.
Clin.Pharmacol.Ther. 23, 371-4 (1978)

1838. Reiffenstuhl,G.
Über die Anwendung von Valium während der Geburt und die Möglichkeiten seiner relaxierenden Wirkung auf die Uterusmuskulatur.
III. Sympos. Bern, Basel: S. Karger 1963, Fortschr.d.Geburtsh.u.Gynäk. 19, 254 (1964)

1839. Reisine,T.D., Wastek,G.J., Yamamura,H.I.
Alterations in benzodiazepine-binding-sites in huntington disease.
Pharmacology 20, 240 (1978)

1840. Rett,A.
Möglichkeiten und Grenzen der Clonazepam-Therapie im Kindesalter.
Wien.Klin.Wschr. 83, 725 (1971)

1841. Richards,D.J.
Clinical profile of lorazepam - new benzodiazepine tranquilizer.
J.Clin.Psych. 39, 58-66 (1978)

1842. Rickels,K.
Predictors of response to benzodiazepines in anxious outpatients.
In: 362. pp. 391-404

1843. Rickels,K., Case,W.G., Csanalosi,I., Pereira-Ogan, J.A., Parish,L., Bell,P.J.
Lorazepam in anxiety: A controlled study.
J.Int.Med.Res. 2, 20-5 (1974)

1844. Ridley,C.M.
Bullous lesions in nitrazepam overdosage.
Brit.Med.J. 3, 28 (1971)

1845. Ried,W., Teubner,R.
H-3-1,5-Benzodiazepines from ethynyl ketones and ortho-phenylendiamines.
Il.Ann.Chem. 1978, 741-4 (1978)

1846. Rieder,J., Wendt,G.
Pharmacokinetics and metabolism of the hypnotic nitrazepam.
In: 362. pp. 99-128

1847. Riley,A.L., Lovely,R.H.
Chlordiazepoxide-induced reversal of an amphetamine-established aversion - dipsogenic effects.
Physiol.Psych. 6, 488-92 (1978)

1848. Roberts,J.C.
A double blind study comparing promethazine-pethidine with diazepam.
In: P.F.Knight, C.G.Burges (Ed.) : Diazepam in Anaesthesia. J.Wright and Sons Ltd., Bristol 1968

1849. Roberts,R.K., Wilkinson,G.R., Branch,R.A. et al.
Effect of age and cirrhosis on the disposition and elimination of chlordiazepoxide (Librium[R]).
Gastroenterology 73, 1243 (1977)

1850. Roberts,R.K., Wilkinson,G.R., Branch,R.A., Schenker,S.
Effect of age and parenchymal liver-disease on disposition and elimination of chlordiazepoxide (librium).
Gastroenterology 75, 479-85 (1978)

1851. Robinson.D.S., Amidon,E.L.
Interactions of benzodiazepines with warfarin in man.
In: 362. pp. 641-6

1852. Roche Laboratories
Irritant properties of diazepam (reply to a letter)
Brit.Dent.J. 124, 295 (1968)

1853. Roden,S., Harvey,P., Mitchard,M.
The influence of alcohol on the persistent effects on human performance of the hypnotics mandrax and nitrazepam.
Int.J.Clin.Pharmacol. (München) 15, 350-5 (1977)

1854. Roma,G., Vigevani,E., Balbi,A., Ermili,A.
Research on 1,5-benzodiazepines. 3. Synthesis of 2,4-bisdialkylamino-3H-1,5-benzodiazepine.
Farmaco Sci. 34, 62-71 (1979)

1855. Root,B., Loveland,J.P.
Pediatric premedication with diazepam or hydroxyzine: Oral versus intramuscular route.
Anesth.Analg. 52, 717-23 (1973)

1856. Ross,F.H., Sermons,A.L., Walker,C.A.
Influence of diazepam on circadian-rhythm of glycine in rodent brain.
Pharmacology 20, 241 (1978)

1857. Rossi,G.F., DiRocco,C., Maira,G., Meglio,M.
Experimental and clinical studies of the anticonvulsant properties of a benzodiazepine derivative, clonazepam (RO 5-4023).
In: 362. pp. 461-88

1858. Rowlatt,R.J.
Effect of maternal diazepam on the newborn.
Brit.Med.J. 1, 985 (1978)

1859. Rucki,R., Ross,A., Donahue,J., Moros,S.
Effect of amitriptyline on polarography of chlordiazepoxide.
J.Pharm.Sci. 67, 1297-1300 (1978)

1860. Rudolf,M., Geddes,D.M., Turner,J.A., Saunders,K.B.
Depression of central respiratory drive by nitrazepam.
Thorax 33, 97-100 (1978)

1861. Rudzik,A.D., Hester,J.B., Tang,A.H., Straw,R.N., Friis,W.
Triazolobenzodiazepines, a new class of central nervous system-depressant compounds.
In: 362. pp. 285-98

1862. Rushton,R., Steinberg,H., Tomkiewicz,M.
Effects of chlordiazepoxide alone and in combination with amphetamine on animal and human behavior.
In: 362. pp. 355-66

1863. Rutherford,D.M., Okoko,A., Tyrer,P.J.
Plasma concentrations of diazepam and desmethyldiazepam during chronic diazepam therapy.
Brit.J.Clin.Pharmacol. 6, 69-73 (1978)

1864. Saario,I., Seppala,T.
Dose-response effect of bromazepam on psychomotor-skills.
Eur.J.Clin.Pharmacol. 13, 419-22 (1978)

1865. Saba,G., Boero,G.C.
The clinical use of chlordiazepine in pre-operative anxiety states.
Minerva Anestesiologica (Torino) 31, 643 (1965)

1866. Sagen,N., Haram,K.
Diazepam (Valium) as an anaesthetic for operative vaginal delivery.
Acta Obstet.Gynecol.Scand. 52, 153-6 (1973)

1867. Saletu,B., Gruenberger,J., Linzmayer,L., Nitsche,V.
Assessment of psychoactivity and long-term efficacy of a retard preparation of oxazepam by blood level determinations and quantitative EEG and psychometric analysis.
Wien.Klin.Wschr. 90, 382-9 (1978)

1868. Salkind,M.R., Silverstone,T.
A clinical and psychometric evaluation of flurazepam.
Brit.J.Clin.Pharmacol. 2, 223-6 (1975)

1869. Sallé,J.
Expertise pharmacologique et toxicologique du chlorazepate dipotassique.
Clin-Byla N.D.A.-file

1870. Sambrooks,J.E., MacCulloch,M.J.
The thymoleptic action of two salts of flurazepam (Dalmane).
Curr.Med.Res.Opin. 3, 192-8 (1975)

1871. Sankaran,M.
Use of intravenous diazepam in accident department.
Brit.J.Clin.Pathol. 32, 167 (1978)

1872. Sansone,M.
Effects of chlordiazepoxide, amphetamine and their combinations on avoidance behaviour of reserpinized mice.
Pharmacol.Res.Commun. 9, 879-84 (1977)

1873. Sawada,H., Hara,A.
Studies on metabolism of bromazepam. VI. Reduction of 2-(2-Amino-5-bromobenzoyl)pyridine, a metabolite of bromazepam, in rabbit, rat and guinea pig.
Drug Metab.Dispos. 6, 205-12 (1978)

1874. Schallek,W., Kuehn,A.
Effects of trimetadione, diphenylhydantoin, and chlordiazepoxide on after-discharges in brain of cat.
Proc.Soc.Exp.Biol.N.Y. 112, 813-7 (1963)

1875. Schallek,W., Schlosser,W., Randall,L.O.
Recent developments in the pharmacology of the benzodiazepines.
Advanced Pharmacol.Chemotherap. 10, 119-83 (1972)

1876. Scher,J., Hailey,D.M., Beard,R.M.
The effects of diazepam on the fetus.
J.Obstet.Gynecol.Brit.Commonw. 79, 635-8 (1972)

1877. Schlack,H.G.
Erfahrungen mit Clonazepam (Ro 5-4023) in der Therapie kindlicher Epilepsien.
Fortschr.Med. 92, 1176 (1974)

1878. Schmidt,I., Eler,I., Fisenko,V.P.
Effect of clonazepam on neuronal-activity of sensomotor brain cortex in rats.
Farmakol.T. 41, 673-6 (1978)

1879. Schmitt,J., Comoy,P., Suguet,M., Callef,G., Le Muer,J., Clim,T., Brunaud,M., Salle,J., Srov,G.
Sur des nouvelles benzodiazepines hydrosolubles douées d'une puissante activité sur le système nerveux central.
Chim.Thér. 4, 239 (1969)

1880. Schmitz,J.E., Lotz,P., Bock,K.H., Fisseler,A., Ahnefeld,F.W.
Auswirkungen des Flunitrazepam auf die Atmung. Effects of flunitrazepam on respiration.
Klin.Anaesthesiol.Intensivther. 17, 67-81 (1978)

1881. Schneider,J., Kamm,G.
Klinische Pharmakologie. Gibt es eine relevante Arzneimittelinteraktion zwischen Oxazepam und Phenprocoumon.
Clinical Pharmacology. Is there such a thing as a relevant drug interaction between oxazepam and phenprocoumon.
Verh.Dtsch.Ges.Inn.Med. 83, 1577- (1977)

1882. Schoenemeyer,J.
Die Stellung von Kaliumdichlorazepat in der modernen Tranquilizer-Therapie unter besonderer Berücksichtigung der abendlichen Einmaldosis (Tranxilium[R] 20).
In: Langzeittherapie neuropsychiatrischer Erkrankungen, Verlag Dr. med. D. Straube, Erlangen 1978

1883. Schoenhals-Abrahamsohn,M., Schoenhals,M., Wesslau,W.
Methoden und Probleme einer psychopharmakologischen Wirkungsuntersuchung dargestellt anhand eines neuartigen Pyridilbenzodiazepines im Vergleich zu Diazepam.
Methods and problems of investigation of psychopharmacological effect illustrated by the comparison of a novel pyridylbenzodiazepine with diazepam.
Münch.Med.Wschr. 120, 1029-32 (1978)

1884. Schulz,P., Dayer,P.
Students-attitudes concerning therapeutic image of 4 benzodiazepines and 2 antibiotics.
J.Clin.Pharm. 3, 225-7 (1978)

1885. Schwandt,H.J., Sadée,W., Beyer,K.-H.
Metabolic rearrangements of 1,4-benzodiazepine derivatives.
Xenobiotica 4 , 733-41 (1974)

1886. Schwartz,M.A.
Pathways of metabolism of the benzodiazepines.
In: 362. pp. 53-74

1887. Scrollini,F., Pizzi,A., Amigoni,S.
The psychopharmacological properties of pinazepam, a new benzodiazepine derivative.
Arzneim.-Forsch. (Drug Res.) 28, 423-6 (1978)

1888. Sedgwick,P.R.
Benzodiazepines, Type A Procedure.
In: Methodology of Analytical Toxicology, I.Sunshine,ed., CRC Press, Cleveland, 1975, pp. 45-7

1889. Sehgal,H., Wadhwa,S., Lal,C.
Evaluation of diazepam as an anticonvulsant in treatment of tetanus neonatorum.
J.Pediatr. 15, 161-5 (1978)

1890. Sellers,E.M.
Clinical pharmacology and therapeutics of benzodiazepines.
Can.Med.A.J. 118, 1533-8 (1978)

1891. Sellers,E.M., Greenblatt,D.J., Zilm,D.H.
Decline in chlordiazepoxide plasma-levels during fixed-dose therapy of alcohol withdrawal.
Bit.J.Clin.Pharmacol. 6, 370-2 (1978)

1892. Sellman,R., Kanto,J., Raijola,E., Pekkarinen,A.
Induction effect of diazepam in its own metabolism.
Acta Pharmacol.Toxicol. 37, 345-51 (1975)

1893. Sellman,R., Pekkarinen,A., Raijola,E.
Reduces plasma diazepam concentrations in chronic alcoholic patients following an oral absorption test of diazepam.
Acta physiol.Scand. 396, 224 (1973)

1894. Seppälä,T., Korttila,K., Häkkinen,S., Linnoila,M.
Residual effects and skills related to driving after a single oral administration of diazepam, medazepam or lorazepam.
Brit.J.Clin.Pharmacol. 3,831-41(1976)

1895. Sereny,G., Kalant,H.
Comparative clinical evaluation of chlordiazepoxide and promazine in treatment of alcohol-withdrawal syndrome.
Brit.Med.J. 1, 92 (1965)

1896. Serfontein,W.J., Botha,D., DeVilliers,L.S.
A rapid and comprehensive system for the routine identification of drugs in biological material based on microphase extraction and drug colour profiles.
J.Chromatogr. 115, 507-18 (1975)

1897. Shader,R.I., Ciraulo,D.A., Greenblatt,D.J.
Drug interactions involving psychotropic-drugs.
Psychosomat. 19, 671 (1978)

1898. Shader,R.I., DiMascio,A., Harmatz,J.S.
Single versus repeated dosage of the minor tranquilizer chlordiazepoxide (Librium).
Amer.J.Psychiatry 128, 1576-7 (1972)

1899. Shader,R.I., Georgota,A., Greenblatt,D.J., Harmatz,J.S., Allen,M.D.
Impaired absorption of desmethyldiazepam from chlorazepate by magnesium aluminium hydroxyde.
Clin.Pharm. 24, 308-15 (1978)

1900. Shannon,R.W., Fraser,G.P., Aitken,R.G., Harper,J.R.
Diazepam in preeclamptic toxaemia with special reference to its effect on the newborn infant.
Brit.J.Clin.Pract. 26, 271-5 (1972)

1901. Shira,R.B.
A technique for investigating the intensity and duration of human psychomotor impairment after intravenous diazepam.
Oral Surg. 45, 493-502 (1978)

1902. Shusterman,N.H.
Treatment of anxiety - phenobarbital versus benzodiazepines.
Del.Med.J. 50, 605-7 (1978)

1903. Siassi,I., Thomas,M., Vanov,S.K.
Evaluation of the safety and therapeutic effects of lorazepam on long-term use.
Curr.Ther.Res. 18, 163-71 (1975)

1904. Sice,J. Rees,R.M., Tyler,T.L., Arnold,J.D.
Psychomotor function, memory, and subjective feelings, after sleep induced by a benzodiazepine.
Pharmacology 20, 171 (1978)

1905. Sigg,H.P., Toth,A.
Über die Struktur der Phenazin-N-Oxide.
Helv.Chim.Acta 50, 716-9 (1967)

1906. Singh,H., Gupta,V.K.
Chlordiazepoxide poisoning: A case report.
Curr.Med.Pract. 7, 519-20 (1963)

1907. Singh,A.N., Saxena,B.
A comparison of lorazepam, diazepam and placebo in the treatment of anxiety-states.
Curr.Ther.Res. 16, 149-62 (1974)

1908. Sita,F., Krizala,J.F., Dite,P., Krupar,V.
Nachweis einiger Heilmittel in der Kniegelenk-synovialflüssigkeit.
Arch.Toxikol. 27, 242-7 (1971)

1909. Skellern,G.G., Meier,J., Knight,B.I., Whiting,B.
Application of HPLC to determination of some 1,4-benzodiazepines and their metabolites in plasma.
Brit.J.Clin.Pharm. 5, 483-7 (1978)

1910. Skolimowski,J., Maciejewska,M., Prochacka,K.
Assessment of volumetric and gasometric values during induction of general anesthesia with intravenous rohypnol.
Wid.Lek. 31, 167-70 (1978)

1911. Skolnick,P., Goodwin,F.K., Paul,S.M.
Rapid and sensitive radioreceptor assay for benzodiazepine in plasma.
Arch.General Psychiatry 36, 78-80 (1979)

1912. Skolnick,P., Marangos,P.J., Goodwin,F.K., Edwards,M., Paul,S.
Identification of inosine and hypoxanthine as endogenous inhibitors of ^{3}H-diazepam-binding in central nervous-system.
Life Sci. 23, 1473-80 (1978)

1913. Skolnick,P., Syapin,P.J., Paugh,B.A., Paul,S.M.
Reduction in benzodiazepine receptors associated with purkinje-cell degeneration in nervous mutant mice.
Nature 277, 397-9 (1979)

1914. Skupin,G., Franzke,H.G.
Tranxilium 20 (Dikalium-chlorazepat) als 24-Stunden-Tranquilizer.
Med.Welt 26, 956-9 (1975)

1915. Smith,M.E.
Suicidal attempt by oral ingestion of chlordiazepoxide (Librium).
Clin.Med. 8, 72-4 (1961)

1916. Smith,R.C., Dekirmenjian,H., Davis,J., Casper,R., Gosenfeld,L., Tsai,C.
Blood level, mood and MHPG response to diazepam in man.
In: Gottschalk,L.A., Merlis,D. editors; Pharmacokinetics of psychoactive drugs: Blood levels and clinical response. Flushing, N.Y., 1976, Spectrum Publications, pp. 141-56

1917. Smyth,D., Pennington,G.W.
The detection and excretion of chlordiazepoxide (Librium) in human plasma and urine.
Arch.Int.Pharmacodyn. 145, 154-65 (1963)

1918. Smyth,W.F., Smyth,M.R., Groves,J.A., Tan,S.B.
Polarographic method for the identification of 1,4-benzodiazepines.
Analyst 103, 497-508 (1978)

1919. Solomon,K.
High-dose benzodiazepines in treatment of severe neurotic anxiety.
J.Clin.Psy. 39, 610-3 (1978)

1920. Solomon,K.
High-dose benzodiazepines in the treatment of severe neurotic anxiety - reply.
J.Clin.Psych. 40, 54 (1979)

1921. Solomon,K., Hart,R.
Pitfalls and prospects in clinical research on antianxiety drugs - benzodiazepines and placebo-research reviews.
J.Clin.Psych. 39, 823-31 (1978)

1922. Soubrie,P., Jobert,A., Thiebot,M.H.
Picrotoxin-diazepam interaction in a behavioral schedule of differential reinforcement of low rates.
Experientia 34, 1621-2 (1978)

1923. Spark,H., Goldman,A.S.
Diazepam intoxication in a child.
Amer.J.Dis.Child. 109, 128-9 (1965)

1924. Speight,A.N.P.
Diazepam in pre-eclamptic toxemia.
Brit.Med.J. 1, 1420-1 (1978)

1925. Speth,R.C., Wastek,G.J., Johnson,P.C., Yamamura,H.I.
Benzodiazepine binding in human brain: Characterization using ^{3}H-Flunitrazepam.
Life Sci. 22, 859-66 (1978)

1926. Staak,M., Moosmayer,A.
Pharmakokinetische Untersuchungen über Wechselwirkungen zwischen Dikalium-chlorazepat und Alkohol nach oraler Applikation.
Arzneim.-Forsch. (Drug Res.) 28, 1187-91 (1978)

1927. Steen,S.N., Hahl,D.
Controlled evaluation of parenteral diazepam as preanesthic medication.
Anesth.Analg.Curr.Res. 48, 549 (1969)

1928. Stein,L., Berger,B.D.
Psychopharmacology of 7-chloro-5-(o-chlorphenyl)-1,3-dihydro-3-hydroxy-2H-1,4-benzodiazepin-2-one (lorazepam) in sqirrel monkey and rat.
Arzneim.-Forsch. (Drug Res.) 21, 1073 (1971)

1929. Stein,L., Wise,C.D., Berger,B.D.
Antianxiety action of benzodiazepines: Decrease in activity of serotonin neurons in the punishment system.
In: 362. pp. 299-326

1930. Sternbach,L.H.
Chemistry of 1,4-benzodiazepines and some aspects of the structure-activity-relationship.
In: 362. pp. 1-26

1931. Sternbach,L.H.
Benzodiazepine story.
J.Med.Chem. 22, 1-7 (1979)

1932. Sternbach,L., Fryer,R.I., Metlesics,W., Sach,G., Stempel,A.
Quinazolines and 1,4-Benzodiazepines. V. O-aminobenzophenones.
J.Org.Chem. 27, 3781 (1962)

1933. Stevens,H.M.
Use of a color reagent for the detection and estimation of benzodiazepines and their benzophenone derivatives.
J.Forens.Sci. 18, 69-73 (1978)

1934. Stewart,C.P., Stolman,A.
Toxicology: Mechanisms and Analytical Methods. Vol. I
Academic Press, New York 1960

1935. Stewart,C.P., Stolman,A.
Toxicology: Mechanisms and Analytical Methods. Vol. II
Academic Press, New York 1961

1936. Stewart,F.H.C., Rivett,D.E.
Formation of a tricyclic 1,4-benzodiazepine derivative from benzoyl-DL-kynurenylglycine.
Chem.Ind.L. 1978, 347-8 (1978)

1937. Stoebner,R.C., Kiser,R.W., Decherd,J.F. et al.
Diazepam (Valium) in the treatment of tetanus: A report of five cases.
South Med.J. 63, 445-7 (1970)

1938. Stone,W.E., Javid,M.J.
Benzodiazepines and phenobarbital as antagonists of dissimilar chemical convulsants.
Epilepsia 19, 361-8 (1978)

1939. Stovehill,E., Lee,H., Ban,T.A.
A comparative study with benzodiazepines in chronic psychotic patients.
Dis.Nerv.Syst. 27, 411 (1966)

1940. Stovner,J., Endresen,R., Osterud,A.
Intravenous anaesthesia with a new benzodiazepine Ro 5-4200.
Acta Anaesthesiol.Scand. 17, 163-9 (1973)

1941. Straughan ,J.L., Cathcart-Rake,W.F., Shoeman,D.W., Azarnoff,D.L.
Quantitation of chlordiazepoxide and its metabolites in biological-fluids by thin-layer chromatography.
J.Chromatogr. 146, 473-80 (1978)

1942. Street,H.V.
Gas-Liquid Chromatography of submicrogram amounts of drugs. III. Analysis of alkaloids in biological media.
J.Chromatogr. 29, 68-79 (1967)

1943. Subbaraman,L.R., Subbaraman,J., Behrman,E.J.
The reaction of nucleic acid components with m-chloroperoxybenzoic acid.
Biochemistry 8, 3059-66 (1969)

1944. Sugimoto,J., Nagata,M., Ikeda,Y.
Effects of diazepam on rat isolated heart-muscle.
Clin.Exp.Pharm. 5, 655-63 (1978)

1945. Sun,S.R.
Rapid gas-liquid-chromatographic determination of chlordiazepoxide in serum.
J.Chromatogr. 166, 604-8 (1978)

1946. Sun,S.R.
Quantitative determination of chlordiazepoxide and its metabolites in serum by fluorescence TLC-densitometry.
J.Pharm.Sci. 67, 639-41 (1978)

1947. Sun,S.R.
Fluorescence-TLC densitometric determination of diazepam and other 1,4-benzodiazepines in serum.
J.Pharm.Sci. 67, 1413-5 (1978)

1948. Sun,S.R., Hoffman,D.J.
Rapid GLC-Determination of chlordiazepoxide and metabolite in serum using on-column methylation.
J.Pharm.Sci. 67, 1647-8 (1978)

1949. Sunshine,A.
Comparison of the hypnotic activity of triazolam, flurazepam hydrochloride, and placebo.
Clin.Pharmacol.Ther. 17, 573 (1975)

1950. Sunshine,I.
Methodology of Analytical Toxicology.
CRC-Press, Cleveland, 1975

1951. Suonio,S., Kauppila,A., Jouppila,P., Linna,O.
The effect of intravenous diazepam on fetal and maternal acid-base balance during and after delivery.
Ann.Chir.Gynaecol.Fenn. 60, 52 (1972)

1952. Tachikaw ,R., Miyadera,T., Tamura,C., Terada,A., Naruto,S., Nagamats ,E.
Studies of oxazolobenzodiazepines. - 7. Synthesis of 3-methyl-oxazolo (3,2-D)-1,4-benzodiazepines and configurational studies of their ketimine intermediates.
J.Chem.Soc. 1978, 1524-9 (1978)

1953. Takano,K., Student,J.C.
Effect of diazepam on the gamma motor system indicated by the response of the muscle spindle of the triceps surae muscle of the decerebrate cat to the muscle stretch.
Naunyn-Schmied.-Arch.Pharmacol. 302, 91-101 (1978)

1954. Tallman,J.F., Thomas,J.W., Gallager,D.W.
Gabaergic modulation of benzodiazepine-binding site sensivity.
Nature 274, 383-5 (1978)

1955. Tanaka,M., Isozaki,H., Inanaga,K., Ogawa,N.
Effects of a new benzodiazepine-derivative - ID 540- on averaged photopalpebral reflex in man.
Psychopharmacology 58, 217-22 (1978)

1956. Tansella,M., Siciliani,O., Burti,I., Schiavon,M., Zimmermann-Tansella,C., Gerna,M., Tognoni,G., Morselli,P.L.
N-desmethyldiazepam and amylobarbitone-sodium as hypnotics in anxious patients, plasma levels, clinical efficacy and residual effects.
Psychopharmacologia 41, 81-5 (1975)

1957. Tansella,M., Zimmermann-Tansella,C., Ferrario,L., Preziati,L., Tognoni,G., Lader,M.
Plasma concentrations of diazepam, nordiazepam, and amylobarbitone after short-term treatment of anxious patients.
Pharmakopsychiatr.Neuropsychopharmakol. 11, 68-75 (1978)

1958. Tarnow,J., Hess,W., Schmidt,D., Eberlein,H.J.
Wirkung von Flunitrazepam und Diazepam auf den Kreislauf koronarchirurgischer Patienten bei der Narkoseeinleitung und während der extrakorporalen Zirkulation.
The effect of flunitrazepam and diazepam on circulation in coronary surgical patients after anesthesia induction and during extracorporeal circulation.
Klin.Anaesthesiol.Intensivther. 17, 119-29 (1978)

1959. Tartara,A., Moglia,A., Bono,G., Bruni,G.C., Loreti,P., Tallone,G., Ghirardi,P.
Hypnotic activity of flurazepam in solution and in capsules.
Curr.Ther.Res. 24, 853-7 (1978)

1960. Tateishi,M., Suzuki,S., Shimizu,H.
The metabolism of bromazepam in the rat - identification of mercapturic acid and its conversion in vitro to methyl-thio-bromazepam.
Biochem.Pharmacol. 27, 809-10 (1978)

1961. Tavares,F., Massoud,N.
Effectiveness of flurazepam and chloral hydrate as hypnotics in the acutely disturbed psychiatric patient.
Can.J.Pharm.Sci. 13, 104 (1978)

1962. Taws,E.R., Brunning,J., Arenillas,L.
A clinical evaluation of flurazepam (Dalmane) as a hypnotic in psychiatric patients.
J.Int.Med.Res. 3, 417-22 (1975)

1963. Taylor,K.M., Laverty,R.
The interaction of chlordiazepoxide, diazepam, and nitrazepam with catecholamines and histamine in regions of the rat brain.
In: 362. pp. 191-202

1964. Taylor,M.A., Spero,M., Simeon,J., Fink,M.
High dose chlordiazepoxide therapy of anxiety.
Curr.Ther.Res. 11, 9-14 (1969)

1965. Tehrani,J.B., Cavanaugh,A.
Diazepam infusion in the treatment of tetanus.
Drug Intell.Clin.Pharm. 11, 491 (1977)

1966. Terhaag,B., Ackerman,E.
About influence of benzodiazepines on fluorescence of tryptophan on human-serum albumin, hemoglobin and ghosts.
Act.Bio.Med. 37, 387-91 (1978)

1967. Tewari,S.N., Shukla,S.K.
Studies on identification of 1,4-benzodiazepine drugs by micro-crystal tests.
Pharmazie 33, 372-3 (1978)

1968. Thearle,M.J., Dunn,P.M., Hailey,D.M.
Exchange transfusion for diazepam intoxication at birth followed by jejunal stenosis.
Proc.R.Soc.Med. 66, 349-50 (1973)

1969. Thomas,J., Aubry,P., Rosso,A.M., Herault,L., Marie-Nelly,A., Lhoste,F.
Tétanos néonatal. Traitment par l'administration orale du diazépam et l'alimentation précoce par sonde nasogastrique.
Bull.Soc.Pathol.exot. 3, 373 (1972)

1970. Thomson,J., Glen,A.I.M.
A large overdose of chlordiazepoxide.
Lancet 2, 722-3 (1961)

1971. Thong,Y.H., Abramson,D.C.
Continuous infusion of diazepam in infants with severe recurrent convulsions.
Med.Ann.D.C. 43, 63-5 (1974)

1972. Timonen,S., Hagner,M.
Benzodiazepines in unselected obstetrical series.
Ann.Chir.Gynaecol.Fenn. 55, 65 (1966)

1973. Tognoni,G., Gomeni,R., DeMaio,D., Alberti,G.G., Franciosi,P., Scieghi,G.
Pharmacokinetics of N-desmethyldiazepam in patients suffering from insomnia and treated with nortriptyline.
Brit.J.Clin.Pharmacol. 2, 227-32 (1975)

1974. Tomson,G., Lunell,N.O., Sundwall,A., Rane,A.
Pharmacokinetics of oxazepam given during labor.
Acta Psych.Scand. 1978, 75-81 (1978)

1975. Tomson,G., Lunell,N.O., Sundwall,A., Rane,A.
Placental passage of oxazepam and its metabolism in mother and newborn.
Clin.Pharm. 25, 74-81 (1979)

1976. Toulouse,R., Maffei,J.L.
Utilisation du Valium en obstétrique.
Rev.Franc.Gynecol.Obstet. 60, 263-70 (1965)

1977. Trka,A., Frigerio,A., Nardi,D., Tajana,A., Rapp,U.
Mass-spectrometric studies on 1,5-benzodiazepine derivatives. 2.
Farmaco Sci. 33, 885-900 (1978)

1978. Tsuchiya,T., Fukushima,H.
Effects of benzodiazepines and pentobarbitone on the GABA-ergic recurrent inhibition of hippocampal neurons.
Eur.J.Pharmacol. 48, 421-4 (1978)

1979. Tsuchiya,T., Kurita,J.
Studies on Diazepines. - 4. 3H-1,2-benzodiazepines.
Chem.Pharm. 26, 1890-5 (1978)

1980. Tsuchiya,T., Kurita,J.
Studies on Diazepines. 5. Synthesis of 3-substituted 1H-1,2-benzodiazepines.
Chem.Pharm. 26, 1896-1900 (1978)

1981. Tsuchiya,T., Kurita,J., Takayama,K.
Photosensitized oxygenation of 1H-1,2-benzodiazepines.
Heterocycles 9, 1549-54 (1978)

1982. Ueki,S., Watanabe,S., Fujiwara,M., Yamamoto,T., Araki,H., Ohmori,K.
Behavioral and EEG effects of triazolam in comparison with those of diazepam.
Fol.Pharm.J. 74, 597-614 (1978)

1983. Uges,D.R.A., Bouma,P.
A simple determination of clonazepam in serum by high pressure liquid chromatography.
Pharm.Weekbl. 111, 877 (1976)

1984. Ungerer,M.J., Erasmus,F.R.
Evaluation of a new benzodiazepine, flunitrazepam (Ro 5-4200) as an anaesthetic induction agent.
S.Afr.med.J. 47, 787-90 (1973)

1985. Valentour,J.
Chlordiazepoxide, Type C Procedure.
In: Methodology for Analytical Toxicology, I.Sunshine,ed., CRC Press, Cleveland, 1975, pp. 79-80

1986. Vallner,J.J., Needham,T.E., Jun,H.W., Brown,W.J., Stewart,J.T., Kotzan,J.A., Honigberg,I.L.
Plasma levels of clobazam after three oral dosage forms in healthy subjects.
J.Clin.Pharm. 18, 319-24 (1978)

1987. Valzelli,L.
Activity of benzodiazepines on aggressive behavior in rats and mice.
In: 362. pp. 405-18

1988. Van der Kleijn,E.
Discussion Summary.
In: 362. pp. 667-8

1989. Van der Kleijn,E.
Pharmacokinetics of ataractic drug.
Thesis, University of Nijmegen, The Netherlands, 1969

1990. Van der Kleijn,E.
Pharmacokinetics of diazepam in dogs, mice and humans.
Acta Pharmacol.Toxicol. 29, 109 (1971)

1991. Van der Kleijn,E., Guelen,P.J.M., van Wijk,C.G.W.M., Baars,I., Tree,T.B.
Clinical pharmacokinetics of benzodiazepines, barbiturates, and short chain fatty acids.
In: Clinical pharmacokinetics, Ed.: G.Levy, APhA, Washington,DC, 1974, pp. 79

1992. van Rossum,J.M.
Pharmacokinetics of accumulation.
J.Pharm.Sci. 57, 2162 (1968)

1993. Varano,C.
Intravenous diazepam administration.
Am.J.Hosp.P. 35, 779 (1978)

1994. Vasella,F. et al.
Treatment of infantile spasms and Lennox-Gastaut-syndrome with clonazepam (Rivotril[R]).
Epilepsia 14, 165 (1973)

1995. Vega,D.E.
Induction of anaesthetic sleep by means of a new benzodiazepine derivative.
Rev.Urug.Anesth. 5, 41-4 (1971)

1996. Verbeeck,R., Tjandramaga,T.B., Verberckmoes,R., DeSchepper,P.J.
Biotransformation and excretion of lorazepam in patients with chronic renal failure.
Brit.J.Clin.Pharmacol. 3, 1033 (1975)

1997. Verma,R.S., Chatterj ,S., Mathur,N.
Diazepam and succinylcholine-induced muscle pains.
Anesth.Anal. 57, 295-7 (1978)

1998. Vessman,J., Alexanderson,B., Sjöqvist,F., Strindberg,B., Sundwall,A.
Comparative pharmacokinetics of oxazepam and nortriptyline after single oral dose in man.
In: 362. pp. 165-74

1999. Viala,A., Cano,J.P., Angeletti-Philippe,A.
Recherche toxicologique des benzodiazepines dans le sang et l'urine.
Eur.J.Toxicol. 3, 197 (1971)

2000. Villarre,J.A., Grubbs,E.J.
Investigation of intermolecularity versus intramolecularity of thermal rearrangement of N-benzhydryl-alpha,alpha-diphenylnitrone to benzophenone o-benzhydryloxime.
J.Org.Chem. 43, 1896-9 (1978)

2001. Voegtlin,W.L.
Management of functional gastrointestinal disorder with diazepam.
Appl.Ther. 6, 801-5 (1964)

2002. Voigt,S., Elkousy,S., Schwelle,N., Nover,L., Luckner,M.
Activities invitro and invivo of enzymes of benzodiazepine alkaloid biosynthesis during development of penicillium-cyclopium.
Phytochem. 17, 1705-9 (1978)

2003. Volke,J., Ellaithy,M.M., Manousek,O.
Spectrophotometric and polarographic investigation of 3 new cyclohexene-substituted benzodiazepines.
Talanta 25, 209-13 (1978)

2004. Vontin,H., Heller,W.
Stoffwechselveränderungen unter Flunitrazepam.
Metabolic Changes from flunitrazepam.
Klin.Anaesthesiol.Intensivther. 17, 108-18 (1978)

2005. Vycudilik,W.
Die Derivatisierung in der gaschromatographischen Analyse.
Z.Rechtsmedizin 80, 197-203 (1977)

2006. Wade,P.C., Kissick,T.P., Vogt,B.R., Toeplitz,B.
Synthesis of the triazolo (5,1-A)-2,4-benzodiazepine-ring-system.
J.Org.Chem. 44, 84-8 (1978)

2007. Waddington,J.L.
Behavioral evidence for gabaergic activity of benzodiazepine flurazepam.
Eur.J.Pharmacol. 51, 417-22 (1978)

2008. Waddington,J.L., Owen,F.
Stereospecific benzodiazepine receptor binding by the enantiomers of oxazepam sodium hemisuccinate.
Neuropharmacology 17, 215-6 (1978)

2009. Wagner,J.G.
Fundamentals of clinical pharmacokinetics.
Hamilton, Ill., Drug Intelligence Publ., 1975

2010. Wagner,J.G., Northam,J.I., Always,C.D., Carpenter,O.S.
Blood levels of drugs at equilibrium state after multiple dosing.
Nature 207, 1301-2 (1965)

2011. Walberg,C.B.
The determination of diazepam, type C procedure.
In: Manual of Analytical Toxicology, I.Sunshine, Ed. CRC Press, Cleveland, Ohio, 1971, pp. 123-6

2012. Walser,A., Flynn,T., Fryer,R.I.
Quinazolines and 1,4-benzodiazepines. 85. Syntheses of 3-substituted imidazo-1,5-alpha-1,4-benzodiazepines.
J.Heterocycl.Chem. 15, 577-83 (1978)

2013. Walser,A., Lauer,R.F., Fryer,R.I.
Quinazolines and 1,4-benzodiazepines. 87. Synthesis of 1-phenylimidazo and 3-phenyl-imidazo (1,5-alpha)-1,4-benzodiazepines.
J.Heterocycl.Chem. 15, 855-8 (1978)

2014. Wang,R.I.H., Stockdale,S.L.
The hypnotic efficacy of triazolam.
J.Int.Med.Res. 1, 600-7 (1973)

2015. Wang,R.I.H., Stockdale,S.L., Hieb,E.
Hypnotic efficacy of lorazepam and flurazepam.
Clin.Pharmacol.Ther. 19, 191-5 (1976)

2016. Weir,J.H.
Prazepam in treatment of anxiety. Placebo-controlled multicenter evaluation.
J.Clin.Psychiatry 39, 841-7 (1978)

2017. Wesseling,H.
Comparative study of the efficacy of diazepam, pentobarbital, and fentanyl-droperidol (THALAMONAL) against toxicity induced by local anesthesics in mice.
In: 362. pp. 655-66

2018. Weyer,U.
Gaschromatographische Simultanbestimmung von Diazepam, Ketamin und deren Metaboliten.
- Pharmakokinetische Verlaufskontrolle -
Inaug.Dissertation Gießen 1979

2019. Whiting,B., Lawrence,J.R., Skellern,G.G., Meier,J.
Effect of acute alcohol intoxication on the metabolism and plasma kinetics of chlordiazepoxide.
Brit.J.Clin.Pharm. 7, 95-100 (1979)

2020. Wilensky,A.J., Levy,R.H., Troupin,A.S., Moretti-Ojemann,L.
Chlorazepate kinetics in treated epileptics.
Clin.Pharmacol.Ther. 24, 22-30 (1978)

2021. Wilkinson,G.R.

Effects of liver-disease and aging on the disposition of diazepam, chlordiazepoxide, oxazepam and lorazepam in man.

Acta Psych.Scand. 1978, 56-74 (1978)

2022. Williamson,M.J., Paul,S.M., Skolnick,P.

Labeling of benzodiazepine receptors invivo.

Nature 275, 551-3 (1978)

2023. Williamson,M.J., Paul,S.M., Skolnick,P.

Demonstration of ^{3}H-diazepam binding to benzodiazepine receptors in vivo.

Life Sci. 23, 1935-40 (1978)

2024. Wilson,J.

Lorazepam as a premedicant for general anaesthesia.

Curr.Med.Res.Opinion 1, 308 (1973)

2025. Wilson,J., Ellis,F.R.

Oral premedication with lorazepam (Ativan): A comparison with heptabarbitone (Medomin) and diazepam (Valium).

Brit.J.Anaesth. 45, 738-44 (1973)

2026. Windorfer,A., Pringsheim,W.

Investigations on the influence of a tocolytic treatment of pregnant-women with diazepam and fenoterol on the bilirubin levels and apgar score of newborn.

Klin.Pädiatr. 191, 51-60 (1979)

2027. Winfield,D.L., Aivazian,G.H.

Librium therapy and electroencephalographic correlates.

J.Nerv.Ment.Dis. 133, 240 (1961)

2028. Winstead,D.K., Lawson,T., Abbott,D.

Diazepam use in military sick call.

Military Med. 141, 180-1 (1976)

2029. Witkop,H.-J.

Zur Frage der Placentarpassage von Ketamin und Diazepam: Quantitative Untersuchungen mit Hilfe der Gaschromatographie.

Dissertation Gießen 1973

2030. Wolf,P., Haas,H.L.

Effects of diazepines and barbiturates of hippocampal recurrent inhibition.

Arch.Pharm. 299, 211-8 (1977)

2031. Woods,D.L., Malan,A.F.

Side-effects of maternal diazepam on newborn-infant.

S.Afr.Med.J. 54, 636 (1978)

2032. Worthington,D., Piercy,W.N., Smith,B.T.

Modification of ovine fetal respiratory-like activity by chronic diazepam administration.

Amer.J.Obstet.Gynecol. 131, 749-54 (1978)

2033. Wright,W.B., Brabande,H.J., Greenblatt,E.N., Day,I.P., Hardy,R.A.

Derivatives of 1,2,3,11A-tetrahydro-5H-pyrrolo-2-1-c-1,4-benzodiazepines-5,11(10H)-dione as anxiolytic agents.

J.Med.Chem. 21, 1087-9 (1978)

2034. Wulff,O.

Sönderfallstid och upplösningshastighed av tabletter innehallande diazepam.

Farm.Rev. 68, 97-104 (1973)

2035. Zackova,P., Vlkova,A., Kvetina,J., Zamazalova,I.

Comparison of the effect of some benzodiazepines with the "staircase method".

Act.Nerv.super. (Praha) 20, 75-6 (1978)

2036. Zackova,P., Zamazalova,I., Laznicek,M.

Influence of ethylalcohol on the effect of benzodiazepines in rats and mice.

Activ.Nerv. 20, 242-4 (1978)

2037. Zagar,J.B., Van Lenten,F.J., Chrekian,G.P.

High pressure liquid chromatographic separation and quantitation of chlordiazepoxide x HCl and two of its related compounds.

J.Assoc.Off.Anal.Chem. 61, 678-82 (1978)

2038. Zileli,M.S., Telatar,F., Deniz,S., Ilter,B., Adalar,N.

Pseudohyperosmolar non-ketoacitotic coma due to oxazepam intoxication.

Clin.Tox. 5, 337-41 (1972)

Alphabetical List 3

2039. Abel,R.M., Reis,R.L.
Intravenous diazepam for sedation following cardiac operations. Clinical and hemodynamic assessments.
Anesth.Analg.Curr.Res. 50, 244-8 (1971)

2040. Abel,R.M., Reis,R.L., Staroscik,R.N.
Coronary vasodilation following diazepam (valium).
Brit.J.Pharmacol. 38, 620-31 (1970)

2041. Abel,R.M., Reis,R.L., Staroscik,R.N.
The pharmacological basis of coronary and systemic vasodilator actions of diazepam (valium).
Brit.J.Pharmacol. 39, 261-74 (1970)

2042. Abel,R.M., Staroscik,R.N., Reis,R.L.
The effects of diazepam on left ventricular contractility an coronary blood flow.
Circulation 40, 33 (1969)

2043. Abel,R.M., Staroscik,R.N., Reis,R.L.
The effects of diazepam (valium) on left ventricular function and systemic vascular resistance.
J.Pharmacol.exp.Ther. 173, 364-70 (1970)

2044. Ackermann,E., Richter,K.
Diazepam metabolism in human foetal and adult liver.
Eur.J.Clin.Pharmacol. 11, 43-9 (1977)

2045. Albanus,L., Jönsson,M., Sparf,B.
Multiple oral dose of diazepam, oxazepam and phenobarbital to dogs - behavioural effects and correlation with antipyrine half-life.
Acta Pharmacol.Toxicol. 40, Suppl. 1, 63-9 (1977)

2046. Allen,R.E., Pitts,F.N.
Drug modification of ECT - methohexital and diazepam.
Biol.Psychiatr. 14, 69-76 (1979)

2047. Amrein,R., Cano,J.P., Hügin,W.
Pharmakokinetische und pharmakodynamische Befunde nach einmaliger intravenöser, intramuskulärer und oraler Applikation von "Rohypnol".
In: W.Hügin, G.Hossli, M.Gemperle (eds), Bisherige Erfahrungen mit "Rohypnol" (Flunitrazepam) in der Anästhesiologie und Intensivtherapie. F.Hoffmann-La Roche & Co. AG, Basel, 1976, pp. 39-56

2048. Anderson ,W., McLaughlin,C.L., Baile,C.A.
Hypothalamic injections of barbiturates, benzodiazepines and cannabinols and food-intake in rats.
Fed.Proc. 38, 257 (1979)

2049. Andreas,K.
Effects of benzodiazepines on evoked potentials in the gyrus dentatus hippocampi of rats by stimulation on the enthorhinal cortex.
Acta biol.med.Ger. 37, 371-3 (1978)

2050. Asano,T., Spector,S.
Identification of inosine and hypoxanthine as andogenous ligands for the brain benzodiazepine-binding sites.
Proc.Nat.Acad.Sci.USA 76, 977-81 (1979)

2051. Austen,D.P., Gilmartin,B.A.
The effect of chlordiazepoxide on visual field, extracular muscle balance, colour matching ability and hand-eye co-ordination in man.
Brit.J.Physiol.Optics 26, 161-5 (1971)

2052. Ayd,jr.,J.J.
A critical appraisal of chlordiazepoxide.
J.Neuropsychiat. 3, 177 (1962)

2053. Bacellar,B.B.
The treatment of acute anxiety states in neurotic patients with intravenous lorazepam. A placebo controlled trial.
Curr.Med.Res.Opin. 3, 16 (1975)

2054. Bacellar,B.B.
Intravenous lorazepam in the treatment of acute anxiety states in neurotic patients. Comparison of two dosages in a placebo-controlled trial.
Pharmacotherapeutica 1, 8 (1976)

2055. Ban,T.A., Lehmann,H.E., Matthews,V., Conald,M.
Comparative study of chlorpromazine and chlordiazepoxide withdrawal symptoms.
Clin.Med. 72, 59 (1965)

2056. Baraldi,M., Costa,E., Schwartz,J.P., Guidotti,A.
Interaction between benzodiazepine and GABA-receptors in clonal cell-lines.
Fed.Proc. 38, 687 (1979)

2057. Barankay,A.
Diazepam in cardiac surgery.
Brit.J.Anaesth. 51, 74 (1979)

2058. Barrett,J.W., Smyth,F., Davidson,I.E.
An examination of acid-base equilibria of 1,4-benzodiazepines by spectrophotometry.
J.Pharm.Pharmacol. 25, 387-93 (1973)

2059. Bartenbach,D.E.
Clorazepate dipotassium.
Amer.Fam.Physician 18, 43 (1978)

2060. Barthalmus,G.T., Leander,J.D., McMillan,D.E.
Combined effects of ethanol and diazepam on performance and aquisition of serial position sequences by pigeons.
Psychopharmacology 59, 101-2 (1978)

2061. Baumgarten,K.
Die klinische Bedeutung der Benzodiazepine bei der Behandlung des Abortus imminens (und der drohenden Frühgeburt).

In: Relaxation und Sedation des menschlichen Uterus, pp. 362-74, Ed. W.Neuweiler, M.Berger, Basel,New York: Karger, 1964

2062. Baxter,M.T., McKenzie,D.D., Mikish,R.A.
Dilution of diazepam in intravenous fluids.
Amer.J.Hosp.Pharm. 34, 124 (1977)

2063. Becker,C.E., Roe,R., Scott,R., Tong,T., Boerner,U., Luce,J.
Rational drug therapy of alcoholism with sedative hypnotic drugs! Is it possible?
Ann.N.Y.Acad.Sci. 252, 379-84 (1975)

2064. Beer,B., Klepner,C.A., Lippa,A.S., Squires,R.F.
Enhancement of diazepam-H-3 binding by SQ 65,396 - novel anti-anxiety agent.
Pharm.Biol.Behavior 9, 849-51 (1978)

2065. Bell,R.W., Dickie,D.S., Stewart-Jones,J., Turner,P.
Lorazepam on visuo-motor co-ordination and visual function in man.
J.Pharm.Pharmacol. 25, 87-8 (1973)

2066. Benke,A., Balogh,A., Reichhilf,B.
Solubilizer of diazepam (valium) - its action on respiration.
Anaesthesis 28, 24-8 (1979)

2067. Bennett,N.R., Thornton,J.A., Pearson,I.B., Allen,J.G.
Blood-concentrations of diazepam following parenteral administration of Ro 03-7355, a new benzodiazepine prodrug.
Brit.J.Anaesth. 51, 64-5 (1979)

2068. Bennett,P.N., Davies,P., Frigo,G.M., Weerasinghe, W.M.T., Lennard-Jones,J.E.
Effect of diazepam on unstimulated and on stimulated gastric secretion.
Scand.J.Gastroenterol. 10, 101 (1975)

2069. Benson,W.H. jr.
Comparative evaluation of diazepam (valium) and phenobarbital. For the relief of anxiety-related symptoms in patients hospitalized for acute myocardial infarction.
J.med.Ass.Ga. 1971, 276-8

2070. Bepko,F., Lear,E., Waxman,B.
Relief of the emotional factor in labor with parenterally administered diazepam.
Obstet.Gynecol. 26, 6-10 (1965)

2071. Berg,W., Flegel,H.
EEG-Untersuchung mit Medazepam, einem neuen Benzodiazepin-Derivat.
Arzneim.-Forsch. (Drug Res.) 19, 740 (1969)

2072. Bergmann,H., Borg,S., Hogman,B., Larsson,H., Linde,C.J., Tengroth,B.
Effect of oxazepam on ocular re-adaptation time.
Acta Ophth.K. 57, 145-50 (1979)

2073. Bernheim,J., Michiels,W.
Effects psycho-physiques du diazépam (Valium) et d'une faible dose d'alcool chez l'homme.
Schweiz.med.Wschr. 103, 863-70 (1973)

2074. Berry,P.A., Grubb,D.J.
Effects of oxypertine and chlordiazepoxide on human motor co-ordination.
J.Int.Med.Res. 2, 177-88 (1974)

2075. Besser,G.M.
Time course of action of diazepam.
Nature 214, 428 (1967)

2076. Besser,G.M., Duncan,C.
The time course of action of single dose of diazepam, chlorpromazine and some barbiturates as measured by auditory flutter fusion and visual flicker fusion thresholds in man.
Brit.J.Pharmacol.Chemother. 30, 341-8 (1967)

2077. Betts,T.A., Clayton,A.B., MacKay,G.M.
Effects of four sommenly-used tranquillizers on low-speed driving performance tests.
Brit.Med.J. 4, 580-4 (1972)

2078. Bianco,J.A., Shanahan,E.A., Ostheimer,G.W. et al.
Cardiovascular effects of diazepam.
J.thorac.cardiovasc.Surg. 62, 125-30 (1971)

2079. Birnbaum,D., Karmeli,F., Tefera,M.
The effect of diazepam on human gastric secretion.
Gut 12, 616 (1971)

2080. Biscaldi,G.P., Hattab,J., Montanaro,N., Scoz,R.
Quantitative polygraphic evaluation of emotional tension in the study of a new benzodiazepine.
Curr.Ther.Res. 13, 606-15 (1971)

2081. Bissell,L.
The treatment of alcoholism: what do we do about long-term sedatives?
Ann.N.Y.Acad.Sci. 252, 396-9 (1975)

2082. Blackwell,B.
Psychotropic drugs in use today. The role of diazepam in medical practice.
J.Amer.Med.Ass. 225, 1637-41 (1973)

2083. Bloor,C.M., Leon,A.S., Walker,D.E.
Coronary and systemic hemodynamic effects of diazepam (valium) in the unanesthetized dog.
Res.Commun.Chem.Pathol. and Pharmacol. 6, 1043-51 (1973)

2084. Blustein,J., Rhéaume,S., Sendbuehler,J.M.
A pilot study of injectable diazepam in a general hospital setting.
Laval.méd. 41, 490-4 (1970)

2085. Boethius,G., Westerholm,B.
Is the use of hypnotics, sedatives and minor tranquillizers really a major health problem?
Acta Med.Scand. 199, 507-12 (1976)

2086. Bogatsky,A.V., Davidenko,T.I., Bondaren ,G.I., Kotlyar,I.I.
Enzymatic reduction of nitrazepam.
Dop.Ukr.B. 1979, 130-2 (1979)

2087. Bolesch,J.
Zur Behandlung des Abortus imminens, der drohenden Frühgeburt und der Placenta praevia mit Librium[R] und Valium[R] Roche.
Ther.d.Gegenw. 108, 1020-6 (1969)

2088. Bond,A.J., Lader,M.H.
Residual effects of hypnotics.
Psychopharmacologia 25, 117-32 (1972)

2089. Bond,A.J., Lader,M.H.
Residual effects of a new benzodiazepine: flurazepam.
Brit.J.Pharmacol. 44, 343P-4P (1972)

2090. Bond,A.J., Lader,M.H.
Residual effects of flunitrazepam.
Brit.J.Clin.Pharmacol. 2, 143 (1975)

2091. Bonnichsen,R., Meahly,A.C., Aqvist,S.
Arzneimittel und Fahrtüchtigkeit. III. Mitteilung Benzodiazepinderivate.
Blutalkohol 7, 1-12 (1970)

2092. Borland,R.G., Nicholson,A.N.
Residual effects of potassium chlorazepate, a precursor of nordiazepam.
Brit.J.Clin.Pharmacol. 4, 86-9 (1977)

2093. Boucsein,W.
Experimentalpsychologische Untersuchungen zur Wirkung von Tranquillizern (Diazepam und einer Prüfsubstanz) unter Berücksichtigung von Persönlichkeitsmerkmalen.
Arzneim.-Forsch. (Drug Res.) 26, 1138-41 (1976)

2094. Bourrinet,P., Sommaire,P.A.
Effect of acute and chronic alcoholization upon the activity of clobazam in mouse.
Ann.Pharm.France 36, 237-42 (1978)

2095. Bowden,C.L.
Recent advances in the benzodiazepines.
Tex.Med. 75, 51-4 (1979)

2096. Boxenbaum,K.A., Geitner,M.L.J., Dixon,W.R. et al.
Pharmacokinetic and biopharmaceutic profile of chlordiazepoxide - HCl in healthy subjects: Multiple dose oral administration.
J.Pharmacokinet.Biopharm. 5, 25-39 (1977)

2097. Braestrup,C., Nielsen,M., Squires,R.F.
No changes in rat benzodiazepine receptors after withdrawal from continous treatment with lorazepam and diazepam.
Life Sci. 24, 347-50 (1979)

2098. Brassier,J., Eben-Moussi,E., Allain,P. et al.
Action du diazépam sur la pression sanguine et sur la réactivité cardio-vasculaire du chien à l'adrénaline et à noradrénaline.
Thérapie 21, 379-85 (1966)

2099. Brimer,A., Schmieden,H., Simon,A.
The effect of chlorpromazine and chlordiazepoxide on cognitive functioning.
Brit.J.Psychiat. 110, 723-5 (1964)

2100. Brown,A.S.
Never intravenous anaesthetics: diazepam.
Int.Anaesthesiol.Clin. 7, 159 (1969)

2101. Brown,P.R.H., Main,D.M.G., Lawson,J.I.M.
Diazepam in dentistry.
Brit.Dent.J. 125, 498-501 (1968)

2102. Brown,Z.W., Amit,Z., Smith,B., Rockman,G.
Disruption of taste-aversion learning by pretreatment with diazepam and morphine.
Pharm.Biochem.Behav. 10, 17-20 (1979)

2103. Browne,T.R.
Clonazepam A review of a new anticonvulsant drug.
Arch.Neurol. 33, 326-32 (1976)

2104. Brüner,H., Jory,D., Klein,K.E.
Der Einfluß einiger verkehrsmedizinisch wichtiger Pharmaka auf die menschliche Leistungsbereitschaft.
Arzneim.-Forsch. (Drug Res.) 11, 995-1000 (1961)

2105. Burger,E.
Beeinflussung der Alkoholwirkung durch Librium im Straßenverkehr.
Hefte z. Unfallheilkunde 75, 256-8 (1963)

2106. Cailar,J.D., Kienlen,J.
Pharmacology of Flunitrazepam.
Ann.Anesth. 19, 1-9 (1978)

2107. Caldeyro-Barcia,R.
Action du Valium en obstétrique (Résumé critique).
Bull.Féd.Soc.Gynéc.Obstét.franc. 17, 451-7 (1965)

2108. Campan,L., Espagno,M.T.
Note sur le diazépam en anesthésiologie.
Ann.Anesthésiol.Franc. 5, 711-20 (1964)

2109. Cano Puerta,G., Angulo Estrada,D.
Accion del diazepam en la dinamica cardio-vascular. Efecto protector sobre el miocardio. Informe preliminar.
Sem.méd. (B.Aires) 141, 645-8 (1972)

2110. Castro,A., Malkus,H.
Radioimmunoassay of drugs of abuse in humans: a review.
Res.Commun.Chem.Pathol.Pharmacol. 16, 291-309 (1977)

2111. Catz,C.S.
Diazepam in breast milk.
Drug Ther. 3, 72-3 (1973)

2112. Chai,C.Y., Wang,S.C.
Cardiovascular actions of diazepam in the cat.
J.Pharmacol.exp.Ther. 154, 271-80 (1966)

2113. Chan,M.L., Whetsell,C., McChesney,J.D.
Use of high pressure liquid chromatography for the separation of drugs of abuse.
J.Chromatogr.Sci. 12, 512-6 (1974)

2114. Chassaing,C., Duchene-Marullaz,P.
Diazépam et fréquence cardiaque du chien non narcosé.
J.Pharmacol. (Paris) 4, 465-70 (1973)

2115. Cheesman,A.D.
Experience with the use of intravenous diazepam in outpatient procedures.
J.Laryngol.Otol. 87, 1249-52 (1973)

2116. Cheeseman,G.W., Greenberg,S.G.
Synthesis of 5,6-dihydro-4H-pyrrolo (1,2-A)-4-benzodiazepines.
J.Heterocycl.Chem. 16, 241-4 (1979)

2117. Chiu,T.H., Rosenberg,H.C.
GABA-receptor mediated modulation of diazepam binding.
Fed.Proc. 38, 687 (1979)

2118. Clarke,R.S.J., Dundee,J.W., Lyons,S.M.
Some cardiovascular and respiratory effects of four non-barbiturate anaesthetic induction agents.
Naunyn Schmiedebergs Arch.Pharmacol. 279, R 47 (1973)

2119. Cohen,M.M., Hirschhorn,K., Frosch,W.A.
Cytogenetic effects of tranquilizing drugs in vivo and in vitro.
J.Amer.med.Ass. 207, 2425-6 (1969)

2120. Cole,A.P., Hailey,D.M.
Diazepam and active metabolite in breast milk and their transfer to the neonate.
Arch.Dis.Childhood 50, 741-2 (1975)

2121. Collins,M., Evans,L., Tyrer,J.H., Eadie,M.J.
Pharmacokinetics of prazepam in man.
Clin.Exp.Pharm. 6, 213 (1979)

2122. Constant,G.A., Gruver,F.A.
Preliminary evaluation of diazepam in psychiatric disorders.
Psychosomatics 4, 80-4 (1963)

2123. Cooper,S.J., Crummy,Y.M.
Enhanced choice of familiar food in a food preference test after chlordiazepoxide administration.
Psychopharmacology 59, 51-6 (1978)

2124. Copperstock,R.
Psychotropic drug use among women.
Canad.Med.Assoc.J. 115, 760-3 (1976)

2125. Costa,E., Greengard,P.
Mechanism of action of benzodiazepines.
Raven Press, New York 1975

2126. Cotler,S., Gustafson,J.H., Okamoto,M.
Comparative blood level profile of diazepam and nordiazepam in normal cats and in pentobarbital-addicted cats during withdrawal.
Fed.Proc. 38, 366 (1979)

2127. Covi,L., Lipman,R.S., Pattison,J.H., Derogatis,L.R., Uhlenhuth,E.H.
Length of treatment with anxiolytic sedatives and response to their sudden withdrawal.
Acta Psychiat.Scand. 49, 51-64 (1973)

2128. Cunningham,M.L.
Acute hepatic necrosis following treatment with amitriptyline and diazepam.
Brit.J.Psychiat. 3, 1107-9 (1965)

2129. Dalen,J.E., Evans,G.L., Banas,J.S. et al.
Hemodynamic and respiratory effects of intravenous diazepam in man.
Clin.Res. 16, 226 (1968)

2130. D'Amelio,G., Dalla Volta,S., Stritoni,P. et al.
Acute cardiovascular effects of diazepam in patients with mitral valve disease.
Europ.J.clin.Pharmacol. 6, 61-3 (1973)

2131. Danechmand,L., Casier,H., Hebbelinck,M., De Schaepdryver,A.
Combined effects of ethanol and psychotropic drugs on muscular tone in mice.
Quart.J.Stud.Alcohol 28, 424-9 (1967)

2132. Dardel,von,O., Mebius,C., Mossberg,T.
Diazepam in emulsion form for intravenous usage.
Acta Anesth.Scand. 20, 221 (1976)

2133. De Bard,M.L.
Diazepam withdrawal syndrome: A case with psychosis seizures and coma.
Amer.J.Psychiatry 136, 104-5 (1979)

2134. Deberdt,R.
Lorazepam in the treatment of severe anxiety and anxiety associated with psychotic conditions.
Curr.Med.Res.Opinion 1, 296-300 (1973)

2135. DeCastro,J.
L'utilisation en anesthesiologie du Ro 5-4200. Premieres observations cliniques.
Ars medici 8, 1233 (1972)

2136. Dechene,J.P., Desrosiers,R.
Diazepam in pulmonary surgery.
Canad.Anaesth.Soc.J. 16, 162-6 (1969)

2137. de Jong,R.H., Heavner,J.E.
Diazepam and lidocaine-induced cardiovascular changes.
Anesthesiology 6, 633-8 (1973)

2138. Denham,J.
Psychotherapy of obsessional neurosis assisted by Librium. Topical problems of psychotherapy.
Acta Psychother.Psychosomat. 4, 195 (1963)

2139. Desmond,P., Roberts,R., Wilkinson,G., Wood,A., Dunn,D., Schenker,S.
Effect of heparin on benzodiazepin binding in plasma.
Fed.Proc. 38, 743 (1979)

2140. Dhar,A.K., Kutt,H.
Blood level monitoring of benzodiazepines by using nitrogen sensitive detectors.
Pharmacologist 19, 182 (1977)

2141. Dickel,H.A., Dixon,H.H., Shanklin,J.G., Dixon,jr.,H.H.
A clinical double-blind comparison of librium, meprobamate and phenobarbital.
Psychosomatics 3, 129 (1962)

2142. DiStefano,P., Case,K.R., Collelo,G.D., Bosmann,H.B.
Increased specific binding of ^{3}H-diazepam in rat-brain following chronic diazepam administration.
Cell.Biol. 3, 163-7 (1979)

2143. Dixon,H.R., Tilton,B.E., Briggs,B.D.
A comparison of the sedative and cardiorespiratory effects of diazepam and pentazocine for premedication.
Anaesth.Analg.Curr.Res. 49, 546-50 (1970)

2144. Dixon,R.A., Hatt,S.D., Rowse,C.W.
Intravenous diazepam in dentistry: Operating conditions in a controlled clinical trial.
J.Dentistry 1, 2 (1972)

2145. Dixon,R., Lucek,R., Earley,J., Perry,C.
Chlordiazepoxide - new, more sensitive and specific radioimmunoassay.
J.Pharm.Sci. 68, 261 (1979)

2146. Dixon,W.R., Brooks,M.A., Postma,E., Hackman,M.R., Schwartz,M.A.
Identification and determination of N-desmethyl-diazepam in plasma following chronic administration of chlordiazepoxide hydrochloride (Librium) to man.
Fed.Proc. 33, 472 (1974)

2147. Dixon,W.R., Young,R.L., Ning,R., Liebman,A.
Radioimmunoassay of the anticonvulsant agent: Clonazepam.
The Pharmacologist 17, 251 (1975)

2148. Döring,G,K., Kauka,E.
Kasuistische Mitteilung über die Gabe hoher Dosen von Valium Roche in der Schwangerschaft.
Med.Welt (Stuttg.) 1964, 1855

2149. Dorn,M., Haag,T., Lange-Löhrs,M., Mallach,H.J., Wilk,G.
Statistische Untersuchungen über die Beeinträchtigung der Fahrtüchtigkeit durch Alkohol- und Arzneimittel-einwirkungen sowie Alkoholeinfluß und Begleitkrank-heiten.
Med.Monatsschr. 24, 285-91 (1970)

2150. Driscoll,E.J., Smilack,Z.H., Lightbody,P.M., Fiorucci,R.D.
Sedation with intravenous diazepam.
J.Oral.Surg. 30, 332-43 (1972)

2151. Drury,K.A.D., Spalding,E., Donaldson,D., Rutherford,D.
Floppy-infant syndrome:
Is prazepam the answer?
Lancet 2, 1126-7 (1977)

2152. Dundee,J.W., Haslett,W.H.K., Keilty,S.R., Pandit,S.K.
Studies of drugs given before anaesthesia.
XX. Diazepam-containing mixtures.
Anaesthesia 30, 164 (1975)

2153. Dundee,J.W., Howard,H.J., Isaac,M.
Alcohol and the benzodiazepines. The interaction between intravenous ethanol and chlordiazepoxide and diazepam.
Quart.J.Stud.Alcohol 32, 960-8 (1971)

2154. Dundee,J.W., Isaac,M.
Interaction of alcohol with sedatives and tran-quilizers (a study of blood levels at loss of consciousness following rapid infusion).
Med.Sci.Law 10, 220-4 (1970)

2155. Dundee,J.W., Isaac,M.
Interaction between intravenous alcohol and some sedatives and tranquillizers.
Med.Sci.Law 11, 49-50 (1971)

2156. Dundee,J.W., Isaac,M.
Interaction between intravenous alcohol and some sedatives and tranquillizers.
Brit.J.Pharmacol. 39, 199P-200P

2157. Eadie,M.J., Tyrer,J.H., Smith,G.A., McKauge,L.
Pharmacokinetics of drugs used for petit mal "absence" epilepsy.
Proc.Aust.Assoc.Neurol. 14, 172-83 (1977)

2158. Ebel,S.
Synthetische Arzneimittel.
- Ein Lehr- und Handbuch.
pp. 225-47
Verlag Chemie - Weinheim - 1979

2159. Erbguth,P.H., Reiman,B., Klein,R.L.
The influence of chlorpromazine, diazepam and droperidol on emergence from ketamine.
Anesth.Analg. 51, 693- (1972)

2160. Erkkola,R., Kanto,J., Kangas,L., Piiroinen,O.
Feto-maternal concentration of diazepam and N-demethyldiazepam after intra-amniotic diazepam injection.
Int.J.Gynaecol.Obstet. 14, 213-6 (1976)

2161. Essig,C.F.
Addiction to nonbarbiturate sedative and tranquilizing drugs.
Clin.Pharmacol.Ther. 5, 334-43 (1964)

2162. Essig,C.F.
Newer sedative drugs that can cause states of intoxication and dependence of barbiturate type.
JAMA 196, 714-7 (1966)

2163. Fabre,L.F., McLendon,D.M., Borgen,L.A.
Comparison of trebenzomine with chlordiazepoxide and placebo in the treatment of anxious-depressed outpatients.
Curr.Ther.Res. 25, 311-9 (1979)

2164. Feldman,R.S., Smith,W.C.
Chlordiazepoxide-fluoxetine interactions on food intake in free-feeding rats.
Pharmacol.Biochem.Behav. 8, 749-52 (1978)

2165. Femi-Pearse,D.
Experience with diazepam in tetanus.
Brit.med.J. 1966/2, 862-5

2166. Fernandez,F.A.
Target indications and the psychodynamic action of chlordiazepoxide (Librium) as an antialcoholic psychopharmacological agent.
Arch.Neurol.Psychiat. 93, 150 (1964)

2167. Ferrara,S.D., Tedeschi,L., Marigo,M., Castagna,F.
Concentrations of phenobarbital, flurazepam, and flurazepam metabolites in autopsy cases.
J.Forens.Sci. 24, 61-9 (1979)

2168. Field,D.E., Malpass,C.A., Frank,M.J.
Hemodynamic and electrocardiographic effects following the acute administration of chlorpromazine and diazepam.
Clin.Res. 19, 313 (1971)

2169. Field,G.F., Sternbach,L.H.
Quinazolines and 1,4-benzodiazepines: XLII: Photochemistry of some N-Oxides.
J.Org.Chem. 33, 4438 (1968)

2170. Fink,M.
Convulsive Therapy: Theory and Practice.
Raven Press, New York 1979

2171. Fink,M., Irwin,P., Weinfeld,R.E., Schwartz,M.A., Co-ney,A.H.
Blood levels and electroencephalographic effects of diazepam and bromazepam.
Clin.Pharmacol.Ther. 20, 184-91 (1976)

2172. Flowers,C.E., Facog,A.J.R., Desmond,M.M.
Diazepam (Valium) as an adjunct in obstetric analgesia.
Obstet.Gynecol. 34, 68-81 (1969)

2173. Fransisco,N., Lebowitz,W.B.
Intravenous diazepam in the cardiovascular laboratory. A Physiologic study.
St.Vincent's Hosp.Med.Bull. 10, 8-12 (1968)

2174. Frost Jr.,D.J., Carrie,J.R.G., Borda,R.P., Kellaway,P.
The effects of dalmane (flurazepam hydrochloride) on human EEG characteristics.
Electroenceph.Clin.Neurophysiol. 34, 171-5 (1973)

2175. Fuccella,L.M., Bolcioni,G., Tamassia,V., Ferrario, L., Tognoni,G.
Human pharmacokinetics and bioavailability of temazepam administered in soft gelatine capsules.
Eur.J.Clin.Pharmacol. 12, 383-6 (1977)

2176. Gaillard,J.M., Schulz,P., Tissot,R.
Effects of three benzodiazepines (nitrazepam, flunitrazepam and bromazepam) on sleep of normal subjects, studies with an automatic sleep-scoring system.
Pharmakopsychiat.Neuropsychopharmakol. 6, 207-17 (1973)

2177. Garattini,S., Marcucci,F., Mussini,E.
Biotransformation of drugs to pharmacologically active metabolites.
In: Eichler, Farah, Herken and Welch (eds.). Handbook of Experimental Pharmacology, Vol. 28, pp. 113-9 (Springer Verlag, Berlin - Heidelberg - New York, 1975)

2178. Gebhart,G.F., Plaa,G.L., Mitchell,C.L.
The effects of ethanol alone and in combination with phenobarbital, chlorpromazine, or chlordiazepoxide.
Toxicol.Appl.Pharmacol. 15, 405-14 (1969)

2179. Gelbke,H.P., Schlicht,H.J., Schmidt,Gg.
Radioimmunologische Serienbestimmung und gaschromatographische Identifizierung von Diazepam in Blut und Serum.
Unfall-Sicherh.-Forsch.Straßenverkehr 10, 436-40 (1977)

2180. Gentles,W., Thomas,E.L.
Effect of benzodiazepines upon saccadic eye movements in man.
Clin.Pharmacol.Ther. 12, 563-74 (1971)

2181. George,K.A., Dundee,J.W.
Relative amnesic actions of diazepam, flunitrazepam und lorazepam in man (benzodiazepine amnesia).
Brit.J.clin.Pharmacol. 4, 45-50 (1976)

2182. Georgiev,V.
Effects of imidazole, papaverine and theophylline on the picrotoxin convulsion-seizure threshold. The correlation with GABA and diazepam).
Eksp.Med.Morfol. 17, 139-44 (1978)

2183. Gerchow,J.
Medikamente und Verkehrssicherheit.
Caritas 78, Heft 3 (1977)

2184. German,L.J.
Basal sedation with intravenous diazepam for instrumental vaginal deliveries.
In: Psychosomatic Medicine in Obstetrics and Gynaecology, 3rd. Int. Congr. (ed. N.Morris), p. 244, London 1971

2185. Ghoneim,M.M., Mewaldt,S.P.
Effects of diazepam and scopolamine on the storage, retrieval and organizational processes in memory.
Psychopharmacologia 44, 257-62 (1975)

2186. Ghoneim,M.M., Mewaldt,S.P.
Studies on human memory: the interactions of diazepam, scopolamine, and physostigmine.
Psychopharmacologia 52, 1-6 (1977)

2187. Ghoneim,M.M., Mewaldt,S.P., Thatcher,J.W.
The effect of diazepam and fentanyl on mental, psychomotor and electroencephalographic functions and their rate of recovery.
Psychopharmacologia 44, 61-6 (1975)

2188. Ghoneim,M.M., Petersen,R.C.
Diazepam (Valium) and memory-effects on acquisition, retrieval, and state-dependent learning in man.
Fed.Proc. 38, 861 (1979)

2189. Glasser,H., Krieglstein,J.
Die Eiweißbindung einiger Psychopharmaka mit tricyclischem Ringsystem in Abhängigkeit von ihrer chemischen Konstitution.
Naunyn-Schmied.-Arch.Toxicol. 265, 321-34 (1969)

2190. Glazko,A.J., Chang,T., Peterson,F.E., Johnson,E.L., Young,R.M., Hayes,A.G., Goulet,R.J., Smith,T.C.
Metabolic disposition of diazepam and prazepam in man-multiple dose studies.
Fed.Proc. 38, 742 (1979)

2191. Glover,W., Dixon,R.
Radioimmunoassay for the hypnotic, flurazepam (Dalmane), in plasma.
Fed.Proc. 38, 443 (1979)

2192. Gluckman,M.I., Stein,L.
Pharmacology of lorazepam.
J.Clin.Psychiatry 39, 3-10 (1978)

2193. Gold,R.L., Dribben,I.S.
Diazepam therapy of depressed patients.
J.Neuropsychiat. 5, 366-9 (1964)

2194. Gomita,Y., Gomita,H., Nakaebisu,H., Kataoka,Y., Ueki,S.
Effects of triazolam on coditioned behavior in rats.
Nippon Yakurigaku Zasshi 74, 615-28 (1978)

2195. Gottschalk,L.A.
Effects of certain benzodiazepine derivates on disorganization of thought as manifested in speech.
Curr.Ther.Res. 21, 192-206 (1977)

2196. Greenblatt,D.J., Shader,R.I., Franke,K., Koch-Weser,J.
Pharmacokinetics of intravenous chlordiazepoxide.
Clin.Pharmacol.Ther. 17, 235 (1975)

2197. Gurman,G.
Notre expérience de l'utilisation du diazépam (Valium) dans l'induction de l'anesthésie générale.
Ann.Anesth.Franc. 11, 419-29 (1970)

2198. Gylys,J.A., Chamberlain,J.H., Wright,R.N., Doran,K.M.
Interaction between diazepam and naloxone in conflict, novel food-intake and anti-metrazol tests.
Fed.Proc. 38, 863 (1979)

2199. Haefelfinger,P.
Determination of the 7-amino-metabolites of the 7-nitro-benzodiazepines in human plasma by thin-layer chromatography.
J.of High Resolution Chrom.and Chrom.Comm. 1, 39-42 (1979)

2200. Hahn,J.
Vorläufige Ergebnisse bei der Behandlung des Abortus imminens und der drohenden Frühgeburt mit Valium.
In: Relaxation und Sedation des menschlichen Uterus, pp. 345-9. Ed. W.Neuweiler, M.Berger, Basel, New York: Karger, 1964

2201. Haider,J.
Evaluation of a new tranquilizer - WY 4036 - in the treatment of anxiety.
Brit.J.Psychiat. 119, 597-8 (1971)

2202. Hamilton,J.
Muscle-relaxant activity of chlordiazepoxide and diazepam.
Can.J.Physiol. 45, 191-9 (1967)

2203. Hanna,S., Diana,F., Slevinski,J., Veronich,K., Lachman,L.
Differential pulse polarographic determination of clorazepate monopotassium and dipotassium.
J.Pharm.Sci. 67, 1723-5 (1978)

2204. Hara,T., Inami,M., Kaneko,T.
The effect of clonazepam on plasma diphenylhydantoin levels in epileptic patients.
In: Abstracts. Seventh International Symposium on Epilepsy, p. 45, Berlin, June 19-21, 1975

2205. Hardin,T.C., Evens,R.P.
Benzodiazepine use in glaucoma.
Drug Intell. 13, 109 (1979)

2206. Harrison Snyder,C.
Myoclonic epilepsy in children: short-term comparative study of two benzodiazepine derivates in treatment.
Sth.med.J. 61, 17-20 (1968)

2207. Harry,T.W.A., Richards,D.J.
Lorazepam - a study on psychomotor depression.
Brit.J.Clin.Practice 26, 371-3 (1972)

2208. Hart,J., Hill,H.M., Bye,C.E., Wilkinson,R.T., Peck,A.W.
The effects of low doses of amylobarbitone sodium and diazepam on human performance.
Brit.J.Clin.Pharmacol. 3, 289-98 (1976)

2209. Havard,C.W.H., Salhanda,V.F., Bird,R., Gardner,R.
The effect of diazepam on pituitary function in man.
J.Endocr. 52, 79 (1972)

2210. Havard,J.D.J.
Drugs and driving.
Brit.J.Hosp.Med. 4, 455-8 (1970)

2211. Healy,T.E.J., Hamilton,M.C.
Intravenous diazepam in the apprehensive child.
Brit.dent.J. 130, 25 (1971)

2212. Healy,T.E.J., Robinson,J.S., Vickers,M.D.
Physiological responses to intravenous diazepam sedation for outpatient dentistry.
Brit.med.J. 3, 10-13 (1970)

2213. Hedges,A., Turner,P., Harry,T.V.A.
Preliminary studies on the central lorazepam, a new benzodiazepine.
J.Clin.Pharmacol. 11, 423-7 (1971)

2214. Heermann,J.
Flunitrazepam with anterograde amnesia and reduction of blood-pressure before local-anesthesia without intubation in 3000 operations.
Laryng.Rhinol.Otol. 58, 162-4 (1979)

2215. Hendel,J., Elsass,P., Buch-Andreasen,P., Gymoese,E., Hvidberg,E.F.
Neuropsychological effects of diazepam related to single dose kinetics and liver function.
Psychopharmacology 48, 11-7 (1976)

2216. Hindmarch,I.
A 1,4-benzodiazepine, temazepam (K 3917), its effect on some psychological parameters of sleep and behaviour.
Arzneim.-Forsch. (Drug Res.) 25, 1836-9 (1975)

2217. Hindmarch,I.
A sub-chronic study of the subjective quality of sleep and psychological measures of performance the morning following night-time medication with temazepam.
Arzneim.-Forsch. (Drug Res.) 26, 2113-6 (1976)

2218. Hindmarch,I., Parrott,A.C., Arenillas,L.
A repeated dose comparison of dichloralphenazone, flunitrazepam and amylobarbitone sodium on some aspects of sleep and early morning behaviour in normal subjects.
Brit.J.Clin.Pharmacol. 4, 229-33 (1977)

2219. Ho,I.K., Flint,B.A., Gillilani,T.
Comparative effect of diazepam and valproate on pentylenetetrazol induced convulsions in pento-barbital dependent mice.
Fed.Proc. 38, 434 (1979)

2220. Hollis,D.A.
Diazepam as an induction agent II
In: Knight,P.F., Burgess,C.G.: Diazepam in Anaesthesia. Proc.Symp.Roy.Soc.Med., Bristol/Eng. 1968

2221. Holzman,P.S., Levy,D.L., Uhlenhuth,E.H., Proctor,L.R., Freedman,D.X.
Smooth-pursuit eye movements, and diazepam, CPZ, and secobarbital.
Psychopharmacologia 44, 111-5 (1975)

2222. Hoyer,J.
Action of benzodiazepines: Electrophysiological analysis on neurones of the sea hare, aplysia california.
Pharmakopsychiatr.Neuropsychopharmacol. 10, 271-80 (1977)

2223. Hromatka,O., Knollmüller,M., Binder,D.
Über die Synthese von 1,3-Dihydro-2,1,4-benzothiadiazepinen.
Monatsh.Chem. 100, 872 (1969)

2224. Huck,S., Stacher,G., Gogolák,G., Stumpf,C.
Action of six commonly used benzodiazepines on isolated guinea-pigs ileum preparation.
Arch.Int.Pharmacodyn.Ther. 218, 77-83 (1975)

2225. Ideström,C.M., Cadenus,B.
Chlordiazepoxide, dipiperon, amobarbital. Dose effect studies on human beings.
Psychopharmacologia 4, 235-46 (1963)

2226. Ikram,H., Rubin,A.P., Jewkes,R.F.
Effect of diazepam on myocardial blood flow of patients with and without coronary artery disease.
Brit.Heart J. 35, 626-30 (1973)

2227. Isaac,M., Bovill,J.G., Dundee,J.W., Pandit,S.K.
Clinical studies of induction agents. XXXV: studies on combination of ethanol with methohexitone and diazepam.
Brit.J.Anaesth. 42, 521-3 (1970)

2228. Janke,W., Stoll,K.D.
Untersuchungen zur Wirkung eines Tranquilizers auf emotional labile Personen unter verschiedenen Versuchsbedingungen.
Arzneim.-Forsch. (Drug Res.) 15, 366-74 (1965)

2229. Jeavons,P.M.
The effect of chlordiazepoxide on the electroencephalogram.
Epilepsia 3, 110 (1962)

2230. Jitsukon,N., Sapantup ,S., Kasemsup,K.
Clonazepam in epilepsy.
J.Med.Ass.Thailand 62, 47-9 (1979)

2231. Johannessen,S.I., Strandjord,R.E., Munthe-Kaas,A.W.
Lack of effect of clonazepam on serum levels of diphenylhydantoin, phenobarbital and carbamazepine.
Acta Neurol.Scand. 55, 506-12 (1977)

2232. Johns,M.W., Masterton,J.P.
Effect of flurazepam on sleep in the laboratory.
Pharmacology 11, 358-64 (1974)

2233. Johnson,D.A.W.
Double-blind comparison of flupenthixol, nortriptyline and diazepam in neurotic depression.
Act.Psych.Sci. 59, 1-8 (1979)

2234. Kaegi,H.H.

Synthesis of 7-chloro-2,3-dihydro-1-methyl-5-phenyl-1H-1,4-benzodiazepine-5-^{14}C-hydrochloride.

J.Labelled Comp. 4, 363-7 (1968)

2235. Kaldor,A.

Pattern and problems of drug consumption in a developing country.

Clin.Pharmacol.Ther. 19, 657-62 (1976)

2236. Kanjilal,G.C.

A clinical evaluation of valium (Ro 5-2807) in cerebral palsy.

Brit.J.clin.Pract. 18, 21-2 (1964)

2237. Kanto,J., Erkkola,R., Sellman,R.

Distribution and metabolism of diazepam in early and late human pregnancy. Postnatal metabolism of diazepam.

Acta Pharmacol.Toxicol. 35, 36 (1974)

2238. Kaplan,S.R., Murkofsky,C.

Oral-buccal dyskinesia symptoms associated with low-dose benzodiazepine treatment.

Amer.J.Psychiatry 135, 1558-9 (1978)

2239. Karle,J., Karle,I.L.

The crystal and molecular structure of 7-chloro-5-(2,4-dichlorophenyl)-4,5-dihydro-1,4-dimethyl-3H-1,4-benzodiazepin-2-one, $C_{17}H_{15}Cl_3N_2O$.

J.Amer.Chem.Soc. 89, 804-7 (1969)

2240. Karobath,M., Sperk,G.

Stimulation of benzodiazepine-receptor-binding by GABA.

Proc.Nat.Acad.Sci.USA 76, 1004-6 (1979)

2241. Kasich,A.M.

Clinical evaluation of doxepin and diazepam in patients with gastrointestinal diseases and anxiety. A controlled double-blind study and long-term evaluation.

Psychosomatics 10, 18-20 (1969)

2242. Katz,J., Finestone,S.C., Pappas,T.

Circulatory response to tilting after intravenous diazepam in volunteers.

Anesth.Analg.Curr.Res. 46, 243-6 (1967)

2243. Kelley,J.W.

Management of psychiatric disorders with diazepam.

Clin.Med. 69, 1789 (1962)

2244. Kelly,D., Pik,R., Chen,C.

A psychological and physiological evaluation of the effects of intravenous diazepam.

Brit.J.Psychiat. 121, 445 (1972)

2245. Kernohan,R.J.

Diazepam in cardioversion of supraventricular arrhythmias.

J.Irish Coll.Phys.Surg. 1, 88-90 (1972)

2246. Keskinder,A., Lloyd-Smith,D.L.

Effect of intravenous chlordiazepoxide on the electroencephalogram with some clinical observations.

J.Nerv.Ment.Dis. 134, 218 (1962)

2247. Khan,A.U., Forney,R.B., Hughes,F.W.

Effect of tranquilizers on the metabolism of ethanol.

Arch.Int.Pharmacodyn. 150, 171-6 (1964)

2248. Kibrick,E., Smart,R.G.

Psychotropic drug use and driving risk: a review and analysis.

J.Safety Res. 2, 73-85 (1970)

2249. Kielholz,P., Goldberg,L., Im Obersteg,J., Pöldinger,W., Ramseyer,A., Schmid,P.

Fahrversuche zur Frage der Beeinträchtigung der Verkehrstüchtigkeit durch Alcohol, Tranquilizer und Hypnotika.

Dtsch.med.Wschr. 94, 301-6 (1969)

2250. Kissin,B.

The use of psychoactive drugs in the longterm treatment of chronic alcoholics.

Ann.N.Y.Acad.Sci. 252, 385-95 (1975)

2251. Klebovich,I., Vereczkey,L.

Comparative bioavailability studies on two oral diazepam preparations.

Acta Pharm.Hung. 48, 216-20 (1978)

2252. Kleinknecht,R.A., Donaldson,D.

A review on the effects of diazepam on cognitive and psychomotor performance.

J.Nerv.Ment.Dis. 161, 399-411 (1975)

2253. Knapp,R.B., Dubow,H.S.

Diazepam as induction agent for patients with cardiopulmonary disease.

Sth.med.J. 63, 1451-3 (1970)

2254. Knapp,R.B., Dubow,H.

Comparison of diazepam with thiopental as an induction agent in cardiopulmonary disease.

Anesth.Analg.Curr.Res. 49, 722-6 (1970)

2255. Kobiela,A.

Spectrofluorometric determination of clonazepam and its metabolites in the serum.

Brom.Ch.Tok. 11, 439-44 (1978)

2256. Kodama,H., Takahashi,H., Takomura,I., Nobuto,H.

Clinical experience with chlordiazepoxide on epilepsy.

Brain Nerve 13, 1027 (1961)

2257. Kohlschmidt,K.

18 Monate Erfahrung mit Valium Roche in der ärztlichen Allgemeinpraxis.

Forsch.Prax.Fortbild. 17, 308-10 (1966)

2258. Korttila,K., Levaenen,J.
Untoward effects of ketamine combined with diazepam for supplementing conduction anaesthesia in young and middle-aged adults.
Acta Anaesthesiol.Scand. 22, 640-8 (1978)

2259. Kramer,M.S.
Use of diazepam in gastrointestinal endoscopy.
S.Afr.Med.J. 55, 195 (1979)

2260. Krieglstein,J., Kuschinsky,G.
Quantitative Bestimmung der Eiweißbindung von Pharmaka durch Gelfiltration.
Arzneim.-Forsch. (Drug Res.) 18, 287-9 (1968)

2261. Kudrin,A.N., Koroza,G.S., Gersamiia,T.V.
Action of fentanyl, droperidol and diazepam on the contractile function of the isolated human myometrium.
Farmakol.Toksikol. 41, 548-52 (1978)

2262. Küster,J.
Increased creatine-kinase concentrations after intramuscular injection of diazepam.
German Medicine 2, 154-5 (1972)

2263. Kuftinec,J., Klasinc,L., Kajfez,F., Mihalic,M., Decorte,E., Sunjic,V.
Kinetics of cyclization of 2-(N-Beta-bromoethyl)-amino-5-substituted benzophenones into 1,4-benzo-diazepines.
Croat.Chem. 51, 213 (1978)

2264. Kuschinsky,G.
Medikamente und Straßenverkehr.
Dtsch.Ärztebl. 73, 1977-9 (1977)

2265. Kvetina,J., Guaitani,A., Publiatti,C.
Effect of diazepam on liver function of rats.
Pharmacology 2, 17-21 (1969)

2266. Laepple,O., Rothlin,M.
Kreislaufverhältnisse während der Narkoseeinleitung mit Diazepam und Thiopental vor Herzoperationen.
Anaesthesist 19, 23-31 (1970)

2267. Landauer,A.A., Pocock,D.A., Prott,F.W.
The effect of medazepam and alcohol on cognitive and motor skills used in car driving.
Psychopharmacologia 37, 159-68 (1974)

2268. Landon,J., Moffat,A.C.
The radioimmunoassay of drugs.
Analyst 101, 225-43 (1976)

2269. Lauer,R.F., Zenchoff,G.
2-(Aminomethyl)-phthylimide - new reagent for the synthesis of 2,4-benzodiazepines.
J.Heterocycl.Chem. 16, 339-40 (1979)

2270. Lawton,M.P., Cahn,B.
The effects of diazepam (Valium[R]) and alcohol on psychomotor performance.
J.Nerv.Ment.Dis. 136, 550-4 (1963)

2271. Levenson,A.J. (Ed.)
Aging. Vol. 9: Neuropsychiatric Side Effects of Drugs in the Elderly.
Raven Press, New York 1979

2272. Levine,I.M., Jossmann,P.B., Friend,D.G., DeAngelis,V., Kane,M.
Diazepam in the treatment of spasticity.
J.chron.Dis. 22, 57-62 (1969)

2273. Lilburn,J.K., Dundee,J.W., Moore,J.
Lorazepam-ketamine: Preliminary report.
Brit.J.Anaesth. 48, 1125 (1976)

2274. Liljequist,R., Linnoila,M., Mattila,M.J., Saario,I., Seppälä,T.
Effect of two weeks' treatment with thioridazine, chlorpromazine, sulpiride and bromazepam, alone or in combination with alcohol, on learning and memory in man.
Psychopharmacologia 44, 205-8 (1975)

2275. Lind,N.A., Turner,P.
The effect of chlordiazepoxide and fluphenazine on critical flicker frequency.
J.Pharm.Pharmacol. 20, 804 (1968)

2276. Lindley,T.N.
Temperature-dependence of electron-capture detector responses in the analysis of chlorpromazine, diazepam, and clonazepam.
J.Anal.Toxicol. 3, 18-20 (1979)

2277. Linnoila,M.
Drug interaction on psychomotor skills related to driving: hypnotics and alcohol.
Ann.Med.Exp.Biol.Fenn. 51, 118-24 (1973)

2278. Linnoila,M.
Effects of drugs and alcohol on psychomotor skills related to driving.
Ann.Clin.Res. 6, 7-18 (1974)

2279. Linnoila,M.
Tranquilizers and driving.
Accid.Anal.Prev. 8, 15-9 (1976)

2280. Linnoila,M., Liljeqvist,R., Olkoniemi,J., Saario,I.
Effect of alcohol and benzodiazepines on performance as related to personality characteristics. Personality characteristics among healthy "placebo reactors" and nonreactors.
Pharmakopsychiat. 10, 246-53 (1977)

2281. Linnoila,M., Mäki,M.
Acute effects of alcohol, diazepam, thioridazine, flupenthixole and atropine on psychomotor per-formance profiles.
Arzneim.-Forsch. (Drug Res.) 24, 565-9 (1974)

2282. Linnoila,M., Mattila,M.J.
Drug interaction on driving skills as evaluated by laboratory rests and by a driving simulator.
Pharmakopsychiat. 6, 127-32 (1973)

2283. Linnoila,M., Saario,I., Mattila,M.J.
Drug alcohol interaction on psychomotor skills during subacute treatment with benzodiazepines, flupenthixole, or lithium.
Brit.J.Clin.Pharmacol. 1, 176 P (1974)

2284. Lion,J.R.
Benzodiazepines in the treatment of aggressive patients.
J.Clin.Psych. 40, 70-1 (1979)

2285. Lippa,A.S., Klepner,C.A., Yunger,L., Sand,M.C., Smith,W.V., Beer,B.
Relationship between benzodiazepine receptors and experimental anxiety in rats.
Pharm.Biol.Behavior 9, 853-6 (1978)

2286. Lipton,M.A., DiMascio,A., Killam,K.F. (Eds.)
Psychopharmacology. A Generation of Progress.
Raven Press, New York 1978

2287. Lockwood,W.R., Allison,F.
Injectable diazepam: a new drug for the treatment of tetanus.
J.Miss.med.Ass. 8, 66-70 (1967)

2288. Lutze,J., Gelbke,H.P., Schmidt,Gg.
Zur Leistungsbeeinträchtigung durch Alkohol und Diazepam.
Impairment of Performance by Alcohol and Diazepam.
Z.Rechtsmed. 82, 327-36 (1979)

2289. Mackerer,C.R., Lydigsen,J.L., Bierschenk,B.A., Kochman,R.L., Clay,G.A.
Correlation between prevention of pentylenetetrazole induced lethality and inhibition of ^{3}H-diazepam-binding.
Fed.Proc. 38, 754 (1979)

2290. Maier,L.
Relaxation und Geburtsverkürzung durch Benzodiazepinderivate.
Wien.Klin.Wschr. 75, 611-2 (1963)

2291. Malpas,A., Rowan,A.J., Joyce,C.R.B., Scotts,D.F.
Persistent behavioural and electroencephalographic changes after single doses of nitrazepam and amylobarbitone sodium.
Brit.Med.J. 2, 762-4 (1970)

2292. Manheimer,D.I., Davidson,S.T., Balter,M.B., Mellinger,G.D., Cisin,I.H., Parry,H.J.
Popular attitudes and beliefs about tranquilizers.
Am.J.Psychiat. 130, 1246-53 (1973)

2293. Mansikka,M., Kanto,J., Kangas,L., Allonen,H.
Oral oxazepam as a premedicant in minor surgery.
Anaesthesis 28, 36-8 (1979)

2294. Marangos,P.J., Paul,S.M., Parma,A.M., Goodwin,F.K., Syapin,P., Skolnick,P.
Purinergic inhibition of diazepam binding to rat-brain (invitro).
Life Sci. 24, 851-7 (1979)

2295. Marjerrison,G., Neufeld,A.H., Holmes,V., Ho,T.
Comparative psychophysiological and mood effects of diazepam and dipotassium chlorazepate.
Biol.Psychiat. 7, 31-41 (1973)

2296. Mattila,M.A.K., Larni,H.M., Nummi,S.E., Pekkola,P.O.
Effect of diazepam on emergence from ketamine anesthesia - double-blind-study.
Anaesthesis 28, 20-3 (1979)

2297. McClish,A.
Diazepam as an intravenous induction agent for general anaesthesia.
Can.Anesthes.Soc.J. 13, 562-75 (1966)

2298. McCurdy,L.
Lorazepam, a new benzodiazepine derivative, in the treatment of anxiety - double-blind clinical evaluation.
Amer.J.Psychiatry 136, 187-90 (1979)

2299. McMillan,D.E., Leander,J.D.
Chronic chlordiazepoxide and pentobarbital interactions on punished and unpunished behavior.
J.Pharmacol.Exp.Ther. 207, 515-20 (1978)

2300. Meléndez,L.J., Eugenio Gonzales,L., Moisés Katz,W.
La medication sedante en el infarto miocardio. Resultados obtenidos con diazepam (Valium).
Univ.med. 12, 143-8 (1970)

2301. Mendelson,W.B., Goodwin,D.W., Hill,S.Y., Reichman,J.D.
The morning after: residual EEG effects of triazolam and flurazepam, alone and in combination with alcohol.
Curr.Ther.Res. 19, 155-63 (1976)

2302. Miller,A.I., D'Agostino,A., Minsky,R.
Effects of combined chlordiazepoxide and alcohol in man.
Quart.J.Stud.Alcohol 24, 9-13 (1963)

2303. Milner,G.
The effect of antidepressants and "tranquillizers" on the response of mice to ethanol.
Brit.J.Pharmacol. 34, 370-6 (1968)

2304. Milner,G.
Interaction between barbiturates, alcohol and some psychotropic drugs.
Med.J.Austr. 1, 1204-7 (1970)

2305. Mörsdorf,O.
Physikalische Kreislaufmessungen über den Einfluß von Diazepam.
Dissertation, Homburg/Saar, 1973

2306. Mofid,M., Brinkman,C.R., Assali,N.S.
Effects of diazepam on uteroplacental hemodynamics and metabolism.
Obstet. and Gynec. 41, 364-8 (1973)

2307. Moore,N.C.
Medazepam and the driving ability of anxious patients.
Psychopharmacology 52, 103-6 (1977)

2308. Müller,W.E.
Über die Bedeutung der Plasmaproteinbindung für Verteilung und Wirkung von Tranquillantien vom Benzodiazepintyp.
Klin.Wschr. 55, 105-10 (1977)

2309. Muller,P., Dellenbach,P., Szwarcberg,R.
Les effects du diazépam dans le menaces d'interruption de grossesse.
Bull.Féd.Soc.Gynéc.Obstét.franc. 17, 261-4 (1965)

2310. Münzel,K.
The desorption of medicinal substances from adsorbents in oral pharmaceutical suspensions.
Acta Pharmacol.Toxicol. 29, 81-7 (1971)

2311. Murray,N.
Methaminodiazepoxide.
JAMA 173, 1760-1 (1960)

2312. Nagy,J., Decsi,L.
Further studies on the site of action of diazepam anticonvulsant effect in the rabbit.
Neuropharm. 18, 39-45 (1979)

2313. Nair,S.G., Gamble,J.A.S., Dundee,J.W., Howard,P.J.
The influence of three antacids on the adsorption and clinical action of oral diazepam.
Brit.J.Anaesth. 48, 1175-80 (1976)

2314. Nakano,S., Ogawa,N., Kawazu,Y., Osato,E., Miyamato,M.
Effects of bromazepam, diazepam and placebo on subjective feeling, psychomotor performance and heart rate in normal volunteers - a double blind controlled study.
J.Japan.Psychosom.Soc. 13, 111-8 (1973)

2315. Nayal,S., Castleden,C.M., George,C.F., Marcer,D.
The effects of an hypnotic with a short half-life on hangover effect in old patients.
Age Ageing, Suppl. 50-4 (1978)

2316. Nesbitt,R., Bauess,S., Kantor,H.
Diazepam (Valium) during labor.
Obstet.Gynecol. 29, 5-9 (1967)

2317. Nestoros,J.N., Nistri,A.
A presynaptic component of the action of iontophoretically applied flurazepam on feline cortical neurones.
Can.J.Physiol.Pharmacol. 56, 889-92 (1978)

2318. Nicholson,A.N., Stone,B.M., Clarke,C.H.
Effect of diazepam and fosazepam (a soluble derivative of diazepam) on sleep in man.
Brit.J.clin.Pharmacol. 3, 533-43 (1976)

2319. Nisbet,R., Boulas,S.H., Kantor,H.I.
Diazepam (valium) during labor.
Obstet.Gynecol. 29, 726-9 (1967)

2320. Norio,N., Ioaho,R., Idäpään-Heikkilä,J.
Interaction of benzodiazepines and ethanol on sleeping time in rats.
Scand.J.Clin.Lab.Invest. 27, Suppl. 116, 76 (1971)

2321. Oelschläger,H., Hoffmann,H.
Ringverengung bei der elektrochemischen Reduktion eines 1,4-Benzodiazepin-Derivates.
Arch.Pharm. 300, 816-22 (1967)

2322. Okamoto,K., Sakai,Y.
Augmentation by chlordiazepoxide of the inhibitory effects of taurine, beta-alanine and gamma-aminobutyric acid on spike discharges in guinea-pig cerebellar slices.
Brit.J.Pharmacol. 65, 277-85 (1979)

2323. O'Neill,R., Verrill,P.J.
Intravenous diazepam in minor oral surgery.
Brit.J.Oral Surg. 7, 12-4 (1969)

2324. Parkes,M.W.
The pharmacology of diazepam.
In: Knight,P.F., Burgess,C.G. (eds.). Diazepam in anesthesia. Wright & Sons, Bristol 1968

2325. Parrott,A.C., Hindmarch,I.
Clobazam, a 1,5-benzodiazepine derivative: Effects on anxiety, arousal and performance compared with those of CNS stimulants, sedatives and tranquilizers.
IRCS Med.Sci.Clin.Pharmacol.Ther. 3, 177 (1975)

2326. Patay,M., Le Clec'h,G., Henry,P., Van Den Drissche,J.
Recherche de l'influence de clorazépate dipotassique sur des réactions psychomotrices.
Thérapie 30, 679-84 (1975)

2327. Pax,R., Bennett,J.L., Fetterer,R.
A benzodiazepine derivative and praziquantel: Effects on musculature of schistosoma mansoni and schistosoma japonicum.
Naunyn-Schmied.Arch.Pharmacol. 304, 309-15 (1978)

2328. Peat,M.A., Chem,C., Kopjak,L.
Screening and quantitation of diazepam, flurazepam, chlordiazepoxide, and their metabolites in blood and plasma by electron-capture gas-chromatography and high-pressure liquid-chromatography.
J.Forens.Sci. 24, 46-54 (1979)

2329. Peirson,G.A., Fowlks,E.W., King,P.S.
Long-term follow-up on the use of diazepam in the treatment of spasticity.
J.phys.Med. 47, 143-9 (1968)

2330. Perry,H.J.
Use of psychotropic drugs by U.S. adults.
Publ.Health Report 83, 799-809 (1968)

2331. Petro,W.
Camazepam (Albego) in psychovegetative disorders and psychosomatic diseases.
Ther.Gegenw. 118, 362 (1979)

2332. Pevzner,L.Z., Iakoubek,B.
Protein concentration in the neuron-neuroglia system of the anterior horns of the spinal cord in rats following exposure to the tranquilizer diazepam against a background of anticipation stress.
Tsitologiia 20, 225-8 (1978)

2333. Pfister,W.R., Yim,G.K.W.
Effects of chlordimeform, chlordiazepoxide and 2-deoxy-D-glucose on feeding and glycemic responses in mice and rats.
Fed.Proc. 38, 863 (1979)

2334. Phatak,A.T., Shah,S.H.
Diazepam as adjuvant therapy in childhood tetanus.
Clin.Pediatrics 9, 573-6 (1970)

2335. Phillips,M.T., Wilson,R.D.
Comparative studies of cardiopulmonary effects of two parenteral benzodiazepins.
Feder.Proc. 33, 510 (1974)

2336. Pittrich,W., Bochnik,H.J.
Aktuelle experimentelle und forensische Aspekte relativ niedriger Blutalkoholwerte in Kombination mit Beruhigungsmitteln.
Z.Verkehrssicherheit 17, 34-47 (1971)

2337. Podiwinsky,F.
Erfahrungen mit dem Benzodiazepinderivat Valium.
Wien.med.Wschr. 115, 649-52 (1965)

2338. Pöldinger,W., Sutter,W.
Die Beeinflussung der Verkehrstüchtigkeit durch psychotrope Pharmaka.
Pharmakopsychiat. 3, 223-31 (1968)

2339. Ponce,P.L.
Clonazepam: Preliminary results of a clinical trial.
In: Antiepileptic Drugs, D.M.Woodbury, J.K.Penry and R.P.Schmidt (eds.), Raven Press, New York, p. 517 (1972)

2340. Prevec,T.S.
Effects of valium on evoked cerebral cortex activity.
Neurologija 25, 77-80 (1977)

2341. Przybyla,A.C., Wang,S.C.
Studies on the locus of CNS action of diazepam.
Pharmacologist 9, 188 (1967)

2342. Raft,D., Davidson,J., Toomey,T.C., Spencer,R.F., Lewis,B.F.
Inpatient and outpatient patterns of psychotropic drug prescibing by nonpsychiatrist physicians.
Am.J.Psychiat. 132, 1309-12 (1975)

2343. Ramanujam,V.M., Trieff,N.M.
Structure activity relation for some 1,4-benzodiazepinones: Correlation between rate constants for reduction by sodium borohydride and antileptazol ED 50.
J.Pharm.Pharmacol. 30, 542-6 (1978)

2344. Rao,S., Sherbaniuk,R.W., Prasad,K. et al.
Cardiorespiratory effects of diazepam in patients undergoing endoscopy.
Clin.Pharmacol.Ther. 13, 150 (1972)

2345. Rattray,I.J.
Observations on the use of diazepam in general dental practice.
Brit.Dent.J. 125, 495-8 (1968)

2346. Rees,W.D.
Psychotropic drugs and the motorist.
Practitioner 196, 704-6 (1966)

2347. Rendic,S., Klasinc,L., Sunjic,V., Kajfez,F., Kramer,V., Mildner,P.
Mass spectrometry of 1,4-benzodiazepines.
Biomed.Mass Spectrometry 2, 97 (1975)

2348. Rice,A.J., Gruhn,S.W., Gibson,T.P. et al.
Effect of saline infusion on the renal excretion of secobarbital, meprobamate, and chlordiazepoxide.
J.Lab.Clin.Med. 80, 56-62 (1972)

2349. Richter,R., Hobi,V.
Die persönlichkeitsspezifische Wirkung eines Tranquilizers.
Arzneim.-Forsch. (Drug Res.) 26, 1136-8 (1976)

2350. Ritchie,J.A., Truelove,S.C.
Treatment of irritable bowel syndrome with lorazepam, hyoscine butylbromide and ispaghula husk.
Brit.Med.J. 1, 376-8 (1979)

2351. Robertson,H.A., Martin,I.L., Candy,J.M.
Differences in benzodiazepine-receptor binding in maudsley reactive and maudsley non-reactive rats.
Eur.J.Pharmacol. 50, 455-7 (1978)

2352. Rogers,E.J.
Double-blind comparative study of diazepam and methocarbamol in treatment of skeletal muscle spasm.
Western Med. 4, 11-5 (1963)

2353. Rosenberg,H.C., Chiu,T.H.
Decreased ^{3}H-diazepam binding is a specific response to chronic benzodiazepine treatment.
Life Sci. 24, 803-7 (1979)

2354. Roth,H.J., Adomeit,M.
Photochemische Reduktion des 7-Nitro-5-phenyl-2,3-dihydro-1H-1,4-benzodiazepin-2-on und der drei isomeren N-Acetyl-nitraniline.
Tetrahedron Lett. 37, 3201 (1969)

2355. Ruelius,H.W.
Comparative metabolism of lorazepam in man and four animal species.
J.Clin.Psychiatry 39, 11-5 (1978)

2356. Ruoss,C.
The management of eclampsia and severe pre-eclampsia with diazepam and dihydrallazine.
S.Afr.Med.J. 48, 1459 (1974)

2357. Ruskin,J., Greenfield,J.C., Durham,N.C.
Comparison of diazepam and sodium thiopental in cardioversion.
N.C.Med.J. 31, 84-6 (1970)

2358. Saario,I.
Psychomotor skills during subacute treatment with thioridazine and bromazepam, and their combined effects with alcohol.
Ann.Clin.Res. 8, 117-23 (1976)

2359. Saario,I., Linnoila,M.
Effect of subacute treatment with hypnotics, alone or in combination with alcohol, on psychomotor skills related to driving.
Acta Pharmacol.Toxicol. 38, 382-92 (1976)

2360. Saario,I., Linnoila,M., Mattila,M.J.
Modification by diazepam or thioridazine of the psychomotor skills related to driving: a subacute trial in neurotic outpatients.
Brit.J.Clin.Pharmacol. 3, 843-8 (1976)

2361. Sahgal,A., Iversen,S.D.
The effects of chlordiazepoxide on a delayed pair comparison task in pigeons.
Psychopharmacology 59, 57-64 (1978)

2362. Sambrooks,J.E., MacCulloch,M.J., Birtles,C.J., Sullman,C.
Assessment of the effects of flurazepam and nitrazepam on visuo-motor performance using an automated assessment technique.
Acta Psychiat.Scand. 48, 443-54 (1972)

2363. Sambrooks,J.E., MacCulloch,M., Rooney,J.F.F.
The automated assessment of the effect of flurazepam and nitrazepam on mood state.
Acta Psychiat.Scand. 51, 201-9 (1975)

2364. Sanghavi,N.M., Jivani,N.G.
Colorimetric method for the determination of nitrazepam.
Talanta 26, 63-4 (1979)

2365. Sawada,H., Hara,A.
Identification of new urinary metabolites and biotransformation of nitrazepam.
Yakugaku Zasshi 99, 30-7 (1979)

2366. Schallek,W., Kuehn,A.
Effects of benzodiazepines on spontaneous EEG and arousal responses of cats.
Progr.Brain Res. 18, 231 (1965)

2367. Schallek,W., Thomas,J., Kuehn,A., Zabransky,F.
Effects of mogadon on response to stimulation of sciatic nerve, amygdala and hypothalamus of cat.
Int.J.Neuropharmacol. 4, 317 (1965)

2368. Schapira,K., McClelland,H.A., Newell,D.J.
A comparison of high- and low-dose lorazepam with amylobarbitone in patients with anxiety states.
Amer.J.Psychiat. 134, 25-8 (1977)

2369. Schenberg,L.C., Graeff,F.G.
Role of the periaqueductal gray substance in the antianxiety action of benzodiazepines.
Pharmacol.Biochem.Behav. 9, 287-95 (1978)

2370. Schenker,S.
Effects of liver disease and of aging on the disposition and elimination of sedatives.
Trans.Amer.Clin.Climatol.Assoc. 89, 91-9 (1977)

2371. Schillings,R.T., Russel,P.B., Ruelius,H.W.
The binding of ^{14}C-lorazepam (^{14}C-Wy-4036) to human plasma proteins.
Wyeth General Technical/Medical Report 5393 (1975)

2372. Schlicht,H.J., Schmidt,Gg., Gelbke,H.P.
Häufigkeit positiver Diazepam-Befunde bei Sektionsfällen.
Frequency of Positive Diazepam-samples in Postmortem Examinations.
Z.Rechtsmed. 82, 271-7 (1979)

2373. Schmid,W., Staiger,G.R.
Chromosome studies on bone marrow from chinese hamsters treated with benzodiazepine tranquillizers and cyclophosphamide.
Mutation Res. 7, 99-108 (1969)

2374. Schubert,B., Malmgren,G.
Diazepam - en klinisk-analytisk undersökning.
Opuscula Med. 8, 288 (1969)

2375. Schüppel,R.
Pharmakokinetische Wechselwirkungen von Alkohol mit Arzneimitteln - Beiträge zur Pathogenese von Kombinationswirkungen.
Unfall- und Sicherheitsforschung Straßenverkehr, 10, 81-92 (1977)
(Kongreßbericht 1977 der Deutschen Gesellschaft für Verkehrsmedizin)

2376. Schultze,K.W., Patt,V.
Zur Behandlung der Abortus imminens mit Valium, einem Benzodiazepinpräparat.
Geburtsh.u.Frauenheilk. 23, 1003-9 (1963)

2377. Schwandt,H.J., Sadée,W., Beyer,K.H., Hildebrandt,A.G.
Effects of enzyme induction and inhibition on microsomal oxidation of 1,4-benzodiazepines.
Naunyn-Schmiedeberg's Arch.Pharmakol. 294, 91-7 (1976)

2378. Schweitzer,H.
Die visuelle Wahrnehmung bei Kombination von Alkohol mit Valium.
Aktuelle Fragen der gerichtlichen Medizin, Bd. III, 218-27 (1968)

2379. Scollo-Lavizzari,G., Pralle,W., De la Cruz,N.
Clinical experience with clonazepam (Rivotril) in the treatment of epilepsy in adults.
Europ.Neurol. 11, 340-4 (1974)

2380. Seitzinger,R.W.T.
Chemisch-analytisch onderzoek van benzodiazepinen in farmaceutische bereidingen (II).
Pharm.Weekbl. 110, 1109 (1975)

2381. Seixas,F.A.
Alcohol and its drug interactions.
Ann.Internal Med. 83, 86-92 (1975)

2382. Sellers,E.M., MacLeod,S.M., Greenblatt,D.J., Giles,H.G.
Inhibition of chlordiazepoxide biotransformation by disulfiram.
Clin.Res. 24, 652 A (1976)

2383. Sellers,E.M., MacLeod,S.M., Greenblatt,D.J., Giles,H.G.
Influence of disulfiram and disease on benzodiazepine disposition.
Clin.Pharmacol.Ther. 21, 117 (1977)

2384. Seppälä,T., Saario,I., Mattila,M.J.
Two weeks treatment with chlorpromazine, thioridazine, sulpiride, or bromazepam: actions and interactions with alcohol on psychomotor skills related to driving.
In: Modern Problems of Pharmacopsychiatry, Vol. 11, Alcohol, Drugs and Driving, S. Karger, Basel 1976, S. 85-90

2385. Shepherd,M.
The benzodiazepines.
Prescribers' J. 12, 144-7 (1972)

2386. Sherliker,J.
A comparison of lorazepam and diazepam in general practice.
Curr.Med.Res.Opinion 1, 308-16 (1973)

2387. Shershin,P.H., Katz,S.S.
Diazepam in the treatment of tetanus. Report of a case following tooth extraction.
Clin.Med. 71, 362-6 (1964)

2388. Shimizu,S., Yamauchi,Y., Ikuta,J., Ishii,T., Ueki,S.
Effects of prazepam on electroencephalogram and pressor response to hypothalamic stimulation.
Igaku Kenkyu 48, 220-30 (1978)

2389. Shimizu,S., Yamauchi,Y., Ueki,S.
Behavioral effects of prazepam.
Igaku Kenkyu 48, 189-209 (1978)

2390. Smart,R.G., Schmidt,W., Bateman,K.
Psychoactive drugs and traffic accidents.
J.Safety Res. 1, 67-73 (1969)

2391. Smith,C.M.
Interactions of drugs of abuse with alcohol.
Ann.N.Y.Acad.Sci. 281, 384-92 (1976)

2392. Smith,J.M., Misiak,H.
Critical flicker frequency (CFF) and psychotropic drugs in normal human subjects - a review.
Psychopharmacology 47, 175-82 (1976)

2393. Smyth,D., Pennington,G.W., Jackson,N.
Identification reactions of chlordiazepoxide (Librium) and the product of acid hydrolysis 2-amino-5-chloro-benzophenone.
Arch.Int.Pharmacodyn. 145, 147-53 (1963)

2394. Snider,W.D., Demaria,A.A., Mann,J.D.
Diazepam and dialysis encephalopathy.
Neurology 29, 414-5 (1979)

2395. Soares,E.L., Costa,M.H., Massa,L., Costa,S., Tavares,R.
Flunitrazepam (Ro 5-4200) como agente de induccion anesthesia.
Rev.Esp.Anest. 21, 489 (1974)

2396. Sokol,G.H., Greenblatt,D.J., Lloyd,B.L., Georgotas, A., Allen,M.D., Harmatz,J.S., Smith,T.W., Shader,R.I.
Effect of abdominal radiation therapy on drug absorption in humans.
J.Clin.Pharmacol. 18, 388-96 (1978)

2397. Soubrie,P., Thiebot,M.H., Simon,P., Boissier,J.R.
Benzodiazepines and behavioral effects of reward (water) omission in the rat.
Psychopharmacology 59, 95-100 (1978)

2398. Speth,R.C., Wastek,G.J., Yamamura,H.I.
Benzodiazepine receptors - temperature-dependence of ^{3}H-Flunitrazepam binding.
Life Sci. 24, 351-7 (1979)

2399. Speth,R.C., Yamamura,H.I.
Alterations in benzodiazepine receptors in cerebellar of mutant mice.
Fed.Proc. 38, 687 (1979)

2400. Staak,M., Gottwald,K., Mallach,H.J., Schubring,G.
Pharmakopsychiologische Untersuchungen über Wechselwirkungen zwischen Alkohol und Oxazepam im Hinblick auf das Reaktionsverhalten. I. Mitteilung: Veränderungen der psychomotorischen Koordination und des Reaktionsverhaltens.
Int.J.Clin.Pharmacol. 14, 48-65 (1976)

2401. Staak,M., Gottwald,K., Mallach,H.J., Schubring,G.
Pharmakopsychiologische Untersuchungen über Kombinationswirkungen von Alkohol und Oxazepam auf das Reaktionsverhalten.
II. Mitteilung: Subjektive Befindlichkeit und Reaktionsverhalten.
Int.J.Clin.Pharmacol. 15, 234-44 (1977)

2402. Staak,M., Raff,G., Moosmayer,A.
Experimentelle Untersuchungen über die Auswirkungen von Dikaliumchlorazepat auf das Reaktionsverhalten.
Unfall- und Sicherheitsforschung Straßenverkehr, 10 (1977), 173-7
(Kongreßbericht 1977 der Deutschen Gesellschaft für Verkehrsmedizin)

2403. Staiger,G.R.
Chlordiazepoxide and diazepam: absence of effects on the chromosomes of diploid human fibroblast cells.
Mutation Res. 7, 109-15 (1969)

2404. Staiger,G.R.
Studies on the chromosomes of human lymphocytes treated with diazepam in vitro.
Mutation Res. 10, 635-44 (1970)

2405. Starley,J.W., Fangman,T.R., Michie,D.D.
Cardiovascular response of injectable diazepam in conscious dogs.
Clin.Res. 17, 518 (1969)

2406. Starley,J.W., Michie,D.D.
Hemodynamic alterations produced by intravenous diazepam in conscious, unrestrained dogs.
Curr.Ther.Res.Clin.Exp. 11, 796-801 (1969)

2407. Stefko,P.L., Zbinden,G.
Effect of chlorpromazine, chlordiazepoxide, diazepam and chlorprothixene on bile flow and intrabiliary pressure on cholecystectomized dogs.
Amer.J.Gastroent. 39, 410-7 (1963)

2408. Stenchever,M.A., Frankel,R.B.
Some effects of diazepam in human cells in vitro.
Amer.J.Obstet.Gynec. 103, 836-42 (1969)

2409. Stenchever,M.A., Frankel,R.S., Jarvis,J.A.
Effect of diazepam on chromosomes of human leukocytes in vivo.
Amer.J.Obstet.Gynec. 107, 456-60 (1970)

2410. Sternbach,L.H.
The discovery of Librium.
Agents and Actions 2, 193-6 (1972)

2411. Sternbach,L.H.
The benzodiazepine story.
Progr.Drug Res. 22, 229-66 (1978)

2412. Stika,L.
Arzneimittelverbrauch und pharmakotherapeutische Gruppen.
Die Pharmazie (Pharmazeutische Praxis) 38-42 (1977)

2413. Stimmel,B.
Cardiovascular Effects of Mood-Altering Drugs.
Raven Press, New York 1979

2414. Stovner,J., Vangen,O.
Diazepam compared to thiopentone as induction agent for Caesarean sections.
Acta Anaesth.Scand. 18, 264 (1974)

2415. Sturdee,D.W.
Diazepam: Routes of administration and rate of absorption. A study of woman with preclampsia.
Brit.J.Anaesth. 48, 1091-6 (1976)

2416. Tansella,M., Burti,L., Siciliani,O., Zimmermann,C., Schiavon,M., Gerna,M., Tognoni,G., Morselli,P.L.
N-desmethyldiazepam and amylobarbitone sodium as hypnotics in anxious patients: Correlations between plasma levels and behavioral test.
Psychopharmacologia

2417. Tansella,M., Zimmermann-Tansella,C., Lader,M.
The residual effects of N-desmethyldiazepam in patients.
Psychopharmacologia 38, 81-90 (1974)

2418. Tarnow,J., Hess,W., Schmidt,D., Eberlein,H.J.
Induction of anesthesia in patients with coronary-artery disease - flunitrazepam, diazepam, ketamine, fentanyl - hemodynamic study.
Anaesthesis 28, 9-19 (1979)

2419. Taylor,P.L., Daniell,H.B., Bagwell,E.E.
Studies on the myocardial hemodynamic and metabolic effects of diazepam in the dog.
Pharmacologist 12, 233 (1970)

2420. Tolksdorf,W., Berlin,J., Bethke,U., Striebel,J.P., Westphal,K.T., Lutz,H.
Sedative and amnesic effects of flunitrazepam during regional anesthesia.
Prakt.Anästh. 14, 59-70 (1979)

2421. Tolksdorf,W., Rohowsky,R., Klose,R., Lutz,H.
Influence of sedation with diazepam and flunitrazepam during regional anesthesia upon post-operative pulmonary performance.
Prakt.Anästh. 14, 52-8 (1979)

2422. Tosi,G.C., Tosi,E.C., Hattab,J.R.
The use of N-demethyldiazepam in outpatients suffering from insomnia.
Curr.Ther.Res. 15, 460-4 (1973)

2423. Touchard,P., Bobin,P.
Contribution á l'étude du diazépam en anesthesiologie.
Anaesth.Analg.Reanim. 23, 599-631 (1966)

2424. Toulouse,R.
Utilisation du diazépam intraveineux au cours de menaces d'avortements ou d'accouchements prématurés.
Bull.Féd.Soc.Gynéc.Obstét.franc. 17, 529-31 (1965)

2425. Towler,M.L.
The clinical use of diazepam in anxiety states and depressions.
J.Neuropsychiat. 3, Suppl. 1, 68-72 (1962)

2426. Tyrer,P.J., Lader,M.H.
Physiological and psychiological effects of ± propanol, + propanol and diazepam in induced anxiety.
Brit.J.Clin.Pharmacol. 1, 379-85 (1974)

2427. Vandemark,F.L., Adams,R.F.
Determination of some benzodiazepines in serum utilizing gas chromatography and a nitrogen detector.
Chromatogr.Newsletter 5, 4-7 (1977)

2428. Vapaatalo,H., Karppanen,H.
Influence of ethanol on the toxicity of some psychotropic drugs.
Scand.J.Clin.Lab.Invest. 23, 77 (1969)

2429. Vesell,E.S., Passananti,G.T., Viau,J.P. et al.
Effects of chronic prazepam administration on drug metabolism in man and rat.
Pharmacology 7, 197-206 (1972)

2430. Venzlaff,U.
Über Valium-Mißbrauch und Valium-Sucht.
Tägl.Praxis 13, 349 (1972)

2431. Vietor,K.W.
Diazepam gestattet beim Säugling Herzkatheterisierung ohne Narkose.
Med.Trib. (Wiesbaden) 7, No. 3a, 6 (1972)

2432. Votova,Z., Vojtechovsky,M.
An experimental and clinical contribution to interaction of alcohol and diazepam.
Activites Nervosa Superior 13, 197-8 (1971)

2433. Wastek,G.J., Speth,R.C., Reisine,T.D., Yamamura,H.I.
The effect of GABA on ^{3}H-flunitrazepam binding in rat brain.
Eur.J.Pharmacol. 50, 445-7 (1978)

2434. Wehlage,D.F.
Diazepam phlebitis.
J.Amer.Med.Ass. 224, 128 (1973)

2435. Wendt,G.
Schicksal des Hypnotikums Flunitrazepam im menschlichen Organismus.
In: W.Hügin, G.Hossli, M.Gemperle (eds.), Bisherige Erfahrungen mit "Rohypnol" (Flunitrazepam) in der Anästhesiologie und Intensivtherapie, F.Hoffmann-La Roche & Co.AG, Basel, 1976, pp. 27-38

2436. Wesley,W.H., Yakatan,G.J., Maness,D.D.
Kinetics and mechanisms of hydrolysis of 1,4-benzodiazepines. I: Chlordiazepoxide and Demoxepam.
J.Pharm.Sci. 65, 1198 (1976)

2437. Whitman,E.N., Stern,M.M.
Correlation of serum levels with EEG effects of chlordiazepoxide in man.
J.Newark City Hosp. 3, 3-10 (1966)

2438. Wickström,E.
Flunitrazepam (Ro 5-4200)-ett nytt hypnoticum.
Tids.Norske Laegeforen 93, 1494 (1973)

2439. Wickstrom,M.E.
Clinical trial of flurazepam.
In: Sleep, W.P.Koella and P.Levin (eds.). Karger, Basel 1973

2440. Wiechman,B.E., Spratto,G.R.
Interactions of diazepam and cocaine in morphine-treated rats.
Fed.Proc. 38, 682 (1979)

2441. Wiersum,J.
Psychotropic drugs in addiction.
JAMA 227, 79 (1974)

2442. Wilkinson,I.M.S.
The influence of drugs and alcohol upon human eye movement.
Proc.Roy.Soc.Med. 69, 479-80 (1976)

2443. Williams,M., Risley,E.A.
Enhancement of the binding of ^{3}H-diazepam to rat-brain membranes invitro by SQ-20009, a novel anxiolytic, GABA and muscimol.
Life Sci. 24, 833-41 (1979)

2444. Winstead,D., Anderson,A., Eilers,K., Blackwell, B., Zaremba,A.L.
Diazepam on demand: drug seeking behaviour in psychiatric in-patients.
Arch.Gen.Psychiatry 30, 349-51 (1974)

2445. Wise,C.D.
Benzodiazepines: Anxiety reducing activity by reduction of serotonin turnover in the brain.
Science 177, 180 (1972)

2446. Witten,G.L.
The use and abuse of psychic drugs.
General Practitioner 34, 175 (1966)

2447. Wittenborn,J.R., Flaherty,C.F., Hamilton,L.W., Schiffman,H.R., McGough,W.E.
The effect of minor tranquilizers on psychomotor performance.
Psychopharmacologia 47, 281-6 (1976)

2448. Wong,H.Y.C., Nighting ,T.E., Richardi,J.C., David,S.N., Orimilik ,S.O.
Long-term effect of diazepam (valium) on plasma-lipids, aortic artherosclerosis and blood pressures of atherogenic-fed roosters.
Fed.Proc. 38, 445 (1979)

2449. Woody,G.E., O'Brien,C.P., Greenstein,R.
Misuse and abuse of diazepam: An increasingly common medical problem.
Int.J.Addict. 10, 843-8 (1975)

2450. Yamauchi,Y., Shimizu,S., Nakamura,M., Ishihama,H., Sano,N., Ueki,S.
Behavioral effects of prazepam and its metabolites.
Igaku Kenkyu 48, 210-9 (1978)

2451. Young,W.S., Kuhar,M.J.
Auto-radiography of opiate and benzodiazepine receptors - invitro labeling of tissue-sections.
Fed.Proc. 38, 687 (1979)

2452. Zimmermann,A.M.
Comparative effects of flurazepam hydrochloride (Dalmane) and placebo in patients with insomnia.
Curr.Ther.Res. 13, 18-22 (1971)

2453. Zimmermann-Tansella,C., Tansella,M., Lader,M.
The effects of chlordesmethyldiazepam on behavioral performance and subjective judgement in normal subjects.
J.Clin.Pharmacol. 16, 481-8 (1976)

2454. Zsoter,T.T., Gospodarowicz,M.
The effect of diazepam and pentazocine on the venomotor reflexes in man.
J.Clin.Pharmacol.N.Drugs 12, 89-94 (1972)

2455. Zuccaro,G.M., Delfino,U., Graziani,M. et al.
Influenzy del metildiazepione ad alte dosie sull'apparato cardiovasculare del coniglio.
Minerva Anesth. 35, 406-15 (1969)

2456. Unpublished Data

2457. Personal Communication

Addendum 1

2458. Boehringer Ingelheim (Firmenschrift)
Albego^R - Albego^R forte - Tranquilizer.
15 S., Ingelheim am Rhein 1978

2459. Hoechst AG (Firmenschrift)
Frisium^R 10 - Frisium^R 20.
62 S., Frankfurt/Main 1977

2460. Biehl,P.
Studies of clobazam and car-driving.
Brit.J.Clin.Pharmacol. 7, 85-90 (1979)

2461. Fielding,S., Hoffmann,I.
Pharmacology of anti-anxiety drugs with special reference to clobazam.
Brit.J.Clin.Pharmacol. 7, 7-15 (1979)

2462. Gerhards,H.J.
Neuro-pharmacological profile of clobazam, a new 1,5-benzodiazepine.
Brit.J.Clin.Pharmacol. 7, 23-4 (1979)

2463. Hindmarch,I.
Some aspects of the effects of clobazam on human psychomotor performance.
Brit.J.Clin.Pharmacol. 7, 77-82 (1979)

2464. Hunt,P.
Assay of clobazam in human-serum by a radio-receptor technique.
Brit.J.Clin.Pharmacol. 7, 37-40 (1979)

2465. Meldrum,B.S., Chapman,A.G., Horton,R.W.
Clobazam - anticonvulsant action in animal-models of epilepsy.
Brit.J.Clin.Pharmacol. 7, 59-60 (1979)

2466. Rupp,W., Badian,M., Christ,O., Hajdu,P., Kulkarni,R.D., Taeuber,K., Uihlein,M., Bender,R., Vanderberg,O.
Pharmacokinetics of single and multiple doses of clobazam in humans.
Brit.J.Clin.Pharmacol. 7, 51-7 (1979)

2467. Schuetz,E.
Toxicology of clobazam.
Brit.J.Clin.Pharmacol. 7, 33-5 (1979)

2468. Taeuber,K., Badian,M., Brettel,H.F., Royen,T., Rupp,W., Sittig,W., Uihlein,M.
Kinetic and dynamic interaction of clobazam and alcohol.
Brit.J.Clin.Pharmacol. 7, 91-7 (1979)

2469. Volz,M., Christ,O., Kellner,H.M., Kuch,H., Fehlhaber, H.W., Gantz,D., Hajdu,P., Cavagna,F.
Kinetics and metabolism of clobazam in animals and man.
Brit.J.Clin.Pharmacol. 7, 41-50 (1979)

2470. Celli,L., Santagostino,C.
Camazepam versus diazepam: a double-blind study during endoscopy insepction.
Curr.Ther.Res. 16, 457-60 (1974)

2471. Cesa-Bianchi,M., Ghirardi,P., Ravaccia,F.
A preliminary double-blind study with SB 5833 (camazepam), a new benzodiazepine derivative.
Arzneim.-Forsch. (Drug Res.) 24, 2032-5 (1974)

2472. Ferrini,R., Miragoli,G., Taccardi,B.
Neuropharmacological studies on SB 5833, a new psychotherapeutic agent of the benzodiazepine class.
Arzneim.-Forsch. (Drug Res.) 24, 2029-32 (1974)

2473. Galli,G.
Camazepam (SB 5833) in preparation for endoscopy inspection: open and double-blind study versus diazepam.
Curr.Ther.Res. 19, 316-9 (1976)

2474. Merlo,L., Noseda,V., Ferrini,R., Miragoli,G., Marchetti, G.
Effect of camazepam (SB 5833), a new antianxious drug, on cardiac contractility and coronary hemodynamics.
Arzneim.-Forsch. (Drug Res.) 24, 1759-62 (1974)

2475. Tammaro,A., Picceo,M.T., Gemmellaro,P., Bonaccorso, O.
Camazepam versus placebo. A double-blind clinical study on geriatric patients suffering from psychic complaints.
Arzneim.-Forsch. (Drug Res.) 27, 2177-8 (1977)

2476. Aderjan,R., Schmidt, Gg.
Ein Screening-Radioimmunoassay für 1,4-Benzodiazepine in menschlichem Blut, Serum und Urin mit Antikörpern gegen Oxazepamhemisuccinat.
Z.Rechtsmed. 83, 191-200 (1979)

2477. Battista,H.-J., Udermann,H., Henning,G., Vycudilik,W.
Zum Nachweis der Benzodiazepine in der forensischen Chemie.
Beitr.gerichtl.Med. 37, 5-28 (1979)

2478. Caccia,S., Ballabio,M., Guiso,G., Zanini,M.G.
Gas-liquid chromatographic determination of clobazam and N-desmethylclobazam in plasma.
J.Chromatogr. 164, 100-5 (1979)

2479. Emery,M., Kowtko,J.
High-performance liquid chromatography of benzodiazepines. I: Stability-indicating assay of diazepam tablets.
J.Pharm.Sci. 68, 1185-7 (1979)

2480. Higuchi,S., Urabe,H., Shiobara,Y.
Simplified determination of lorazepam and oxazepam in biological fluids by gas-chromatography - mass spectrometry.
J.Chromatogr. 164, 55-61 (1979)

2481. Hunt,P., Husson,J.-M., Raynaud,J.-P.
A radioreceptor assay for benzodiazepines.
J.Pharm.Pharmacol. 31, 448-51 (1979)

2482. Kelly,R.C., Anthony,R.M., Krent,L., Thompson,W.L., Sunshine,I.
Toxicological determination of benzodiazepines in serum: Methods and concentrations associated with high-dose intravenous therapy with diazepam.
Clin.Toxicology 14, 445-57 (1979)

2483. Lund,W., Hannisdal,M., Greibrokk,T.
Evaluation of amperometric detectors for high-performance liquid chromatography: Analysis of benzodiazepines.
J.Chromatogr. 173, 249-61 (1979)

2484. MacKichan,J.J., Jusko,W.J., Duffner,P.K., Cohen, M.E.
Liquid-chromatographic assay of diazepam and its major metabolites in plasma.
Clin.Chem. 25, 856-9 (1979)

2485. McCurdy,H.H., Slightom,E.L., Harrill,J.C.
Diazepam and desmethyldiazepam quantitation in whole blood by nitrogen-sensitive detector after derivatization.
J.Anal.Toxicol. 3, 195-8 (1979)

2486. Min,B.H., Garland,W.A., Khoo,K.-C., Torres,G.S.
Determination of clonazepam and its amino and acetamido metabolites in human plasma by combined gas chromatography chemical ionization mass spectrometry and selected ion monitoring.
Biomed.Mass Spectrometry 5, 692-8 (1978)

2487. Noggle,F.T.,jr., Clark,C.R.
Identification of some benzodiazepines of forensic interest.
J.Assoc.Off.Anal.Chem. 62, 799-807 (1979)

2488. Owen,F., Lofthouse,R., Bourne,R.C.
A radioreceptor assay for diazepam and its metabolites in serum.
Clin.Chim.Acta 93, 305-10 (1979)

2489. Rosenblatt,J.E., Bridge,T.P., Wyatt,R.J.
A novel method for measuring benzodiazepines in saliva.
Comm.Psychopharmacology 3, 49-53 (1979)

2490. Smith,M.T., Evans,L.E.J., Eadie,M.J., Tyrer,J.H.
Pharmacokinetics of prazepam in man.
Eur.J.Clin.Pharmacol. 16, 141-7 (1979)

2491. Stewart,J.T., Honigberg,I.L., Tsai,A.Y., Hajdu,P.
Fluorometric determination of clobazam, a 1,5-benzodiazepine in human plasma.
J.Pharm.Sci. 68, 494-6 (1979)

2492. Vree,T.B., Baars,A.M., Hekster,Y.A., Van Der Kleijn,E.
Simultaneous determination of diazepam and its metabolites N-desmethyldiazepam, oxydiazepam and oxazepam in plasma and urine of man and dog by means of high-performance liquid chromatography.
J.Chromatogr. 162, 605-14 (1979)

2493. Wallace,J.E., Schwertner,H.A., Shimek,E.L.,jr.
Analysis for diazepam and nordiazepam by electron-capture gas chromatography and by liquid chromatography.
Clin.Chem. 25, 1296-1300 (1979)

2494. Cuisinaud,G., Peillon,E., Ferry,N., Deruaz,D., Sassard,J.
Simple and sensitive gas chromatographic method for the determination of camazepam in human plasma.
J.Chromatogr. 178, 314-9 (1979)

2495. Aderjan,R., Schmidt,Gg.
Die Bedeutung der quantitativen Benzodiazepin-Analyse in Urin- und Blutproben - Pharmakokinetischer Ansatz zur gutachterlichen Beurteilung von Dosis und Wirkung bei Diazepam.
Med.Sachverst. 76, 92-6 (1980)

2496. Aderjan,R., Fritz,P., Mattern,R.
Zur Bedeutung des Nachweises und der Pharmakokinetik von Flurazepam-Metaboliten in menschlichem Blut.
Arzneim.-Forsch. (Drug Res.) 30, 1944-7 (1980)

2497. Aderjan,R., Mattern,R.
Eine tödlich verlaufene Monointoxikation mit Flurazepam (Dalmadorm[R]).
Arch.Toxicol. 43, 69-75 (1979)

2498. Harrer,G., Leutner,V., Leickert,K.H.
Schlaf und Pharmakon - Symposion 1978
Editiones Roche Basel 1979

2499. Priest,R.G., Pletscher,A., Ward,J.
Sleep Research - Proceedings of the Northern European Symposium on Sleep Research.
MTP Press Limited, International Medical Publishers Basle 1978

2500. Hügin,W., Hossli,G., Gemperle,M.
Bisherige Erfahrungen mit Rohypnol (Flunitrazepam) in der Anästhesiologie und Intensivtherapie.
Editiones Roche Basel 1976

2501. Rohypnol (Flunitrazepam). Pharmakologische Grundlagen - Klinische Anwendung.
hrsg. von Ahnefeld,F.W., Bergmann,H., Burri,C., Dick,W., Hålmagyi,M., Hossli,G., Rügheimer,E.
Springer - Berlin Heidelberg New York 1978

2502. Wickstrøm,E., Amrein,R., Haefelfinger,P., Hartmann,D.
Pharmacokinetic and clinical observations on prolonged administration.
Eur.J.Clin.Pharmacol. 17, 189-96 (1980)

2503. Adams,W.J.
Specific and sensitive high performance liquid chromatographic determination of alprazolam or triazolam.
Anal.Lett. 12, 657-71 (1979)

2504. Breimer,D.D.
Pharmacokinetics and metabolism of various benzodiazepines used as hypnotics.
Brit.J.Clin.Pharm. 8, 7S-13S (1979)

2505. Cooper,S.J., Francis,R.L.
Water intake and time course of drinking after single or repeated chlordiazepoxide injections.
Psychopharmacology 65, 191-5 (1979)

2506. Cornelissen,P.J.G., Beijersbergen,G.M.J., Gerritsma,K.W.
Photochemical decomposition of 1,4-benzodiazepines. Chlordiazepoxide.
Int.J.Pharm. 3, 205-20 (1979)

2507. De Gier,J.J., t'Hart,B.J.
Sensitive gas chromatographic method for the determination of diazepam and N-desmethyl-diazepam in plasma.
J.Chromatogr. 163, 304-9 (1979)

2508. Gasparic,J., Zamak,J., Sedmera,P., Breberova,Z., Volke,J.
Products of the acid hydrolysis of 7-chloro-1,3-dihydro-3-hydroxy-5-phenyl-2H-1,4-benzo - diazepin-2-one (oxazepam).
Coll.Czech.Chem.Commun. 44, 2243-9 (1979)

2509. Giusti,G.V., Chiarotti,M.
Lethal nitrazepam intoxications - report of two cases.
Z.Rechtsmed. 84, 75-8 (1979)

2510. Hailey,D.M., Baird,E.S.
Plasma concentrations of medazepam and its metabolites after oral administration.
Brit.J.Anaesth. 51, 493-6 (1979)

2511. Jatlow,P., Dobular,K., Bailey,D.
Serum diazepam concentrations in overdose. Their significance.
Amer.J.Clin.Path. 72, 571-7 (1979)

2512. Kangas,L.
Urinary elimination of nitrazepam and its main metabolites.
Acta pharmacol.et toxicol. 45, 16-9 (1979)

2513. Kangas,L., Allonen,H., Lammintausta,R., Salonen,M., Pekkarinen,A.
Pharmacokinetics of nitrazepam in saliva and serum after a single oral dose.
Acta pharmacol.et toxicol. 45, 20-4 (1979)

2514. Kangas,L., Iisalo,E., Kanto,J., Lehtinen,V., Pynnönen,S., Ruikka,J., Salminen,J., Sillanpää, M., Syvälahti,E.
Human pharmacokinetics of nitrazepam: Effect of age and diseases.
Eur.J.Clin.Pharmacol. 15, 163-70 (1979)

2515. Kanto,J., Aaltonen,L., Kangas,L., Erkkola,R., Pitkänen,Y.
Placental transfer and breast milk levels of flunitrazepam.
Curr.Ther.Res. 26, 539-46 (1979)

2516. Kiereś,H.
Metoda spektrofotometryczna dla oznaczania niektórych pochodnych benzodwuazepiny w przypadkach zatruc.
Bromat.Chem.Toksykol. 12, 289-92 (1979)

2517. MacKichan,J., Duffner,P.K., Cohen,M.E.
Adsorption of diazepam to plastic tubing.
N.Engl.J.Med. 301, 332-3 (1979)

2518. Miller,F., Nulsen,J.
Diazepam (Valium) detoxification.
J.Nerv.Ment.Dis 167, 637-8 (1979)

2519. Müller,W.E.
Der Benzodiazepinrezeptor.
Dtsch.Med.Wschr. 105, 69-71 (1980)

2520. Smyth,M.R., Beng,T.S., Smyth,W.F.
A spectral and polarographic study of the acid-base and complexing behaviour of bromazepam.
Anal.Chim.Acta 92, 129-38 (1977)

2521. Palva,E.S., Linnoila,M., Saario,I., Mattila,M.J.
Acute and subacute effects of diazepam on psychomotor skills: Interaction with alcohol.
Acta pharmacol.et toxicol. 45, 257-64 (1979)

2522. Peat,M.A., Finkle,B.S., Deyman,M.E.
High-pressure liquid chromatographic determination of chlordiazepoxide and its major metabolites in biological fluids.
J.Pharm.Sci. 68, 1467-8 (1979)

2523. Proudfoot,A.T., Park,J.
Suizidale Arzneimittelvérgiftungen. Benzodiazepine verdrängen Barbiturate.
Dtsch.Apoth.-Ztg. 118, 1015 (1978)

2524. Peat,M.A., Kopjak,L., Finkle,B.S.
Screening of benzodiazepines and metabolites.
J.Forens.Sci. 24, 719-21 (1979)

2525. Singlas,E.
Pharmacocinêtique du flunitrazêpam.
Nouv.Presse Med. 8, 2519-23 (1979)

2526. Thoma,J.J.
Screening of benzodiazepines and metabolites.
J.Forens.Sci. 24, 719 (1979)

2527. Tom,H., Schneider,R.S., Ernst,R., Khan,W., Singh,P., Kabakoff,D.
Homogenous enzyme immunoassays for barbiturates and benzodiazepines in serum.
Clin.Chem. 25, 1094 (1979)

2528. Wouters,I., Roets,E., Hoogmartens,J.
Thin-layer chromatographic identification of nineteen benzodiazepine derivatives.
J.Chromatogr. 179, 381-9 (1979)

2529. McBride,R.J., Dundee,J.W., Moore,J., Toner,W., Howard,P.J.
A study of the plasma concentrations of lorazepam in mother und neonate.
Brit.J.Anaesth. 51, 971-8 (1979)

2530. Greenblatt,D.J., Shader,R.R.
Blood Levels of Benzodiazepines: Applications in Medicine and Toxicology.
in: Clinical Pharmacology of Psychoactive Drugs, p. 87-104

2531. HALCION[R] - Triazolam.
Firmenschrift Upjohn GmbH, 6148 Heppenheim/Bergstraße 1980

2532. Bittencourt,P., Richens,A., Toseland,P.A., Wicks,J.F.C., Latham,A.N.
Pharmacokinetics of the hypnotic benzodiazepine, temazepam.
Brit.J.Clin.Pharmacol. 8, 37 S-38 S (1979)

2533. Cano,J.P., Lindoulsi,T., Sumirtapura,Y., Hot,B., Gouezo,F., Viala,A.
Considerations generales sur la methodologie et les cinetiques de deux benzodiazepines: Le clonazepam (Rivotril[R]) et le clobazam (Urbanyl[R]).
Lyon Mêdical 242, 535-44 (1979)

2534. Garland,W.A., Min,B.H.
Determination of clonazepam in human plasma by gas chromatography-negative ion chemical ionization mass spectrometry.
J.Chromatogr. 172, 279-86 (1979)

2535. Kangas,L.
Determination of nitrazepam and its main metabolites in urine by gas-liquid chromatography: Use of electron capture and nitrogen-selective detectors.
J.Chromatogr. 172, 273-8 (1979)

2536. Kuriyama,T., Shibata,M.
A study on Y-6047 (clotiazepam) - absorption, metabolism and excretion in men.
Unpublished

2537. Leutner,V., Müller-Clemm,H.
Ein neuer Weg in der Behandlung von schweren Schlafstörungen: Rohypnol®.
Therapiewoche 29, 5670-82 (1979)

2538. Leutner,V., Müller-Clemm,H.
Rohypnol parenteral das Benzodiazepin für die Anästhesiologie.
Med.Welt 30, 1276-82 (1979)

2539. Nakanishi,M., Setoguchi,M.
Studies on psychotropic drugs.
XX: Effects of Y-6047 (clotiazepam) on the metabolism of biogenic amines.
Arzneim.-Forsch. (Drug Res.) 22, 1914-8 (1972)

2540. Nakanishi,M., Tsumagari,T., Takigawa,Y., Shuto,S., Kenjo,T., Fukuda,T.
Studies on psychotropic drugs.
XIX: Psychopharmacological studies of Y-6047 (clotiazepam).
Arzneim.-Forsch. (Drug Res.) 22, 1905-14 (1972)

2541. Nakazawa,Y., Kotorii,M., Ohshima,M., Horikawa,S., Tachibana,H.
Effects of thienodiazepine derivatives on human sleep as compared to those of benzodiazepine derivatives.
Psychopharmacologia (Berl.) 44, 165-71 (1975)

2542. Oelschläger,H.
Ideales Schlafmittel in Sicht ? - Referat eines Vortrages.
Dtsch.Apoth.-Ztg. 118, 835-7 (1978)

2543. Rambeck,B., Meijer,J.W.A.
Comprehensive method for the determination of antiepileptic drugs using a novel extraction technique and a fully automated gas chromatograph.
Arzneim.-Forsch. (Drug Res.) 29, 99-103 (1979)

2544. Sanjuan,M., Rovei,V.
Methode simple et sensible de dosage du clonazepam.
Lyon Médical 242, 545-9 (1979)

2545. Breiter,J., Helger,R., Lang,H.
Evaluation of column extraction: A new procedure for the analysis of drugs in body fluids.
Forensic Sci. 7, 131-40 (1976)

2546. Helmsing,P.J., van der Woude,J., van Eupen,O.M.
A micromethod for simultaneous estimation of blood levels of some commonly used antiepileptic drugs.
Clin.Chim.Acta 89, 301-9 (1978)

2547. Klotz,U.
Klinische Pharmakokinetik.
Gustav Fischer Verlag, Stuttgart (1979)

2548. Schütz,H., Ebel,S.
Reaktionen auf der DC-Platte.
Pharmazie in unserer Zeit 9, 139-51 (1980)

2549. Trecalmo® (Clotiazepam) - Beipackzettel.
Troponwerke 500 Köln 1979

2550. Paget,G.E.
Quality Control in Toxicology.
MTP Press Ltd. 1977

2551. Drasch,G., v. Meyer,L., Kauert,G.
Veränderungen im Spektrum verkehrsmedizinisch relevanter Arzneimittel in den letzten Jahren.
Kongreßbericht Deutsche Gesellschaft für Verkehrsmedizin e.V., Jahrestagung 1980, Münster, S. 3-6

2552. Möller,M.R.
Klinische und toxikologische Untersuchungen von Blutproben verkehrsauffälliger Verkehrsteilnehmer.
Kongreßbericht Deutsche Gesellschaft für Verkehrsmedizin e.V., Jahrestagung 1980, Münster, S. 46-48

2553. Aaltonen,L., Kanto,J., Salo,M.
Cerebrospinal-fluid concentrations and serum-protein binding of lorazepam and its conjugate.
Acta Pharmacol.Toxicol. 46, 156-8 (1980)

2554. Aaronson,L., Hinman,D.J., Okamoto,M.
Effectiveness of diazepam on ethanol and barbiturate withdrawal.
Fed.Proc. 39, 542 (1980)

2555. Abel,J.G., Sellers,E.M., Naranjo,C.A., Shaw,J., Kadar,D., Romach,M.K.
Inter- and intrasubject variation in diazepam free fraction.
Clin.Pharmacol.Ther. 26, 247-55 (1979)

2556. Aberneth.,D.R., Greenblatt,D.J., Allen,M.D.
Diazepam kinetics in obesity.
Clin.Res. 28, 233 (1980)

2557. Acevesfl.,I.
Comparative clinical-trial of clobazam versus diazepam in menopausal patients.
Inv.Med.Int. 6, 230-9 (1979)

2558. Acevesfl.,I.
Comparative clinical-study of clobazam 20 mg as against lorazepam 2 mg in gynecology.
Inv.Med.Int. 7, 251-60 (1980)

2559. Achté,K.
Anwendung von Benzodiazepinen bei stationären, psychiatrischen Patienten.
Use of Benzodiazepines in Psychiatric In-patients.
New Perspectives in Benzodiazepine Therapy - International Symposium Heidelberg 1979
Arzneim.-Forsch. (Drug Res.) 30, 902-5 (1980)

2560. Acosta,J.R., Lugo,V.M.W., Rios,B.G. Habib,G.L.
Injectable lorazepam as premedication in general-anesthesia - sedative effect, recall of events and safety compared to diazepam.
Rev.Inv.Clin. 31, 369-76 (1979)

2561. Acuda,S.W., Muhangi,J.
Diazepam addiction in Kenya.
E.Afr.Med.J. 56, 76-9 (1979)

2562. Adams,D.
A study of the effects of diazepam (Valium) on the brain-STEM evoked-response.
Clin.Otolar. 5, 351 (1980)

2563. Adams,W.J., Rykert,U.M., Bombardt,P.A.
High performance liquid chromatographic determination of triazolam in human serum.
Analyt.Lett. 13, 149-61 (1980)

2564. Aden,G.C., Ohair,D.E.
Effectiveness of bedtime dosing of benzodiazepines - a placebo-controlled comparison of halazepam and clorazepate.
Clin.Ther. 3, 209-18 (1980)

2565. Aden,G.C., Thein,S.G. Jr.
Alprazolam compared to diazepam and placebo in the treatment of anxiety.
J.Clin.Psychiatry 41, 245-8 (1980)

2566. Adeoshun,I.O., Healy,T.E., Patrick,J.M.
Ventilatory pattern following diazepam and lorazepam.
Anaesthesia 34, 450-2 (1979)

2567. Agoston,S., Salt,P.J., Erdmann,W., Hilkemei., T.
Antagonism of ketamine-diazepam anesthesia by 4-aminopyridine in human volunteers.
Brit.J.Anaest. 52, 367-70 (1980)

2568. Agricola,A., Mazzarini,M., Agriola,R., Urani,R., Fresia,P.
A double-blind, crossover clinical-trial of chlordesmethyldiazepam versus lorazepam in neurotic inpatients - activity on anxiety-depression symptoms.
Clin.Ther. 2, 399-408 (1980)

2569. Ajlouni,K., Elkhatee.,M.
Growth-hormone response to diazepam in diabetics.
Clin.Res. 28, 645 (1980)

2570. Ajlouni,K., Khatib,M.
The effect of glucose on the growth-hormone response to diazepam in normal subjects.
Clin.Res. 28, 384 (1980)

2571. Ali,S.L.
High-performance liquid-chromatographic separation and determination of chlordiazepoxide hydrochloride and 2 of its decomposition products.
Int.J.Pharm. 5, 85-9 (1980)

2572. Allen,M.D., Greenblatt,D.J.
Comparative protein-binding of diazepam and desmethyldiazepam.
Clin.Res. 27, 598 (1979)

2573. Allen,M.D., Greenblatt,D.J.
Desmethyldiazepam kinetics following oral prazepam in the elderly.
Clin.Pharm. 27, 244 (1980)

2574. Allen,M.D., Greenblatt,D.J.
Alcohol does not enhance diazepam absorption.
Clin.Res. 28, 587 (1980)

2575. Allen,M.D., Greenblatt,D.J., Arnold,J.D.
Single- and multiple-dose kinetics of estazolam, a triazolo benzodiazepine.
Psychopharmacology (Berlin) 66, 267-74 (1979)

2576. Allen,M.D., Greenblatt,D.J., Harmatz,J.S., Shader,R.I.
Single-dose kinetics of prazepam, a precursor of desmethyldiazepam.
J.Clin.Pharm. 19, 445-50 (1979)

2577. Allen,M.D., Greenblatt,D.J., Harmatz,J.S., Shader,R.I.
Desmethyldiazepam kinetics in the elderly after oral prazepam.
Clin.Pharm. 28, 196-202 (1980)

2578. Allen,M.D., Greenblatt,D.J., Lacasse,Y., Shader,R.I.
Pharmacokinetic study of lorazepam overdosage.
Amer.J.Psychiatry 137, 1414-5 (1980)

2579. Allen,M.D., Greenblatt,D.J., Noel,B.J.
Self-poisoning with over-the-counter hypnotics.
Clin.Toxicol. 15, 151-68 (1979)

2580. Allen,M.D., Greenblatt,D.J., Shader,R.I.
Single-dose kinetics of oral prazepam.
Clin.Pharm. 25, 211-2 (1979)

2581. Ananth,J., Vandenst.,N.
Clobazam in the treatment of anxiety neurosis - double-blind-study.
Curr.Ther.Res. 26, 119-26 (1979)

2582. Anderson-Baker,W.C., McLaughlin,C.L., Baile,C.A.
Oral and hypothalamic injections of barbiturates, benzodiazepines and cannabinoids and food intake in rats.
Pharmacol.Biochem.Behav. 11, 487-91 (1979)

2583. Anezaki,K., Ando,R., Sakurada,T., Tadano,T., Sakurada, Kisara,K.
Effects of diazepam on rage reaction elicited by the lateral hypothalamus (LH) and on single unit activities in the LH and the basal medial amygdaloid nucleus (ABM) in cats.
Nippon Yakurigaku Zasshi 75, 391-7 (1979)

2584. Anhalt,H.S., Young,R., Roginsky,M.
Double-blind comparison of ketazolam, diazepam and placebo in once-a-day versus t.i.d. dosing.
J.Clin.Psych. 41, 386-92 (1980)

2585. Antoniadis,A., Müller,W.E., Wollert,U.
Central nervous system stimulating and depressing drugs as possible ligands of the benzodiazepine receptor.
Neuropharmacology 19, 121-4 (1980)

2586. Antoniadis,A., Müller,W.E., Wollert,U.
Inhibition of GABA and benzodiazepine receptor-binding by penicillins.
Neurosci. Lett. 18, 309-12 (1980)

2587. Antoniadis,A., Müller,W.E., Wollert,U.
Benzodiazepine receptor interactions may be involved in the neurotoxicity of various penicillin derivatives.
Ann.Neurol. 8, 71-3 (1980)

2588. Arnone,M., Dantzer,R.
Effects of diazepam on extinction induced aggression in pigs.
Pharmacol.Biochem.Behav. 13, 27-30 (1980)

2589. Arnt,J., Christensen,A.V., Scheel-Krueger,J.
Benzodiazepines potentiate GABA-dopamine stereotyped dependent gnawing in mice.
J.Pharm.Pharmacol. 31, 56-8 (1979)

2590. Aromaa,U., Korttila,K., Tammisto,T.
Role of diazepam and fentanyl in the product of balanced anestesia.
Acta Anaesth.Scand. 24, 36-40 (1980)

2591. Arrate,J.K., Ugidos,M., Garciaro.,S., Saitua,G., Degarate,J.
Neonatal tetanum treatment with high-doses of diazepam.
An.Esp.Ped. 13, 243-6 (1980)

2592. Asano,T., Ogasawara,N.
Solubilization of the benzodiazepine receptor from rat brain.
Life Sci. 26, 607-13 (1980)

2593. Ascalone,V.
Determination of chlordiazepoxide and its metabolites in human plasma by reversed-phase high-performance liquid-chromatography.
J.Chromatogr. 181, 141-6 (1980)

2594. Assumpca.,J.A., Bernardi,N., Brown,J., Stone,T.W.
Selective antagonism by benzodiazepines of neuronal responses to excitatory amino-acids in the cerebral-cortex.
Brit.J.Pharmacol. 67, 563-8 (1979)

2595. Ator,N.A.
Differential effects of chlordiazepoxide on comparable rates of responding maintained by food and shock avoidance.
Psychopharmacology (Berlin) 66, 227-31 (1979)

2596. Attwood,D.A.
Effect of moderate levels of alcohol and diazepam on closed-course driving performance.
Ergonomics 22, 757 (1979)

2597. Austin,T.R.
Low-dose ketamine and diazepam during spinal analgesia.
Anaesthesia 35, 391-2 (1980)

2598. Avant,G.R., Speeg,K.V., Freemon,F.R., Schenker,S., Berman,M.L.
Physostigmine reversal of diazepam-induced hypnosis study in human volunteers.
Ann.Int.Med. 91, 53-5 (1979)

2599. Aversa,M.C., Giannett.,P., Romeo,G., Vigorita,M.G.
Nuclear magnetic-resonance of 1,4-benzodiazepine - spatial coupling of 1-substituted 2,3-dihydro-1H-1,4-benzodiazepine.
Chim.Ind.M. 61, 155 (1979)

2600. Aversa,M.C., Romeo,G., Gianett.,P., Ficarra,P., Vigorita,M.G.
Nuclear magnetic-resonance spectra of psychotherapeutic agents. 3. Stereochemistry of 1-methyl-5-phenyl-2,3,4,5-tetrahydro-1H-1,5-benzodiazepine-2,4-diones.
J.Heterocycl.Chem. 17, 551-4 (1980)

2601. Ayd,F.J.
Benzodiazepines - dependence and withdrawal.
J.Amer.Med.Ass. 242, 1401-2 (1979)

2602. Babbini,M., Gaiardi,M., Bartoletti,M.
Anxiolytic versus sedative properties in the benzodiazepines series: Differences in structure-activity relationships.
Life Sci. 25, 15-22 (1979)

2603. Backes,C.R., Cordero,L.
Withdrawal symptoms in the neonate from presumptive intrauterine exposure to diazepam - report of case.
J.Amer.Osteop. 79, 584-5 (1980)

2604. Bailie,G.R., Calder,I.T., Kesson,C.M., Lawson,D.H.
A comparison of temazepam with nitrazepam and with placebo as a hypnotic in medical patients in hospital.
J.Clin.Hosp. 5, 311-7 (1980)

2605. Baker,T., Riker,W.F., Zeldes,G.
A benzodiazepine-anticholinergic drug synergism in the prevention of stress-induced gastric mucosal erosion in mice.
J.Clin.Pharmacol. 19, 409-14 (1979)

2606. Balfour,D.J.K.
Effects of GABA and diazepam on serotonin-H-3 release from hippocampal synaptosomes.
Eur.J.Pharmacol. 68, 11-6 (1980)

2607. Ball,H.A., Davies,J.A., Nicholson,A.N.
Effect of diazepam and its metabolites on the binding of L-tryptophan to human serum albumin.
Brit.J.Pharmacol. 66, 92P-93P (1979)

2608. Ban,T.A., Amin,M.M.
Clobazam: Uncontrolled and standard controlled clinical trials.
Brit.J.Clin.Pharmacol. 7, 135S-138S (1979)

2609. Bantutova,I., Ovcharov,R., Koburova,K.
Changes in the convulsion threshold and in the level of brain biogenic amines in rats chronically treated with phenobarbital or diazepam.
Acta Physiol.Pharmacol.Bulg. 4, 26-9 (1978)

2610. Baraldi,M., Guidotti,A., Schwartz,J.P., Costa,E.
GABA receptors in clonal cell lines: A model for study of benzodiazepine action at molecular level.
Science 205, 821-3 (1979)

2611. Barbato,F., Grieco,C., Silipo,C., Vittoria,A.
A reanalysis of acid-base equilibria of 1,4-benzodiazepines in nonaqueous media.
Farmaco (Prat) 34, 187-201 (1979)

2612. Barclay,A., Houlton,P.C., Downing,J.W.
Total intravenous anesthesia - technique using flunitrazepam, ketamine, muscle-relaxants and controlled ventilation of the lung.
Anaesthesia 35, 287-90 (1980)

2613. Barry,H., Krimmer,E.C.
Differential stimulus attributes of chlordiazepoxide and pentobarbital.
Neuropharmacology 18, 991-8 (1979)

2614. Baselt,R.C.
Analytical Procedures for Therapeutic Drug Monitoring and Emergency Toxicology.
Biomedical Publications - Davis (Calif.) 1980
John Wiley & Sons, New York - Chichester - Brisbane - Toronto (1980)

2615. Battersby,M.K., Richards,J.G., Moehler,H.
Benzodiazepine receptor: Photoaffinity labeling and localization.
Eur.J.Pharmacol. 57, 277-8 (1979)

2616. Baudon,J.J., Blanc,A.M., Berger,J.P., Costil,J., Taburet,A.M., Aymard,P.
Plasma levels of diazepam and N-desmethyldiazepam after intramuscular administration in newborn.
Arch.Fr.Ped. 36,(S1) R 101- R 102 (1980)

2617. Beattie,B.L., Sellers,E.M.
Psychoactive drug-use in the elderly - pharmacokinetics.
Psychosomat. 20, 474-9 (1979)

2618. Beckmann,H., Haas,S.
High-dose diazepam in schizophrenia.
Psychopharmacology 71, 79-82 (1980)

2619. Belkin,J.
Atropine in physostigmine reversal of diazepam.
Anesth.Analg. (Cleve) 59, 459 (1980)

2620. Bell,E.F.
Naloxone reversal of diazepam effects.
Anesthesiol. 53, 264 (1980)

2621. Bellantuono,C., Reggi,C., Tognoni,G., Garattini,S.
Benzodiazepines: Clinical pharmacology and therapeutic use.
Drugs 19, 195-219 (1980)

2622. Bender,A.S., Phillis,J.W., Wu,P.H.
Diazepam and flurazepam inhibit adenosine uptake by rat brain synaptosomes.
J.Pharm.Pharmacol. 32, 293-4 (1980)

2623. Benzer,D., Cushman,P.,Jr.
Alcohol and benzodiazepines: withdrawal syndromes.
Cancer Chemother.Pharmacol. 4, 243-7 (1980)

2624. Berg,S., Dehlin,O., Falkhede.,T., Gatzinsk.,R., Nordqvis.,P.
Long-term study of hypnotic medication in geriatric-patients - a study of dixyrazine, nitrazepam and amylobarbitone.
Scand.J.Soc.Med. 1980, 85-96 (1980)

2625. Berman,M.L.
Diazepam reversal by physostigmine.
Anesth.Anal. 59, 805-6 (1980)

2626. Berntman,L., Welsh,F.A., Bianrosa,J.J., Harp,J.R.
Diazepam fails to protect brain-tissue in hypoxic stress.
Anesthesiol. 51, S 202 (1979)

2627. Bertler,A., Lindgren,S., Malmgren,H.
Pharmacokinetics of dipotassium chlorazepate in patients after repeated 50-mg oral doses.
Psychopharmacology 71, 165-7 (1980)

2628. Besancon,G., Guillore.,A.M., Tuffreau,R.
Clinical-trial of flunitrazepam in a hospital department of general psychiatry.
Nouv.Presse 8, 2538-40 (1979)

2629. Bhattacharyya,P.K.
NMR spectral study of proton transfer in amitriptyline hydrochloride-chlordiazepoxide hydrochloride combinations in dipolar aprotic solvent.
J.Pharm.Sci. 69, 180-3 (1980)

2630. Bhotina.,B., McGarry,J.
Treatment of spasmodic torticollis with clonazepam.
J.Med.Ass.Thailand 62, 395-7 (1979)

2631. Biagi,G.L., Barbaro,A.M., Guerra,M.C., Babbini,M., Gaiardi,M., Bartoletti,M, Borea,P.A.
RM values and structure-activity relationship of benzodiazepines.
J.Med.Chem. 23, 193-201 (1980)

2632. Bianchi,S., Cattaneo,G., Cervi,E., Merluzzi,F., Cassitto,G.
Studio comportamentale di lavoratori addetti alla produzione di benzodiazepine.
Behavioral study of workers engaged in production of benzodiazepines.
Med.Lav. 70, 8-15 (1979)

2633. Bibracher,C.
Camazepam - medicamentous treatment of the psycho-vegetative syndrome.
Med.Welt 31, 855-6 (1980)

2634. Bidwai,A.V., Stanley,T.H.
Antagonism of diazepam by physostigmine - reply
Anesthesiol. 52, 372-3 (1980)

2635. Bidwai,A.V., Stanley,T.H., Rogers,C., Riet,E.K.
Reversal of diazepam-induced postanesthetic somnolence with physostigmine.
Anesthesiol. 51, 256-9 (1979)

2636. Biggio,G., Corda,M.G., De Montis,G., Gessa,G.L.
Differential effects of kainic acid on benzodiazepine receptors, GABA receptors, and GABA-modulin in the cerebellar cortex.
Adv.Biochem.Psychopharmacol. 21, 265-70 (1980)

2637. Biggio,G., Corda,M.G., De Montis,G., Stefanini,E., Gessa,G.L.
Kainic acid differentiates GABA receptors from benzodiazepine receptors in the rat cerebellum.
Brain Res. 193, 589-93 (1980)

2638. Biggio,G., Corda,M.G., Lamberti,C., Gessa,G.L.
Changes in benzodiazepine receptors following GABA-ergic denervation of substantia nigra.
Eur.J.Pharmacol. 58, 215-6 (1979)

2639. Billings.,M., Suria,A., Williams,J.
Effects of picrotoxin, naloxone, and vagotomy on chlordiazepoxide-induced respiratory depression.
Arch.Int.Pharmacodyn.Ther. 242, 95-103 (1979)

2640. Binder,M.
Wirkungsmechanismen psychotroper Drogen.
Med.Mo.Pharm. 4, 10-5 (1981)

2641. Birkmayer,W.
Clinical experiences with clobazam (proceedings).
Brit.J.Clin.Pharmacol. 7, 121S-122S (1979)

2642. Bismuth,C., Dally,S., Lagier,G.
Benzodiazepine physical-dependence - 5 cases.
Intens.Care Med. 6, 68 (1980)

2643. Bismuth,C., Lebellec,M., Dally,S.
Benzodiazepine physical dependance - 6 cases.
Nouv.Presse 9, 1941-5 (1980)

2644. Blanchard,J.C., Boireau,A., Garret,C., Julou,L.
In vitro and in vivo inhibition by zopiclone of benzodiazepine binding to rodent brain receptors.
Life Sci. 24, 2417-20 (1979)

2645. Blaschke,G., Markgraf,H.
Chromatographic resolutions of racemates. 9. Chlorotalidone-enantiomers, chlorotalidone methyl ether-enantioners, and oxazepam-enantiomers.
Chem.Ber. 113, 2031-5 (1980)

2646. Blot,P.
Pharmacology of diazepam and atropine.
Soins 25, 41-3 (1980)

2647. Blume,H.
Reduction of nitrazepam by rat-liver mitochondria.
Arzneim.-Forsch. (Drug Res.) 30, 1566-71 (1980)

2648. Blumenthal,M., Byring,R., Koivula,K.
Comparison of nitrazepam 5 mg with triazolam 0.5 mg in young psychiatric insomniac inpatients - double-blind single night crossover study.
Acta Psych.Scand. 62, 519-24 (1980)

2649. Boakes,R.J., Weston,S.B.
Use of an in vitro hippocampal slice preparation in studies of the actions of the benzodiazepines (proceedings).
Brit.J.Pharmacol. 66, 507P (1979)

2650. Bodnar,R.J., Kelly,D.D., Thomas,L.W., Mansour,A., Brutus,M., Glusman,M.
Chlordiazepoxide antinociception: cross-tolerance with opiates and with stress.
Psychopharmacology (Berlin) 69, 107-10 (1980)

2651. Bogatskii,A.V., Davidenko,T.I., Sevastianov,O.V.
Application of immobilized animal liver microsomal fraction to the reaction of 1,4-benzodiazepine-2-one conversion.
Ukr.Biokhim.Zh. 51, 382-6 (1979)

2652. Bogatskii,A.V., Golovenko,N.I.A., Zinkovskii,V.G.
Intrahepatic circulation of ^{14}C-phenazepam and its metabolites in albino rats.
Biull.Eksp.Biol.Med. 89, 27-9 (1980)

2653. Bogatskii,A.V., Serdyuk,V.V., Nazarov,E.I., Golovenko,N.Y.
Changes in postsynaptic excitation processes in the presence of the soviet benzodiazepine derivative phenazepam.
Biull.Eksp.Biol.Med. 87, 318-21 (1979)

2654. Boghen,D.
Successful treatment of restless legs with clonazepam.
Ann.Neurol. 8, 341 (1980)

2655. Bolelouc.,Z., Boriova,M., Synkova,J., Nahunek,K.
The use of clorotepin and diazepam in a complex therapy of neuroses (controlled comparison).
Activ.Nerv. 22, 180-1 (1980)

2656. Bonaduce,D., Spirito,G., Romano,M., Ferrara,N., Petretta,M., Rengo,F.
Medical evaluation of left-ventricular function in cardiopathic patients during short and longterm treatment with flurazepam.
Minerva Car. 27, 793-800 (1979)

2657. Bonkowski,H.L., Sinclair,P.R., Emery,S., Sinclair,J.F.
Seizure management in acute hepatic porphyria - risks of valproate and clonazepam.
Neurology 30, 588-92 (1980)

2658. Bonnet,M., Kramer,M, Rosa,R.
The hypnotic effectiveness of ketazolam in anxious subjects.
Curr.Ther.Res. 28, 284-93 (1980)

2659. Bonnet,M.H., Webb,W.B., Barnard,G.
Effect of flurazepam, pentobarbital, and caffeine on arousal threshold.
Sleep 1, 271-9 (1979)

2660. Borbe,H.O., Müller,W.E., Wollert,U.
The identification of benzodiazepine receptors with brain-like specificity in bovine retina.
Brain Res. 182, 466-9 (1980)

2661. Borchert,H.H., Schuster,S., Pfeifer,S.
Beeinflussung der UDP-Glucuronyltransferaseaktivität durch Carbamazepin und Clonazepam.
The influence of carbamazepine and clonazepam on UDP-glucuronyltransferase activity.
Pharmazie 34, 450 (1979)

2662. Borea,P.A., Gilli,G., Bertolas.,V.
Application of the free-wilson model to the analysis of 3 different pharmacological activity tests in benzodiazepines.
Farmaco Sci. 34, 1073-82 (1979)

2663. Borenstein,P., Gekiere,F., Allegre,G., Brindeau,F., Cleau,M.
Action of pentobarbital and nitrazepam on the sleep-wakefulness cycle of the cat.
Adv.Biosci. 21, 261-3 (1978)

2664. Bosmann,H.B., Penney,D.P., Case,K.R., Averill,K.
Diazepam receptor: Specific nuclear binding of ^{3}H-flunitrazepam.
Proc.Natl.Acad.Sci.USA 77, 1195-8 (1980)

2665. Botter,P.A.
Single daily dose treatment of anxiety with clobazam - a double-blind-study versus normal multiple-dose treatment with diazepam.
Curr.Med.Res.Opin. 6, 593-7 (1980)

2666. Boulenger,J.P.
Mechanism of action of the benzodiazepines.
New biological data.
Nouv.Presse Med. 8, 2513-8 (1979)

2667. Bourin,M., Breteau,M.
Acute overdosage with benzodiazepine derivatives.
Toxicol.Eur.Res. 2, 163-7 (1979)

2668. Boxenbaum,H.
Interspecies variation in liver weight, hepatic blood-flow, and antipyrine intrinsic clearance-extrapolation of data to benzodiazepines and phenytoin.
J.Pharmacok.Biopharm. 8, 165-76 (1980)

2669. Bradshaw,E.G., Dodson,M., Soden,P.
Diazepam and the neuro-muscular function.
Brit.J.Anaest. 52, 960 (1980)

2670. Bradshaw,E.G., Maddison,S.
Effect of diazepam at the neuromuscular function.
A clinical study.
Brit.J.Anaesth. 51, 955-60 (1979)

2671. Braestrup,C., Nielsen,M.
Benzodiazepin-Rezeptoren.
Benzodiazepine Receptors.
New Perspectives in Benzodiazepine Therapy - International Symposium Heidelberg 1979.
Arzneim.-Forsch. (Drug Res.) 30, 852-7 (1980)

2672. Braestrup,C., Nielsen,M.
Searching for endogenous benzodiazepine receptor ligands.
Trends Pharm. 1, 424-7 (1980)

2673. Braestrup,C., Nielsen,M.
Strychnine as a potent inhibitor of the brain GABA-benzodiazepine receptor complex.
Brain Res.Bull. 5, 681-4 (1980)

2674. Braestrup,C., Nielsen,M., Biggio,G., Squires,R.F.
Neuronal localization of benzodiazepine receptors in cerebellum.
Neurosci.Lett. 13, 219-24 (1979)

2675. Braestrup,C., Nielsen,M., Krogsgaard-Larsen,P., Falch,E.
Partial agonists for brain GABA/benzodiazepine receptor complex.
Nature 280, 331-3 (1979)

2676. Braestrup,C., Nielsen,M., Krogsgaard-Larsen,P., Falch,E.
Two or more conformations of benzodiazepine receptors depending on GABA receptors and other variables.
Adv.Biochem.Psychopharmacol. 21, 301-12 (1980)

2677. Braestrup,C., Nielsen,M., Nielsen,E.B., Lyon,M.
Benzodiazepine receptors in the brain as affected by different experimental stresses: the changes are small and not undirectional.
Psychopharmacology (Berlin) 65, 273-7 (1979)

2678. Braunstein,M.C.
Apnea with maintenance of consciousness, following intravenous diazepam.
Anesth.Analg. (Cleve) 58, 52-3 (1979)

2677. Breimer,D.D., Jochemsen,R., von Albert,H.H.
Pharmakokinetik der Benzodiazepine / Lange gegen kurze Wirkungsdauer.
Pharmacokinetics of Benzodiazepines / Short-acting versus long-acting.
New Perspectives in Benzodiazepine Therapy - International Symposium Heidelberg 1979
Arzneim.Forsch. (Drug Res.) 30, 875-81 (1980)

2678. Brendel,R.
Clobazam - neuer Tranquilizer-Typ.
In: Offizinpharmazie, Hrsg. H. Morck, H. Liekfeld und L. Schneider, Bd. 2, S. 61-4 (1980)
Thieme - Stuttgart

2679. Briggs,R.S., Castleden,C.M., Kraft,C.A.
Improved hypnotic treatment using chlormethiazole and temazepam.
Brit.Med.J. 280, 601-4 (1980)

2680. Brisson,C., Durand,M., Jugie,G., Padelou.,M.
^{35}Cl nuclear-quadrupole resonance-spectra in diazepam and its 1-1 complex with chloral hydrate.
J.Mol.Struct. 68, 137-43 (1980)

2681. Brockutn.,J.G., Norbury,A.G., Holloway,A.M., Downing,J.W.
Flunitrazepam for the intravenous induction of anesthesia in children.
S.Afr.Med.J. 57, 986-7 (1980)

2682. Brogden,R.N., Heel,R.C., Speight,T.M., Avery,G.S.
Clobazam - a review of its pharmacological properties and therapeutic use in anxiety.
Drugs 20, 161-78 (1980)

2683. Brown,C.R., Sarnquist,F.H., Canup,C.A., Pedley,T.A.
Clinical, electroencephalographic, and pharmacokinetic studies of a water-soluble benzodiazepine, midazolam maleate.
Anesthesiol. 50, 467-70 (1979)

2684. Brown,N.D., Lofberg,R.T., Gibson,T.P.
A study of the Bratton-Marshall hydrolysis procedure utilizing high performance liquid chromatography.
Clin.Chim.Acta 70, 239-45 (1976)

2685. Brown,Z.W., Amit,Z., Smith,B., Rockman,G.
Disruption of taste aversion learning by pretreatment with diazepam and morphine.
Pharmacol.Biochem.Behav. 10, 17-20 (1979)

2686. Browne,T.R.
Interaction between clonazepam and sodium valproate.
N.Engl.J.Med. 300, 679 (1979)

2687. Brucato,A., Coppola,A., Gianguzza,S., Provenzano,P.M.
Triazolam: characteristics of its depressive action.
Boll.Soc.Ital.Biol.Sper. 54, 1051-7 (1978)

2688. Brucato,A.F., Coppola,A., Provenzano,P.M.
Depressive and disinhibitory effects of triazolam following brief continous administration.
Boll.Soc.Ital.Biol.Sper. 54, 1822-7 (1978)

2689. Bruni,G., Dalpra,P., Dotti,M.T., Segre,G.
Plasma ACTH and cortisol levels in benzodiazepine treated rats.
Pharmacol.Res.Commun. 12, 163-75 (1980)

2690. Brunner,H., Patris,M.F., Baudry,P., Feugere,T., Wertensc.,H.
Clinical-trial of flunitrazepam in the hospital practice of psychiatry.
Nouv.Presse 8, 2541-3 (1979)

2691. Budd,R.D., Walkin,E.
Mass-screening and confirmation of diazepam in urine by EMIT - thin-layer-chromatography.
Clin.Toxicol. 16, 201-7 (1980)

2692. Budd,R.D., Walkin,E., Jain,N.C., Sneath,T.C.
Frequency of use of diazepam in individuals on probation and in methadone maintenance programs.
Amer.J.Drug Alcohol Abuse 6, 511-4 (1979)

2693. Budden,M.G.
Comparative-study of haloperidol and diazepam in the treatment of anxiety.
Curr.Med.Res. 5, 759-65 (1979)

2694. Bueno,J.R.
Hypnotic effects of triazolam - comparison with flurazepam.
Rev.Bras.Med. 36, 584-6 (1979)

2695. Burch,T.P., Ticku,M.K.
Ethanol enhances diazepam-H-3 binding at the benzodiazepine-GABA-receptor-ionophore complex.
Eur.J.Pharmacol. 67, 325-6 (1980)

2696. Burdette,S., Delorenz.,R.
Benzodiazepine inhibition of calcium-dependent protein-phosphorylation in synaptosome and synaptic vesicle preparations.
Neurology 30, 449 (1980)

2697. Burgschat,H., von Bruchhausen,V.
Camazepam.
In: Offizinpharmazie, Hrsg. H. Morck, H. Liekfeld und L. Schneider, Bd. 2, S. 65-8 (1980)
Thieme - Stuttgart

2698. Burke,D., Sokoloff,H.
Simultaneous high-performance liquid-chromatographic determination of chlordiazepoxide and amitriptyline hydrochloride in two-component tablet formulations.
J.Pharm.Sci. 69, 138-40 (1980)

2699. Burton,M.J., Cooper,S.J., Posadasa.,A.
Interactions between chlordiazepoxide and food-deprivation determining choice in a food-preference test.
Brit.J.Pharm. 68, P157-P158 (1980)

2700. Busto,U., Kaplan,H.L., Sellers,E.M.
Benzodiazepine-associated emergencies in Toronto.
Amer.J.Psychiatry 137, 224-7 (1980)

2701. Buttar,H.S.
Effects of the combined administration of ethanol and chlordiazepoxide on the prenatal and postnatal-development of rats.
Teratology 21, A32-A33 (1980)

2702. Caccia,S., Carli,M., Garattini,S., Poggesi,E., Rech,R., Samanin,R.
Pharmacological activities of clobazam and diazepam in the rat: relation to drug brain levels.
Arch.Int.Pharmacodyn.Ther. 243, 275-83 (1980)

2703. Caccia,S., Guiso,G., Garattini,S.
Brain concentrations of clobazam and N-desmethyl-clobazam and antileptazol activity.
J.Pharm.Pharmacol. 32, 295-6 (1980)

2704. Caccia,S., Guiso,G., Samanin,R., Garattini,S.
Species differences in clobazam metabolism and antileptazol effect.
J.Pharm.Pharmacol. 32, 101-3 (1980)

2705. Cananzi,A.R., Costa,E., Guidotti,A.
Potentiation by intraventricular muscimol of the anticonflict effect of benzodiazepines.
Brain Res. 196, 447-53 (1980)

2706. Candy,J.M., Martin,I.L.
Is the benzodiazepine receptor coupled to a chloride anion channel.
Nature 280, 172-3 (1979)

2707. Candy,J.M., Martin,I.L.
The postnatal development of the benzodiazepine receptor in the cerebral cortex and cerebellum of the rat.
J.Neurochem. 32, 655-8 (1979)

2708. Cano,J.P., Gouezo,F., Lindoulsi,T., Viala,A.
Direct determination of clonazepam (Rivotril) and 7-amino clonazepam in plasma by gas-chromatography.
Toxicol.Eur.Res. 2, 25-33 (1979)

2709. Cara,M., Salauen,C., Saly,S.T., Vodhin,J., Debras,C.
Dipotassic chlorazepate premedication. Its effects on preoperative narcosis: a double-blind study.
Anesth.Analg. (Paris) 35, 1101-13 (1978)

2710. Carnie,J.
Diazepam and the neuro-muscular function.
Brit.J.Anaest. 52, 960 (1980)

2711. Carranza,J.
Long-term use and abuse of benzodiazepines.
Pharmakopsych. 13, 254-8 (1980)

2712. Carrigan,P.J., Bartenbach,D.
Elimination half-life of nordiazepam.
South Med.J. 72, 769-70 (1979)

2713. Castillo-Fernando,J.R., Garcia,M., Carmona,J.
Digoxin levels and diazepam.
Lancet 2, 368 (1980)

2714. Chan,A.W.K., Heubusch,P.
The combined effect of chlordiazepoxide and ethanol on brain cyclic-nucleotides.
Alc.Clin.Ex. 4, 211 (1980)

2715. Chan,A.W.K., Schanley,D.L., Strauss,W.
Combined effect of chlordiazepoxide and ethanol on brain gamma-aminobutyric acid levels.
Res.Commun.Psych. 4, 277-84 (1979)

2716. Chananon.,P., Hamor,T.A., Martin,I.L.
Structure of 7-chloro-2,3-dihydro-1-methyl-5-phenyl-1H-1,4-benzodiazepine hydrochloride (medazepam hydrochloride).
Acta Cryst.(B) 36, 898-902 (1980)

2717. Chang,R.S., Tran,V.I., Snyder,S.H.
Neurotransmitter receptor localizations: brain lesion induced alterations in benzodiazepine, GABA, beta-adrenergic and histamine H1-receptor binding.
Brain Res. 190, 95-110 (1980)

2718. Chantela.,E.A., Schneider,J.
Advantageous effect of clonazepam in the treatment of delirium tremens.
Med.Welt 31, 451-4 (1980)

2719. Charbonneau,P., Lecacheux,C., Bazin,C.
Meprobamate and benzodiazepine poisoning.
Rev.Prat. 28, 4533-41 (1978)

2720. Chasseaud,L.F., Taylor,T., Brodie,R.R.
Prazepam metabolism in female subjects (technical note).
J.Pharm.Pharmacol. 32, 652-3 (1980)

2721. Chiarenz.,G.A., Rho,M., Resele,L.
Hangover effects of some benzodiazepines studied by means of the contingent negative-variaton (CNV) and neuropsychological tests.
Res.Comm.Psych. 4, 371-82 (1979)

2722. Chick,J.
Hypnotics and hangover.
Brit.Med.J. 280, 1322 (1980)

2723. Chiu,T.H., Rosenberg,H.C.
GABA receptor-mediated modulation of 3H-diazepam binding in rat cortex.
Eur.J.Pharmacol. 56, 337-45 (1979)

2724. Chiu,T.H., Rosenberg,H.C.
Differential effects of triton X-100 on benzodiazepine and GABA binding in a frozen-thawed synaptosomal fraction of rat brain.
Eur.J.Pharmacol. 58, 335-8 (1979)

2725. Chiu,T.H., Rosenberg,H.C.
Studies of digitonin-solubilized benzodiazepine receptor system.
Fed.Proc. 39, 1006 (1980)

2726. Christen.,K.N., Huttel,M.
Naloxone does not antagonize diazepam-induced sedation.
Anesthesiol. 51, 187 (1979)

2727. Chung Hwang,E., van Woert,M.H.
Antimyoclonic action of clonazepam: the role of serotonin.
Eur.J.Pharmacol. 60, 31-40 (1979)

2728. Church,M.W., Johnson,L.C.
Mood and performance of poor sleepers during repeated use of flurazepam.
Psychopharmacology 61, 309-16 (1979)

2729. Cierpka,G., Prott,V., Grellman.,A., Dorghoty,A.H., Zanker,R.
Experience obtained from use of Faustan (diazepam)-ketamine combination in anesthesia for minor gynecological surgery.
Zbl.Gynäkol. 101, 704-8 (1979)

2730. Clanachan,A.S., Marshall,R.J.
Therapeutic concentrations of diazepam potentiate the effects of adenosine on isolated cardiac and smooth muscle.
Brit.J.Pharmacol. 68, 148P-149P (1980)

2731. Clanachan,A.S., Marshall,R.J.
Diazepam potentiates the coronary vasodilator actions of adenosine in anesthetized dogs.
Brit.J.Pharmacol. 70, P66-P67 (1980)

2732. Clark,E.O., Glanzer,M., Turndorf,H.
The pattern of memory loss resulting from intravenously administered diazepam.
Arch.Neurol. 36, 296-300 (1979)

2733. Clarke,P.R.F., Bennett,N.R., Milne,B.R., Thornton,J.A.
Gone but not forgotten - benzodiazepine-induced amnesia.
Brit.J.Anaest. 52, P231 (1980)

2734. Clarke,R.S.J., Dundee,J.W., McGowan,W.A.W., Howard,P.J.
Comparison of the subjective effects and plasma-concentrations following oral and i.m. administration of flunitrazepam in volunteers.
Brit.J.Anaest. 52, 437-45 (1980)

2735. Clement,J., Durand,G., Gruselle,G.
Flunitrazepam in hospital psychiatry.
Nouv.Presse 8, 2554-8 (1979)

2736. Cloyd,J.C.
Diluting diazepam injection.
Amer.J.Hosp.Pharm. 38, 32 (1981)

2737. Cloyd,J.C., Vezeau,C., Miller,K.W.
Availability of diazepam from plastic containers.
Amer.J.Hosp.Pharm. 37, 492-6 (1980)

2738. Coassolo,P., Sarrazin,M., Sari,J.C., Briand,C.
Microcalorimetric studies on the binding of some benzodiazepine derivatives to human serum albumin.
Biochem.Pharmacol. 27, 2787-92 (1978)

2739. Cohen.A.R.
Chlorazepate for premedication - reply.
Brit.J.Anaest. 51, 263 (1979)

2740. Cohn,J.B., Gittschalk,L.A.
Double-blind comparison of ketazolam and placebo using once-a-day dosing.
J.Clin.Pharmacol. 20, 676-80 (1980)

2741. Colburn,W.A., Bekersky,I., Min,B.H., Hodwhon,B.J., Garland,W.A.
Contribution of gut contents, intestinal wall and liver to the first-pass metabolism of clonazepam in the rat.
Res.Commun.Chem.Pathol.Pharmacol. 27, 73-90 (1980)

2742. Colello,G.D., Hockenbery,D.M., Bosmann,H.B., Fuchs,S., Folkers,K.
Competitive inhibition of benzodiazepine binding by fractions from porcine brain.
Proc.Natl.Acad.Sci.USA 75, 6319-23 (1978)

2743. Collard,M., Paille,R.
Double-blind trial of flunitrazepam in insomnia.
Nouv.Presse 8, 2559-60 (1979)

2744. Comar,D., Maziere,M., Godot,J.M., Berger,G., Soussali.,F., Menini,C., Arfel,G., Naquet,R.
Visualization of flunitrazepam-C-11 displacement in the brain of the live baboon.
Nature 280, 329-31 (1979)

2745. Congdon,P.J., Forsythe,W.I.
Intravenous clonazepam in the treatment of status epilepticus in children.
Epilepsia 21, 97-102 (1980)

2746. Conti,L., Pinder,R.M.
Controlled comparative trial of mianserin and diazepam in the treatment of anxiety-states in psychiatric out-patients.
J.Int.Med.Res. 7, 285-9 (1979)

2747. Cook,L., Sepinwall,J.
Relationship of GABA to the anxiolytic effects of benzodiazepines.
Brain Res.Bull. 4, 692 (1979)

2748. Cook,L., Sepinwall,J.
Relationship of anticonflict activity of benzodiazepines to brain receptor binding, serotonin, and GABA.
Psychopharmacol.Bull. 16, 30-2 (1980)

2749. Cook,P.S., Notelovitz,M., Kalra,P.S., Kalra,S.P.
Effect of diazepam on serum testosterone and the ventral prostate gland in male rats.
Arch.Androl. 3, 31-5 (1979)

2750. Cooke,J.
Benzodiazepine pharmacokinetics.
Brit.Med.J. 1, 752 (1979)

2751. Cooper,S.J.
Effects of chlordiazepoxide and diazepam on feeding performance in a food-preference test.
Psychopharmacology (Berlin) 69, 73-8 (1980)

2752. Cooper,S.J., Francis,R.L.
Feeding parameters in the rat: interactions of chlordiazepoxide with (+)-amphetamine or fenfluramine
Brit.J.Pharmacol. 64, 378P-379O (1978)

2753. Cooper,S.J., Francis,R.L.
Feeding parameters with two food textures after chlordiazepoxide administration, alone or in combination with D-amphetamine or fenfluramine.
Psychopharmacology (Berlin) 62, 253-9 (1979)

2754. Cooper,S.J., Francis,R.L.
Food-choice in a food-preference test: comparison of two mouse strains and the effects of chlordiazepoxide treatment.
Psychopharmacology (Berlin) 65, 89-93 (1979)

2755. Cooper,S.J., Francis,R.L.
Effects of acute or chronic administration of chlordiazepoxide on feeding parameters using two food textures in the rat.
J.Pharm.Pharmacol. 31, 743-6 (1979)

2756. Cooper,S.J., McClelland,A.
Effects of chlordiazepoxide, food familiarization, and prior shock experience on food choice in rats.
Pharmacol.Biochem.Behav. 12, 23-8 (1980)

2757. Cooper,S.J., Posadas-Andrews,A.
Food and water intake in the non-deprived pigeon after chlordiazepoxide administration.
Psychopharmacology (Berlin) 65, 99-101 (1979)

2758. Corall,I.M., Strunin,L., Ward,M.E., Mason,S.A., Alcalay,M.
Sedation for outpatient conservative dentistry - trial of pentazocine supplementation to diazepam and local analgesia techniques.
Anaesthesia 34, 855-8 (1979)

2759. Cornelissen,P.J., Beijersbergen,G.M.J.
Photo-chemical decomposition of 1,4-benzodiazepines - nitrazepam.
Photochem.Photobiol. 30, 337-41 (1979)

2760. Cornelissen,P.J., Beijersbergen,G.M.J., Mohn,G.R.
Structure and photobiological activity of 7-chloro-1,4-benzodiazepines - studies on the phototoxic effects of chlordiazepoxide, desmethylchlordiazepoxide and demoxepam using a bacterial indicator system.
Photochem.Photobiol. 32, 653-9 (1980)

2761. Corradetti,R., Moroni,F., Pepeu,G.
Pharmacological effects of benzodiazepines in the leech; benzodiazepine and GABA receptors and GABA level.
Pharmacol.Res.Commun. 12, 581-5 (1980)

2762. Corwin,H., Demyer,W.
Failure of chlorazepate to cause malformations or fetal wastage in the rat.
Arch.Neurol. 37, 347-9 (1980)

2763. Costa,E.
Role of gamma-aminobutyric acid in the action of 1,4-benzodiazepines.
Trends Pharm. 1, 41-4 (1979)

2764. Costa,E.
Benzodiazepine und Neurotransmitter.
Benzodiazepines and Neurotransmitters.
New Perspectives in Benzodiazepine Therapy - International Symposium Heidelberg 1979.
Arzneim.-Forsch. (Drug Res.) 30, 858-61 (1980)

2765. Costa,E., Guidotti,A.
Molecular mechanisms in the receptor action of benzodiazepines.
Ann.Rev.Pharmacol.Toxicol. 19, 531-45 (1979)

2766. Costa,E., Guidotti,A.
Recent studies on the mechanism whereby benzodiazepines facilitate GABA-ergic transmission.
Adv.Exp.Med.Biol. 123, 371-8 (1979)

2767. Coutosal.,S., Rey,E., Radvanyi,M.F., Dreyfusb.,C. Rapon,L., Castex,M.
Effects of therapy (diazepam, phenobarbital) on the EEG in newborn babies during the 1st 24 hours of treatment.
Rev.EEG.Neur. 9, 26-34 (1979)

2768. Coutosal.,S., Rey,E., Radvanyi,M.F., Dreyfusb.,C.
Effects of therapy (diazepam, phenobarbital) on the EEG in newborn babies during the first 24 h of treatment.
EEG.Clin.Neur. 49, P102-P103 (1980)

2769. Crawley,J., Goodwin,F.K.
Preliminary-report of a simple animal behavior model for the anxiolytic effects of benzodiazepines.
Pharm.Bio.B. 13, 167-70 (1980)

2770. Crayton,J.W.
The effect of diazepam on the spinal mono-synaptic (H-) reflex in man.
Neuropharm. 19, 915-8 (1980)

2771. Cronau,P.F., Zebisch,P., Tilkorn,P.
Short duration anesthesia in horses with diazepam-xylazin-ketamine.
Tier Umsch. 35, 393-4 (1980)

2772. Crossman,A.R., Lee,L.A., Longman,D.A., Slater,P.
Effects of benzodiazepines and barbiturates in a GABA-dependent animal model: interactions with muscimol in the globus pallidus.
Brit.J.Pharmacol. 66, 493P-494P (1979)

2773. Crowley,T.J., Hydinger-MacDonald,M.
Bedtime flurazepam and the human circadian rhythm of spontaneous motility.
Psychopharmacology (Berlin) 62, 157-61 (1979)

2774. Cuka,D.J., Edelman,J.D.
Atropine in physostigmine reversal of diazepam.
Anesth.Analg. (Cleve) 59, 459 (1980)

2775. Currin,M.R.
Which benzodiazepine, why and how?
S.Afr.Med.J. 56, 464-5 (1979)

2776. Curry,S.H., Smith,C.M.
Diazepam-ethanol interaction in humans: addition or potentiation?
Commun.Psychopharmacol. 3, 101-13 (1979)

2777. Curry,S.H., Whelpton,R.
Pharmacokinetics of closely related benzodiazepines.
Brit.J.Clin.Pharmacol. 8, 15S-21S (1979)

2778. Cushman,P., Benzer,D.
Alcohol and benzodiazepines - withdrawal syndromes.
Alc.Clin.Exp. 4, 212 (1980)

2779. Cutler,R.E., Blair,A.D.
Pharmacokinetics of diazepam in normal and uremic humans.
Clin.Pharm. 25, 219-20 (1979)

2780. Dalbo,L., Marcucci,F., Mussini,E., Perbelli.,D., Castella.,A., Fresia,P.
Plasma-levels of chlorodesmethyldiazepam in humans.
Biopharm.Dr. 1, 123-6 (1980)

2781. Damm,H.W., Müller,W.E., Wollert,U.
Is the benzodiazepine receptor purinergic?
Eur.J.Pharmacol. 55, 331-3 (1979)

2782. Das,S., Datta,S.C., Guin,A.K., Dey,S., Sengupta,D.
Studies on the invitro effect of different benzodiazepines on cholinesterase activity of human-fetal brain.
Current Sci. 48, 979-82 (1979)

2783. Das,S., Dey,S., Datta,S.C., Guin,A.K., Sengupta,D.
In vitro effects of diazepam, desmethyldiazepam and nitrazepam on atpase activity of human fetal brain.
Indian J.Exp.Biol. 17, 895-8 (1979)

2784. Dasberg,H.H., Shalif,I.
Brief treatment with oxazepam in crisis-intervention - with a symptom-profile study in acute anxiety patients.
Isr.Ann.Psych. 17, 201-8 (1979)

2785. Dasta,J., Mackichan,J., Lima,J., Altman,M.
Diazepam-cimetidine interaction - a preliminary report.
Drug Intel. 14, 633 (1980)

2786. Davies,L.P., Cook,A.F., Poonian,M., Taylor,K.M.
Displacement of (3H) diazepam binding in rat brain by dipyridamole and by 1-methylisoguanosine, a marine natural product with muscle relaxant activity.
Life Sci. 26, 1089-95 (1980)

2787. Davis,D., Grossman,S.H., Kitchell,B.B., Shand,D.G., Routledge,P.A.
Age-related changes in the plasma-protein binding of lidocaine and diazepam.
Clin.Res. 28, A234 (1980)

2788. Davis,L.G., Cohen,R.K.
Identification of an endogenous peptide-ligand for the benzodiazepine receptor.
Biochem.Biophys.Res.Commun. 92, 141-8 (1980)

2789. Davis,L.G., Cohen,R.K.
Inhibition of (3H) diazepam binding by an endogenous fraction from rat brain synaptosomes.
J.Pharm.Pharmacol. 32, 218-9 (1980)

2790. Davis,M.
Diazepam and flurazepam: effects on conditioned fear as measured with the potentiated startle paradigm.
Psychopharmacology (Berlin) 62, 1-7 (1979)

2791. De Angelis,L., File,S.E.
Acute and chronic effects of three benzodiazepines in the social interaction anxiety test in mice.
Psychopharmacology (Berlin) 64, 127-9 (1979)

2792. Debard,M.L.
Maintenance treatment with benzodiazepines.
Amer.J.Psychiat. 137, 130 (1980)

2793. Deberdt,R.
Triazolam, a benzodiazepine hypnotic used continuously for one year - further communication.
Curr.Ther.Res. 28, 31-3 (1980)

2794. Debruyne,D., Moulin,M.A., Camsonne,R., Bigot,M.C.
Wall-coated open tubular column coupled with nitrogen-selective detector for routine GLC determination of diazepam, meprobamate, phenylbutazone, and thioridazine in serum.
J.Pharm.Sci. 69, 835-8 (1980)

2795. Defayolle,M., Petresou,L., Liegeois,J.M.
Clinical pharmacology of the hypnotics. Comparison of changes in the modifications of the vigilance under the influence of the estazolam and the nitrazepam.
Therapie 33, 447-54 (1978)

2796. Degos,J.D., Meyrigna.,C., Kammerer,J., Houin,G., Jarry,G.G.
Effects of diazepam on EEG in cirrhotic patients - detection of the hepatic encephalopathy risk.
Nouv.Presse 9, 1097-8 (1980)

2797. Delafuen.,J.R., Rosenbaum,A.H.., Martin,H.R., Niven,R.G.
Lorazepam-related withdrawal seizures.
Mayo Clin.Proc. 55, 190-2 (1980)

2798. Della-Fera,M.A., Baile,C.A., McLaughlin,C.L.
Feeding elicited by benzodiazepine-like chemicals in puppies and cats: structure-activity relationships.
Pharmacol.Biochem.Behav. 12, 195-200 (1980)

2799. Demailly,P., Paycha,F.
Chlorazepate and glaucomas.
Bull.Soc.Ophthalmol.Fr. 78, 585-8 (1978)

2800. De Groof,R.C.
Effect of solvents on the in vitro uptake and distribution of diazepam.
Proc.West Pharmacol.Soc. 22, 351-4 (1979)

2801. Desarmenien,M., Lamour,Y., Feltz,P.
Effects of diazepam on GABA-evoked depolarization in rat dorsal root ganglia in vivo.
Prog.Neuropsychopharmacol. 4, 31-6 (1980)

2802. Desmond,P.V., Patwardhan,R.V., Schenker,S., Hoyumpa,H.M.
Short-term ethanol administration impairs the elimination of chlordiazepoxide (Librium) in man.
Eur.J.Clin.Pharm. 18, 275-8 (1980)

2803. Desmond,P.V., Patwardhan,R.V., Schenker,S., Hoyumpa,A.
Acute ethanol ingestion impairs chlordiazepoxide (Librium) elimination in man.
Clin.Res. 28, A482 (1980)

2804. Desmond,P.V., Patwardhan,R.V., Schenker,S., Speeg,K.V.,jr.
Cimetidine impairs elimination of chlordiazepoxide (Librium) in man.
Ann.Intern.Med. 93, 266-8 (1980)

2805. Desmond,P.V., Roberts,R.K., Wood,A.J., Dunn,G.D., Wilkinson,G.R., Schenker,S.
Effect of heparin administration on plasma binding of benzodiazepines.
Brit.J.Clin.Pharmacol. 9, 171-5 (1980)

2806. Desmond,P.V., Schenker,S.
Chlordiazepoxide in acute alcoholism.
Brit.J.Clin.Pharmacol. 8, 85 (1979)

2807. Deshmukh,P.P., Yamamura,H.I.
Localization of benzodiazepine receptor in human and rat-brain by light and electron-microscopic autoradiography following photoaffinity-labeling.
Fed.Proc. 39, 387 (1980)

2808. De Wet,B.S.
The benzodiazepines - friends, but also strangers.
S.Afr.Med.J. 55, 494 (1979)

2809. De Wet,B.S.
Which benzodiazepine, why and how?
S.Afr.Med.J. 56, 464-5 (1979)

2810. D'Hollander,A., Hennart,D., Primo-Dubois,J., Dewachter,B., Massaut,J.
Hemodynamic effects of flunitrazepam in the coronary patient under moderated analgesic anesthesia.
Acta Anaesthesiol.Belg. 30, 79-80 (1979)

2811. Dick,W., Knoche,E., Milewski,P., Schmitz,J.E.
Influence of flunitrazepam on body functions.
S.Afr.Med.J. 55, 277-9 (1979)

2812. Dick,W., Knoche,E., Milewski,P., Schmitz,J.E., Eisele,G.
The influence of flunitrazepam on different body functions.
Acta Anaesthesiol.Belg. 30, 175-82 (1979)

2813. Din,G.M., Epstein,B.H., Cohen,L.E.
Hemodilution as a preventive measure against thrombophlebitis resulting from intravenous administration of diazepam (Valium).
Gastroin.Ent. 26, 65-6 (1980)

2814. Dixon,R.A., Bennett,N.R., Harrison,M.J., Kenyon,C., Thornton,J.A.
I.v. flunitrazepam and i.v. diazepam in conservative dentistry - a crossover trial.
Brit.J.Anaest. 52, 517-26 (1980)

2815. Dixon,R.A., Edwards,I.R., Pilcher,J.
Diazepam in immediate post-myocardial infarct period - a double-blind trial.
Brit.Heart J. 43, 535-40 (1980)

2816. Dixon,R., Glover,W., Earley,J., Delaney,M.
Desmethyldiazepam: a specific radioimmunoassay.
J.Pharm.Sci. 68, 1471 (1979)

2817. Dixon,R., Lucek,R., Earley,J., Perry,C.
Chlordiazepoxide: a new, more sensitive and specific radioimmunoassay.
J.Pharm.Sci. 68, 261 (1979)

2818. Dixon,R., Lucek,R., Young,R., Ning,R., Darragh,A.
Radioimmunoassay for nitrazepam in plasma.
Life Sci. 25, 311-6 (1979)

2819. Doenicke,A., Kugler,J., Kropp,M., Laub,M., Kalbfleisch,G.
Hypnotic effect of the new benzodiazepine derivative lormetazepam when given intravenously.
Anaesthesis 28, 578-83 (1979)

2820. Doenicke,A., Kugler,J., Suttmann,H., Grote,B., Donner,W.
Midazolam - dependence of depth of sleep on length of injection and dosage.
Anaesthesis 29, 637-8 (1980)

2821. Domino,L.E., Domino,E.F., Zsigmond,E.K.
Enhancement of ketamine plasma-levels by diazepam in man.
Clin.Res. 27, A716 (1979)

2822. Donaldson,D., Gibson,G.
Local complications with intravenous diazepam.
Can.Dent.Assoc.J. 45, 337-41 (1979)

2823. Donaldson,D., Gibson,G.
Systemic complications with intravenous diazepam.
Oral Surg. 49, 126-30 (1980)

2824. Donlon,P.T., Singer,J.M.
Clobazam versus placebo for anxiety and tension in psychoneurotic outpatients. A multicenter collaborative study.
J.Clin.Pharmacol. 19, 297-302 (1979)

2825. Doongaji,D.R., Sheth,A., Apte,J.S., Lakdawala,P.D., Khare,C.B., Thatte,S.S.
Clobazam versus diazepam: a double-blind study in anxiety neurosis.
Brit.J.Clin.Pharmacol. 7, 119S (1979)

2826. Dordain,G., Puech,A.J., Hecquet,S., Paturaud,J.P., Simon,P.
Clinical-trial of a new hypnotic agent (triazolam) realized by a group of general-practice - methodological difficulties.
Therapie 35, 119-24 (1980)

2827. Douglas,J.G., Nimmo,W.S., Wanless,R., Jarvie,D.R., Heading,R.C., Finlayso.,N.D.
Sedation for upper gastrointestinal endoscopy - a comparison of oral temazepam and i.v. diazepam.
Brit.J.Anaest. 52, 811-5 (1980)

2828. Driscoll,E.J., Gelfman,S.S., Sweet,J.B., Butler,D.P., Wirdzck,P.R., Medlin,T.
Thrombophlebitis after intravenous use of anesthesia and sedation: its incidence and natural history.
J.Oral Surg. 37, 809-15 (1979)

2829. Drost,R.A.
The halcion story.
Lancet 1, 1027-8 (1980)

2830. Du Cailar,J., Kienlein,J.
Pharmacology of flunitrazepam.
Ann.Anesthesiol.Fr. 19, 10-90 (1978)

2831. Ducreuzet,C.
Study of flunitrazepam in the insomnia of the aged.
Sem.Hop.Pharm. 56, 2005-7 (1980)

2832. Dudai,Y.
Modulation of benzodiazepine binding sites in calf cortex by an endogenous factor and GABAergic ligands.
Brain Res. 167, 422-5 (1979)

2833. Dudai,Y., Yavin,Z., Yavin,E.
Binding of (3H)flunitrazepam to differentiating rat cerebral cells in culture.
Brain Res. 177, 418-22 (1979)

2834. Duka,T., Hoellt,V., Herz,A.
In vivo receptor occupation by benzodiazepines and correlation with the pharmacological effect.
Brain Res. 179, 147-56 (1979)

2835. Duka,T., Wuester,M., Herz,A.
Rapid changes in enkephalin levels in rat striatum and hypothalamus induced by diazepam.
Naunyn Schmied.Arch.Pharmacol. 309, 1-5 (1979)

2836. Duka,T., Wuester,M., Herz,A.
Benzodiazepines modulate striatal enkephalin levels via a GABAergic mechanism.
Life Sci. 26, 771-6 (1980)

2837. Dumont,D., Mathê,D., Piva,C.
Intoxication par une nouvelle benzodiazepine l'estazolam.
Med.Leg.Toxicol. 23, 161-5 (1980)

2838. Dundee,J.W., McGowan,W.A., Lilburn,J.K., McKay,A.C., Hegarty,J.E.
Comparison of the actions of diazepam and lorazepam.
Brit.J.Anaesth. 51, 439-46 (1979)

2839. Dundee,J.W., Samuel,I.O., Wilson,D.B., Toner,W., Howard,P.J.
Midazolam maleate: a water-soluble benzodiazepine-preliminary results.
Brit.J.Clin.Pharmacol. 9, 305P-306P (1980)

2840. Dundee,J.W., Samuel,I.O., Toner,W., Howard,P.J.
Midazolam - a water-soluble benzodiazepine - studies in volunteers.
Anaesthesia 35, 454-8 (1980)

2841. Dundee,J.W., Wilson,D.B.
Amnesic action of midazolam.
Anaesthesia 35, 459-61 (1980)

2842. Dunkasem,K., Sutthiwa.,P.
Clinical-trial of flunitrazepam as an intravenous induction agent.
J.Med.Ass.Thail. 63, 374-81 (1980)

2843. Dykstra,L.A.
Effects of morphine, diazepam and chlorpromazine on discrimination of electric shock.
J.Pharmacol.Exp.Ther. 209, 297-303 (1979)

2844. Earley,J.V., Fryer,R.I., Ning,R.Y.
Quinazolines and 1,4-benzodiazepines. LXXXIX: Haptnes useful in benzodiazepine immunoassay development.
J.Pharm.Sci. 68, 845-50 (1979)

2845. Ebel,S., Schütz,H.
Biotransformation of benzodiazepine derivatives.
Pharm.Unserer Zeit 8, 87-93 (1979)

2846. Eberts,F.S., Philopoulos,V., Vliek,R.W.
Disposition of ^{14}C-triazolam, a short acting hypnotic in man.
Pharmacologist 21, 168 (1979)

2847. Edwards,J.D., Eckerman,D.A.
Effects of diazepam and ethanol alone and in combination on conditioned suppression of key-pecking in the pigeon.
Pharmacol.Biochem.Behav. 10, 217-21 (1979)

2848. Edwards,R.A., Medlicot.,R.W.
Advantages and disadvantages of benzodiazepine prescription.
N.Zeal.Med.J. 92, 357-9 (1980)

2849. Eiden,F., Schmiz,E.
Clobazam (Frisium^{R}). Ein Beitrag zur Analyse von Psychopharmaka.
Dtsch.Apoth.-Ztg. 120, 933-7 (1980)

2850. Einarson,T.R.
Lorazepam withdrawal seizures.
Lancet 1, 151 (1980)

2851. Einarson,T.R.
Hostility reaction to flurazepam.
Drug Intell. 14, 291-2 (1980)

2852. Einarson,T.R.
Hallucinations from triazolam.
Drug Intell. 14, 714-5 (1980)

2853. Einarson,T.R.
Systematic review of the benzodiazepines.
Brit.Med.J. 281, 1009 (1980)

2854. Eisenberg,M., Balsley,S., Katz,R.L.
Effects of diazepam on succinylcholine-induced myalgia, potassium increase, creatine phosphokinase elevation, and relaxation.
Anesth.Analg. (Cleve) 58, 314-7 (1979)

2855. Eliander,H., Pekkarinen,A.
Enzyme inducing effects of phenobarbital on nitrazepam metabolism in dogs.
Acta Pharmacol.Toxicol. 47, 171-4 (1980)

2856. El-Mikatty,N., Shalaby,M.M., El Khodary,M., Gaafar,M.I.
Evaluation of intra-venous diazepam anaesthesia on liver functions.
J.Egypt.Med.Assoc. 60, 745-58 (1977)

2857. Elrabbat,N.A., Youssef,A.F., Omar,N.M.
Study of certain 1,5-benzodiazepine derivatives as acid-base indicators.
Analyst 105, 165-9 (1980)

2858. Elsass,P., Hendel,J., Hvidberg,E.F., Hansen,T.
Kinetics and neuropsychologic effects of i.v.-diazepam in the presence and absence of its active N-desmethyl metabolite in humans.
Psychopharmacology 70, 307-12 (1980)

2859. Enkelmann,R.
Klinische Erprobung und Vorstellung eines neuen Schlafmittels auf Benzodiazepin-Basis.
Clinical testing and presentation of a new hypnotic on the basis of benzodiazepines.
Fortschr.Med. 97, 1377-82 (1979)

2860. Epstein,R.S.
Benzodiazepine withdrawal symptoms - reply.
Amer.J.Psychiatr. 137, 751 (1980)

2861. Erdmann,W., Salt,P.J., Agoston,S., Langrehr,D.
Antagonism of the cardiovascular effects of ketamine by diazepam in volunteers.
Acta Anaesthesiol.Belg. 30, 239-45 (1979)

2862. Escuret,E., Roquefeu.,B., Lapaglia,M.A., Chapron,C., Baldymou.,M.
Hemodynamic and cerebral metabolic study of diazepam in neurosurgical intensive-care.
Neuro-Chire 25, 47-51 (1979)

2863. Euvrard,P., Chapalai.,J.C., Contasso.,J.C., Tolot,F.
Double-blind test of a new tranquilizer - cloxazolam - comparison with lorazepam.
Lyon Med. 244, 419-21 (1980)

2864. Fabre,L.F., McLendon,D.M.
Ketazolam administered once-a-day compared to clorazepate t.i.d. and placebo in a double-blind study to anxious out-patients.
Curr.Ther.Res. 25, 710-20 (1979)

2865. Fabre,L.F., McLendon,D.M.
Double-blind comparison of chlorazepate mono-potassium (Azene) with diazepam (Valium) in the treatment of anxious outpatients.
Curr.Ther.Res. 26, 1019-26 (1979)

2866. Fabre,L.F., McLendon,D.M.
A double-blind-study comparing the efficacy and safety of alprazolam with impramine and placebo in primary depression.
Curr.Ther.Res. 27, 474-82 (1980)

2867. Fabre,L.F., McLendon,D.M.
Long-term (6 month) safety and efficacy study of the benzodiazepines ketazolam and diazepam.
Clin.Res. 28, A588 (1980)

2868. Fabre,L.F., McLendon,D.M., Mallette,A.
Double-blind comparison of prazepam with diazepam, chlorazepate dipotassium and placebo in anxious out-patients.
J.Int.Med.Res. 7, 147-51 (1979)

2869. Fabre,L.F., McLendon,D.M., Mallette,A.
Prazepam efficacy in anxiety - double-blind comparative-study with diazepam, chlorazepate dipotassium and placebo.
Curr.Ther.Res. 25, 527-33 (1979)

2870. Fabre,L.F., McLendon,D.M., Mallette,A.
Phase-i.v. outpatient comparison study of prazepam against placebo, diazepam and clorazepate dipotassium in anxiety.
Curr.Ther.Res. 28, 784-91 (1980)

2871. Fahmy,N.R., Malek,S., Lappas,D.G.
Diazepam prevents some adverse-effects of succinylcholine.
Clin.Pharmacol.Ther. 26, 395-8 (1979)

2872. Feeney,D.W.
Benzodiazepine hypnotics.
N.Zeal.Med.J. 92, 256 (1980)

2873. Fehske,K.J., Müller,W.E., Wollert,U.
A highly reactive tyrosine residue as part of the indole and benzodiazepine binding site of human serum albumin.
Biochim.Biophys.Acta 577, 346-59 (1979)

2874. Fehske,K.J., Müller,W.E., Wollert,U., Velden,L.M.
Lone tryptophan residue of human-serum albumin as part of the specific warfarin-binding site - binding of dicoumarol to the warfarin, indole and benzodiazepine binding-sites.
Molec.Pharm. 16, 778-89 (1979)

2875. Feighner,J.P.
Ketazolam once-a-day in the treatment of anxiety - a double-blind comparison with diazepam and placebo.
Curr.Ther.Res. 28, 425-31 (1980)

2876. Ferko,A.P., Bobyock,E., Chernick,W.S.
A study on diazepam and postwithdrawal drinking of ethanol solution in rats.
Toxicol.Appl.Pharmacol. 50, 355-63 (1979)

2877. Fernholm,B., Nielsen,M., Braestrup,C.
Absence of brain specific benzodiazepine receptors in cyclostomes and elasmobranchs.
Comp.Biochem.Physiol. (C) 62C, 209-11 (1979)

2878. Ferreira,J.A.
The role of diazepam in skin hyper-pigmentation.
Aes.Plas.Su. 4, 343-8 (1980)

2879. Ffoulkes.,D.J., Okeowo,O.O., Johnson,T.O.
Objektive evaluation of premedicants - effect of medazepam on adrenocortical function in the pre-operative state.
Niger.Med.J. 9, 215-20 (1979)

2880. File,S.E.
The use of social-interaction as a method for detecting anxiolytic activity of chlordiazepoxide-like drugs.
J. Neurosci.Med. 2, 219-38 (1980)

2881. File,S.D., Bond,A.J.
Impaired performance and sedation after a single dose of lorazepam.
Psychopharmacology (Berlin) 66, 309-13 (1979)

2882. File,S.E., Hyde,J.R.
A test of anxiety that distinguishes between the actions of benzodiazepines and those of other minor tranquilisers and of stimulants.
Pharmacol.Biochem.Behav. 11, 65-9 (1979)

2883. Filippi,G., Trebbi,A.
Physicochemical profile of a new tranquillizer: pinazepam.
Boll.Chim.Farm. 118, 105-14 (1979)

2884. Finkle,B.S., McCloskey,K.L., Goodman,L.S.
Diazepam and drug-associated deaths - survey in the United States and Canada.
J.Amer.Med.Ass. 242, 429-34 (1979)

2885. Flaherty,C.F., Lombardi,B.R., Wrightson,J., Deptula,D.
Conditions under which chlordiazepoxide influences gustatory contrast.
Psychopharmacology (Berlin) 67, 269-77 (1980)

2886. Flaherty,C.F., Wrightson,J., Deptula,D., Duston,C.
Chlordiazepoxide does not influence simultaneous gustatory contrast.
Bull.Psychonomic Soc. 14, 216-8 (1979)

2887. Fleckens.,L., Lifshay,A.
Respiratory depression from intravenous alphaprodine and diazepam.
Clin.Pharmacol.Ther. 25, 224 (1979)

2888. Ford,R.D., Rech,R.H., Commissaris,R.L., Meyer,L.Y.
Effects of acute and chronic interactions of diazepam and D-amphetamine on punished behavior of rats.
Psychopharmacology (Berlin) 65, 197-204 (1979)

2889. Foreman,J.M., Griffith,W.C., Dextraze,P.G., Diamond,I.
Simultaneous assay of diazepam, chlordiazepoxide, N-desmethyldiazepam, N-desmethylchlordiazepoxide, and demoxepam in serum by high-performance liquid-chromatography.
Clin.Biochem. 13, 122-5 (1980)
Ann.Clin.Lab. 10, 443 (1980)

2890. Forster,A., Gardaz,J.P., Suter,P.M., Gemperle,M.
I.v. midazolam as an induction agent for anesthesia - a study in volunteers.
Brit.J.Anaest. 52, 907-11 (1980)

2891. Forster,A., Gardaz,J.P., Suter,P.M., Gemperle,M.
Respiratory depression by midazolam and diazepam.
Anesthesiol. 53, 494-7 (1980)

2892. Francis,R.L., Cooper,S.J.
Chlordiazepoxide-induced disruption of discrimination behavior - signal-detection analysis.
Psychopharmacology 63, 307-10 (1979)

2893. Francois,G., Blache,J.L., Granthil,C., Sumintap.,I., Rigault,J.P., Cano,J.P.
Pharmacokinetics of flunitrazepam (Narcozep) after repeated i.v. injections - preliminary-results.
Intens.Care Med. 6, 69 (1980)

2894. Frecker,R.C., Gander,R.E., Giles,H.G., Beeching,M., Sellers,E.M.
Differentiation of central nervous-system (CNS) effects of ethanol and diazepam by the measurement of flicker sensitivity using 2 psychophysical methods.
Clin.Pharmacol.Ther. 27, 255 (1980)

2895. Frecker,R.C., Giles,H.G.
Concurrent kinetic and dynamic measurements to correlate plasma and saliva diazepam levels with changes in visual flicker fusion frequency.
Clin.Pharmacol.Ther. 25, 226 (1979)

2896. Frei,K.
Vergleichsuntersuchung zur Sedierung geriatrischer Patienten während der Spinalanaesthesie.
Comparative study on the sedation of geriatric patients during spinal anesthesia.
Anaesthesiol.Intensivmed.Prax. 16, 23-7 (1979)

2897. Freund,G.
Loss of benzodiazepine receptors from brains of mice after 6 months of ethanol-consumption.
Alcohol Clin.Exp.Res. 4, 214 (1980)

2898. Froehlich,E.M., Fritz-Niggli,H.
The effect of valium anaesthesia on the radiosensitivity of the skin of the mouse foot.
Experientia 36, 340-1 (1980)

2899. Frost,J.D., Delucchi,M.R.
Insomnia in the elderly - treatment with flurazepam hydrochloride.
J.Amer.Ger.Soc. 27, 541-6 (1979)

2900. Frye,G., Vogel,R., Mailman,R., Ondrusek,G., Kilts,C., Wilson,J., Müller,R., Breese,G.
Comparison of the central effects of ethanol and benzodiazepines.
Alcohol Clin.Exp.Res. 3, 278 (1979)

2901. Fuccella,L.M.
Bioavailability of temazepam in soft gelatin capsules.
Brit.J.Clin.Pharmacol. 8, 31S-35S (1979)

2902. Fujimoto,M., Tsukinoki,Y., Hirose,K., Hirai,K., Okabayashi,T.
Interaction of peptido-aminobenzophenones with benzodiazepine receptors.
Chem.Pharm.Bull. 28, 1374-7 (1980)

2903. Fujimoto,M., Tsukinoki,Y., Hirose,K., Kuruma,K., Konaka,R., Okabayashi,T.
Detection and determination of pharmacologically active benzodiazepines in rat brain after the administration of 2-o-chlorobenzoyl-4-chloro-N-methyl-N'-glycylglycianilide, using a combination of high-pressure liquid chromatography and radioreceptorassay.
Chem.Pharm.Bull. (Tokyo) 28, 1378-86 (1980)

2904. Fukuda,H.
Effects of diazepam and baclofen on the anemic decerebrate rigidity in rats.
Nippon Yakurigaku Zasshi 75, 535-42 (1979)

2905. Fukuda,H., Kudo,Y., Takeuchi,E.
Effects of benzodiazepine derivatives on gamma-motor system in rats.
Nippon Yakurigaku Zasshi 75, 315-9 (1979)

2906. Fukumoto,M.
Spectrophotometric determination of bromazepam.
Chem.Pharm. 28, 3678-81 (1980)

2907. Gajewska,M., Ciszewsk.,M., Lugowska,E., Kwiatkow.,B.
Complex-compounds of benzodiazepine derivatives.
1. Preparation, physicochemical and analytical properties of complex-compounds of diazepam, nitrazepam, oxazepam with lead picrate.
Chem.Anal. 24, 119-27 (1979)

2908. Galinsky,D.E.
Caution on use of benzodiazepines in the elderly.
N.Engl.J.Med. 300, 1054-5 (1979)

2909. Gall,J.M.
Reader questions the safety of flurazepam.
Can.Fam.Phys. 25, 786 (1979)

2910. Gall,M., Hester,J.B., Rudzik,A.D.,jr., Lahti,R.A.
Synthesis and pharmacology of novel anxiolytic agents derived from 2-(dialkylamino)-methyl-4H-triazol-4-yl-benzophenones and related heterocyclic benzophenones.
J.Med.Chem. 19, 1057 (1976)

2911. Gall,M., Kamdar,B.V., Collins,R.J.
Pharmacology of some metabolites of triazolam, alprazolam and diazepam prepared by a simple,one-step oxidation of benzodiazepines.
J.Med.Chem. 21, 1290-4 (1978)

2912. Gall,M., Lahti,R.A., Rudzik,A.D.
Novel anxiolytic agents derived from o-amino-o-phenyl-o-tolyl-4H-triazoles and -imidazoles.
J.Med.Chem. 21, 542 (1978)

2913. Gallager,D.W.
Functional importance of benzodiazepine binding in brain.
Brain Res.Bull. 5, 833-8 (1980)

2914. Gallager,D.W., Mallorga,P.
Diphenylhydantoin: pre- and postnatal administration alters diazepam binding in developing rat cerebral cortex.
Science 208, 64-6 (1980)

2915. Gallager,D.W., Mallorga,P., Tallman,J.F.
Interaction of diphenylhydantoin and benzodiazepines in the CNS.
Brain Res. 189, 209-20 (1980)

2916. Gallager,D.W., Mallorga,P., Thomas,J.W., Tallman,J.F.
GABA-benzodiazepine interactions - physiological, pharmacological and developmental aspects.
Fed.Proc. 39, 3043-9 (1980)

2917. Gallager,R.M.
Impact of benzodiazepines on clinical practice - considerations for therapeutic use.
Minn.Med. 62, 580-5 (1979)

2918. Gamble,J.A.S., Dundee,J.W., Kawar,P.
Midazolam - an alternative to thiopentone.
Brit.J.Anaest. 52, P951-P952 (1980)

2919. Garanti,L., Testoni,G., Zecchi,G.
Synthesis of 3-unsubstituted and 3-alkyl-substituted H-1-1,2-benzodiazepines
Synthesis S1979, 380-1 (1979)

2920. Garanti,L., Zecchi,G.
Synthesis and thermochemical behavior of 1H-1,2-benzodiazepine-3-carboxylic acids.
J.Heterocycl.Chem. 16, 1061-2 (1979)

2921. Garber,J.G., Ominsky,A.J., Orkin,F.K.
Physostigmine reversal of diazepam sedation.
Anesthesiol. 51, S37 (1979)

2922. Garber,J.G., Ominsky,A.J., Orkin,F.K.
Atropine in physostigmine reversal of diazepam.
Anesth.Analg. (Cleve) 59, 459-60 (1980)

2923. Garber,J.G., Ominsky,A.J., Orkin,F.K., Quinn,P.
Physostigmine-atropine solution fails to reverse diazepam sedation.
Anesth.Analg. (Cleve) 59, 58-60 (1980)

2924. Garcia,O., Echecerr.,F., Letelier,M.E., Delvilla.,M.E., Sanchez,E.
Differential effects of diazepam and N-desmethyl-diazepam on morphine glucuronidation in rats liver-microsomes.
Arch.Biol.Med. 12, 515 (1979)

2925. Gastaut,H., Low,M.D.
Antiepileptic properties of clobazam, a 1,5-benzodiazepine, in man.
Epilepsia 20, 437-46 (1979)

2926. Gaszynaki,W., Chmielewski,O.
Ketamine-diazepam anesthesia in gynecologic surgery.
Ginekol.Pol. 50, 421-6 (1979)

2927. Gates,M.
New synthesis of diazepam.
J.Org.Chem. 45, 1675-81 (1980)

2928. Gavish,M., Chang,R.S.L., Snyder,S.H.
Solubilization of histamine H-1, GABA and benzodiazepine receptors.
Life Sci. 25, 783-9 (1979)

2929. Gavish,M., Snyder,S.H.
Soluble benzodiazepine receptors: GABAergic regulation.
Life Sci. 26, 579-82 (1980)

2930. Gavish,M., Snyder,S.H.
Properties of soluble gamma-aminobutyric acid (GABA) and benzodiazepine receptors.
Fed.Proc. 39, 1098 (1980)

2931. Gavish,M., Snyder,S.H.
Benzodiazepine recognition sites on GABA receptors.
Nature 287, 651-2 (1980)

2932. Gekiere,F., Allegre,G., Brindeau,F., Borenstein,P.
Benzodiazepines and limbic system. Anxiety and vigilance.
Pathol.Biol. (Paris) 28, 63-7 (1980)

2933. Gelfman,S.S., Gracely,R.H., Driscoll,E.J., Wirdzek, P.R., Butler,D.P., Sweet,J.B.
Comparison of recovery tests after intravenous sedation with diazepam-methohexital and diazepam-methohexital and fentanyl.
J.Oral.Surg. 37, 391-7 (1979)

2934. Geller,H.M.
Water-soluble benzodiazepines with agonistic and antagonistic actions on GABA-induced inhibition in cultured hypothalamus.
Neurosci.Lett. 15, 313-8 (1979)

2935. Geller,H.M., Hoffer,B.J., Taylor,D.A.
Electro-physiological actions of benzodiazepines.
Fed.Proc. 39, 3016-23 (1980)

2936. Ghoneim,M.M.
Antagonism of diazepam by physostigmine.
Anesthesiol. 52, 372 (1980)

2937. Ghoneim,M.M., Mewaldt,S.P., Berie,J.L., Hinrichs,J.V.
Memory effects of single and 3-weeks administration of diazepam (Valium).
Fed.Proc. 39, 519 (1980)

2938. Giasi,R.M., Covino,B.G., Dagostin.,E.
Pharmacokinetic interaction of local-anesthetics and diazepam.
Anesth.Analg.Curr.Res. 59, 540-1 (1980)

2939. Gielsdorf,W., Herper,M.
Gaschromatographisch-massenspektrometrische Untersuchungen zur Analytik von Clobazam (FRISIUM[R]).
Z.Rechtsmed. 85, 295-303 (1980)

2940. Gier,J.J.D., Thart,B.J., Wilderin.,P.F., Nelemans,F.A.
Comparison of plasma and saliva levels of diazepam.
Brit.J.Clin.Pharm. 10, 151-5 (1980)

2941. Giles,H.G., Kadar,G., Macleod,S.M., Sellers,E.M.
Use of the overturn end point in goldfish to measure the interaction of diazepam and ethanol and the effects of the binding of diazepam to bovine serum albumin.
Can.J.Physiol.Pharmacol. 57, 1186-8 (1979)

2942. Giles,H.G., Miller,R., Macleod,S.M., Sellers,E.M.
Diazepam and N-desmethyldiazepam in saliva of hospital inpatients.
J.Clin.Pharmacol. 20, 71-6 (1980)

2943. Gillin,J.C., Mendelson,W.B., Dement,W.C., Solomon,F.
Flurazepam and insomnia.
Science 205, 954-5 (1979)

2944. Giner-Sorolla,A., Greenbaum,J., Last-Barney,K., Anderson,L.M., Budinger,J.M.
Lack of carcinogenic effect of nitrosochlordiazepoxide and of nitrosomethylphenidate given orally to mice.
Food Cosmet.Toxicol. 18, 81-3 (1980)

2945. Girkin,R., Baldock,G.A., Chasseaud,L.F., Huempel,M., Hawkins,D.R., Mayo,B.C.
The absorption, distribution and excretion of ^{14}C-lormetazepam in dogs, rabbits, rats and rhesus monkeys.
Xenobiotica 10, 401-11 (1980)

2946. Gisselma.,A.
Insomnia in recently disintoxicated alcoholics - treatment using flunitrazepam.
Nouv.Presse 8, 2544-7 (1979)

2947. Glover,W., Dixon,R.
Radioimmunoassay for the hypnotic, flunitrazepam, in plasma.
Fed.Proc. 39, 537 (1980)

2948. Glover,W., Earley,J., Delaney,M., Dixon,R.
Radioimmunoassay of flurazepam in human plasma.
J.Pharm.Sci. 69, 601-2 (1980)

2949. Goetestam,K.G., Andersson,B.E.
Subjective effects and vigilance after diazepam and oxazepam in normal subjects.
Acta Psychiatr.Scand. (Suppl) 274, 117-21 (1978)

2950. Goldberg,H.L., Finnerty,R.J.
Double-blind-study of prochlorperazine, chlordiazepoxide and placebo in psychoneurotic outpatients with dominant symptoms of anxiety.
Int.Pharmacopsych. 14, 264-77 (1979)

2951. Goldberg,M.A., Todoroff,T.
Benzodiazepine receptors - the contribution of lipids and calcium.
Neurology 30, 421 (1980)

2952. Goransso.,A.M.
Premedication for gastroscopy - comparative-study of diazepam, dixyrazine, and placebo.
Scand.J.Gastr. 14, 961-7 (1979)

2953. Gouffier,E., Monteiro,I., Schnurma.,D., Voiry,A.M.
Treatment of alcohol withdrawal syndromes by intravenous administration of large doses of diazepam.
Med.Chir.Dig. 9, 361-3 (1980)

2954. Gouffier,E., Monterio,I., Schnurma.,D., Voiry,A.M.
Treatment of delirium tremens with large intravenous doses of diazepam.
Nouv.Presse 9, 2748 (1980)

2955. Govaerts,M.J.
Double-blind-study of rectal flunitrazepam in pediatric premedication.
Anaesthesia 35, 1132 (1980)

2956. Gran,L., Kaufmann,P., Bennett,P.B.
High-pressure, diazepam and pH influences on ketamine anesthesia in the rat.
Acta Anaesth.Scand. 24, 310-3 (1980)

2957. Greeff,O.B.W.
Diazepam in the treatment of children with drug-induced extrapyramidal symptoms.
S.Afr.Med.J. 55, 820 (1979)

2958. Greenblatt,D.J.
Electron-capture GLC-determination of clobazam and desmethylclobazam in plasma.
J.Pharm.Sci. 69, 1351-2 (1980)

2959. Greenblatt,D.J.
Phenobarbital and diazepam treatment of isolated seizures.
J.Amer.Med.Ass. 244, 1380 (1980)

2960. Greenblatt,D.J., Allen,M.D., Harmatz,J.S., Shader,R.I.
Diazepam disposition determinants.
Clin.Pharmacol. 27, 301-12 (1980)

2961. Greenblatt,D.J., Allen,M.D., Locniscar,A., Harmatz, J.S., Shader,R.I.
Lorazepam kinetics in the elderly.
Clin.Pharmacol. 26, 103-13 (1979)

2962. Greenblatt,D.J., Allen,M.D., Locniskar,A., Shader,R.I.
Lorazepam kinetics in the elderly.
Clin.Pharmacol. 25, 227 (1979)

2963. Greenblatt,D.J., Allen,M.D., Locniskar,A., Shader,R.I.
Age, sex and diazepam kinetics.
Clin.Pharmacol. 25, 227 (1979)

2964. Greenblatt,D.J., Allen,M.D., MacLaughlin,D.S., Huffman,D.H., Harmatz,J.S., Shader,R.I.
Single-dose and multiple-dose kinetics of oral lorazepam in humans - predictability of accumulation.
J.Pharm.Biopharm. 7, 159-79 (1979)

2965. Greenblatt,D.J., Divoll,M., Harmatz,J.S., Shader,R.I.
Oxazepam kinetics - effects of age and sex.
J.Pharm.Exp. 215, 86-91 (1980)

2966. Greenblatt,D.J., Ochs,H.R., Lloyd,B.L.
Entry of diazepam and its major metabolite into cerebrospinal-fluid.
Psychopharmacol. 70, 89-93 (1980)

2967. Greenblatt,D.J., Shader,R.I.
Effekte des Alters und anderer Medikamente auf die Kinetik der Benzodiazepine.
Effects of Age and other Drugs on Benzodiazepine Kinetics.
New Perspectives in Benzodiazepine Therapy - International Symposium Heidelberg 1979
Arzneim.-Forsch. (Drug Res.) 30, 886-90 (1980)

2968. Greenblatt,D.J., Shader,R.I.
Pharmacokinetic aspects of anxiolytic drug-therapy.
Can.J.Neur. 7, 269-70 (1980)

2969. Greenblatt,D.J., Shader,R.I., Harmatz,J.S., Georgotas,A.
Self-rated sedation and plasma concentrations of desmethyldiazepam following single doses of clorazepate.
Psychopharmacology (Berlin) 66, 289-90 (1979)

2970. Greiss,K.C., Fogari,R.
Double-blind clinical-assessment of alprazolam, a new benzodiazepine derivative, in the treatment of moderate to severe anxiety.
J.Clin.Pharmacol. 20, 693-9 (1980)

2971. Greizerstein,H.B., McLaughlin,I.G.
The high-pressure liquid-chromatographic determination of chlordiazepoxide and its N-demethyl-metabolite in mouse-brain.
J.Liqu.Chrom. 3, 1023-30 (1980)

2972. Griauzde,M.L., Chen,E.H., Radulovacki,M.
Effects of diazepam on sleep, temperature, 5-hydroxyindoleacetic and homovanillic acids in cisternal cerebrospinal fluid of cats.
Pharmacology 19, 149-55 (1979)

2973. Griffe,O., Griffe,H., Du Cailar,J.
Effects of diazepam on oxygen consumption.
Ann.Anesthesiol.Fr. 20, 37-40 (1979)

2974. Griffith,P.A.
Experience with lorazepam (Ativan) in the treatment of status epilepticus.
EEG Clin.Neur. 49, P75 (1980)

2975. Griffith,P.A., Karp,H.R.
Lorazepam in therapy for status epilepticus.
Ann.Neurol. 7, 493 (1980)

2976. Grijalba,A., Fos,D., Valls,L.M., Idoate,A., Vega,F.A.
Densitometric evaluation of diazepam in pharmaceutical preparations.
J.Chromatogr. 178, 443-51 (1979)

2977. Grille,W., Kolenda,K.D.
Wechselwirkungen von Digitoxin und Diazepam auf Stoffwechselebene. Untersuchungen über die Dosisabhängigkeit am Modell der isoliert-perfundierten Meerschweinchenleber.
Reciprocal effects of digitoxin and diazepam on metabolism. Study of the dose response relationship in the model isolated perfused guinea pig liver.
Pharm.Unserer Zeit 9, 75-80 (1980)

2978. Grishin,B.S.
Effect of dipidolor, diazepam, pipilphen and their combinations on the vasomotor reflex and respiration.
Farmakol.Tox. 43, 661-4 (1980)

2979. Groof,R.C.D.
Effect of solvents on the invitro uptake and distribution of diazepam.
Proc.West Pharmacol.Soc. 22, 351-4 (1979)

2980. Grossman,S.H., Davis,D., Kitchell,B.B., Shand,D.G., Routledge,P.A.
Plasma-protein binding of diazepam and lidocaine in renal-disease.
Clin.Res. 27, A738 (1979)

2981. Grote,B., Doenicke,A., Kugler,J., Suttmann,H., Laub,M.
Midazolam - dosage with the aid of encephalograms.
Anaesthesis 29, 635-6 (1980)

2982. Groves,J.A., Smyth,W.F.
Studies of the acid-base equilibria of some 7-fluoro-1,4-benzodiazepines in aqueous-solutions.
Spect.Act.A. 35, 603-11 (1979)

2983. Grundy,B.L., Brown,R.H., Greenberg,P.S.
Diazepam alters cortical evoked-potentials.
Anesthesiol. 51, 38 (1979)

2984. Guaitani,A., Carli,M., Rocchetti,M., Garattini,S.
Diazepam and experimental tumour growth.
Lancet 1, 1147-8 (1979)

2985. Gudgeon,A.C., Hindmarch,I.
The effects of 1,4-benzodiazepines and 1,5-benzodiazepines on aspects of car driving behavior - a preliminary investigation.
IRCS-Biochem. 8, 709-10 (1980)

2986. Guerre-Millo,M., Rey,E., Challier,J.C., Turquais,J.M., D'Athis,P., Olive,G.
Transfer in vitro of three benzodiazepines across the human placenta.
Eur.J.Clin.Pharmacol. 15, 171-3 (1979)

2987. Guidotti,A.
Pharmacological and biochemical evidence for an interaction between the benzodiazepine and GABA receptors.
Adv.Biochem.Psychopharmacol. 21, 271-5 (1980)

2988. Guidotti,A., Baraldi,M.
Modulation by benzodiazepines of GABA-coupled Cl-ionophore in neuro-blastoma NB2A cells.
Fed.Proc. 39, 1098 (1980)

2989. Guidotti,A., Baraldi,M., Costa,E.
1,4-benzodiazepines and gamma-aminobutyric acid: pharmacological and biochemical correlates.
Pharmacology 19, 267-77 (1979)

2990. Guidotti,A., Baraldi,M., Leon,A., Costa,E.
Benzodiazepines - a tool to explore the biochemical and neurophysiological basis of anxiety.
Fed.Proc. 39, 3039-42 (1980)

2991. Guidotti,A., Baraldi,M., Schwartz,J.P., Costa,E.
Molecular mechanisms regulating the interactions between the benzodiazepines and GABA receptors in the central nervous system.
Pharmacol.Biochem.Behav. 10, 803-7 (1979)

2992. Gupta,S.M., Takkar,V.P., Verma,A.K.
Retrospective study of tetanus neonatorum and comparative-assessment of diazepam in its treatment.
Ind.Pediatries 16, 343-6 (1979)

2993. Haas,S., Moises,H.W., Gattaz,W.F., Beckmann,H.
High-doses of diazepam in schizophrenia - an open study.
Arzneim.-Forsch. (Drug Res.) 30, 1214-5 (1980)

2994. Haefely,W.E.
GABA and the anticonvulsant action of benzodiazepines and barbiturates.
Brain Res.Bull. 5, 873-8 (1980)

2995. Haidukewych,D., Rodin,E.A., Davenport,R.
Monitoring clorazepate dipotassium as desmethyl-diazepam in plasma by electron-capture-gas-liquid-chromatography.
Clin.Chem. 26, 142-4 (1980)

2996. Hajdú,P., Uihlein,M., Damm,D.
Quantitative determination of clobazam in serum and urine by gas-chromatography, thin-layer chromatography and fluorometry.
J.Clin.Chem.Clin.Biochem. 209-14 (1980)

2997. Halcion - the unmasking of a myth.
Ned.Tijdschr.Geneeskd. 123, 1653-5 (1979)

2998. Hall,J.H., Marshall,P.C.
Clonazepam therapy in reading epilepsy.
Neurology 30, 550-1 (1980)

2999. Hallstroem,C., Lader,M.H., Curry,S.H.
Diazepam and N-desmethyldiazepam concentrations in saliva, plasma and CSF.
Brit.J.Clin.Pharm. 9, 333-9 (1980)

3000. Hammer,R., Koss,F.W.
The pharmacokinetic profile of pirenzepine.
Scand.J.Gastroenterol. Suppl 57, 1-6 (1979)

3001. Hammer,R., Koss,F.W.
Zum Wirkungsmechanismus des Magensekretionshemmers Pirenzepin.
Mechanism of action of the gastric secretion inhibitor pirenzepin.
Fortschr.Med. 98, 549-54 (1980)

3002. Hamouz,W., Pinder,R.M., Stulemei.,S.M.
Double-blind group comparative trial of mianserin and diazepam in depressed out-patients.
Curr.Med.Res. 6, 72-80 (1980)

3003. Hamouz,W., Pinder,R.M. Stulemei.,S.M.
A double-blind group comparative trial of mianserin and diazepam in depressed outpatients.
Pharmakopsych. 13, 79-83 (1980)

3004. Hanekamp,H.B., Voogt,W.H., Bos,P., Frei,R.W.
A pulse polarographic detector for HPLC-determination of nitrazepam.
J.Liqu.Chrom. 3, 1205-17 (1980)

3005. Hanks,G.W.
Clobazam: pharmacological and therapeutic profile.
Brit.J.Clin.Pharmacol. 7, 151S-155S (1979)

3006. Hara,T.
Syntheses and CNS activity of 1,4-benzodiazepines with a nitrogen atom-containing 5-membered ring fused to the 1,2-position of the diazepine ring.
Jap.Syn.Org.J. 38, 1105-18 (1980)

3007. Haram,K., Bakke,O.M.
Diazepam as an induction agent for caesarean section: a clinical and pharmacokinetic study of fetal drug exposure.
Brit.J.Obstet.Gynaecol. 87, 506-12 (1980)

3008. Haram,K., Bakke,O.M., Sandvei,R., Lund,T.
Foetal drug exposure following intravenous injection of diazepam immediately before breech delivery.
Ann.Chir.Gynaecol. 68, 104-8 (1979)

3009. Haran,R., Tuchague.,J.P.
C-13 and proton NMR-studies of 1,4-benzodiazepines.
J.Heterocycl.Chem. 17, 1483-8 (1980)

3010. Harris,R.A., Case,J.
Effects of maternal consumption of ethanol, barbital, or chlordiazepoxide on the behavior of the offspring.
Behav.Neural.Biol. 26, 234-47 (1979)

3011. Harry,T.V., Latham,A.N.
Hypnotic and residual effects of temazepam in volunteers.
Brit.J.Clin.Pharmacol. 9, 618-20 (1980)

3012. Hartley,L.
Diazepam: human learning of different materials.
Prog.Neuropsychopharmacol. 4, 193-7 (1980)

3013. Haward,L.R.C.
Multivariate symptom analysis related to response to lorazepam treatment.
Curr.Med.Res. 6, 20-3 (1979)

3014. Heinzl,H., Axhausen,C., Bahler,U., Gehrer,H.
Comparison of effects of triazolam (Halcion) and flunitrazepam (Rohypnol) in a double-blind cross-over study of patients in the preoperative stage.
Schweiz.Med.Wschr. 110, 1745-8 (1980)

3015. Hendel,J., Elsass,P., Sorensen,K.H., Moller,I.W., Hvidberg,E.F., Hansen,T.
Anxiety and sedation during a stressful situation after single dose of diazepam versus N-desmethyl-diazepam - a controlled trial.
Psychopharmacology 70, 303-5 (1980)

3016. Hendler,N., Cimini,C., Ma,T., Long,D.
A comparison of cognitive impairment due to benzo-diazepines and to narcotics.
Amer.J.Psychiatry 137, 828-30 (1980)

3017. Henn,F.A.
Relationship of GABA and diazepam receptors in cerebellar purkinje-cells.
Brain Res.Bull. 5, 879-83 (1980)

3018. Herink,J., Fusek,J., Bajgar,J., Hrdina,V.
The effect of diazepam on EEG changes following intraseptal administration of atropine.
Act.Nerv.Super. (Praha) 21, 184-5 (1979)

3019. Herink,J., Fusek,J., Hrdina,V.
The effect of clonazepam on atropine spikes in the limbic system.
Activ.Nerv. 22, 209-10 (1980)

3020. Herr,G.P., Conner,J.T., Katz,R.L., Larmand,J., Schehl,D.
Diazepam and droperidol as i.v. premedicants.
Brit.J.Anaest. 51, 537-42 (1979)

3021. Herrnstadt,C., Mootz,D., Wunderlich,H., Mohrle,H.
Protonation sites of organic-bases with several nitrogen functions - crystal-structures of salts of chlordiazepoxide, dihydralazine, and phenformin.
J.Chem.Soc. P21979, 735-40 (1979)

3022. Hertz,L., Mukerji,S.
Diazepam receptors on mouse astrocytes in primary cultures: displacement by pharmacologically active concentrations of benzodiazepines or barbiturates.
Can.J.Physiol.Pharmacol. 58, 217-20 (1980)

3023. Hester,J.B.,jr., von Voiglander,P.
6-aryl-4H-S-triazolo(4,3-A)(1,4)benzodiazepines. Influence of 1-substitution on pharmacological activity.
J.Med.Chem. 22, 1390-8 (1979)

3024. Hilfiker,O., Larsen,R., Stafforst,D., Kettler,D.
The effects of midazolam on the general, coronary and cerebral circulation.
Anaesthesist 29, 337-8 (1980)

3025. Hindmarch,I.
Benzodiazepines and traffic accidents.
Brit.Med.J. 2, 671 (1979)

3026. Hindmarch,I.
A preliminary study of the effects of repeated doses of clobazam on aspects of performance, arousal and behaviour in a group of anxiety rated volunteers.
Eur.J.Clin.Pharmacol. 16, 17-21 (1979)

3027. Hindmarch,I., Clyde,C.A.
The effect of triazolam and nitrazepam on sleep quality, morning vigilance and psychomotor performance.
Arzneim.-Forsch. (Drug Res.) 30, 1163-6 (1980)

3028. Hindmarch,I., Gudgeon,A.C.
The effects of clobazam and lorazepam on aspects of psychomotor performance and car handling ability.
Brit.J.Clin.Pharmacol. 10, 145-50 (1980)

3029. Hindmarch,I., Parrott,A.C.
The effects of repeated nocturnal doses of clobazam, dipotassium chlorazepate and placebo on subjective ratings of sleep and early morning behaviour and objective measures of arousal, psychomotor performance and anxiety.
Brit.J.Clin.Pharmacol. 8, 325-9 (1979)

3030. Hirai,K., Ishiba,T., Sugimoto,H., Fujishit.,T., Tsukinok.,Y, Hirose,K.
Open-ring derivatives of 1,4-benzodiazepines.
Abs.Pap.Acs. 1979, 6 (1979)

3031. Hockel,S.H.J., Müller,W.E., Wollert,U.
Diazepam increases L-tryptophan uptake into various regions of the rat-brain.
Res.Comm.Psych. 4, 467-75 (1979)

3032. Hodshon,B.J., Garland,W.A.
Plasma-concentration of flurazepam in man following a 30-mg dose of Dalmane.
Fed.Proc. 39, 758 (1980)

3033. Horber,M., Baldauf,A., Poupier,G., Sichel,J.P.
Study of flunitrazepam in 41 cases of severe insomnia in patients hospitalized in psychiatry.
Nouv.Presse 8, 2535-7 (1979)

3034. Horsky,J.
Effect on the climacteric syndrome of natural estrogens and diazepam individually and in combination.
Münch.Med.Wschr. 121, 765-6 (1979)

3035. Hosein,I.N., Defreita.,R., Beaubrun,M.H.
Intramuscular oral lorazepam in acute alcohol withdrawal and incipient delirium tremens.
West Ind.Med.J. 28, 45-8 (1979)

3036. Hossmann,V., Maling,T.J., Hamilton,C.A., Reid,J.L., Dollery,C.T.
Sedative and cardiovascular effects of clonidine and nitrazepam.
Clin.Pharmacol.Ther. 28, 167-76 (1980)

3037. Hossmann,V., Maling,T., Reid,J.L., Dollery,C.T.
Double-blind, placebo controlled, cross-over comparison of the sedative and haemodynamic effect of single doses of clonidine and nitrazepam.
Brit.J.Clin.Pharmacol. 8, 401P (1979)

3038. Hovivian.,M., Kangas,L., Kanto,J.
A comparative-study of the clinical effects of pentobarbital and diazepam given orally as preoperative-medication.
J.Oral Surg. 38, 188-90 (1980)

3039. Howe,J.G.
Lorazepam withdrawal seizures.
Brit.Med.J. 280, 1163-4 (1980)

3040. Howells,R.D., Hiller,J.M., Simon,E.J.
Benzodiazepine binding sites are present in retina.
Life Sci. 25, 2131-6 (1979)

3041. Hoyumpa,A.M.,jr., Desmond,P.V., Roberts,R.K., Nichols,S., Johnson,R.F., Schenker,S.
Effect of ethanol on benzodiazepine disposition in dogs.
J.Lab.Clin.Med. 95, 310-22 (1980)

3042. Hoyumpa,A., Patwardhan,R., Maples,M., Desmond,P., Johnson,R., Schenker,S.
Effect of short-term ethanol administration on lorazepam metabolism.
Gastroenty. 79, 1027 (1980)

3043. Hrbek,J., Komenda,S., Macakova,J., Siroka,A., Navratil,J.
The acute effect of diazepine derivatives on the higher nervous activity in man.
Agressologie 19, 189-91 (1978)

3044. Huang,A., Barker,J.L., Paul,S.M., Moncada,V., Skolnick,P.
Characterization of benzodiazepine receptors in primary cultures of fetal mouse brain and spinal cord neurons.
Brain Res. 190, 485-91 (1980)

3045. Huber,J.W., Raymond,G.G.
Additional conclusions on diazepam injectable precipitate: GC-MS confirmation.
Clin.Toxicol. 14, 439-44 (1979)

3046. Hudson,I.N., Davidson,I.A., Hider,C.F., Wright,A.D.G.
Use of lorazepam in cardiac bypass surgery - comparative-study.
Curr.Med.Res. 6, 303-8 (1979)

3047. Hümpel,M., Illi,V., Milius,W., Wendt,H., Kurowski,M.
The pharmacokinetics and biotransformation of the new benzodiazepine lormetazepam in humans. I. Ab-

sorption, distribution, elimination and metabolism of lormetazepam-5-^{14}C.
Eur.J.Drug Metab.Pharmacokinet. 4, 237-43 (1979)

3048. Hümpel,M., Nieuweboer,B., Milius,W., Hanke,H., Wendt,H.
Kinetics and biotransformation of lormetazepam. II. Radioimmunological determinations in plasma and urine of young and elderly subjects - first-pass-effects.
Clin.Pharmacol. 28, 673-9 (1980)

3049. Huettel,M.S., Christensen,K.N.
Naloxone as antidote in benzodiazepine poisoning.
Ugeskr.Laeger 141, 1979-81 (1979)

3050. Huettel,M.S., Schou Olesen,A., Stoffersen,E.
Complement-mediated reactions to diazepam with cremophor as solvent (Stesolid mr.).
Brit.J.Anaesth. 52, 77-9 (1980)

3051. Hug,R., Richou,H.
4 years experience of a hypno-inducer in psychiatry - 200 patients treated with flunitrazepam.
Nouv.Presse 8, 2548-9 (1979)

3052. Hunninghake,D.B., Wallace,R.B., Reiland,S., Barrettc.,E., Hoover,J., Mackenth.,A., Wahl,P., Heiss,G.
Alterations in plasma-lipid and lipoprotein levels associated with the use of benzodiazepine tranquilizers - the lipid research clinics program.
Amer.J.Epidem. 112, 451 (1980)

3053. Hwang,E.C., Vanwoert,M.H.
Anti-myoclonic action of clonazepam - role of serotonin.
Pharmacologist 21, 183 (1979)

3054. Hwang,E.C., Vanwoert,M.H.
Anti-myoclonic action of clonazepam - role of serotonin.
Eur.J.Pharmacol. 60, 31-40 (1979)

3055. Illingworth,R.
Systematic review of benzodiazepines.
Brit.Med.J. 280, 1085 (1980)

3056. Imoto,R.M.
Benzodiazepine withdrawal reaction.
Drug Intell. 14, 187 (1980)

3057. Inaba,M., Kamata,K., Kamide,M.
Diurnal -variation of polyphagic effect of diazepam and its mechanism.
J.Pharmacol. 3, 3 (1980)

3058. Inaba,M., Kamata,K., Kamide,M.
Diazepam-induced polyphagia - diurnal-variation of polyphagic effect and inverse relationship between decrease in the polyphagic effect and increase in serum corticosterone level.
Fol.Pharm.Jap. 76, 122 (1980)

3059. Inotsume,N., Nakano,M.
Reversible azomethine bond-cleavage of 2'-fluoro derivatives of benzodiazepines in acidic solutions at body-temperature.
Int.J.Pharm. 6, 147-54 (1980)

3060. Inotsume,N., Nakano,M.
Reversible ring-opening reactions of nimetazepam and nitrazepam in acidic media at body-temperature.
J.Pharm.Sci. 69, 1331-4 (1980)

3061. Inotsume,N., Nakano,M., Sekikawa,H., Juni,K., Kohri,N., Arita,T.
Hydrolysis of drugs in acidic media - reversible ring-opening reactions of benzodiazepine anti-anxiety agents.
J.Pharmacol. 3, 3 (1980)

3062. Iriki,A., Ikezono,E., Toda,K., Tanaka,H.
Diazepam-induced suppression of jaw opening reflex in rats.
Bull.Tokyo Med.Dent.Univ. 27, 1-7 (1980)

3063. Ishida,Y., Dalri,H., Schmidt,G., Vetterlein,F.
Actions of diazepam on the discharge pattern of phrenic motoneurones in rats.
Neuropharmacology 18, 679-87 (1979)

3064. Iversen,L.L.
Der gegenwärtige Status der Benzodiazepine in der Psychopharmakologie.
The Present Status of Benzodiazepines in Psychopharmacology.
New Perspectives in Benzodiazepine Therapy - International Symposium Heidelberg 1979.
Arzneim.-Forsch. (Drug Res.) 30, 907-10 (1980)

3065. Iversen,S.D.
Tiermodelle für die Prüfung von Angst und Benzodiazepin-Wirkung.
Animal Models of Anxiety and Benzodiazepine Actions.
New Perspectives in Benzodiazepine Therapy - International Symposium Heidelberg 1979.
Arzneim.-Forsch. (Drug Res.) 30, 862-68 (1980)

3066. Iversen,L.L.
The present state of tranquility.
Nature 285, 285-6 (1980)

3067. Jackson,M.R., Harris,P.A.
Absence of effect of diazepam on tumors.
Lancet 1, 104 (1981)

3068. Jacobsen,D., Kjeldsen,S.E., Bredesen,J.E.
Hazards of benzodiazepine poisoning.
Tidsskr.Nor.Laegeforen 99, 1707-8 (1979)

3069. Jakoubek,B., Pevzer,L.Z., Pavlik,A.
Changes of the protein-metabolism in rat spinal motoneurons and perineuronal glial-cells induced by anticipation stress and the administration of diazepam - cytospectrophotometric and autoradiographic study.
Neuroscience 4, 1179-86 (1979)

3070. James,R.T.D., Dean,B.C.
A comparison of a single night-time and a divided daily dosage regimen of a chlordiazepoxide-amitriptyline combination.
Curr.Med.Res. 6, 573-5 (1980)

3071. James,T.A., Macleod,N.K., Mayer,M.L.
A functional antagonisms between benzodiazepines and ACTH?
Brit.J.Pharmacol. 66, 115P-116P (1979)

3072. Javors,M., Erwin,V.G.
Effects of benzodiazepines and valproic acid on brain aldehyde reductase and a proposed mechanism of anticonvulsant action.
Biochem.Pharmacol. 29, 1703-8 (1980)

3073. Jeal,D.E.
Chlorazepate for premedication.
Brit.J.Anaest. 51, 263 (1979)

3074. Jeffery,D.R., Barrett,J.E.
Effects of chlordiazepoxide on comparable rates of punished and unpunished responding.
Psychopharmacology (Berlin) 64, 9-11 (1979)

3075. Jenner,P., Marsden,C.D., Pratt,J., Reynolds,E.H.
Altered serotoninergic activity in mouse brain induced by clonazepam.
Brit.J.Pharmacol. 64, 432P (1978)

3076. Jepsen,P.W., Haastrup,S.
Withdrawal reactions after benzodiazepine treatment.
Ugeskr.Laeger 141, 1121-5 (1979)

3077. Jessel,H.J.
Wirkungsfall und Verträglichkeit eines neuen Tranquilizers (Clobazam) im Rahmen einer Langzeitstudie.
Therapiewoche 29, 4348-53 (1979)

3078. Johansson,B.W.
Comparative-study of cardioselective beta-blockade and diazepam in patients with acute myocardial-infarction and tachycardia.
Act.Med.Scand. 207, 47-53 (1980)

3079. Johanson,C.E., Uhlenhut.,E.H.
Drug preference and mood in humans - diazepam.
Psychopharmacology 71, 269-73 (1980)

3080. Johnson,B.W., Kramer,M., Bonnet,M., Roth,T., Jansen,T.
The effect of ketazolam on ocular motility during rem-sleep.
Curr.Ther.Res. 28, 792-9 (1980)

3081. Johnson,L.C., Church,M.W., Seales,D.M., Rossiter,V.S.
Auditory arousal thresholds of good sleepers and poor sleepers with and without flurazepam.
Sleep 1, 259-70 (1979)

3082. Johnson,L.C., Seales,D.M., Naitoh,P., Church,M.W., Sinclair,M.
The effects of flurazepam hydrochloride on brain electrical activity during sleep.
Electroencephalogr.Clin.Neurophysiol. 47, 309-21 (1979)

3083. Johnson,R.F., Schenker,S., Roberts,R.K., Desmond, P.V., Wilkinson,G.R.
Plasma binding of benzodiazepines in humans.
J.Pharm.Sci. 68, 1320-2 (1979)

3084. Johnson,R.W., Yamamura,H.I.
Photoaffinity labeling of the benzodiazepine receptor in bovine cerebral cortex.
Life Sci. 25, 1613-20 (1979)

3085. Johnson,R.W., Yamamura,H.I.
Photoaffinity-labeling, solubilization and partial-purification of benzodiazepine receptors from mammalian brain.
Fed.Proc. 39, 387 (1980)

3086. Jonen,H.G.
Enhancement of reductive metabolism of p-nitrobenzoate and nitrazepam in isolated perfused rat liver by ethanol.
Drug Metab.Dispos. 7, 176-80 (1979)

3087. Jones,D.J., Stehling,L.C., Zauder,H.L.
Cardiovascular responses to diazepam and midazolam maleate in the dog.
Anesthesiology 51, 430-4 (1979)

3088. Jones,D.M., Jones,M.E., Lewis,M.J., Spriggs,T.L.
Drugs and human memory: effects of low doses of nitrazepam and hyoscine on retention.
Brit.J.Clin.Pharmacol. 7, 479-83 (1979)

3089. Jordan,C., Lehane,J.R., Jones,J.G.
Effect of naloxone on respiratory changes after diazepam.
Brit.J.Anaest. 51, P570 (1979)

3090. Jordan,C., Tech,B., Lehane,J.R., Jones,J.G.
Respiratory depression following diazepam - reversal with high-dose naloxone.
Anesthesiol. 53, 293-8 (1980)

3091. Jost,U., Bortel,H.J., Schmitt,M., Hoyer,S.
Beeinflussung der cerebralen Glycolyse und Atmungskettenoxidation (dem neuronalen energieliefernden Stoffwechsel) durch Thiopental, Flunitrazepam und Etomidate im steady state einer standardisierten Inhalationsnarkose.
The effects of thiopentone, etomidate and flunitrazepam on cerebral energy metabolism in the rat.
Anaesthesist 29, 12-7 (1980)

3092. Kageyama,H., Kurosawa,A.
Effect of diazepam on rat cerebellar GABAergic mechanisms.
Fol.Pharm.Jap. 75, 90 (1979)

3093. Kageyama,H., Kurosawa,A.
A probable site of action of diazepam in rat cerebellar GABA system.
Life Sci. 27, 1783-9 (1980)

3094. Kales,A., Scharf,M.B., Kales,J.D., Soldatos,C.R.
Rebound insomnia. A potential hazard following withdrawal of certain benzodiazepines.
J.Amer.Med.Ass. 241, 1692-5 (1979)

3095. Kales,A., Scharf,M.B., Soldatos,C.R., Bixler,E.O., Bianchi,S.B., Schweitzer,P.K.
Quazepam, a new benzodiazepin hypnotic. - Intermediate-term sleep laboratory evaluation.
J.Clin.Pharm. 20, 184-92 (1980)

3096. Kamioka,T., Nakayama,I., Hara,T., Takagi,H.
Pharmacological studies on CS-430, a new psychotropic agent.
Arzneim.-Forsch. (Drug Res.) 28, 838-47 (1978)

3097. Kanfer,I., Holmes,J., Zwarenstein,H.
Benzodiazepine-cholinesterase interactions.
S.Afr.J.Sci. 75, 318-9 (1979)

3098. Kangas,L., Erkkola,R., Kanto,J., Eronen,M.
Transfer of free and conjugated oxazepam across the human placenta.
Eur.J.Clin.Pharmacol. 17, 301-4 (1980)

3099. Kangas,L., Kanto,J., Lehtinen,V., Salminen,J.
Long-term nitrazepam treatment in psychiatric out-patients with insomnia.
Psychopharmacology 63, 63-6 (1979)

3100. Kaniewska,T., Wejman,W.
Gas-chromatographic determination of bromo and fluoro derivatives of benzodiazepine in human body fluid.
J.Chromatogr. 182, 81-7 (1980)

3101. Kanto,J., Aaltonen,L., Liukko,P., Maenpaeae,K.
Transfer of lorazepam and its conjugate across the human placenta.
Acta Pharmacol.et Toxicol. 47, 130-4 (1980)

3102. Kanto,J., Iisalo,E.U., Hovi-Viander,M., Kangas,L.
A comparative study on the clinical effects of oxazepam and diazepam: relationship between plasma level and effect.
Int.J.Clin.Pharmacol.Biopharm. 17, 26-31 (1979)

3103. Kanto,J., Iisalo,E., Kangas,L., Valovirta,E.
A comparative-study on the clinical effects of rectal diazepam and pentobarbital on small children - relationship between plasma-level and effect.
Int.J.Clin.Pharmacol. 18, 348-51 (1980)

3104. Kanto,J., Kangas,L., Mansikka,M.
Flunitrazepam versus placebo premedication for minor surgery.
Acta Anaesth.Scand. 23, 561-6 (1979)

3105. Kanto,J., Maeenpaeae,M., Maentylae,R., Sellman,R., Valovirta,E.
Effect of age on the pharmacokinetics of diazepam given in conjunction with spinal anesthesia.
Anesthesiology 51, 154-9 (1979)

3106. Kaplan,S.R.
Benzodiazepine withdrawal symptoms.
Amer.J.Psychiatry 137, 750-1 (1980)

3107. Karapety.,A.A., Andriano.,V.G., Struchko.,Y.T., Bogatsky,A.V., Andronat.,S.A., Korotenk.,T.I.
Crystal and molecular-structure of 7-bromo-5-(o-chlorophenyl)-1,3-dihydro-2H-1,4-benzodiazepine-2-one.
Bioorg.Khim. 5, 1684-90 (1979)

3108. Karch,F.E.
Rage reaction associated with clorazepate dipotassium.
Ann.Intern.Med. 91, 61-2 (1979)

3109. Karlicze.,G., Birks,R.J.S., Brenken,U., Agnew,M.
Termination of anesthesia - do we pay enough attention to its consequences - hemodynamic-studies following the use of piritramide, flunitrazepam and nitrous-oxide anesthesia for open-heart surgery.
Anaesthesis 29, 370-5 (1980)

3110. Karmali,R.A.
Inhibition of prostaglandin synthesis by diazepam in macrophages.
Eur.J.Cell. 22, 573 (1980)

3111. Karmali,R.A., Volkman,A., Muse,P., Louis,T.M.
Effects of diazepam on tumor growth and plasma prostaglandin E2 in rats.
Adv.Prostaglandin Thromboxane Res. 6, 523-4 (1980)

3112. Karobath,M.
Molecular-basis of benzodiazepine actions.
Trends Neur. 2, 166-8 (1979)

3113. Karobath,M., Drexler,G., Supavila.,P.
Modulation by picrotoxin and IPTBO of flunitrazepam-H-3 binding to the GABA-benzodiazepine receptor complex of rat cerebellum.
Life Sci. 28, 307-13 (1981)

3114. Karobath,M., Lippitsch,M.
Thip and isoguvacine are partial agonists of GABA-stimulated benzodiazepine receptor binding.
Eur.J.Pharmacol. 58, 485-8 (1979)

3115. Karobath,M., Placheta, P.
Pharmacological characterization of GABA-stimulated benzodiazepine receptor-binding.
Naunyn-Schmied.Arch.Pharmacol. 307, 62 (1979)

3116. Karobath,M., Placheta,P., Lippitsch,M., Krogsgaard-Larsen,P.
Is stimulation of benzodiazepine receptor binding mediated by a novel GABA receptor?
Nature 278, 748-9 (1979)

3117. Karobath,M., Placheta,P., Lippitsch,M., Krogsgaard-Larsen,P.
Characterization of GABA-stimulated benzodiazepine receptor binding.
Adv.Biochem.Psychopharmacol. 21, 313-20 (1980)

3118. Karobath,M., Rogers,J., Bloom,F.E.
Benzodiazepine receptors remain unchanged after chronic ethanol administration.
Neuropharmacology 19, 125-8 (1980)

3119. Kawahara,R., Houri,D., Tanabe,K., Kimishim.,K.
Correlation between anticonvulsive activity and antianxiety action of benzodiazepines.
Fol.Pharm.Jap. 75, P67-P68 (1979)

3120. Keinanen.,S., Simila,S., Lucma,P., Kangas,L., Saukkone.,A.L.
Anti-pyretic effect and plasma-concentrations of rectal acetaminophen and diazepam in children.
Epilepsia 20, 607-12 (1979)

3121. Kellermann,G.H., Luyten-Kellermann,M.
On the regulation of antipyrine and oxazepam metabolism in man.
Res.Commun.Chem.Pathol.Pharmacol. 23, 287-96 (1979)

3122. Kellner,R., Rada,R.T., Andersen,T., Pathak,D.
Effects of chlordiazepoxide on self-rated depression, anxiety, and well-being.
Psychopharmacology 64, 185-91 (1979)

3123. Kellogg,C., Tervo,D., Ison,J., Parisi,T., Miller,R.K.
Prenatal exposure to diazepam alters behavioral development in rats.
Acience 207, 205-7 (1980)

3124. Kemper,N., Poser,W., Poser,S.
Benzodiazepine dependence - addiction potential of the benzodiazepines is greater than previously assumed.
Deut.Med.Wschr. 105, 1707-12 (1980)

3125. Kennedy,B. , Leonard,B.E.
Similarity between the action of nicotinamide and diazepam on neurotransmitter metabolism in the rat.
Biochem.Soc.Trans. 8, 59-60 (1980)

3126. Khan,A.A.
Preliminary in vitro study of diazepam and droperidol on oestrus rat uterus.
Brit.J.Anaesth. 52, 349-54 (1980)

3127. Khan,A., Joyce,P., Jones,A.V.
Benzodiazepine withdrawal syndromes.
New Zeal.Med.J. 92, 94-6 (1980)

3128. Khoo,K.C., Mendels,J., Rothbart,M., Garland,W.A., Colburn,W.A., Min,B.H., Lucek,R., Carbone,J.J., Boxenbaum,H.G., Kaplan,S.A.
Influence of phenytoin and phenobarbital on the disposition of a single oral dose of clonazepam.
Clin.Pharm.Ther. 28, 368-75 (1980)

3129. Killam,E.K., Suria,A.
Benzodiazepines.
Adv.Neurol. 27, 597-615 (1980)

3130. Kim,K.K., Sirman,A., Trainor,F.S., Lee,B.Y.
Anxiolytic efficacy and safety of ketazolam compared with diazepam and placebo.
Clin.Ther. 3, 9-14 (1980)

3131. Kissin,I.
Diazepam anesthesia and myocardial-contractility.
Anesthesiol. 53, 78 (1980)

3132. Kitagawa,H., Esumi,Y., Kurosawa,S., Sekine,S., Yokoshima,T.
Metabolism of 8-chloro-6-(o-chlorophenyl)-1-methyl-4H-S-triazolo (4,3-alpha) (1,4) benzodiazepine, triazolam, a new central depressant. I. Absorption, distribution and excretion in rats, dogs and monkeys.
Xenobiotica 9, 415-28 (1979)

3133. Kitagawa,H., Esumi,Y., Kurosawa,S., Sekine,S., Yokoshima,T.
Metabolism of 8-chloro-6-(o-chlorophenyl)-1-methyl-4H-S-triazolo (4,3-alpha) (1,4) benzodiazepine, triazolam, a new central depressant. II. Identification and determination of metabolites in rats and dogs.
Xenobiotica 9, 429-39 (1979)

3134. Kleber,R.J.
Double-blind comparative-study of desipramine hydrochloride and diazepam in the control of mixed anxiety-depression symptomatology.
J.Clin.Psych. 40, 165-70 (1979)

3135. Kleber,R.J.
Ketazolam compared to diazepam and placebo in the treatment of anxiety.
J.Int.Med.Res. 8, 439-45 (1980)

3136. Kleindienst,W., Frangenh.,H.
Ketamine-HCl-diazepam anesthesia for laparoscopy.
J.Repro.Med. 23, 299-303 (1979)

3137. Klepner,C.A., Lippa,A.S., Benson,D.I., Sano,M.C., Beer,B.
Resolution of two biochemically and pharmacologically distinct benzodiazepine receptors.
Pharmacol.Biochem.Behav. 11, 457-62 (1979)

3138. Klotz,U.
Effect of age on levels of diazepam in plasma and brain of rats.
Naunyn Schmied.Arch.Pharmacol. 307, 167-9 (1979)

3139. Klotz,U., Anttila,V.J., Reimann,T.
Cimetidine/diazepam interaction.
Lancet 2, 699 (1979)

3140. Klotz,U., Kangas,L., Kanto,J.
Clinical Pharmacokinetics of Benzodiazepines.
Gustav Fischer Verlag, Stuttgart-New York 1980

3141. Klotz,U., Mueller-Seydlitz,P.
Altered elimination of desmethyldiazepam in the elderly.
Brit.J.Clin.Pharmacol. 7, 119-20 (1979)

3142. Klotz,U., Reimann,I.
Delayed clearance of diazepam due to cimetidine.
N.Engl.J.Med. 302, 1012-4 (1980)

3143. Klotz,U., Reimann,I.
Effect of cimetidine on the clearance of benzodiazepines - reply.
N.Engl.J.Med. 303, 754 (1980)

3144. Klotz,U., Reimann,I.
Influence of cimetidine on the pharmacokinetics of desmethyldiazepam and oxazepam.
Eur.J.Clin.Pharmacol. 18, 517-20 (1980)

3145. Knobel,M.
Hypnotic effect of triazolam.
Rev.Bras.Med. 36, 518-24 (1979)

3146. Knudsen,F.U.
Rectal administration of diazepam in solution in the acute treatment of convulsions in infants and children - anticonvulsant effect and side-effects.
Arch.Dis.Ch. 54, 855-7 (1979)

3147. Ko,H., Royer,M., Hester,J.B., Johnston,K.T.
Radioimmunoassay of triazolam.
Analyt.Lett. 10, 1019 (1977)

3148. Kober,A., Sjoeholm,I., Borga,O., Odar-Cederloef,I.
Protein binding of diazepam and digitoxin in uremic and normal serum.
Biochem.Pharmacol. 28, 1037-42 (1979)

3149. Koeppen,D.
Review of clinical studies on clobazam.
Brit.J.Clin.Pharmacol. 7, 139S-150S (1979)

3150. Korttila,K., Aromaa,U.
Venous complications after intravenous-injection of diazepam, flunitrazepam, thiopentone and etomidate.
Acta Anaesth.Scand. 24, 227-30 (1980)

3151. Korttila,K., Levanen,J., Auvinen,J.
Failure of intramuscularly administered lorazepam and scopolamine-morphine premedication to produce amnesic effects to supplement conduction anesthesia.
Acta Anaesth.Scand. 24, 325-330 (1980)

3152. Korttila,K., Tammisto,T., Aromaa,U.
Comparison of etomidate in combination with fentanyl or diazepam, with thiopentone as an induction agent for general-anesthesia.
Brit.J.Anaest. 51, 1151-7 (1979)

3153. Kotzan,J.A., Meedham,T.E., Honigberg,I.L., Vallner, J.J., Stewart,J.T., Brown,W.J., Jun,H.W.
Examination of blood clobazam levels and several pupillary measures in humans.
J.Pharm.Sci. 68, 1002-4 (1979)

3154. Kramp, P., Rnsted,P., Hansen,T.
Barbital and diazepam plasma levels during treatment of delirium tremens.
Acta Psychiatr.Scand. 59, 263-75 (1979)

3155. Krimmer,E.C., Barry,H.
Pentobarbital and chlordiazepoxide differentiated from each other and from nondrug.
Commun.Psychopharmacol. 3, 93-9 (1979)

3156. Krimmer,E.C., Barry,H.
Relationship among pentobarbital, chlordiazepoxide and alcohol tested by their discriminative effects.
Fed.Proc. 39, 402 (1980)

3157. Krogsgaard,P., Arnt,J.
Pharmacological studies of the interactions between GABA and benzodiazepine receptors.
Brain Res.Bull. 4, 706 (1979)

3158. Krogsgaard,P., Arnt,J.
Pharmacological studies of interactions between benzodiazepines and GABA receptors.
Brain Res.Bull. 5, 867-72 (1980)

3159. Krzysko,K., Wichlinski,L.M.
Pharmacokinetics and bioavailability of chlordiazepoxide in humans.
Mater.Med.Pol. 11, 15-8 (1979)

3160. Kuch,H.
Clobazam: chemical aspects of the 1,4- and 1,5-benzodiazepines.
Brit.J.Clin.Pharmacol. 7 Suppl 1, 17S-21S (1979)

3161. Kuhar,M.J., Palacios,J.M., Young,W.S.
Radio-histochemical studies of the GABA and benzodiazepine receptors.
Brain Res.Bull. 4, 700 (1979)

3162. Kuhn,H.
Autoradiographic evidence for binding of 3H-flunitrazepam (Rohypnol) to melanin granules in the cat eye.
Experientia 36, 863-5 (1980)

3163. Kumar,S.M., Kothary,S.P., Zsigmond,E.K.
Lack of cardiovascular stimulation during endotracheal intubation in cardiac surgical patients anesthetized with diazepam-ketamine-pancuronium.
Clin.Ther. 3, 43-8 (1980)

3164. Kurokawa,T., Yokota,K., Mitsudom.,A., Shibata,R., Takashim.,S., Goya,N.
Diagnostic and prognostic significance of electroencephalography with intravenous diazepam in epilepsy.
Fol.Psychiatr. 33, 15-20 (1979)

3165. Kuruvilla,A., Uretsky,N.
The interaction of chlordiazepoxide and sodium valproate in the nucleus accumbens of the rat.
Life Sci. 28, 393-9 (1981)

3166. Kusaka,M., Horikawa,A., Meshi,T., Maruyama,Y.
Interaction of triazolam with desipramine - effects of single and repeated treatment on certain pharmacologic responses and brain catecholamine levels.
Psychopharmacology 70, 255-61 (1980)

3167. Laakmann,G., Blaschke,D., Buttermann,M., Hippius,H., Schewe,S., Uberla,K.
Double-blind study with the benzodiazepine derivative KA-2547 in out-patients with anxiety neurosis.
Arzneim.-Forsch. (Drug Res.) 30, 1233-4 (1980)

3168. Lader,M.
Der gegenwärtige Status der Benzodiazepine in Psychiatrie und Medizin.
The Present Status of the Benzodiazepines in Psychiatry and Medicine.
New Perspectives in Benzodiazepine Therapy - International Symposium Heidelberg 1979.
Arzneim.-Forsch. (Drug Res.) 30, 910-3 (1980)

3169. Lader,M.H., Curry,S., Baker,W.J.
Physiological and psychological effects of clorazepate in man.
Brit.J.Clin.Pharmacol. 9, 83-90 (1980)

3170. Ladewig,D.
Is there rebound insomnia following benzodiazepine administration.
Deut.Med.Wschr. 105, 1483-4 (1980)

3171. Ladimer,I.
Trials and tribulations of triazolam.
J.Clin.Pharmacol. 20, 159-61 (1980)

3172. Ladimer,I.
Trials and tribulations of triazolam.
J.Clin.Pharmacol. 20, 701-2 (1980)

3173. Lahti,R.A., Gall,M.
Conversion of N-alkylaminobenzophenones to benzodiazepines in vivo.
J.Med.Chem. 19, 1064-7 (1976)

3174. Lai,A.A., Levy,R.H.
Pharmacokinetic description of drug interactions by enzyme induction: carbamazepine-clonazepam in monkeys.
J.Pharm.Sci. 68, 416-21 (1979)

3175. Lai,A.A., Min,B.H., Garland,W.A., Levy,R.H.
Kinetics of biotransformation of clonazepam to its 7-amino metabolite in the monkey.
J.Pharm.Biopharm. 7, 87-95 (1979)

3176. Laisi,U., Linnoila,M., Seppälä,T., Himberg,J.J., Mattila,M.J.
Pharmacokinetic and pharmacodynamic interactions of diazepam with different alcoholic beverages.
Eur.J.Clin.Pharm. 16, 263-70 (1979)

3177. Lal,H., Shearman,G.T., Fielding,S., Dunn,R., Kruse,H., Theurer,K.
Evidence that GABA mechanisms mediate the anxiolytic action of benzodiazepines - a study with valproic acid.
Neuropharm. 19, 785-9 (1980)

3178. Landauer,A.
Diazepam and traffic accidents.
Brit.Med.J. 2, 207 (1979)

3179. Lang,B., Barnard,E.A., Chang,L.R., Dolly,J.O.
Putative benzodiazepine receptor: a protein solubilised from brain.
FEBS Lett. 104, 149-53 (1979)

3180. Larmand,J., Vredevoe,L.A., Conner,J.T., Herr,G.P., Schehl,D.
Lorazepam and morphine for i.v. surgical premedication.
Brit.J.Anaest. 52, 1259-63 (1980)

3181. Lasagna,L.
The Halcion story - trial by media.
Lancet 1, 815-6 (1980)

3182. Lasagna,L.
The Halcion story.
Lancet 1, 1304-5 (1980)

3183. Lasserre,E.
Insomnia at altitude - efficacy of flunitrazepam.
Nouv.Presse 8, 2577-8 (1979)

3184. Laudano,O.
Clinical study of clobazam in patients with gastro-intestinal disorders.
Brit.J.Clin.Pharmacol. 7, 129S (1979)

3185. Laughren,T.P.
Maintenance treatment with benzodiazepines.
Amer.J.Psychiatry 137, 130 (1980)

3186. Lavielle,S., Tassin,J.P., Thierry,A.M., Blanc,G., Herve,D., Barthele.,C., Glowinsk.,J.
Blockade by benzodiazepines of the selective high increase in dopamine turnover induced by stress in mesocortical dopaminergic-neurons of the rat.
Brain Res. 168, 585-94 (1979)

3187. Leander,J.D.
Chronic diazepam pretreatment reduces the behavior suppressing effects of meperidine and normeperidine.
Pharmacology 21, 160 (1979)

3188. Lebellec,M., Bismuth,C., Lagier,G., Dally,S.
Strong withdrawal syndrome with benzodiazepines (6 cases).
Therapie 35, 113-8 (1980)

3189. Leclert,A., Lacassin,G., Marceau,J.F., Gavaldon,E.
Study of flunitrazepam in orthopedic-surgery and traumatology.
Nouv.Presse 8, 2567-8 (1979)

3190. Le Fur,G., Guilloux,F., Mitrani,N., Mizoule,J., Uzan,A.
Relationships between plasma corticosteroids and benzodiazepines in stress.
J.Pharmacol.Exp.Ther. 211, 305-8 (1979)

3191. Lehmann,K., Schmidt,J.
Beeinflussung somatosensorisch ausgelöster Kortex-potentiale durch Psychopharmaka.
Effect of psychotropic drugs on somatosensory evoked cortical potentials.
Acta Biol.Med.Ger. 38, 619-25 (1979)

3192. Leutner,V., Müller-Clemm,H.
Rohypnol parenterally - benzodiazepine for the anesthesiology.
Med.Welt 30, 1276-82 (1979)

3193. Liddiard,C., Egger,H.J., Nau.H.
Placental-transfer and invitro fetal hepatic-metabolism of prazepam and diphenylhydantoin in humans during the 1st-half of pregnancy.
Naunyn-Schmied.Arch.Pharmacol. 307, 16 (1979)

3194. Liljequist,R., Mattila,M.J.
Acute effects of temazepam and nitrazepam on psychomotor skills and memory.
Acta Pharmacol.Toxicol. (Copenh) 44, 364-9 (1979)

3195. Liljequist,R., Palva,E., Linnoila,M.
Effects on learning and memory of 2-week treatments with chlordiazepoxide lactam, N-desmethyldiazepam, oxazepam and methyloxazepam, alone or in combination with alcohol.
Int.Pharmacopsychiatry 14, 190-8 (1979)

3196. Lindgren,L., Saarniva.,L., Himberg,J.J.
Comparison of oral triclofos, diazepam and flunitrazepam as premedicants in children undergoing otolaryngological surgery.
Brit.J.Anaest. 52, 283-90 (1980)

3197. Lindgren,L., Saarniva.,L., Himberg,J.J.
Comparison of i.m. pethidine, diazepam and flunitrazepam as premedicants in children undergoing otolaryngological surgery.
Brit.J.Anaest. 51, 321-7 (1979)

3198. Linnoila,M., Erwin,C.W., Brendle,A., Skinner,T., Routledge,P.A.
Pharmacodynamics and pharmacokinetics of diazepam in an abuser.
Acta Pharmacol.Toxicol. 47, 75-7 (1980)

3199. Linnoila,M., Erwin,C.W., Logue,P.E.
Efficacy and side-effects of flurazepam and combination of amobarbital and secobarbital in insomniac patients.
J.Clin.Pharmacol. 20, 117-23 (1980)

3200. Linnoila,M., Viukari,M., Lamminsi.,U., Auvinen,J.
Efficacy and side-effects of lorazepam, oxazepam, and temazepam as sleeping aids in psychogeriatric inpatients.
Int.Pharmacopsych. 15, 129-35 (1980)

3201. Lippa,A.S., Coupet,J., Greenblatt,E.N., Klepner,C.A., Beer,B.
A synthetic non-benzodiazepine ligand for benzodiazepine receptors: a probe for investigating neuronal substrates of anxiety.
Pharmacol.Biochem.Behav. 11, 99-106 (1979)

3202. Lippa,A.S., Critchett,D., Sano,M.C., Klepner,C.A., Greenblatt,E.N., Coupet,J., Beer,B.
Benzodiazepine receptors: cellural and behavioral characteristics.
Pharmacol.Biochem.Behav. 10, 831-43 (1979)

3203. Lippa,A.S., Klepner,C.A., Benson,D.I., Critchet.,D.J., Sano,M.C., Beer,B.
The role of GABA in mediating the anticonvulsant properties of benzodiazepines.
Brain Res.Bull. 5, 861-5 (1980)

3204. Livingstone,S.
Phenobarbital and diazepam treatment of isolated seizures.
J.Amer.Med.Ass. 244, 1380 (1980)

3205. Loehning,R.W., Kerber,C.W.
Value of lorazepam in gas encephalography - preliminary-report.
Neuroradiol. 18, 37-40 (1979)

3206. Login,I.S.
Clonazepam therapy in reading epilepsy.
Neurology 31, 115 (1981)

3207. Longstreth,G.F., Obrien,P.M., Youkeles,L.F.
Determinants of the intravenous diazepam dose required for gastroscopy.
Gastrointest.Endoscopy 26, 92-4 (1980)

3208. Loo,H., Moussaou.,D., Guillou,S., Sechter,D.
Questionnaire comparing the hypnotic effects of flunitrazepam and a placebo in a psychiatric setting.
Rev.Med.Parm. 21, 517-23 (1980)

3209. Lossius,R., Dietrich.,P., Lunde,P.K.M.
Effect of diazepam and desmethyldiazepam in spasticity and rigidity - a quantitative study of reflexes and plasma-concentrations.
Acta Neurol.Sci. 61, 378-83 (1980)

3210. Lovell,D.K., Bedford,J.A., Grove,L., Wilson,M.C.
Effects of d-amphetamine and diazepam on paired and grouped primate food competition.
Pharmacol.Biochem.Behav. 13, 177-81 (1980)

3211. Lucek,R., Dixon,R.
Chlordiazepoxide concentrations in saliva and plasma measured by radioimmunoassay.
Res.Comm.Chem.Path.Pharmacol. 27, 397-400 (1980)

3212. Lukovits,I., Otvos,L.
Correlation between the protein-binding, biological-activity and the energy of the highest occupied molecular-orbital of benzodiazepine.
Acta Physiol.Hung. 52, 235 (1978)

3213. MacDonald,R.L., Barker,J.L.
Enhancement of GABA-mediated postsynaptic inhibition in cultured mammalian spinal-cord neurons - common-mode of anticonvulsant action.
Brain Res. 167, 323-36 (1979)

3214. MacDonald,J.F., Barker,J.L., Paul,S.M., Marangos,P.J., Skolnick,P.
Inosine may be an endogenous ligand for benzodiazepine receptors on cultured spinal neurons.
Science 205, 715-7 (1979)

3215. MacKichan,J.J., Duffner,P.K., Cohen,M.E.
Disposition of intravenous diazepam in epileptic children.
Drug Intell. 14, 636 (1980)

3216. Macklon,A.F., James,O., Rawlins,M.D.
Hepatic-metabolism of diazepam in relation to age.
Clin.Sci. 56, 14 (1979)

3217. Macleod,N., Kratochvil,C.H.
Behavioural reactions to triazolam.
Lancet 2, 638-9 (1979)

3218. Macleod,S.M., Giles,H.G., Porter,B., Kaplan,H.L., Frecker,R.C., Sellers,E.M.
Gender-related differences in diazepam dynamics.
Clin.Pharmacol. 25, 236 (1979)

3219. Macnew,B.A., Finnegan,L.P.
Diazepam in the treatment of neonatal methadone abstinence.
Pediat.Res. 14, 469 (1980)

3220. Macphail,I., Ogilvie,W.A., Purvis,C.R.
Comparison of diazepam and flurazepam in the treatment of insomnia in general-practice.
J.Int.Med.Res. 7, 401-3 (1979)

3221. Madsen,P.E., Grove,O., Jensen,K.B., Lauritsen,K., Marner,I.L.
Thrombophlebitis after intravenous injection of diazepam. Prevention with dilution or flushing with isotonic saline evaluated in a randomized clinical trial.
Ugeskr.Laeger 142, 643-4 (1980)

3222. Maekawa,T., Oshibuch.,T., Imamura,A., Takeshit.,H.
Effects of psychotropic-drugs on the cerebral energy-state and glycolytic metabolism in the rat - diazepam, clomipramine and chlorpromazine.
Biochem.Pharmacol. 29, 15-8 (1980)

3223. Magelund,C.G., Marck,H.I.
Gynecomastia during benzodiazepine abuse.
Ugeskr.Laeger 141, 2677 (1979)

3224. Maggi,A., Satinove.,J., Oberdorf.,M., Mann,E., Enna,S.J.
Phylogenetic characteristics of muscimol-activated benzodiazepine receptor-binding.
Brain Res.Bull. 5, 167-71 (1980)

3225. Magnussen,I., Oxlund,H.R., Alsbirk,K.E., Arnold,E.
Absorption of diazepam in man following rectal and parenteral administration.
Acta Pharmacol.Toxicol. (Copenh) 45, 87-90 (1979)

3226. Maher,J.
Intravenous lorazepam to prevent nausea and vomiting associated with cancer-chemotherapy.
Lancet 1, 91-2 (1981)

3227. Maksay,G., Tegyey,Z., Kemeny,V., Lukovits,I., Otvos,L., Palosi,E.
Oxazepam esters. 1. Correlation between hydrolysis rates and brain appearance of oxazepam.
J.Med.Chem. 22, 1436-43 (1979)

3228. Maksay,G., Tegyey,Z., Otvos,L.
Oxazepam esters. 2. Correlation of hydrophobicity with serum binding, brain penetration, and excretion.
J.Med.Chem. 22, 1443-7 (1979)

3229. Male,C.G., Lim,Y.T., Male,M., Stewart,J.M., Gibbs,J.M
Comparison of 3 benzodiazepines for oral premedication in minor gynecological surgery.
Brit.J. Anaesth. 52, 429-36 (1980)

3230. Maletzky,B.M.
Anxiolytic efficacy of alprazolam compared to diazepam and placebo.
J.Int.Med.Res. 8, 139-43 (1980)

3231. Malick,J.B., Enna,S.J.
Comparative effects of benzodiazepines and non-benzodiazepine anxiolytics on biochemical and behavioral tests predictive of anxiolytic activity.
Commun.Psychopharmacol. 3, 245-52 (1979)

3232. Malizia,E., Cerbo,R., Smerigli.,M., Ambrosin.,M., Russo,A.
Naloxone treatment of alcoholic and benzodiazepine intoxication.
Tox.Lett. 1980, 158 (1980)

3233. Mallorga,P., Hamburg,M., Tallman,J.F., Gallager,D.W.
Ontogenetic changes in GABA modulation of brain benzodiazepine binding.
Neuropharmacology 19, 405-8 (1980)

3234. Maltby,J.R., Hamilton,R.C., Phillips,R.
Comparison of flunitrazepam and thiopentone for induction of general-anesthesia.
Can.Anaest.Soc.J. 27, 331-7 (1980)

3235. Mansikka,M., Kangas,L., Kanto,J.
A comparative-study on the clinical effects of flunitrazepam and lorazepam.
Int.J.Clin.Pharmacol. 18, 320-1 (1980)

3236. Marangos,P.J., Clark,R., Martino,A.M., Paul,S.M., Skolnick,P.
Demonstration of 2 new endogenous benzodiazepine-like compounds from brain.
Psychiatr.Res. 1, 121-30 (1979)

3237. Marangos,P.J., Paul,S.M., Goodwin,F.K., Skolnick,P.
Putative endogenous ligands for the benzodiazepine receptor.
Life Sci. 25, 1093-102 (1979)

3238. Marcu,P., Grecu,I.
Thermogravimetric study of some benzodiazepine derivatives with complex chromium(III)-compounds.
Pharmazie 34, 432-3 (1979)

3239. Marcucci,F., Garbagna,L., Monti,F., Bonazzi,P., Canobbio,L., Zuccato,E., Mussini,E.
Gas-chromatographic determination of 2 fluorinated benzodiazepines in rats and mice.
J.Chromatogr. 198, 180-4 (1980)

3240. Marczyk-Barya,I.
Analysis of urinary concentrations of the metabolites of various neurohormones in cases of acute poisoning with hypnotic and psychotropic drugs and carbon monoxide.
Wiad.Lek. 33, 695-9 (1980)

3241. Marks,J.
Benzodiazepine - Gebrauch und Mißbrauch.
The Benzodiazepines - Use and Abuse.
New Perspectives in Benzodiazepine Therapy - International Symposium Heidelberg 1979.
Arzneim.-Forsch. (Drug Res.) 30, 898-901 (1980)

3242. Martin,I.L., Candy,J.M.
Facilitation of specific benzodiazepine binding in rat brain membrane fragments by a number of anions.
Neuropharmacology 19, 175-9 (1980)

3243. Martin,I.L., Mitchell,P.R.
Diazepam facilitates the potassium-stimulated release of (3H)-dopamine from rat striatal tissue.
Brit.J.Pharmacol. 66, 107 (1979)

3244. Martin,R.S.
Binding of diazepam and phenytoin to plasma-albumin and lipoproteins by gel-filtration and ultra-centrifugation.
Clin.Res. 27, 720 (1979)

3245. Martin,R.
The use of flunitrazepam and ketamine in the dog.
Kleintier-Praxis 25, 91 (1980)

3246. Martini,C., Lucacchi.,A.
Benzodiazepine binding-proteins studied by affinity chromatography.
Ital.J.Bioch. 29, 216-7 (1980)

3247. Masso,M., Perez,H.
Double-blind clinical-trial of bromazepam and alpha-methyldopa in arterial-hypertension.
Pharmatherap. 2, 195-204 (1979)

3248. Massotti,M., Alleva,F., Balazs,T.
Biochemical and pharmacological aspects of fetal exposure to diazepam.
Tox.Lett. 1980, 125 (1980)

3249. Massotti,M., Alleva,F.R., Balazs,T., Guidotti,A.
GABA and benzodiazepine receptors in the offspring of cams receiving diazepam - ontogenetic studies.
Neuropharm. 19, 951-6 (1980)

3250. Massotti,M., Balazs,T., Guidotti,A., Costa,E.
Modulation of H-3-GABA and diazepam-H-3 binding in different brain-areas.
Pharmacolog. 21, 179 (1979)

3251. Massotti,M., Guidotti,A.
Endogenous regulators of benzodiazepine recognition sites.
Life Sci. 27, 847-54 (1980)

3252. Matsui,Y., Kamioka,T.
Potentiation of muscimol-induced hyperactivity by benzodiazepines.
J.Pharm.Pharmacol. 31, 427-8 (1979)

3253. Matthews,W.B.
Treatment of the restless legs syndrome with clonazepam.
Brit.Med.J. 1, 751 (1979)

3254. Mattila,M.A.K., Larni,H.M.
Flunitrazepam - a review of its pharmacological properties and therapeutic use.
Drugs 20, 353-74 (1980)

3255. Mattila,M.A., Ruoppi,M., Korhonen,M., Larni,H.M., Valtonen,L., Heikkinen,H.
Prevention of diazepam-induced thrombophlebitis with cremophor as a solvent.
Brit.J.Anaest. 51, 891-4 (1979)

3256. Mattila,M.A.K., Saila,K., Kokko,T., Karkkain.,T.
Comparison to general-anesthesia in preventing arousal following surgical stimuli.
Brit.J.Anaest. 51, 329-37 (1979)

3257. Maurer,R.
The GABA agonist thip a muscimol analogue, does not interfere with the benzodiazepine binding site on rats cortical membranes.
Neurosci.Lett. 12, 65-8 (1979)

3258. Mayo,B.C., Hawkins,D.R., Huempel,M., Chasseaud,L.F., Girkin,R.
The biotransformation of ^{14}C-lormetazepam in dogs, rabbits, rats and rhesus monkeys.
Xenobiotica 10, 413-20 (1980)

3259. Maziere,M., Godot,J.M., Berger,G., Prenant,C., Comar,D.
High specific activity C-11 labeling of benzodiazepines - diazepam and flunitrazepam.
J.Rad.Chem. 56, 229-35 (1980)

3260. Maziere,M., Godot,J.M., Menini,C., Berger,G., Comar,D.
Benzodiazepines-C-11 - labeling procedure and invivo pharmacodynamics.
Int.J.Nuc.Med. 7, 204 (1980)

3261. McAllister,C.B.
Placental transfer and neonatal effects of diazepam when administered to women just before delivery.
Brit.J.Anaesth. 52, 423-7 (1980)

3262. McBride,R.J., Dundee,J.W., Moore,J., Toner,W., Howard,P.J.
Placental-transfer of lorazepam.
Brit.J.Clin.Pharm. 7, P420 (1979)

3263. McCammon,R.L., Hilgenberg.J.C., Stoelting,R.K.
Hemodynamic effects of diazepam and diazepam-nitrous oxide in patients with coronary artery disease.
Anesth.Analg. (Cleve) 59, 438-41 (1980)

3264. McCurdy,H.H., Slightom,E.L., Harrill,J.C.
Diazepam and desmethyldiazepam quantitation whole-blood by nitrogen-sensitive detector after derivatization.
J.Anal.Tox. 3, 195-8 (1979)

3265. McCurdy,L.
Die kurzzeitige Anwendung von Benzodiazepinen.
The Short-term Use of Benzodiazepines.
New Perspectives in Benzodiazepine Therapy - International Symposium Heidelberg 1979
Arzneim.-Forsch. (Drug Res.) 30, 895-7 (1980)

3266. McClain,R.M., Hoar,R.M.
The effect of flunitrazepam on reproduction in the rat. The use of cross-fostering in the evaluation of postnatal parameters in rat reproduction studies.
Toxicol.Appl.Pharmacol. 53, 92-100 (1980)

3267. McGowan,W.A.W., Dundee,J.W., Clarke,R.S.J., Howard,P.J.
Comparison of the subjective effects and plasma-concentrations following oral and i.m. administration of flunitrazepam in patients.
Brit.J.Anaest. 52, 447-51 (1980)

3268. McKay,A.C., Dundee,J.W.
Effect of oral benzodiazepines on memory.
Brit.J.Anaest. 52, 1247-57 (1980)

3269. McLaughlin,C.L., Baile,C.A.
Cholecystokinin, amphetamine and diazepam and feeding in lean and obese zucker rats.
Pharmacol.Biochem.Behav. 10, 87-93 (1979)

3270. McLendon,D.M., Fabre,L.F.
Double-blind comparison of the anxiolytic efficacy of alprazolam and chlordiazepoxide hydrochloride in the chronic withdrawal period from alcohol.
Curr.Ther.Res. 26, 430-9 (1979)

3271. McLendon,D.M., Fabre,L.F.
A double-blind comparison of the efficacy of alprazolam, chlordiazepoxide hydrochloride and placebo in the chronic withdrawal period from alcohol.
Curr.Ther.Res. 28, 447-55 (1980)

3272. McNamara,J.O., Peper,A.M., Patrone,V.
Repeated seizures induce long-term increase in hippocampal benzodiazepine receptors.
Proc.Natl.Acad.Sci.USA 77, 3029-32 (1980)

3273. McNamara,J.O., Peper,A., Patrone,V.
Repeated seizures induce increased numbers of hippocampal benzodiazepine receptors.
Neurology 30, 421 (1980)

3274. Medd,B.H.
Sleeping pills and insomnia.
Science 205, 6-7 (1979)

3275. Medd,B.H.
Sleeping pills.
N.Engl.J.Med. 301, 214 (1979)

3276. Meldrum,B.S., Horton,R.W.
Anticonvulsant activity in photosensitive baboons, papio papio, of two new 1,5 benzodiazepines.
Psychopharmacology (Berlin) 60, 277-80 (1979)

3277. Memo,M., Spano,P.F., Trabucch.,M.
Brain benzodiazepine receptor changes during aging.
J.Pharm.Pharmacol. 33, 64 (1981)

3278. Menuck,M.
Use of benzodiazepines.
Can.Med.Ass.J. 122, 152 (1980)

3279. Mery,C., Martin,J.C.
Clinical study of clobazam in alcohol detoxification.
Brit.J.Clin.Pharmacol. 7, 133S (1979)

3280. Miczek,K.A., O'Donnell,J.M.
Alcohol and chlordiazepoxide increase suppressed aggression in mice.
Psychopharmacology (Berlin) 69, 39-44 (1980)

3281. Mignee,C.
Results of a 9-month survey of Rohypnol (flunitrazepam) at the Paris Poison Control Center.
Med.Leg.Tox. 23, 166-7 (1980)

3282. Mignee,C., Garnier,R., Conso,F., Efthymio.,M.L., Fournier,E.
Acute overdosage with flunitrazepam.
Therapie 35, 581-9 (1980)

3283. Mikkelsen,H., Hoel,T.M., Bryne,H., Krohn,C.D.
Local reactions after i.v. injections of diazepam, flunitrazepam and isotonic saline.
Brit.J.Anaest. 52, 817-9 (1980)

3284. Miller,F., Nulsen,J.
Single case study. Diazepam (Valium) detoxification.
J.Nerv.Ment.Dis. 167, 637-8 (1979)

3285. Mimaki,T., Deshmukh,P.P., Yamamura,H.I.
Decreased benzodiazepine receptor density in rat-brain following chronic phenytoin administration.
Ann.Neurol. 8, 230 (1980)

3286. Minter,R., Murray,G.B.
Diazepam withdrawal: a current problem in recognition.
J.Fam.Pract. 7, 1233-5 (1978)

3287. Mitchell,P.F.
Diazepam-associated thrombophlebitis - a review and discussion of possible prevention.
J.Amer.Dent.Ass. 101, 492-5 (1980)

3288. Mitchell,R.
Benzodiazepines modify the agonist responses at a presynaptic GABA receptor.
Eur.J.Pharmacol. 68, 369-72 (1980)

3289. Mittal,S.K., Khanna,S.R., Gupta,A.
Diazepam therapy in post neonatal pediatric tetanus.
Ind.Pediatr. 16, 255-7 (1979)

3290. Miyasato,K.
Experimental study on development of physical dependence on alcohol and cross physical dependence liability of diazepam and barbital to alcohol in rhesus monkeys.
Seishin Shinkeigaku Zasshi 80, 657-67 (1978)

3291. Modras,Z., Sekura,M.
Effects of visible and ultraviolet-radiation on chloroform solutions of oxazepam.
Act.Pol.Pharm. 37, 451-6 (1980)

3292. Moehler,H., Battersby,M.K., Richards,J.G.
Benzodiazepine receptor protein identified and visualized in brain tissue by a photoaffinity label.
Proc.Natl.Acad.Sci.USA 77, 1666-70 (1980)

3293. Möhler,H., Battersby,M.K., Richards,J.G.
Benzodiazepine receptors in rat-brain - localization in regions of synaptic contacts.
Brain Res.Bull. 5, 155-9 (1980)

3294. Möhler,H., Battersby,M.K., Richards,J.G., Polc,P., Cumin,R., Pieri,L., Kettler,R.
Benzodiazepine receptor: localization by photo-affinity labeling and isolation of a possible endogenous ligand.
Adv.Biochem.Psychopharmacol. 21, 295-9 (1980)

3295. Möhler,H., Polc,P., Cumin,R., Pieri,L., Kettler,R.
Nicotinamide is a brain constituent with benzo-diazepine-like actions.
Nature 278, 563-5 (1979)

3296. Mörck,H.J., Magelund,G.
Gynaecomastia and diazepam abuse.
Lancet 1, 1344-5 (1979)

3297. Montarolo,P.G., Raschi,F., Strata,P.
Interactions between benzodiazepines and GABA in the cerebellar cortex.
Brain Res. 162, 358-62 (1979)

3298. Monti,J.M., Altier,H., D'Angelo,L.
The effects of the combined administration of gamma-hydroxybutyrate and diazepam on sleep parameters in the rat.
J.Neural.Transm. 45, 177-83 (1979)

3299. Monti,J.M., Altier,H., D'Angelo,L.
Diazepam, GABA agonists and antagonists and the sleep-wakefulness cycle.
Adv.Biosci. 21, 65-73 (1978)

3300. Moolenaar,F., Bakker,S., Visser,J., Huizinga,T.
Biopharmaceutics of rectal administration of drugs in man. 9. Comparative biopharmaceutics of diazepam after single rectal, oral, intramuscular and intravenous administration in man.
Int.J.Pharmacol. 5, 127-37 (1980)

3301. Morozov,I.S.
Stress-protective effect of diazepam and its combinations with adrenergic and dopaminergic substances as measured by the operative activity test in rats.
Farmakol.T. 43, 540-3 (1980)

3302. Morris,M.D., Burger,A.B., Gebhart,G.F.
Effect of chlordiazepoxide on conditioned and unconditioned fear in rats.
Progr.Neuropsychopharmacol. 4, 153-60 (1980)

3303. Mosset,A., Tuchague.,J.P., Bonnet,J.J., Haran,R., Sharrock,P.
Solution and solid-state structural study of the copper(II) complex of diazepam.
Inorg.Chem. 19, 290-4 (1980)

3304. Mueller,H., Voit,E., Schwarz,R.
Klinische Untersuchungen über das Verhalten von Atmung und Kreislauf bei Verwendung von Rohypnol zur Basissedierung für hals-nasen-ohrenärztliche Eingriffe in Lokalanästhesie.
Clinical investigations about the behaviour of pulmonary respiration and cardiovascular circulation after the application of Rohypnol for basis-sedation for microsurgical operations in otolaryngology in local anaesthesia.
Laryngol.Rhinol.Otol. (Stuttg.) 58, 165-8 (1979)

3305. Murie,J.A., Mackay,C.
The effect of lorazepam on human gastric-secretion.
Clin.Ther. 2, 387-9 (1980)

3306. Murray,T.G., Koepke,H.H., Walker,B.R., Chiang,S.T., Knowles,J.A., Ruelius,H.W., Goldberg,M.
Effect of renal-disease and age on oxazepam pharmacokinetics in man.
Clin.Res. 27, 545 (1979)

3307. Nagy,J., Decsi,L.
Physostigmine as an antidote in acute diazepam intoxication.
Acta Physiol.Hung. 53, 197 (1979)

3308. Nahas,G., Goujard,J.
Phenothiazines, benzodiazepines, and the fetus.
Rev.Perinat.Med. 3, 243-80 (1979)

3309. Naidu,K.R.
A clinical study of local reactions following intravenous diazepam.
J.Assoc.Physicians India 27, 649-50 (1979)

3310. Nair,N.P., Schwartz,G.
Comparison of the hypnotic activity of triazolam and flurazepam.
Union Med.Can. 108, 187-92 (1979)

3311. Naitoh,P., Seales,D.M., Johnson,L.C., Church,M.W.
Flurazepam-induced changes in cerebral electrical-activity.
EEG Clin.Neur. 49, 11 (1980)

3312. Nakano,M., Inotsume,N., Kohri,N., Arita,T.
Reversible ring-opening reaction of diazepam in acid-media around body-temperature.
Int.J.Pharm. 3, 195-204 (1979)

3313. Nakano,M., Kohri,N., Arakawa,Y., Arita,T.
Pharmaceutical studies on benzodiazepines. 1. Permeation of benzodiazepines through synthetic membranes.
Chem.Pharm. 27, 573-7 (1979)

3314. Nakano,S., Ogawa,N., Kawazu,Y.
Influence of neuroticism on oral absorption of diazepam.
Clin.Pharmacol.Ther. 27, 370-4 (1980)

3315. Nakano,S., Watanabe,H., Ogawa,N.
Circadian effect on diazepam kinetics in man.
Clin.Pharmacol. 27, 274 (1980)

3316. Nakazawa,Y., Kotorii,T., Horikawa,S., Kotorii,M., Ohshima,M., Hasuzawa,H.
Individual variations in the effects of flurazepam, clorazepate, l-dopa and thyrotropin-releasing hormone on REM sleep in man.
Psychopharmacology (Berlin) 60, 203-6 (1979)

3317. Naranjo,C.A., Abel,J.G., Sellers,E.M., Giles,H.G.
Unaltered diazepam plasma binding using indwelling heparinized cannulae for sampling.
Brit.J.Clin.Pharmacol. 9, 103-5 (1980)

3318. Naranjo,C.A., Sellers,E.M., Giles,H.G., Abel,J.G.
Diurnal variations in plasma diazepam concentrations associated with reciprocal changes in free fraction.
Brit.J.Clin.Pharmacol. 9, 265-72 (1980)

3319. Naranjo,C.A., Sellers,E.M., Khouw,V.
Fatty-acids modulation of meal-induced cariations in diazepam free fraction.
Brit.J.Clin.Pharmacol. 10, 308-10 (1980)

3320. Nau,H., Brendel,K., Liddiard,C.
Benzodiazepine metabolism in cultures of isolated hepatocytes and liver fragments of human fetus.
Drug Metab.Rev. 9, 131-46 (1979)

3321. Nau,H., Liddiard,C.
Postnatal development of sex-dependent differences in the metabolism of diazepam by rat liver.
Biochem.Pharmacol. 29, 447-9 (1980)

3322. Nawojski,A., Nawrocka,W., Wilimowski,M., Orzechowska-Juzwenko,K., Barczynska,J., Kedzierska,L., Wojewodzki,W., Przybylska,E., Felsztynska,J.
1,5-benzodiazepine derivatives with expected psychotropic activity.
Pol.J.Pharmacol.Pharm. 31, 615-22 (1979)

3323. Nayel,S.A., Elhabash.,M.A., Said,S., Darwish,E., Osman,M., Abdelaal,A.
Bed rest and diazepam versus methyl dopa in the treatment of EPH gestosis.
Sing.J.Ob.G. 11, 25-31 (1980)

3324. Nestoros,J.N.
Electro-physiological evidence that GABA potentiation invivo correlates with benzodiazepine receptor affinity.
Brain Res.Bull. 5, 849-51 (1980)

3325. Nestoros,J.N., Nistri,A.
Effects of microiontophoretically applied flurazepam on response of cerebral cortical neurones to putative neurotransmitters.
Can.J.Physiol.Pharmacol. 57, 1324-9 (1979)

3326. Newton,D.W.
pka of 2-methylamino-5-chlorobenzophenone, a diazepam hydrolysis product.
J.Pharm.Sci. 68, 937-8 (1979)

3327. Newton,D.W., Kauffman,J.M.
Plausible stepwise reaction mechanism for the acid catalyzed hydrolysis of diazepam.
Amer.J.Pharm.Educ. 44, 46-9 (1980)

3328. Ng,S.S., Bhattacharyya,P.K.
Solvent effects on IR spectra of flurazepam.
J.Pharm.Sci. 69, 270-3 (1980)

3329. Nicholson,A.N.
Proceedings of a symposium on temazepam and related 1,4-benzodiazepines - effects on sleep and on performance, october 1978.
Brit.J.Clin.Pharmacol. 8, 3 (1979)

3330. Nicholson,A.N.
Differential effects of the 1,4 and 1,5 benzodiazepines on performance in healthy man.
Brit.J.Clin.Pharmacol. 7, 83S-84S (1979)

3331. Nicholson,A.N.
Performance studies with diazepam and its hydroxylated metabolites.
Brit.J.Clin.Pharmacol. 8, 39S-42S (1979)

3332. Nicholson,A.N., Stone,B.M.
Diazepam and 3-hydroxydiazepam (temazepam) and sleep of middle age.
Brit.J.Clin.Pharmacol. 7, 463-8 (1979)

3333. Nicholson,A.N., Stone,B.M.
Activity of the hypnotics, flunitrazepam and triazolam, in man.
Brit.J.Clin.Pharmacol. 9, 187-94 (1980)

3334. Nicholson,A.N., Stone,B.M., Pascoe,P.A.
Efficacy of some benzodiazepines for daytime sleep.
Brit.J.Clin.Pharmacol. 10, 459-63 (1980)

3335. Nielsen,M., Braestrup,C.
Ethyl beta-carboline-3-carboxylate shows differential benzodiazepine receptor interaction.
Nature 286, 606-7 (1980)

3336. Nielsen,M., Gredal,O., Braestrup,C.
Some properties of 3H-diazepam displacing activity from human urine.
Life Sci. 25, 679-86 (1979)

3337. Nielsen,M., Schou,H., Braestrup,C.
Propyl-H-3 beta-carboline-3-carboxylate binds specifically to brain benzodiazepine receptors.
J.Neurochem. 36, 276-85 (1981)

3338. Nielsen-Kudsk,F., Jakobsen,P.
Disposition pharmacokinetics of lorazepam in the rabbit.
Acta Pharmacol.Toxicol. (Copenh.) 46, 388-91 (1980)

3339. Nikolaev,V.I., Marusov,I.V.
Antistress effects of diazepam and activation of the positive reinforcing system upon changes on corticosteroid excretion and lipid level after peripheral electric pain stimulation.
Biull.Eksp.Biol.Med. 88, 289-91 (1979)

3340. Nixon,J.C., Woolf,J.H.
Isolation of a peptide which displaces diazepam-H-3 from brain benzodiazepine receptors.
Pharmacology 21, 242 (1979)

3341. O'Brien,R.A., Spirt,N.M.
The inhibition of GABA-stimulated benzodiazepine binding by a convulsant benzodiazepine.
Life Sci. 26, 1441-5 (1980)

3342. Ochs,H.R., Busse,J., Greenblatt,D.J., Allen,M.D.
Entry of lorazepam into cerebrospinal-fluid.
Brit.J.Clin.Pharmacol. 10, 405-6 (1980)

3343. Ochs,H.R., Greenblatt,D.J., Allen,M.D., Harmatz,J.S., Shader,R.I., Bodem,G.
Effect of age and billroth gastrectomy on absorption of desmethyldiazepam from clorazepate.
Clin.Pharmacol.Ther. 26, 449-56 (1979)

3344. Offerhans,L.
Trials and tribulations of triazolam
J.Clin.Pharmacol. 20, 700-1 (1980)

3345. Ogata,H., Horii,S., Shibazaki,T., Aoyagi,N., Kaniwa,N., Ejima,A.
Salivary excretion of barbital and diazepam in human.
Eisei Shikenjo Hokoku 96, 27-32 (1978)

3346. Ogura,C., Nakazawa,K., Majima,K., Nakamura,K., Ueda,H., Umezawa,Y., Wardell,W.M.
Residual effects of hypnotics: triazolam, flurazepam, and nitrazepam.
Psychopharmacology (Berlin) 68, 61-5 (1980)

3347. Ohnhaus,E.E., Park.B.K., Colombo,J.P., Heizmann,P.
The effect of enzyme induction on diazepam metabolism in man.
Brit.J.Clin.Pharmacol. 8, 557-63 (1979)

3348. Oka,J.I., Fukuda,H., Kudo,Y.
The interaction between GABA-diazepam and benzodiazepine binding-sites in the frog spinal-cord.
Fol.Pharm.Jap. 76, 181-2 (1980)

3349. Okawara,H.
Clobazam in the treatment of anxiety in female patients with functional sexual disorders - double-blind trial against placebo.
Rev.Bra.Med. 37, 38-41 (1980)

3350. Okazawa,M., Ono,Y., Nishimura,N.
Flunitrazepam as an induction agent.
Masui 29, 373-80 (1980)

3351. Okimura,T., Tsuji,J.I., Yamamoto,I.
Stress and immune-responses suppression of immune-responses by restraint and its restoration by diazepam.
Fol.Pharm.Jap. 76, 111 (1980)

3352. Okumura,T., Nagaoka,T.
Separation of benzodiazepine minor tranqulizers by means of reversed-phase thin-layer chromatography.
Bunseki Kag. 28, 584-7 (1979)

3353. Olive,G., Rey,E.
Benzodiazepine levels.
Gaz.Med.Franc. 87, 4275 (1980)

3354. Olive,G., Rey,E.
Benzodiazepine levels.
Gaz.Med.Franc. 87, 4291 (1980)

3355. Ollivier,A., Taburet,A.M., Richarde.,J.M., Aymard,P.
Diazepam and N-demethyldiazepam levels in infants treated orally.
Arch.France Ped. 37, 60 (1980)

3356. Ortiz,M., Ruiz,I., Naranjo,C.A.
Efficacy and adverse reactions of benzodiazepines.
Arch.Biol.Med. 13, 94 (1980)

3357. Osborne,N.N.
Benzodiazepine binding to bovine retina.
Neurosci.Lett. 16, 167-70 (1980)

3358. Oshtory,M.A., Vijayan,N.
Clonazepam treatment of insomnia due to sleep myoclonus.
Arch.Neurol. 37, 119-20 (1980)

3359. Ostrovskaia,G.Z.
Effect of high and low environmental temperature on benzodiazepine tranquilizer activity.
Farmakol.Toksikol. 42, 349-51 (1979)

3360. Oswald,I., Adam,K.
Chlormethiazole and temazepam.
Brit.Med.J. 280, 860-1 (1980)

3361. Oswald,I., Adam,K.
Benzodiazepines cause small loss of body-weight.
Brit.Med.J. 281, 1039-40 (1980)

3362. Pakkanen,A., Kanto,J., Kangas,L., Mansikka,M.
Comparative-study of the clinical effects of tofizopam, nitrazepam and placebo as oral premedication.
Brit.J.Anaest. 52, 1009-12 (1980)

3363. Palacios,J.M., Niehoff,D.L., Kuhar,M.J.
Ontogeny of GABA and benzodiazepine receptors: effects of triton X-100, bromide and muscimol.
Brain Res. 179, 390-5 (1979)

3364. Parker,J.L.
Potassium clorazepate (Tranxene)-induced jaundice.
Postgrad.Med.J. 55, 908-10 (1979)

3365. Parker,W.A., MacCara,M.E.
Compatibility of diazepam with intravenous fluid containers and administration sets.
Amer.J.Hosp.Pharm. 37, 496-500 (1980)

3366. Parker,W.A., Morris,M.E., Shearer,C.A.
Incompatibility of diazepam injection in plastic intravenous bags.
Amer.J.Hosp.Pharmacy 36, 505-7 (1979)

3367. Parkes,J.D., Schate.,M.
Clomipramine and clonazepam in cataplexy.
Lancet 2, 1085-6 (1979)

3368. Pasch,T., Bugsch,L.A.
Influence of narcotics analgesics, droperidol, diazepam, and flunitrazepam on the smooth muscles of small arteries.
Anaesthesis 28, 283-9 (1979)

3369. Pascuzzi Jackson,V., Demyer,W., Hingtgen,J.
Delayed maze-learning in rats after prenatal exposure to clorazepate.
Arch.Neurol. 37, 350-1 (1980)

3370. Patel,D.A., Patel,A.R.
Clorazepate and congenital malformations.
J.Amer.Med.Ass. 244, 135-6 (1980)

3371. Patel,J.B., Ciofalo,V.B., Iorio,L.C.
Benzodiazepine blockade of passive-avoidance task in mice - state-dependent phenomenon.
Psychopharmacology 61, 25-8 (1979)

3372. Patel,J.B., Malick,J.B.
Effects of isoproterenol and chlordiazepoxide on drinking and conflict behaviors in rats.
Pharmacol.Biochem.Behav. 12, 819-21 (1980)

3373. Patrick,J.M., Sempik,A.K., Bennett,T.
The effect of diazepam on the threshold of the ventilatory response to CO_2.
Brit.J.Pharmacol. 64, 454-5 (1978)

3374. Patwardhan,R.V., Yarborou.,G.W., Desmond,P.V., Johnson,R.F., Schenker,S., Speeg,K.V.
Cimetidine spares the glucuronidation of lorazepam and oxazepam.
Gastroenty. 79, 912-6 (1980)

3375. Paul,A.K., Bhattacharya,B.
Influence of premedication with diazepam, prochlorperazine and triflupromazine on blood glucose level.
J.Indian Med.Assoc. 71, 144-6 (1978)

3376. Paul,H.H., Sapper,H., Lohmann,W.
H-NMR investigations of a hammet-type substituent effect on the hydrogen bond interaction of some 1,4-benzodiazepines.
Biochem.Pharmacol. 29, 137-40 (1980)

3377. Paul,S.M., Marangos,P.J., Goodwin,F.K., Skolnick,P.
Brain-specific benzodiazepine receptors and putative endogenous benzodiazepine-like compounds.
Biol.Psychiatry 15, 407-28 (1980)

3378. Paul,S.M., Marangos,P.J., Skolnick,P., Goodwin,F.K.
Brain-specific benzodiazepine receptors and putative endogenous benzodiazepine-like compounds.
Psychopharmacol.Bull. 16, 9-20 (1980)

3379. Paul,S.M., Skolnick,P., Zatz,M.
Avermectin B1A - an irreversible activator of the gamma-aminobutyric acid-benzodiazepine-chloride-ionophore receptor complex.
Biochem.Biophys.Res.Comm. 96, 632-8 (1980)

3380. Paul,S.M., Syapin,P.J., Paugh,B.A., Moncada,V., Skolnick,P.
Correlation between benzodiazepine receptor occupation and anticonvulsant effects of diazepam.
Nature 281, 688-9 (1979)

3381. Paul,S.M., Zatz,M., Skolnick,P.
Demonstration of brain-specific benzodiazepine receptors in rat retina.
Brain Res. 187, 243-6 (1980)

3382. Peat,M.A., Kopjak,L.
The screening and quantitation of diazepam, flurazepam, chlordiazepoxide, and their metabolites in blood and plasma by electron-capture gas chromatography and high pressure liquid chromatography.
J.Forensic Sci. 24, 46-54 (1979)

3383. Peel,E.T., James,O., Macklon,A.F., Rawlins,M.D., Skillen,A.W.
Plasma protein-binding sites of diazepam in normal subjects and patients with alcoholic cirrhosis.
Clin.Sci. 58, 15-6 (1980)

3384. Peel,H.W., Perrigo,B.J.
Toxicological analysis of benzodiazepine-type compounds in postmortem blood by gas-chromatography.
J.Anal.Tox. 4, 105-13 (1980)

3385. Pegram,V., Hyde,P., Linton,P.
Chronic use of triazolam: the effects on the sleep patterns of insomniacs.
J.Int.Med.Res. 8, 224-31 (1980)

3386. Pelicier,Y.
Use and abuse of benzodiazepine.
Ann.Med.Psych. 137, 1033-5 (1979)

3387. Petersen,R.C., Ghoneim,M.M.
Diazepam and human memory: influence on acquisition, retrieval, and state-dependent learning.
Prog.Neuropsychopharmacol. 4, 81-9 (1980)

3388. Peyton,J.C., Borowitz,J.L.
Chlordiazepoxide and theophylline alter calcium levels in subcellular fractions of rat brain cortex.
Proc.Soc.Exp.Biol.Med. 161, 178-82 (1979)

3389. Phillis,J.W.
Diazepam potentiation of purinergic depression of central neurons.
Can.J.Physiol.Pharmacol. 57, 432-5 (1979)

3390. Phillis,J.W., Bender,A.S., Wu,P.H.
Benzodiazepines inhibit adenosine uptake into rat brain synaptosomes.
Brain Res. 195, 494-8 (1980)

3391. Phillis,J.W., Siemens,R.K., Wu,P.H.
Effects of diazepam on adenosine and acetylcholine-release from rat cerebral-cortex - further evidence for a purinergic mechanism in action of diazepam.
Brit.J.Pharmacol. 70, 341-8 (1980)

3392. Phillis,J.W., Wu,P.H.
Interactions between the benzodiazepines, methylxanthines and adenosine.
Can.J.Neur. 7, 247-9 (1980)

3393. Piccione,P., Zorick,F., Lutz,T., Grissom,T., Kramer,M., Roth,T.
The efficacy of triazolam and chloral hydrate in geriatric insomniacs.
J.Int.Med.Res. 8, 361-7 (1980)

3394. Pichlmayr,I., Lips,U.
Diazepam-Effekte im Elektroencephalogramm. Klinische Studie an 16 Patienten.
EEG effects of diazepam. Studies on 16 patients.
Anaesthesist 29, 317-27 (1980)

3395. Placheta,P., Karobath,M.
Regional distribution of Na^+-independent GABA and benzodiazepine binding sites in rat CNS.
Brain Res. 178, 580-3 (1979)

3396. Poddar,M.K., Urquhart,D., Sinha,A.K.
Diazepam binding in brain after sleep and wakefulness.
Brain Res. 193, 519-28 (1980)

3397. Podiwins.,F., Jellinge.,K.
Bromazepam in the treatment of somatized psychogenic disorders.
Wien.Klin.Wschr. 91, 240-4 (1979)

3398. Poitras,R.
Episodes of anterograde amnesia associated with triazolam - report of 3 cases.
Un.Med.Can. 109, 427-9 (1980)

3399. Polzin,R.L., Barnes,C.D.
Effect of diazepam on GABAergic cuneate neurons.
Neuropharmacology 18, 431-4 (1979)

3400. Pond,S.M., Phillips,M., Benowitz,N.L., Galinsky,R.E., Ting,T.G., Becker,C.E.
Diazepam kinetics in acute alcohol withdrawal.
Clin.Pharmacol.Ther. 25, 832-6 (1979)

3401. Pop,R., Moldovan,O., Fodorean.,L., Leucuta,S.
Estimation of diazepam bioavailability from tablets by the measurement of its clinical effect.
Drug.Exp.Clin. 6, 45-52 (1980)

3402. Porot,M., Perol,Y.
Clinical use of bromazepam on a long period.
Ann.Med.Psych. 137, 516-8 (1979)

3403. Preti,C., Tosi,G.
Novel series of palladium(II) and platinum(II) complexes with 1,4-benzodiazepines as ligands.
J.Coord.Chem. 8, 223-9 (1979)

3404. Preti,C., Tosi,G.
Complexing behavior of diazepam towards some bivalent 1st row transition-metals.
J.Inorg.Nuc. 41, 263-6 (1979)

3405. Priest,R.G.
Systematic review of the benzodiazepines.
Brit.Med.J. 280, 1085 (1980)

3406. Rainierp.,C.R.
Treatment with diazepam of children with drug-induced extrapyramidal symptoms.
S.Afr.Med.J. 55, 328-30 (1979)

3407. Raisys,V.A., Friel,P.N., Graaff,P.R., Opheim,K.E., Wilensky,A.J.
High-performance liquid-chromatographic and gas-liquid-chromatographic determination of diazepam and nordiazepam in plasma.
J.Chromatogr. 183, 441-8 (1980)

3408. Rajtar,G.
Influence of chlorpromazine, diazepam, imipramine and pyrazole on ethanol-induced changes in activity of some enzymes in isolated rat-liver.
Arch.Immun. 27, 329-37 (1979)

3409. Ramsay,R.E., Hammond,E.J., Perchalski,R.J., Wilder,B.J.
Brain uptake of phenytoin, phenobarbital, and diazepam.
Arch.Neurol. 36, 535-9 (1979)

3410. Rastogi,R.B., Lapierre,Y.D., Singhal,R.L.
Diazepam modifies 1-triiodothyronine-stimulated changes in behavior and the metabolism of brain norepinephrine, dopamine and 5-hydroxytryptamine - possible mechanism of action.
J.Psych.Res. 15, 7-20 (1979)

3411. Rastogi,R.B., Lapierre,Y.D., Singhal,R.L., Nair,N.P.
Evidence for involvement of dopamine in the action of diazepam: potentiation of haloperidol and chlorpromazine action in the brain.
Adv.Biochem.Psychopharmacol. 24, 283-9 (1980)

3412. Raymond,G.G., DeGennaro,M.D., Yau,M., Buice,R.G.
Effect of hyperbilirubinemia on the pharmacokinetics of diazepam in the rat.
Res.Commun.Chem.Pathol.Pharmacol. 28, 133-44 (1980)

3413. Rees,M., Dormandy,J.
Accidental intra-arterial injection of diazepam.
Brit.Med.J. 281, 289-90 (1980)

3414. Regan,J.W., Roeske,W.R., Berens,E.S., Yamamura,H.I.
Characteristics of flunitrazepam-H-3 binding to bovine retinae.
Fed.Proc. 39, 387 (1980)

3415. Regan,J.W., Roeske,W.R., Yamamura,H.I.
The benzodiazepine receptor: its development and its modulation by gamma-aminobutyric acid.
J.Pharmacol.Exp.Ther. 212, 137-43 (1980)

3416. Regan,J.W., Roeske,W.R., Yamamura,H.I.
3H-flunitrazepam binding to bovine retina and the effect of GABA thereon.
Neuropharmacology 19, 413-4 (1980)

3417. Regan,J.W., Roeske,W.R., Yamamura,H.I.
The effect of GABA on the binding of flunitrazepam-H-3 in mouse brains during development.
Brain Res.Bull. 5, 857-60 (1980)

3418. Reilly,J.
The prevention of laryngeal spasm by diazepam.
Anaesth.Int.Care 8, 365 (1980)

3419. Reisine,T.D., Azari,J., Johnson,P.C., Barbeau,A., Huxtable,R., Yamamura,H.I.
Brain neurotransmitter receptors in Friedreich's ataxia.
Can.J.Neurol.Sci. 6, 259-62 (1979)

3420. Reisine,T.D., Overstreet,D., Gale,K., Rossor,M., Iversen,L., Yamamura,H.I.
Benzodiazepine receptors: the effect of GABA on their characteristics in human brain and their alteration in Huntington's disease.
Brain Res. 199, 79-88 (1980)

3421. Reisine,T.D., Wastek,G.J., Speth,R.C., Bird,E.D., Yamamura,H.I.
Alterations in the benzodiazepine receptor of Huntington's diseased human brain.
Brain Res. 165, 183-7 (1979)

3422. Reves,J.G., Samuelson,P.N., Lewis,S.
Midazolam maleate induction in patients with ischaemic heart disease: haemodynamic observations.
Can.Anaesth.Soc.J. 26, 402-9 (1979)

3423. Reves,J.G., Vinik,R., Hirschfield,A.M., Holcomb,C., Strong,S.
Midazolam compared with thiopentone as a hypnotic component in balanced anaesthesia: a randomized, double-blind study.
Can.Anaesth.Soc.J. 26, 42-9 (1979)

3424. Rey,E., D'Athis,P., Giraux,P., De Lauture,D., Turquais,J.M., Chavinie,J., Olive,G.
Pharmacokinetics of clorazepate in pregnant and non-pregnant women.
Eur.J.Clin.Pharmacol. 15, 175-80 (1979)

3425. Rey,E., Giraux,P., D'Athis,P., Turquais,J.M., Chavinie, J., Olive,G.
Pharmacokinetics of the placental transfer and distribution of clorazepate and its metabolite nordiazepam in the feto-placental unit and in the neonate.
Eur.J.Clin.Pharmacol. 15, 181-5 (1979)

3426. Rey,E., Turquais,J.M., Olive,G.
Determination of dipotassium clorazepate in the plasma by gas chromatography.
Ann.Biol.Clin. (Paris) 36, 355-8 (1978)

3427. Riboulet.,G., Falcy,M., Efthymio.,M.L., Fournier,E.
Acute-poisoning with prazepam.
Med.Leg.Tox. 23, 631-5 (1980)

3428. Rice,K.C., Brossi,A., Tallman,J., Paul,S.M., Skolnick,P.
Irazepine, and noncompetitive, irreversible inhibitor of 3H-diazepam binding to benzodiazepine receptors.
Nature 278, 854-5 (1979)

3429. Rice,K.C., Williams,E., Skolnick,P.
Synthesis and biological characterization of specific, irreversible inhibitors of benzodiazepine receptors.
Abs.Pap.Acs. 1979, 11 (1979)

3430. Richard,P., Mak,D., Deligne,P.
Competitive effect of 2 benzodiazepines: flunitrazepam and diazepam. Demonstration in humans.
Nouv.Presse Med. 8, 1945 (1979)

3431. Richards.,F.J., Manford,M.L.M.
Comparison of flunitrazepam and diazepam for oral premedication in older children.
Brit.J.Anaest. 51, 313-9 (1979)

3432. Rickels,K., Csanalos.,I., Greisman,P., Mirman,M.J., Morris,R.J., Weise,C.C., Weiss,G.
Ketazolam and diazepam in anxiety - a controlled-study.
J.Clin.Pharmacol. 20, 581-9 (1980)

3433. Rizzo,P.A., Caporali,M., Spadaro,M., Zanasi,M.
Slow cerebral potentials following administration of flunitrazepam to patients with sleep disturbances.
Minerva Med. 71, 425-8 (1980)

3434. Roberts,R.K., Desmond,P.V., Wilkinson,G.R., Schenker,S.
Disposition of chlordiazepoxide - sex-differences and effects of oral-contraceptives.
Clin.Pharm. 25, 826-31 (1979)

3435. Robertson,H.A.
Benzodiazepine receptors in emotional and non-emotional mice; comparison of four strains.
Eur.J.Pharmacol. 56, 163-6 (1979)

3436. Robertson,H.A.
Harmaline-induced tremor - the benzodiazepine receptor as a site of action.
Eur.J.Pharmacol. 67, 129-32 (1980)

3437. Robertson,H.A.
The benzodiazepine receptor - the pharmacology of emotion.
Can.J.Neur. 7, 243-5 (1980)

3438. Robinson,J.H., Wang,S.C.
Unit activity of limbic system neurons: effects of morphine, diazepam and neuroleptic agents.
Brain Res. 166, 149-59 (1979)

3439. Robinson,K., Rutterford,M.G., Smith,R.N.
A sensitive benzodiazepine radioimmunoassay of broad specificity.
J.Pharm.Pharmacol. 32, 773-7 (1980)

3440. Robles,L.E.
Continuous intravenous drip flunitrazepam and ketamine in cardiovascular-surgery.
Inv.Med.Int. 6, 207-13 (1979)

3441. Rockoff,M., Ingvar,M., Gagnon,R., Ray,K., Naughton,K.V., Marshall,L.F., Shapiro,H.M.
Cerebral circulatory and metabolic responses to intravenously administered lorazepam.
Anesthesiol. 51, 42 (1979)

3442. Rockoff,M., Naughton,K.V., Shapiro,H.M., Ingvar,M., Ray,K.F., Gagnon,R.L., Marshall,L.F.
Cerebral circulatory and metabolic responses to intravenously administered lorazepam.
Anesthesiol. 53, 215-8 (1980)

3443. Rodbard,D., Costa,T., Pert,C.B.
Is the benzodiazepine receptor coupled to a chloride anion channel - reply.
Nature 280, 173-4 (1979)

3444. Rodgers,T., Powel,B., Vasiliades,J.
The determination of diazepam in serum by gas-chromatography and gas-chromatography-mass-spectrometry.
Clin.Chem. 26, 1005 (1980)

3445. Roets,E., Hoogmartens,J.
Thin-layer chromatography of the acid hydrolysis products of nineteen benzodiazepine derivatives.
J.Chromatogr. 194, 262-9 (1980)

3446. Romeo,G., Aversa,M.C., Gianett.,P., Vigorita,M.G., Ficarra,P.
Nuclear magnetic-resonance of 1,4-benzodiazepines. 2. Stereochemistry of 1,3-dihydro-2H-1,4-benzo-diazepin-2-ones by lanthanide shift-reagents.
NMR-Org.Mag. 12, 593-7 (1979)

3447. Rommelspacher,H., Nanz,C., Borbe,H.O., Fehske,K.J., Müller,W.E., Wollert,U.
1-methyl-beta-carboline (Harmane), a potent endogenous inhibitor of benzodiazepine receptor-binding.
Naunyn-Schmied.Arch.Pharmacol. 314, 97-100 (1980)

3448. Rosenbaum,A.H., de la Fluente,J.R.
Benzodiazepines and tardive dyskinesia.
Lancet 2, 900 (1979)

3449. Rosenberg,H.C.
Central excitatory actions of flurazepam.
Pharm.Bio.Bull. 13, 415-20 (1980)

3450. Rosenberg,H.C., Chiu,T.H.
Decreased 3H-diazepam binding is a specific response to chronic benzodiazepine treatment.
Life Sci. 24, 803-7 (1979)

3451. Rosenberg,H.C., Chiu,T.H.
Benzodiazepine binding after in vivo elevation of GABA.
Neurosci.Lett. 15, 277-81 (1979)

3452. Rosenberg,K.R., Korberly,B.H., Graziani,L.J.
Combination of clonazepam and sodium valproate in the treatment of refractory epileptic seizures in 12 children.
Amer.J.Hosp.Pharmacy 36, 736 (1979)

3453. Rosoff,M., Serajudd.,A.T.
Solubilization of diazepam in bile-salts and in sodium cholate-lecithin-water phases.
Int.J.Pharmacol. 6, 137-46 (1980)

3454. Rosser,W.M.
Patterns of benzodiazepine usage in a family medicine center.
Can.Fam.Phys. 26, 718-20 (1980)

3455. Roth,T., Hartse,K.M., Saab,P.G., Piccione,P.M., Kramer,M.
The effects of flurazepam, lorazepam, and triazolam on sleep and memory.
Psychopharmacology 70, 231-7 (1980)

3456. Roth,T., Hartse,K.M., Zorick,F.J., Kaffeman,M.E.
Differenzierte Effekte von kurz- und langwirksamen Benzodiazepinen auf Nachtschlaf und Tagesleistung.
The differential Effects of Short- und Long-acting Benzodiazepines upon Nocturnal Sleep and Daytime Performance.
New Perspectives in Benzodiazepine Therapy - International Symposium Heidelberg 1979
Arzneim.-Forsch. (Drug Res.) 30, 891-4 (1980)

3457. Roth,T., Piccione,P., Salis,P., Kramer,M., Kaffeman,M.
Effects of temazepam, flurazepam and quinalbarbitone on sleep: psychomotor and cognitive function.
Brit.J.Clin.Pharmacol. 8, 47-54 (1979)

3458. Rousson.,S.H., Rudolf,N.D.M.
A long-term electro-clinical study of clonazepam in children with intractable seizures.
EEG Clin.Neur. 49, 90 (1980)

3459. Routledge,P.A., Kitchell,B.B., Bjornsson,T.D., Skinner,T., Linnoila,M., Shand,D.G.
Diazepam and N-desmethyldiazepam redistribution after heparin.
Clin.Pharmacol.Ther. 27, 528-32 (1980)

3460. Routledge,P.A., Stargel,W.W., Kitchell,B.B., Shand,D.G.
Determinants of plasma-protein binding of diazepam.
Clin.Pharm. 27, 282 (1980)

3461. Rovei,V., Sanjuan,M.
Simple and specific high-performance liquid-chromatographic method for the routine monitoring of clonazepam in plasma.
Ther.Drug.Monit. 2, 283-7 (1980)

3462. Rubin,A., Allen,G.D., Everett,G.B.
Induction of general anesthesia with diazepam or thiopental: a comparison of the cardiorespiratory effects.
Anesth.Progr. 25, 39-44 (1978)

3463. Rubin,J., Schweggm.,I., Uys,P.
Lorazepam as a premedicant in dental surgery.
S.Afr.Med.J. 58, 124-6 (1980)

3464. Ruelius,H.W., Tio,C.O., Knowles,J.A., Mchugh,S.L., Schillings,R.T., Sisenwine,S.F.
Diastereoisomeric glucuronides of oxazepam. Isolation and stereoselective enzymic hydrolysis.
Drug Metab.Dispos. 7, 40-3 (1979)

3465. Ruffalo,R.L., Thompson,J.F.
Effect of cimetidine on the clearance of benzodiazepines.
N.Engl.J.Med. 303, 753-4 (1980)

3466. Ruiz,I., Ortiz,M., Naranjo,C.A.
Efficacy and adverse reactions of benzodiazepines.
Arch.Biol.Med. 13, 106 (1980)

3467. Rupreht,J.
Physostigmine reversal of diazepam.
Anesthesiol. 53, 180-1 (1980)

3468. Rushnak,M.J., Leevy,C.M.
Effect of diazepam on the lower esophageal sphincter. A double-blind controlled study.
Amer.J.Gastroenterol. 73, 127-30 (1980)

3469. Ruskin,P., Averbukh,I., Belmaker,R.H., Dasberg,H.
Benzodiazepines in chronic-schizophrenia.
Biol.Psychiat. 14, 557-8 (1979)

3470. Rutterford,M.G., Smith,R.N.
Radioimmunoassay of diazepam in samples of forensic interest.
J.Pharm.Pharmacol. 32, 449-52 (1980)

3471. Saad,S.F., Jawad,F.H., Hafed,K.
Effect of aminooxyacetic acid on the anticonvulsant actions of clonazepam and the relationship to cerebral gamma-aminobutyric acid content in mice.
IRCS-Bioch. 8, 104-5 (1980)

3472. Sadée,W., Beelen,G.C.M.
Drug Level Monitoring - Analytical Techniques, Metabolism, and Pharmacokinetics.
John Wiley & Sons, New York - Chichester - Brisbane - Toronto (1980)

3473. Sakai,Y.
Comparative study on the depressive action of several benzodiazepine minor tranquilizers.
Nippon Yakurigaku Zasshi 75,777-87 (1979)

3474. Saleh,A.M., Khalil,S.A., Elkhorda.,L.K.
Solubility and stability of diazepam in sodium-salicylate solution.
Int.J.Pharmacol. 5, 161-4 (1980)

3475. Saletu,B., Grunberg.,J.
Changes in clinical symptomatology and psychometric assessments in depressed-patients during mianserin and combined amitriptyline-chlordiazepoxide therapy -
double-blind comparison.
Curr.Med.Res. 6, 52-62 (1980)

3476. Saletu,B., Lippler,I., Grunberg.,J.
Nocturnal traffic noise and sleep - effects and countereffects by oxazolam.
Arzneim.-Forsch. (Drug Res.) 30, 1231 (1980)

3477. Salkind,M.R., Hanks,G.W., Silverstone,J.T.
Evaluation of the effects of clobazam, a 1,5 benzodiazepine, on mood and psychomotor performance in clinically anxious patients in general practice.
Brit.J.Clin.Pharmacol. 7, 113-118 (1979)

3478. Sallstro.,G., Maasing,R.
Swedish company doctors attitudes to benzodiazepines and neuroleptics used as minor tranquilizers.
Pharmatherap. 2, 380-6 (1980)

3479. Salomon,C.
Study of flunitrazepam in psychiatric-treatment.
Nouv.Presse 8, 2571-6 (1979)

3480. Salzman,C., Vanderko.,E.
Psychotropic-drug prescriptons for elderly patients in a general-hospital.
J.Amer.Ger.Soc. 28, 18-22 (1980)

3481. Samet,C.M., Geller,R.D.
Anxiety associated with cardiovascular disorders - study using lorazepam.
Psychosomat. 20, 709-13 (1979)

3482. Samuelson,P.N., Lell,W.A., Kouchouk.,N.T., Strong,S.D., Dole,K.M.
Hemodynamics during diazepam induction of anesthesia for coronary-artery bypass grafting.
South Med.J. 73, 332-4 (1980)

3483. Saner,A., Pletscher,A.
Effect of diazepam on cerebral 5-hydroxytryptamine synthesis.
Eur.J.Pharmacol. 55, 315-8 (1979)

3484. Sansone,M.
Effects of chlordiazepoxide-scopolamine combinations on shuttle-box avoidance performance of mice.
Arch.Int.Pharmacodyn.Ther. 235, 93-102 (1978)

3485. Sansone,M.
Effects of chlordiazepoxide, amitriptyline, imipramine, and their combinations on avoidance behaviour in mice.
Psychopharmacology (Berlin) 59, 151-5 (1978)

3486. Sansone,M.
Facilitating effects of chlordiazepoxide on locomotor activity and avoidance behaviour of reserpinized mice.
Psychopharmacology (Berlin) 59, 157-60 (1978)

3487. Sansone,M.
A further investigation on the effects of chlordiazepoxide given during avoidance training in two inbred strains of mice.
Pharmacol.Res.Commun. 11, 365-70 (1979)

3488. Sansone,M.
Effects of repeated administration of chlordiazepoxide on spontaneous locomotor activity in mice.
Psychopharmacology (Berlin) 66, 109-10 (1979)

3489. Sansone,M.
Influence of benzodiazepine tranquilizers on scopolamine-induced locomotor stimulation in mice.
Psychopharmacology 71, 243-5 (1980)

3490. Sansone,M., Hano,J.
Enhancement by chlordiazepoxide of the anticholinergic-induced locomotor stimulation in mice.
Psychopharmacology (Berlin) 64, 181-4 (1979)

3491. Sansone,M., Vetulani,J.
Facilitation of avoidance-behavior by chlordiazepoxide and chlordiazepoxide-amphetamine combination - effect on performance.
Pol.J.Pharm. 32, 125-31 (1980)

3492. Sarnquist,F.H., Gustafson,J., Blaschke,T.
Steady-state pharmacokinetics of midazolam maleate.
Clin.Pharm. 27, 283-4 (1980)

3493. Sarnquist,F.H., Nathers,W.D., Brockutn.,J., Carr,E., Canup,C., Brown,C.R.
Bioassay of a water-soluble benzodiazepine against sodium thiopental.
Anesthesiol. 52, 149-53 (1980)

3494. Sarrazin,M., Sari,J.C., Bourdeaux-Pontier,M., Briand,C.
NMR study of the interactions between flurazepam and human serum albumin. The nature of the complexation site on the benzodiazepine molecule.
Mol.Pharmacol. 15, 71-7 (1979)

3495. Saxena,B.M., Singh,A.N., Nelson,H.L., Mahutte,G.
Clinical-experience with oral and parenteral lorazepam - review of our studies.
Curr.Ther.Res. 25, 150-64 (1979)

3496. Saxena,B.M., Singh,A.N., Porter,W.R.
Clinical and experimental comparison of intramuscular lorazepam, diazepam, and placebo - psychometric tests and psychiatric rating-scales in the assessment of benzodiazepines.
Curr.Ther.Res. 28, 260-76 (1980)

3497. Schallek,W., Horst,W.D., Schlosser,W.
Mechanism of action of benzodiazepines (review or bibliography).
Adv.Pharm.Chemother. 16, 45-87 (1979)

3498. Scharf,M.B., Bixler,E.O., Kales,A., Soldatos,C.R.
Long-term sleep laboratory evaluation of flunitrazepam.
Pharmacol. 19, 173-81 (1979)

3499. Schecker,H.G., Zinner,G.
Zur "sogenannten Polonovski-Reaktion der 1,4-Benzodiazepin-4-oxide".
Chemiker-Ztg. 103, 317-9 (1979)

3500. Schecker,H.G., Zinner,G.
The oxidoreductive 1,3-rearrangement of 3H-1,4-benzodiazepines with semicyclic hydroxyamide structure to 2-alkylamino-3-acyloxy-3H-1,4-benzodiazepines.
Arch.Pharm. (Weinheim) 313, 926-36 (1980)

3501. Schieken,R.M.
The effect of diazepam upon the development of hypertension in the spontaneously hypertensive rat.
Pediatr.Res. 13, 992-6 (1979)

3502. Schjonsby,H.P., Gordon,A.E., Koeppen,D.
A three-month double-blind study of clobazam versus diazepam in out-patients suffering from neurotic disturbances.
J.Int.Med.Res. 7, 404-10 (1979)

3503. Schlosser,W., Franco,S.
Modification of GABA-mediated depolarization of the cat ganglion by pentobarbital and two benzodiazepines.
Neuropharmacology 18, 377-81 (1979)

3504. Schlosser,W., Franco,S.
Reduction of gamma-aminobutyric and (GABA)-mediated transmission by a convulsant benzodiazepine.
J.Pharmacol.Exp.Ther. 211, 290-5 (1979)

3505. Schmidt,D.
Benzodiazepines in status epilepticus and nodding spasms
Dtsch.Med.Wschr. 105, 1142 (1980)

3506. Schoenfe.,R.I.
Symposium on recent developments in the study of the mechanisms of benzodiazepine actions - Maui Hawaii December, 1978.
Pharm.Bio.Bull. 10, 801 (1979)

3507. Schohn,D., Jahn,H.
Action of flunitrazepam on organic and functional sleep disturbances.
Nouv.Presse 8, 2550-3 (1979)

3508. Schouole.,A., Huttel,M.S.
Local reactions to i.v. diazepam in 3 different formulations.
Brit.J.Anaest. 52, 609-11 (1980)

3509. Schütz,H.
Screening, detection and biotransformation of lormetazepam (Noctamid[R]), a new hypnotic agent from the 1,4-benzodiazepine group.
Arch.Toxicol. (in the press)

3510. Schütz,H.
Analytik und Biotransformation von Triazolam (Halcion[R]), einem neuen Benzodiazepin mit forensisch relevanten Nebenwirkungen.
Beitr.gerichtl.Med. (im Druck)

3511. Schütz,H.
Einflußmöglichkeiten verschiedener Parameter auf die Höhe einer Fremdstoffkonzentration in Körperflüssigkeiten, dargestellt am Beispiel der Benzodiazepine.
Dtsch.Apoth.-Ztg. (im Druck)

3512. Schwarz,H.J.
Pharmacokinetics and metabolism of temazepam in man and several animal species.
Brit.J.Clin.Pharmacol. 8, 23-29 (1979)

3513. Schwartz,S.E., Fazio,T.L.
Pre-endoscopic medication - randomized double-blind trial of atropine and meperidine as a supplement to diazepam.
Scand.J.Gastroenterol. 14, 747-51 (1979)

3514. Sellers,E.M., Giles,H.G., Greenblatt,D.J., Naranjo,C.A.
Differential effects on benzodiazepine disposition by disulfiram and ethanol.
Arzneim.-Forsch. (Drug Res.) 30, 882-6 (1980)

3515. Sellers,E.M., Greenblatt,D.J., Giles,H.G., Naranjo,C.A., Kaplan,H., MacLeod,S.M.
Chlordiazepoxide and oxazepam disposition in cirrhosis.
Clin.Pharm. 26, 240-6 (1979)

3516. Sellers,E.M., Jacob,M.S.
Use of benzodiazepines.
Can.Med.Ass.J. 122, 152 (1980)

3517. Sellers,E.M., Naranjo,C.A., Abel,J.G., Khouw,V., Sandor,P., Alexander,P.
Fatty-acid modulation of reciprocal variation in diazepam (D-alpha) and warfarin free fraction (W-alpha).
Clin.Pharm. 27, 285-6 (1980)

3518. Sellers,E.M., Naranjo,C.A., Abel,J.G., Khouw,V., Sandor,P., Alexander,P.
Changes in fatty-acids modulate reciprocal variations in diazepam (D-alpha) and warfarin free fraction (W-alpha).
Clin.Res. 28, 666 (1980)

3519. Sellers,E.M., Naranjo,C.A., Giles,H.G., Frecker,R.C., Beeching,M.
Intravenous diazepam and oral ethanol interaction.
Clin.Pharm. 28, 638-45 (1980)

3520. Sellers,E.M., Naranjo,C.A., Giles,H.G., Frecker,R.C., Khouw,V., Beeching,M., Fan,T.
Mechanism of ethanol-diazepam pharmacokinetic interaction.
Clin.Pharm. 27, 286 (1980)

3521. Sepinwall,J., Cook,L.
Relationship of gamma-aminobutyric acid (GABA) to antianxiety effects of benzodiazepines.
Brain Res.Bull. 5, 839-48 (1980)

3522. Sepinwall,J., Cook,L.
Mechanism of action of the benzodiazepines - behavioral-aspect.
Fed.Proc. 39, 3024-31 (1980)

3523. Seppala,T., Palva,E., Mattila,M.J., Korttila,K., Shrotriy.,R.C.
Tofisopam, a novel 3,4,-benzodiazepine - multiple-dose effects on psychomotor-skills and memory - comparison with diazepam and interactions with ethanol.
Psychopharmacology 69, 209-18 (1980)

3524. Serratri.,G.
Value of nitrazepam in the treatment of insomnia in a department of neurology.
Nouv.Presse 8, 2533-4 (1979)

3525. Shader,R.I., Greenblatt,D.J.
Clinical indications for plasma-level monitoring of psychotropic-drugs.
Amer.J.Psychiat. 136, 1590-1 (1979)

3526. Shah,N.S., Patel,V.O., Donald,A.G.
Effect of diazepam, desmethylimipramine, and SKF 525-A on the disposition of levo-methadone in mice after single or double injection.
Drug.Metab.Dispos. 7, 241-2 (1979)

3527. Shah,P.G., Sheth,A.R., Sheth,U.K.
Mode of action of pentobarbital and diazepam on hypothalamo-pituitary function in adult male rats.
Indian J.Exp.Biol. 17, 776-8 (1979)

3528. Shah,R.M., Donaldson,D., Burdett,D.
Teratogenic effects of diazepam in the hamster.
Can.J.Physiol.Pharmacol. 57, 556-61 (1979)

3529. Shakir,R.A., Nanda,R.N., Lambie,D.G., Johnson,R.H.
Comparative trial of valproate sodium and clonazepam in chronic epilepsy.
Arch.Neurol. 36, 301-4 (1979)

3530. Shearman,G.T., Lal,H., Fielding,S., Dunn,R., Kruse,H., Theurer,K.
Possible involvement of GABA mechanisms in the anxiolytic action of benzodiazepines - study with valproic acid.
Fed.Proc. 39, 753 (1980)

3531. Sherman-Gold,R., Dudai,Y.
Solubilization and properties of a benzodiazepine receptor from calf cortex.
Brain Res. 198, 485-90 (1980)

3532. Shibuya,H., Gale,K., Pert,C.B.
Supersensitivity to GABA's effect on benzodiazepine receptors develops after striatonigral lesions.
Eur.J.Pharmacol. 62, 243-4 (1980)

3533. Shija,A.B., Wosornu,L.
Evaluation of flurazepam (Dalmane) in surgical patients.
Med.J.Zamb. 12, 152-3 (1979)

3534. Shugars,K.D., Linet,O.I., Metzler,C.M., Rudzik,A.D.
A multiclinic comparison of the hypnotic efficacy of triazolam and placebo in insomniac outpatients.
Clin.Ther. 2, 390-8 (1980)

3535. Sieberns,S.
Clotiazepam.
In: Offizinpharmazie, hrsg. v. H. Morck, H. Liekfeld und L. Schneider, Bd. 2, S. 69-73 (1980), Thieme - Stuttgart

3536. Sieberns,S.
Therapeutische Erfahrungen mit Clotiazepam (Trecalmo), einem neuen Anxiolytikum aus der Gruppe der Thieno-diazepine. Ergebnisse eines Feldversuchs bei 186 Patienten).
Therapeutic experiences with clotiazepam (Trecalmo), a new anxiolytic drug from the thienodiazepine group. Results of a field study on 186 patients.
Fortschr.Med. 97, 1705-8 (1979)

3537. Sieghart,W., Karobath,M.
Molecular heterogeneity of benzodiazepine receptors.
Nature 286, 285-7 (1980)

3538. Sieghart,W., Karobath,M.
Molecular heterogeneity of benzodiazepine receptors.
Hoppe-Seylers Z.Physiol. 361, 1346-6 (1980)

3539. Silber,W.
Diazepam in gastrointestinal endoscopy.
S.Afr.Med.J. 55, 782 (1979)

3540. Silbernagel,W., Netter,P.
The assessment of anterograde amnesia induced by various benzodiazepines.
Arzneim.-Forsch. (Drug Res.) 30, 1232-3 (1980)

3541. Silva,J.A.C.E.
Nomifensin associated to clobazam in the treatment of anxious depression - a comparative double-blind trial against amitriptyline associated to chlor-diazepoxide.
Rev.Bra.Med. 37, 573-84 (1980)

3542. Simmonds,M.A.
A site for the potentiation of GABA-mediated responses by benzodiazepines.
Nature 284, 558-60 (1980)

3543. Simonyi,M., Fitos,I., Tegyey,Z.
Stereoselective labeling of racemic oxazepam acetate and its use in studying stereoselective binding to human-serum albumin.
J.Chem.Soc. 1980, 1105-6 (1980)

3544. Singer,L., Danion,J.M.
Insomnia in clinical-psychiatry - treatment using flunitrazepam.
Nouv.Presse 8, 2529-32 (1979)

3545. Singh,A.N., Psych,M.R.C., Saxena,B.
Intramuscular lorazepam, diazepam and placebo in the treatment of acute anxiety - double-blind controlled-study.
Curr.Ther.Res. 26, 260-74 (1979)

3546. Singh,A.N., Saxena,B.
Double-blind crossover comparison of triazolam and flurazepam in hospitalized psychiatric-patients with insomnia.
Curr.Ther.Res. 27, 627-34 (1980)

3547. Singh,H.C., Singh,R.H., Udupa,K.N.
Effect of diazepam on acetylcholine content in rat brain following electric shock.
Indian J.Exp.Biol. 18, 415-6 (1980)

3548. Singh,M.M., Nasralla.,H.A., Lal,H., Pitman,R.K., Becker,R.E., Kucharsk.,T., Karkalas,J., Fox,R.
Treatment of tardive-dyskinesia with diazepam - indirect evidence for the involvement of limbic, possibly GABA-ergic mechanisms.
Brain Res.Bull. 5, 673-80 (1980)

3549. Skolnick,P., Lock,K.L., Paugh,B., Marangos,P., Windsor,R., Paul,S.
Pharmacologic and behavioral effects of EMD 28422: a novel purine which enhances (3H) diazepam binding to brain benzodiazepine receptors.
Pharmacol.Biochem.Behav. 12, 685-9 (1980)

3550. Skolnick,P., Lock,K.L., Paul,S.M., Marangos,P.J., Jones,R., Irmscher,K.
Increased benzodiazepine receptor number elicited invitro by a novel purine, EMD-28422.
Eur.J.Pharmacol. 67, 179-86 (1980)

3551. Skolnick,P., Marangos,P.J., Syapin,P., Goodwin,F.K., Paul,S.M.
CNS benzodiazepine receptors: physiological studies and putative endogenous ligands.
Pharmacol.Biochem.Behav. 10, 815-23 (1979)

3552. Skolnick,P., Paul,S.M., Barker,J.L.
Pentobarbital potentiates GABA-enhanced (3H)-diazepam binding to benzodiazepine receptors.
Eur.J.Pharmacol. 65, 125-7 (1980)

3553. Skolnick,P., Paul,S.M., Marangos,P.J.
Brain benzodiazepine levels following intravenous administration of (3H)diazepam: relationship to the potentiation of purinergic depression of central nervous system neurons.
Can.J.Physiol.Pharmacol. 57, 1040-2 (1979)

3554. Skolnick,P., Paul,S.M., Marangos,P.J.
Purines as endogenous ligands of the benzodiazepine receptor.
Fed.Proc. 39, 3050-5 (1980)

3555. Skolnick,P., Paul,S., Zatz,M., Eskay,R.
Brain-specific benzodiazepine receptors are localized in the inner plexiform layer of rat retina.
Eur.J.Pharmacol. 66, 133-6 (1980)

3556. Skolnick,P., Syapin,P.J., Paugh,B.A., Moncada,V., Marangos,P.J., Paul,S.M.
Inosine, an endogenous ligand of the brain benzodiazepine receptor, antagonizes pentylenetetrazole-evoked seizures.
Proc.Natl.Acad.Sci.USA 76, 1515-8 (1979)

3557. Skolnick,P., Syapin,P.J., Paugh,B.A., Paul,S.M.
Reduction in benzodiazepine receptors associated with Purkinje cell degeneration in 'nervous' mutant mice.
Nature 277, 397-9 (1979)

3558. Slater,P., Longman,D.A.
Effects of diazepam and muscimol on GABA-mediated neurotransmission: interactions with inosine and nicotinamide.
Life Sci. 25, 1963-7 (1979)

3559. Smith,M.T., Eadie,M.J., Orourkeb.,T., Smith,T.C.
The pharmacokinetics of midazolam in man.
Clin.Exp.Pharm. 7, 680 (1980)

3560. Snell,E.S.
Systematic review of the benzodiazepines.
Brit.Med.J. 280, 1053-4 (1980)

3561. Solomon,F., Mendelson,W.B.
Sleeping pills.
N.Engl.J.Med. 301, 214-5 (1979)

3562. Sonnenberg,A., Koelz,H.R., Herz,R., Benes,I., Blum,A.L.
Der Einfluß oraler Kontrazeptiva auf die Demethylierung von Diazepam und Dimethyl-N-aminoantipyrin.
Effect of oral contraceptives on the demethylation of diazepam and dimethyl-N-aminoantipyrine.
Verh.Dtsch.Ges.Inn.Med. 84, 1485-8 (1978)

3563. Sorel,L., Mechler,L., Harmant,J.
A comparative-study of intravenous lorazepam and clonazepam in the treatment of status epilepticus.
Act.Neur.Belg. 80, 368-79 (1980)

3564. Soroker,D., Barzilay,E., Konichezky,S., Bruderman,I.
Respiratory function following premedication with droperidol or diazepam.
Anesth.Analg. (Cleve) 57, 695-9 (1978)

3565. Soubrie,P., Thiebot,M.H., Jobert,A., Montastruc,J.L., Hery,F., Hamon,M.
Decreased convulsant potency of picrotoxin and pentetrazol and enhanced (3H)flunitrazepam cortical binding following stressful manipulations in rats.
Brain Res. 189, 505-17 (1980)

3566. Speeg,K.V., Avant,G.R., Schenker,S.
Inhibition of cerebral benzodiazepine binding by cimetidine and other antihistamines.
Clin.Res. 27, 684 (1979)

3567. Speeg,K.V.,jr., Wang,S., Avant,G.R., Berman,M.L., Schenker,S.
Antagonism of benzodiazepine binding in brain by antilirium, benzyl alcohol, and physostigmine.
J.Neurochem. 34, 856-65 (1980)

3568. Speeg,K.V.,jr., Wang,S., Avant,G.R., Berman,M.L., Schenker,S.
Antagonism of benzodiazepine binding in rat and human brain by antilirium.
Life Sci. 24, 1345-50 (1979)

3569. Speth,R.C., Johnson,R.W., Regan,J., Reisine,T., Kobayash.,R.M., Bresolin,N., Roeske,W.R., Yamamura,H.I.
The benzodiazepine receptor of mammalian brain.
Fed.Proc. 39, 3032-8 (1980)

3570. Spencer,J.
Use of injectable lorazepam in alcohol withdrawal.
Med.J.Aust. 2, 211-2 (1980)

3571. Sperk,G., Schloegl,E.
Reduction of number of benzodiazepine binding sites in the caudate nucleus of the rat after kainic acid injections.
Brain Res. 170, 563-7 (1979)

3572. Speth,R.C., Bresolin,N., Yamamura,H.I.
Acute diazepam administration produces rapid increases in brain benzodiazepine receptor density.
Eur.J.Pharmacol. 59, 159-60 (1979)

3573. Speth,R.C., Wastek,G.J., Reisine,T.D., Yamamura,H.I.
Benzodiazepine receptors: effects of tissue preincubation at 37°C.
Neurosci.Lett. 13, 243-7 (1979)

3574. Speth,R.C., Yamamura,H.I.
Benzodiazepine receptors: alterations in mutant mouse cerebellum.
Eur.J.Pharmacol. 54, 397-9 (1979)

3575. Spyraki,C., Papadopoulou,Z., Zis,B., Varonos,D.
Effects of diazepam-infrasounds combination on locomotor activity and avoidance behaviour of rats.
Pharmacol.Biochem.Behav. 12, 767-71 (1980)

3576. Squires,R.F., Benson,D.I., Braestrup,C., Coupet,J., Klepner,C.A., Myers,V., Beer,B.
Some properties of brain specific benzodiazepine receptors: new evidence for multiple receptors.
Pharmacol.Biochem.Behav. 10, 825-30 (1979)

3577. Squires,R.F., Klepner,C.A., Benson,D.I.
Multiple benzodiazepine receptor complexes: some benzodiazepine recognition sites are coupled to GABA receptors and ionophores.
Adv.Biochem.Psychopharmacol. 21, 285-93 (1980)

3578. Squires,R., Naquet,R., Riche,D., Braestrup,C.
Increased thermolability of benzodiazepine receptors in cerebral-cortex of a baboon with spontaneous seizures - case report.
Epilepsia 20, 215-21 (1979)

3579. Staak,M., Raff,G., Nusser,W.
Pharmacopsychological investigations concerning the combined effects of dipotassium clorazepate and ethanol.
Int.J.Clin.Pharmacol.Biopharm. 17, 205-12 (1979)

3580. Staak,M., Raff,G., Strohm,H.
Pharmacopsychological investigation of changes in mood induced by dipotassium chlorazepate with and without simultaneous alcohol administration.
Int.J.Clin.Pharmacol.Biopharm. 18, 283-91 (1980)

3581. Standish,L.J., Feldman,R.S.
Differential effects of chlordiazepoxide on conditioned and unconditioned behavior in mice with septal lesions.
Psychopharmacology (Berlin) 61, 293-7 (1979)

3582. Stark,R.D., Gambles,S.A.
Effects of diazepam and promethazine on breathlessness induced by exercise or raised CO_2 in healthy-subjects.
Clin.Resp.P. 16, 220-1 (1980)

3583. Stein,L.
Neurochemie der Beeinflussung des Verhaltens durch Benzodiazepine.
Behavioral Neurochemistry of Benzodiazepines.
New Perspectives in Benzodiazepine Therapy - International Symposium Heidelberg 1979
Arzneim.-Forsch. (Drug Res.) 30, 868-73 (1980)

3584. Stella,L., Torri,G., Castiglioni,C.L.
The relative potencies of thiopentone, ketamine, propanidid, alphaxalone and diazepam. A statistical study in man.
Brit.J.Anaesth. 51, 119-22 (1979)

3585. Stensrud,P., Sjaastad,O.
Clonazepam (Rivotril) in migraine prophylaxis.
Headache 19, 333-4 (1979)

3586. Stephens.,O.K.
Socratic dialog clarifies benzodiazepine debate.
Penn.Med. 82, 39-40 (1979)

3587. Stewart,R.B., Salem,R.B., Springer,P.K.
A case-report of lorazepam withdrawal.
Amer.J.Psychiat. 137, 1113-4 (1980)

3588. Stewart,R.C.
Respiratory depression with diazepam: potential complications and contraindications.
Anesth.Prog. 25, 117-8 (1978)

3589. Stockmann, R., Sidiropoulos,D., Wendt,G.
The effects on neonatal hyperbilirubinaemia of parenteral administration of Valium to women in labour.
J.Int.Med.Res. 6, 468-70 (1978)

3590. Stone,B.M.
Diazepam and its hydroxylated metabolites: studies on sleep in healthy man.
Brit.J.Clin.Pharmacol. 8, 57 (1979)

3591. Stone,M.A., Topham,L.D., Greenwood,D.T.
Does binding to the high and low affinity GABA binding-sites represent binding to benzodiazepine receptor linked and non-benzodiazepine receptor linked GABA receptors.
Brit.J.Pharmacol. 69, 326-7 (1980)

3592. Straughan,J.L.
Which benzodiazepine, why and how?
S.Afr.Med.J. 55, 1110-4 (1979)

3593. Strittmatter,W.J., Hirata,F., Axelrod,J., Mallorga,P., Tallman,J.F., Henneberry,R.C.
Benzodiazepine and beta-adrenergic receptor ligands independently stimulate phospholipid methylation.
Nature 282, 857-9 (1979)

3594. Studd,C., Eltringh.,R.J.
Lorazepam as night sedation and premedication - comparison with diazepam.
Anaesthesia 35, 60-4 (1980)

3595. Stumpf,C., Jindra,R., Huck,S., Ewers,H.
Wechselwirkungen zwischen Stickoxydul und zentral dämpfend wirkenden Pharmaka.
Interactions between nitrous and central depressants.
Anaesthesist 28, 3-8 (1979)

3596. Sugasawa,T., Adachi,M., Toyoda,T., Sasakura,K.
New simple synthesis of 1,4-benzodiazepines.
J.Heterocycl.Chem. 16, 445-8 (1979)

3597. Sunjic,V., Oklobdzi.,M., Lisini,A., Sega,A., Kajfez,F.

Chiral 1,4-benzodiazepines. 11. Kinetics of degenerate nucleophilic exchange of C(3)-hydroxy group.
Tetrahedron 35, 2531-7 (1979)

3598. Supavilai,P., Karobath,M.
Stimulation of benzodiazepine receptor binding by SQ 20009 is chloride-dependent and picrotoxin-sensitive.
Eur.J.Pharmacol. 60, 111-3 (1979)

3599. Supavilai,P., Karobath,M.
Interaction of SQ 20009 and GABA-like drugs as modulators of benzodiazepine receptor binding.
Eur.J.Pharmacol. 62, 229-33 (1980)

3600. Supavilai,P., Karobath,M.
The effect of temperature and chloride-ions on the stimulation of flunitrazepam-H-3 binding by the muscimol analogs thip and piperidine-4-sulfonic acid.
Neurosci.Lett. 19, 337-41 (1980)

3601. Svensson,C.K.
Lorazepam withdrawal.
Drug Intell. 14, 628 (1980)

3602. Svensson,E., Persson,L.O., Sjoeberg,L.
Mood effects of diazepam and caffeine.
Psychopharmacology (Berlin) 67, 73-80 (1980)

3603. Swift,C.G., Haythorne,J.M., Clarke,P., Stevenson,I.H.
Chlormethiazole and temazepam.
Brit.Med.J. 280, 1322 (1980)

3604. Swift,C.G., Hewick,D.S., Ogg,G., Stevenson,I.H.
Acetylator phenotype, nitrazepam plasma concentrations and residual effects.
Brit.J.Clin.Pharmacol. 9, 312-3 (1980)

3605. Swinyard,E.A., Shenoy,A.K., Kupferberg,H.J.
Anticonvulsant profiles of clobazam, diazepam, phenobarbital and valproate.
Fed.Proc. 39, 1100 (1980)

3606. Syapin,P.J., Skolnick,P.
Characterization of benzodiazepine binding sites in cultured cells of neural origin.
J.Neurochem. 32, 1047-51 (1979)

3607. Tajana,A., Pennini,R., Nardi,D.
New 2-monoalkylamino and 2-dialkylamino-4-phenyl-3H-1,5-benzodiazepines.
Farmaco Sci. 35, 181-90 (1980)

3608. Takahash.,N., Ando,R., Sakurada,S., Kisara,K.
Effect of diazepam on unit-activity of amygdaloid neurons.
Fol.Pharm.Jap. 76, 35-6 (1980)

3609. Takasu,T., Matsuda,H., Sato,K., Hayashi,M., Aizawa,K., Shieh,M.T., Shibuya,T.
Pharmacological consideration of substitute-F of diazepam.
Fol.Pharm.Jap. 76, 1 (1980)

3610. Tallman,J.F.
Interaction between benzodiazepines and GABA.
Brain Res.Bull. 4, 710 (1979)

3611. Tallman,J.F.
Interactions between GABA and benzodiazepines.
Brain Res.Bull. 5, 829-32 (1980)

3612. Tallman,J.F., Gallager,D.W.
Modulation of benzodiazepine binding site sensitivity.
Pharmacol.Biochem.Behav. 10, 809-13 (1979)

3613. Tallman,J.F., Gallager,D.W., Mallorga,P., Thomas,J.W., Strittmatter,W., Hirata,F., Axelrod,J.
Studies on benzodiazepine receptors.
Adv.Biochem.Psychopharmacol. 21, 277-83 (1980)

3614. Tallman,J.F., Paul,S.M., Skolnick,P., Gallager,D.W.
Receptors for the age of anxiety: pharmacology of the benzodiazepines.
Science 207, 274-81 (1980)

3615. Tallman,J.F., Thomas,J.W., Gallager,D.W.
Identification of diazepam binding in intact animals.
Life Sci. 24, 873-9 (1979)

3616. Tallone,G., Ghirardi,P., Cesabian.,M., Ravaccia,F., Bruni,G., Loreti,P.
Reaction-time to acoustic or visual-stimuli after administration of camazepam and diazepam in man.
Arzneim.-Forsch. (Drug Res.) 30, 1021-4 (1980)

3617. Taniguchi,T., Wang,J.K., Spector,S.
Properties of (3H) diazepam binding to rat peritoneal mast cells.
Life Sci. 27, 171-8 (1980)

3618. Tansella,C.Z.
The long-term treatment with benzodiazepines. - Suggestions for further research.
Int.Pharmacopsych. 15, 99-104 (1980)

3619. Tarnow,J., Hess,W.
Flunitrazepam-pretreatment for prevention of adverse cardiovascular effects following ketamine.
Anaesthesis 28, 468-73 (1979)

3620. Teal,J.S.
Comments on benzodiazepine reaction.
Drug Intell. 14, 723 (1980)

3621. Tegyey,Z., Maksay,G., Otvos,L.
Synthesis of 2-C-14-labeled 3H-1,4-benzodiazepines.
J.Label.Chem.Res. 16, 377-85 (1979)

3622. Teller,C., Kinawi,A.
Bestimmung der Bindung von Chlordiazepoxid, Diazepam, Nitrazepam und Phenprocoumon an Human- und Rinder-serumalbumin.
Determination of the binding of chlordiazepoxide, diazepam, nitrazepam and phenprocoumon to human and bovine serum albumin.
Arch.Pharm. (Weinheim) 312, 295-8 (1979)

3623. Tenen,S.S., Hirsch,J.D.
Beta-carboline-3-carboxylic acid ethyl-ester antagonizes diazepam activity.
Nature 288, 609-10 (1980)

3624. Teo,K.K., Kelly,J.G., Horgan,J.J.
Lack of effect of diazepam on the ST segment of the electrocardiogram during maximal exercise stress testing in normal subjects.
J.Cardiovasc.Pharmacol. 2, 337-8 (1980)

3625. Tessore,A.
Double blind study of clobazam (HR 376) in pre- and postoperative anxiety states.
Clin.Ter. 87, 141-50 (1978)

3626. Tewari,S.N., Shukla,S.K.
Paper chromatographic separation and identification of 1,4-benzodiazepines and Mandrax.
Pharmazie 34, 567 (1979)

3627. Thakuria,S.P.
Prevention of pain and phlebitis due to diazepam injection.
Anaesthesia 35, 392 (1980)

3628. Thiebot,M.H., Jobert,A., Soubrie,P.
Conditioned suppression of behavior - its reversal by intra raphe micro-injection of chlordiazepoxide and GABA.
Neurosci.Lett. 16, 213-7 (1980)

3629. Thompson,D., Hohenwar.,M.
Haloperidol and diazepam - dangerous look-alikes.
Amer.Pharmacy 20, 6 (1980)

3630. Thorn,I.
Prophylactic treatment of febrile convulsions with continuous phenobarbital contra intermittent diazepam.
Develop.Med. 22, 267-8 (1980)

3631. Thornton,J.A., Bennett,N.R., Dixon,R.
The use of flunitrazepam for controlled sedation in dentistry.
J.Dent.Res. 59, 1796 (1980)

3632. Thorsen,T., Gran,L.
Ketamine/diazepam infusion anaesthesia with special attention to the effect on cerebrospinal fluid pressure and arterial blood pressure.
Acta Anaesthesiol.Scand. 24, 1-4 (1980)

3633. Tjaden,U.R., Meeles,M.T., Thys,C.P., van der Kaay,M.
Determination of some benzodiazepines and metabolites in serum, urine and saliva by high-performance liquid chromatography.
J.Chromatogr. 181, 227-41 (1980)

3634. Toda,K., Tanaka,H., Iriki,A.
Effects of diazepam (Cercine) on the somatosensory evoked responses following tooth pulp stimulation in rat.
Bull.Tokyo Med.Dent.Univ. 26, 85-9 (1979)

3635. Todt,H., Wuensche,W.
Provokation tonischer Anfälle unter intravenöser Faustaninjektion.
Provocation of tonic seizures during intravenous faustan administration.
Kinderaerztl.Prax. 46, 580-2 (1978)

3636. Tolbert,L.C.
Mechanism of action of benzodiazepines.
Ala.J.Med.Soc. 17, 168-70 (1980)

3637. Tolksdorf,W., Hartung,H.J., Kammerer,T., Rohowsky,R., Lutz,H.
The influence of benzoctamin and flunitrazepam as sedative drugs during spinal-anesthesia in patients with preoperative decreased lung-function.
Anaesthesis 29, 434-8 (1980)

3638. Tonczar,L.
The influence of flunitrazepam on the blood-gases during subarachnoid block in geriatric patients.
Anaesthesis 29, 487-9 (1980)

3639. Tormey,W.P., Dolphin,C., Darragh,A.S.
Effects of diazepam on sleep, and on the nocturnal release of growth-hormone, prolactin, ACTH and cortisol.
Brit.J.Clin.Pharmacol. 8, 90-2 (1979)

3640. Trauner,D.A., Clayman,M.
Dialysis encephalopathy treated with clonazepam.
Ann.Neurol. 6, 555-6 (1979)

3641. Traversa,U., Newman,M.
Stereospecific influence of oxazepam hemisuccinate on cyclic AMP accumulation elicited by adenosine in cerebral cortical slices.
Biochem.Pharmacol. 28, 2363-5 (1979)

3642. Triazolam (Halcion): psychological disturbances.
Drug Ther.Bull. 17, 76 (1979)

3643. Trillet,M., Chazot,G.
The effectiveness of benzodiazepines (clobazam) in cerebellar and postural tremor.
Lyon Med. 244, 31-4 (1980)

3644. Tsuchiya,T., Enkaku,M., Okajima,S.
Studies on diazepines. 12. Photochemical-synthesis of novel 1H-1,3-benzodiazepines from isoquinoline N-imides.
Chem.Pharm. 28, 2602-8 (1980)

3645. Tsuchiya,T., Kurita,J.
Synthesis of the first examples of 5H-1,2-benzodiazepines.
J.Chem.Soc. 1979, 803-4 (1979)

3646. Tunnicliff,G., Smith,J.A., Ngo,T.T.
Competition for diazepam receptor binding by diphenylhydantoin and its enhancement by gamma-aminobutyric acid.
Biochem.Biophys.Res.Commun. 91, 1018-24 (1979)

3647. Tye,N.C., Iversen,S.D., Green,A.R.
The effects of benzodiazepines and serotonergic manipulations on punished responding.
Neuropharmacology 18, 689-95 (1979)

3648. Tyrer,P.
Lorazepam withdrawal seizures - reply.
Lancet 1, 151 (1980)

3649. Ushirogo.,A., Tominaga,Y., Matsuda,Y., Kobayashi,G.
Synthesis of 1,5-benzodiazepines.
Heterocycles 14, 7-10 (1980)

3650. Vaille,C., Souchard,M., Chariot,J.
Action of diazepam on biliary secretion in the rat.
Ann.Pharm.Franc. 37, 5-11 (1979)

3651. Valdman,A.V., Marusov,I.V.
Role of GABA-ergic brain systems in the activating effect of diazepam.
Bull.Exp.Biol.Med. 87, 576-8 (1979)

3652. Valli,M., Pringuey,D.
New trends on biochemical-mechanism of action of benzodiazepines.
Therapie 35, 561-9 (1980)

3653. Vallner,J.J., Kotzan,J.A., Stewart,J.T., Honigberg, I.L., Needham,T.E., Brown,W.J.
Plasma-levels of clobazam after 10-mg, 20-mg, and 40-mg tablet doses in healthy-subjects.
J.Clin.Pharm. 20, 444-51 (1980)

3654. van der Kroef,C.
Halcion, an innocent hypnotic?
Ned.Tijdschr.Geneeskd. 123, 1160-1 (1979)

3655. van der Kroef,C.
Reactions to triazolam.
Lancet 2, 526 (1979)

3656. Vane,F.M., Benz,W.
M/Z 91 rearrangement ion in the mass-spectra of some 1,4-benzodiazepines.
Org.Mass Spectr. 14, 233-8 (1979)

3657. van Geijn,H.P., Jongsma,H.W., Doesburg,W.H., Lemmens,W.A., de Haan,J., Eskes,T.K.
The effect of diazepam administration during pregnancy or labor on the heart rate variability of the newborn infant.
Eur.J.Obstet.Gynaecol.Reprod.Biol. 10, 187-201 (1980)

3658. Vasiliades,J., Owens,C.
Determination of midazolam in serum by gas chromatography with a nitrogen-selective detector.
J.Chromatogr. 182, 439-44 (1980)

3659. Vasiliades,J., Owens,C., Ogletree,F.
The determination of midazolam by gas-chromatography, liquid-chromatography and gas-chromatography mass-spectrometry.
Clin.Chem. 26, 985 (1980)

3660. Vassella,F.
Benzodiazepines in the treatment of epilepsy - a review.
Schweiz.Rundsch.Med.Prax. 69, 827-34 (1980)

3661. Vellucci,S.V., File,S.E.
Chlordiazepoxide loses its anxiolytic action with long-term treatment.
Psychopharmacology (Berlin) 62, 61-5 (1979)

3662. Vesell,E.S.
Elucidation of the pharmacokinetic interaction between acutely administered ethanol and benzodiazepines.
J.Lab.Clin.Med. 95, 305-9 (1980)

3663. Vetulani,J., Sansone,M.
Stimulatory effect of chlordiazepoxide on locomotor activity in mice: importance of noradrenergic transmission.
Pol.J.Pharmacol.Pharm. 30, 791-8 (1978)

3664. Villegas,A.N., Ramirez,D.A.
Effects of diazepam (Valium) on human-chromosomes.
Kalikasan 8, 1-12 (1979)

3665. Violon,C., Vercruysse,A.
Screening-procedure for therapeutic benzodiazepines by high-performance liquid-chromatography of their benzophenones.
J.Chromatogr. 189, 94-7 (1980)

3666. Vogel,R.A., Frye,G.D., Wilson,J.H., Kuhn,C.M., Koepke, K.M., Mailman,R.B., Mueller,R.A., Breese,G.R.
Attenuation of the effects of punishment by ethanol - comparisons with chlordiazepoxide.
Psychopharmacology 71, 123-9 (1980)

3667. Voronina,T.A., Garibova,T.L.
Role of GABA-ergic and dopaminergic mechanisms in the withdrawal syndrome after discontinuation of long-term phenazepam administration.
Biull.Eksp.Biol.Med. 89, 41-3 (1980)

3668. Voronina,T.A., Littrov,K.V.
Comparison of clonazepam and diazepam in experimental studies.
Farmakol.Toxikol. 43, 296-9 (1980)

3669. Vyborova,L., Balastik.,B., Misurec,J., Drtilkov.,I., Nahunek,K.
Controlled-study with bromazepam and clorotepin in child instability.
Activ.Nerv. 22, 181-2 (1980)

3670. Walker,C.R., Bandman,E., Strohman,R.C.
Diazepam induces relaxation of chick embryo muscle fibers in vitro and inhibits myosin synthesis.
Exp.Cell.Res. 123, 285-91 (1979)

3671. Walker,J.E., Homan,R.W., Vasko,M.R., Crawford,I.L., Bell,R.D., Tasker,W.G.
Lorazepam in status epilepticus.
Ann.Neurol. 6, 207-13 (1979)

3672. Wallace,J.E., Harris,S.C., Shimek,E.L.
Evaluation of an enzyme immunoassay for determining diazepam and nordiazepam in serum and urine.
Clin.Chem. 26, 1905-7 (1980)

3673. Wallace,R.B., Hunningh.,D.B., Reiland,S., Barrettc.,E., Hoover,J., Mackenth.,A., Heiss,G.
Alterations in plasma-lipid and lipoprotein levels associated with the use of benzodiazepine tranquilizers - the lipid research clinics program.
Clin.Res. 28, 228 (1980)

3674. Wallis,T.D., Valle-Jones,J.C., Craven,J.R., Hanks,G.W., Stonier,P.D.
Single daily dose treatment of anxiety with clobazam or dipotassium clorazepate.
Brit.J.Clin.Pharmacol. 7, 123-7 (1979)

3675. Walters,F.J., Pearce,D.J., Hanks,G.W.
Clinical and biochemical evaluations of premedicants. A double-blind assessment of clobazam, a new 1,5-benzodiazepine.
Anaesthesia 34, 444-9 (1979)

3676. Walther,M.
The treatment of insomnia - a contribution to the evaluation of a new benzodiazepin triazolam.
Schweiz.Rev.Med. 69, 460-7 (1980)

3677. Walz,M.A., Davis,W.M.
Experimental diazepam intoxication in rodents: physostigmine and naloxone as potential antagonists.
Drug Chem.Toxicol. 2, 257-67 (1979)

3678. Wang,C.M., James,C.A.
An analysis of the direct effect of chlordiazepoxide on mammalian cardiac tissues and crayfish and squid giant axons: possible basis of antiarrhythmic activity.
Life Sci. 24, 1357-65 (1979)

3679. Ward,J.
Allgemeine chemische Betrachtungen über die Benzodiazepine.
In: Offizinpharmazie, hrsg. von H. Morck, H. Liekfeld und L. Schneider, Bd. 2, S. 55-60 (1980), Thieme - Stuttgart

3680. Warren,J.W., Shah,K.A., Benmaman,J.D., Freeman,D.B., Lewkowic.,R.T., Friend,C.G.
Variations among 10 chlordiazepoxide HCL 10-mg capsule products.
Curr.Ther.Res. 25, 172-9 (1979)

3681. Watson,B.
Absence status and the concurrent administration of clonazepam and valproate sodium.
Amer.J.Hosp.Pharm. 36, 887 (1979)

3682. Watson,P.J., Short,M.A., Huenink,G.L., Hartman,D.F.
Diazepam effects on hypothalamically elicited drinking and eating.
Physiol.Behav. 24, 39-44 (1980)

3683. Watson,W.A.
Interaction between clonazepam and sodium valproate.
N.Engl.J.Med. 300, 678-9 (1979)

3684. Weihrauch,T.R., Foerster,C.F., Koehler,H., Ewe,K., Krieglstein,J.
Effect of intravenous diazepam on human lower oesophageal sphincter pressure under controlled double blind crossover conditions.
GUT 20, 64-7 (1979)

3685. Weizman,R., Weizman,A., Tyano,S., Wijsenbe.,H., Bendavid,M.
Biphasic effect of gradually increased doses of diazepam on prolactin secretion in acute schizophrenic-patients.
Isr.Ann.Psy. 17, 233-40 (1979)

3686. Wetherell,A.
Individual and group effects of 10 mg diazepam on drivers' ability, confidence and willingsness to act in a gap-judging task.
Psychopharmacology (Berlin) 63, 259-67 (1979)

3687. Whelpton,R.
Data compilation - benzodiazepine compounds.
Biopharm.Drug Disp. 1, 37-45 (1979)

3688. Whiting,B., Lawrence,J.R., Skellern,G.G.
Chlordiazepoxide in acute alcoholism.
Brit.J.Clin.Pharmacol. 8, 85-6 (1979)

3689. Whitwam,J.G., Scott,W.A.C., Kurimoto,S., Orchard,C., Chakraba.,M.K.
Cardiovascular effects of midazolam (RO 21-3981) in the dog.
Brit.J.Anaest. 52, 954 (1980)

3690. Wiatt,A.L., Ornato,J.P.
Outpatient utilization of diazepam in a military hospital.
Milit.Med. 145, 394-6 (1980)

3691. Wichlins.,L.M., Sieradzk.,E.
Comparative studies of the influence of elevated serum-lipid levels on the pharmacokinetics of diazepam in rabbits and humans.
Drug Intell. 14, 765-8 (1980)

3692. Wickstroem,E., Giercksk.,K.E.
Comparative-study of zopiclone, a novel hypnotic, and 3 benzodiazepines.
Eur.J.Clin.Pharmacol. 17, 93-9 (1980)

3693. Wieck,H.H.
Mode of action of modern tranquillizers from the benzodiazepine group: a clinical view.
Brit.J.Clin.Pharmacol. 7, 107-8 (1979)

3694. Wieck,H.H., Blaha,L., Heerklotz,B.
A clinical view of clobazam.
Brit.J.Clin.Pharmacol. 7, 109-12 (1979)

3695. Wieck,H.H., Heerklotz,B.
The mode of action of modern tranquilizers from the benzodiazepine group: a clinical view.
J.Int.Med.Res. 7, 573-82 (1979)

3696. Williams,A., Gillespi.,M.
Clonazepam-induced incontinence.
Ann.Neurol. 6, 86 (1979)

3697. Williams,E.F., Rice,K.C., Paul,S.M., Skolnick,P.
Heterogeneity of benzodiazepine receptors in the central nervous-system demonstrated with kenazepine, an alkylating benzodiazepine.
J.Neurochem. 35, 591-7 (1980)

3698. Williams,M., Risley,E.A.
Enhancement of the binding of 3H-diazepam to rat brain membranes in vitro by SQ 20009, a novel anxiolytic, gamma-aminobutyric acid (GABA) and muscimol.
Life Sci. 24, 833-41 (1979)

3699. Williams,M., Yarbrough,G.G.
Enhancement of in vitro binding and some of the pharmacological properties of diazepam by a novel anthelmintic agent, avermectin B1A.
Eur.J.Pharmacol. 56, 273-6 (1979)

3700. Williams,R.C.
Automated sample extraction of benzodiazepine drugs and their metabolites in blood-serum with analysis by LC.
Clin.Chem. 26, 1002 (1980)

3701. Williams,R.C.
Application of an automated sample processor to the analysis of benzodiazepine drugs and their metabolites in blood-serum by HPLC.
Z.Anal.Chem. 301, 116-7 (1980)

3702. Williams,T.H., Sasso,G.J., Ryan,J.J., Schwartz,M.A.
Novel application of proton nuclear magnetic resonance spectroscopy in the identification of 2'-chloronor-diazepam metabolites in the dog.
J.Med.Chem. 22, 436-40 (1979)

3703. Willow,M., Morgan,I.G.
Retinal benzodiazepine receptors are destroyed by kainic acid lesions.
Neurosci.Lett. 20, 147-52 (1980)

3704. Wilson,E.A.
Diazepam and local-anesthetic spray versus general-anesthesia for gastroduodenoscopy.
S.Afr.Med.J. 57, 111-3 (1980)

3705. Wilson,J.D., King,D.J., Sheridan,B.
Tranquillisers and plasma prolactin.
Brit.Med.J. 1, 123-4 (1979)

3706. Wilson,J.M., Raisys,V.A.
Determination of clonazepam by GC-MS.
Clin.Chem. 25, 1090 (1979)

3707. Wilson,W.H., Freemon,F.R., Ban,T.A., Petrie,W.M., Clinton,C.L.
Acute effects of viloxazine HCl and flurazepam when given alone and in combination on sleep EEG - a double-blind interaction study with normals.
Pav.J.Biol. 15, 68-73 (1980)

3708. Winokur,A., Rickels,K., Greenblatt,D.J., Snyder,P.J., Schatz,N.J.
Withdrawal reaction from long-term, low-dosage administration of diazepam. A double-blind, placebo-controlled case study.
Arch.Gen.Psychiatry 37, 101-5 (1980)

3709. Wittenborn,J.R.
Effects of benzodiazepines on psychomotor performance.
Brit.J.Clin.Pharmacol. 7, 61-7 (1979)

3710. Wittenborn,J.R., Flaherty,C.F., McGough,W.E., Nash,R.J.
Psychomotor changes during the initial day of benzodiazepine medication.
Psychopharmacol.Bull. 15, 39-40 (1979)

3711. Wittenborn,J.R., Flaherty,C.F., McGough,W.E., Nash,R.J.
Psychomotor changes during initial day of benzodiazepine medication.
Brit.J.Clin.Pharmacol. 7, 69-76 (1979)

3712. Wittwer,J.D.
Application of high-pressure liquid-chromatography to the forensic analysis of several benzodiazepines.
J.Liqu.Chrom. 3, 1713-24 (1980)

3713. Wong,D.T., Bymaster,F.P., Lane,P.T.
GABA activation of benzodiazepine receptors in native and triton-treated membranes.
Brain Res.Bull. 5, 853-6 (1980)

3714. Wong,G.B., Sellers,E.M.
Intravascular factors affecting diazepam binding to human serum albumin.
Biochem.Pharmacol. 28, 3265-70 (1979)

3715. Woo,E., Greenblatt,D.J.
Massive benzodiazepine requirements during acute alcohol withdrawal.
Amer.J.Psychiat. 136, 821-3 (1979)

3716. Wood,A.J.J., Robertson,D., Robertson,R.M., Wilkinson, G.R., Wood,M.
Elevated plasma-free drug concentrations of propranolol and diazepam during cardiac-catheterization.
Circulation 62, 1119-22 (1980)

3717. Wood,A.J.J., Robertson,R.M., Wilkinson,G.R., Wood,N.
Effect of cardiac-catheterization on the free levels of diazepam and propranolol.
Circulation 60, 264 (1979)

3718. Wu,P.H., Phillis,J.W., Bender,A.S.
Inhibition of (3H) diazepam binding to rat brain cortical synaptosomal membranes by adenosine uptake blockers.
Eur.J.Pharmacol. 65, 459-60 (1980)

3719. Wuester,M., Duka,T., Herz,A.
Diazepam effects on striatal met-enkephalin levels following long-term pharmacological manipulations.
Neuropharmacology 19, 501-5 (1980)

3720. Yamaguchi,N., Makihara,M., Kubota,M., Yoshimot.,H., Nakamura,K.
Influences of benzodiazepine derivatives on the hippocampal rhythmical slow activity during wakefulness and paradoxical sleep in chronically prepared cats.
EEG Clin.Neurol. 47, 9 (1979)

3721. Yamahira,Y., Noguchi,T., Noguchi,T., Takenaka,H., Maeda,T.
Absorption of diazepam from a lipid-containing oral dosage form.
Chem.Pharm.Bull. (Tokyo) 27, 1190-8 (1979)

3722. Yamamoto,K., Kuze,S., Murakami,S.
Clinical pharmacology of pentazocine-diazepam anesthesia.
Correlation between the order of drug administration and the plasma diazepam levels.
Masui 27, 1580-6 (1978)

3723. Yamamura,H.I., Reisine,T.D., Beaumont,K.
Huntingtons-disease - alterations in GABA and benzodiazepine receptors in the human brain.
Brain Res.Bull. 5, 773-5 (1980)

3724. Yang,J.C., Clark,W.C., Ngai,S.H., Berkowitz,B.A., Spector,S.
Analgesic action and pharmacokinetics of morphine and diazepam in man: an evaluation by sensory decision theory.
Anesthesiology 51, 495-502 (1979)

3725. Yehia,B.M., Oliver,J.S., Mackay,A.
The detection and measurement of diazepam in plasma by gas chromatography - mass fragmentography.
Vet.Hum.Tox. 21 (S), 167-9 (1979)

3726. Young,W.S., Kuhar,M.J.
Autoradiographic localisation of benzodiazepine receptors in the brains of humans and animals.
Nature 280, 391-4 (1979)

3727. Young,W.S., Kuhar,M.J.
Radiohistochemical localization of benzodiazepine receptors in rat brain.
J.Pharmacol.Exp.Ther. 212, 337-46 (1980)

3728. Yuasa,H., Banno,T., Oda,M., Watanabe,S.
Influence of diazepam in the thalamic neurons.
EEG Clin.Neurol. 47, 8 (1979)

3729. Yutrzenk.,G.J., Parmar,S.S., Davis,J.S.
Mediation by catecholamines of the anticonvulsant activity of diazepam.
Res.Comm.Pharm. 4, 79-88 (1979)

3730. Yutrzenk.,G.J., Davis,J.S., Parmar,S.S.
Catecholamine mediation of the anticonvulsant activity of flurazepam.
Res.Comm.Pharm. 5, 2-12 (1980)

3731. Zaidan,J.R., Kaplan,J.A., Sumpter,R.M.
Cardiovascular effects of dimethyl tubocurarine in patients with aortic valvular disease during morphine-diazepam-oxygen anesthesia.
Anesthesiol. 51, 137 (1979)

3732. Zarifian,B.
Benzodiazepine cerebral receptors and concept of endogenous ligand.
Rev.Prat. 30, 1561 (1980)

3733. Zarowny,D.P.
Clinical pharmacology and therapeutics of benzodiazepines.
Can.Med.Assoc.J. 121, 1571 (1979)

3734. Zetier,G.
Anticonvulsant effects of careulein and cholecystokinin octapeptide, compared with those of diazepam.
Eur.J.Pharmacol. 65, 297-300 (1980)

3735. Zilm,D.H., Jacob,M.S., MacLeod,S.M., Sellers,E.M., Ti,T.Y.
Propranolol and chlordiazepoxide effects on cardiac-arrhythmias during alcohol withdrawal.
Alc.Clin.Ex. 4, 400-5 (1980)

3736. Zimmer,S., Taub,H., Marks,G.S.
A comparison of the porphyrin-inducing activity of barbiturates and benzodiazepines in chick-embryo liver-cells.
Can.J.Physl. 58, 991-5 (1980)

3737. Zimmermann,C., Tansella,M., Lader,M.
Psychological performance in anxious patients treated with diazepam.
Progr.Neurol. 3, 361-8 (1979)

3738. Zimmermann,C., Tansella,M., Lader,M.
Comparison of the clinical and psychological effects of diazepam and amylobarbitone in anxious patients.
Brit.J.Clin.Pharmacol. 7, 605-11 (1979)

3739. Zsigmond,E.K., Kothary,S.P., Kumar,S.M., Kelsch,R.C.
Counteraction of circulatory side-effects of ketamine by pretreatment with diazepam.
Clin.Ther. 3, 28-32 (1980)

3740. Allen,M.D., Greenblatt,D.J.
Comparative protein-binding of diazepam and desmethyldiazepam.
J.Clin.Pharmacol. 20, 639-43 (1980)

3741. Barazi,S., Bonini,M.
Determination of 11 benzodiazepine derivatives in acetone solution by gaschromatography utilizing nitrogen as a specific detector.
J.Chromatogr. 202, 473-7 (1980)

3742. Cotler,S., Puglisi,C.V., Gustafson,J.H.
Determination of diazepam and its major metabolites in man and in the cat by high-performance liquid-chromatography.
J.Chromatogr. 222, 95-106 (1981)

3743. Dhar,A.K., Kutt,H.
Improved gas-chromatographic procedure for the determination of clonazepam levels in plasma using a nitrogen-sensitive detector.
J.Chromatogr. 222, 203-11 (1981)

3744. Divoll,M., Greenblatt,D.J.
Plasma-concentrations of temazepam, a 3-hydroxy benzodiazepine, determined by electron-capture gas-liquid-chromatography.
J.Chromatogr. 222, 125-8 (1981)

3745. Dixon,R., Glover,W., Earley,J.
Specific radioimmunoassay for flunitrazepam.
J.Pharm.Sci. 70, 230-1 (1981)

3746. Greenblatt,D.J.
Clinical pharmacokinetics of oxazepam and lorazepam.
Clin.Pharmacokin. 6, 89-105 (1981)

3747. Greenblatt.D.J., Divoll,M., Harmatz,J.S., Shader,R.I.
Desalkylflurazepam kinetics in the elderly following single and multiple doses of flurazepam (Dalmane).
Clin.Pharmacol.Ther. 29, 249 (1981)

3748. Greenblatt,D.J., Laughren,T.P., Allen,M.D., Harmatz, J.S., Shader,R.I.
Plasma diazepam and desmethyldiazepam concentrations during long-term diazepam therapy.
Brit.J.Clin.Pharm. 11, 35-40 (1981)

3749. Greenblatt,D.J., Shader,R.I., Divoll,M., Harmatz, J.S.
Benzodiazepines - a summary of pharmacokinetic properties.
Brit.J.Clin.Pharm. 11, 11-6 (1981)

3750. Hall,R.C.W., Zisook,S.
Paradoxical reactions to benzodiazepines.
Brit.J.Clin.Pharm. 11, 99-104 (1981)

3751. Holzbech.,M., Ellenber.,H.A.
Simultaneous determination of diphenhydramine, methaqualone, diazepam and chlorpromazine in liver by use of enzyme digestion - a comparison of digestion procedures.
J.Anal.Toxicol. 5, 62-4 (1981)

3752. Klotz,U.
Determination of bromazepam by gas-liquid-chromatography and its application for pharmacokinetic studies in man.
J.Chromatogr. 222, 501-6 (1981)

3753. Martinez,D., Gimenez,P.
Determination of benzodiazepines by derivative spectroscopy.
J.Anal.Toxicol. 5, 10-3 (1981)

3754. Maurer,H., Pfleger,K.
Determination of 1,4-benzodiazepines and 1,5-benzodiazepines in urine using a computerized gas chromatographic-mass spectrometric technique.
J.Chromatogr. 222, 409-19 (1981)

3755. Morgan,D.D., Robinson,J.D., Mendenha.,C.L.
Clinical pharmacokinetics of chlordiazepoxide in patients with alcoholic hepatitis.
Eur.J.Clin.Pharmacol. 19, 279-85 (1981)

3756. Riva,R., Deanna,M., Albani,F., Baruzzi,A.
Rapid quantitation of flurazepam and its major metabolite, N-desalkylflurazepam, in human-plasma by gas-liquid-chromatography with electron-capture detection.
J.Chromatogr. 222, 491-5 (1981)

3757. Schütz,H.
Benzodiazepine - Dünnschicht- und gaschromatographische Trennungen unter besonderer Berücksichtigung der Benzophenonderivate.
Bericht über das Symposium "Psychopharmaka und Suchtstoffe", Mosbach 1980 (S. 64-84)

3758. Schütz,H.
Einflußmöglichkeiten verschiedener Parameter auf die Höhe einer Fremdstoffkonzentration in Körperflüssigkeiten, dargestellt am Beispiel der Benzodiazepine.
Dtsch.Apoth.-Ztg. 121, 1059-65 (1981)

3759. Schütz,H., Fitz,H.
Screening, Nachweis und Biotransformation von Lormetazepam (Noctamid[R]), einem neuen Hypnotikum aus der Reihe der 1,4-Benzodiazepine.
Arch.Toxicol. (Manuskript eingereicht)

3760. Schütz,H., Fitz,H.
Analytik und Biotransformation von Triazolam (Halcion[R]), einem neuen Benzodiazepin mit forensisch relevanten Nebenwirkungen.
Beitr.gerichtl.Med. (im Druck)

3761. Schütz,H., Fitz,H.
Screening auf Benzodiazepine.
Dtsch.Apoth.-Ztg. (Manuskript eingereicht)

3762. Smith,M.T., Eadie,M.J., Brophy,T.O.
The pharmacokinetics of midazolam in man.
Eur.J.Clin.Pharmacol. 19, 271-8 (1981)

3763. Smyth,W.F., Groves,J.A.
The solvent-extraction of flurazepam and its major metabolites and their determination by polarography.
Analyt.Chim. 123, 175-86 (1981)

3764. Sumirtapura,Y.C., Aubert,C., Cano,J.P.
Highly specific and sensitive method for the determination of flunitrazepam in plasma by electron-capture gas-liquid chromatography.
Arzneim.-Forsch. (Drug Res.) (in the press)

3765. Troschutz,J.
Fluorometric-determination of some 1,4-benzodiazepines.
Arch.Pharm. 314, 204-9 (1981)

3766. Van der Kleijn,E., Vree,T.B., Baars,A.M., Wijsman,R., Edmunds,L.C., Knop,H.J.
Factors influencing the activity and fate of benzodiazepines in the body.
Brit.J.Clin.Pharmacol. 11, 85-98 (1981)

3767. Wallace,J.E., Shimek,E.L., Harris,S.C.
Determination of tricyclic antidepressants by high-performance liquid chromatography.
J.Anal.Toxicol. 5, 20-3 (1981)

3768. CONTAMEX[R] - Ketazolam.
Firmenschrift Johann A. Wülfing, Neuss, 45 S.

3769. Eberts,F.S., Philopoulos,Y., Reineke,L.M., Vliek,R.W., Metzler,C.M.
Disposition of ketazolam, a new anxiolytic agent, in man.
Pharmacologist 19, 165 (1977)

3770. Gottschalk,L.A., Cohn,J.B.
The relationship of diazepam and ketazolam blood levels to anxiety and hostility in chronic alcoholics.
Psychopharmacol.Bull. 14, 39-43 (1978)

3771. Szmuszkovicz,J., Chidester,C.G., Duchamp,D.J., MacKellar,F.A., Slomp,G.
Synthesis and proof of structure of a novel 1,4-benzodiazepine (ketazolam).
Tetrahedron Lett. 39, 3665-8 (1971)

3772. MUSARIL[R] - Tetrazepam.
Firmenschrift Mack-Midy Arzneimittel GmbH, 8000 München 2

3773. Arendt,R., Ochs,H.R., Greenblatt,D.
Electron-capture GLC analysis of the thienodiazepine clotiazepam (Trecalmo[R]): Preliminary pharmacokinetic studies.
Arzneim.-Forsch. (Drug Res.) (in the press)

3774. Ardrey,R.E., Moffat,A.C.
Gas-liquid chromatographic retention indices of 1318 substances of toxicological interest on SE-30 or OV-1 stationary phase.
Subject to be published

3775. Metzler,C.M., Ko,H., Royer,M.E., Veldkamp,W., Linet, O.I.
Bioavailability and pharmacokinetics of orally administered triazolam in normal subjects.
Clin.Pharm.Ther. 21, 111 (1977)

3776. Müller,W.E.
Der Benzodiazepinrezeptor: Eigenschaften und Bedeutung für Pharmakologie, Psychiatrie und Neurologie.
Med.Mo.Pharm. 4, 174-84 (1981)

3777. Pretsch,E., Clerc,T., Seibl,J., Simon,W.
Tabellen zur Strukturaufklärung organischer Verbindungen mit spektroskopischen Methoden.
Springer Verlag, Berlin Heidelberg New York 1976

3778. Seyffart,G.
Giftindex - Dialyse und Hämoperfusion bei Vergiftungen.
Fresenius-Stiftung - Bad Homburg 1975

Subject Index

Sachregister

Abbreviations XII

Absorption 245-246

Absorption Half-Life
(see Pharmacokinetic Data)

Absorption Maxima (UV-Spectra) 91-122

7-Acetamido-Clonazepam (Subst.Nr. 24)
- Analytical Methods 155,183,187,188
- Biotransformation 7
- GLC 25
- IR 51
- Levels 231
- MS 51
- TLC 22
- UV 105

7-Acetamido-Flunitrazepam (Subst.Nr. 39)
- Biotransformation 9
- GLC 25
- IR 66
- MS 66
- TLC 22
- UV 112

7-Acetamido-Nitrazepam (Subst.Nr. 12)
- Analytical Methods 174
- Biotransformation 5
- GLC 24
- IR 39
- Levels 221
- MS 39
- TLC 22
- UV 99

3-Acetoxy-Diazepam (Subst.Nr. 50)
- IR 77
- MS 77
- TLC 23

3-Acetoxy-Prazepam (Subst.Nr. 52)
- IR 79
- MS 79
- TLC 23

Acid Hydrolysis 4,253

Adumbran®
(see Oxazepam)

Adverse Effects 268-270

Albego®
(see Camazepam)

Aminobenzophenones (Formation) 13-16

2-(2-Amino-5-brom-benzoyl)-pyridine (Subst.Nr. 35)
- Analytical Methods 130, 194,195
- Biotransformation 8
- Formation 13
- GLC 25
- IR 62
- MS 62
- TLC 22
- UV 110

2-Amino-5-chlor-benzophenone (Subst.Nr. 4)
- Analytical Methods 130,165,176
- Biotransformation 4,5,6
- Formation 13,14
- GLC 24
- IR 31
- MS 31
- TLC 21
- UV 95

2-Amino-5-chlor-2'-fluor-benzophenone (Subst.Nr. 31)
- Formation 13,15
- GLC 25
- IR 58
- MS 58
- TLC 22
- UV 108

7-Amino-Clonazepam (Subst.Nr. 23)
- Analytical Methods 155,171,183,186,187,188
- Biotransformation 7
- GLC 25
- IR 50
- Levels 230,231
- MS 50
- TLC 22
- UV 104

2-Amino-5,2'-dichlor-benzophenone (Subst.Nr. 18)
- Analytical Methods 130,178
- Biotransformation 6
- Formation 13,15
- GLC 25
- IR 45
- MS 45
- TLC 22
- UV 102

7-Amino-Flunitrazepam (Subst.Nr. 38)
- Analytical Methods 171
- Biotransformation 9
- GLC 25
- IR 65

7-Amino-Flunitrazepam (Subst.Nr. 38)
- Levels 236,237
- MS 65
- TLC 22
- UV 112

2-Amino-3-hydroxy-5-chlor-benzophenone (Subst.Nr. 45)
- Biotransformation 6
- GLC 25
- IR 72
- MS 72
- TLC 23
- UV 115

7-Amino-Nitrazepam (Subst.Nr. 11)
- Analytical Methods 171,174
- Biotransformation 5
- GLC 24
- IR 38
- Levels 221
- MS 38
- TLC 22
- UV 98

2-Amino-5-nitro-benzophenone (Subst.Nr. 13)
- Analytical Methods 130,168,169,171,172
- Biotransformation 5
- Formation 13,15
- GLC 24
- IR 40
- MS 40
- TLC 22
- UV 99

2-Amino-5-nitro-2'-chlor-benzophenone (Subst.Nr. 25)
- Biotransformation 7
- Formation 13,15
- GLC 25
- IR 52
- MS 52
- TLC 22
- UV 105

2-Amino-5-nitro-2'-fluor-benzophenone (Subst.Nr. 42)
- Analytical Methods 130,197,198
- Formation 13,15
- GLC 25
- IR 69
- MS 69
- TLC 22
- UV 114

7-Amino-Nor-Flunitrazepam (Subst.Nr. 40)
- Biotransformation 9
- GLC 25
- IR 67
- Levels 236
- MS 67
- TLC 22
- UV 113

Analytical Methods (Mono-Methods)
- Bromazepam 194-196
- Camazepam 204
- Chlordiazepoxide 144-148
- Clobazam 201-203
- Clonazepam 182-189
- Clorazepate 176-177
- Diazepam 149-164
- Flunitrazepam 197-200
- Flurazepam 190-193
- Lorazepam 178-180
- Medazepam 175
- Nitrazepam 168-174
- Oxazepam 165-167
- Prazepam 181

Analytical Methods (Simultaneous Methods) 123-143

Apparent Volume of Distribution
(see Pharmacokinetic Data)

Ativan[R]
(see Lorazepam)

Base-Peaks (MS) 17-20

Benzodiazepine Receptor 272-275

Benzodiazepines in Relation to Mother,Fetus,Newborn, Infant and Child 246-247

Benzophenones (Formation) 13-16)

Bioavailability Studies 247

Biotransformation 4-11,247-248
- Bromazepam 8
- Camazepam 10
- Chlordiazepoxide 4
- Clobazam 9
- Clonazepam 7
- Clorazepate 7
- Clotiazepam 11
- Diazepam 5
- Flunitrazepam 9
- Flurazepam 8
- Ketazolam 10
- Lorazepam 6
- Lormetazepam 11
- Medazepam 6
- Nitrazepam 5
- Oxazepam 5
- Prazepam 6
- Temazepam 5
- Tetrazepam 11
- Triazolam 10

Blood Concentrations
(see Levels)

Body-Fluid Levels
(see Levels)

BRATTON-MARSHALL-Reaction 14,21-23

Breast-Feeding 246-247

Bromazepam (Subst.Nr. 33)
- Analytical Methods 124,128,130,131,134,194-196,199

- Biotransformation 8
- GLC 25
- IR 60
- Levels 235,244
- MS 60
- Pharmacokinetic Data 235
- TLC 22
- UV 109

Bromazepam-N(Py)-Oxide (Subst.Nr. 56)
- Biotransformation 8
- GLC 26
- IR 83
- MS 83
- TLC 23
- UV 119

Camazepam (Subst.Nr. 48)
- Analytical Methods 130,131,135,204
- Biotransformation 10
- GLC 26
- IR 75
- Levels 239
- MS 75
- Pharmacokinetic Data 239
- TLC 23
- UV 117

Capillary - GLC 251-252

Chlorazepate
(see Clorazepate)

Chlordiazepoxide (Subst.Nr. 1)
- Analytical Methods 123-138, 140-148
- Biotransformation 4
- GLC 24
- IR 28
- Levels 205-208,243
- MS 28
- Pharmacokinetic Data 208
- TLC 21
- UV 93

Clearance
(see Pharmacokinetic Data)

Cleavage of Conjugates 4

Clinical Investigations 257-265

Clobazam (Subst.Nr. 46)
- Analytical Methods 131,134,138,139,201-203
- Biotransformation 9
- GLC 25
- IR 73
- Levels 238
- MS 73
- Pharmacokinetic Data 238
- TLC 23
- UV 116

Clofazin
(see Nor-Clobazam)

Clonazepam (Subst.Nr. 22)
- Analytical Methods 124,125,128-131,134,136,143,155,170,171,182-189
- Biotransformation 7
- GLC 25
- IR 49
- Levels 230-232
- MS 49
- Pharmacokinetic Data 232
- TLC 22
- UV 104

Clorazepate (Subst.Nr. 16)
- Analytical Methods 128-131,134-136,141,176-177
- Biotransformation 7
- GLC 25
- IR 43
- Levels 225-226
- MS 43
- Pharmacokinetic Data 226
- TLC 22
- UV 101

Clotiazepam (Subst.Nr. 59)
- Biotransformation (assumed) 11
- GLC 26
- IR 86
- MS 86
- TLC 23
- UV 120

Colorimetry 146,172

Concentrations
(see Levels)

Conjugates (Cleavage) 4

Contamex^R
(see Ketazolam)

2-Cyclopropyl-methylamino-5-chlor-benzophenone (Subst.Nr. 21)
- Analytical Methods 130
- Formation 13,15
- GLC 25
- IR 48
- MS 48
- TLC 22
- UV 103

Dalmadorm^R
(see Flurazepam)

Dalmane^R
(see Flurazepam)

Demetrin^R
(see Prazepam)

Demoxepam (Subst.Nr. 2)
- Analytical Methods 127,135,138,145,146,147,148
- Biotransformation 4
- GLC 24
- IR 29
- Levels 205-207

Demoxepam (Subst.Nr. 2)
- MS 29
- TLC 21
- UV 94

Densitometry 135,145,191

Desalkyl-
(see also Nor-)

Desalkyl-Flurazepam (Subst.Nr. 28)
- Analytical Methods 127,128,129,138,190,191,192
- Biotransformation 8
- GLC 25
- IR 55
- Levels 233,234
- MS 55
- TLC 22
- UV 107

Desmethyl-
(see also Nor-)

Desmethyl-Chlordiazepoxide (Subst.Nr. 3)
- Analytical Methods 127,135,142,145,147,148
- Biotransformation 4
- GLC 24
- IR 30
- Levels 205-207
- MS 30
- TLC 21
- UV 94

Desmethyl-Clobazam
(see Nor-Clobazam)

Desmethyl-Diazepam
(see Nor-Diazepam)

Desmethyl-Flunitrazepam
(see Nor-Flunitrazepam)

Desmethyl-Medazepam (Subst.Nr. 53)
- Biotransformation 6
- GLC 26
- IR 80
- Levels 224
- MS 80
- TLC 23
- UV 117

Desmethyl-Tetrazepam
(see Nor-Tetrazepam)

Detection 14,21-23,443-444

2,5-Diamino-benzophenone (Subst.Nr. 14)
- Formation 13,15
- GLC 24
- IR 41
- MS 41
- TLC 22
- UV 100

2,5-Diamino-2'-chlor-benzophenone (Subst.Nr. 26)
- Formation 13,15
- GLC 25
- IR 53
- MS 53
- TLC 22
- UV 106

2,5-Diamino-2'-fluor-benzophenone (Subst.Nr. 44)
- Formation 13,16
- GLC 25
- IR 71
- MS 71
- TLC 23
- UV 115

Diazepam (Subst.Nr. 5)
- Analytical Methods 123-139,141-143,149-164,187
- Biotransformation 5,6,10
- GLC 24
- IR 32
- Levels 209-218, 224,240,243,244
- MS 32
- Pharmacokinetic Data 217-218
- TLC 21
- UV 95

Diazepam-N-Oxide (Subst.Nr. 49)
- IR 76
- MS 76
- TLC 23

Diazotization 14,443-444

Didesethyl-Flurazepam (Subst.Nr. 55)
- Analytical Methods 192
- Biotransformation 8
- GLC 26
- IR 82
- MS 82
- TLC 23
- UV 118

2-Diethylamino-ethylamino-5-chlor-2'-fluor-benzophenone (Subst.Nr. 30)
- Formation 13,15
- GLC 25
- IR 57
- MS 57
- TLC 22
- UV 108

Differential Pulse Polarography (DPP) 137,147,156,177,180, 188,192,196

Disposition 248

Distribution Half-Life
(see Pharmacokinetic Data)

Distribution Volume
(see Pharmacokinetic Data)

Drug Monitoring
(see Levels)

Effects and Interactions with other Compounds 248-250

Elimination Half-Life
(see Pharmacokinetic Data)

Emergency Drug Analysis 250-251

EMIT[R] 160

Enzymatic Hydrolysis 4

Extraction from biological Samples 4,251

Faustan[R]
(see Diazepam)

Fetus 246-247

Flunitrazepam (Subst.Nr. 36)
- Analytical Methods 123,128-131,134,171,197-200
- Biotransformation 9
- GLC 25
- IR 63
- Levels 236-237
- MS 63
- Pharmacokinetic Data 237
- TLC 22
- UV 111

Fluorescence 251

Fluorescence Densitometry 145,155,156

Fluorometry 145,146,155,156,173,191,202,203

Flurazepam (Subst.Nr. 27)
- Analytical Methods 123-131,134,136,137,141-143,190-193
- Biotransformation 8
- GLC 25
- IR 54
- Levels 233-234
- MS 54
- Pharmacokinetic Data 234
- TLC 22
- UV 106

Forensic Cases
- Diazepam 211
- Nitrazepam 222
(see also Poisoning 265-266)

Formula Index 1-3

Frisium[R]
(see Clobazam)

GABA 272-275

Gas-Chromatography 24-26, 251-252

Gas-Liquid-Chromatography 24-26, 251-252
(see GLC)

General Analytical Data 252

General Treatment in Books and Reviews 253-254

Generic Names 1-3

GLC-Data 24-26

GLC-ECD 123-128,144,145,149-151,165,166,168-170,175-186, 190,194,195,197-199,201,202,204

GLC-FID 129-131,134,152,167,171

GLC-Literature 251-252

GLC/MS 153,167,187,255

GLC-NFID 132,175,199,201

GLC-NPD 154

Halcion[R]
(see Triazolam)

Helogaphen[R]
(see Chlordiazepoxide)

High-Pressure Liquid Chromatography (see HPLC)

HPLC 136,141-143,148,160-164,174,189,200
- Literature 253

Hydrolysis of Benzodiazepines 4, 253

Hydrolysis Procedures 4, 253

Hydrolysis Products 13,14-16

3-Hydroxy-Bromazepam (Subst.Nr. 34)
- Analytical Methods 194,196
- Biotransformation 8
- GLC 25
- IR 61
- MS 61
- TLC 22
- UV 110

3-Hydroxy-Diazepam = Temazepam (Subst.Nr. 7)
- Analytical Methods 128,134,148,149,154,155,163,175
- Biotransformation 5,6,7,10
- GLC 24
- IR 34
- Levels 214-217
- MS 34
- TLC 21
- UV 96

2-Hydroxyethylamino-5-chlor-2′-fluor-benzophenone (Subst.Nr. 32)
- Formation 13,15
- GLC 25
- IR 59
- MS 59
- TLC 22
- UV 109

N-1-Hydroxyethyl-Flurazepam (Subst.Nr. 29)
- Analytical Methods 190-192
- Biotransformation 8
- GLC 25
- IR 56

N-1-Hydroxyethyl-Flurazepam (Subst.Nr. 29)
- Levels 233,234
- MS 56
- TLC 22
- UV 107

3-Hydroxy-Prazepam (Subst.Nr. 20)
- Analytical Methods 181
- Biotransformation 7
- GLC 25
- IR 47
- MS 47
- TLC 22
- UV 103

i.m.-Administration
- Chlordiazepoxide 207,208
- Diazepam 213, 218
- Flunitrazepam 237
- Lorazepam 227,228

Imeson[R]
(see Nitrazepam)

Impairment of Skills related to Driving 276,277

Important Data 17-20

Index of Treated Substances 12

Infant 246-247

Infrared-Spectra (including important metabolites and hydrolysis derivatives)
- Bromazepam 60-62, 83
- Camazepam 75
- Chlordiazepoxide 28-31
- Clobazam 73-74
- Clonazepam 49-53
- Clorazepate 43
- Clotiazepam 86
- Diazepam 32-36
- Flunitrazepam 63-71
- Flurazepam 54-59,81,82
- Ketazolam 33-36,84
- Lorazepam 44-45
- Lormetazepam 87-88
- Medazepam 42,72,80
- Nitrazepam 37-41
- Oxazepam 35
- Prazepam 46-48
- Temazepam 34
- Tetrazepam 89-90
- Triazolam 85

Interactions 248-250, 268-270

Interpretation of Infrared-Spectra 27

Interpretation of Mass-Spectra 27

intramuscular Administration
(see i.m. Administration)

intravenous Administration
(see i.v. Administration)

IR - Literature 253

IR - Spectra
(see Infrared-Spectra)

i.v.-Administration
- Bromazepam 235
- Camazepam 239
- Chlordiazepoxide 206,208
- Clonazepam 230,232
- Diazepam 211,212,217,218
- Flunitrazepam 236,237
- Lorazepam 227,228
- Nitrazepam 221,223

Ketazolam (Subst.Nr. 57)
- Biotransformation 10
- GLC 26
- IR 84
- Levels 240
- MS 84
- Pharmacokinetic Data 240
- TLC 23
- UV 119

KOVATS-Index 24-26

Labour 246,247

Lactation Period 246,247

Lamra[R]
(see Diazepam)

Levels (Blood-, Serum-, Plasma-)
- Bromazepam 235,244
- Camazepam 239
- Chlordiazepoxide 205-208,243
- Clobazam 238
- Clonazepam 230-232
- Clorazepate 225-226
- Diazepam 209-218,243,244
- Flunitrazepam 236-237
- Flurazepam 233-234
- Ketazolam 240
- Lorazepam 227-228,244
- Lormetazepam 242
- Medazepam 224,244
- Nitrazepam 221-223,243
- Oxazepam 219-220,243
- Prazepam 229
- Triazolam 241

Levels (Literature) 254,255

Lexotan[R]
(see Bromazepam)

Lexotanil[R]
(see Bromazepam)

Librax[R]
(see Chlordiazepoxide)

Librium^R
(see Chlordiazepoxide)

Limbatril^R
(see Chlordiazepoxide)

Literature 279

Lorazepam (Subst.Nr. 17)
- Analytical Methods 123,124,128,130,131,134,136,138, 141,167,178-180
- Biotransformation 6,11
- GLC 25
- IR 44
- Levels 227,228,244
- MS 44
- Pharmacokinetic Data 228
- TLC 22
- UV 101

Lormetazepam (Subst.Nr. 60)
- Biotransformation 11
- GLC 26
- IR 87
- Levels 242
- MS 87
- TLC 23
- UV 121

Mass-Spectra (including important metabolites and hydrolysis derivatives)
- Bromazepam 60-62,83
- Camazepam 75
- Chlordiazepoxide 28-31
- Clobazam 73-74
- Clonazepam 49-53
- Clorazepate 43
- Clotiazepam 86
- Diazepam 32-36
- Flunitrazepam 63-71
- Flurazepam 54-59,81,82
- Ketazolam 32-36,84
- Lorazepam 44-45
- Lormetazepam 87-88
- Medazepam 42,72,80
- Nitrazepam 37-41
- Oxazepam 35
- Prazepam 46-48
- Temazepam 34

Mass-Spectra (continued)
- Tetrazepam 89-90
- Triazolam 85

Mass-Spectra Literature 255

Mass-Spectra Peaks 17-20

Maximum Concentrations 243-244

Medazepam (Subst.Nr. 15)
- Analytical Methods 124,128-131,134,138,141,143,175
- Biotransformation 6
- GLC 25
- IR 42
- Levels 224,244
- MS 42
- Pharmacokinetic Data 224
- TLC 22
- UV 100

Melting Points 1-3

Metabolism
(see Biotransformation)

2-Methylamino-5-amino-2'-fluor-benzophenone (Subst.Nr. 43)
- Formation 13,15
- GLC 25
- IR 70
- MS 70
- TLC 22
- UV 114

2-Methylamino-5-chlor-benzophenone (Subst.Nr. 9)
- Analytical Methods 130,149,152
- Biotransformation 6
- Formation 13,14
- GLC 24
- IR 36
- MS 36
- TLC 21
- UV 97

2-Methylamino-2',5-dichlor-benzophenone (Subst.Nr. 61)
- Formation 13,16
- GLC 26
- IR 88
- MS 88
- TLC 23
- UV 121

2-Methylamino-5-nitro-2'-fluor-benzophenone (Subst.Nr. 41)
- Analytical Methods 130, 197,198
- Formation 13,15
- GLC 25
- IR 68
- MS 68
- TLC 22
- UV 113

Milk-Levels 246-247

Mogadan^R
(see Nitrazepam)

Mogadon^R
(see Nitrazepam)

Molecular Formulas 17-20

Molecular Weights 17-20

Monitoring (Single Ion Monitoring) 27

Mono Demetrin^R
(see Prazepam)

Mono-Desethyl-Flurazepam (Subst.Nr. 54)
- Analytical Methods 192
- Biotransformation 8
- GLC 26

Mono-Desethyl-Flurazepam (Subst.Nr. 54)
- IR 81
- MS 81
- TLC 23
- UV 118

MS
(see Mass-Spectra)

Multiple Administration
- Bromazepam 235
- Chlordiazepoxide 207
- Clobazam 238
- Clonazepam 230-232
- Clorazepate 225
- Diazepam 214-217
- Flunitrazepam 237
- Flurazepam 233
- Lorazepam 228
- Medazepam 224
- Nitrazepam 222
- Oxazepam 220
- Triazolam 241

Multum[R]
(see Chlordiazepoxide)

Musaril[R]
(see Tetrazepam)

N-Desalkyl-
(see Desalkyl- or Nor-)

N-1-Desalkyl-Flurazepam
(see Desalkyl-Flurazepam)

N-Descyclopropylmethyl-Prazepam
(see Nor-Prazepam)

N-Desmethyl-
(see Desalkyl- or Nor-)

N-Desmethyl-Chlordiazepoxide
(see Desmethyl-Chlordiazepoxide)

N-Desmethyl-Clobazam
(see Nor-Clobazam)

N-Desmethyl-Diazepam
(see Nor-Diazepam)

N-Desmethyl-Flunitrazepam
(see Nor-Flunitrazepam)

N-Desmethyl-Medazepam
(see Desmethyl-Medazepam)

N-Desmethyl-Tetrazepam
(see Nor-Tetrazepam)

Newborn 246-247

Nitrazepam (Subst.Nr. 10)
- Analytical Methods 123,128-131,134,136,138-141,143, 168-174
- Biotransformation 5
- GLC 24
- IR 37
- Levels 221-223,243
- MS 37
- Pharmacokinetic Data 222-223
- TLC 21
- UV 98

NMR-Spectra 255

N-(1-Naphthyl)-ethylenediamine 14

Nobrium[R]
(see Medazepam)

Noctamid[R]
(see Lormetazepam)

Nomenclature XI and XII

Nor-Clobazam (Subst.Nr. 47)
- Analytical Methods 201-203
- Biotransformation 9
- GLC 26
- IR 74
- Levels 238
- MS 74
- TLC 23
- UV 116

Nor-Diazepam (Subst.Nr. 6)
- Analytical Methods 125-129,135,148,149-156,160-164, 175-177,181
- Biotransformation 4,5,6,7,10
- GLC 24
- IR 33
- Levels 209-217,224,225,229,244
- MS 33
- TLC 21
- UV 96

Nor-Flunitrazepam (Subst.Nr. 37)
- Analytical Methods 197,198
- Biotransformation 9
- GLC 25
- IR 64
- Levels 236
- MS 64
- TLC 22
- UV 111

Nor-Flurazepam
(see N-1-Desalkyl-Flurazepam)

Nor-Medazepam
(see Desmethyl-Medazepam)

Nor-Prazepam
(see Nor-Diazepam)

Nor-Tetrazepam (Subst.Nr. 63)
- Biotransformation 11
- GLC 26
- IR 90
- MS 90
- TLC 23
- UV 122

Oral Administration
- Bromazepam 235,244
- Camazepam 239
- Chlordiazepoxide 205-207,208,243
- Clobazam 238
- Clonazepam 230-232
- Clorazepate 225-226
- Diazepam 209-211, 214-217,243,244
- Flunitrazepam 236-237
- Flurazepam 233-234
- Ketazolam 240
- Lorazepam 227-228,244
- Lormetazepam 242
- Medazepam 224,244
- Nitrazepam 221-222,243
- Oxazepam 219-220,243
- Prazepam 229
- Triazolam 241

Other Themes 277-278

Overdose Levels
(see Levels)

Oxazepam (Subst.Nr. 8)
- Analytical Methods 124-126,128-132,134-141,143, 165-167
- Biotransformation 4,5,6,7,10
- GLC 24
- IR 35
- Levels 215-217,219-220,243
- MS 35
- Pharmacokinetic Data 220
- TLC 21
- UV 97

Pantrop^R - retard
(see Chlordiazepoxide)

Peak Concentrations 243-244

Peak Levels 243-244

Perinatal Period (Levels) 246-247

Pharmacokinetic Data (e.g. Half-Lifes)
- Bromazepam 235
- Camazepam 239
- Chlordiazepoxide 208
- Clobazam 238
- Clonazepam 232
- Clorazepate 226
- Diazepam 217-218
- Flunitrazepam 237
- Flurazepam 234
- Ketazolam 240
- Lorazepam 228
- Lormetazepam 242
- Medazepam 224
- Nitrazepam 222-223
- Oxazepam 220
- Prazepam 229
- Triazolam 241

Pharmacokinetics (Literature) 255-257

Pharmacology and Clinical Investigations 257 - 265

Placental Passage 246-247

Planum^R
(see Temazepam)

Plasma Concentrations
(see Levels)

Poisoning (Treatment, Reports, Cases) 265-266

Polarography 137,147,156,173,177,180,188,192,196,266

Praxiten^R
(see Oxazepam)

Prazepam (Subst.Nr. 19)
- Analytical Methods 128-131,134,136,138,141,143,181
- Biotransformation 7
- GLC 25
- IR 46
- Levels 229
- MS 46
- Pharmacokinetic Data 229
- TLC 22
- UV 102

Prazepam-N-Oxide (Subst.Nr. 51)
- IR 78
- MS 78
- TLC 23

Pregnancy 246-247

Prenatal Period 246-247

Proteinbinding 266
(see also Pharmacokinetic Data)

Radioactive-Labelled Benzodiazepines 267

Radioimmunoassay
(see RIA)

Radioimmunoassay (Literature) 267-268

Radioreceptor Assay 139,140,158,159

Rearrangements 24

Receptor 272-275

Receptor Theory 272-275

Rectal Administration
- Diazepam 214,218
- Flunitrazepam 237
- Oxazepam 219

Repeated
(see Multiple)

Residual Effects 268-270

Retention Index 24-26

Retention Time 24-26

R_f-Values 21-23

RIA 138,147,148,157,158,159,188,193,199

Ring Nomenclature XI

Rivotril[R]
(see Clonazepam)

Rohypnol[R]
(see Flunitrazepam)

Screening Findings 443-444

Screening Procedure 268

Serax[R]
(see Oxazepam)

Serenal[R]-D
(see Oxazepam)

Serum Concentrations
(see Levels)

Side-, Adverse-, Residual- and Withdrawal-Effects 268-270

Simultaneous Methods 123-143

Single i.m. Administration
(see i.m. Administration)

Single-Ion-Monitoring Values 27

Single i.v. Administration
(see i.v. Administration)

Single Oral Administration
(see oral Administration)

Single Rectal Administration
(see rectal Administration)

Skills related to Driving 276-277

Sleep Effects and Studies 271

Solvent Systems 21

Spectrophotodensitometry 135

Staurodorm[R]
(see Flurazepam)

Survey of Benzodiazepine Literature 245

Symbols XII

Synthesis 271-272

Tabulation of UV-Maxima 91-93

Tavor[R]
(see Lorazepam)

Temazepam (Subst.Nr. 7)
- Analytical Methods 128,134,138,148,149,154,155,163,175
- Biotransformation 5,6,10
- GLC 24
- IR 34
- Levels 214-217
- MS 34
- TLC 21
- UV 96

Temesta[R]
(see Lorazepam)

Tetrazepam (Subst.Nr. 62)
- Biotransformation 11
- GLC 26
- IR 89
- MS 89
- TLC 23
- UV 122

Theory of Action 272-275

Thermolysis 24

Thin Layer Chromatography 21-23, 275-276

TLC 21-23,130,131,133,135,145,154-156,171,187,191,195,203

TLC-Data 21-23

Toxic Levels
(see Levels)

Toxicity 276

Toxicology 276

Traffic Medicine 276-277

Tranquase[R]
(see Diazepam)

Tranquo-Buscopan[R]
(see Oxazepam)

Tranquo-Tablinen[R]
(see Diazepam)

Tranxene[R]
(see Clorazepate)

Tranxilium[R]
(see Clorazepate)

Trecalmo[R]
(see Clotiazepam)

Triazolam (Subst.Nr. 58)
- Analytical Methods 138
- Biotransformation 10
- GLC 26
- IR 85
- Levels 241
- MS 85
- Pharmacokinetic Data 241
- TLC 23
- UV 120

Ultraviolet-Spectra (including important metabolites and hydrolysis derivatives)
- Bromazepam 109-110
- Camazepam 117
- Chlordiazepoxide 93-95
- Clobazam 116
- Clonazepam 104-106
- Clorazepate 101
- Clotiazepam 120
- Diazepam 95-97
- Flunitrazepam 111-115
- Flurazepam 106-109
- Ketazolam 119
- Lorazepam 101
- Lormetazepam 121
- Medazepam 100
- Nitrazepam 98-99
- Oxazepam 97
- Prazepam 102-103
- Temazepam 96
- Tetrazepam 122
- Triazolam 120

Ultraviolet-Spectra (Literature) 277

UV-Photometry 146, 277

UV-Spectra
(see Ultraviolet-Spectra)

Valium[R]
(see Diazepam)

Verstran[R]
(see Prazepam)

Volume of Distribution
(see Pharmacokinetic Data)

Withdrawal Effects 268-270

Benzodiazepin-Screening im Harn

Typische positive Befunde

Verfahren:

Saure Hydrolyse und Extraktion entsprechend der auf Seite 4 beschriebenen Methodik.

DC-Trennung (s. Seite 21 zu den DC-Bedingungen)

Detektion a) Photolytische Desalkylierung N-1-substituierter Aminobenzophenone (Bestrahlen mit UV-Licht, z. B. Höhensonne, Bestrahlungsdauer 30 min, Entfernung 30 cm, Literatur (279).
b) Kaltluftstrom (15 min)
c) Diazotierung durch Begasen mit Stickoxiden in einer Kammer (3–5 min) oder Besprühen mit einer Lösung von 1 g Natriumnitrit in 100 ml HCl (2 mol/l).
d) Kaltluftstrom (15 min)
e) Azokupplung nach BRATTON und MARSHALL (s. Formelschema auf Seite 14). Sprühen mit einer Lösung von 1 g N-(1-Naphthyl)-ethylendiammoniumdichlorid in 50 ml Dimethylformamid und 50 ml HCl (4 mol/l).

Anmerkungen:
Die vollständigen Metabolitenmuster sind oft erst in Fällen der Überdosierung zu erkennen.
Die Nummern neben den DC-Flecken bezeichnen die Substanznummern (s. Seite 1–3 bezüglich der Namen).
Abbildung auf Seite 444: Fließmittel Toluol
Abbildung auf Seite 443: Fließmittel Chloroform/Aceton (80+20)

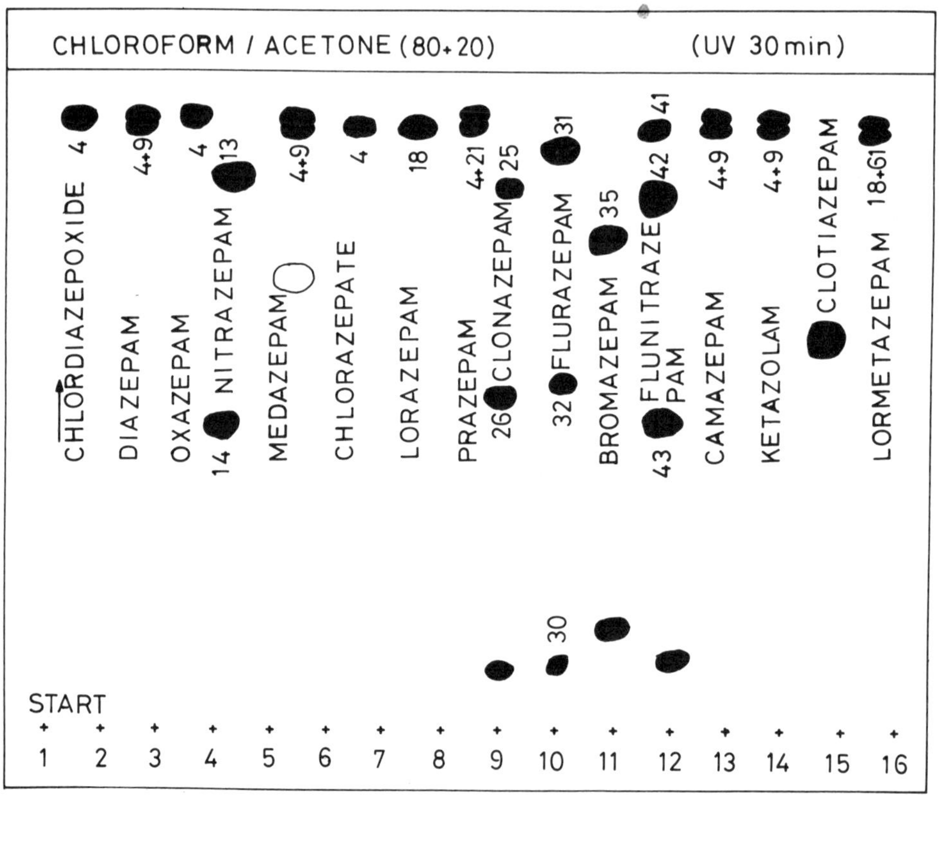